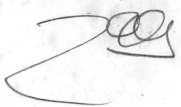

Pathophysiology

**Concepts
of Altered
Health
States**

Carol Mattson Porth

R.N., M.S.N., Ph.D. (Physiology)

Associate Professor
School of Nursing
University of Wisconsin, Milwaukee

Adjunct Assistant Professor
Department of Physiology
Medical College of Wisconsin
Milwaukee, Wisconsin

With eleven contributors

Illustrated by *Carole Russell Hilmer*
and others

J. B. Lippincott

Philadelphia
London
Mexico City
New York
St. Louis
São Paulo
Sydney

Pathophysiology

Concepts of Altered Health States

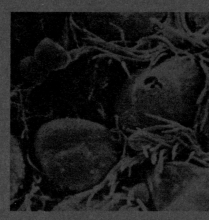
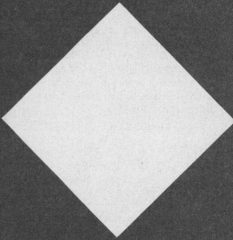
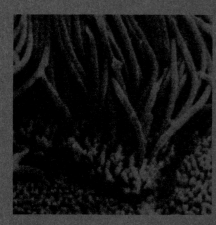
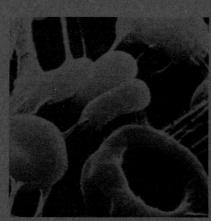
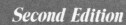
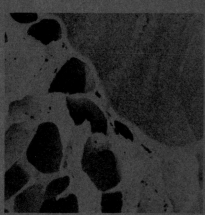

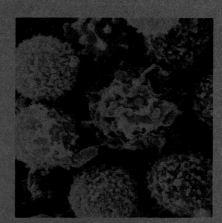

Second Edition

Sponsoring Editor: Jeanne H. Wallace
Manuscript Editor: Martha Hicks-Courant
Indexer: Ruth Elwell
Art Director: Tracy Baldwin
Design Coordinator: Charles W. Field
Designer: Arlene Putterman
Production Supervisor: J. Corey Gray
Production Assistant: Charlene Catlett Squibb
Compositor: John C. Meyer & Son, Inc.
Printer/Binder: Murray Printing Company

2nd Edition

Copyright © 1986, by J. B. Lippincott Company.

6 5

Library of Congress
Cataloging-in-Publication Data

Porth, Carol.
    Pathophysiology—concepts of altered health states.

    Includes bibliographies and index.
    1. Physiology, Pathological.   2. Nursing.
I. Title.   [DNLM: 1. Disease—nurses' instruction.
2. Pathology—nurses' instruction.   3. Physiology—nurses'
instruction.   QZ 4 P851p]
RB113.P67   1986   616.07   85-16053
ISBN 0-397-54481-2

The authors and publisher have exerted every
effort to ensure that drug selection and dosage
set forth in this text are in accord with current
recommendations and practice at the time of
publication. However, in view of ongoing
research, changes in government regulations, and
the constant flow of information relating to drug
therapy and drug reactions, the reader is urged to
check the package insert for each drug for any
change in indications and dosage and for added
warnings and precautions. This is particularly
important when the recommended agent is a
new or infrequently employed drug.

Contributors

Debbie L. Cook, C.R.N., M.S.N., C.N.M.
Certified Nurse Midwife, Group Health Cooperative of
Puget Sound
Tacoma, Washington

Robin L. Curtis, Ph.D.
Associate Professor, Department of Anatomy and Cellular
Science and Department of Physical Medicine and
Rehabilitation
Medical College of Wisconsin
Milwaukee, Wisconsin

Sheila M. Curtis, R.N., M.S.
Doctoral student, Marquette University
Milwaukee, Wisconsin

Kathleen E. Gunta, R.N., M.S.N.
Clinical Nurse Specialist, Orthopedics
St. Luke's Hospital
Milwaukee, Wisconsin

Linda S. Hurwitz, R.N., M.S.N.
Associate Director of Nursing, Presbyterian Hospital
Columbia-Presbyterian Medical Center
The Center for Women and Children (Babies' Hospital
and Sloan Hospital for Women)
New York, New York

Stephanie MacLaughlin, R.N., M.S.N.
Assistant Professor, Cardinal Stritch College
Milwaukee, Wisconsin

Pamela M. Schroeder, R.N., M.S.N.
Clinical Nurse Specialist, Rheumatology
St. Luke's-Samaritan Health Care, Inc.
Milwaukee, Wisconsin

Gladys Simandl, R.N., M.S.N.
Doctoral student, School of Nursing
University of Wisconsin
Milwaukee, Wisconsin

Darlene Gene Thornhill, R.N., M.S.N., D.S.
Formerly, Hypertension Clinician
Milwaukee County Medical Complex;
Currently, Program Specialist
University of Wisconsin
Milwaukee, Wisconsin

Mary Wierenga, *R.N., Ph.D.*
Associate Professor, School of Nursing
University of Wisconsin
Milwaukee, Wisconsin

E. Ronald Wright, *Ph.D.*
Associate Professor of Microbiology
Frances Payne Bolton School of Nursing
Case Western Reserve University
Cleveland, Ohio

CONSULTANT IN PHARMACOLOGY

Mary S. Rice, *Pharm. D.*
Director of Drug Information, Columbia Hospital
Milwaukee, Wisconsin

Preface

The meaning of *pathophysiology,* or *altered health,* as it is referred to in this book, reflects not so much the pathologic processes that take place as the physiologic changes that produce the signs and symptoms. It is these changes that determine, to a large extent, whether a disease will be disabling. Furthermore, it is the maintenance of adequate levels of functioning with which most health care professionals concern themselves.

The second edition of this text has been greatly expanded and revised to provide a comprehensive pathophysiology book that can be used both as a student text and as a reference source. The chapters on stress and adaptation, infectious processes, alterations in urine elimination, sexually transmitted diseases, alterations in special sensory function, skeletal disorders, and alterations in skin integrity are new.

A major aim in writing the second edition, as in the first, was to relate normal body functioning to the physiologic changes that occur as a result of illness, as well as to the body's remarkable ability to compensate for these illness-related changes. A conceptual model that integrates developmental and preventive aspects of illness was used. Selection of content was based on common health problems, including the special health problems of children and the elderly. The book provides the rationale for health care, but not the "how to's" of health care, the specifics of drug therapy, or the particulars of diagnostic methods. It is assumed that those using the book have access to more complete reference sources in these areas than this book could provide.

A second aim was to present the content in a manner that could be easily understood. Diagrams to aid in visualizing the content and tables to aid in identifying and summarizing essential information have been liberally placed throughout the text. The study guide that appears at the end of each chapter serves as a quick review of chapter content and chapter objectives. The additional references provided in many chapters were carefully selected because of their accuracy and comprehensiveness and the quality of their bibliographies.

A word of explanation is needed about the organization of the book. The book is divided into units, the first of which deals with the cellular aspects of disease, the second with body defenses, and the others with alterations in organ or system function. The book has been organized into three areas of focus based on the health–illness continuum: (1) *control* of normal body function; (2) pathophysiology, or *alterations* in body function; and (3) system *failure* regardless of pathologic state (*e.g.,* heart failure and renal failure). The material presented in chapters that deal with the control of normal body function is information that some students may have learned in other courses, and teachers may want to use these chapters as optional review assignments.

Although intended primarily for nurses and nursing students, the text is general enough to be used in other health professions. By focusing on physiologic responses to actual and potential health problems, the book helps facilitate the development and use of nursing diagnoses. The book can also be used as a source of information for patient education; many of the diagrams are suitable for this purpose.

Every effort was made to make the text as accurate and up-to-date as possible. This was accomplished through an extensive review of the literature and through the use of critiques provided by students, faculty, and clinical specialists. As this vast amount of information was processed, inaccuracies or omissions may have occurred. Readers are encouraged to contact us about such errors. Such feedback is essential to the continued development of the book.

Carol Mattson Porth, R.N., M.S.N., Ph.D.

Acknowledgments

It is difficult to consider the preparation of a new edition of a book such as this without considerable help. The reactions and suggestions of colleagues and students regarding the first edition were essential to the development of this edition, and I wish to thank all of the people who were willing to share their reactions and ideas.

A number of persons were kind enough to review parts of the text and make helpful suggestions: Laura Burke, R.N., M.S.N.; Michael C. Collopy, M.D.; Michelle J. Gieger-Bronsky, R.N., M.S.N.; Paul B. Halverson, M.D.; Julie Kuenzi, R.N., M.S.N.; Patricia Mehring, R.N., M.S.N.; Susan Nuccio, R.N., M.S.N.; and Betty Pearson, R.N., Ph.D.

The contributors to the book also deserve special mention, for they worked long hours to supply essential content. Mary Rice read all of the pharmacology content and supplied information for a number of the tables that dealt with drug content. Carole Hilmer not only developed sketches and finished art work, but also made many helpful suggestions about illustration selection.

Several other persons deserve special recognition. Georgianne Heymann, R.N., B.S.N., served as my local editor for the book. She provided not only excellent editorial services, but also encouragement, humor, and support when the tasks associated with manuscript preparation became most dismal. Elisabeth Allen performed a number of essential services: she did manuscript typing and copying, kept my files organized, and assisted with library research. Jerry Baumgarten also helped with library research. I also wish to express my appreciation to the editorial and production staff of the J. B. Lippincott Company. All of these people gave help well above and beyond the call of duty.

Contents

Unit I

Alterations
in Cell Function
and Growth

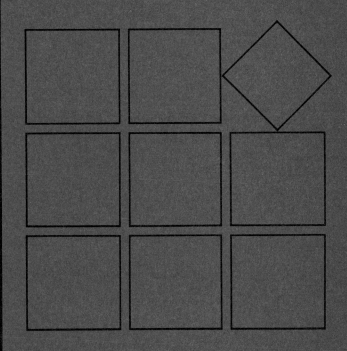

Chapter 1

Cell and Tissue Characteristics

Robin L. Curtis

Carol Mattson Porth

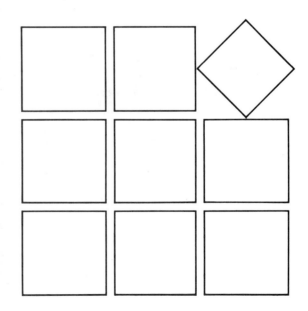

In order to understand the functioning of the human body in health and disease, it is necessary to understand how the individual cells of the body are structured and how they function. The cell is the smallest functional unit that an organism can be divided into and still retain the characteristics of life. Cells, in turn, are organized into larger functional units called *tissue,* and it is the tissues that form body structures and organs. Although the cells of different tissues and organs vary in structure and function, there are certain general characteristics that are common to most cells. Cells are remarkably similar in their ability to exchange materials with their immediate environment, in obtaining energy from organic nutrients, in synthesizing complex molecules, and in duplicating themselves. It is at the level of the cell that most disease processes exert their effects. Some diseases affect the cells of a single organ, others affect the cells of a particular tissue type, and still others affect the cells of the entire organism.

The substances that make up cells of living organisms are collectively referred to as *protoplasm.* Protoplasm is composed of water, electrolytes, proteins, lipids, and carbohydrates. Water makes up 70% to 85% of the cell's protoplasm. The second most abundant constituent (10–20%) of protoplasm is the cell proteins, that form cell structures and the enzymes necessary for cellular reactions. Lipids constitute 2% to 3% of most cells and are insoluble in water. They combine with proteins to form the membranes that separate the various compartments of the cell and serve as a cellular storage form for foodstuffs. Only small amounts of carbohydrates are found in the cell, and these are used primarily for fuel. The major intracellular electrolytes are potassium, magnesium, phosphate, sulfate, and bicarbonate. There are also smaller quantities of sodium, chloride, and calcium. These electrolytes facilitate the generation and transmission of electrochemical impulses in nerve and muscle cells. Intracellular electrolytes participate in reactions that are necessary for cellular metabolism. In this chapter, we discuss the functional components of the cell, cellular energy metabolism, tissue types, and membrane potentials and properties of excitable tissue.

■ Functional Components of the Cell

Although diverse in their organization, all cells have common structures that perform unique and special functions. When seen under a light microscope, three major components of the cell become evident: the nucleus, the cytoplasm, and the cell membrane (Fig. 1-1). Within the cytoplasm are a number of physical structures generally called the *organelles.*

The Nucleus

The nucleus is the control center for the cell. It contains the individual units of heredity—*the genes*—which are strung along the chromosomes. In a resting cell the chromosomes appear as darkly stained granules known as *chromatin material.* Chemically, each gene consists of deoxyribonucleic acid (DNA). Genes control not only cellular replication but also cellular activity, by determining the type of proteins and other substances that are made by the cell. In addition to the chromosomes, the nucleus also contains one or two rounded bodies called

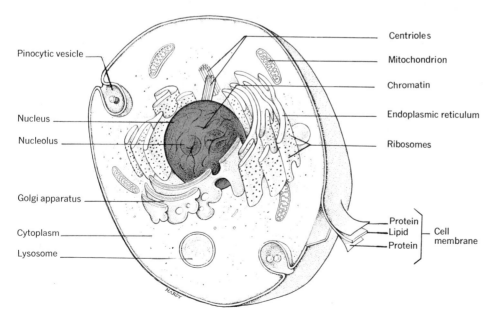

Pinocytic vesicle

Nucleus

Nucleolus

Golgi apparatus

Cytoplasm

Lysosome

Centrioles

Mitochondrion

Chromatin

Endoplasmic reticulum

Ribosomes

Protein
Lipid — Cell
Protein   membrane

Figure 1-1   A composite cell designed to show, in one cell, all of the various components of the nucleus and cytoplasm. (Chaffee EE, Greisheimer EM; Basic Physiology and Anatomy, 3rd ed. Philadelphia, JB Lippincott, 1974)

nucleoli. It is here that ribonucleic acid (RNA), which is part of the elaborate messenger system that allows DNA to communicate with the protein-building ribosomes in the cytoplasm, is synthesized. The nuclear contents are surrounded by a double-walled nuclear membrane. The pores present in this membrane allow fluids, electrolytes, RNA, and other materials to move between the nuclear and cytoplasmic compartments.

The Cytoplasm and Its Organelles

The cytoplasm surrounds the nucleus, and it is here that the work of the cell takes place. The cytoplasm is essentially a colloidal solution that contains water, electrolytes, suspended proteins, neutral fats, and glycogen molecules. Although they do not contribute to the cell's function, pigments may also accumulate in the cytoplasm. Some pigments, such as melanin, which gives skin its color, are normal constituents of the cell. Others, such as carbon and coal dust, which are commonly found in the lungs of coal miners and persons living in polluted environments, are abnormal.

Embedded within the cytoplasm are the *organelles,* or inner organs of the cell. These include the ribosomes, endoplasmic reticulum, mitochondria, lysosomes, microtubules, and microfilaments.

Ribosomes

The ribosomes serve as sites of protein synthesis in the cell. They are small particles of nucleoproteins (rRNA and proteins) that are synthesized in the cell nucleus and can be found attached to the wall of endoplasmic reticulum or as free ribosomes (Fig. 1-2). The free ribosomes are scattered singly in the cytoplasm or joined to form functional units called *polyribosomes.* The free ribosomes are involved in the synthesis of proteins, such as intracellular enzymes, that are used within the cell. The ribosomes that are attached to the endoplasmic reticulum synthesize proteins that are exported from the cell.

Endoplasmic reticulum

The endoplasmic reticulum (ER) is an extensive system of paired parallel membranes that connects various parts of the inner cell (see Fig. 1-2). The space between the paired membrane layers is connected with the space between the two membranes of the double-layered nuclear membrane, allowing for transport between the nucleus and the cytoplasm. There are two types of ER— rough and smooth. The rough ER is studded with ribosomes and functions in the synthesis of proteins. Hormone synthesis by glandular cells and plasma protein production by liver cells take place in the rough ER. The smooth ER is free of ribosomes but is often attached

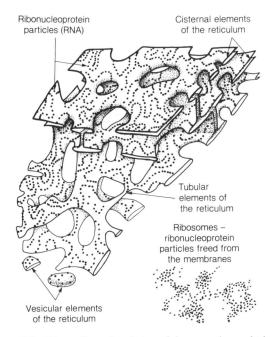

Figure 1-2 *Three-dimensional view of the granular endoplasmic reticulum with ribosomal RNA. (Modified from Bloom W, Faucett DW: Histology, 10th ed. Philadelphia, WB Saunders, 1975)*

to the rough ER. The functions of the smooth ER vary in different cells. The sarcoplasmic reticulum of skeletal and cardiac muscle cells is a form of smooth ER. Calcium ions needed for muscle contraction are stored and released from cisterns located in the sarcoplasmic reticulum of these cells.

In the liver, the smooth ER is involved in glycogen storage and drug metabolism. An interesting form of adaptation occurs in the smooth ER of the liver cells responsible for metabolizing certain drugs such as phenobarbital. It is known that repeated administration of phenobarbital leads to a state of increased tolerance to the drug, such that the same dose of drug no longer produces the same degree of sedation. This response has been traced to increased drug metabolism due to increased synthesis of drug-metabolizing enzymes by the ER membrane. This system is sometimes called the *microsomal system* because the ER can be fragmented in the laboratory, and when this is done, small vesicles called *microsomes* are formed. The microsomal system responsible for metabolizing phenobarbital has a crossover effect that influences the metabolism of other drugs that use the same metabolic pathway.

Golgi complex

The Golgi complex (or apparatus) consists of flattened membranous saccules and cisterns that communicate with the ER and acts as a receptacle for hormones and

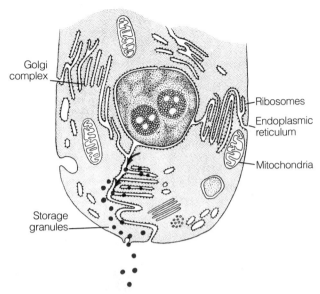

Golgi complex

Ribosomes

Endoplasmic reticulum

Mitochondria

Storage granules

Figure 1-3 *Hormone synthesis and secretion. In hormone secretion, the hormone is synthesized by the ribosomes. It moves from the rough endoplasmic reticulum to the Golgi complex where it is stored as secretory granules. These leave the Golgi complex and are stored within the cytoplasm until released from the cell in response to an appropriate signal.*

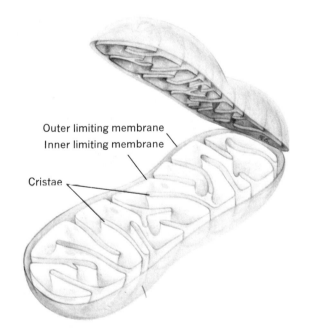

Outer limiting membrane
Inner limiting membrane

Cristae

Figure 1-4 *Mitochondrion. The inner membrane forms transverse folds called cristae. It is here that the enzymes needed for the final step in adenosine triphosphate (ATP) production (oxidative phosphorylation) are located. (Chaffee EE, Lytle IM: Basic Physiology and Anatomy, 4th ed. Philadelphia, JB Lippincott, 1980)*

other substances that the ER produces. It then collects and packages these substances into secretory granules and vesicles capable of exocytosis. The secretory granules move out of the Golgi complex, into the cytoplasm, and, following an appropriate signal, are then released from the cell through the process of exocytosis or reverse phagocytosis. Figure 1-3 is a diagram of the synthesis and movement of a hormone through the endoplasmic reticulum and Golgi complex. In addition to secreting proteins, the Golgi complex is thought to produce some of the large carbohydrate molecules that are needed to combine with proteins produced in the rough ER to form glycoproteins.

Mitochondria

The mitochondria are literally the "power plants" of the cell, for it is here that the energy-rich compound adenosine triphosphate (ATP), which powers the various cellular activities, is generated. The mitochondria capture energy contained in foodstuffs and convert it into the high-energy bonds of ATP. The enzymes involved in oxidative metabolism are present only in the mitochondria.

The mitochondria are encased in a double membrane. An outer membrane encloses the periphery of the mitochondria and an inner membrane is enfolded to form the cristae, which aid in the production and temporary storage of ATP (Fig. 1-4). The mitochondria are located close to the site of energy consumption in the cell, for example, near the myofibrils in muscle cells. The number of mitochondria in a given cell type is largely determined by the type of activity that the cell performs and the amount of energy that is needed to perform this activity.

Lysosomes

The lysosomes essentially form the digestive system of the cell. They consist of small membrane-enclosed vesicles or sacs that contain hydrolytic enzymes capable of breaking down worn-out cell parts and foreign material that enters the cell. The enzymes contained in the lysosomes are so powerful that they are often called "suicide bags," because under abnormal conditions their contents can be released, causing lysis and the destruction of cellular contents. Under other conditions their contents can be released into the extracellular spaces, destroying the surrounding cells. One theory of irreversible shock suggests that this stage of shock is caused, at least in part, by widespread release of lysosomal enzymes from cells that have been damaged by lack of oxygen.

Microtubules and microfilaments

The *microtubules* are long, rigid, threadlike structures dispersed throughout the cytoplasm. Cells use microtubules for a number of purposes. Within the cell, microtubules (1) maintain the shape of cells—long cell processes like the axons of nerve cells exist only because they are reinforced by numerous microtubules; (2) serve as a transport system for the movement of compounds and organelles within the cell; (3) construct the mitotic spindle; and (4) provide for the support and movement of cilia and flagella. Because they control cell shape and movement, the microtubules and microfilaments are often called the *cytoskeletal system*.

In cilia and sperm, the microtubules occur in doublets. The centrioles, which will be discussed next, contain microtubules arranged in triplets. It appears that microtubules can be rapidly assembled and disassembled according to the needs of the cell. The assembly of microtubules is halted by the action of the plant alkaloid colchicine. In the laboratory this compound is used to halt cell mitosis. It is also used in the treatment of gout. It is thought that the drug interferes with microtubular function and leukocyte motility and, therefore, leads to a decrease in the inflammatory reaction that occurs with this condition.

The *microfilaments* occur in association with the microtubules. The contractile proteins—actin, myosin, and troponin—are examples of microfilaments found in muscle cells.

Abnormalities of the cytoskeletal system may constitute important causes of alterations in cellular function. For example, proper functioning of the microfilaments and microtubules is essential for various stages of leukocyte migration. In certain disease conditions such as diabetes mellitus, alterations in leukocyte mobility and migration may interfere with the chemotaxis and phagocytosis of the inflammatory response and predispose to the development of bacterial infection.[1]

The *centrioles,* found in cells capable of reproducing themselves, are composed of nine bundles of microfilaments, each of which contains three microfilaments. The microfilaments aid the separation and movement of the chromosome's daughter cells during cell division.

Cell Membrane

The cell is enclosed in a thin membrane that separates the intracellular contents from the extracellular environment. To distinguish it from the other cell membranes, such as the mitochondrial or nuclear membranes, the cell membrane is often called the *plasma membrane*. In many respects, the plasma membrane is one of the most important parts of the cell. The functions of the cell membrane include (1) acting as a semipermeable membrane that separates the intracellular and extracellular environments; (2) carrying receptors for hormones and other biologically active substances; (3) participating in the electrical events that occur in nerve and muscle cells; and (4) aiding in the regulation of growth and proliferation. It is also thought that the cell membrane may play an important role in the behavior of cancer cells,[2] which function will be discussed in Chapter 5.

The cell membrane consists of an organized arrangement of lipids, carbohydrates, and proteins (Fig. 1-5). According to current theories, the lipids form a

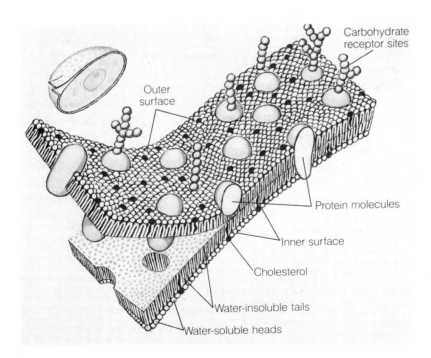

Figure 1-5 *Cell membrane. The right end is intact, but the left end has been split along the plane of the lipid tails. (Chaffee EE, Lytle IM: Basic Physiology and Anatomy, 4th ed. Philadelphia, JB Lippincott, 1980)*

bilayer structure that is essentially impermeable to all but the lipid-soluble substances. It is believed that globular proteins are embedded in this lipid bilayer and that these proteins participate in the transport of lipid-insoluble particles through the plasma membrane. According to this schema, some of the globular proteins move within the membrane structure acting as carriers, some are attached to either side of the membrane, and others pass directly through the membrane communicating with both the inside and the outside of the cell. It is probable that these latter proteins form channels that permit passage of substances such as water and specific ions such as sodium, hydrogen, and chloride. There are different membrane channels for different ion species. For example, one set of pores, called the *sodium channels,* are selectively permeable to sodium.

The cell surface has been observed, under the electron microscope, to be surrounded by a fuzzy-looking layer called the *cell coat,* or *glycocalyx.* This layer is made up of glycolipid and glycoprotein molecules that participate in cell membrane interactions. The cell coat contains the sites for hormone recognition, the ABO blood group, and other tissue antigens.

Microvilli are elongated protrusions of the cell membrane that are arranged as a series of tubular extensions. These extensions greatly increase the surface area of the cell membrane. This specialized cell membrane arrangement facilitates the absorption of fluids and other materials. Microvilli are found in the lumen of the small intestine and renal tubules.

Cilia are long protuberances of the cell membrane with the tapered ends that are characteristic of many cell types, particularly the epithelium. They are anchored in the cytoplasm by a structure similar to the centriole, and extending from this structure is a series of microtubules that are surrounded by the cell membrane. By sliding the microfilaments on each other, the cilia are capable of a sweeping type of movement. Longer cilia are called *flagella.* The cilia provide a mechanism for cell movement or, if the location of the cell is fixed, as in the respiratory tract, for the movement of adjacent fluids.

Membrane junctions

With the exception of blood cells, most cells are organized into tissues and organs. In these tissues or organs, cells are held together by the intercellular adhesions that connect the membranes of adjacent cells.

There are at least three classes of adhesions that hold cells together: *electrostatic interactions,* which are the weakest and develop between the charged cell surfaces; *aggregation proteins,* which bind specific types of cells together; and *intercellular junctions.* The binding together of cells by aggregation proteins depends on specific binding sites on the cell membrane. Both the formation of aggregation proteins and binding sites appear to be genetically determined during the process of cell differentiation. Thus, the aggregation proteins and binding sites of heart cells are different from those of liver cells.

There are at least three types of cell junctions that join the cell membranes of adjacent cells to form a unit. One type of intercellular junction, known as a *desmosome,* is disk shaped and can be likened to a rivet. A second type, the *zona occludens* or *tight junction,* actually fuses the membranes of adjacent cells together. This type of intercellular connection is found in tissues such as the skin that are subject to considerable stretching and in epithelial tissues that separate two compartments with different chemical compositions (*e.g.,* bladder and gastrointestinal tract lining). A third and less common form of intercellular junction involves the close approximation of the cell membranes with the formation of apparent pores between the cytoplasms of the two cells. These *nexus,* or *gap, junctions* possess low electrical-resistance properties and permit electrical communication between cells. The type of cell junction varies with the function of the tissue type. Tissues that facilitate the absorption of fluid usually have cells that are connected by tight junctions. The intercollated disks that join the myocardial fibers of the heart muscle are nexus with low-resistance electrical properties.

Membrane transport

There is a constant movement of molecules and ions across the cell membrane. This movement is facilitated by osmosis, diffusion, facilitated diffusion, active transport, exocytosis, and endocytosis (Fig. 1-6).

Osmosis. Osmosis is concerned with the passage of water across a semipermeable membrane. It is regulated by the concentration of osmotically active particles present on either side of the membrane. For example, when a greater number of osmotically active particles is present on one side of a semipermeable membrane, water will move down its concentration gradient from the side that has the lesser number of particles to the side with the greater number of particles. This movement of water will continue until the solute particles on both sides of the membrane are equally diluted or until the hydrostatic pressure created by the movement of water opposes its flow.

Diffusion. Diffusion refers to the process whereby molecules of gases and other substances move from an area of higher concentration to an area of lower concentration and become equally distributed across the cell membrane. Lipid-soluble molecules such as oxygen, carbon dioxide, alcohol, and fatty acids become dissolved in

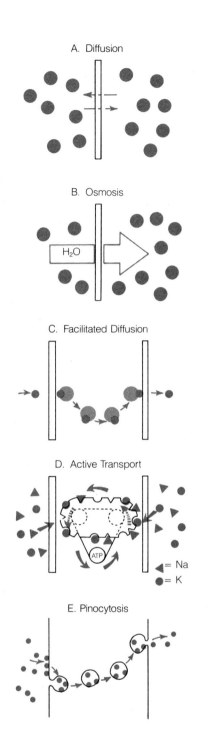

A. Diffusion

B. Osmosis

H₂O

C. Facilitated Diffusion

D. Active Transport

ATP

◄ = Na
● = K

E. Pinocytosis

Figure 1-6 *Mechanisms of membrane transport. A represents diffusion, in which particles move to become equally distributed across the membrane. In B the osmotically active particles regulate the flow of water. In C, facilitated diffusion uses a carrier system. D represents active transport, in which selected molecules are transported across the membrane using the energy-driven (ATP) pump. The membrane forms a vesicle in E that engulfs the particle and then transports it across the membrane where it is released. This is called pinocytosis.*

the lipid matrix of the cell membrane and diffuse through the membrane in the same manner that diffusion occurs in water. Other substances diffuse through minute pores in the cell membrane.

Facilitated diffusion. Facilitated diffusion involves a carrier system. Some substances, such as glucose, cannot pass through the cell membrane because they are not lipid soluble or they are too large to pass through the membrane's pores. These substances combine with a special lipid-soluble carrier at the membrane's outer surface, are carried across the membrane attached to the carrier, and are then released at the inner surface of the membrane. In facilitated diffusion a substance can move only from an area of higher concentration to an area of lower concentration. The rate at which a substance moves across the membrane through the process of facilitated diffusion depends on the difference in concentration between the two sides of the membrane, the amount of carrier that is available for transport, and the rapidity with which the carrier binds and releases the substances that are being transported.[2] It is thought that insulin, which increases glucose transport, may increase either the amount of carrier that is present or the rate at which the reactions between glucose and the carrier take place.

Active transport. Whereas diffusion and facilitated diffusion move substances from an area of higher concentration to one of lower concentration, active transport can move substances across the cell membrane against a concentration gradient, from a lower to a higher concentration. Active transport requires expenditure of energy from the hydrolysis of adenosine triphosphate (ATP). The sodium and potassium membrane transport system, sometimes called the *sodium–potassium pump,* is an example of active transport. The sodium–potassium pump moves sodium from the inside to the outside of the cell, where its concentration is about 14 times greater than inside, and then returns potassium to the inside, where its concentration is about 35 times greater than it is outside the cell. Were it not for the activity of the sodium–potassium pump, sodium would accumulate within the cell, causing cellular swelling as water moves into the cell along an osmotic gradient.

Pinocytosis. Pinocytosis is a mechanism by which the cell membrane engulfs particles and forms a vesicle. The vesicle then breaks away from the inner surface of the cell membrane and moves into the cytoplasm, where it is eventually freed by the action of lysosomes or other cytoplasmic enzymes. Pinocytosis refers to the ingestion of small amounts of extracellular fluid and dissolved particles; it is important in the transport of proteins and strong solutions of electrolytes.

Phagocytosis. Phagocytosis is a mechanism similar to pinocytosis, except that larger indentations occur in the cell membrane. This mechanism allows the cell to ingest large particles such as bacteria and cell debris.

Exocytosis. Exocytosis is the mechanism for the secretion of intracellular substances into the extracellular spaces. It is the reverse of pinocytosis in that a fluid-filled vacuole fuses to the inner side of the cell membrane and an opening occurs to the outside of the cell surface. This opening allows the contents of the vacuole to be released into the extracellular fluid. Exocytosis is important in removing cellular debris from the cell and releasing substances such as hormones, which have been synthesized within the cell.

Membrane potentials

Electrical potentials exist across the membranes of most, if not all, cells in the body. In excitable tissues such as nerve or muscle cells, changes in the membrane potential are necessary for generation and conduction of impulses. In other types of cells, such as glandular cells, changes in the membrane potential contribute to other functions.

An electrical potential describes the ability of separated electrical charges of opposite polarity (+ and −) to do work; it is measured in volts (V). The terms *potential difference* and *voltage* are synonymous. Voltage is always measured with respect to two points in a system. For example, the potential difference between the two terminals in a car battery is 6 V or 12 V. Since the total amount of charge that can be separated by a biological membrane is very small, the potential differences are very

small. Membrane potentials are measured in millivolts. (A *millivolt* is $\frac{1}{1000}$ of a volt.) The voltage difference between the inside and the outside of a cell can be measured in the laboratory by inserting a very fine electrode into the cell and another into the extracellular fluid surrounding the cell and connecting the two electrodes to a voltmeter (Fig. 1-7). The movement of charge between two points is called *current;* it occurs when a potential difference has been established and the charged particles are able to move between the two points.

Both extracellular and intracellular fluids are electrolyte solutions containing about 150 mEq to 160 mEq of positively charged ions and equal concentration of negatively charged ions; these are the *current-carrying ions* responsible for generating and conducting the electrical potentials of the cell. Generally, there is a minute excess of positive ions outside the cell and an equal amount of negative ions inside the cell. Because of the extreme thinness of the cell membrane, these charges accumulate on either side of the membrane, contributing to the establishment of a membrane potential.

Origin of the membrane potential. The uneven distribution of the various ions in the extra- and intracellular fluids is required for the existence of a membrane potential. Three factors contribute to the origin of the membrane potential: (1) the selective permeability of the resting cell membrane to the positively charged potassium ion; (2) the presence of large numbers of nondiffusible intracellular anions, such as protein ions, sulfate ions, and phosphate ions; and (3) the sodium–potassium membrane pump (Fig. 1-8). Most resting membranes are 50 to 100 times more permeable to potassium ions than to sodium ions; because of this, there is limited movement of sodium ions to the inside of the cell. On the other hand, the potassium ion, which can diffuse easily across the cell membrane, remains inside the cell, attracted by the nondiffusible intracellular anions and repelled by the positively charged extracellular sodium ions. Although the cell membrane is relatively impermeable to the sodium ion, some sodium ions do cross the membrane and are extruded by the sodium–potassium membrane pump. In the process of removing sodium ions from inside the membrane, the sodium–potassium pump extrudes three positively charged sodium ions for every two positively charged potassium ions that are returned to the inside of the membrane, resulting in a net removal of positive charges.

There is no pump for the chloride ion. Although the membrane is permeable to the ion, it remains on the outside of the membrane because it is attracted by the positively charged sodium ions and repelled from moving to the inside of the membrane by the nondiffusible intracellular anions.

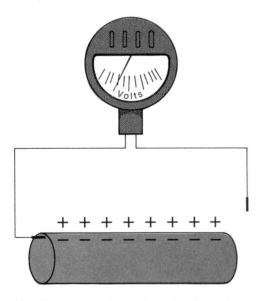

Figure 1-7 *Alignment of charge along the cell membrane. The electrical potential is negative on the inside of the cell membrane in relation to the outside.*

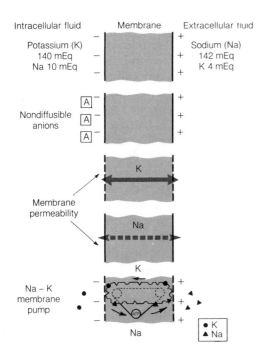

Intracellular fluid | **Membrane** | **Extracellular fluid**

Potassium (K)
140 mEq
Na 10 mEq

Sodium (Na)
142 mEq
K 4 mEq

Nondiffusible
anions

Membrane
permeability

Na – K
membrane
pump

● K
▲ Na

Figure 1-8 *Mechanisms in the development of membrane potentials. Three factors contribute to the difference in electrical potential (negative on the inside and positive on the outside) and Na⁺ and K⁺ concentration across the cell membrane: (1) the presence of nondiffusible anions on the inside of the membrane, which attract the positively charged K⁺ ions; (2) selective permeability of the resting membrane to Na⁺ and K⁺ (the resting membrane is about 100 times more permeable to K⁺ than to Na⁺) so that K⁺ diffuses and remains inside the membrane and Na⁺ remains outside; and (3) the Na⁺–K⁺ membrane pump, which extrudes three Na⁺ ions for every two K⁺ ions, resulting in a net removal of positive charge from inside the membrane.*

Diffusion potentials. The effects of the major electrolytes (sodium and potassium) on body membranes is determined by the electrolytes' concentrations on the inside and outside of the membrane and by the membrane's permeability to the electrolytes. A membrane potential produced by diffusion of an ion reflects the driving force of the ion's concentration gradient across the membrane and the electrical forces that oppose its movement. At the level of the cell membrane, the concentration of potassium ions inside of the cell is about 35 times that on the outside of the cell. The diffusion gradient caused by this concentration difference would cause potassium ions to move out of the cell were it not for the opposing force provided by the positively charged sodium ions on the outside of the membrane. An *equilibrium potential* is one in which there is no net movement of ions because the diffusion and electrical forces are exactly balanced. The equilibrium potentials

for sodium and potassium can be calculated using the following equation:

$$E \text{ (millivolts)} = -61 \log \frac{\text{ion concentration inside}}{\text{ion concentration outside*}}$$

where E is the equilibrium potential for the ion and -61 is a constant derived from the gas constant, the absolute temperature, the valence of the ion, and a term for converting natural logarithms to base 10. For example, if the inside of the membrane contains 100 millimols (mM) of an ion and the outside contains 0.1 mM (100/0.01 = 10 and the log of 10 is 1), and the equilibrium potential for that ion would be 61. It would take 61 mV of charge on the outside of the membrane to balance the diffusion gradient created by the concentration difference across the membrane for this ion. Two conditions are necessary for a membrane potential to occur as a result of diffusion: (1) the membrane must be semipermeable, allowing ions of one type of charge to diffuse through the pores while ions of the opposite charge cannot pass through the pores, and (2) the concentration of the diffusible ion must be greater on one side of the membrane than on the other.

If the membrane were permeable only to potassium and there were no pumping of ions across the membrane, the equilibrium potential for the potassium ion would be -94 mV ($-61 \times \log 140$ mEq inside/4 mEq outside), which approximates the -70 mV to -90 mV resting membrane potential that has been reported for nerve fibers. If the same conditions held true for sodium, the equilibrium potential would be about $+61$ mV ($-61 \times \log 14$ mEq inside/140 mEq outside). This value approaches the $+45$ mV reported for the fraction of a second that occurs at the peak of the action potential when the membrane is much more permeable to sodium than to potassium.

When the membrane is permeable to several different ions, the diffusion potential that develops depends on the concentration difference for each of the ions, their charges, and the permeability of the membrane to each of these ions.

Action potentials. Action potentials are abrupt, pulselike changes in the membrane potential that last a few ten-thousandths to a few thousandths of a second. In a nerve fiber an action potential can be elicited by any factor that suddenly increases the permeability of the membrane to sodium. It is thought that there are pores or channels in the cell membrane through which the current-carrying ions flow. Sodium and potassium use different channels as they move through the membrane, allowing the membrane to change its permeability dur-

*Known as the Nernst equation.

ing different phases of the action potential. It is also thought that these channels are guarded by electrically charged "gates" that open and close with changes in the membrane potential (Fig. 1-9). There are similar channels for calcium in the membrane, and it is these channels that are blocked by the calcium channel-blocking drugs used in treatment of cardiovascular disease.

When charges of opposite polarity ($+$ and $-$) are aligned across the membrane, it is said to be polarized. The changes that occur in excitable tissue during an action potential can be divided into three phases—the resting or polarized state, depolarization, and repolarization (Fig. 1-10).

The *resting membrane potential* is characterized by the relatively low permeability of the membrane to the rapid flow of charged ions. During this phase, there is about 70 mV less charge on the inside of the membrane (-70 mV) compared to the outside. This difference in concentration of charge is necessary for the establishment of current flow once the membrane becomes permeable to the flow of charged ions.

The *threshold potential* (about -60 mV) represents the membrane potential at which the neuron is stimulated to fire. Stimuli that excite a neuron produce marked increases in membrane permeability and an increased flow of sodium through the membrane, causing it to become less negative and moving it toward the threshold potential. When the threshold level is reached, the sodium gates swing open and there is a rapid inflow of positively charged sodium ions through the membrane and into the cell. In neurons, the sodium ion gate remains open for only about a quarter of a millisecond, and then closes quickly. During this period, the membrane potential rapidly shifts toward zero and beyond so that the membrane is positively charged. At the same time, a slower operating increase in outflow of potassium ions moves the potential back toward zero. Once a neuron reaches the minimal threshold for excitation, it is committed to fire and its response will be maximal. This is called the *all or none law*.

Depolarization represents the phase of the action potential during which the membrane is highly permeable to the sodium ions. During this phase, there is reversal of the membrane potential and the inside of the membrane becomes positive (about $+20$ mV).

The third phase of the action potential is called *repolarization*. During this phase, the polarity of the resting membrane potential is reestablished. This is accomplished as sodium permeability quickly returns to normal while potassium permeability increases. The outflowing positively charged potassium ions return the membrane potential toward negativity. The sodium gates close. The sodium–potassium pump gradually reestablishes the resting ionic concentrations on each side of the membrane.

The membrane of excitable tissue must be sufficiently repolarized before it can be reexcited. In the process of repolarization, the membrane remains refractory (will not fire) until the repolarization is about one-third complete. This period of approximately one-half millisecond is called the *absolute refractory period*. There is an additional period of time during the recovery period in which the membrane can be excited, but only by a stronger-than-normal stimulus. This period is called the *relative refractory period*.

The excitability of a neuron or muscle fiber depends on the amount of change that must occur in the membrane potential to reach the threshold level needed for initiation of an action potential. When the resting membrane potential becomes extremely negative, the membrane is said to be hyperpolarized (see Fig. 1-10). When this happens, reexcitation becomes more difficult or does not occur. *Hypopolarization*, on the other hand, represents the situation in which the resting membrane potential *becomes less negative*. When it approaches the threshold potential, the membrane becomes extremely excitable and may undergo spontaneous depolarization.

Alterations in membrane excitability. There are a number of factors that alter membrane excitability.

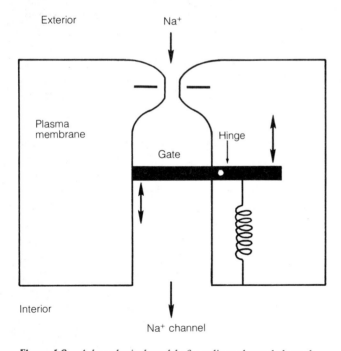

Figure 1-9 A hypothetical model of a sodium channel through the plasma membrane of an axon. A narrow pore (0.3 nm × 0.5 nm) with a negatively charged wall provides selectivity to hydrated sodium ions. When the gate is opened during the initial stage of depolarization, the flow of sodium is greatly increased.

Among these are (1) changes in the resting membrane potential and (2) changes in the permeability of the membrane.

Serum levels of potassium exert a strong influence on repolarization (and the resting membrane potential) of excitable tissue. In situations in which there is a decrease in serum levels of potassium, the resting membrane potential becomes more negative, and nerve and muscle fibers become hyperpolarized, sometimes to the extent that they cannot be reexcited. *Familial periodic paralysis* is a hereditary condition in which extracellular potassium levels periodically fall to low levels, causing muscle paralysis (Chap. 25). An increase in potassium, on the other hand, interferes with the repolarization of the membrane; it causes hypopolarization, and the resting membrane potential moves closer to threshold levels and then to zero. When this happens, the strength of the action potential is decreased. This is because there is a decrease in the concentration of charge between the two sides of the membrane, and consequently less charge is available to move through the membrane during each action potential. Should the resting potential be reduced so that it approaches zero, the membrane will remain depolarized. This situation is similar to what happens when the car battery goes dead and needs to be recharged. Elevations in serum potassium exert their greatest effect on the conduction system of the heart. The force of cardiac contractions becomes weaker until eventually repolarization is inadequate to maintain excitability, and the heart stops in diastole.

Neural excitability is markedly altered by changes in membrane permeability. Calcium ions decrease membrane permeability to sodium ions. If there are not sufficient calcium ions available, the permeability of the membrane becomes increased and, as a result, membrane excitability increases—sometimes to the extent that spontaneous muscle movements (tetany) occur. *Local anesthetic agents* (such as procaine or cocaine) act directly on the membrane to decrease its permeability to sodium.

In summary, the cell is a remarkably autonomous structure that functions in a manner strikingly similar to that of the total organism. The cell nucleus controls cell function and is the mastermind of the cell, whereas the cytoplasm contains the cell's inner organs and is the cell's work site. Cells contain other structures such as microtubules and microfilaments, which are needed for the special function that they perform. Cells are separated from their external environment by a semipermeable cell membrane that aids in regulating the osmotic and ionic homeostasis of the cell's interior. Semipermeability to Na^+ and K^+, impermeability to larger negative cytoplasmic ions, and the action of an $Na^+–K^+$ pumping mechanism results in a net electrical charge differen-

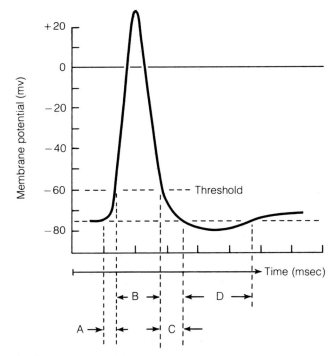

A = Generator potential that exceeds threshold
B = Absolute refractory period (active potential and partial recovery)
C = Negative-relation refractory period
D = Positive-relation refractory period

Figure 1-10 *The time course of the action potential recorded at one point of an axon with one electrode inside and one on the outside of the plasma membrane. The generator potential is the stimulus-induced change in membrane potential that initiates the action potential. The rising part of the action potential is called the spike. The rising phase plus approximately the first half of the repolarization phase is equal to the absolute refractory period. The remaining portion of the repolarization phase to the resting membrane potential is equal to the negative after potential. Hyperpolarization is equal to the positive after potential.*

tial (negative inside) across the plasma membrane. Electrical potentials (negative on the inside and positive on the outside) exist across the membranes of most, if not all, cells in the body. These electrical potentials result from the selective permeability of the cell membrane to Na^+ and K^+, the presence of nondiffusible anions inside the cell membrane, and the activity of the $Na^+–K^+$ membrane pump, which extrudes Na^+ from the inside of the membrane and returns K^+ to the inside. In the resting state, excitable tissues such as neurons and muscle cells are impermeable to the flow of electrical charge. An action potential is an abrupt, pulselike change in the membrane potential. It consists of a depolarization phase during which the membrane is permeable to the rapid inflow of charge, causing the reversal (positive on the inside and negative on the outside) of the membrane potential, and a repolarization phase during which the resting membrane potential is reestablished. The threshold potential is the change in membrane potential that is sufficient to produce an action potential.

■ Cellular Energy Metabolism

Energy is defined as the ability to do work. Cells utilize oxygen and the breakdown products of the foods we eat to produce the energy needed for muscle contraction, transport of ions and molecules, and synthesis of enzymes, hormones, and other macromolecules. *Energy metabolism* refers to processes by which fats, proteins, and carbohydrates from the foods we eat are converted into energy or complex energy sources in the cell. There are two phases of metabolism, *catabolism* and *anabolism*. Catabolism consists of the breaking down of substances, particularly the breaking down of food and body tissues with the resultant liberation of energy. Anabolism is a building-up process in which more complex molecules are formed from simpler ones.

The special carrier for cellular energy is *adenosine triphosphate* (ATP). The ATP molecule consists of adenosine, a nitrogenous base; ribose, a five-carbon sugar; and three phosphate groups (Fig. 1-11). The phosphate groups contain two high-energy bonds that store seven calories each; free energy from foodstuffs is transformed into energy that is stored in these bonds. ATP is often referred to as the "energy currency" of the cell; energy can be "saved or spent" using ATP as an exchange currency.

There are two sites of energy production in the cell: (1) the anaerobic (without oxygen) glycolytic pathway, which is located in the cytoplasm, and (2) the aerobic (with oxygen) pathways in the mitochondria.

Anaerobic Metabolism

Glycolysis is the process by which energy is liberated from glucose. It occurs in the cytoplasm of the cell and can proceed anaerobically, or without the presence of oxygen. Glycolysis is an important energy provider for cells that lack mitochondria, the cell structure in which aerobic metabolism occurs. The process also provides energy in situations when delivery of oxygen to the cell is either delayed or impaired. The process involves a sequence of reactions that converts glucose to pyruvate with the concomitant production of ATP. The net gain of energy from the glycolysis of one molecule of glucose is two ATP molecules and two molecules of pyruvate. If oxygen is present, the two molecules of pyruvate move into the mitochondria, where they enter the citric acid cycle (Fig. 1-12). When oxygen is lacking, pyruvate is converted to lactic acid and released into the extracellular fluid as a means of removing glycolytic end products from the cell so that glycolysis can proceed. Indeed, glycolysis could proceed for only a few seconds if pyruvic acid were not removed from the cytoplasm. The conversion of pyruvate to lactic acid is reversible, so that once the oxygen supply has been restored, lactic acid is converted back either to pyruvic acid or to glucose. Heart cells are particularly efficient in converting lactic acid to pyruvic acid and then using this as a fuel source. While relatively inefficient in terms of energy yield, the glycolytic pathway is important during periods of decreased oxygen delivery, such as occurs in skeletal muscle during the first few minutes of exercise.

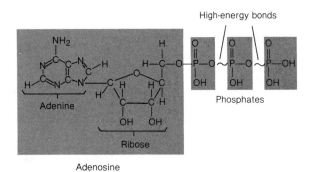

Figure 1-11 *Structure of the adenosine triphosphate (ATP) molecule.*

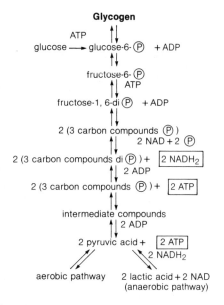

Figure 1-12 *The glycolytic pathway.*

Aerobic Metabolism

Aerobic metabolism occurs in the cell's mitochondria. The mitochondria are oval-shaped organelles located in the cell's cytoplasm (see Fig. 1-4). The oxidative processes responsible for the production of energy occur in the mitochondria, and it is here that hydrogen and carbon molecules from the fats, proteins, and carbohydrates in our diet are broken down and combined with molecular oxygen to form carbon dioxide and water as energy is released. Unlike lactic acid, which is an end product of anaerobic metabolism, carbon dioxide and water are relatively harmless and easily eliminated from the body. The mitochondria have two membrane systems: an outer membrane and an inner membrane with a series of ridges called the *cristae*. Hence, the mitochondria have two compartments; there is an intermembrane space between the inner and outer membrane and an internal matrix, which is bounded by the inner membrane. The reactions of the citric acid cycle and fatty acid oxidation occur in the internal matrix, whereas the respiratory assembly for oxidative phosphorylation is an integral part of the inner membrane.

The citric acid cycle

The citric acid cycle, sometimes called the *tricarboxylic acid* or *Kreb's cycle*, provides the final common pathway for the metabolism of nutrients. In the citric acid cycle, an activated two-carbon molecule of acetyl-coenzyme A (CoA) condenses with a four-carbon molecule of oxaloacetic acid and then moves through a series of enzyme-mediated steps in which hydrogen and carbon dioxide are formed. The hydrogen atoms become attached to one of two special carriers, favin adenine dinucleotide (FAD) or nicotinamide adenine dinucleotide (NAD), for transfer to the electron transport system. The carbon dioxide molecules are carried to the lungs and then exhaled. Two carbon atoms are lost in one turn of the cycle, neither from the original acetyl-CoA; these two are then lost as carbon dioxide in the second revolution of the cycle. In the citric acid cycle, shown in Figure 1-13, each of the two pyruvate molecules that were formed in the cytoplasm from one molecule of glucose yield another molecule of ATP along with two molecules of carbon dioxide and five hydrogen atoms. These hydrogen molecules are transferred to the electron transport system on the inner mitochondrial membrane for oxidation. In addition to pyruvate from the glycolysis of glucose, products of amino acid and fatty acid degradation enter the citric acid cycle.

Oxidative phosphorylation

Oxidative metabolism, which supplies 90% of the body's energy needs, is the process in which inorganic phosphorylation is coupled with adenosine diphosphate (ADP) to form ATP as hydrogen electrons are transferred from $FADH_2$ and NADH to molecular oxygen by a series of electron carriers that are present in the inner

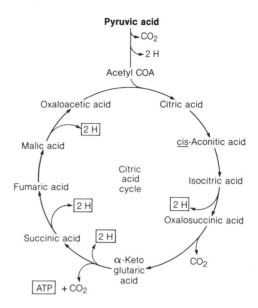

Figure 1-13 *The citric acid cycle. (Chaffee EE, Lytle IM: Basic Physiology and Anatomy, 4th ed. Philadelphia, JB Lippincott, 1980)*

mitochondrial membrane. As molecular oxygen combines with the electrons from the hydrogen atom, water is formed. In a 24-hour period of time, oxidative metabolism supplies the body with 300 ml to 500 ml of water.

In summary, cellular energy metabolism is the process whereby the carbohydrates, fats, and proteins from the foods we eat are broken down and converted into energy that is stored in the form of ATP's high-energy bonds. There are two sites of energy metabolism in cells: the mitochrondria and the cytoplasmic matrix. The most efficient of these pathways are those that are located in the mitochondria. These pathways require oxygen and produce carbon dioxide and water as end products. The glycolytic pathway, which is located in the cytoplasm, involves the breakdown of glucose to form ATP. The formation of lactic acid allows this process to proceed in the absence of oxygen.

■ Tissue Types

In the preceding sections we discussed the individual cell and its metabolic processes. Although cells are similar, their structure and function vary according to the needs of the tissues. There are four categories of specialized tissue: epithelium, connective tissue, nerve, and muscle. This section provides a brief overview of these tissue types as preparation for understanding the subsequent chapters in this and other units.

Cell Differentiation

The formation of different types of cells and the disposition of these cells into tissue types is called *cell differentiation*. Following conception, the fertilized ovum divides and subdivides and ultimately forms over a hundred different cell types. The process of cell differentiation normally moves forward and is irreversible, producing cells that are more specialized than their predecessors. This means that once differentiation has occurred, the tissue type does not move backward to an earlier stage of differentiation. Usually, a highly differentiated cell loses its ability to undergo cell division.

Although most cells proceed through differentiation into specialized cell types, many tissues contain a few cells that apparently are only partially differentiated. These cells are still capable of cell division and serve as a stem cell, or reserve source, for continued production of specialized cells throughout the life span of the organism. This is one of the major processes by which regeneration is possible in some but not all tissues. Skeletal muscle, for example, has relatively few undifferentiated cells to serve as a reserve supply. Cancer cells are thought to originate from undifferentiated stem cells (see Chap. 5 for further discussion).

Embryonic Origin of Tissue Types

The four basic tissue types are often described in terms of embryonic origin. The very young embryo is essentially a three-layered tubular structure (Fig. 1-14). The outer layer of the tube is called the *ectoderm;* the middle layer, the *mesoderm;* and the inner layer, the *endoderm.* All of the adult body tissues originate from these three cellular layers. Epithelium has its origin in all three embryonic layers, connective tissue and muscle develop from the mesoderm, and nervous tissue develops from the ectoderm. Mesenchymal tissue is a precursor to connective tissue and has its origin in the mesoderm. The epithelial lining of the gut, the respiratory tract, and much of the urinary system is derived from the endoderm.

All of the more than 100 different types of body cells can be classified under four basic or primary tissue types: epithelial, connective, muscle, and nervous. Each of the primary tissue types has various subdivisions. The four tissue types and the major subdivisions are summarized in Table 1-1.

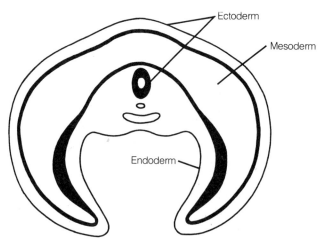

Figure 1-14   *The embryonic tissue layers.*

Table 1-1   Classification of Tissue Types

Tissue Type	Location*
Epithelium	
Covering and lining of body surfaces	
Simple epithelium	
Squamous	Lining of blood vessels and body cavities
Cuboidal	Covering of ovaries and thyroid gland
Columnar	Lining of intestine and gallbladder
Pseudostratified epithelium	Trachea and respiratory passages
Stratified epithelium	
Squamous keratinized	Skin
Squamous nonkeratinized	Mucous membranes of mouth, esophagus, and vagina
Transitional	Bladder
Glandular	
Endocrine	Pituitary, thyroid, adrenal, others
Exocrine	Sweat glands and glands in gastrointestinal tract
Connective	
Loose	Fibroblasts, adipose tissue, endothelial vessel lining
Hematopoietic	Blood cells, myeloid tissue (bone marrow), lymphoid tissue
Supporting tissues	Connective tissue and cartilage, bone and joint structures
Muscle	
Striated	Skeletal muscles
Cardiac	Myocardium
Smooth	Gastrointestinal tract, blood vessels, bronchi, bladder, others
Nervous	
Neurons	Central and peripheral neurons and nerve fibers
Supporting cells	Glia in central nervous system, Schwann and satellite cells in peripheral nervous system

*Not inclusive.

Epithelial tissue

Epithelial tissue covers the body's outer surface, lines the internal surface, and forms the glandular tissues. The epithelium protects (skin and mucous membranes), secretes (glandular tissue and goblet cells), absorbs (intestinal mucosa), and filters (renal glomeruli). The epithelial cells are avascular, that is, they have no blood vessels of their own and must receive oxygen and nutrients from the capillaries of the connective tissue on which the epithelium rests (Fig. 1-15). To survive, the epithelial cells must be kept moist. Even the seemingly dry skin epithelium is kept moist by a nonvitalized water-proof layer of keratin that prevents evaporation of moisture from the deeper living cells. Epithelium is able to regenerate quickly when injury occurs.

Epithelial cells are classified into three types according to the shape of the cells and the number of layers that are present: simple, stratified, and pseudostratified. The terms *squamous* (thin and flat), *cuboidal* (cube shaped), and *columnar* (resembling a column) refer to the cell shapes (Fig. 1-16).

Simple types of epithelium.   Simple epithelium contains a single layer of cells. *Squamous epithelium* is adapted for filtration; it is found lining the blood vessels, lymph nodes, and alveoli of the lungs. The single layer of squamous epithelium that lines the inside of the heart and blood vessels is known as the *endothelium*. A similar type of layer, called the *mesothelium*, is found in the serous

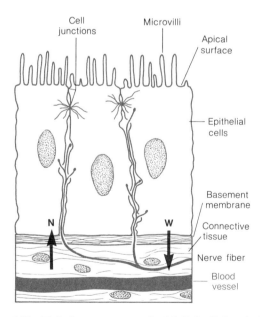

Figure 1-15   *Typical arrangement of epithelial cells in relation to underlying tissues and blood supply. Epithelial tissue has no blood supply of its own, but relies on the blood vessels in the underlying connective tissue for nutrition (N) and elimination of wastes (W).*

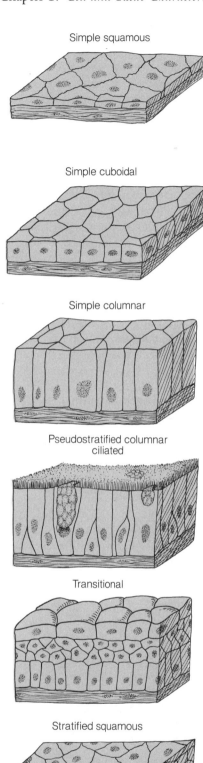

Figure 1-16   *Representation of the various epithelial tissue types.*

membranes that line the pleura and the pericardial and peritoneal cavities. *Simple cuboidal epithelium* is found on the surface of the ovary and in the thyroid. *Simple columnar epithelium* lines the intestine. One form of simple columnar epithelium has hairlike projections called *cilia,* and another produces mucous and is called a *goblet* cell.

Stratified epithelium. Stratified epithelium contains more than one layer of cells and is designed to protect the body surface. *Keratin* is a tough, fibrous protein that is formed from flattened dead cells. *Stratified squamous keratinized epithelium* makes up the epidermis of the skin, and *nonkeratinized cells* are found on wet surfaces such as the mouth and tongue.

Pseudostratified epithelium. Pseudostratified columnar epithelium is a mixture of columnar cell types. Because some of these do not reach the surface of the tissue, it gives the appearance of stratified epithelium. Pseudostratified columnar ciliated epithelium with goblet cells forms the lining of most of the upper respiratory tract.

Glandular epithelium. Glandular epithelium can be divided into two types: exocrine and endocrine. The *exocrine glands* have ducts and discharge their secretions directly onto the epithelial surface where they are located. Sweat glands and alveolar glands are examples of exocrine glands. The *endocrine glands* produce secretions that move directly into the bloodstream.

Connective tissue

Connective tissue is the most abundant tissue in the body. As its name indicates, it connects and holds tissues together. Connective tissue is unique in that it includes nonliving forms of intracellular substances such as collagen fibers and the tissue gel that fills the intercellular spaces. Connective tissue can be divided into three types: loose connective tissue, hematopoietic types of connective tissue, and strong supporting types of tissue.

Loose connective tissue (Fig. 1-17). The loose connective tissue is soft and pliable and consists of fibroblasts, mast cells, adipose tissue, the intracellular lining of blood vessels, and intracellular substances. The fibroblasts secrete collagen and produce the intracellular substances. These intracellular substances are of two types: the *amorphous type,* which fills the tissue spaces, and the fibrous form, which includes collagen, elastin, and reticular fibers. *Collagen* is the most common protein in the body;

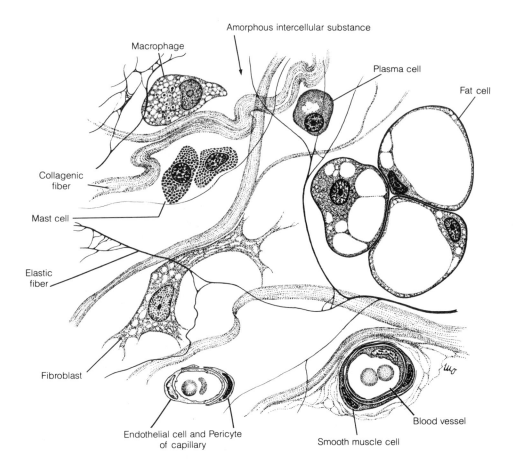

Figure 1-17 *Diagrammatic representation of cells that may be seen in loose connective tissue. The cells lie in an intercellular matrix that is bathed in tissue fluid that originates in capillaries. (Ham AW, Cormack DH: Histology, 8th ed. Philadelphia, JB Lippincott, 1979)*

it is a tough, nonliving white fiber that serves as the structural framework for skin, ligaments, tendons, and numerous other structures. *Elastin* acts like a rubber band, for it can be stretched and then return to its original form. Elastin fibers are abundant in structures such as the aorta that are subjected to frequent stretching. *Reticular fibers* made of collagen form networks that join connective tissue to other tissues. Loose connective tissue supports the epithelial tissues and provides the means by which these tissues are nourished. In an organ that contains both epithelial and connective tissue, the term *parenchymal* tissue refers to the functioning epithelium in contradistinction to its connective tissue framework.

Hematopoietic tissue.   The hematopoietic types of connective tissue include the blood cells, bone marrow, and lymphatic tissue. The role of the hematopoietic system in inflammation and immunity is discussed in Chapters 8 and 9; the reticulocyte, or red blood cell, is discussed in Chapter 13.

Strong supporting connective tissue.   The third form of connective tissue—the strong supporting form—consists of dense connective tissue, cartilage, and bone. The dense connective tissues are rich in collagen and form the tendons and ligaments that join muscle to bones and bones to bones. A layer of dense connective tissue also forms a capsule for many organs and body structures such as the kidney and heart. Dense connective tissue does not require many capillaries because it is composed largely of nonliving collagen fibers. Cartilage and bone are discussed in Chapter 50.

Muscle tissue

There are three types of muscle tissue: skeletal, cardiac, and smooth muscle. Skeletal and cardiac muscles are striated muscles. The actin and myosin filaments in these muscle types are arranged in striations, giving the muscle fibers a striped appearance.

Skeletal muscle is the largest tissue in the body, accounting for 40% to 45% of the total body weight. Most skeletal muscle is attached to bones, and its contraction is responsible for movement of the skeleton. It differs from cardiac and smooth muscle in that it is under voluntary control and is innervated by the somatic nervous system.

Cardiac muscle is found in the myocardium. Myocardial muscle is designed to pump blood continuously. It has inherent properties of automaticity, rhythmicity, and conductivity. The pumping action of the heart is controlled by impulses originating in the cardiac conduction system and is modified by blood-borne neural mediators and impulses from the autonomic nervous system.

Smooth muscle is found in many organs, including the blood vessels, the iris of the eye, and tubes such as the ureters and bile ducts that connect many internal organs.

Neither skeletal nor cardiac muscle is able to undergo the mitotic activity needed to replace injured cells. Smooth muscle, however, may proliferate and undergo mitotic activity. Some increases in smooth muscle are physiologic, such as occurs in the uterus during pregnancy. Others, such as the increase in smooth muscle that occurs in the arteries of persons with chronic hypertension, are pathologic.

Although the three types of muscle tissue differ significantly in structure, contractile properties, and control mechanisms, they have many similarities. The structural properties of skeletal muscle are presented as a prototype of muscle tissue, followed by a discussion of smooth muscle and the ways in which it differs from skeletal muscle. Cardiac muscle is described in Chapter 18.

Structural properties.   Muscle tissue is highly specialized for contractility and producing movement of internal and external body structures. Most muscle cells are long and narrow, a characteristic that allows the two ends of the cell to shorten and pull closer together during contraction. Because of their length, muscle cells are called *fibers.* The cell membrane of a muscle fiber is called the *sarcolemma,* and the cytoplasm is referred to as the *sarcoplasm.* Embedded in the sarcoplasmic reticulum are the contractile elements, *actin* and *myosin* (Fig. 1-18). The sarcoplasmic reticulum, which is comparable to the endoplasmic reticulum, is composed of longitudinal tubules that run parallel to the muscle fiber and surrounds the actin and myosin filaments. The sarcoplasmic reticulum ends in enlarged, saclike regions called the *lateral sacs.* The lateral sacs store calcium to be released during muscle contraction. A second system of tubules consists of the *transverse,* or *T-tubules,* which run perpendicular to the muscle fiber. The lumen of the transverse tubule is continuous with the extracellular fluid; and the membrane of the T-tubule is able to propagate action potentials, which are rapidly conducted over the surface of the muscle fiber and into the sarcoplasmic reticulum. As the action potential moves through the lateral sacs, the sacs release calcium, which initiates muscle contraction. The membrane of the sarcoplasmic reticulum also has an active transport mechanism for pumping the calcium ions back into the reticulum as a means of removing it from the vicinity of the actin and myosin cross-bridges on termination of muscle contraction.

Molecular mechanisms of contractions.   In striated muscle the thin, lighter filaments and the thick, darker filaments are arranged in striations that give the muscle a striped appearance. Although the striated pattern

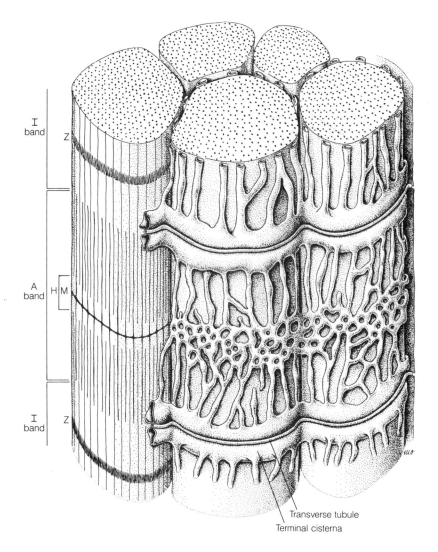

I band

Z

A band H M

I band Z

Transverse tubule
Terminal cisterna

Figure 1-18 *Part of a mammalian striated muscle fiber, illustrating the layout of the sarcoplasmic reticulum surrounding its myofibrils. In the myofibril at the left the A, I, and other bands and Z lines are indicated. The sarcoplasmic reticulum surrounding the myofibrils is illustrated at the middle and right. Note that in mammalian striated muscle fibers two transverse (T) tubules supply a sarcomere. Each T tubule is located close to the junction between an A and an I band, where it is associated with two terminal cisternae of sarcoplasmic reticulum, one on each side of it. Each terminal cisterna connects with more or less longitudinal sarcotubules of the reticulum located around the A band and these, in turn, anastomose to form a network in the more central region of the band (extending across the H band). (Courtesy of C. P. Leblond. In Ham AW, Cormack DH: Histology, 8th ed. Philadelphia, JB Lippincott, 1979)*

appears to be continuous across a single fiber, the fiber is actually composed of a number of independent cylindrical elements called *myofibrils* (Fig. 1-19). The myofibril, in turn, consists of smaller filaments that form a regular repeating pattern along the length of the myofibril; each of these units is called a *sarcomere*. The sarcomeres, which contain the thin actin and thick myosin filaments, are the functional units of the contractile system in muscle. A sarcomere extends from one Z line to another Z line. The dark A bands contain the thick myosin filaments and the lighter I bands contain the thin actin filaments. The Z lines consist of short elements that interconnect and provide the thin filaments from two adjoining sarcomeres with an anchoring point. The H zone in the center of the sarcomere corresponds to the space between the thin filaments; only thick filaments are found in this area. In the center of the H zone is a thin, dark band known as the *M line;* it is produced by linkages between the thick filaments.

During muscle contraction, the thick myosin and the thin actin filaments slide past each other, causing shortening of the muscle fiber while the length of the individual thick and thin filaments remains unchanged. The structures that produce the sliding of the filaments are the myosin cross-bridges. When activated by ATP, the cross-bridges swivel in a fixed arc, much like the oars of a boat, as they become attached to the actin filament. During contraction, each cross-bridge undergoes its own cycle of movement, forming a bridge attachment and releasing it, and then moving to another site where the same sequence of movement occurs. This has the effect of pulling the thin and thick filaments past each other.

Myosin is the chief constituent of the thick filament; it consists of a thin tail, which provides the structural backbone for the filament, and a globular head. Each globular head contains a binding site able to bind a complementary site on the actin molecule. In addition to the binding site for actin, each myosin head has a separate active site that catalyzes the breakdown of ATP to provide the energy needed to activate the myosin head so that it can form a cross-bridge with actin. Following

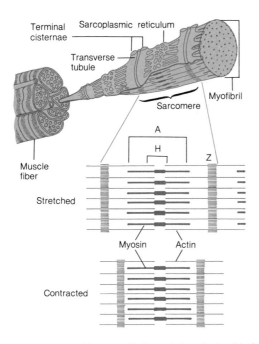

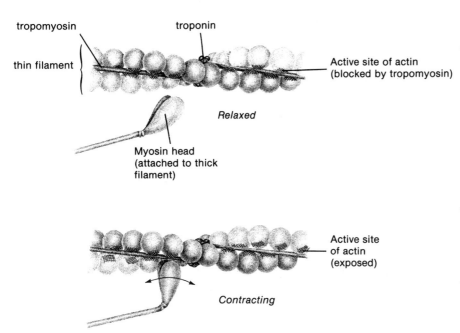

Figure 1-19 Muscle fiber, myofibril, and the relationship between actin and myosin filaments during relaxation and contraction.

contraction, myosin also binds ATP as a means of breaking the linkage between actin and myosin. The myosin molecules are bundled together side by side in the thick filaments so that half have their heads toward one end of the filament and their tails toward the other end, while the other half are arranged in the opposite manner.

The thin filaments are composed mainly of actin, a globular protein that is lined up in two rows that coil around each other to form a long helix strand. Associated with each actin filament are two regulatory proteins, tropomyosin and troponin (Fig. 1-20). *Tropomyosin,* which lies in grooves of the actin strand, provides the site for attachment of the globular heads of the myosin filament. In the noncontractile state, *troponin* covers the tropomyosin binding sites and prevents formation of cross-bridges between the actin and myosin. The binding of calcium to troponin during an action potential uncovers the actin binding sites for formation of cross-bridges with the myosin molecule. Following breaking of the linkage between actin and myosin, the concentration of calcium around the myofibrils decreases as calcium is actively transported into the sarcoplasmic reticulum by a membrane pump that uses energy derived from ATP.

Smooth muscle. Smooth muscle is often called *involuntary muscle* because its activity arises either spontaneously or through activity of the autonomic nervous

Figure 1-20 Structure of a thin filament of striated muscle at the molecular level, illustrating how in contraction the double head region of a myosin molecule of a thick filament (not shown) becomes able to interact with the actin molecules in the thin filament. As shown here, a thin filament comprises a double-stranded helix of G-actin molecules, with tropomyosin molecules (shown as rods) and units of troponin complex (shown in black) lying along the grooves between the strands. (Top) Note that the position of the tropomyosin molecules during relaxation is such that they block the active sites on the actin molecules so as to prevent myosin heads from interacting with them. (Bottom) The configuration of the troponin complex is altered by calcium ions during contraction. This, in turn, causes the tropomyosin molecules to move away from the active sites on the actin molecules so that these sites become exposed and able to interact with myosin heads of thick filaments. (Ham AW, Cormack DH: Histology, 8th ed. Philadelphia, JB Lippincott, 1979)

system. On the whole, smooth muscle contraction tends to be slower and more sustained than skeletal or cardiac muscle contraction. Its cells are spindle shaped and considerably smaller than skeletal muscle fibers. There are no Z or M lines in smooth muscle fibers, and the cross-striations are absent. The contractile filaments of actin and myosin are scattered throughout the cytoplasm. The lack of Z lines and regular overlapping of the contractile elements provide for a greater range of tension development. This is important in hollow organs that undergo changes in volume and length of the smooth muscle fibers in their walls. Even at large increases in volume the smooth muscle fiber retains some ability to develop tension, whereas such distention would have stretched skeletal muscle beyond the area where the thick and thin filaments overlap. Smooth muscle is generally arranged in sheets or bundles. In hollow organs, such as the intestines, the bundles are organized into two layers—an outer, longitudinal layer and an inner, circular layer. In blood vessels, the bundles are arranged in a circular or helical manner around the vessel wall.

Smooth muscle differs from skeletal muscle in the way its cross-bridges are formed. In smooth muscle, calcium binds to a smooth muscle cytoplasmic protein, calmoudulin; the calcium–calmoudulin complex binds to and activates the myosin-containing thick filaments, which then interact with actin. The sarcoplasmic reticulum is less well developed in smooth muscle than in skeletal muscle, and there are no transverse tubules connected to the cell membrane. Thus, smooth muscle relies on the entrance of extracellular calcium across the cell membrane as well as release of calcium from the sarcoplasmic reticulum for muscle contraction. This dependence on movement of extracellular calcium across the cell membrane during muscle contraction contributes to the effectiveness of calcium-blocking drugs that are used in treatment of cardiovascular disease.

Smooth muscle may be divided into two broad categories according to the mode of activation: multiunit and single-unit smooth muscle. *Multiunit* smooth muscle has no inherent activity, but depends on the autonomic nervous system for its activation. This type of smooth muscle is found in the large airways of the lungs, in large arteries, and attached to hairs in the skin. *Single-unit* smooth muscle is able to contract spontaneously in the absence of either nerve or hormnal stimulation. Normally, a large number of muscle fibers contract synchronously, hence the term *single-unit*. The action potentials originating from pacemaker cells show regular slow waves of depolarization and are transmitted from cell to cell by nexus formed by the fusion of adjacent cell membranes. The intensity of contraction increases with the frequency of the action potential. Certain hormones, other agents, and local factors can modify smooth mus-

cle activity by either depolarizing or hyperpolarizing the membrane. The smooth muscle of the intestinal tract, the uterus, and small-diameter blood vessels are examples of single-unit smooth muscle.

Nervous tissue

Nervous tissue is a specialized form of tissue designed for communication purposes. The nervous tissue develops from the ectoderm of the embryo and includes the neurons, the supporting cells of the nervous system, and the ependymal cells that line the ventricular system. The structure and organization of the nervous system are discussed in Chapter 45.

In summary, body cells are organized into four basic tissue types: epithelial, connective, muscle, and nervous. The epithelium covers the body surfaces and forms the functional components of the glandular structures. Connective tissue supports and connects body structures; it forms the bones and skeletal system, the joint structures, the blood cells, and the intercellular substances. Muscle tissue is a specialized tissue that is designed for contractility. There are three types of muscle tissue: skeletal, cardiac, and smooth. Nervous tissue is designed for communication purposes and includes the neurons, the supporting neural structures, and the ependymal cells that line the ventricles of the brain and the spinal canal.

■ Study Guide

After you have studied this chapter, you should be able to meet the following objectives:

☐ List the components of the cell nucleus and the function of each.

☐ State the composition of the ribosomes.

☐ Differentiate rough ER and smooth ER according to function.

☐ State the function of the Golgi complex.

☐ State the composition of the cytoplasm.

☐ Explain why the mitochondria are described as the power plants of the cell.

☐ State a possible role of the lysosomes in irreversible shock.

☐ Define *microtubule, microfilament,* and *centriole* on the basis of function.

☐ State four functions of the cell membrane.

☐ State the mechanisms of membrane transport.

☐ Explain the function of the intercellular junctions.

☐ Describe the process of cell differentiation.

☐ Use the Nernst equation to explain how an increase or decrease in serum potassium affects the resting membrane potential.

☐ Describe the movement of charge and changes in membrane potential that occur during an action potential.

☐ Explain why the basic tissue types are described in terms of their embryonic origin.

☐ Define the three types of epithelium.

☐ State the function of each of the three types of connective tissue.

☐ Describe the properties of muscle tissue.

☐ State the general function of nervous tissue.

■ References

1. Robbins SL, Cotran RS: Pathologic Basis of Disease, 2nd ed, p 11. Philadelphia, WB Saunders, 1979
2. Guyton A: Medical Physiology, 6th ed. p 43. Philadelphia, WB Saunders, 1981

Chapter 2

Cellular Adaptation and Injury

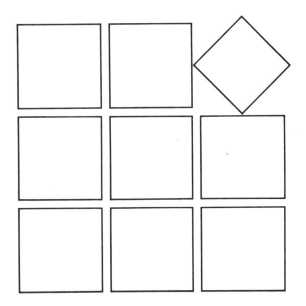

When confronted with stresses that tend to disrupt its normal structure and function, the cell undergoes adaptive changes that permit survival and maintenance of function. This chapter addresses cellular responses to stress, injury, and death.

■ Cellular Adaptation

Cells adapt to changes in the internal environment just as the total organism adapts to changes in the external environment. Cells may adapt by undergoing changes in size, number, and type. These changes, acting singly or in combination, may lead to atrophy, hypertrophy, hyperplasia, metaplasia, and dysplasia. In contrast to abnormal adaptive responses, normal adaptive responses occur in response to need and an appropriate stimulus. Once the need has been removed, the adaptive response ceases.

Atrophy

Atrophy refers to a decrease in the size of a body part brought about by shrinkage in the size of its cells. When confronted with a decrease in work demands or adverse environmental conditions, most cells are able to revert to a smaller size and a lower and more efficient level of functioning that is compatible with survival. The size of all the structural components of the cell usually decreases as the cell atrophies.

The general causes of atrophy can be grouped into the following categories: (1) disuse, (2) denervation, (3) lack of endocrine stimulation, (4) decreased nutrition, and (5) ischemia. Cell size, particularly in muscle tissue, is related to work load. As the work load of a cell diminishes there is a general decrease in oxygen consumption and protein synthesis. The cell conserves energy by decreasing the number and size of its organelles and other structures. Disuse atrophy is seen in the muscles of extremities that have been encased in plaster casts. Denervation atrophy is a form of disuse atrophy that occurs in the muscles of paralyzed limbs. Lack of endocrine stimulation causes the involutional changes that occur in the reproductive structures during menopause. During prolonged periods of interference with general nutrition, such as occurs during starvation or other disease conditions, the body undergoes a more or less generalized wasting of tissue mass. *Ischemia* results from localized lack of blood flow and delivery of oxygen and nutrients to the affected tissues. In peripheral vascular disease there is often atrophy of the muscles and skin in the affected extremities due to ischemia.

In some situations, a collection of yellow-brown pigment called *lipofuscin* accompanies the retrogressive changes that occur with atrophy. This form of atrophy is referred to as *brown atrophy*. The discoloration is thought to represent an accumulation of indigestible residues from within the cell. It is seen more commonly in heart, nerve, and liver cells than in other forms of tissue. Lipofuscin itself is not injurious to cell structure or function.[1] The accumulation of lipofuscin increases with age and is sometimes referred to as the wear-and-tear pigment.

Hypertrophy

Hypertrophy is an increase in the amount of functioning tissue mass of an organ or part caused by an increase in cell size. It results from increased functional demands and is most commonly seen in cardiac and skeletal muscle tissue. This type of tissue cannot adapt to an increase in work load by mitotic division and formation of more cells. In hypertrophy there is an increase in the functional components of the cell that allows equilibrium between demand and the functional capacity to be reached by the cell. For example, as muscle cells hypertrophy synthesis of additional microfilaments, cell enzymes, and ATP occurs. The mechanism of increased cell components is not completely understood. It is thought to be related to a decreased rate of protein degradation with a slightly increased rate of protein synthesis.[1] Whatever the mechanism, a limit is eventually reached beyond which further enlargement of the tissue mass is no longer able to compensate for the increased work demands. The limiting factors for continued hypertrophy may be related to limitations in blood flow.[1]

Hypertrophy may be either physiologic or pathologic. The increase in muscle mass associated with exercise is an example of physiologic hypertrophy. Pathologic hypertrophy may be adaptive or compensatory. Examples of adaptive hypertrophy are the thickening of the urinary bladder due to long-continued obstruction of urinary outflow and myocardial hypertrophy that results from valvular heart disease or hypertension. Compensatory hypertrophy is the enlargement of a remaining organ or tissue after a portion has been surgically removed or rendered inactive. For instance, if one kidney is removed, the remaining kidney enlarges to compensate for the loss.

Hyperplasia

Hyperplasia is an increase in the number of cells of a part. Hyperplasia occurs in cells that are capable of mitotic division, such as those of the epidermis, intestinal epithelial layer, and glandular tissue. Nerve cells and skeletal and cardiac muscle do not divide and therefore have no capacity for hyperplastic growth. As with other normal adaptive cellular responses, hyperplasia is a controlled process that occurs in response to an appropriate stimulus and ceases once the stimulus has been removed. There are two types of stimuli that are generally associated with hyperplasia—physiologic and nonphysiologic. Breast and uterine enlargement during pregnancy is an example of a physiologic hyperplasia that is hormonally regulated. An example of a nonphysiological form of hyperplasia occurs in response to abnormal hormonal stimulation of target cells. Hyperplasia of target cells in the endometrium occurs with excessive estrogen production; the abnormally thickened uterine layer may bleed excessively and frequently.

Metaplasia

Metaplasia is the conversion from one adult cell type to another adult cell type. It allows for substitution of cells that are better able to tolerate environmental stresses. The conversion of cell types never oversteps the boundaries of the primary groups of tissue (epithelial or connective). In metaplasia, one type of epithelial cell may be converted to another type of epithelial cell but not to a connective tissue cell. An example of a metaplasia is the adaptive substitution of stratified squamous epithelial cells for the ciliated columnar epithelial cells in the trachea and large airways in the person who is a habitual cigarette smoker. Metaplasia of epithelial tissue occurs in chronic irritation and inflammation. For unknown reasons, a vitamin A deficiency tends to cause squamous metaplasia of the respiratory tract. Metaplasia occurs in response to a stimulus and is potentially reversible.

Dysplasia

Dysplasia is deranged cell growth of a specific tissue that results in cells with variations in size, shape, and appearance. Minor degrees of dysplasia occur in association with chronic irritation or inflammation. Although dysplasia is abnormal, it is adaptive in that it is potentially reversible once the irritating cause has been found and removed. Dysplastic tissue changes may progress to neoplastic disease, and it is at this point that displasia gains its importance.

In summary, cells adapt to changes in their environment and in their work demands by changing size, number, and character. Changes include atrophy—a shrinking of tissue due to a decrease in cell size and functional components within the cell; hypertrophy—an increase in tissue size brought about by an increase in cell size and functional components within the cell; hyperplasia—an increase in cell number; metaplasia—the conversion of one adult cell type to another adult cell type; and dysplasia—disordered cell growth resulting in altered cell structure. Normal adaptive changes are consistent with the needs of the cell and occur in response to an appropriate stimulus. The changes are reversed once the stimuli have been withdrawn.

◼ Cell Injury

The extent to which any injurious agent can cause cell injury and death is dependent, in large measure, on the intensity and duration of the injury and the type of cell that is involved. When cells are injured or the need to adapt becomes overwhelming, degenerative changes begin to appear. Degeneration is a retrogressive process in which there is a cellular deterioration along with changes in both the chemical structure and microscopic appearance of the cell. Degeneration can follow many paths and eventually leads to cell changes, which may be reversible or irreversible. Irreversible changes consist of necrosis (cell death) and tissue dissolution. Frequently, however, the final outcome is not reached because somewhere along the way the process is reversed, allowing cells and tissues to return to their normal state.

Reversible Cell Injury

The manifestations of reversible cell injury fall into three main categories: cellular swelling, fatty changes, and intracellular accumulations.

Cellular swelling
An accumulation of water within the cell is an early manifestation of almost all types of cell injury. When this happens, the cytoplasm of the cell develops a cloudy appearance (*cloudy swelling*). It has been postulated that the swelling is caused by a decrease in ATP and impaired function of the sodium pump. This leads to an accumulation of intracellular sodium and subsequent waterlogging of the cell, with the appearance of vacuoles if water continues to accumulate. These vacuoles probably represent the collection of water in the endoplasmic reticulum.

Fatty changes
Fatty cellular changes are linked to intracellular accumulation of fat. When fatty changes occur, small vacuoles of fat disperse throughout the cytoplasm. The process is usually more ominous than cloudy swelling, and although it is reversible, its presence usually indicates severe injury. These fatty changes may occur because normal cells are presented with an increased fat load or because injured cells are unable to metabolize the fat properly. In obesity, fatty infiltrates often occur within and between the cells of the liver and heart because of an increased fat load. Impairment of metabolic pathways for

fat metabolism may occur during cell injury and fat may accumulate within the cell as production exceeds use and export. The liver, where most fats are synthesized and metabolized, is particularly susceptible to fatty change, but fatty change may also occur in the kidney, the heart, and other organs.

Intracellular accumulations

Under certain conditions, various substances may accumulate in both normal and abnormal cells. Robbins has grouped these substances into three categories: (1) normal cellular constituents, such as lipids, proteins, and carbohydrates, which are present in large amounts; (2) abnormal substances such as those resulting from inborn errors of metabolism; and (3) pigments.[1] The previously described fatty changes are an example of intracellular accumulation of a normal cell constituent.

There are a number of genetic disorders that disrupt the metabolism of selected substances. A normal enzyme may be replaced with an abnormal one, resulting in the formation of a substance that cannot be utilized or eliminated from the cell; or an enzyme may be missing, so that an intermediate product piles up in the cell. For example, there are at least ten inborn errors of glycogen metabolism, most of which lead to the accumulation of intracellular glycogen stores. In the most common form of this disorder, von Gierke's disease, large amounts of glycogen accumulate in the liver and kidneys because of a deficiency of the enzyme glucose-6-phosphatase. Without this enzyme, glucose-6-phosphate stored in the form of glycogen cannot be broken down to form glucose. In a similar manner, other enzyme defects lead to the accumulation of other substances.

Pigments are colored substances that may accumulate within cells. They can be either endogenous (arising from within the body) or exogenous (arising from outside the body) in origin. Icterus, or jaundice, is a yellow discoloration of tissue caused by the retention of endogenous bile pigments. This condition may result from increased bilirubin production due to red blood cell destruction, obstruction of bile passage into the intestine, or toxic diseases that affect the liver's ability to remove bilirubins from the blood. One of the most common exogenous pigments is carbon in the form of coal dust. In coal miners or individuals exposed to heavily polluted environments, the accumulation of carbon or other environmental dusts may cause serious lung disease. Lung disease associated with coal dust is termed *anthracosis* and that associated with silica (sand dust) is called *silicosis*. The formation of a blue lead line along the margins of the gum is one of the diagnostic features of lead poisoning.

Whatever the nature or cause of the abnormal accumulation, it implies storage of some substance by a cell. If the accumulation is due to a correctable systemic disorder such as hyperbilirubinemia, which causes jaundice, the accumulation is reversible. If the disorder cannot be corrected, as often occurs in many inborn errors of metabolism, the cells become overloaded, causing cell injury and death.

Irreversible Cell Injury and Death

Necrosis means death of the cell, organ, or tissue that is still a part of the body. Widespread necrosis can occur without somatic (body) death. With cell death there are marked changes in the appearance of both the cytoplasmic contents and the nucleus. These changes are often not visible, even under the microscope, for hours following cell death. The dissolution of the necrotic cell or tissue can follow several paths: the cell can undergo liquefaction (liquefaction necrosis); it can be transformed to a gray, firm mass (coagulation necrosis); or it can be converted to a cheesy material by infiltration of fatlike substances (caseous necrosis). *Liquefaction necrosis* occurs when some of the cells die, but their catalytic enzymes are not destroyed. An example of liquefaction necrosis is the softening of the center of an abscess with discharge of its contents. During *coagulation necrosis*, acidosis denatures the enzymatic proteins along with the structural proteins of the cell. This type of necrosis is characteristic of hypoxic injury and is seen in infarcted areas. An infarction occurs when the artery that supplies an organ or part of the body becomes occluded and no other source of blood supply exists. As a rule, the infarct is conical in shape and corresponds to the distribution of the artery and its branches. An artery may be occluded by an embolus, a thrombus, disease of the arterial wall, or pressure on the vessel from without. *Caseous necrosis*, or cheesy necrosis, is associated with tubercular lesions.

Gangrene

The term *gangrene* is applied when a considerable mass of tissue undergoes necrosis (Fig. 2-1). Gangrene may be classified as either dry or moist. Dry gangrene is usually due to interference with arterial blood supply to a part without interference of venous return. Strictly speaking, it is a form of coagulation necrosis. Moist, or wet, gangrene is primarily due to interference with the venous return from the part. Bacterial invasion plays an important role in the development of wet gangrene and is responsible for many of its prominent symptoms. Dry gangrene is confined almost exclusively to the extremities, whereas moist gangrene may affect either the internal organs or the extremities.

In dry gangrene, the part becomes dry and shrinks; the skin wrinkles, and its color changes to dark brown or black. The spread of dry gangrene is slow, and its symp-

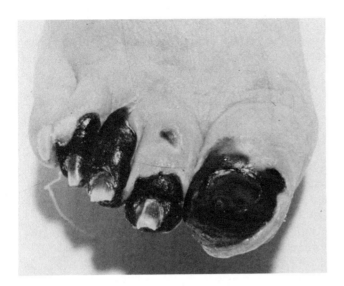

Figure 2-1 *Photograph of a foot with dry gangrene of the first four toes. Note the sharp line of demarcation between the normal and necrotic tissue. (Courtesy of M. Wagner, M.D. The Anatomy Department, Medical College of Wisconsin)*

toms are not as marked as those of wet gangrene. The irritation caused by the dead tissue produces a line of inflammatory reaction (line of demarcation) between the dead tissue and the gangrenous area and the healthy tissue. If bacteria invade the necrotic tissue, dry gangrene is converted to wet gangrene.

In moist gangrene, the area is cold, swollen, and pulseless. The skin is moist, black, and under tension. Blebs form on the surface, liquefaction occurs, and a foul odor (due to bacterial action) is present. There is no line of demarcation between the normal and diseased tissues and the spread of tissue damage is rapid. Systemic symptoms are usually severe, and death may occur unless the condition can be arrested.

Gas gangrene is a special type of gangrene that is due to infection of devitalized tissues by one of several clostridial bacteria. These anaerobic bacteria produce toxins that cause shock, hemolysis, and death of muscle cells. Characteristic of this disorder are the bubbles of gas that form in the muscle. Gas gangrene is a serious and potentially fatal disease. Treatment includes administration of gas gangrene antitoxin. Because the organism is anaerobic, oxygen is sometimes administered in a hyperbaric chamber.

In summary, cell injury can be caused by a number of agents. The injury may produce sublethal and reversible cellular damage or may lead to irreversible cell injury and death. Necrosis refers to cell death. There are three forms of cell necrosis: (1) liquefaction necrosis, which occurs when cell death does not result in inactivation of intra-cellular enzymes; (2) coagulation necrosis, which occurs with ischemia; and (3) caseous necrosis, which is associated with tubercular lesions. Necrosis of large areas of tissue leads to gangrene. Gangrene can be classified as dry or wet gangrene. Dry gangrene is essentially a form of coagulation necrosis, and wet gangrene is due to bacterial invasion of the necrotic area.

■ Types of Cell Injury

There are many ways in which cell damage can occur. The common forms of injury tend to fall into several categories: (1) hypoxic cell injury, (2) cell injury due to physical agents, (3) radiation injury, (4) chemical injury, (5) injury due to biologic agents, and (6) injury associated with nutritional imbalances. Genetic derangements such as inborn errors of metabolism predispose to cell injury, inflammation, and immune responses. Although these mechanisms are normally protective in nature, they can cause cell injury and death.

Hypoxic Injury

One of the most common causes of tissue injury is hypoxia. Hypoxia deprives the cell of oxygen and interrupts oxidative metabolism and the generation of ATP. The actual time necessary to produce irreversible cell damage depends on the degree of oxygen deprivation and the metabolic needs of the cell. Well-differentiated cells such as those in the heart, brain, and kidney require large amounts of oxygen to provide energy for their special functions. Brain cells, for example, begin to undergo permanent damage following 4 to 6 minutes of oxygen deprivation. Furthermore, there is often a fine margin between the time involved in reversible and irreversible cell damage. In one study it was found that the epithelial cells of the proximal tubule of the kidney in the rat could survive 20 but not 30 minutes of ischemia.[2]

Hypoxia can result from an inadequate amount of oxygen in the air, disease of the respiratory system, alterations in circulatory function, anemia, or inability of the cells to utilize oxygen. In edema, the distance for diffusion of oxygen may become a limiting factor. In hypermetabolic states the cells may require more oxygen than can be supplied by normal respiratory function and oxygen transport. Hypoxia also serves as the ultimate cause of cell death in other injuries. For example, toxins from certain microorganisms interfere with cellular utilization of oxygen, and a physical agent such as cold causes severe vasoconstriction and impairs blood flow.

Hypoxia literally causes a power failure within the cell with widespread effects on the cell's function and structural components. As oxygen tension within the cell falls, oxidative metabolism ceases, and the cell reverts to anaerobic metabolism, using the cell's limited glycogen stores in an attempt to maintain vital cell functions. Cellular pH falls as lactic acid and inorganic phosphates resulting from hydrolysis of ATP accumulate within the cell. This reduction in pH can have profound effects on intracellular structures. Clumping of the nuclear chromatin occurs, and myelin figures, which are derived from destructive changes in cell membranes and intracellular structures, are seen within the cytoplasm and extracellular spaces.

One of the earliest effects of reduced ATP is acute cellular swelling caused by failure of the energy-dependent sodium-potassium membrane pump, which extrudes sodium and returns potassium to the cell. With impaired function of this pump, intracellular potassium decreases, and sodium and water accumulate within the cell. The movement of fluid and ions into the cell is associated with dilatation of the endoplasmic reticulum, increased membrane permeability, and decreased mitochondrial function.[1]

To this point, the cellular changes are reversible if oxygenation is restored. If the oxygen supply is not restored, however, there is a continued loss of essential enzymes, proteins, and ribonucleic acid through the hyperpermeable membrane of the cell. Injury to the lysosomal membranes results in leakage of destructive lysosomal enzymes into the cytoplasm of the cell with enzymatic digestion of cell components. The leakage of intracellular enzymes through the permeable cell membrane into the extracellular fluid is used as an important clinical indicator of cell injury and death. These enzymes enter the blood and can be measured by laboratory tests. For example, heart muscle liberates glutamine oxaloacetic transaminase (GOT), creatine phosphokinase (CPK), and lactate dehydrogenase (LDH) when injured. Because different types of tissue have different enzymes, the presence of elevated levels of specific enzymes provides information about the location of tissue injury due to hypoxia.

Injury Due to Physical Agents

Physical agents responsible for cell and tissue injury include mechanical forces, extremes of temperature, and electrical forces. Injury due to mechanical forces occurs as the result of body impact with another object. Either the body or the mass can be in motion, or, as sometimes happens, both can be in motion at the time of impact. These types of injuries split and tear tissue, fracture bones, injure blood vessels, and disrupt blood flow.

Extremes of heat and cold cause damage to the cell, its organelles, and its enzyme systems. Exposure to low-intensity heat (43° to 46°C), such as occurs with partial-thickness burns and severe heat stroke, causes cell injury by inducing vascular injury, accelerating cell metabolism, inactivating temperature-sensitive enzymes, and disrupting the cell membrane.[1] With more intense heat, coagulation of blood vessels and tissue proteins occurs.

Exposure to cold induces vasoconstriction by direct action on blood vessels and also by reflex sympathetic nervous system activity. The resultant decrease in blood flow may lead to hypoxic tissue injury, depending on the degree and duration of cold exposure. Injury due to freezing is probably a combination of ice crystal formation and vasoconstriction. The decreased blood flow leads to capillary stasis and arteriolar and capillary thrombosis. Edema results from increased capillary permeability.

Electrical injuries can affect the body in two ways—through extensive tissue injury and disruption of neural and cardiac impulses. The effect of elecricity on the body is mainly determined by (1) the type of circuit (direct or alternating), (2) its voltage, (3) its amperage, (4) resistance of the intervening tissue, (5) the pathway of the current, and (6) the duration of exposure.

Alternating current (AC) is usually more dangerous than direct current (DC) because it causes violent muscle contractions, preventing release of the electrical source and sometimes resulting in fractures and dislocations. In electrical injuries, the body acts as a conductor of the electrical current; that is, the current enters the body from an electrical source such as an exposed wire and then passes through the body and exits to another conductor, such as the moisture on the ground or a piece of metal the person is holding. The pathway that a current takes is of critical importance because the electrical energy disrupts impulses in excitable tissues. Electrical flow through the brain may interrupt respiratory impulses from medullary centers, and flow of current through the chest may cause fatal cardiac arrhythmias.

In electrical circuits, resistance to the flow of current transforms electrical energy into heat. This is why the elements in electrical heating devices are made of highly resistant metals. Much of the tissue damage produced by electrical injuries is due to heat production that occurs in tissues that have the highest electrical resistance. Resistance to electrical current varies from the greatest to the least as follows: bone, fat, tendons, skin, muscles, blood, and nerves. Maximum tissue injury usually occurs at the skin sites where the current enters and leaves the body. After electricity has penetrated the skin, it passes rapidly through the body along the lines of least resistance—through body fluids and nerves. Degeneration of vessel walls may occur and thrombi may form as current flows along the blood vessels. This can cause extensive muscle and deep tissue injury. Thick, dry skin is more resistant to the flow of electricity than thin, wet skin. It is generally believed that the greater the skin resistance, the greater the amount of local skin burn; the less the resistance, the greater the deep and systemic effects.

Radiation Injury

Electromagnetic radiation comprises a wide spectrum of wave-propagated energy ranging from ionizing gamma rays to radiofrequency waves (Fig. 2-2). A photon is a particle of radiation energy. Radiation energy above the visible ultraviolet range is called *ionizing radiation* because the photons have enough energy to knock electrons off atoms and molecules. Radiation energy in a frequency range that is less than visible light is often referred to as *nonionizing radiation*. Ultraviolet radiation represents the visible spectrum of electromagnetic radiation. It contains increasingly energetic rays that are powerful enough to disrupt intracellular bonds and cause sunburn (Chap. 54).

Ionizing radiation

The spectrum of ionizing radiation includes two distinct forms of energy propagation: electromagnetic waves and fast-moving particles. Gamma waves and x-rays are similar in their interaction with body tissues but differ in their origin; x-rays are machine-generated, and gamma rays are emitted from the spontaneous decay of radioactive materials. Both of these forms of radiation are very energetic and extremely penetrating, and they assume characteristics of both waves and particles.

Particulate radiation involves particles of definite mass and charge given off by both naturally occurring and artificially produced radioactive elements, processes of fission (atomic reactors), and particle accelerators. Naturally occurring substances (*e.g.*, radium) and artificially produced radioisotopes undergo spontaneous decay emitting radiant energy. This rate of decay varies greatly and is expressed in terms of the half-life of the product, or the time necessary to reduce its radioactivity to one-half its initial value. The half-life of a radioisotope may be as short as a fraction of a second, or it may be as long as 1638 years (radium).[3]

Ionizing radiation affects cells by causing ionization of molecules and atoms within the cells either by directly hitting the target molecules or by producing free radicals that interact with critical cell components. It can immediately kill cells, interrupt cell replication, or cause a variety of mutations, which may or may not be lethal. During an initial radiation response, cell swelling, disruption of the mitochondria and other organelles, alterations in the cell membrane, and marked nuclear changes occur. Because of inhibition of DNA synthesis and interference with the mitotic process, rapidly dividing cells

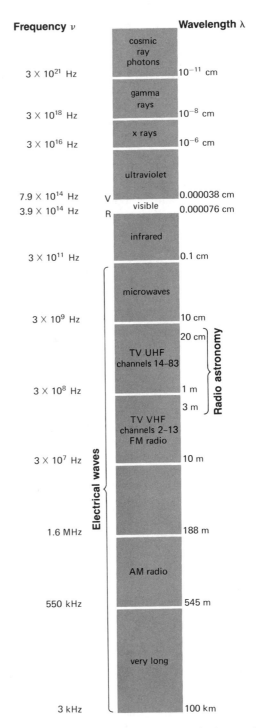

Figure 2-2 *The electromagnetic spectrum. The frequencies are shown on the left side of the diagram, and the corresponding wavelengths appear on the right. The frequencies and wavelengths are related by* $C = \nu\lambda$, *where* C = *the speed of light in free space* $(3 \times 10^8 \ m/sec)$ *and is the same for all wavelengths of the electromagnetic spectrum. (Hooper HO, Gwynne P: Physics and the Physical Perspectives. New York, Harper & Row, 1980)*

such as those of the bone marrow and gastrointestinal epithelium are more susceptible to radiation injury than nondividing cells. Cancer cells are rapidly proliferating cells; therefore, radiation therapy is often used in treating cancer.

Dose-dependent vascular changes occur in all irradiated tissues. During the immediate postirradiation period, only vessel dilatation takes place (*e.g.,* the initial erythema of the skin after radiotherapy). Later, or with higher levels of radiation, destructive changes occur in small blood vessels such as the capillaries and venules.

At relatively low doses, both normal cells and cancer cells are able to repair radiation damage. If, however, cell recovery is not complete at the time of the next exposure, there may be additional damage. The importance of cell repair in protecting against radiation injury is evidenced by the vulnerability of persons who lack repair enzymes to ultraviolet-induced skin cancer. In a disease called xeroderma pigmentosum, an enzyme needed for DNA replication to repair sunlight-induced defects is lacking, and this results in the development of a mutant cancer cell line.

Nonionizing radiation

Nonionizing radiation includes infrared light, ultrasound, microwaves, and laser energy. Unlike ionizing radiation, which can directly break chemical bonds, nonionizing radiation exerts its effects by causing vibrations and rotations of atoms and molecules. Essentially, all of this vibrational and rotational energy is eventually converted to thermal energy. Because all of these types of radiation are finding increasing usage for industrial, domestic, and medical purposes, there is increasing concern about the safety, dosimetry, and long-term effects of exposure to these types of radiation. In laboratory animals, for example, cataracts and lymphocyte dysfunction have been associated with exposure to microwave radiation.[4] Unquestionably, much of this damage was due to local and general hyperthermia.[5] A number of epidemiologic studies on the ocular effects of occupational exposure have not found an increase in lens opacity in humans.[4]

Ultrasound, too, has been shown to alter nerve transmission in lower animals; but, again, this was related to the thermal effects.[1] Questions regarding the safety of ultrasound during pregnancy as a routine screening method have prompted the National Institutes of Health and the Federal Drug Administration to sponsor a consensus development conference on diagnostic ultrasound in pregnancy. The group advised that "data on the clinical efficacy and safety do not allow a recommendation for routine screening of the fetus at this time." They further cautioned that "ultrasound examinations performed solely to satisfy the family's desire to know fetal sex, or obtain a picture of the fetus should be discouraged."[6]

Chemical Injury

Chemical agents are numerous and can cause injury to the cell membrane and other cell structures, block enzymatic pathways, cause coagulation of cell proteins, and disrupt the osmotic and ionic balance of the cell. Even excessive amounts of simple table salt (sodium chloride) can cause cell damage by disrupting the cell's osmotic and ionic homeostasis. Chemicals can destroy cells at the site of contact. Corrosive substances such as strong acids and alkalies destroy cells as they come into contact with the body. Other chemicals may injure cells in the process of metabolism or elimination. Carbon tetrachloride (CCl_4, for example, causes little damage until it is metabolized by liver enzymes to a highly reactive free radical (CCl_3)). Carbon tetrachloride is extremely toxic to liver cells. Still other types of chemicals are selective in their sites of action. Carbon monoxide has a special affinity for the hemoglobin molecule.

Injury Due to Biologic Agents

Biologic agents differ from other injurious agents in that they are able to replicate and thus can continue to produce their injurious effects. These agents range from submicroscopic viruses to the larger parasites. Biologic agents cause cell injury by a number of diverse mechanisms: viruses enter the cell and become incorporated into its synthetic machinery. Certain bacteria elaborate exotoxins that interfere with cellular production of ATP. Other bacteria such as the gram-negative bacilli release endotoxins that cause cell injury and increased capillary permeability. Still other microorganisms produce their effects through inflammatory or immune mechanisms. Infectious processes are discussed in Chapter 7.

Injury Associated with Nutritional Imbalances

Both nutritional excesses and deficiencies predispose to cell injury. Obesity and diets high in saturated fats are thought to predispose to atherosclerosis. More than 50 to 60 organic and inorganic substances are required by the body, in amounts ranging from micrograms to grams. These nutrients include minerals, vitamins, certain fatty acids, and specific amino acids. Dietary deficiencies can occur in the form of starvation in which there is a deficiency of all nutrients and vitamins, or it may occur because of a selective deficiency of a single nutrient or vitamin. Iron-deficiency anemia, scurvy, beriberi, and pellagra are examples of injury caused by the lack of specific vitamins or minerals. The protein and calorie deficiencies that occur with starvation cause widespread tissue damage.

In summary, the causes of cell injury are many and diverse. One common cause is hypoxia. It can result from inadequate oxygen in the air, cardiorespiratory disease, anemia, or the inability of the cells to use oxygen. The impairment of blood flow to an area of the body is called *ischemia*. It produces a state of localized hypoxia. Among the physical agents that produce cell injury are mechanical forces that produce tissue trauma, extremes of temperature, electricity, and radiation. Chemical agents can cause cell injury through several mechanisms; they can block enzymatic pathways, cause coagulation of tissues, or disrupt the osmotic or ionic balance of the cell. Biologic agents differ from other injurious agents in that they are able to replicate and continue to produce injury. Among the nutritional factors that contribute to cell injury are excesses and deficiencies of nutrients, vitamins, and minerals.

■ Study Guide

After you have studied this chapter, you should be able to meet the following objectives:

☐ State the general purpose of changes in cell structure and function that occur as the result of normal adaptive processes.

☐ State the relationship between changes in cell structure and function that occur as a result of normal adaptive processes and the stimuli producing these changes.

☐ Describe cell changes that occur with atrophy, hypertrophy, hyperplasia, metaplasia, and dysplasia.

☐ State the general conditions under which atrophy, hypertrophy, hyperplasia, metaplasia, and dysplasia occur.

☐ Describe three types of reversible cell changes that can occur with cell injury.

☐ State the difference in outcome between intracellular accumulations due to systemic disorders and those due to inborn errors of metabolism.

☐ Cite the rationale for the changes that occur with the wet and dry forms of gangrene.

☐ Describe cell changes that occur with hypoxia, electrical injury, and thermal injury.

☐ Explain how injurious effects of biologic agents differ from those produced by physical and chemical agents.

☐ Differentiate between the effects of ionizing and nonionizing radiation in terms of their ability to cause cell injury.

☐ State how nutritional imbalances contribute to cell injury.

■ References

1. Robbins SL, Cotran RS, Kumar V: Pathologic Basis of Disease, 3rd ed, pp 23, 31, 47, 6, 462, and 470. Philadelphia, WB Saunders, 1984
2. Vogt MT, Farber E: On the molecular pathology of ischemic renal cell death. Reversible and irreversible cellular and mitochondrial metabolic alterations. Am J Pathol 53: 1, 1968
3. Robbins SL, Cotran RS, Kumar V: Pathologic Basis of Disease, 3rd ed, p 551. Philadelphia, WB Saunders, 1979
4. Erwin DN: An overview of the biological effects of radiofrequency radiation. Milit Med 148, No. 2: 113—117, 1983
5. Djordjevic Z, Kolak A, Djokovic V et al: Results of our 15-year study on biological effects of microwave exposure. Aviat Space Environ Med 54, No. 6:539—542, 1983
6. Ultrasound use in pregnancy. FDA Drug Bull 14, No. 1:6, 1984

Chapter 3

Genetic Control of Cell Function and Inheritance

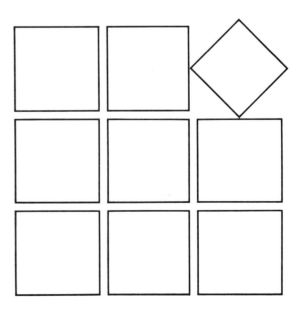

The word *gene* is defined somewhat differently by the various scientific disciplines. There are breeding genetic units, cellular chromosomal or cytogenetic genes, functional polypeptide genes, and nucleoprotein structural unit genes, as well as others. In all of these terms, the word gene stands for the *fundamental unit of information storage*. This information is stored in the structure of an extremely stable macromolecule within the nucleus of each cell. Because of this stable structure, the genetic information survives the many processes of reduction division of the gametes (ovum and sperm), fertilization, and the many cell divisions involved in the formation of a new organism from the single-celled zygote formed by the union of an ovum and sperm.

Genes determine the types of proteins and enzymes that are made by the cell, and hence control not only inheritance but the day-to-day function of all the cells in the body. For example, genes control the type and quantity of hormones that a cell produces, the antigens and receptors that are present on the cell membrane, and the synthesis of enzymes needed for metabolism. More than 3000 genes have been identified. Although there are some exceptions, each gene provides the instructions for the synthesis of a single protein. This chapter includes a discussion of genetic regulation of cell function, chromosomal structure, patterns of inheritance, and gene mapping.

■ Genetic Control of Cell Function

The genetic information needed for protein synthesis is inscribed on *deoxyribonucleic acid (DNA)* contained in the cell nucleus. A second type of nucleic acid, *ribonucleic acid (RNA)*, is involved in the actual synthesis of cellular enzymes and proteins. *Messenger RNA* transcribes the instructions for protein synthesis from the DNA molecule and carries them into the cytoplasm, whereas *ribosomal RNA* translates the message into production language that can be used by the cell's polypeptide building machinery. *Transfer RNA* delivers the appropriate amino acids to the ribosome, where they are incorporated into the protein being synthesized. This process for the control of cell function is described in Figure 3-1.

The nuclei of all the cells in an organism contain the same accumulation of genes derived from the gametes of the two parents. This means that liver cells contain the same genetic information as skin and muscle cells. For this to be true, the molecular code must be duplicated prior to each succeeding cell division, or mitosis. Theoretically, although not yet achieved in humans, any of the highly differentiated cells of an organism could be used to produce a complete genetically identical organism, or clone. From this it becomes evident that each particular tissue uses only some of the information stored on the genetic code. Although information required for the function of other types of tissues is still present, it is repressed.

Gene Structure

The stable structure that stores the genetic information within the nucleus is a very long, double-stranded, chainlike molecule of DNA coiled around a common axis to form a double helix. The DNA molecule is composed of nucleotides, which consist of (1) phosphoric acid, (2) a five-carbon sugar called deoxyribose, and (3) one of four nitrogenous bases. The four bases can be divided into two groups: the purine bases of adenine and guanine, which have two nitrogen ring structures, and the pyrimidine bases thymine and cytosine, which have one ring. Alternating groups of sugar and phosphoric acid form the backbone of the molecule, whereas the paired bases project inward from the sides of the sugar molecule. The entire chain is like a spiral staircase, with the paired bases representing the steps (Fig. 3-2).

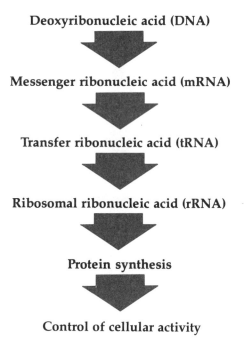

Deoxyribonucleic acid (DNA)

↓

Messenger ribonucleic acid (mRNA)

↓

Transfer ribonucleic acid (tRNA)

↓

Ribosomal ribonucleic acid (rRNA)

↓

Protein synthesis

↓

Control of cellular activity

Figure 3-1 *DNA-directed control of cellular activity through synthesis of cellular proteins. Messenger RNA carries the transcribed message, which directs protein synthesis from the nucleus to the cytoplasm. Transfer RNA translates the message and selects the appropriate amino acids and carries them to ribosomal RNA, where assembly of the proteins takes place.*

There is a precise pairing of the nucleotides in the double-stranded DNA molecule. The nucleotides exist in complementary pairs of a purine and pyrimidine base: adenine is paired with thymine and guanine with cytosine (Fig. 3-3). Each nucleotide in a pair is on one strand of the DNA molecule, with the bases of the pair loosely bound by a hydrogen bond. Because of the looseness of the bond, the two strands can pull apart with ease so that the genetic information can be duplicated or transcribed.

A gene can be regarded as being represented by several hundred to a thousand base pairs. Of the two DNA strands, only one is used in transcribing the information for the cell's polypeptide-building machinery. If the genetic information of one strand is meaningful, then the complementary code of the other strand will not make sense and will therefore be ignored. Both strands, however, are involved in DNA duplication. Prior to cell division, the two strands of the helix separate and a complementary molecule is organized next to each original strand. Thus, two strands make four strands, with each strand joined to a new complementary strand (Fig. 3-4). During cell division, the newly duplicated double-helix molecules are separated and placed in each daughter cell by the mechanics of mitosis. As a result, each of the daughter cells again contains the meaningful strand and the complementary strand joined in the form of a double helix. Replication of DNA has been termed *semiconservatism* because both parental strands are conserved in the next generation.

The very long DNA molecule is combined with several types of protein and small amounts of RNA into a complex known as *chromatin*. Chromatin is the more readily stainable portion of the cell nucleus. Some of these proteins form binding sites for repressor molecules and hormones that regulate genetic transcription. Other proteins may themselves block genetic transcription by preventing access of nucleotides to the surface of the DNA molecule. A specific group of proteins, called *histones*, are thought to control the folding of the DNA strands. As will be discussed later, the chromatin coils and folds over to form chromosomes during cell division.

The Genetic Code

The four bases (guanine, adenine, cytosine, and uracil) make up the alphabet of the genetic code. A sequence of three bases constitutes the fundamental triplet code for transmission of genetic information needed for protein synthesis; this triplet code is called a *codon*. An example is the nucleotide sequence GCU (guanine, cytosine, and uracil), which is the triplet RNA code for the amino acid

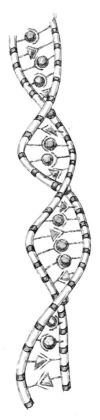

Figure 3-2 *Schematic representation of a long, double-stranded DNA molecule, which is a repeating arrangement of nucleotides. It is thought that from 500 to 1000 nucleotides make up a single gene and that there are over 1000 genes in a chromosome. (Chaffee EE, Lytle IM: Basic Physiology and Anatomy, 4th ed. Philadelphia, JB Lippincott, 1980)*

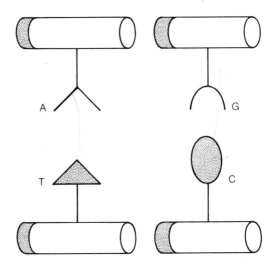

Figure 3-3 *Pairing of the nucleotides in DNA. Thymine pairs with adenine and cytosine with guanine.*

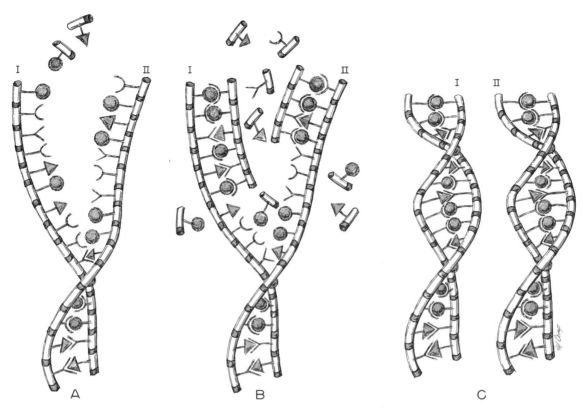

Figure 3-4   *Schematic representation of the replication of DNA. (A) Prior to cell division, the bonds between the nitrogenous bases are broken, the two strands separate, and each strand takes with it the bases attached to its side. (B) The bases attached to each single strand attract free-floating nucleotide units and pair off in the usual way: adenine with thymine, guanine with cytosine. (C) The end result is two exact replicas of the original DNA molecule, and the cell is ready to undergo division. (Chaffee EE, Lytle IM: Basic Physiology and Anatomy, 4th ed. Philadelphia, JB Lippincott, 1980)*

alanine. The genetic code is a universal language used by all living cells, that is, the code for the amino acid tryptophan is the same in a bacterium, a plant, and a human being. There are also start and stop codes, which signal the beginning and end of a protein molecule. Mathematically, the 4 bases can be arranged in 64 different combinations ($4 \times 4 \times 4 = 64$). This means 64 combinations are used to specify amino acids and, because there are 20 amino acids that can be used in protein synthesis, there must be several codes for the same amino acid. It has been discovered that 18 of the amino acids have more than one code word.

Protein Synthesis

Although DNA determines the type of biochemical product that is to be synthesized by the cell, the transmission and decoding of information needed for protein synthesis are carried out by RNA, the formation of which is directed by DNA. The general structure of RNA differs from DNA in three respects: (1) RNA is a single- rather than a double-stranded molecule; (2) the sugar in each nucleotide of RNA is ribose instead of deoxyribose; and (3) the pyridimine base, thymine, in DNA is replaced by uracil in RNA. As previously mentioned, there are three types of RNA: messenger RNA (mRNA), transfer RNA (tRNA), and ribosomal RNA (rRNA).

Messenger RNA

Messenger RNA is a long molecule containing several hundred to several thousand nucleotides, which are codons that are exactly complementary to code words on the genes. Messenger RNA is formed by a process called *transcription*, in which the weak hydrogen bonds of the DNA are broken so that free RNA nucleotides can pair with their exposed DNA counterparts on the meaningful strand of the DNA molecule. As with the base pairing of the DNA strands, complementary RNA bases will pair with the DNA bases (uracil, which replaces thymine in

RNA, pairs with adenine). The joining together of the RNA molecule is catalyzed by the transcriptase enzyme, which is active only in the presence of DNA.

Transfer RNA

Transfer RNA transfers amino acids to protein molecules as they are being synthesized; it has two recognition sites: one for the mRNA codon for the amino acid and a second for the amino acid itself. There are many different types of tRNA, but each type combines with only one type of amino acid.

Ribosomal RNA

Ribosomal RNA constitutes 60% of the ribosome in which protein synthesis occurs. The remainder of the ribosome is structural proteins and enzymes needed for protein synthesis. Ribosomal RNA uses the "blueprint" transcribed on mRNA in assembling proteins. This process is called *translation*. There is no specificity of ribosomes for synthesis of a particular protein; a particular mRNA can direct protein synthesis in any ribosome. During protein synthesis most ribosomes become attached to the endoplasmic reticulum. This attachment facilitates transport of the protein end product and is particularly important in cells that produce products, such as hormones, that are released from the cell.

Proteins are made from a standard set of 20 amino acids, which are joined end to end to form the long polypeptide chains of protein molecules. Each polypeptide may have as many as 100 to more than 300 amino acids in it. During protein synthesis, mRNA comes in contact with and then passes through the ribosome— much in the same manner that a tape moves through a tape player. As mRNA passes through the ribosome, rRNA translates the message into assembly language, and tRNA delivers the appropriate amino acids for attachment to the growing polypeptide chain. The long mRNA molecule usually travels through and directs protein synthesis in more than one ribosome at a time. As the first part of the mRNA is read by the first ribosome, it moves on to a second, and then a third; as a result, ribosomes that are actively involved in protein synthesis are often found in clusters called *polyribosomes*. The process of protein synthesis is depicted in Figure 3-5.

Regulation of Gene Expression

Although all cells contain the same genes, not all genes are active all of the time, nor are the same genes active in all cell types. On the contrary, only a small, select group of genes is active in directing protein synthesis in the cell, and this group varies from one cell type to another. In order for different types of cells to develop in the body as a result of cell differentiation, the protein synthesis in

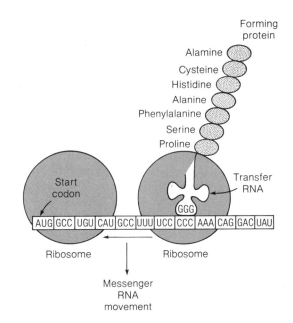

Figure 3-5 *Postulated mechanism by which a protein molecule is formed in ribosomes in association with messenger RNA and ribosomal RNA. (Guyton A: Medical Physiology, 6th ed. Philadelphia, WB Saunders, 1981)*

some cells must be different from that in others. Furthermore, in order to adapt to an ever changing environment, certain cells may need to produce different amounts and types of proteins. In addition, there are certain enzymes, such as carbonic anhydrase, that all cells must synthesize for the fundamental metabolic process on which life depends.

At present there are believed to be at least two types of genes that control protein synthesis: (1) structural genes that specify the amino acid sequence of a polypeptide chain and (2) genes that serve a regulatory function without stipulating the structure of protein molecules. The degree to which a gene or particular group of genes is active is referred to as *gene expression*. A phenomenon termed *induction* seems to be an important process in turning genes on that are responsible for the synthesis of proteins needed for cell differentiation. Except in early embryonic development, induction is produced by some external influence. A *repressor* is a substance produced by a regulatory gene that acts to prevent protein synthesis. Some genes are normally dormant and can be activated by inducer substances, and other genes are naturally active and can be inhibited by repressor substances.

Genetic mechanisms for the control of protein synthesis are much better understood in microorganisms that in humans. It can be assumed, however, that many of the same principles apply. The mechanism that has been most extensively studied is the one by which the synthesis of particular proteins can be turned on and off. In

Escherichia coli (E. coli) grown in a nutrient medium containing the disaccharide lactose, an enzyme (galactosidase) can be isolated that catalyzes the splitting of lactose into a molecule of glucose and a molecule of galactose; this is necessary if lactose is to be metabolized by *E. coli*. On the other hand, if the *E. coli* is grown in a medium that does not contain lactose, very little of the enzyme is produced. From these and other studies, it is theorized that the synthesis of a particular protein, such as galactosidase, requires a series of reactions, each of which is catalyzed by a specific enzyme. The formation of all of the enzymes needed for the synthetic process is controlled by a sequence of genes that are located on adjacent sites on the same chromosome. This area of the DNA strand is called an *operon*. The rate at which the operon functions to transcribe RNA, and therefore sets into motion the enzymatic system for the synthetic process, is controlled by a small adjacent segment of the DNA molecule. This small segment functions as a control unit for the operon; it can activate or repress the function of the operon. The control unit for the operon often monitors levels of the synthesized product and regulates the activity of the operon in a negative feedback manner; whenever there is enough of the required product, the operon becomes inactive. The operon can also be activated by an inducer substance. For example, some of the steroid hormones perform their hormonal action by activating operons in this manner. Regulatory genes located elsewhere in the genetic complex can exert control over an operon through activator or repressor substances, as can the availability of the transcriptase enzyme needed for transcription of RNA. Not all genes are subject to induction and repression; many appear to lack control genes and are continually active.

Gene Mutations

Rarely, accidental errors in duplication or destruction of parts of the genetic code occur. Such changes are called *mutations*. Many of these mutations are caused by environmental agents, chemicals, and radiation. If the duplicating cell line that contains such a change forms gametes, or germ cells, then the mutation can be transmitted to the offspring. Much more frequently, the affected cell line differentiates into one or more of the many tissues of the body and thus is not transmissible to the next generation. These are *somatic mutations* and they result in genetic differences between the cells and tissues of the same organism, producing what is called a *genetic mosaic*. Occasionally, a person is born with one brown eye and one blue eye as a result of a somatic mutation. The change or loss of gene information is just as likely to affect the fundamental processes of cell function or organ differentiation. Such somatic mutations in the early embryonic period can result in embryonic death or congenital malformations. Somatic mutations are important causes of cancer and other tumors in which cell differentiation and growth get out of hand. Fishermen, farmers, and others who are excessively exposed to the ultraviolet radiation of sunlight have an increased risk of developing skin cancer resulting from potential radiation damage to the genetic structure of the skin-forming cells.

In summary, genes are the fundamental unit of information storage in the cell. They determine the types of proteins and enzymes that are made by the cell and therefore control not only inheritance but day-to-day cell function. Genes store information in the form of a very stable macromolecule called DNA. Genes transmit information in the form of a triplet code, which uses the nitrogenous bases of the four nucleotides (adenine, guanine, thymine, and cytosine) of which the DNA molecule is composed. The transfer of stored information into production of cell products is accomplished through a second type of macromolecule called RNA. Messenger RNA transcribes the instructions for product synthesis from the DNA molecule and carries it into the cell's cytoplasm, where ribosomal RNA utilizes the information to direct product synthesis. Transfer RNA acts as a carrier system for delivering the appropriate amino acids to the ribosomes, where the synthesis of cell products occurs. Although all cells contain the same genes, only a small, select group of genes are active in a given cell type. In all cells some genetic information is repressed while other information is expressed. Gene mutations represent accidental errors in duplication or destruction of parts of the genetic code.

■ Chromosomes

The genetic information of a cell is organized, stored, and retrieved in the form of small cellular structures called *chromosomes*. There are 46 human chromosomes—22 pairs of autosomes and 1 pair of sex chromosomes.

Autosomes
Each of the autosomes appears to be identical to its partner, but each is different in genetic content and appearance from the other pairs. These 22 pairs are the same in all individuals and have been given a numerical designation for classification purposes.

Sex Chromosomes
The 23rd pair of chromosomes are the sex chromosomes (Fig. 3-6). They determine the sex of an individual. There are two sex chromosomes: the Y coming from the father and the X from the mother. All normal females have two X chromosomes, one from each parent. It is believed that

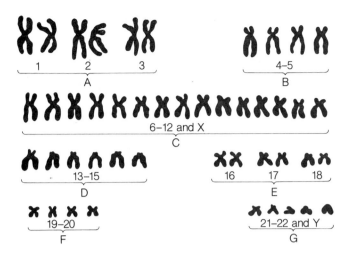

Figure 3-6 *Normal male karyotype. The first 22 pairs of chromosomes are the autosomes and the last 2 chromosomes are the sex chromosomes, in this case an X and Y chromosome. (Singer S: Human Genetics. San Francisco, WH Freeman and Co., Copyright © 1978)*

with two X chromosomes in the female only one is active in controlling the expression of genetic traits. Both X chromosomes are involved, however, in transmission to the offspring. In the female the active X chromosome is invisible, whereas the inactive X chromosome can be demonstrated by nuclear staining techniques such as the *chromatin mass* or *Barr body.* Thus the genetic sex of a child can be determined by microscopic study of cell or tissue samples. The total number of X chromosomes is equal to the number of Barr bodies (inactive X chromosomes) plus one (active X chromosome). For example, the cells of a normal female will have one Barr body and two X chromosomes. A male will have no Barr bodies. In the female, whether the X chromosome derived from the mother or that derived from the father is active is determined within a few days after conception; the selection is random for each postmitotic cell line. This is called the Lyon principle (after Mary Lyon, the British geneticist who developed it).

Chromosome Studies

Cytogenetics is the study of the structure and numerical characteristics of the cell's chromosomes. Chromosome studies can be done on any tissue or cell that will grow and divide in culture. The lymphocytes from venous blood are frequently used for this purpose. Once the cultured cells have been fixed and spread on a slide, they are stained to demonstrate banding patterns so that they can be identified. The chromosomes are then photographed, and each chromosome is cut from the photograph and arranged according to the standard set by the 1971 Paris Chromosome Conference to form the

karyotype (or chromosome picture) of the individual.[1] This arrangement is called an *idiogram.*

In summary, the genetic information in a cell is organized, stored, and retrieved in the form of small cellular structures called chromosomes. There are 46 chromosomes arranged in 23 pairs. Twenty-two of these pairs are autosomes. The 23rd pair contains the sex chromosomes, which determine the sex of an individual. A karyotype is a photograph of an individual's chromosomes. It is prepared by special laboratory techniques in which body cells are cultured, fixed, stained to demonstrate identifiable banding patterns, and photographed.

■ Patterns of Inheritance

The main feature of inheritance is predictability: given certain conditions, the likelihood of the occurrence or recurrence of a specific trait is remarkably predictable. The units of inheritance are the genes, and the pattern of single-gene expression can be predicted using Mendel's laws, with some modification as the result of knowledge accumulated since 1865, the date of Mendel's publication.

Definitions

Genetics has its own set of definitions. The *genotype* of an individual is a term for the genetic information stored in the base sequence triplet code. The *phenotype* refers to the recognizable traits, physical or biochemical, that are associated with a specific genotype. There are many instances in which the genotype is not evident by available detection methods. Thus, more than one genotype may have the same phenotype. Some brown-eyed people are carriers of the code for blue eyes and other brown-eyed persons are not. Phenotypically, these two types of brown-eyed people are the same, but genotypically they are different.

When it comes to a genetic disorder, not all individuals with a mutant gene are affected to the same extent. *Expressivity* refers to the expression of the gene in the phenotype, which can range from mild to severe. *Penetrance* means the ability of a gene to express its function. Seventy-five percent penetrance means that only 75% of the individuals of a particular genotype will demonstrate a recognizable phenotype.

A locus is the location or site on a chromosome (*i.e.,* along the DNA molecule) where an allele or group of alleles is located. When only a pair of alleles are involved in the transmission of information, the term *single-gene* is used. Single-gene traits follow the mendelian laws of inheritance. Polygenic inheritance involves multiple genes, each exerting a small additive effect in determining a trait. At present it appears there are multiple alleles, or alternative codes, in about one-half of the genetic loci in humans, accounting for some of the dissimilar forms that occur with certain genetic disorders. Polygenic traits share the feature of predictability but to a lesser degree than single-gene traits.

Mendel's Laws

At a particular point on the DNA molecule, the genetic code may be capable of controlling the production of an observable trait. Such a segment of the DNA molecule is called a *gene locus*. Alternative forms of the gene code are possible (one inherited from the mother and the other from the father) and each form may produce a different aspect of the trait. Alternative codes at one gene locus are called *alleles*. A cell contains two and only two alleles at each locus.

It was Mendel who, in 1865, discovered the basic pattern of inheritance by conducting carefully planned experiments with simple garden peas. From his experiments with wrinkled and round peas, Mendel proposed that inherited traits are transmitted from parents to off-spring by means of independently inherited factors—now known as genes—and that these factors are transmitted as recessive and dominant traits. Mendel labeled dominant factors (his round peas) "A" and recessive (his wrinkled peas) "a." Geneticists continue to use capital letters to designate dominant traits and lower-case letters to identify recessive traits. The possible combinations that can occur with transmission of single-gene dominant and recessive traits can be described by constructing a figure using capital and lower-case letters (Fig. 3-7).

The observable traits are inherited from one's parents. During maturation, the germ cells (sperm and ovum) of both parents undergo meiosis, or reduction division, in which the number of chromosomes is divided in half (from 46 to 23). At this time, the two alleles from a gene locus separate so that each germ cell gets one allele from each pair. According to Mendel's laws, the alleles from the different gene loci segregate independently and then recombine in a random fashion in the zygote that is formed by the union of the two germ cells (Fig. 3-8). Individuals in whom the two alleles of a given pair are the same (AA or aa) are called *homozygotes*. *Heterozygotes* have different (Aa) alleles at a gene locus.

A *recessive trait* is one that is expressed only in a homozygous pairing; a *dominant trait* is one that is expressed in either a homozygous or a heterozygous pairing. All persons with a dominant allele inherit that trait. A *carrier* is a person who is heterozygous for a recessive trait and does not manifest the trait. For example, if the genes for blond hair were determined to be recessive and those for brunet hair dominant, then only persons with a genotype with two alleles for blond hair would be blond, and all persons with either one or two brunet alleles would have dark hair.

Pedigree

A pedigree is a graphic method for portraying a family history of an inherited trait (Fig. 3-9). It is constructed from a carefully obtained family history and is useful for tracing the pattern of inheritance for a particular trait.

In summary, inheritance represents the likelihood of the occurrence or recurrence of a specific genetic trait. The genotype refers to information that is stored on the genetic code of an individual. The phenotype represents the recognizable traits, physical and biochemical, that are associated with the genotype. Expressivity refers to the expression of a gene in the phenotype, and penetrance is the ability of a gene to express its function. The point on the DNA molecule that controls the inheritance of a particular trait is called a gene locus. Alternate codes at one gene locus are called alleles. According to Mendel's law, the two alleles at a gene locus can transmit recessive or dominant traits. A recessive trait is one that is expressed only when there is homozygous pairing of the alleles. A dominant trait is expressed with either homozygous or heterozygous pairing of the alleles. A pedigree is a graphic method for portraying a family history of an inherited trait.

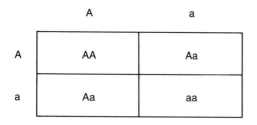

Figure 3-7 *Possible combinations for dominant, A, and recessive, a, observable traits.*

■ Gene Mapping

Gene mapping is the assignment of genes to specific chromosomes or parts of the chromosome. The initial assignment of a gene to a particular chromosome was made in 1911 for the color blindness gene that followed the X-linked pattern of inheritance.[2] In 1968 the specific location of the Duffy blood group on the long arm of chromosome 1 was determined.[3] At present the location

Patterns of Single-gene Inheritance

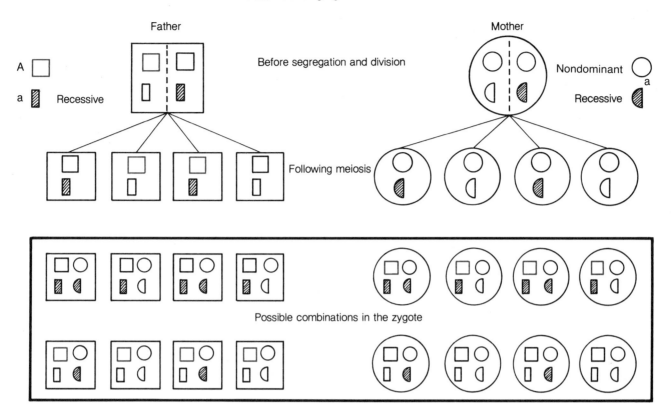

Figure 3-8 *Segregation of gene pairs during meiosis and the possible recombinations in the zygote. If a represents a recessive mutant gene, then only 25% of the offspring will be affected with the trait; 50% of the offspring will be carriers; and 25% of the offspring will be free of the mutant gene.*

of about 300 autosomal and 115 X-linked genes have been assigned.[4]

A number of methods have been used for gene mapping. The most important ones currently used are somatic cell hybridization, which has accounted for 60% of genes that have been mapped, and family linkage studies, which have accounted for 25% of mapped genes.[5] Another method of assigning chromosomes involves the use of recombinant DNA. Often, the specific assignment of a gene is made possible by the use of information from several mapping techniques.

Somatic cell hybridization involves the fusion of a mouse or Chinese hamster cell line with human leukocyte or fibroblasts to produce a rodent–human somatic cell. These hybrids preferentially lose human chromosomes in a random manner during cell mitosis, so it is possible to obtain cells with different partial combinations of human chromosomes. In this way, the correlation of the expression of human gene markers, such as production of a specific enzyme, can be linked to a particular chromosome.

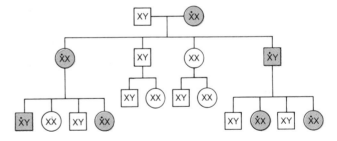

Figure 3-9 *Simple pedigree showing the inheritance of a dominant genetic trait.*

Linkage studies assume that genes occur in a linear array along the chromosomes. During meiosis, the paired chromosomes of the diploid germ cell exchange genetic material in a phenomenon called *crossing over*. This exchange involves not individual, but large blocks of genes, each accounting for a sizable fraction of the chromosome. Although the point at which one block separates from another occurs randomly, the closer together two genes are on the same chromosome, the greater the chance they will be passed on to the offspring. When two inherited traits occur together at a rate significantly greater than would occur by chance, they are said to be linked. Any gene that is already assigned to a chromosome can be used as a marker to assign other linked genes. For example, it was found that both an extra long 1 chromosome and the Duffy blood group were inherited as a dominant trait, placing the position of the blood group close to the extra material on the 1 chromosome. Color blindness has been linked to hemophilia A in some pedigrees, hemophilia to glucose-6-phosphatase deficiency in others, and color blindness and glucose-6-phosphatase deficiency in still others. Therefore, all three genes must be located in a small section of the X chromosome. Linkage analysis can be used clinically to identify affected persons in a family with a known genetic defect. Two autosomal recessive disorders successfully diagnosed prenatally (using amniocentesis) by linkage studies are congenital adrenal hyperplasia (due to 21-hydroxylase deficiency and linked to an HLA type) and hemophilia A (which is linked to glucose-6-phosphatase deficiency in some families). Postnatally, linkage studies have been used in diagnosing hemochromatosis, which is closely linked to another immune-response gene or HLA type (see discussion in Chap. 9). Persons with this disorder are unable to metabolize iron, and it accumulates in the liver and other organs. It cannot be diagnosed by conventional means until irreversible damage has been done. Given a family history of the disorder, HLA typing can determine if the gene is present; if it is present, dietary restriction of iron intake may be used to prevent organ damage.

Recombinant DNA research is used to locate genes that do not express themselves in cell culture. It begins with extraction of specific cell types of mRNA for a specific protein. The mRNA is then used as a template for synthesis of the complementary DNA strand. The complementary DNA, labeled with a radioisotope, binds to the gene to which it is complementary and is used as a probe for gene location. For example, mRNA for two components of the hemoglobin A molecule (Hb a and Hb b) have been extracted from the red blood cell, and it was through this method that the location of the Hb a gene was found to be located on chromosome 16 and the gene for the Hb b on chromosome 11.

In summary, gene mapping is a method used to assign genes to particular chromosomes or parts of the chromosome. Methods currently used in gene mapping are somatic cell hybridization and the use of recombinant DNA. Somatic cell hybridization is a method used to obtain cells with partial combinations of human chromosomes and involves the fusion of mouse or Chinese hamster cell lines with human leukocytes or fibroblasts. It is used in linkage studies that assign a chromosomal location to genes based on their close association with other genes of known location. Recombinant DNA studies involve the extraction of specific types of messenger RNA that are used in the synthesis of complementary DNA strands. The complementary DNA strands, labeled with a radioisotope, bind with the genes for which they are complementary and are used as gene probes.

■ Study Guide

After you have studied this chapter, you should be able to meet the following objectives:

☐ State the definition of a gene.

☐ Describe the structure of a gene.

☐ Explain the mechanisms whereby genes control cell function.

☐ Explain how genetic information is transferred from one generation to another generation.

☐ Compare the functions of messenger RNA, transfer RNA, and ribosomal RNA.

☐ Describe the concept of induction and repression in terms of gene function.

☐ Describe the pathogenesis of gene mutation.

☐ Construct a hypothetical pedigree according to Mendel's law.

☐ Contrast genotype and phenotype.

☐ Define gene mapping.

☐ List the steps in the construction of a karyotype using cytogenetic studies.

■ References

1. ISCN (1981): An International System for Human Cytogenetic Nomenclature—High Resolution Banding (1981). Birth Defects 17, No. 5, 1981

2. Wilson EB: The sex chromosomes. Arch Mikrosc Anat 77:249, 1911

3. McKusick, VA: The anatomy of the human genome. Hosp Pract 16, No. 4:82, 1981

4. Oslo Conference (1982): Human Gene Mapping 6. Birth Defects. 18, No. 2, 1982

5. Sparkes RS, Spence MA, Mohandas T et al: Human gene mapping, genetic linkage, and clinical application. Ann Intern Med 93: 469, 1980

Chapter 4

Genetic and Congenital Disorders

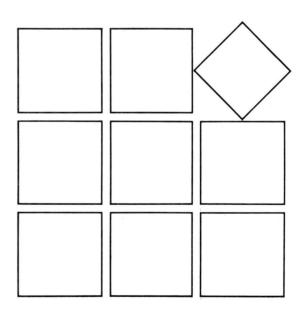

Genetic and congenital disorders are important at all levels of health care because they affect all age groups and can involve any of the body organs and tissues. A congenital defect has been described as any structural, functional, or biochemical abnormality in development that originated prior to birth or shortly after and causes an immediate or a delayed abnormality in the structure and function of an organ.[1] There are two general categories of congenital defects: (1) those that have a hereditary basis, such as single-gene and polygenic abnormalities or chromosomal aberrations, and (2) abnormalities that are caused by environmental agents such as maternal disease, radiation, or drugs. One-quarter million infants are born with physical or mental damage in the United States each year.[2] More than 60,000 Americans die of birth defects annually. It has been estimated that 80% of birth defects arise as the result of genetic disorders, and the remaining 20% represent the effects of agents such as infection, drugs, and physical injury to the fetus.[3]

This chapter is designed to provide an overview of genetic and congenital disorders and is divided into three parts: (1) genetic and chromosomal disorders, (2) disorders due to environmental agents, and (3) diagnosis and counseling.

■ Genetic and Chromosomal Disorders

A mutant gene is inferred by the sudden appearance of a genotype in a demonstrably noncarrier pedigree. Genetic disorders represent changes (or mutations) in gene function or changes in chromosomal structure. A genetic disorder can involve a single-gene trait or it can involve a polygenic trait. Polygenic traits are observable characteristics that result from the additive interactions of more than one, and sometimes many, gene loci. The shape of the nose, body height, native intelligence, and other characteristics involve polygenic inheritance. Almost all of the hereditary traits that are of importance in most individuals result from the interaction between multiple, independently associated gene loci and the environment.

The expression of the effects of a genetic trait may be present at birth or may not become apparent until later in life. Huntington's chorea, for example, has its onset between 20 and 30 years of age. Some diseases tend to run in families and it is thought that the combined effects of a genetic predisposition and environmental factors influence the development of these diseases. This is true of some types of diabetes mellitus, hypertension, and cancer.

Every individual probably has five to eight recessive genes that would cause defects if present in the homo-

Table 4-1	Some Disorders of Mendelian or Single-Gene Inheritance

Autosomal Dominant
Achondroplasia (short-limb dwarfism)
Adult polycystic kidney disease
Huntington's chorea
Hypercholesterolemia
Marfan's syndrome
Multiple neurofibromatosis (von Recklinghausen's disease)
Osteogenesis imperfecta
Spherocytosis
von Willebrand's disease (bleeding diathesis)
Autosomal Recessive
Color blindness
Cystic fibrosis
Glycogen storage diseases
Oculocutaneous albinism
Phenylketonuria (PKU)
Renal glycosuria
Sickle cell disease
Tay-Sachs disease
Wilson's disease
X-Linked Recessive
Bruton-type agammaglobulinemia
Classic hemophilia
Duchenne muscular dystrophy

zygous state.[4] About 80% to 85% of these abnormal genes are from the pedigree and the remainder represent new mutations. Either autosomal genes (those located on the nonsex chromosomes) or those located on the sex chromosomes can be affected in single-gene disorders. At last count there were more than 3000 single-gene disorders—including autosomal dominant, autosomal recessive, and X-linked disorders.[5] Table 4-1 lists some of the more common defects in each of these classifications.

Single-Gene Disorders

Single-gene disorders involve dominant or recessive traits. They may involve a gene locus on an autosome (nonsex chromosome) or a sex chromosome. Disorders of the Y, or male, chromosome are extremely rare.

Autosomal dominant

In autosomal dominant disorders, an affected parent has a single mutant gene that is transmitted to the offspring regardless of sex. The unaffected relatives of the parent or siblings of the affected offspring do not transmit the disorder. The affected individual has a 50% chance of transmitting the disorder to each offspring.

Autosomal recessive

Autosomal recessive disorders are manifested only when both members of the gene pair are mutant alleles. Both parents are usually unaffected but are carriers for the defective gene. The disorder affects persons of both sexes. The recurrence risk in each pregnancy is one in four for an affected child, two in four for a carrier child, and one in four for a normal, homozygous child.

X-linked recessive

Sex-linked inheritance is almost always associated with the X, or female, chromosome and is predominantly recessive. The common pattern of inheritance is seen in an unaffected mother who carries one normal and one mutant allele on the X chromosome. This means that she will have a 50% chance of transmitting the defect to her sons and that her female children will have a 50% chance of being carriers of the mutant gene (Fig. 4-1). When the affected male procreates, he will transmit the defect to all of his daughters, who will then become carriers of the mutant gene. Since the genes of the Y chromosome are unaffected, the affected male will not transmit the defect to any of his sons and they will not be carriers or transmit the disorder to their children.

Manifestations of single-gene disorders

Many single-gene disorders result in inborn errors of metabolism. These biochemical defects involve the formation of abnormal structural proteins, abnormal biochemical mediators or enzymes, or abnormal diffusible or membrane-bound transport or receptor proteins.

Structural protein defects are usually manifested as autosomal dominant disorders. *Marfan's syndrome*, for example, is a disorder of the connective tissues that is manifested by changes in the skeleton, the eyes, and the cardiovascular system. Characteristics of the skeletal defects are a long thin body, hyperextensive joints, arachnodactyly (spider fingers), and scoliosis. Defects of the eye include the upward displacement of the lens and the potential for retinal detachment. Involvement of connective tissue in the cardiovascular system may lead to mitral valve disease and a tendency for development of a dissecting aortic aneurysm. Abraham Lincoln's extremely long legs and the unequal lengths of his thumbs suggest that he may have been mildly affected by Marfan's syndrome. Both Abraham Lincoln and a distant male cousin, who was diagnosed as having Marfan's syndrome, are descendants of Mordecai Lincoln II. Although Mordecai almost certainly had the gene for Marfan's syndrome, he showed no signs of the disorder, probably because in him the gene had low expressivity.[6]

Primary enzyme defects are usually autosomal recessive. These enzyme defects may result in any of the following: (1) deficiency of a metabolic endproduct, (2) production of harmful intermediates or toxic by-products of metabolism, or (3) accumulation of destructive substances within the cell. In *albinism,* the basic biochemical defect is the absence or nonfunctioning of the

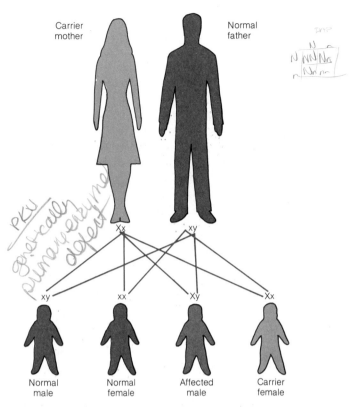

How X − Linked Inheritance Works

In the most common form, the female sex chromosome of an unaffected mother carries one faulty gene (X) and one normal one (x). The father has normal male x and y chromosome complement.

Carrier mother   Normal father

Xx   xy

xy   xx   Xy   Xx

Normal male   Normal female   Affected male   Carrier female

The odds for each *male* child are 50/50:
1. 50% risk of inheriting the faulty X and the disorder
2. 50% chance of inheriting normal x and y chromosomes

For each *female* child, the odds are:
1. 50% risk of inheriting one faulty X, to be a carrier like mother
2. 50% chance of inheriting no faulty gene

Figure 4-1 *Pattern of inheritance for an X-linked recessive trait. (From Department of Health, Education, and Welfare: What Are the Facts About Genetic Disease? Washington, DC, 1977)*

enzyme tyrosinase. This enzyme is necessary for the production of melanin, the pigment that gives skin its color.

Phenylketonuria (PKU) is another genetically inherited primary enzyme defect. In this disorder, there is a deficiency of phenylalanine hydroxylase, the enzyme needed for conversion of phenylalanine to tyrosine, and as a result of this deficiency, toxic levels of phenylalanine accumulate in the blood. Like other inborn errors of metabolism, PKU is inherited as a recessive trait and is manifested only in the homozygote. It is possible to identify carriers of the trait by subjecting them to a phenylalanine test in which a large dose of phenylalanine is administered orally and the rate at which it disappears from the bloodstream is measured. PKU occurs once in approximately 10,000 births, and damage to the developing brain almost always results when the concentrations of phenylalanine and other metabolites persist in the blood. Presently, a screening test is widely used for detection of abnormal levels of serum phenylalanine in newborn infants. Infants with the disorder are treated with a special diet that restricts phenylalanine intake. Dietary treatment must be started early in neonatal life because the untreated affected child may have evidence of arrested brain development by 4 months of age.[7]

Tay-Sachs disease is caused by an accumulation of ganglioside GM_2 (a glycolipid) in body tissues due to an enzyme deficiency (hexosaminidase A), resulting in gangliosidosis. The disease is particularly prevalent among eastern European (Ashkenazi) Jews. Infants with Tay-Sachs appear normal at birth but begin to manifest neurologic signs at about 6 months of age. These neurologic manifestations eventually lead to muscle flaccidity, dementia, and finally death at about 2 to 3 years of age. Although there is no cure for the disease, analysis of the blood serum for a deficiency of hexosaminidase A allows for accurate identification of the genetic carriers for the disease.

Membrane-associated transport defects can be either dominant or recessive. Hereditary *spherocytosis*, an autosomal dominant trait, is a form of hemolytic anemia that is caused by a defect in sodium transport in the red cell. *Renal glycosuria*, on the other hand, is an autosomal recessive trait that involves glucose transport in the renal tubules.

Polygenic Disorders

Polygenic disorders are conditions in which two or more genes or gene loci are influential in the expression of a gene trait. In some diseases, such as diabetes mellitus and essential hypertension, the genetic component is influenced by multiple environmental influences.

The exact number of genes contributing to polygenic traits is not known, and these traits do not follow the clear-cut pattern of inheritance as do single-gene disorders. Polygenic inheritance has been described as a threshold phenonemon in which the parent's expression of a particular gene trait might be compared to the amount of water contained in a glass of a given capacity (Fig. 4-2).[8] Using this analogy, one might say that the expression of a genetic disorder occurs when the amount of the trait that is in the glass overflows. Some conditions that are thought to arise through polygenic inheritance include the following: allergies, anencephaly, cleft lip or palate, clubfoot, congenital dislocation of the hip, congenital heart disease, diabetes mellitus, hydrocephalus, myelomeningocele, pyloric stenosis, and urinary tract malformation.

Although polygenic traits cannot be predicted with the same amount of accuracy as the mendelian single-gene mutations, characteristic patterns exist. First, polygenic congenital malformations involve a single organ or tissue that is derived from the same embryologic developmental field. Second, the risk of recurrence in future pregnancies is for the same or a similar defect. This means that parents of a child with polygenic cleft palate defect have an increased risk of having another child with a cleft palate, but not with spina bifida. Third, the increased risk (compared with the general population) among first-degree relatives of the affected person is 2% to 5%, and among second-degree relatives it is about one-half that amount.[8] Furthermore, the risk increases

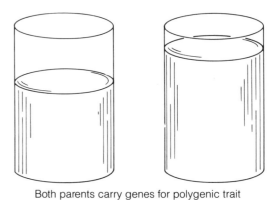

Both parents carry genes for polygenic trait

Trait expressed in offspring

Figure 4-2 *Water glass analogy to explain polygenic inheritance. (Riccardi VM: The Genetic Approach to Human Disease. New York, Oxford University Press, 1977)*

with increasing incidence of the defect among relatives. This means that the risk is greatly increased when a second child with the defect is born to a couple. The risk also increases with severity of the disorder and when the defect occurs in the sex not generally affected by the disorder.

Chromosome Disorders

Chromosome disorders involve a change in chromosome number or structure that results in damage to sensitive genetic mechanisms or in reproductive disorders.[9] During the process of germ cell (sperm and ovum) formation, a special form of cell division called *meiosis* takes place. During this division, the double sets of 22 autosomes and the 2 sex chromosomes (normal diploid number) become reduced to single sets (haploid number) in each gamete. In cell division in nongerm cells (mitosis), replication of the chromosomes occurs, so that each cell receives a full diploid number. At the time of conception, the haploid number in the ovum and that in the sperm join and restore the diploid number of chromosomes. Chromosome defects usually develop because of defective movement during meiosis or breakage of a chromosome with loss or translocation of genetic material.

Alterations in chromosome duplication
Mosaicism. Mosaicism is the presence in one individual of two or more cell lines characterized by distinctive karyotypes. This defect results from a chromosomal duplication accident. Sometimes mosaicism consists of an abnormal karyotype and a normal one, in which case the physical deformities caused by the abnormal cell line are usually less severe.

Alterations in chromosome number
A change in chromosome number is called *aneuploidy*. Among the causes of aneuploidy are failure of separation of the chromosomes during oogenesis or spermatogenesis. This can occur in either the autosomes or the sex chromosomes and is called *nondisjunction*. Nondisjunction gives rise to germ cells that have an even number of chromosomes (22 or 24). The products of conception that are formed from this even number of chromosomes will have an uneven number of chromosomes, either 45 or 47. *Monosomy* refers to the presence of only one member of a chromosome pair. The defects associated with monosomy of the autosomes are severe and usually cause abortion. Monosomy of the X chromosome (45, X/O), or Turner's syndrome, causes less severe defects. *Polysomy*, or the presence of more than two chromosomes to a set, occurs when a germ cell

containing more than 23 chromosomes is involved in conception. This defect has been described for both the autosomes and the sex chromosomes. Trisomy of chromosomes 8, 13, 18, and 21 is the more common form of polysomy of the autosomes. There are several forms of polysomy of the sex chromosomes in which one or more extra X or Y chromosomes are present.

Trisomy 21 (Down's syndrome). Trisomy 21, or Down's syndrome, is the most common form of chromosome disorder. It has an incidence of 1 in 800 births.[10] The condition is usually accompanied by moderately severe mental retardation.

The risk of having a baby with Down's syndrome is greater in women who are 35 years of age or older at the time of delivery (Table 4-2). The sharp rise in incidence of Down's syndrome children born to older women may occur for several reasons. Although males continue to produce sperm throughout their reproductive life, females are born with all the oocytes they will ever have. These oocytes may change as a result of the aging process. Also with increasing age there is a greater chance of a woman having been exposed to damaging environmental agents such as drugs, chemicals, and radiation.

The physical features of a child with Down's syndrome are distinctive, and therefore the condition is usually apparent at birth. These features include a small and rather square head. There is upward slanting of the eyes, small and malformed ears, an open mouth, and a large and protruding tongue. The child's hands are usually short and stubby with fingers that curl inward, and there is usually only a single palmar (simian) crease. There are often accompanying congenital heart defects. Of particular concern is the much greater risk that these children have for the development of acute leukemia—20 times greater than normal children.[10]

Table 4-2 The Relationship Between Maternal Age and the Risk of Down's Syndrome in a Newborn Child

Maternal Age (years)	Approximate Risk of Occurrence
20–24	1 in 1350
25–29	1 in 1175
30–35	1 in 750
36–40	1 in 250
41–45	1 in 65
46–50	1 in 25(?)

(Wisniewski LP, Hirschhorn K: A Guide to Human Chromosome Defects, 2nd ed. White Plains, March of Dimes Birth Defects Foundation, BD: OAS XVI(6), 1980)

Monosomy X (Turner's syndrome). Turner's syndrome describes a monosomy of the X chromosome (45,X/O) with gonadal agenesis, or absence of the ovaries. This disorder is present in about 1 out of every 2500 live births. There are variations in the syndrome, with abnormalities ranging from essentially none to webbing of the neck with redundant skin folds, nonpitting edema of the hands and feet, and congenital heart defects (particularly coarctation of the aorta). Characteristically, the female with Turner's syndrome is short in stature, but her body proportions are normal. She does not menstruate and shows no signs of secondary sex characteristics. Administration of the female sex hormones (estrogens) may cause the secondary sexual characteristics to develop and may produce additional skeletal growth. Infertility of the affected individual cannot be restored. When a mosaic cell line (45,X/O and 46,X/X or 45,X/O and 46,X/Y) is present, the manifestations associated with the chromosomal defect tend to be less severe.

Polysomy X (Klinefelter's syndrome). Klinefelter's syndrome is characterized by an X-chromatin positive (47,X/X/Y) male and is associated with testicular dysgenesis. In rare situations, there may be more than one extra X chromosome, for example, 47,X/X/Y. The incidence of Klinefelter's syndrome is about 1 in 600. The condition may not be detected in the newborn. The infant usually has normal male genitalia, with a small penis and small, firm testicles. Hypogonadism during puberty usually leads to a tall stature with abnormal body proportions in which the lower part of the body is longer than the upper part. Later in life, the body build may become heavy with a female distribution of subcutaneous fat and variable degrees of breast enlargement. There may be deficient secondary male sex characteristics such as a voice that remains feminine in pitch and sparse beard and pubic hair. There may be sexual dysfunction, along with complete infertility and impotence. Personality problems may occur, but the intellect is usually normal. Replacement hormone therapy with testosterone is used to treat the disorder.

Alterations in chromosome structure

Aberrations in chromosome structure occur when there is a break in one or more of the chromosomes followed by rearrangement or deletion of the chromosome parts. Among the factors believed to cause chromosome breakage are the following: (1) exposure to radiation sources, such as x-rays; (2) influence of certain chemicals; (3) extreme changes in the cellular environment; and (4) viral infections.

A number of patterns of chromosome breakage and rearrangement can occur (Fig. 4-3). There can be a *deletion* of the broken portion of the chromosome. When one chromosome is involved, the broken parts may be *inverted*. *Isochromosome formation* occurs when the centromere, or central portion, of the chromosome separates horizontally instead of vertically. *Ring formation* results when deletion is followed by uniting of the chromatids to form a ring. *Translocation* occurs when there are simultaneous breaks in two chromosomes from different pairs with exchange of chromosome parts. With a translocation, no genetic information is lost; therefore, persons with translocations are generally normal. These persons are, however, translocation carriers and may have both normal and abnormal children. A rare form of Down's syndrome is caused by translocation of some segment of chromosome 21 or 22 to another chromosome, often 14 or 15.

The manifestations of aberrations in chromosome strutre will depend to a great extent on the amount of genetic material that is lost. Many cells suffering unrestituted breaks will be eliminated within the next few mitoses because of deficiencies that may in themselves be fatal. This is beneficial because it prevents the damaged cells from becoming a permanent part of the organism or, if it occurs in the gametes, from giving rise to grossly defective zygotes. Some altered chromosomes, such as those that occur with translocations, will be passed on to the next generation.

In summary, genetic and congenital disorders affect all age groups and all body structures. Genetic disorders can affect a single gene (mendelian inheritance) or several genes (polygenic inheritance). Chromosome disorders result from a change in chromosome number or structure. A change in chromosome number is called aneuploidy. Monosomy involves the presence of only one member of a chromosome pair; it is seen in Turner's syndrome, in which there is monosomy of the X chromosome. Polysomy refers to the presence of more than two chromosomes in a set. Klinefelter's syndrome involves polysomy of the X chromosome. Trisomy 21 (Down's syndrome) is the most common form of chromosome disorder. Alterations in chromosome structure involve either deletion or addition of genetic material, which may involve a translocation of genetic material from one chromosome pair to another.

■ Disorders Due to Environmental Agents

The developing embryo is subject to many nongentic influences. Following conception, development is influenced by the environmental factors that the embryo shares with the mother. The physiologic status of the

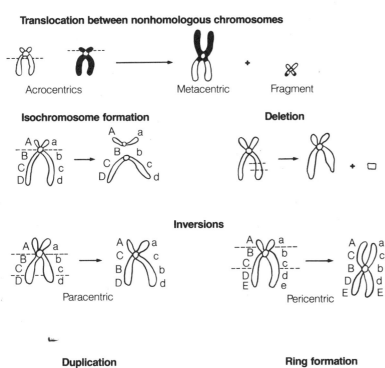

Translocation between nonhomologous chromosomes

Acrocentrics   Metacentric   Fragment

Isochromosome formation   **Deletion**

Inversions

Paracentric   Pericentric

Duplication   **Ring formation**

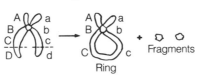

Ring   Fragments

Figure 4-3   *Rearrangement following breaks in chromosome structures. (Robbins SL, Angell M: Basic Pathology, 2nd ed. Philadelphia, WB Saunders, 1976)*

mother—her hormone balance, her general state of health, her nutritional status, and the drugs she takes—undoubtedly influence the development of the unborn child. For example, diabetes mellitus is associated with increased risk of congenital anomalies. Smoking is associated with lower than normal neonatal weight. Alcohol, in the context of chronic alcoholism, is known to cause fetal abnormalities. Some agents cause early abortion. Measles and other infectious agents cause congenital malformations. Other agents, such as radiation, have the potential for causing chromosomal and genetic defects as well as developmental disorders.

Period of Vulnerability

The embryo's development is most easily disturbed during the period when differentiation and development of the organs is taking place. This time interval is often referred to as the period of *organogenesis*; it extends from days 15 to 60 following conception. Environmental influences during the first 2 weeks following fertilization may interfere with implantation and result in abortion or very early resorption of the products of conception. Each organ has a critical period of time during which it is

highly susceptible to environmental derangements (Fig. 4-4). Often the effect is expressed at the biochemical level just before the organ begins to develop. The same agent may affect different organ systems that are developing at the same time.

Teratogenic Agents

A *teratogenic* agent is one that produces abnormalities during embryonic or fetal development. For discussion purposes, teratogenic agents have been divided into three groups: (1) irradiation, (2) drugs and chemical substances, and (3) infectious agents. Table 4-3 lists commonly identified agents in each of these groups.

Irradiation

Heavy doses of ionizing radiation have been shown to cause microcephaly, skeletal malformations, and mental retardation. At present there is no evidence that diagnostic levels of radiation cause congenital abnormalities. Because the question of safety remains, however, many agencies require that the day of a woman's last menstrual period be noted on all radiologic requisitions. Other institutions may require a pregnancy test before any

Highly Sensitive Periods of Development In Terms of Teratogenic Effects

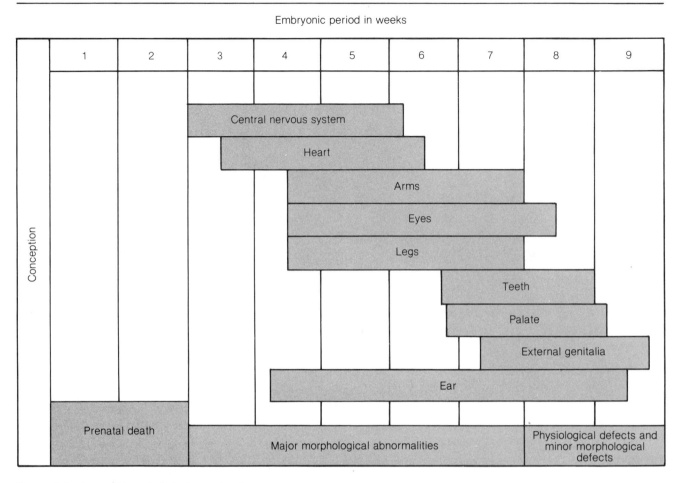

Figure 4-4 *Susceptible periods during embryologic development during which teratogenic agents are most likely to impair development of the various body structures. (Developed from information included in Moore KL: The Developing Human, 2nd ed. Philadelphia, WB Saunders, 1977)*

extensive diagnostic x-ray studies are performed. Radiation is not only teratogenic but also mutagenic, and there is the possibility of effecting inheritable changes in genetic materials. Administration of therapeutic doses of radioactive iodine (I_{131}) during the 13th week of gestation, the time when the fetal thyroid is beginning to concentrate iodine, has been shown to interfere with thyroid development.

Chemicals and drugs

Some of the best-documented chemical teratogens are the organic mercurials, which cause neurologic deficits and blindness. Exposure sources of mercury include contaminated food (fish) and water.

A number of drugs are suspected of being teratogens, but only a few have been documented with certainty. Perhaps the best known of these drugs is thalid-omide, which has been shown to give rise to a full range of malformations, including phocomelia (short flipperlike appendages) of all four extremities. Other drugs known to cause fetal abnormalities are the antimetabolites used in the treatment of cancer, the anticoagulant drug warfarin, several of the anticonvulsant drugs, and ethyl alcohol. Some drugs affect a single developing structure; for example, propylthiouracil can impair thyroid development and tetracycline can interfere with the mineralization phase of tooth development. The progestins, which are included in many birth control pills, can cause virilization of a female fetus depending on their dosage and timing.

Fetal alcohol syndrome.   Only recently have the teratogenic effects of alcohol been described in the literature. Alcohol has widely variable effects on fetal devel-

Table 4-3   Teratogenic Agents

Irradiation
Drugs and Chemical Substances
   Alcohol
   Anticoagulants
     Warfarin
   Anticonvulsants
     Paramethadione
     Phenytoin
     Trimethadione
   Cancer drugs
     Aminopterin
     Methotrexate
     6-mercaptopurine
   Progestins and oral contraceptive drugs
   Propylthiouracil
   Tetracycline
   Thalidomide
Infectious Agents
   Viruses
     Cytomegalovirus
     Herpes simplex virus
     Measles (rubella)
     Mumps
     Chickenpox
   Nonviral factors
     Syphilis
     Toxoplasmosis

opment, ranging from minor abnormalities to a unique constellation of anomalies that has been termed the *fetal alcohol syndrome*.[11] One out of 750 infants born in the United States manifests some characteristics of the syndrome.[12]

The fetal alcohol syndrome is associated with several severe problems: (1) central nervous system dysfunction ranging from hypotonia and poor muscle coordination to moderate mental retardation, (2) craniofacial anomalies that can include microcephaly and a cluster of facial and eye defects, (3) deficient growth, and (4) other problems such as cardiovascular defects. Each of these defects can vary in severity, which probably reflects the amount of alcohol consumed as well as hereditary and environmental influences.

Evidence suggests that the consumption of 89 ml of alcohol per day—equivalent to six hard drinks—constitutes a major risk to the fetus.[11] Although clinical studies have focused on the consequences of chronic maternal alcoholism, there is inadequate information about the possible adverse effects of lower alcohol intake, including social drinking. In studies using pregnant monkeys, alcohol administration produced transient but marked collapse of the umbilical cord, causing severe hypoxia and acidosis in the fetus.[12] If this phenomenon occurs in humans, it could explain the teratogenicity of alcohol. Even in late gestation, the unborn child could be at risk for alcohol-induced hypoxia.

Because many drugs are suspected of causing fetal abnormalities, and even those that were once thought to be safe are now being viewed critically, it seems unwise for women in their childbearing years to use drugs unnecessarily. This pertains to nonpregnant women as well as pregnant ones because many developmental defects occur very early in pregnancy. As happened with thalidomide, the damage to the embryo often occurs before pregnancy is suspected or confirmed.

Infectious agents

Many microorganisms cross the placenta and enter the fetal circulation, often producing multiple malformations. The acronym TORCH stands for *t*oxoplamosis, *o*ther, *r*ubella, *c*ytomegalovirus, and *h*erpes, which are the agents most frequently implicated in fetal anomalies.[13] "Other" stands for type B hepatitis virus, coxsackie B, mumps, poliovirus, rubeola, varicella, listeria, gonorrhea, streptococcus, and treponema. Of these, hepatitis B poses the greatest threat to mother and infant. The TORCH screening test examines the infant's serum for the presence of antibodies to these agents. These infections tend to cause similar clinical manifestations, including microcephaly, hydrocephaly, defects of the eye, and hearing problems. Cytomegalovirus may cause mental retardation and rubella virus may cause congenital heart defects.

Toxoplasmosis is a protozoal infection that can be contracted by eating raw or poorly cooked meat. The domestic cat also seems to carry the organism, excreting the protozoa in its stools. It has been suggested that pregnant women should avoid contact with the excrement from the family cat. *Rubella* (German measles) is a commonly recognized viral teratogen. About 15% to 20% of babies born to women who have had rubella during the first trimester have abnormalities.[14] The epidemiology of the *cytomegalovirus* is largely unknown. Some babies are severely affected at birth and others, though having evidence of the infection, have no symptoms. In some symptom-free babies, brain damage becomes evident over a span of several years. There is also evidence that some babies contract the infection during the first year of life and in some of them the infection leads to retardation a year or two later. *Herpes simplex 2* is considered to be a genital infection and is usually transmitted through sexual contact. The infant acquires this infection either *in utero* or in passage through the birth canal.

In summary, a teratogenic agent is one that produces abnormalities during embryonic or fetal life. It is during the early part of pregnancy (15 to 60 days following conception) that environmental agents are most apt to produce their deleterious effects on the developing embryo. A number of environmental agents can be damaging to the unborn child, including radiation, drugs and chemicals, and infectious agents. The fetal alcohol syndrome is a recently recognized risk for infants of women with regular alcohol consumption during pregnancy. Because many drugs have the potential for causing fetal abnormalities, often at a very early stage of pregnancy, it is recommended that women of childbearing age avoid unnecessary use of drugs.

■ Diagnosis and Counseling

The birth of a defective child is a traumatic event in any parent's life. Usually two issues must be resolved. The first deals with the immediate and future care of the affected child and the second with the possibility of future children in the family having a similar defect.

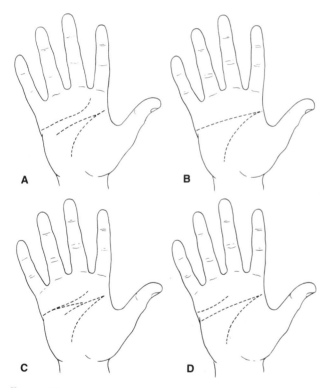

Figure 4-5 *The transverse palmar crease. Hands* A *and* C *are normal. Hand* B *shows the typical transverse or simian crease. It is found in about 4% of the normal population and in about 50% of persons with Down's syndrome and certain other chromosomal defects. The sydney line* D *can be regarded as a variant of* B *and has the same significance. (Valentine GH: The Chromosome Disorders, 3rd ed. Philadelphia, JB Lippincott, 1975)*

Genetic assessment and counseling can help to determine whether the defect was inherited as well as the risk of recurrence. Prenatal diagnosis provides a means of determining whether the unborn child has certain types of abnormalities.

Genetic Assessment

Effective genetic counseling involves accurate diagnosis and communication of the findings along with the risks of recurrence to the parents and other family members who need such information. Counseling may be provided following the birth of an affected child, or it may be offered to persons at risk for having defective children (siblings of persons with birth defects). A team of trained counselors helps the family to understand the problem and stands ready to support their decisions about having more children.

Assessment of genetic risk and prognosis is usually directed by a clinical geneticist, often with the aid of laboratory and clinical specialists. A detailed family history (pedigree), a pregnancy history, and detailed accounts of both the birth process and postnatal health and development are included. A careful physical examination of the affected child and often of the parents and siblings is usually needed. Laboratory work, including chromosomal analysis and biochemical studies, often precedes a definitive diagnosis.

The creases and dermal ridges on the palms and soles are examined in a genetic study called *dermatoglyphic analysis*. This is of value because the dermal ridges are formed by 16 weeks of gestation and any abnormalities will document the time during which the developmental defect occurred. Dermatoglyphic analysis includes examination of the patterns of the arches on the fingertips, the flexion creases of the fifth finger, and the arch pattern of the base of the great toe. One of the most readily identified creases is the palmar (simian) crease (Fig. 4-5). For additional information on dermatoglyphic analysis, the reader is referred to other sources including those listed in the reference section at the end of this chapter.

Prenatal Diagnosis

One form of prenatal diagnosis involves amniocentesis. The test is useful in women over 35 in whom there is an increased risk of giving birth to a baby with Down's syndrome, in parents who have another child with chromosomal abnormalities, and in situations in which either parent is known to be a carrier of an inherited disorder. The procedure involves the withdrawal of a sample of amniotic fluid from the pregnant uterus by means of a needle inserted through the abdominal wall (Fig. 4-6).

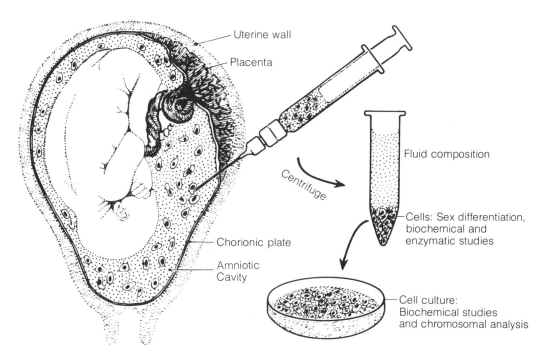

Figure 4-6 *Amniocentesis. A needle is inserted into the uterus through the abdominal wall and a sample of amniotic fluid is withdrawn for chromosomal and biochemical studies. (Department of Health, Education and Welfare: What Are the Facts About Genetic Disease? Washington, DC, 1977)*

Ultrasound is used to gain additional information and as a guide for placement of the amniocentesis needle. The amniotic fluid cells shed by the fetus are then cultured and studied. Amniotic fluid is also useful in biochemical studies. Amniocentesis is currently useful for detecting some 60 genetic disorders, although not all hereditary or developmental defects can be detected in this way. Usually a determination can be made by the 16th to 17th week of pregnancy, and if the fetus is defective, the parents can then decide if they want to terminate the pregnancy. In most cases, the fetus is normal and the fears and anxieties of the prospective parents are relieved.

Ultrasound

Ultrasound is a noninvasive diagnostic method that uses reflections of high-frequency sound waves for visualizing soft tissue structures. Since its introduction in 1958, it has been used during pregnancy to determine fetal size, fetal position, and placental location. Improved resolution of ultrasound scanners and real-time units have enhanced the ability to detect congenital anomalies. With this more sophisticated equipment, it is now possible to obtain information such as measurements of hourly urine output in a high-risk fetus.[15] Ultrasound makes possible the *in utero* diagnosis of hydrocephalus, spina bifida, facial defects, congenital heart defects, con-genital diaphragmatic hernias, disorders of the gastrointestinal tract, and skeletal anomalies. Intrauterine diagnosis of congenital abnormalities permits planning of surgical correction shortly after birth, preterm delivery for early correction, selection of cesarean section to reduce fetal injury, and in some cases *in utero* therapy. At present, 40% of obstetric practices in the United States have all of their patients undergo ultrasound scanning at least once during pregnancy, and 75% of such practices have 50% of their patients undergo sonography.[15] When a congenital abnormality is suspected, a diagnosis made using ultrasound can generally be obtained by weeks 16 to 18 of gestation.

In summary, genetic and prenatal diagnosis and counseling are done in an effort to determine the risk of having a child with a genetic or chromosomal disorder. They often involve a detailed family history (pedigree), examination of any affected and other family members, and laboratory studies including chromosomal analysis and biochemical studies. They are usually done by a genetic counseler and a specially prepared team of health care professionals. Both ultrasound and amniocentesis can be used to screen for congenital defects. Ultrasound is used for determination of fetal size and position and for the presence of structural anomalies. Amniocentesis is used to obtain a specimen of amniotic fluid for cytogenetic and biochemical studies. It is currently used in the prenatal diagnosis of over 60 genetic disorders.

■ Study Guide

After you have studied this chapter, you should be able to meet the following objectives:

- ☐ Define the term congenital defect.
- ☐ Describe three types of single-gene disorders.
- ☐ Contrast polygenic disorders with single-gene disorders.
- ☐ Describe two chromosomal abnormalities that demonstrate aneuploidy.
- ☐ Describe three patterns of chromosomal breakage and rearrangement.
- ☐ Relate maternal age and occurrence of Down's syndrome.
- ☐ Cite the most susceptible period of intrauterine life for development of defects due to environmental agents.
- ☐ State the cautions that should be observed when considering use of drugs during pregnancy.
- ☐ List four infectious agents that cause congenital defects.
- ☐ List types of information that are usually considered when doing an assessment of genetic risk.
- ☐ Cite examples of fetal information that can be obtained with use of amniocentesis and ultrasound.

■ References

1. Goldman AS (Key Consultant): Congenital Defects. Washington, DC, US Department of Health, Education and Welfare, Public Health Service, 1983
2. Facts/1984. White Plains, NY, March of Dimes, 1984
3. National Institutes of Health: What Are the Facts About Genetic Disease? Washington, DC, US Department of Health, Education and Welfare, Public Health Service, 1977
4. Erbe RW: Principles of medical genetics. N Engl J Med 294:381,480, 1976
5. McKusick VA: Mendelian Inheritance in Man: Catalogs of Autosomal Dominant, Autosomal Recessive, and X-linked Phenotypes. Baltimore, Johns Hopkins University Press, 1983
6. Singer S: Human Genetics, p 13. San Francisco, WH Freeman and Co., 1978
7. Vaughn VC, McKay RJ, Nelson WE: Nelson Textbook of Pediatrics, 10th ed, p 132. Philadelphia, WB Saunders, 1975
8. Riccardi VM: The Genetic Approach to Human Disease, pp 92,500. New York, Oxford University Press, 1977
9. A Guide to Chromosome Defects, 2nd ed, The National Foundation—March of Dimes Birth Defects 16, No.6:5, 1980
10. De LaCruz D, Muller JZ: Facts about Down syndrome. Child Today 13, No.6:3, 1983
11. National Institute of Alcohol Abuse and Alcoholism: Critical Review of the Fetal Alcohol Syndrome. Rockville, MD, Alcohol, Drug Abuse, and Mental Health Administration, 1977
12. Mukherjee AB, Hodgen GD: Maternal alcohol exposure induces transient impairment of umbilical circulation and fetal hypoxia in monkeys. Science 218:700, 1982
13. DeVore NE, Jackson VM, Piening SL: TORCH infections. Am J Nurs 83:1660, 1983
14. Dudgeon JA: Infectious causes of human malformations. Br Med J 32:77, 1976
15. Hill LM, Breckle R, Gehrking RT: The prenatal detection of congenital malformations by ultrasonography. Mayo Clin Proc 58:805, 1983

■ Additional References

Clarren SK, Smith DW: The fetal alcohol syndrome. N Engl J Med 298, No. 19:1063, 1978

Dabney BJ: The role of human genetic monitoring in the workplace. J Occup Med 23:626, 1981

Denniston C: Low level radiation and genetic risk estimation in man. Ann Rev Genet 16:329-355, 1982

Erbe RW: Current concepts in genetics: Principles of medical genetics. N Engl J Med 294, No. 7:381, 1976

Erbe RW: Current concepts in genetics: Principles of medical genetics (Part 2). N Engl J Med 294, No. 9:480, 1976

Fabricant JD, Legator MS: Etiology, role and detection of chromosomal aberrations in man. J Occup Med 23, No. 9:617, 1981

Fraser FC: Current concepts in genetics: Genetics as a health care service. N Engl J Med 295, No. 9:486, 1976

Gelehrter TD: The family history and genetic counseling: Tools for preventing and managing genetic disorders. Postgrad Med 73, No. 6:119, 1983

German J: Embryonic stress hypothesis of teratogenesis. Am J Med 76:293, 1984

Golden NL et al: Maternal alcohol use and infant development. Pediatrics 70, No. 6:931, 1982

Hill LM: Effects of drugs and chemicals on the fetus and newborn. Mayo Clin Proc 59:707-716, 1984

Hill LM: Effects of drugs and chemicals on the fetus and newborn (Part 2). Mayo Clin Proc 59:755-765, 1984

Janerich DT, Polednak AP: Epidemiology of birth defects. Epidemiol Rev 5:16-37, 1983

Kalter H, Warkany J: Congenital malformations: Etiological factors and their role in prevention. N Engl J Med 308, No. 8:424-430, 1983

Kalter H, Warkany J: Congenital malformations: Etiological factors and their role in prevention (Part 2). N Engl J Med 308, No. 9:491-497, 1983

Kushnick T: When to refer to the geneticist. JAMA 235, No. 6:623, 1976

Level RR: Ethical Issues Arising in the Genetic Counseling Relationship. National Foundation—March of Dimes Birth Defects 14:9, 1978

Marx JL: Cytomegalovirus: A major cause of birth defects. Science 190:1184, 1975

McKusick VA: The anatomy of the human genome. Hosp Prac 16:82, 1981

Milunsky A: Current concepts in genetics: Prenatal diagnosis of genetic disorders. N Engl J Med 295, No. 7:377, 1976

Mukherjee AB, Hodgen GD: Maternal ethanol exposure induces transient impairment of umbilical circulation and fetal hypoxia in monkeys. Science 218, No. 4573:700-702, 1982

Nitowsky HM: Fetal alcohol syndrome and alcohol-related birth defects. NY State J Med 82, No. 7:1214-1217, 1982

Omenn GS: Prenatal diagnosis of genetic disorders. Science 200, No. 26:952, 1978

Prockop DJ, Kivirikko KI: Heritable diseases of collagen. N Engl J Med 311, No. 6:376-385, 1984

Shiono H Kadowaki J. dermatoglyphics of congenital abnormalities without chromosomal aberrations: A review of clinical applications. Clin Pediatr 14:1003, 1975

Tomasi TB: Structure and function of alpha-fetoprotein. Annu Rev Med 28:453, 1977

Wilson JG: Teratogenic effects of environmental chemicals. Fed Proc 36, No. 5:1698, 1977

Chapter 5

Alterations in Cell Differentiation: Neoplasia

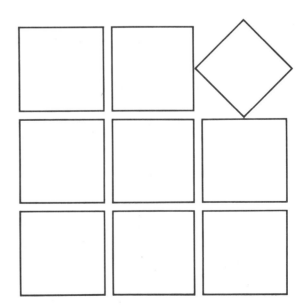

Cancer is the second leading cause of death in the United States, and it affects all age groups. Cancer causes more deaths in children 3 to 14 years of age than any other disease. The American Cancer Society has estimated that over 67 million Americans, or one out of every four alive today, will develop cancer during their lifetimes. In 1985, about 910,000 persons were diagnosed as having cancer.[1] It has been estimated that with present methods of treatment, three out of every eight (38%) persons who develop cancer each year will be alive five years later.

Cancer is not a single disease; rather, the term describes almost all forms of malignant neoplasia. As shown in Figure 5-1, cancer can originate in almost any organ, the lung being the most common site in men and the breast in women. Cancers such as acute lymphocytic leukemia, Hodgkin's disease, testicular and ovarian cancers, and osteogenic sarcoma, which only a few decades ago had a poor prognosis, are today cured in many instances. This is mainly due to advances in chemotherapy. On the other hand, lung cancer, which is the leading cause of death in the United States, is very resistant to therapy, and although some progress has been made in its treatment, mortality rates continue to remain high. This chapter provides a general overview of cancer (malignant neoplasia) along with a brief discussion of benign neoplasia. Specific forms of cancer are discussed elsewhere in the book.

■ Concepts of Cell Growth and Replication

A basic knowledge of cell growth and replication is helpful in understanding the characteristics of neoplasms. Cell division and replication are inherent adaptive mechanisms for many body cells, and in a single day many cells are replaced by new cells. Normally, these cells are identical in structure and function to the cells they replace. When abnormal or mutant cells do develop, they are usually either defective and incapable of survival or are destroyed by the body's immune system.

The Cell Cycle

The life of a cell is called the *cell cycle*. It consists of the interval between the midpoint of mitosis and the subsequent midpoint of mitosis in one or both daughter cells. *Mitosis* is the period of time when cell division is actually taking place. The cell cycle is divided into five distinct phases for which *gap* or *G* terminology is used (Fig. 5-2). G_1 is the first gap, the postmitotic phase during which DNA synthesis ceases while RNA and protein synthesis and cell growth take place. Toward the end of G_1, some critical event occurs that commits the cell to continue through the phases of the gap cycle, and enter mitosis.

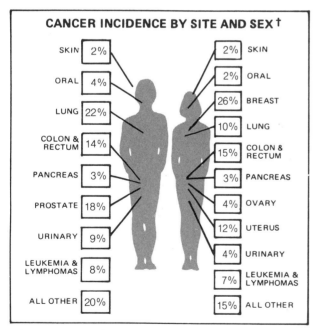

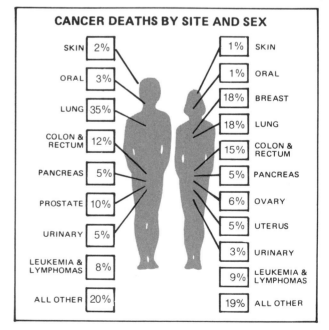

†Excluding non-melanoma skin cancer and carcinoma in situ.

Figure 5-1 *Cancer deaths (1984 estimates) by site and sex. (American Cancer Society: Cancer Facts, New York 1984)*

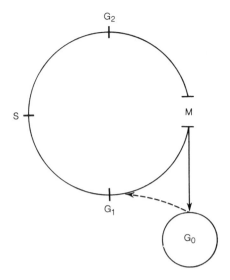

Figure 5-2 *Phases of the cell cycle. The cycle represents the interval between the midpoint of mitosis to the subsequent end point in mitosis in one daughter cell or both. G_1 is the postmitotic phase during which RNA and protein synthesis is increased and cell growth occurs. G_0 is the resting or dormant phase of the cell cycle. The S phase represents synthesis of nucleic acids with chromosome replication in preparation for cell mitosis. During G_2, RNA and protein synthesis occurs as in G_1.*

G_0 is the resting or dormant phase in which the cell performs all activities except those related to proliferation. Cells can leave G_1 and enter G_0. The time spent in G_0 varies according to the cell type, and not all cells spend time in G_0. It is believed that some special growth signal is needed to move cells that have been dormant in G_0 back into the cell cycle.

During the S phase, or synthesis phase, DNA replication occurs, giving rise to two separate sets of chromosomes. G_2 is the premitotic phase. During this phase, as in G_1, DNA synthesis ceases while synthesis of RNA and protein continues.

The M phase represents mitosis. Mitosis is subdivided into four stages: prophase, metaphase, anaphase, and telophase (Fig. 5-3). During *prophase,* the centrioles in the cytoplasm separate and move toward opposite sides of the cell, the chromosomes become shorter and thicker, and the nuclear membrane breaks up so that there is no longer a barrier between the chromosomes and the cytoplasm. *Metaphase* involves the organization of the chromosome pairs in the midline of the cell and the formation of a mitotic spindle composed of the microtubules. *Anaphase* is the period during which splitting of the chromosome pairs occurs, with the microtubules pulling each set of 46 chromosomes toward the opposite cell pole in preparation for cell separation. Cell division is completed during *telophase,*

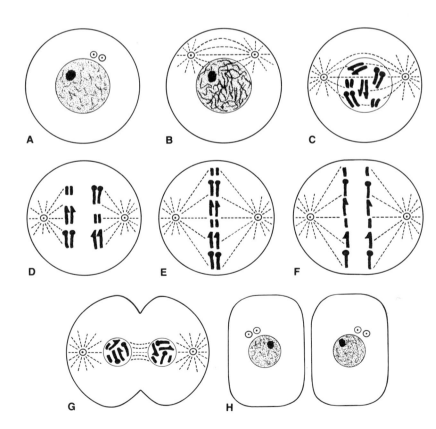

Figure 5-3 *Cell mitosis. A and H represent the nondividing cell; B, C, and D represent prophase; E represents metaphase; F represents anaphase; and G represents telophase. (Chaffee EE, Greisheimer EM: Basic Physiology and Anatomy, 3rd ed. Philadelphia, JB Lippincott, 1974)*

when the mitotic spindles vanish and a new nuclear membrane develops and encloses each of the sets of chromosomes.

Cell Replication

In normal tissue, cell proliferation is regulated, so that the number of cells dividing is equivalent to the number dying or being shed. In terms of cell proliferation, the 100 or more cell types can be divided into two large groups: (1) the well-differentiated neurons and cells of skeletal and cardiac muscle that are unable to divide and reproduce, and (2) the cells that continue to divide and reproduce, such as blood cells, skin cells, and liver cells. The rates of reproduction of these cells vary greatly. White blood cells and the cells that line the gastrointestinal tract live several days and must be replaced constantly. In most tissues, the rate of cell reproduction is greatly increased when tissue is injured or lost. Bleeding, for example, stimulates the rapid reproduction of the blood-forming cells of the bone marrow. Also included in this second group are cells in which reproduction is normally suspended but can be resumed under certain conditions. The liver, for example, has extensive regenerative capabilities under the right conditions.

For very rapidly reproducing cells, the entire cell cycle occupies about 16 hours. For others, such as liver cells, the cycle takes about 400 hours. The durations of the G_2 period (8 hours), S period (2 hours), and mitosis (0.07 hour) are almost identical for all cell types. It is the duration of G_1 and G_0 that determines the duration of the cell cycle.[2] When only a low rate of cell reproduction is needed to maintain the health of tissues, the cells remain dormant in the G_0 phase of G_1; when a more rapid rate of reproduction is needed, the G_0 dormant period is shortened.

Cell Differentiation

Cell differentiation is the process whereby cells are transformed into different and more specialized cell types. The 100 or more cell types in the body are differentiated from a single fertilized ovum. The puzzle of differentiation is that all of the body's cells carry the same information, but only a part of that information is expressed in each differentiated cell type. Differentiation determines what a cell will look like, how it will function, and how long it will live. For example, a red blood cell is programmed to develop as a concave disk that functions as a vehicle for oxygen transport and lives 120 days.

In prenatal and postnatal life, the rates of cell reproduction and differentiation are precisely controlled so that both of these mechanisms cease once the appropriate numbers and kinds of cells are formed and differ-

entiated. As a cell type becomes more specialized, it loses its ability to reproduce. Neurons, which are the most highly specialized cells in the body, lose their ability to divide and reproduce once development of the nervous system is complete. In other tissues with less specialized function, such as skin, blood-forming bone marrow, and the mucosal lining of the gastrointestinal tract, cells continue to reproduce and differentiate throughout life.

Oncogenesis

Cancer cells have two important properties that underlie the nature of the disease: (1) they grow and divide with less restraint than normal cells and (2) they do not differentiate normally. Therefore, they do not function properly and do not die on time. In some types of leukemia, for example, the lymphocytes do not follow the normal developmental process: they do not differentiate fully, they do not acquire the ability to destroy bacteria, and they do not die on schedule. Instead, these long-lived defective cells persist and crowd out normal blood cells, leaving the body less able to defend itself during infection.

In tissues capable of regeneration, new cells derive from undifferentiated reserve cells called stem cells. When a stem cell divides, one daughter cell retains its characteristics. The other daughter cell undergoes multiple mitotic divisions, with each generation of cells becoming more specialized (Fig. 5-4). All of the progeny of each differentiating cell continue along the same genetic program. In this way a single stem cell can give rise to the many cells that are needed for normal tissue repair. When these cells become fully differentiated, they are functional and no longer divide. It is thought that cancer cells develop from mutations that occur during the differentiation process. When the mutation occurs early in the process, the resulting tumor is poorly differentiated and highly malignant. On the other hand, mutations occurring later in the differentiation process give rise to more fully differentiated and less malignant tumors.[2]

In summary, the life of a cell is called the cell cycle. It is divided into five phases: (1) G_1 represents the postmitotic phase during which RNA and protein synthesis occurs; (2) G_2 is the resting or dormant phase of the cell cycle; (3) the S phase is the synthesis phase during which DNA replication occurs; (4) G_2 is the premitotic phase and is similar to G_1 in terms of RNA and protein synthesis; (5) the M phase is the phase during which cell mitosis occurs. Cell proliferation is normally regulated so that the number of cells actively dividing is equal to the number dying or being shed. Stem cells are undifferentiated reserve cells that are

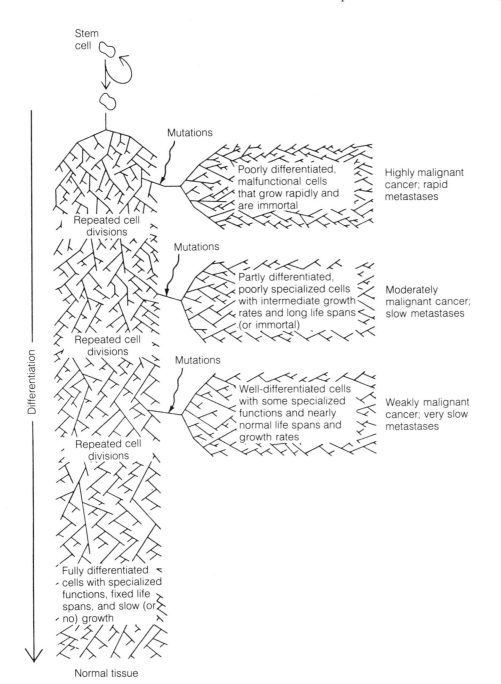

Figure 5-4 *Mutation of a cancer cell line. (Prescott DM, Flexer AS: Cancer, the misguided cell. Sunderland MA, Sinauer Assoc, 1982)*

found in tissues capable of regeneration. Differentiation is the process whereby these stem cells are transformed into a more specialized cell type. Differentiation determines the structure, function, and life span of a cell. As a cell line becomes more differentiated, it becomes more highly specialized in its function and less able to divide. It is thought that cancer cell lines develop from a mutation that occurs during the differentiation process and that cancers developing from mutations occurring early in the differentiation process are more malignant than those that develop from mutations occurring later in the process.

■ Terminology

The term *neoplasm* comes from the Greek word meaning *new formation*. In contrast to tissue growth that occurs with hypertrophy and hyperplasia, a neoplasm serves no useful purpose but tends to increase in size and persist at the expense of the rest of the body. Furthermore, neoplasms do not obey the laws of normal tissue growth. For example, they do not occur in response to an appropriate stimulus, and they continue to grow after the stimulus has ceased or the needs of the organism have been met.

A *tumor* is a swelling that can be caused by a number of conditions, including inflammation and trauma. Although the terms are not synonymous, a neoplasm is often referred to as a tumor. The Latin word *malus* means bad; hence a *malignant tumor* is a "bad" tumor that will cause death if it is not controlled. A *benign tumor* is a "good" tumor—it usually will not cause death unless by its location it interferes with vital functions.

Tumors are usually identified by the addition of the suffix *-oma* to the name of the tissue type from which the growth originated. Thus, a benign tumor of glandular epithelial tissue is called an adenoma, and a benign tumor of bone tissue, an osteoma. If the tumor is malignant, the word *carcinoma* is used with the *epithelial tissue* origin of the tumor; for example, in the case of an adenoma that has become cancerous, the term adenocarcinoma is used. Malignant tumors of *mesenchymal origin* are called *sarcomas,* for example, osteosarcoma. Oncology is the study of tumors and their treatment. Table 5-1 lists the names of selected benign and malignant tumors according to their tissue type. The significance of the system of naming and classifying tumors is that it facilitates communication among researchers and health professionals.

In summary, the term *neoplasm* refers to a new growth. In contrast to normal cellular adaptive processes such as hypertrophy and hyperplasia, neoplasms do not obey the laws of normal cell growth. They serve no useful purpose, they do not occur in response to an appropriate stimulus, and they continue to grow at the expense of the host. Neoplasms may be either benign or malignant. The growth of a benign tumor is restricted to the site of origin and will not cause death unless it interferes with vital functions. Cancer or malignant neoplasms, on the other hand, grow wildly and without organization, spread to distant parts of the body, and cause death unless checked. Tumors are named by the addition of the suffix *-oma* to the name of the tissue type. The term carcinoma refers to a malignant tumor of epithelial cell origin and the term sarcoma to a malignant tumor of mesenchymal cell origin.

■ Characteristics of Neoplasms

Benign versus Malignant Neoplasms

Benign and malignant neoplasms are generally differentiated by their (1) cell characteristics, (2) manner of growth, (3) rate of growth, (4) potential for metastasizing and spreading to other parts of the body, (5) tendency to recur once they have been removed, (6) ability to produce generalized effects, (7) tendency to cause tissue destruction, and (8) capacity to cause death. The characteristics of benign and malignant neoplasms are summarized in Table 5-2.

Benign tumors consist of well-differentiated, mature tissue types. For example, the cells of a uterine leiomyoma resemble uterine smooth muscle. The slow expansive growth of a benign tumor produces pressure on the surrounding tissues leading to formation of a fibrous capsule. Figure 5-5 shows a benign encapsulated tumor. The formation of the capsule is thought to represent the reaction of the surrounding tissues to the tumor. The presence of the capsule is responsible for a sharp line of demarcation between the benign tumor mass and the adjacent tissues, so that benign tumors are usually enucleated more easily than malignant tumors. A benign tumor once removed is not likely to recur.

Benign tumors do not usually undergo degenerative changes as readily as malignant tumors and they do not usually cause death unless by their location they interfere with vital functions. For instance, a benign tumor growing in the cranial cavity can eventually lead to death by compressing the brain. Benign tumors can also cause disturbances in the function of adjacent or distant structures by producing pressure on tissues, blood vessels, or nerves.

Some benign tumors are also known for their ability to cause alterations in body function due to abnormal elaboration of hormones. Examples of hormone-secreting benign tumors are the pheochromocytomas, which produce adrenalin, and parathyroid tumors, which elaborate excessive parathyroid hormone.

In contrast to benign tumors, malignant neoplasms tend to grow more rapidly, spread widely, and kill regardless of their original location. The destructive nature of malignant tumors is related to changes in their rate of growth, lack of cell differentiation, and ability to spread and metastasize. Their malignant potential usually depends on their degree of anaplasia. Because they grow rapidly, they rob normal cells of large quantities of essential amino acids and other nutrients. This rapid growth may also cause compression of blood vessels as well as thrombosis; the tumors outgrow their blood supply, liberating toxins that destroy both tumorous and normal tissue. The end result may be ischemia, degeneration, ulceration, and tissue necrosis. The generalized effects of these changes on body function are discussed later in this chapter.

There are two major categories of cancer—solid tumors and hematologic cancers. *Solid tumors* initially are confined to a specific tissue or organ. The cells shed from the original tumor mass travel through the blood and lymph stream. *Hematologic cancers* involve the blood and lymph systems and are disseminated diseases from the beginning.

Table 5-1   Names of Selected Benign and Malignant Tumors According to Tissue Types

Tissue Type	Benign	Malignant
Epithelial Tumors		
Surface	Papilloma	Squamous cell carcinoma
Glandular	Adenoma	Adenocarcinoma
Connective Tissue Tumors		
Fibrous	Fibroma	Fibrosarcoma
Adipose	Lipoma	Liposarcoma
Cartilage	Chondroma	Chondrosarcoma
Bone	Osteoma	Osteosarcoma
Blood vessels	Hemangioma	Hemangiosarcoma
Lymph vessels	Lymphangioma	Lymphangiosarcoma
Muscle Tumors		
Smooth	Leiomyoma	Leiomyosarcoma
Striated	Rhabdomyoma	Rhabdomyosarcoma
Nerve Cell Tumors		
Nerve cell	Neuroma	
Glial tissue		Glioma
Nerve sheaths	Neurilemmoma	Neurilemic sarcoma
Hematologic Tumors		
Granulocytic		Myelocytic leukemia
Erythrocytic		Erythroleukemia
Plasma cells		Multiple myeloma
Lymphoid		Lymphocytic leukemia

Table 5-2   Characteristics of Benign and Malignant Neoplasms

Characteristics	Benign	Malignant
Cell characteristics	Cells resemble normal cells of the tissue from which the tumor originated	Cells often bear little resemblance to the normal cells of the tissue from which they arose; there is both anaplasia and pleomorphism
Mode of growth	Tumor grows by expansion and does not infiltrate the surrounding tissues; encapsulated	Grows at the periphery and sends out processes that infiltrate and destroy the surrounding tissues
Rate of growth	Rate of growth is usually slow	Rate of growth is usually relatively rapid and is dependent on level of differentiation; the more anaplastic the tumor, the more rapid the rate of growth
Metastasis	Does not spread by metastasis	Gains access to the blood and lymph channels and metastasizes to other areas of the body
Recurrence	Does not recur when removed	Tends to recur when removed
General effects	Is usually a localized phenomenon that does not cause generalized effects unless its location interferes with vital functions	Often causes generalized effects such as anemia, weakness, and weight loss
Destruction of tissue	Does not usually cause tissue damage unless its location interferes with blood flow	Often causes extensive tissue damage as the tumor outgrows its blood supply or encroaches on blood flow to the area; may also produce substances that cause cell damage
Ability to cause death	Does not usually cause death unless its location interferes with vital functions	Will usually cause death unless growth can be controlled

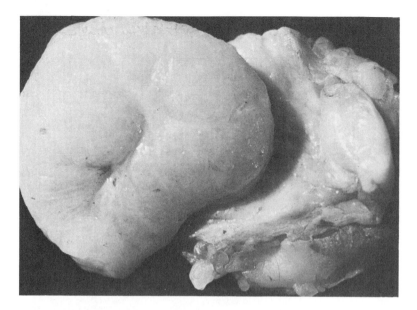

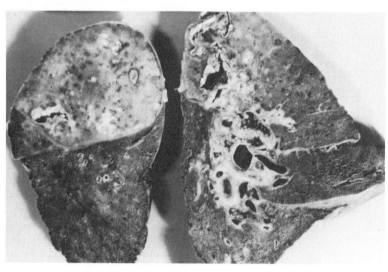

Figure 5-5 *Photograph of a benign encapsuled fibroadenoma of the breast at the top and a bronchogenic carcinoma of the lung at the bottom. Note that the fibroadenoma has sharply defined edges, whereas the bronchogenic carcinoma is diffuse and infiltrates the surrounding tissues.*

Cancer Cell Characteristics

Cancer cells have distinct characteristics that differentiate them from normal cells. These include anaplasia, cell membrane changes, antigenic changes, biochemical changes, and changes in the karyotype.

Anaplasia

In cancerous tissue, the term *differentiation* refers to the extent to which tumor cells resemble the cells of origin and the extent to which they achieve their mature structural and functional characteristics. The term *anaplasia* is used to describe the lack of cell differentiation in cancerous tissue. The process of malignant transformation results in phenotypic changes in cell structure and function that are passed on to all the progeny of the transformed cell line. Cancer cells lack differentiation; they are

altered in appearance, and the size and shape of their nuclei often differ from the tissue cells from which they originated. For example, when examined under the microscope, cancerous tissue that originated in the liver does not have the appearance of normal liver tissue. The degree of anaplasia that a tumor displays varies. Some cancers display only slight anaplasia and others display marked anaplasia. As a general rule, the more undifferentiated the tumor, the more frequent the mitosis and the more rapid the rate of growth. The degree of anaplasia can be determined by a pathologist during tissue studies and is used in the grading of tumors.

Changes in karyotype

Changes in karyotype, or organization of cell chromosomes, can be observed in many cancer cells. Mitosis, in normal cells, yields two identical cells, each with a normal arrangement of chromosomes. In *diploid* cells there is a double set of chromosomes, which, when they divide, form two identical cells. *Polyploidy* is cell division that results in more than two cells. *Aneuploidy* refers to abnormal cell division in which daughter cells receive uneven numbers of chromosomes; one cell may receive 47 chromosomes and another 45. Cancerous tumors often undergo abnormal mitosis and display polyploidy or aneuploidy. These cells often have multiple spindles that result in uneven division of nuclear or cellular contents. The term *pleomorphism* refers to variations in size and shape of cells and cell nuclei.

Membrane changes

In addition to changes in cell growth and differentiation, cancer cells display alteration in surface characteristics related to the cell membrane. These changes include alterations in contact inhibition, cohesiveness, and adhesion; failure to form intercellular connections; and impaired cell-to-cell communication. Contact inhibition is the cessation of growth after a cell comes in contact with another cell. Contact inhibition usually switches off cell growth by blocking RNA and protein synthesis and by blocking DNA synthesis. In wound healing, contact inhibition causes fibrous tissue growth to cease at the point where the edges of the wound come together. Cancer cells, on the other hand, tend to grow rampant without regard for other tissue. Although many of the membrane changes that have been reported for cancer cells have been observed with individual cancer cells in the laboratory, there is reason to believe that these same properties exist in cancer cells in the body, and these changes account for the invasive and destructive nature of cancer cell growth. Changes also occur in the membrane transport of sugars and amino acids by tumor cells. Cancer cells have been called *nitrogen traps* because they tend to rob normal cells of amino acids.

Changes in cell antigens

Many transformed cells produce antigens that are immunologically distinct from normal cell antigens. Possibly it is these antigens that are recognized as foreign by the body's immune system, contributing to the body's defense against the survival of abnormal cell types and the development of cancer. *Fetal antigens* are expressed during intrauterine and early postnatal life that are normally completely repressed in the mature organism. *Serum alpha-fetoprotein* is one such antigen; it can be identified in the plasma of adults with primary liver cell cancer or teratoid cancers of the ovary or testes. *Carcinoembryonic antigen,* another embryonic antigen, can be found in the plasma of adults with endodermally derived cancers of the liver, pancreas, stomach, and lungs.[3] The reappearance of fetal antigens in certain types of cancers represents the undifferentiated nature of these tumors and is thought to result from the expression or enhanced activation of genes coded for these antigens. The presence of these antigens, which can be detected through laboratory studies, is useful in the diagnosis and follow-up treatment of these neoplasms.

Biochemical changes

A number of changes in biochemical behavior are associated with cancer cells; many resemble those associated with the rapid growth of fetal and immature cells. Most cancers elaborate enzymes (proteases and glycosidases) that break down proteins and contribute to the invasiveness of the tumor. Some tumors are transformed into cells that elaborate hormones. For example, some forms of bronchiogenic carcinoma produce antidiuretic hormone (ADH) and adrenocorticotropic hormone (ACTH). As with neoantigens, the biochemical changes displayed by cancer cells are attributed to the expression of genes that are not normally repressed.

Tumor Growth and Spread

The rate of tissue growth in both normal and cancerous tissue depends on three factors: (1) the number of cells actively dividing or moving through the cell cycle, (2) the cell-cycle time, and (3) the number of cells being lost. One of the reasons that cancerous tumors often seem to grow so rapidly is the size of the cell pool that is actively engaged in cycling. It has been shown that the cell-cycle time of cancerous tissue cells is not necessarily shorter than that of normal cells, but rather that cancer cells do not die on schedule. In addition, the growth factors that allow cells to enter G_0 when they are not needed for cell replacement is lacking; therefore, a greater percentage of cells are actively engaged in cycling than in normal tissue.[4]

The ratio of dividing cells to resting cells in a tissue mass is called the *growth factor*. The *doubling time* is the length of time it takes for the total mass of cells in a tumor to double. As the growth factor increases, the doubling time decreases. When normal tissues reach their adult size, an equilibrium between cell birth and cell death is reached. Cancer cells, however, continue to divide and multiply until limitations in blood supply and nutrients retard their growth. As this happens, the doubling time for cancer cells increases.

Experimentally, it is possible to measure the cell-cycle time and the percentage of cells that are cycling during a given period of time and then to estimate the doubling time. From this information, one can then estimate the rate of cell increase per hour for the different types of tumors. Knowledge of cell-cycle time and the rate of cell increase is used in planning cancer therapy.

For example, cancer therapy is most effective during the earlier stages of neoplastic growth when the cells are rapidly dividing and the growth factor is increased.

A tumor is generally undetectable until it has doubled 30 times and contains more than a billion (1×10^9) cells. At this point, it is about 1 cm in size (Fig. 5-6). After 35 doublings the mass contains more than a trillion (1×10^{12}) cells, which may be sufficient to kill the host.

Cancer in situ is a localized preinvasive lesion. Depending on its location, this type of lesion can usually be removed surgically or treated so that the chances of recurrence are small. For example, cancer *in situ* of the cervix is essentially 100% curable.

The spread of cancer can take many forms: direct extension, seeding of cancer cells to adjacent structures, or metastatic spread through the blood or lymph pathways. Growth usually occurs at the tumor periphery with direct extension to or invasion of the surrounding tissue. The word *cancer* is derived from the Latin word meaning crablike, because cancerous growth spreads by sending crablike projections into the surrounding tissues. Unlike benign tumors, which are encapsulated, malignant tumors have no sharp line of demarcation separating them from the surrounding tissue, and this often makes complete surgical removal of the tumor difficult. *Seeding* of cancer cells into body cavities occurs when a tumor erodes into these spaces and tumor cells drop onto the serosal surface. For example, a tumor may penetrate the wall of the stomach and its cells implant on the surfaces of the peritoneal cavity.

Metastatic spread occurs when a malignant tumor invades the vascular or lymphatic channels, and parts of the tumor break loose and travel to distant parts of the body where implantation occurs. When metastasis occurs by way of the lymphatic channels, the tumor cells lodge, first, in the regional lymph nodes that receive their drainage from the tumor site. The regional lymph nodes may contain the tumor cells for a time, but eventually the cells break loose and gain access to more distant nodes and to the bloodstream by way of the thoracic duct. The *lungs* and the *liver* are common sites for secondary growth when a cancer gains access to the venous system. The venous blood from the gastrointestinal tract, the pancreas, and the spleen is routed to the liver through the portal vein before it enters the general circulation. The liver is therefore a common site of metastatic growth for cancers that originate in these organs. Likewise, venous blood from all parts of the body must travel through the lungs before they move to the arterial side of the circulation. On the other hand, the *bone* and the *brain* are common sites of metastasis when cancer cells enter the arterial circulation. This is particularly true of lung cancer; cells from these tumors move directly into the left heart, then out into the systemic circulation.

To a great extent, metastatic tumors retain many of the characteristics of the primary tumor from which they

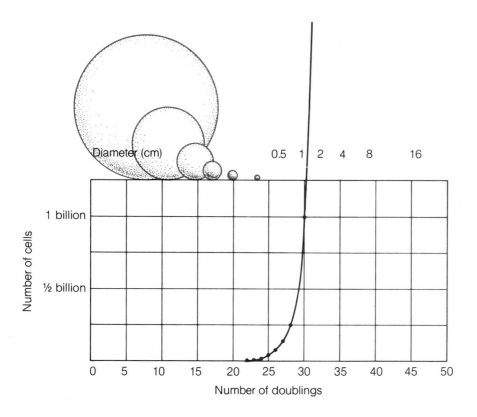

Figure 5-6 *Growth curve of a hypothetical tumor on arithmetic coordinates. Note the number of doubling times before the tumor reaches an appreciable size. (Collins VP et al: Observations of growth rates of human tumors. Am J Roent Rad Ther Nuclear Med 76:988, 1956. Charles C Thomas, Publisher)*

had their origin. Because of this, it is possible in some cases to discover an unsuspected malignancy before the original primary tumor begins to produce symptoms. Some tumors tend to metastasize early in their course, whereas others do not metastasize until late. Occasionally, the metastatic tumor will be far advanced before the primary tumor becomes clinically detectable. Malignant tumors of the kidney, for example, may go completely undetected and be asymptomatic even when a metastasis is found in the lung.

General Effects

There probably is not a single body function that is not affected by the presence of cancer. Table 5-3 summarizes the general associated effects of cancer. Because tumor cells replace normal parenchymal tissue, the primary area involved will manifest the cancer's effects. For example, cancer of the lung impairs respiratory function; then, as the tumor grows and metastasizes, other structures are affected. Metastasis to bone causes bone pain and predisposes the bones to fractures. (Pain, which is common to practically all types of cancer, is discussed in Chap. 49.)

Cancer disrupts tissue integrity. As the tumor grows, it compresses and erodes blood vessels, causing ulceration and necrosis along with frank bleeding and hemorrhage. For example, one early warning sign of cancer of the bowel is blood in the stool. The cancer cells may also produce toxins that are destructive to cells in surrounding tissues and further disrupt tissue integrity. Tissue that has been damaged by cancerous growth does not heal normally. The damaged area usually continues

to increase in size, hence the second warning signal—a sore that will not heal.

Cancer has no regard for normal anatomic boundaries—as it grows, it invades and compresses adjacent structures. Abdominal cancer, for example, compresses the viscera and causes bowel obstruction. When cancer affects the brain, it may interfere with the flow of cerebral spinal fluid as well as other cerebral functions. Cancer can penetrate serous cavities, obstructing lymph flow and causing effusion, such as pleural effusion and ascites.

Because of its undifferentiated nature, cancerous tissue often behaves differently from the normal tissue type. For example, bronchiogenic carcinoma may elaborate (ADH), parathyroid hormone (PTH), ACTH, or other substances that have hormonelike actions. The tumor may also produce coagulation factors—which is one reason that cancer patients frequently develop venous thrombosis. Robbins uses the phrase *paraneoplastic* syndrome to describe symptoms—such as hyponatremia due to excessive levels of ADH—that cannot be explained by either local or distant spread of the disease or by the elaboration of hormones normally produced by tissue from which the tumor arose. Paraneoplastic syndromes are thought to occur in about 15% of persons with advanced malignant disease.[3]

In summary, benign and malignant tumors differ in the following characteristics: (1) cell characteristics, (2) manner of growth, (3) rate of growth, (4) potential for metastasis, (5) tendency to recur, (6) ability to produce generalized effects, (7) tendency to cause tissue destruction, and (8) capacity to cause death. Malignant neo-

Table 5-3   General Effects on Body Function Associated with Cancer Growth

Overall Effect	Related Tumor Action
Altered function of the involved tissue	Destruction and replacement of parenchymal tissue by neoplastic growth
Bleeding and hemorrhage	Compression of blood vessels, with ischemia and necrosis of tissue; or tumor may outgrow its blood supply
Obstruction of hollow viscera or communication pathways	Expansive growth of tumor with compression and invasion of tissues
Effusion in serous cavities	Impaired lymph flow from the serous cavity or erosion of tumor into the cavity
Inappropriate hormone production, *e.g.,* ADH or ACTH secretion by cancers such as bronchiogenic carcinoma	Production by the tumor of hormones or hormonelike substances that are not regulated by normal feedback mechanisms
Ulceration, necrosis, and infection of tumor area	Ischemia associated with rapid growth, with subsequent bacterial invasion
Increased risk of vascular thrombosis	Abnormal production of coagulation factors by the tumor, obstruction of venous channels, and immobility
Anemia	Bleeding and depression of red blood cell production
Bone destruction	Metastatic invasion of bony structures
Hypercalcemia	Destruction of bone due to metastasis and/or production by the tumor of parathyroid hormone or parathyroidlike hormone
Pain	Liberation of pain mediators by the tumor, compression, and/or ischemia of structures
Cachexia, weakness, wasting of tissues	Catabolic effect of the tumor on body metabolism along with selective trapping of nutrients by rapidly growing tumor cells

plasms grow more rapidly, metastasize and spread widely throughout the body, disrupt body functions, and kill regardless of their location. Cancer cells are often poorly differentiated in comparison with normal cells; they display abnormal membrane characteristics, have abnormal antigens, produce abnormal biochemical products, and have abnormal karyotypes.

Staging and Grading of Tumors

At present, there are two basic methods for classifying cancers: (1) grading according to the histologic or cellular characteristics of the tumor and (2) staging according to the spread of the disease. Both methods are used to prognosticate the course of the disease and to aid in selecting an appropriate treatment or management plan. The clinical staging is intended to provide a means by which information related to the progress of the disease, the methods and success of treatment modalities, and the prognosis can be communicated to others. The TNM system, which has evolved from the work of the International Union Against Cancer (IUCC) and the American Joint Committee on Cancer Staging and End Stage Reporting (AJCCS), is used by many cancer facilities. This system, which is briefly described in Table 5-4, quantifies the disease into stages, using three tumor components: (1) T stands for the extent of the primary

tumor, (2) N refers to the involvement of the regional lymph nodes, and (3) M describes the extent of the metastatic involvement. The TNM system further defines each specific type of cancer, such as breast cancer. The rationale for use of the system encompasses the need to classify the disease at various time periods—initial diagnosis, presurgical treatment, postsurgical treatment, and so on.

In summary, there are two basic methods of classifying tumors: (1) grading according to the histologic or tissue characteristics and (2) clinical staging according to the spread of the disease. Histologic studies are done in the laboratory using cells or tissue specimens. The TMN system for clinical staging of cancer uses tumor size, lymph node spread, and presence of metastasis.

Carcinogenesis

Because cancer is thought not to be a single disease, it is reasonable to assume that it does not have a single cause. More likely, cancer occurs because of interaction between multiple risk factors or repeated exposure to a single carcinogenic agent. Among the factors that have been linked with the development of cancer are heredity, chemical and environmental carcinogens, cancer-causing viruses, immunologic defects, and precancerous lesions.

Heredity

Certain types of cancers seem to run in families. Breast cancer, for example, occurs more frequently in women whose grandmothers, mothers, aunts, and sisters also have had a cancerous disease. Cancer is found in approximately 10% of persons having one affected first-degree relative, in approximately 15% of persons having two affected family members, and in 30% of persons having three affected family members.[5]

The genetic predisposition for development of cancer has been documented for a number of cancerous and precancerous lesions that are transmitted by mendelian inheritance (Table 5-5). Fortunately, most of these neoplasms are extremely rare—probably accounting for less than 5% of the cancers that occur in the general population.[3]

Among the inherited forms of cancer are retinoblastoma and multiple polyposis of the colon. In about 40% of cases, retinoblastoma (a form of eye cancer that occurs most frequently in small children) is inherited as an autosomal dominant trait. The penetrance of the genetic trait is high, as evidenced by the fact that the risk of developing the disease is increased 100,000 times

---

Table 5-4 TNM Classification System

T* subclasses
  Tx—tumor cannot be adequately assessed
  T0—no evidence of primary tumor
  TIS—carcinoma *in situ*
  T1, T2, T3, T4—progressive increase in tumor size and
    involvement
N† Nx—regional lymph nodes cannot be assessed clinically
  N0—regional lymph nodes demonstrably abnormal
  N1, N2, N3, N4—increasing degrees of demonstrable
    abnormality of regional lymph nodes
M‡ subclasses
  Mx—not assessed
  M0—no (known) distant metastasis
  M1—distant metastasis present, specify site(s)
Histopathology
  G1—well-differentiated grade
  G-2—moderately well-differentiated grade
  G3, G4—poorly to very poorly differentiated grade

*T = Primary tumor.
†N = Regional lymph nodes.
‡M = Distant metastasis.
(American Joint Committee on Cancer: Manual for Staging of Cancer. Chicago, American Joint Committee, 1977)

Table 5-5 Some Cancers and Cancer Predisposing Diseases with Mendelian Inheritance Patterns

Dominant (Autosomal)	Recessive (Autosomal)
Adenocarcinoma (primarily colon and endometrium)	Albinism
Familial polyposis of colon	Ataxia telangiectasia
Gardner's syndrome (predisposes to colonic cancer)	Bloom's syndrome
Melanocarcinoma	Franconi's aplastic anemia
Multiple endocrine adenomatosis (MEA)	Xeroderma pigmentosum
Neurofibromatosis (von Recklinghausen's disease)	
Retinoblastoma	

(Modified from Robbins SL, Cotran R.S.: Pathologic Basis of Disease, 2nd ed. Philadelphia, WB Saunders, 1979. Fagan-Dubin L: Causes of cancer. Cancer Nurs 2(:6):436, 1979. Copyright © by Masson Publishing USA, Inc., New York.)

when the gene is present from an occurrence rate of 1 in 30,000 in the general population.[6] Familial polyposis of the colon is another example of an autosomal dominant inheritance pattern. Individuals who inherit the gene develop polypoid adenomas of the colon, and almost all are fated to develop cancer by age 50.[3]

Carcinogens

A carcinogen is an agent capable of causing cancer. The role of environmental agents in causation of cancer was first noted in 1775 by Sir Percivall Pott, who related the high incidence of scrotal cancer in chimney sweeps to their exposure to coal soot. In 1915, Yamagiwa and Ichikawa conducted the first experiments in which a chemical agent was used to produce cancer. These investigators found that a cancerous growth developed when they painted a rabbit's ear with coal tar. Coal tar has since been found to contain potent polycyclic aromatic hydrocarbons. Since then, literally hundreds of carcinogenic agents have been identified. In fact, it has been estimated that 80% to 85% of human cancers are associated with exposure to environmental or chemical agents (Table 5-6).[7]

Chemical carcinogens

Literally hundreds of chemical carcinogenic agents exist; some have been found to cause cancers in animals and others are known to cause cancers in humans. These agents include both natural (*e.g.*, aflatoxin B_1) and manmade products (*e.g.*, vinyl chloride). Usually, carcinogenic agents can be divided into two categories: (1)

direct-acting agents and (2) procarcinogens, which are metabolized and converted into carcinogenic agents in the body. Direct-acting agents do not require activation in the body to become carcinogenic. These agents include the alkylating drugs that are used in the treatment of cancer (to be discussed). Procarcinogens, which include the polycyclic hydrocarbons and the azo dyes, are the most potent carcinogens known.[3] With the procarcinogens, cancer usually develops in the organ where the agent is metabolized or stored for elimination, for example, in the bladder in persons exposed to aniline dyes.

Chemical carcinogens form highly reactive ions (electrophiles) that bind with the nucleophilic residues on DNA, RNA, or cellular proteins. The action of these ions tends to cause cell mutation or alteration in synthesis of cell enzymes and structural proteins in a manner that alters cell replication and interferes with cell regulatory controls.

The effects of carcinogenic agents are usually dose dependent—the larger the dose or the longer the duration of exposure, the greater the risk that cancer will develop. There is usually a time delay ranging from 5 to 30 years from the time of exposure to the development of cancer. This is unfortunate, because many persons may have been exposed to the agent and its carcinogenic effects before the association is recognized. This occurred, for example, with the use of diethylstilbestrol, which was widely used in the United States from the mid-1940s to 1970 to prevent miscarriages. But it was

Table 5-6 Some Chemical and Environmental Agents Known to Be Carcinogenic in Humans

Polycyclic Hydrocarbons
Soots, tars, and oils
Cigarette smoke
Industrial Agents
Asbestos
Vinyl chloride
Arsenic compounds
Aniline and azo dyes
Nickel and chromium compounds
Acrylonitrile
a-Naphthylamine
b-Naphthylamine
Benzene
Carbon tetrachloride
Food and Drugs
Smoked foods
Nitrosamines (used in preservation of meats)
Aflatoxin B_1 (mold that grows in nuts and grains)
Phenacetin
Diethylstilbestrol
Estrogens

not until the late 1960s that many cases of vaginal adenosis and adenocarcinoma in young women were found to be a result of their exposure *in utero* to diethylstilbestrol.[8]

Two occupational carcinogens of particular interest are *asbestos* and *vinyl chloride*.[9] Although the history of asbestos disease dates back to the early 1900s, it was not until the late 1960s that the full spectrum of the problem became evident. Exposure to asbestos is associated with cancer of the lung, cancer of the stomach, and a rare form of malignancy (mesothelioma) that affects the pleura and peritoneum. The population groups at increased risk of developing cancer due to asbestos exposure include not only those persons who work directly with the mineral, but also those who live in the vicinity of industrial installations where asbestos is used in one way or another and persons who live in the same household as the asbestos worker. The risk of cancer in these groups is increased even further if they also smoke cigarettes, which points to an additive effect. Until 1973 (when its use was banned), asbestos was frequently used as a fireproofing spray in many high-rise buildings. There is now concern that the air circulating through some buildings in which a dry type of asbestos fireproofing was applied may be contaminated with asbestos fibers. There is also concern about how exposure to asbestos can be controlled when these buildings need to be demolished.

Vinyl chloride, which is used in the rubber industry, is associated with hemangiosarcoma of the liver. As with many other carcinogenic agents, the relationship between vinyl chloride exposure and the development of cancer was not discovered until a large number of workers had been exposed to the chemical. In 1974, the U.S. Department of Labor established regulations for vinyl chloride exposure in industry.

Radiation

Among the well-documented causes of cancer is radiation, including ultraviolet rays from sunlight, x-rays, radioactive chemicals, and other forms of radiation. As with other carcinogens, the effects of radiation are usually additive, and there is usually a long delay between the time of exposure and the time that cancer can be detected. This is true of skin cancer, which is caused by overexposure to the sun and is many years in the making. Skin cancer is an occupational hazard of farmers and sailors, particularly those who work in the southwest United States. Equally hazardous is the practice of sunbathing to achieve a suntan.

Another example of the ultimate consequences of radiation exposure is the therapeutic radiation of the head and neck—particularly in infants and small children—in which there may be a time lag as long as 35 years before thyroid cancer is detected.[10] Even more dramatic are the long-term effects of radiation on the survivors of the atomic blasts in Hiroshima and Nagasaki: between 1950 and 1970, the death rate from leukemia alone in the most heavily exposed population groups in Hiroshima was 147 per 100,000, or 30 times the expected rate.[11]

Viruses

A *virus* is a small particle containing genetic information (DNA and RNA) encased in a protein coat. When viruses enter a cell, called the host, they become incorporated into its chromosomal DNA or take control of the cell's machinery for the purpose of producing viral proteins. Thus, a virus has the potential for effecting a change in the cell's function, or it can insert information into the host cell's chromosomes and thereby alter future generations of cells. Viruses have been shown to produce cancer in animals. In 1908 Ellerman, Bong, and Rous were able to transmit leukemia to chickens through the use of cell-free filtrates of leukemic cells, thereby establishing the role of viral causation of fowl leukemia.[12] The question remains, however, whether or not viruses cause cancer in humans. The Epstein-Barr virus (a herpesvirus known to cause infectious mononucleosis) has been linked with Burkitt's lymphoma, which is endemic in certain areas of Africa. Herpesvirus type II has been associated with carcinoma of the uterine cervix and hepatitis B with hepatocellular carcinoma.[12]

Immunologic Defects

One characteristic of mutant and cancer cells is that they develop neoantigens that attach to the surface of the cell. Immune surveillance is the term often used to describe the mechanism whereby an organism develops an immune response against the antigens expressed by a tumor.[13] The role of the immune system in the destruction of a cancer cell is depicted in Figure 5-7.

It has been suggested that the development of cancer might be associated with impairment or decline in the surveillance capacity of the immune system. For example, increased incidence of cancer in persons with immunodeficiency diseases and in persons with renal transplants who are receiving immunosuppressant drugs has been observed. The incidence of cancer is also increased in the elderly, in whom there is a known decrease in immune activity. The recent association of Kaposi's sarcoma with acquired immune deficiency disease (AIDS) further emphasizes the role of the immune system in preventing malignant cell proliferation. Although seemingly simple, the role of immunity in the development of cancer is still largely uncertain. At present it cannot be said with any certainty that the immune system is able to

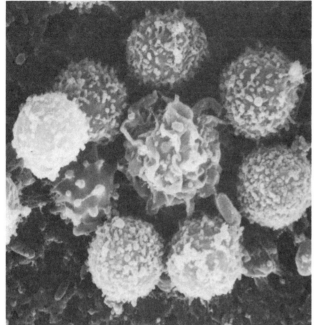

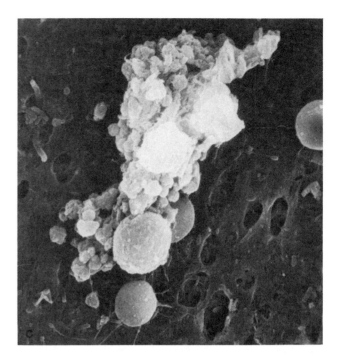

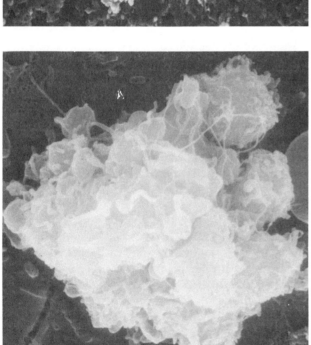

Figure 5-7 *A scanning electron micrograph showing the combination of a cancer cell and lymphocytes removed from the same patient and studied in the laboratory. Photo A shows the lymphocytes surrounding the cancer cell (60 min). Photo B shows the lymphocytes attacking the cancer cell (150 min). In Photo C, the integrity of the cancer cell has been destroyed (240 min). (Courtesy of Kenneth Siegesmund, Ph.D., and Burton A. Waisbren Sr., M.D. The Anatomy Department, The Medical College of Wisconsin.)*

effect protection against all forms of cancer. Many growing tumors appear to suppress the immune response. Furthermore, it is well recognized that some conventional types of cancer treatment—chemotherapy and radiation—tend to suppress the immune response. *Immunotherapy,* which will be discussed later in this chapter, is a cancer treatment modality designed to heighten the patient's general immune responses so as to increase tumor destruction.

Precancerous Lesions

Several types of lesions tend to undergo cancerous transformation. One of these, multiple polyposis of the colon, was described earlier; leukoplakia, a white, patchy lesion of the mucous membrane of the oral mucosa and the genitalia, is a second type of premalignant lesion. Others that may undergo cancerous transformation are fibrocystic disease of the breast, epithelial polyps of the colon, and burn scars.

In summary, the mechanisms involved in cancer development are many and complex. It is likely that cancer occurs because of interactions between multiple-risk factors such as heredity, chemical and environmental carcinogenic agents, cancer-causing viruses, immunologic defects, and precancerous lesions. It has been estimated that carcinogenic agents are involved in 80% to 85% of cancers, probably in association with other risk factors.

■ Diagnosis

Recent advances in technology provide a means whereby many forms of cancer may be successfully treated if discovered early. At present, three out of eight persons diagnosed as having cancer are alive 5 years later. It seems likely that the 5-year survival rate will be improved as people become aware of the early signs of cancer and seek medical attention at that time. One of the best examples of the success of treatment associated with early detection is cervical cancer, which is almost 100% curable if discovered in the *in situ* stage through the use of the Papanicolaou (Pap) test. The overall death rate from cancer of the uterus has decreased more than 70% during the last 40 years, due mainly to the Pap smear and regular checkups.[14]

Responsibility for early detection of cancer rests primarily with the individual. The American Cancer Society, in an effort to help people recognize the early signs of cancer, has developed the *seven warning signals of cancer* (Chart 5-1). Because delay in diagnosis and treatment can significantly alter the course of the disease and the success of treatment, it is suggested that persons who manifest any of these signals see their physician as soon as possible. The Society also recommends that *breast self-examination* and *testicular self-examination* be done regularly on a monthly basis.

The methods used in the diagnosis and staging of cancer are determined largely by the location and type of cancer suspected. A number of diagnostic procedures are used in the diagnosis of cancer, including x-ray studies; endoscopic examinations; blood, urine, and stool tests for blood; bone marrow aspirations; and computed tomography (CT scan). Two diagnostic methods will be discussed in this chapter, the Pap smear and tissue biopsy. The reader is referred to other sources of information regarding other diagnostic procedures.

The Pap smear is an example of the type of test called *exfoliative cytology*. It consists of microscopic examination of a properly prepared slide by a cytotechnologist or pathologist for the purpose of detecting the presence of abnormal cells. The usefulness of exfoliative cytology relies on the lack of the cohesive properties and inter-cellular junctions characteristic of normal tissue in the membranes of cancer cells, which makes them tend to exfoliate and become mixed with the secretions that surround the tumor growth. The routine performance of a Pap smear (once every 3 years after two initial negative tests 1 year apart) in women over age 20 years is recommended as a means of detecting *in situ* cervical cancer.[14] Exfoliative cytology can also be performed on other body secretions, including nipple drainage, pleural or peritoneal fluid, and gastric washings, among others.

A *biopsy* is the removal of a tissue specimen for microscopic study. It can be obtained by needle aspiration (needle biopsy) or by endoscopic methods such as bronchoscopy or cystoscopy, which involve the passage of a scope through an orifice and into the involved structure. In some instances a surgical incision is made. If the tumor is small, this permits the removal of the entire tumor; or if the tumor is too large to be removed, a specimen may be excised for examination. Tissue diagnosis is of critical importance in designing the treatment plan, should cancer cells be found.

In summary, the methods used in the diagnosis of cancer vary with the type of cancer that is present and its location. Because many cancers are curable if diagnosed early, health care practices designed to promote early detection are important. These practices include breast self-examination in the female, testicular self-examination in the male, and consulting a physician when any of the early warning signals of cancer are present. The Pap smear and tissue biopsy are used in detecting the presence of cancer cells and in diagnostic considerations.

■ Cancer Treatment

The goals of current treatment methods fall into three categories: *curative, palliative,* and *adjunctive.* The most common modalities are surgery, radiation, chemotherapy, and endocrinotherapy. In recent years, immunotherapy has been added to the list of treatment modalities. Interferon and hyperthermia are being used on an experimental basis. A current practice in the treatment of cancer is the use of a carefully planned program that combines the benefits of multiple treatment modalities and the expertise of a team of medical specialists such as a medical oncologist, surgical oncologist, and radiologist.

Surgery

Surgery is used for diagnosis, the staging of cancer, the removal of the tumor, and palliation (relief of symptoms) when cure cannot be effected. The type of surgery to be

---

Chart 5-1 Cancer's Seven Warning Signals

Change in bowel or bladder habits
A sore that does not heal
Unusual bleeding or discharge
Thickening or lump in the breast or elsewhere
Indigestion or difficulty swallowing
Obvious change in wart or mole
Nagging cough or hoarseness

---

used is determined by the extent of the disease and the structures involved. When the tumor is small, the total lesion can often be removed; when the tumor is large or involves vital tissues, surgical removal may be impossible.

Surgical techniques have been expanded to include electrosurgery, cryosurgery, chemosurgery, and laser surgery.[15] *Electrosurgery* uses the cutting and coagulating effects of high-frequency current applied by needle, blade, or electrodes. Once considered a palliative type of procedure, it is now being used as an alternative treatment for certain cancers of the skin, oral cavity, and rectum. *Cryosurgery* involves the instillation of liquid nitrogen into the tumor through a probe. It is used in treating cancers of the oral cavity, brain, and prostate. *Chemosurgery* is used in skin cancers. It involves the use of a corrosive paste in combination with multiple frozen sections to ensure complete removal of the tumor. *Laser surgery* uses a laser beam to resect a tumor. It has been used effectively in retinal and vocal cord surgery.

Cooperative efforts between cancer centers throughout the world have helped to standardize and improve surgical procedures, determine which cancers benefit from surgical intervention, and establish in what order surgical and other treatment modalities should be used. Increased emphasis has also been placed on the development of surgical techniques, such as limb salvage surgery, which is used in the treatment of osteogenic sarcoma to preserve functional abilities while permitting complete removal of the tumor.

Radiation Therapy

About 50% of patients with cancer receive radiation therapy, either alone or in combination with other forms of treatment.[16] Radiation can be used singly as the primary method of treatment, as presurgical or postsurgical therapy, with chemotherapy, or with chemotherapy and surgery. Survival rates approaching 90% have been reported with early detection and the use of radiation therapy for seminoma of the testes, Hodgkin's disease, and cancers of the larynx and cervix.[16]

Ionizing radiation was discovered by Marie and Pierre Curie and Wilhelm Conrad Roentgen just before the turn of the century. Development of the first sealed vacuum x-ray tube followed, during the 1920s, along with quantitative methods for measuring radiation dosage. During this same period, Claude Regaud (Foundation Curie in Paris) was able to show that fractionated— small, sublethal—doses of radiation could permanently halt spermatogenesis, whereas no single lethal dose could do so without causing severe damage to the surrounding tissues. It was this observation that linked radiation to the treatment of cancer. Another advance in radiation therapy followed the atomic bomb, with the development of radioactive cobalt. Since then, advances in technology have resulted in the development of sophisticated equipment that produces high-voltage x-ray and electronic beams capable of delivering a therapeutic dose of radiation to the tumor without causing lethal damage to surrounding tissues.

Radiation acts at the cellular level, causing cell death as particles of radioactive energy break chemical bonds, disrupting DNA and interfering with cell activity and mitosis (See Chap. 2). Radiation exerts its greatest effect during certain phases of the cell cycle, particularly during early DNA synthesis of the S phase and in the mitotic or M phase of the cycle. To some extent, radiation is injurious to all cells, but most of all to the poorly differentiated and rapidly proliferating cells of cancer tissue. Radiation also injures such rapidly proliferating cells as those of the bone marrow and the mucosal lining of the gastrointestinal tract. Recovery from sublethal doses of radiation occurs in the interval between the first dose of radiation and subsequent doses. Normal tissue appears to be able to recover from radiation damage more readily than cancerous tissue.

The term *radiosensitivity* describes the sensitivity of cells to radiation, and it varies widely. For example, lymphomas are highly radiosensitive, whereas rhabdomyosarcomas are much less so. The radiation dose that is chosen for treatment of a particular cancer is determined by factors such as the radiosensitivity of the tumor type and the size of the tumor. The *lethal tumor dose* is defined as the dose that achieves 95% tumor control.[17] With external radiation sources, this dose is divided into a series of *smaller fractionated* doses. With the use of fractionated doses, it is more likely that the cancer cells will be dividing and in the vulnerable period of the cell cycle. This dose also allows time for normal tissues to repair the radiation damage. Selecting alternative entrance sites for radiation also helps to spare normal tissue. For example, radiation can be directed at an internal tumor from various points marked off on the front, back, and sides of the body, so that the maximum radiation is directed at the tumor, while the rest of the body receives only minimal radiation.

Administration. Radiation can be administered by using an external machine or an internal source. The machines used to deliver *external radiation* are categorized into the kilovoltage (1000 eV) and megavoltage (1 million eV) range. The early x-ray machines that were used for radiation therapy delivered low penetrance rays in the *kilovoltage (KeV) range*. These rays exert their maximum tumor dose within 1 cm to 2 cm of the skin surface and are now used only in superficial skin lesions or tumors located near the skin surface. *Megavoltage*

(MeV) machines include the cobalt machines, betatrons, and linear accelerators. The MeV machines produce rays that are more penetrating and have more sharply defined edges then the KeV machines; this allows for the delivery of curative doses of radiation without causing damage to skin or other tissues. The rays from the MeV machines also spare bone structures. With the use of KeV machines a marked difference between the absorption in bone and in soft tissue occurred. With the MeV machines this difference does not exist; soft tissue and bone have the same absorption rate—a factor that has allowed delivery of a cancercidal dose of radiation in the vicinity of bone without causing extensive damage to the bone structures.

Internal radiation therapy involves the insertion of radioactive sources within a body cavity, body tissues, or close to the surface being treated. The radioisotopes most commonly used for this purpose are cobalt-60, iridium-192, iodine-125, iodine-131, phosphorus-32, cesium-137, gold-198, and radium-226. Internal radiation can be administered in the form of either sealed or unsealed radiation sources. *Sealed radiation sources* are packed within applicators that can be formed into almost any size or shape. Most commonly they are packed into needles, beads, seeds, ribbons, or catheters, which are then implanted directly into the tumor. Both removable and permanent implants are used. Removable devices make it possible to insert a radioactive material into a tumor area for a period of time (1 or 2 days to a week) and then remove it. The radioactive sources that are used most commonly for this purpose are radium-226, cesium-137, and iridium-192. Cancer of the cervix and uterus is often treated with removable radium implants. Radioactive materials with a relatively short half-life, such as gold-198, radon, or iodine-125, are commonly encapsulated and used in permanent implants. This type of treatment is used for oral, bladder, and prostate cancers. *Unsealed internal radiation sources* are either injected intravenously, administered by mouth, or instilled into a body cavity. Iodine-131, which is given by mouth, is used in the treatment of thyroid cancer. Gold-198 and phosphorus-32 are instilled directly into body cavities to control used effusions (collections of fluid within a serous cavity).

Internal radiation sources are a source of radiation exposure as long as a sealed implant remains in the body or an unsealed implant or injected radioisotope emanates rays of radiant energy. It is essential that the type of ray that is being emitted and the half-life of the radioisotope be considered when care is provided for a person receiving internal radiation. Some radioisotopes such as phosphorus-32 produce only beta rays, which do not create a radiation hazard because of their limited range of beta radiation. Others, such as radium implants, pose a radiation hazard because they emit gamma rays. Institutions that practice nuclear medicine must be licensed by the Atomic Energy Commission and have a radiation protection supervisor, who has the responsibility of establishing policies and maintaining radiation safety within the institution.

Radiation responsiveness. Radiation responsiveness refers to the manner in which a tumor responds to irradiation. Several factors may alter the tumor's response to irradiation. One of these is tumor oxygenation. Many rapidly growing tumors outgrow their blood supply and become deprived of oxygen. It is now recognized that the hypoxic cells of these tumors are more resistant to radiation than normal or well-oxygenated tumor cells. Ways of increasing oxygen delivery to these tumors during radiation therapy are being investigated, as are agents that act as oxygen substitutes. These agents increase the production of free radicals during radiation in a manner similar to oxygen. Another factor is radiosensitivity. Studies are being conducted in hopes of finding ways to increase the radiosensitivity of tumors by altering their DNA in a manner that either makes it more sensitive to radiation or less able to repair radiation damage.

Radioprotectors are substances that selectively protect normal tissue such as bone marrow, salivary glands, and the gastrointestinal mucosa from the effects of radiation without interfering with its effects on cancer tissue. These substances are also being studied.[18]

Adverse effects. Because radiation affects all rapidly proliferating cells, it usually causes some adverse effects. Tissues that are most frequently affected are the skin, the mucosal lining of the gastrointestinal tract, and the bone marrow. Radiation effects are dose dependent: with moderate doses of radiation to the skin, the hair falls out either spontaneously or when being combed, by about the 10th to the 14th day; with larger doses, erythema develops (much like a sunburn) and may turn brown; and at very high doses, the skin is denuded. Fortunately, epithelialization takes place after the treatments have been stopped. The effects of irradiation on the oral and pharyngeal mucous membranes are similar to those that occur on the skin. Radiation-induced bone marrow depression leads to a decrease in white blood cell and platelet production and thus to an increased risk of infection and bleeding tendencies. Other systemic signs associated with irradiation include anorexia, nausea, vomiting, fatigue, profuse perspiration, and even chills. These effects are temporary and reversible.

Protection from radiation is a concern of persons who are in contact with radiation. The three basic mechanisms of protection are time, distance, and shielding. *Shielding* is practiced by persons who are in contact with radiation for long periods of time, such as radiologists and radiologic technicians; they are shielded by special walls or body coverings such as lead aprons, gloves, and throat collars. Increased *time* spent in contact with a radiation source increases exposure. Finally, *distance* must be considered. According to the *inverse square law* that applies to radiation exposure, one can reduce exposure from x-ray or gamma radiation to one-fourth simply by doubling the distance from the radiation source. At a distance of 2 feet from the radiation source, a person receives one-fourth the exposure that he or she would receive at a distance of 1 foot from the source; at a distance of 4 feet, the exposure is one-fourth that received at a distance of 2 feet.

Chemotherapy

In the past three decades, cancer chemotherapy has evolved as a major treatment modality. Drugs may be the chief form of treatment or they may be used adjunctively to other treatments. Chemotherapy is now the primary treatment for most hematologic and some solid tumors, including choriocarcinoma, acute and chronic leukemia, Burkitt's lymphoma, and multiple myeloma.

Cancer chemotherapeutic drugs exert their effects through several mechanisms. At the cellular level, they exert their lethal action by creating adverse conditions that prevent cell growth and replication. These mechanisms include disrupting production of essential enzymes; inhibiting DNA, RNA, and protein synthesis; and preventing cell mitosis. These agents act by first-order kinetics, that is, they kill a percentage rather than a constant number of cells. They are most effective in treating tumors that have a high growth fraction because of their ability to kill rapidly dividing cells.

The anticancer drugs may be classified as either cell-cycle specific or cell-cycle nonspecific. Drugs are cell-cycle specific if they exert their action during a specific phase of the cell cycle. For example, methotrexate, an antimetabolite, acts by interfering with DNA synthesis and thereby interrupts the S phase of the cell cycle. Drugs that are cell-cycle nonspecific affect cancer cells through all the phases of the cell cycle. The alkylating agents, which are cell-cycle nonspecific, act by disrupting DNA when the cells are in the resting state as well as when they are dividing. Chemotherapeutic drugs that have similar structures and effects on cell function are generally grouped together, and these drugs usually have similar toxic and side-effects (Table 5-7). Because they differ in their mechanisms of action, combinations of cell-cycle-specific and cell-cycle-nonspecific agents are often used to treat cancer.

Combination therapy

Combination chemotherapy has been found to be more effective than treatment with a single drug. With this method, multiple drugs with different mechanisms of action, metabolic pathways, time of onsets of action and recovery, side-effects, and onsets of side-effects are used. The regimens for combination therapy are often referred to by acronyms. Two well-known combinations are MOPP (nitrogen mustard, vincristine (Oncovin), procarbazine, and prednisone), used in the treatment of Hodgkin's disease, and CMF (cyclophosphamide, methotrexate, and 5-fluorouracil), used in the treatment of breast cancer. The maximum possible drug doses are usually used to ensure the maximum cell-kill. The routes of administration and dosage schedules are carefully designed to ensure optimal delivery of the active forms of the drugs to a tumor during the sensitive phase of the cell cycle.[19]

Adverse effects.   Because cells are derived from normal cells, they retain many of the latter's properties; thus, chemotherapeutic drugs will affect both the neoplastic and the rapidly proliferating cells of normal tissue. The *nadir* (lowest point) is the point of maximal toxicity for a given adverse effect of a drug and is stated in the time it takes to reach that point. The nadir for leukopenia with Thiotepa occurs at 14 days after the initiation of treatment. Because many toxic effects of chemotherapeutic drugs persist for a period of time after the drug is discontinued, the nadir times and recovery rates are useful guides in evaluating the effects of cancer therapy.

Gastrointestinal tract.   Anorexia, nausea, vomiting, and diarrhea are common problems associated with cancer chemotherapy treatment. They occur within minutes or hours of drug administration and are thought to be due to stimulation of the chemoreceptor trigger zone (vomiting center) in the medulla or the autonomic nervous system. The symptoms usually subside within 24 to 48 hours and often can be relieved by antiemetics. Some drugs cause stomatitis and damage to the rapidly proliferating cells of the gastrointestinal tract mucosal lining.

Bone marrow depression.   Most of the chemotherapeutic drugs depress bone marrow function and the formation of blood cells, leading to anemia, leukopenia, and thrombocytopenia. With severe granulocytopenia there is risk of developing serious infections.

Alopecia.   Many of the cancer drugs impair hair follicle function. The resulting loss of hair is usually temporary and the hair tends to grow back when the treatment is stopped.

Germinal tissues.   The rapidly proliferating structures of the reproductive system are particularly sensitive to the action of cancer drugs. Women may experience changes in menstrual flow or amenorrhea. Men may develop

Table 5-7 Agents Used in Treatment of Cancer

Agent	Mechanism of Action	Major Toxic Manifestations
Alkylating Agents		
Triethylenethiophosphoramide (Thiotepa)	Interfere with DNA replication by attacking DNA synthesis throughout the cell cycle	Bone marrow depression with leukopenia, thrombocytopenia, and bleeding; cyclophosphamide may cause alopecia and hemorrhagic cystitis
Chlorambucil (Leukeran)		
Myleran (Busulfan)		
Cyclophosphamide (Cytoxan)		
Mechlorethamine		
Melphalan (Alkeran)		
Antimetabolites		
Methotrexate (Methotrexate)	Structural analogs of essential metabolites, therefore interfere with synthesis of these metabolites	Bone marrow depression, oral and gastrointestinal ulceration
6-mercaptopurine (6-MP, Purinethol)		
6-thioguanine (6-TG, Thioguan)		
5-fluorouracil (5-FU, Fluorouracil)		
Arabinosylcytosine (Ara-C, Cytosar)		
Antibiotics		
Adriamycin	Interfere with DNA or RNA synthesis, varying with the drug	Stomatitis, gastrointestinal tract disturbances, and bone marrow depression
Bleomycin (Blenoxane)		
Dactinomycin (Cosmegen)		
Daunorubicin (Daunomycin, Cerubidin)		Doxorubicin and daunorubicin cause cardiac toxicity at cumulative doses over 500 mg/m²
Mithramycin (Mithracin)		Bleomycin can cause alopecia and pulmonary fibrosis, but only minimal bone marrow depression
Mitomycin C (Mutamycin)		
Doxorubicin (Adriamycin)		
Plant Alkaloids		
Vinblastine (Velban)	Interfere with cell mitosis	Vinblastine: alopecia, areflexia and bone marrow depression
Vincristine (Oncovin)		Vincristine: neurotoxicity with ataxia and impaired fine motor skills, constipation, and paralytic ileus
Steroid Hormones		
Androgens	Cell-cycle nonspecific	Specific to action of the hormone
Estrogens	Influence cell membrane receptors	
Progestins		
Adrenal glucocorticosteroids		
Others		
L-asparginase	Inhibits protein synthesis	Fever, hypersensitivity
Carmustine	Antimetabolite and alkylating agent	Bone marrow depression
Cisplatin	Inhibits DNA, RNA, protein synthesis	Renal damage
Dacarbazine	Interferes with DNA, RNA synthesis, antimetabolite	Bone marrow depression
Hydroxyrurea	DNA selective antimetabolite	Bone marrow reaction. Allergic reactions to tartrazine dye
Lomustine	Interferes with DNA, RNA synthesis	Bone marrow depression
Procarbazine (Mutulane)	Inhibits DNA, RNA, protein synthesis	CNS depression

oligospermia and azoospermia. Many of these agents may also have teratogenic or mutagenic effects leading to fetal abnormalities.

Oncogenic complications.   Recent epidemiologic studies have shown an increased risk of second malignancies such as acute nonlymphocytic leukemia following long-term use of alkylating agents,[20,21] and semustine[22] for treatment of various forms of cancer. These second malignancies are thought to result from direct cellular changes produced by the drug or from suppression of the immune response.

Endocrine therapy

Endocrine therapy consists of the administration of exogenous hormones in large nonphysiologic doses or the ablation of organs (ovaries, testes, or adrenal glands) responsible for hormone production. This treatment is used in cancers that are responsive to or dependent on hormones for growth. Among the tumors known to be responsive to hormonal manipulations are those of the breast, prostate, thyroid gland, and uterine endometrium. Hormone therapy also involves use of the adrenal corticosteroid hormones. These compounds inhibit mitosis and are cytotoxic to cells of lymphocytic origin. Hormones are cell-cycle nonspecific and are thought to alter the synthesis of RNA and proteins by binding to receptor sites. Unresponsiveness to hormonal manipulation is thought to be related to the absence of specific receptors for the hormone on the tumor.

Immunotherapy

Immunotherapy remains largely investigational and is usually used in conjunction with other forms of treatment. Immunotherapeutic methods fall into three categories. The first is *active nonspecific immune therapy,* whose purpose is to stimulate the immune response. One such agent is BCG (bacillus Calmette-Guérin), an attenuated strain of the bacterium that causes bovine tuberculosis. The second method is *specific immune therapy,* a method that is somewhat similar to immunization in that it involves the use of antigens, from either the patient's tumor or another patient with an antigenically similar tumor, as a challenge to the patient's immune system to produce immune cells against the tumor antigen. The third method is *transfer of passive tumor immunity,* which is accomplished through the administration of antisera or effector substances. Transfer factor is an extract of stimulated lymphocytes that are capable of transferring specific delayed hypersensitivity to other lymphocytes.

Interferon

Interferon is a family of proteins produced by white blood cells and other body cells in response to a variety of stimuli including viral infections (See Chap. 9).

Exposure of cells to interferon triggers intracellular synthesis of antiviral proteins. The antiviral activity of interferon is transferred to neighboring cells by some unknown mechanism without the continued presence of interferon. In addition to its antiviral action, interferon also inhibits cell reproduction, and evidence suggests that it may specifically inhibit the growth of cancer cells. The ultimate value of interferon may be the knowledge gained about a whole new class of compounds called *biologic response modifiers,* which fight cancer by stimulating the body's immune system.[23] The American Cancer Society has allocated more than $6.8 million for interferon research.[28] The first clinical trials of interferon cancer therapy were used with four types of cancer: multiple myeloma, melanoma, breast cancer, and non-Hodgkin's lymphoma. It is still too early to tell what the outcomes of these studies will be. Additional studies involving melanoma, advanced kidney cancer, and nasopharyngeal cancer are now being conducted. Originally, the availability of interferon was limited because it could be obtained only from white blood cells and fibroblasts. Large amounts of interferon can now be produced using techniques of recombinant DNA synthesis.

In summary, treatment plans that use more than one type of therapy, often in combination, are now providing cures for a number of cancers that, a few decades ago, had a poor prognosis and are increasing the life expectancy in patients with other types of cancer. Surgical procedures are now more precise because of improved diagnostic equipment and new techniques such as laser surgery. Radiation equipment and radioactive sources permit greater and more controlled destruction of cancer cells while causing less damage to normal tissues. The use of combination chemotherapy regimens has provided cures for cancers that were previously viewed as incurable. The use of immunotherapy and interferon provides hope of using the body's own defenses in fighting cancer.

■ Study Guide

After you have studied this chapter, you should be able to meet the following objectives:

☐ List the most common sites of cancer in men and women.

☐ Describe the five phases of the cell cycle.

☐ Cite the method used for naming benign and malignant neoplasms.

☐ Define the term *neoplasm* and explain how the behavior of neoplastic growth differs from the normal adaptive changes seen in atrophy, hypertrophy, and hyperplasia.

☐ State at least six ways in which benign and malignant neoplasms differ.

☐ State the difference between solid and hematologic cancers.

☐ Utilize the properties of cell differentiation in describing the development of a cancer cell line and behavior of the tumor.

☐ Utilize the concept of growth fraction and doubling time to explain the growth of cancerous tissue.

☐ Explain the pathogenesis of metastasis.

☐ State the purpose of clinical staging of cancer.

☐ Relate environmental factors to the development of cancer.

☐ Describe the surveillance capacity of the immune system.

☐ Describe the general effects of cancer on body systems.

☐ Compare the methods used in obtaining a Pap smear and tissue biopsy.

☐ Explain the rationale for the use of radiation in the treatment of cancer.

☐ Cite the difference between external beam radiation therapy and radiation therapy using an internal radiation source.

☐ Describe the adverse effects of radiation therapy.

☐ Compare the action of cell-cycle-specific and cell-cycle-nonspecific chemotherapeutic drugs.

■ References

1. Cancer Facts 1985. New York, American Cancer Society, 1985
2. Prescott DM, Flexer AS: Cancer: The Misguided Cell, pp 47, 70. Sunderland, MA, Sinauer Associates, 1982
3. Robbins SL, Cotran RS, Kumar V: Pathologic Basis of Disease, 3rd ed, pp 268, 255, 264, 268. Philadelphia, WB Saunders, 1984
4. Baserga R: The cell cycle. N Engl J Med 304, No. 8:453, 1981
5. Lynch HT: Familial risk and cancer control. JAMA 236, No. 6:585, 1976
6. Knudson, AG: Heredity and human cancer. Am J Pathol 77, No. 1:77, 1974
7. Farber E: Chemical carcinogenesis. N Engl J Med 305:1378, 1981
8. Poskanzer DC, Herbst A: Epidemiology of vaginal adenosis and adenocarcinoma associated with exposure to stilbestrol in utero. Cancer 39, No. 4:1792, 1977
9. Nicholson WJ: Cancer following occupational exposure to asbestos and vinyl chloride. Cancer 39, No. 4:1972, 1977
10. Favus MJ, Schneider AB, Stachura ME, et al: Thyroid cancer occurring as a late consequence of head and neck irradiation: Evaluation of 1056 patients. N Engl J Med 294:1019, 1976
11. Jablon S, Kato H: Studies of the mortality of A-bomb survivors: V. Radiation dose and mortality, 1950—1970. Radiat Res 50:649, 1972
12. Gallo RC: The virus-cancer story. Hosp Pract 18, No. 6:79—89, 1983
13. Burnett FM: Immunologic aspects of malignant disease. Lancet 1:1171, 1967
14. Cancer Facts and Figures, p 16. New York, American Cancer Society, 1981
15. Patterson WB: Principles of surgical oncology. In Rubin P (ed): Clinical Oncology, ed. 6, p 35. New York, American Cancer Society, 1983
16. Bloomer WD, Hellman S: Normal tissue responses to radiation therapy. N Engl J Med 293, No. 2:80, 1975
17. Rubin P, Siemann D: Principles of radiation and cancer radiotherapy. In Rubin P (ed): Clinical Oncology, 6th ed. p 62. New York, American Cancer Society, 1983
18. Phillips TL, Wasserman TH: Promise of radiosensitizers and radioprotectors in treatment of human cancers. Cancer Treat Rep 68:291, 1984
19. Krakoff IRL: Cancer chemotherapeutic agents. CA 31, No. 3:4, 1981
20. Pederson-Bjergaard J, Larsen SO: Incidence of acute non-lymphocytic leukemia, preleukemia and acute myeloproliferative syndrome up to 10 years after treatment of Hodgkin's disease. N Engl J Med 307:964, 1982
21. Coltman CA Jr, Dixon DO: Second malignancies complicating Hodgkin's disease: A Southwest Oncology Group 10 year followup. Cancer Treat Rep 66:1023, 1982
22. Boise JD, Greene MH, Killen JY et al: Leukemia and preleukemia after adjuvant treatment of gastrointestinal cancer with Semustine. N Engl J Med 309:1079, 1983
23. Cancer Facts 1984. p 26. New York, American Cancer Society, 1984

■ Additional References

Bingham CA: The cell cycle and cancer chemotherapy. Am J Nurs 78, No. 7:1201, 1978

Ensminger WD, Gyves JW: Regional cancer chemotherapy. Cancer Treat Rep 68, No. 1:101, 1984

Fagan-Dubin L: Causes of cancer. Cancer Nurs 2, No. 6:435, 1979

Farber E: Chemical carcinogenesis. N Engl J Med 305, No. 23:1379, 1981

Frye RJM, Aninsworth EJ: Radiation injury: Some aspects of the oncogenic effects. Fed Proc 36, No. 5:1703, 1977

Heidelberger C: Chemical carcinogenesis. Annu Rev Biochem 44:79, 1975

Jackson B, Armenaki DW: A tumor classification system. Am J Nurs 76, No. 8:1320, 1976

Krontiris TG: The emerging genetics of human cancer. N Engl J Med 309, No. 7:404, 1983

Lynch HT, Brokley FD, Lynch P et al: Familial risk and cancer control. JAMA 236, No. 6:582, 1976

Lynch HT, Guirgis H, Lynch PM et al: Familial cancer syndromes: A survey. Cancer 39:1967, 1977

McGuire DB: Familial cancer and the role of the nurse. Cancer Nurs 2, No. 6:443, 1979

Richter MP, Kligerman MM: Particle-beam radiation therapy 1983: Evaluation and recommendations. Cancer Treat Rep 68, No. 1:303, 1984

Schmaier AH: Oncologic emergencies. Med Times 111, No. 2:87—99, 1983

Scott RE, Wille JJ: Mechanisms for the initiation and promotion of carcinogenesis: A review and a new concept. Mayo Clin Proc 59:107, 1984

Winters WD: Viruses and cancer. Am J Nurs 78, No. 2:249, 1978

Unit II

Alterations in Body Defenses

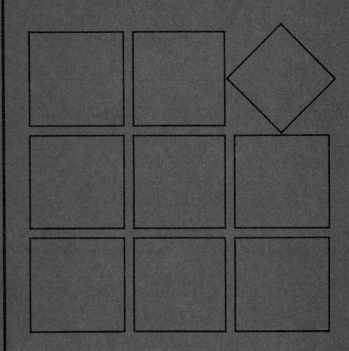

Chapter 6

Stress and Adaptation

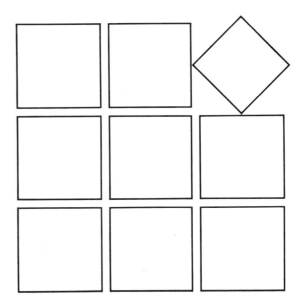

Health is a dynamic state in which a continuous expenditure of energy is required in order to adapt to life stresses. Much of this energy is used to recruit physiologic and psychologic behaviors that oppose or compensate for perceived threats to the maintenance of the internal environment. In this respect, the human body is truly an amazing structure. It is able to withstand exposure to environmental stresses while maintaining its internal environment within the very narrow confines of what is termed *normal*. From astronauts who have traveled to the moon and from explorers of the ocean's depths, we have learned that vital physiologic functions such as heart rate, blood *p*H, and body temperature remain remarkably similar to those observed under normal environmental conditions. Even in advanced disease states, the body maintains much of its adaptive capacity and is able to compensate and maintain the internal environment within relatively normal limits.

■ Stress

In recent years, interest in the roles that stress and altered adaptive processes play in the development of disease has increased. Hypertension, heart disease, and peptic ulcer are but a few of the diseases that have been associated with stress. Stress may contribute directly to the production of disease or it may contribute to the development of behaviors such as smoking, overeating, and drug abuse, which increase the risk of disease.

Stress has been defined in many ways. To the physicist, the term refers to a force, strain, or pressure applied to a system. To the lay person, stress frequently implies exposure to excessive demands or environmental conditions that cause emotional upset and tension. To the psychologist, stress has been described as anything that alters the psychologic homeostatic processes.[1] To the anthropologist, stress is adversity; coercion between people or between the environment and humans, or between history and humankind.[2] Hans Selye, the world-renowned endocrinologist and pioneer in the field of stress research, has described stress as the nonspecific response of the body to any demand made on it.[3] Because the primary focus of this book is physiologic, Selye's theory of stress is used.

Stressors

The events of environmental agents responsible for initiating the stress response are called *stressors*. According to Selye, stressors may be endogenous, arising from within the body, or exogenous, arising from outside the body.[3] Stressors can be physical, psychologic, or sociologic. They include mental and physical effort, extremes of temperature, hunger, thirst, and fatigue, and other everyday experiences. Mason has suggested that

emotional reactions to the stressor serve as the final common pathway for the stress response, emphasizing the need to consider the impact that learning and emotion have on the response.[4]

Stressors can assume a number of patterns in relation to time. They may also be classified as follows: (1) acute time-limiting, (2) event-sequencing, (3) chronic intermittent, or (4) chronic sustained stressors.[5] An acute time-limiting stressor is any event that occurs within a given short period of time and does not usually recur. Event-sequencing stressors are situations in which a stressor initiates a series of stress-producing events (*e.g.*, being fired from a job). Chronic intermittent stress occurs in response to discrete, intermittent stimuli to which a person is habitually exposed. Chronic stressors are those to which a person is continuously exposed. The rapidity or chronicity of events in which the body is asked to respond to a stressor often determines the availability and efficiency of stress responses. The response of the immune system, for example, is more rapid and more efficient on second exposure to a pathogen than it is on first exposure. On the other hand, chronic exposure to a stressor can fatigue the stress response system and impair its effectiveness.

The Stress Response

In explaining the stress response, Selye proposed that two factors determine the nature of the stress response: (1) the properties of the stressor and (2) the conditioning of the individual.[3] Most stressors produce both specific and nonspecific responses. For example, the joy of becoming a new parent and the sorrow of losing a parent are completely different experiences, yet their stressor effect—the nonspecific demand for adjustment to a new situation—can be quite similar. The specific stress responses alert an individual to the presence of the stressor whereas the nonspecific effects, which involve neuroendocrine responses such as increased autonomic nervous system activity, are designed to maintain or reestablish normality and are independent of specific responses. The ability of the same stressor to produce different responses and disorders in different individuals indicates the adaptive capacity of the individual, or what Selye termed *conditioning factors*. These conditioning factors may be internal (genetic predisposition, age, sex, or others) or external (exposure to environmental agents, treatment with certain drugs, or dietary factors).[3]

Manifestation of the Stress Response

The manifestations of the stress response—a pounding headache, cold moist hands, a stiff neck, and increased incidence of infections—reflect, for the most part, the nonspecific aspects of the stress response. They include responses of the autonomic nervous system, the endocrine system, the musculoskeletal system, and the immune system. The integration of these responses, which occurs at the level of the central nervous system, is elusive and complex. It relies on communication between the cerebral cortex, the limbic system, the thalamus, the hypothalamus, and the reticular formation and reticular activating system (Fig. 6-1). The thalamus functions as a relay center for incoming impulses from all parts of the body and is important in sorting out and distributing sensory input. The reticular formation modulates mental alertness, autonomic nervous system activity, and skeletal muscle tone; but it does this using input and output from other neural structures. Likewise, the hypothalamus modulates both the endocrine and the autonomic nervous system function (Fig. 6-1). The limbic system is involved with the emotional components (fear, excitement, rage, anger) of the stress response.

Musculoskeletal responses

Musculoskeletal tension that occurs during the stress response represents the increased activity of the reticular formation and its influence on the muscle spindles and the gamma loop (descending neural pathways, gamma motor neurons, spindle muscle fibers, afferent neurons, and alpha motor neurons), which control muscle tone. Muscle tension can remain as a prolonged manifestation of the stress response and can cause stiffness of the neck, backache, headaches, and other complaints.

Autonomic nervous system responses

The autonomic nervous system manifestation of the stress reaction has been termed the *fight-or-flight response.* This is the most rapid of the stress responses and represents the basic survival response of our primitive ancestors when confronted with the perils of the wilderness and its inhabitants. In the presence of danger, the alternatives were clear—to run away or stand up and fight. The heart and respiratory rates increase, the hands and feet become moist, the pupils dilate, the mouth becomes dry, and the activity of the gastrointestinal tract decreases. The autonomic nervous system is also involved in less-threatening situations. For example, it is the autonomic nervous system that controls the circulatory responses to activities of daily living such as moving from the seated or lying to the standing position.

Hypothalamic-pituitary-adrenal responses

The hypothalamic-pituitary-adrenal response is the mechanism that regulates body levels of adrenocortical hormones (mainly cortisol). The production of cortisol by the adrenal gland is controlled by the adrenocorticotropic hormone (ACTH) from the anterior pituitary. ACTH, in turn, is controlled by the corticotropin-releasing factor from the hypothalamus. The influence of emotion and stress on cortisol production is largely through the central nervous system by means of the hypothalamus. Cortisol is involved in maintaining glucose produc-

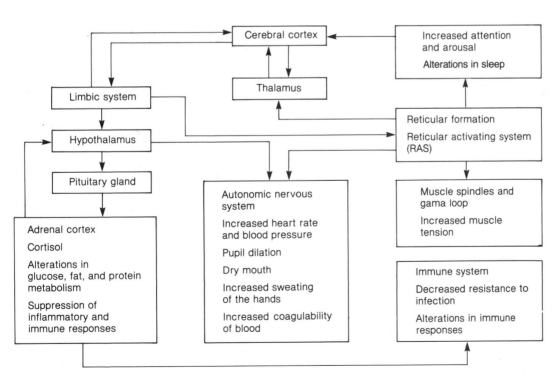

Figure 6-1 *Stress pathways.*

tion from protein, facilitating fat metabolism, supporting vascular responsiveness, and modulating central nervous system (CNS) function.[6] In addition, the hormone affects skeletal turnover, hematopoiesis, muscle function, immune responses, and renal function. The adrenocortical hormones are discussed in Chapter 39. Other hormones (growth hormone, thyroid hormone, vasopressin, the sex hormones, and others) are also involved in the stress response. These hormones are discussed in other sections of this text.

As a young medical student, Selye noted that patients suffering from diverse disease conditions had many signs and symptoms in comon. He noted that "whether a man suffers from a loss of blood, an infectious disease, or advanced cancer, he loses his appetite, his muscular strength, and his ambition to accomplish anything; usually the patient also loses weight, and even his facial expression betrays that he is ill."[3] Selye referred to this as the "syndrome of just being sick." To Selye, the response to stress was a process that enabled the body to resist the stressor in the best possible way by enhancing the function of the system best able to respond to it. He termed this response the *general adaptation syndrome (GAS)*. The GAS involves three stages: (1) the alarm stage, (2) the stage of resistance, and (3) the stage of exhaustion. The hypothalamic-pituitary-adrenal axis assumes a pivotal role in stress homeostasis during the alarm stage. Selye observed a triad of adrenal enlargement, thymus atrophy, and gastric ulcers in the rats used in his original studies. During the alarm stage no one organ system is predominantly active. The most appropriate channels of defense are recruited during the stage of resistance. During this second stage, the increased cortisol levels that were present during the first stage drop, because they are no longer needed. During the third stage—the stage of exhaustion—the reaction spreads because of wear and tear on the most appropriate channel of adaptation.[7]

Selye contended that many ailments such as various emotional disturbances, mildly annoying headaches, insomnia, upset stomach, gastric and duodenal ulcers, and certain types of rheumatic disorders, as well as cardiovascular and kidney diseases, appear to be initiated or encouraged by the "body itself because of its faulty adaptive reactions to potentially injurious agents."[3]

Immunologic responses

There is increasing interest in the effect that stress has on the immunologic responses. The occurrence of the oral disease acute necrotizing gingivitis, in which the normal bacterial flora of the mouth becomes invasive, is well known by dentists to be associated with acute stress, such as final exams.[8] Similarly, herpes simplex I (cold sores) often develop during periods of inadequate rest, fever,

ultraviolet radiation, and emotional upset. In this case, the resident herpesvirus is kept in check by body defenses, most likely by T-lymphocytes, until a stressful event occurs and causes suppression of the immmune system.

The exact mechanism whereby stress produces its effect on the immune response is unknown and probably varies from individual to individual depending on genetic endowment and environmental factors. It is known, however, that the stress response induces changes in a number of hormonal factors that affect the immune response. The hallmark of the stress response, as first described by Selye, is the presence of conditions (increased corticosteroid production and atrophy of the thymus) known to suppress the immune response. The clinical application of this process can occur with administration of pharmacologic preparations of the corticosteroid hormones to suppress the inflammatory and immune response. The existence of a feedback loop between the immune system and the hypothalamic-pituitary-adrenal system offers an intriguing hypothesis for interaction between the two systems in terms of decreasing resistance to infection and the surveilance function of the immune system in terms of preventing neoplastic cell development (Chap. 5). The receptors for a number of CNS-controlled hormones and neuromediators reportedly have been found on lymphocytes. They include receptors for glucocorticoids, insulin, testosterone, catecholamines, estrogens, histamine, acetylcholine, and growth hormone.[9] The presence of a hormone receptor on a cell suggests that the cell's function is influenced by the hormone.

In summary, stress is defined in many ways. Hans Selye, the world-renowned endocrinologist and pioneer in the field of stress research, defines stress as the nonspecific response of the body to any demands made on it. The event or environmental agent that produces the stress is called a stressor. Stressors may be physical, psychologic, or social. They include mental and physical effort, extremes of temperature, hunger, thirst, fatigue, and other everyday experiences. Most stressors produce both specific and nonspecific responses. The specific responses alert the individual to the nature of the stressor and assist in establishing definitive measures to deal with it. The nonspecific responses are designed to maintain or reestablish normality.

■ Adaptation

The ability to adapt to a wide range of environments and stressors is not peculiar to humans. According to René Dubos (a microbiologist noted for his study of human response to the total environment), "adaptability is found throughout life and is perhaps the one attribute that distinguishes most clearly the world of life from the world of inanimate matter."[10] Living organisms, no matter how primitive, do not submit passively to the impact of environmental forces. They attempt to respond adaptively, each in its own unique and most suitable manner. The higher the organism on the evolutionary scale, the larger its repertoire of adaptive mechanisms and its ability to select and limit aspects of the environment to which it will respond. The most fully evolved mechanisms are the social responses through which individuals or groups modify either their environments or their habits, or both, in order to achieve a way of life that is suited to their needs.[10]

Human beings, because of their highly developed nervous system and intellect, usually have alternative mechanisms for adapting and the ability to control many aspects of the environment. Air conditioning and central heating limit the need to adapt to extreme changes in environmental temperature. The control of microbial growth, immunization, and the availability of antibiotics eliminates the need to respond to common infectious agents. On the other hand, modern technology creates new challenges for adaptation and provides new sources of stress such as increased noise, air pollution, exposure to chemicals that reduce the microbial agents in the environment and increase the shelf life of the foods we eat, and changes in the biologic rhythms imposed by shift work and transcontinental flights.

Constancy of the Internal Environment

The environment in which the cells live is not the external environment that surrounds the total organism, but a local fluid environment that surrounds each cell. It is from this internal environment that cells receive their nourishment and it is into this fluid that they secrete their wastes. Even the contents of the gastrointestinal tract and lungs do not become part of the internal environment until they have been absorbed into the extracellular fluid. A multicellular organism is able to survive only as long as the composition of the internal environment is compatible with the survival needs of the individual cells. Even a small change in the *p*H of the body fluids can disrupt the metabolic processes of individual cells. Claude Bernard, the nineteenth-century physiologist, was the first to clearly describe the central importance of a stable internal environment (*milieu interne*). Bernard recognized that body fluids that surround the cells and the various organ systems provide the means for exchange between the external and the internal environments.

Homeostasis

The concept of a stable internal environment was supported by Walter B. Cannon, who emphasized that this kind of stability, which he termed homeostasis, was achieved through a system of carefully coordinated physiologic processes that oppose change. He pointed out that these processes were largely automatic.

Cannon emphasized that homeostasis involves not only resistance to external disturbances, but also resistance to disturbances from within. In his book, *Wisdom of the Body*, published in 1939, Cannon presented four tentative propositions to describe the general features of homeostasis:

1. Constancy in an open system, such as our bodies represent, requires mechanisms that act to maintain this constancy. Cannon based this proposition on insights into the ways by which steady states such as glucose, body temperature, and acid-base balance were regulated.
2. Steady-state conditions require that any tendency toward change be automatically met with factors that resist change. An increase in blood sugar results in thirst as the body attempts to dilute the concentration of sugar in the extracellular fluid.
3. The regulating system that determines the homeostatic state consists of a number of cooperating mechanisms acting simultaneously or successively. Blood sugar is regulated by insulin, glucagon, and other hormones that control its release from the liver or its uptake by the tissues.
4. Homeostasis does not occur by accident, but is the result of organized self-government. With this postulate, Cannon emphasized that when a factor is known to shift homeostasis in one direction, it is reasonable to expect mechanisms that have the opposite effect. In the homeostatic regulation of blood sugar, one would expect to find mechanisms that both raise and lower blood sugar.[11]

Control Systems

The ability of the body to function under conditions of change in the internal and external environment depends on the thousands of control systems that serve to regulate body function. The body's control systems regulate cellular function, control the life processes, and integrate the interrelated functions of the different organ systems.

The most intricate of these control systems are the genetic control systems that regulate cellular function, including cell structure and replication (see Chap. 1). Other control systems regulate function within organs and systems, whereas still others operate throughout the body to integrate the functions of the different organ systems. The concentration of carbon dioxide in the extracellular levels is regulated by the respiratory and nervous systems, and the blood sugar concentration is controlled mainly by the liver and pancreas.

A homeostatic control system is a collection of interconnected components that function to keep a physical or chemical parameter of the body relatively constant. At least three essential components exist in a control system: (1) a *sensor*, which detects changes in product or function, (2) a *comparator*, which compares the sensed value with an acceptable range, and (3) an *effector system*, which returns the function or product to the acceptable range (Fig. 6-2).

System efficiency

The effectiveness of a system is determined by the amount of change (amplification or gain) that occurs in chemical or physical parameters. In his textbook of physiology, Guyton uses the example of a 1-degree Fahrenheit change in body temperature (from 98°F to 99°F) that occurs when environmental temperature is increased from 60°F to 110°F.[12] As body temperature rises because of the change in external temperature, sensors in the system detect the error, and sufficient compensation, in terms of evaporation from the skin with loss of body heat, returns the temperature to within 1 degree Fahrenheit of the set point of the system. Were it not for the efficiency of the control system, the body temperature would have risen 50 degrees Fahrenheit instead of 1 degree Fahrenheit (Fig. 6-3).

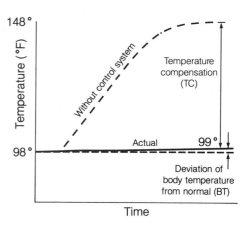

Figure 6-3 *Effects on body temperature of suddenly increasing the air temperature 50° F, showing the hypothetical effect without a control system and the actual effect with a normal control system. (Guyton A: Textbook of Medical Physiology. Philadelphia, WB Saunders, 1981)*

Feedback systems

Most control systems in the body operate by *negative feedback mechanisms*, which function in a manner similar to the thermostat on a heating system. When the monitored function decreases below the set point of the system, the feedback mechanism causes the function to increase, and when the function is increased above the set point, the feedback mechanism causes it to decrease (Fig. 6-4). For example, in the negative feedback mechanism that controls blood glucose levels, an increase in blood glucose stimulates an increase in insulin with the removal of glucose from the blood. When sufficient glucose has left the bloodstream to cause blood glucose levels to fall, the release of glucose from the liver and the recruitment of other counterregulatory mechanisms cause the blood glucose to rise.

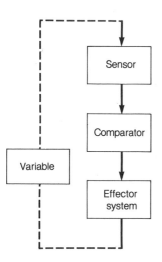

Figure 6-2 *A simple control system consisting of a sensor that monitors a physiological variable, a comparator that compares the actual value of the monitored variable with the set-point of the system, and an effector system that functions to correct the disturbance.*

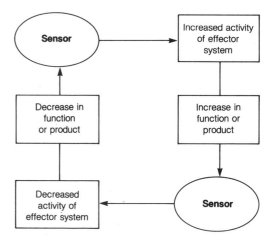

Figure 6-4 *Negative feedback control of a body function, hormone level, or biochemical product.*

The reader is likely to ask why most physiologic control systems function under negative rather than *positive feedback mechanisms** The answer is that a positive feedback mechanism interjects instability rather than stability into a system. It produces a vicious circle in which the initiating stimulus produces more of the same. In a positive feedback system, the previously cited example of exposure to an increase in environmental temperature would lead to compensatory mechanisms designed to increase rather than decrease temperature.

Factors Affecting Adaptation to Stress

Adaptation and homeostasis are only concepts of the ideal. A wide variation and range of responses are available for adjustment to the external and internal environments, and conditions do not always return to their original state.

Generally speaking, adaptation affects the whole person. When adapting to stress, the body uses those behaviors that are most efficient and effective—the body will not use a "baseball bat to kill a mosquito." Nor will the body use long-term mechanisms when short-term adaptation mechanisms are sufficient. The increase in heart rate that accompanies a febrile illness is a temporary response designed to deliver additional oxygen to the tissues during the short period of time that the elevated temperature increases the metabolic needs of the tissues (the increase in heart rate also expedites delivery of heat-carrying blood to the skin surface where the heat can be lost to the external environment). On the other hand, adaptive responses such as hypertrophy of the left ventricle in persons with systemic hypertension are long-term responses.

Adaptation is affected by a number of factors including experience and previous learning, physiologic reserve, genetic endowment, age, the rapidity with which the need to adapt occurs, nutrition, health status, circadian rhythms, and psychosocial factors (Fig.6-5).

Previous experience and learning

Dubos cites the case of an old Chinese fisherman (the type depicted on the scrolls of the Sung era) as an example of the effect that experience and learning have on adaptation:

> The fisherman appears fully at ease and relaxed in his primitive boat, floating on a misty lake, or even a polluted and crowded harbor. He has probably experienced many tribulations in the course of his years of struggle and poverty, but has survived by becoming almost totally identified with his environment. In fact he is so well adapted to

*Some of the amplifying circuits in the nervous system function through positive feedback mechanisms.

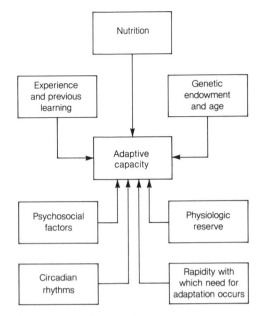

Figure 6-5 *Factors affecting adaptation.*

it that he will probably live for many more years, without modern comfort, sanitation, or medical care, just by letting his existence be ruled by what he considers to be the inalterable laws of the seasons and nature.... In the course of his life, he developed different protective mechanisms that increased his immunologic, physiologic, and psychic resistance to the physico-chemical hardships, the parasites, and the social conflicts which threatened him every day. Finally, he has elected to spend the rest of his life in the environment in which he has evolved and to which he has become adapted. Robust though he appears and really is, he probably would soon become sick if he moved into an area where the parasites, physiologic stresses, and social customs differ from the ones among which he has spent his early life.[10]

Physiologic reserve

The trained athlete is able to increase cardiac output 600- to 700-fold during exercise. The safety margin for adaptation of most body systems is considerably greater than that needed for normal activities. The red blood cells carry more oxygen than the tissues can use, the liver and fat cells store excess nutrients, and bone tissue has an excess storage of calcium in excess of that needed for normal neuromuscular function. The ability of body systems to increase their function given the need to adapt is known as the *physiologic reserve*. It is noteworthy that many of the body organs such as the lungs, kidneys, and adrenal glands are paired to provide not only a physiologic but an *anatomic reserve* as well. Both organs are not needed to ensure the continued existence and maintenance of the internal environment. Many individuals function normally with only one lung or one kidney. In kidney disease, for example, signs of renal failure do not occur until about 90% of the functioning nephrons have been destroyed.

Rapidity of onset

In terms of time, adaptation is most efficient when the changes that occur are gradual rather than sudden. It is possible, for instance, to lose a liter or more of blood through chronic gastrointestinal bleeding over a period of a week without developing signs of shock. However, a sudden hemorrhage that causes loss of an equal amount of blood is apt to cause hypotension and shock.

Genetic endowment and age

Adaptation is further affected by the availability of adaptive responses and flexibility in selecting the most appropriate and economical response. The greater the number of available responses, the more effective the capacity to adapt.

Genetic endowment can ensure an adequate immune system, normal metabolism, elimination of body wastes, and other functions that are essential to adaptation. Even a gene that has deleterious effects may prove adaptive in some environments. In Africa, the gene for sickle cell anemia persists in some populations because it provides some resistance to the parasite that causes malaria.[10]

The adaptive capacity decreases with extremes of age and with disease conditions that limit the availability of adaptive responses. The ability to adapt is impaired by the immaturity of an infant as it is by the decline in functional reserve that occurs with age. For example, the infant has difficulty concentrating urine because of immature renal structures and is therefore less able than an adult to cope with decreased water intake or exaggerated water losses. A similar situation exists in the elderly due to age-related changes in renal function.

Health status

Health status, both physical and mental, determines physiologic and psychologic reserves and is a strong determinant of the ability to adapt. For example, persons with heart disease are less able to adjust to stresses that require the recruitment of cardiovascular responses. Likewise, severe emotional stress often produces disruption of physiologic function and limits the ability to make appropriate choices related to long-term adaptive needs. Those who have worked with acutely ill persons know that the will to live often has a profound influence on survival during life-threatening illnesses.

Nutrition

There are 50 to 60 essential nutrients, including minerals, lipids, certain fatty acids, vitamins, and specific amino acids. Deficiencies or excesses of any of these nutrients can alter one's health status and impair the ability to adapt. The importance of nutrition to enzyme function, the immune response, and wound healing are well known. On a worldwide basis, malnutrition may be one of the most common causes of immunodeficiency. Among the problems associated with dietary excess are obesity and alcohol abuse. Obesity is a common problem. It predisposes to a number of health problems including atherosclerosis and hypertension. Alcohol is a well-known nutrient that is often used in excess. It acutely affects the brain function and with long-term use, can seriously impair the function of the liver, brain, and other vital structures.

Circadian rhythms

Time and rhythms are fundamental properties of life. In the past 20 to 30 years it has become increasingly evident that biologic rhythms play an important role in adaptation to stress, the development of illness, and response to medical treatment.

Although the previously discussed concepts of homeostasis and the constancy of the internal environment hold true, most of the bodily functions are continuously changing, many with a regular oscillatory rhythm. The frequencies of bodily rhythms cover almost every dimension of time (e.g., some brain waves have a rhythm that oscillates once per a fraction of a second, respiration has a rhythm of several seconds, and the menstrual cycle a monthly rhythm. Many rhythms such as sleep, rest and activity, work and leisure, and eating and drinking oscillate with a frequency similar to that of the 24-hour light-dark solar day. The term *circadian*, from the Latin *circa* (about) and *dies* (day) is used to describe these 24-hour diurnal rhythms.

The first studies of endogenous circadian rhythms in human subjecs isolated from time cues were conducted in either underground cellars or caves in which time, light, temperature, noise, and social cues could be controlled or eliminated.[13,14] Subsequent studies have been done in specially constructed isolation rooms. Under these conditions, the fundamental properties of human circadian rhythms have been more thoroughly defined. When a biologic rhythm persists in the absence of any environmental periodicity it is said to be free running. It has been found that human beings have a free-running period of about 25 hours; therefore, if their ciracadian pacemakers were not reset (exposed to environmental cues), they would lose about 1 hour out of the 24-hour clock each day.

Circadian rhythms can arise from within the organism or they can develop as the result of environmental influences. Geographic events such as temperature, light and dark, and seasonal cycles, which occur periodically, serve as regular, predictable environmental synchronizers for circadian rhythms. The process of synchronization of the biologic clock by environmental influences is termed *entrainment*. Hunger can be entrained by meal schedules. The external influences that are capable of entraining the biologic clock have been given the name *zeitgebers* from the German word meaning time-giver or synchronizer. Endogenous circadian rhythms arise from within the individual.

Figure 6-6 shows the normal circadian rhythms for potassium, cortisol, growth hormone, body temperature, and sleep stages. The body temperature is highest in the evening and lowest at the end of sleep time. Adrenocorticotropic hormone (ACTH) and cortisol are secreted in tandem. In persons with a normal sleep-wake cycle, serum cortisol levels reach their peak shortly after rising at about 8 A.M. or 9 A.M. Growth hormone is secreted at the onset of sleep. Evidence suggests that endogenous control of circadian rhythms is vested in neurons that are located in the suprachiasmatic nucleus of the hypothalamus.[15] Presumably, certain hypothalamic-pituitary rhythms such as ACTH-cortisol levels are driven by the suprachiasmatic nucleus in the thalamus.

As was mentioned previously, endogenous circadian rhythms adopt a longer 25-hour day when studied under free-running conditions. The circadian rhythms for body temperature, urine elimination, and cortisol secretion maintain a free-running rhythm when an individual becomes desynchronized from the environment. This has been shown to be true even in blind persons who are not exposed to the usual light-dark stimuli. The sleep-wakefulness cycle has been shown to be weakly entrained. For 20% to 30% of subjects under free-running conditions in one study, the period between awakenings became longer than 25 hours, lengthening to 30 to 33 hours in some subjects.[16] In these individuals the vegetative functions of temperature control, urine elimination, and cortisol secretion remained on a 25-hour rhythm.

Like any physiologic regulatory system, the circadian system occasionally misfunctions. In some disease states, such as Cushing's disease, there is a loss of circadian rhythms for cortisol. Periodic mood swings from mania to hypomania to depression in manic-depressive patients have been linked to changes in phase relationships of circadian rhythms.[16] Internal desynchronization of rhythms may explain some sleep disorders. Aschoff suggests that some of the sleep problems in the elderly may arise from loss of entrainment of the circadian system.[13]

Important questions related to circadian rhythms are whether or not certain pharmacologic agents have different effects when given at different times of the day or night or whether or not the degree of their effective-

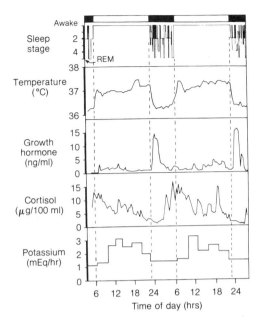

Figure 6-6 *Circadian rhythms in sleep, body temperature, plasma concentration of growth hormone, and of plasma cortisol, and urinary excretion of potassium measured over 48 hr in a normal human subject. Sleep stages include rapid-eye-movement (REM) sleep and non-REM sleep, stages 1 through 4. Body temperature was measured rectally. The light–dark cycle is indicated by the horizontal bar at top. (Moore-Ede MC, Czeisler CA, Richardson GS: Circadian timekeeping in health and disease. N Engl J Med 309, No. 9:330, 1983)*

ness depends on the time of administration. Halberg, using laboratory mice, has shown that the sensitivity of the organism to many stimuli, including ethanol, barbiturates, and exposure to carcinogens, is quite different at different times of the day or night and depends on the phase of the circadian rhythm. In the human, it has been shown that administration of corticosteroid drugs produces less suppression of the hypothalamic-hypophyseal-adrenal axis when synchronized with the normal circadian peaks in cortisol levels.[14]

Shift changes and the time-zone changes associated with transcontinental flights are external influences that affect circadian rhythms. Shift changes usually involve a conflict situation in which the sleep-wakefulness cycle is reversed while social contacts keep the night worker entrained to a day-active cycle. With transcontinental flight, there is a complete phase shift in circadian rhythms. For a time change of 5 to 6 hours it takes several days to become entrained to local time. Less time is usually required to adjust after westward flights than after eastward flights, probably because the endogenous clock adjusts more readily to a longer day than to a shorter day.[17]

Psychosocial factors

A number of studies relate social factors and life events to illness. Scientific interest in the social environment as a cause of stress has gradually broadened to include the social environment as a resource that mediates the relationship between stress and health. For example, married persons have consistently been found to be mentally and physically healthier than unmarried persons, these differences being more pronounced among men than among women.[18,19]

Social networks contribute in a number of ways to an individual's psychosocial and physical integrity. The configuration of significant others that constitutes this network functions to mobilize the resources of the individual; these people share the individual's tasks and provide monetary support, materials and tools, and guidance in improving problem-solving capabilities.[20] There is evidence that persons who have social supports or social assets may live longer and have a lower incidence of somatic illness.[21,22] Social support has been viewed in terms of both the number of relationships a person has and the perons's perception of these relationships. Thus, close relations with others can involve not only positive effects but also the potential for conflict and may, in some situations, leave the individual less able to cope with life stressors. There is also the belief that social supports are likely to be protective only in the presence of stressful circumstances.[23]

Holmes and Rahe (1967) defined *social stressors* as any set of circumstances the advent of which signifies or requires changes in an individual's ongoing life pattern.[24] According to this definition, exposure to social stresses does not cause disease but may alter the individual's susceptibility at a particular time and may therefore serve as a precipitating factor. A Schedule of Recent Experiences, developed by Holmes and Rahe, is an instrument used to measure recent life experiences. The scale lists 43 life changes (*e.g.*, promotion, divorce, being fired) to which subjects respond by indicating how many times in the preceding year each event has occurred. Each event is rated with a score, and the sum of these scores is used to determine the amount of stress associated with recent life change events.

In summary, physiologic adaptation involves the ability to maintain the constancy of the internal environment within a wide range of changes in the internal and external environments. It involves control systems that regulate cellular function, control life's processes, and integrate the function of the different body systems. Adaptation is affected by a number of factors including experience and previous learning, the rapidity with which the need to adapt occurs, genetic endowment and age, health status, nutrition, circadian rhythms, and psychosocial factors.

■ Treatment of Stress

Stress is a normal part of everyday life. However, excessive or inappropriate stress responses can disrupt normal functioning and contribute to the production of disease. Among the nonpharmacologic methods used to assist individuals in controlling the manifestations of the stress response are biofeedback, relaxation, and imagery.

Biofeedback

Biofeedback is a technique in which an individual learns to control physiologic functioning. It involves electronic monitoring of one or more physiologic responses to stress with immediate feedback of the specific response to the person undergoing treatment. Basmajian defined biofeedback as "the technique for using equipment (usually elecronic) to reveal to human beings some of their internal physiological events, normal and abnormal, in the form of visual and auditory signals in order to teach them to manipulate these otherwise involuntary or unfelt events by manipulating the displayed signal."[25]

Several types of responses are currently used: the electromyographic (EMG), electrothermal, and electrodermal (EDR). The EMG response involves the measurement of electrical potentials from muscles, usually the forearm extensor or frontalis. This is used to gain control over contraction of striated skeletal muscles that occurs with anxiety and tension. The electrothermal sensors monitor the skin temperature of the fingers or toes. The sympathetic nervous system exerts significant control over blood flow to the distal parts of the body such as the digits of the hands and feet. Consequently, anxiety is often manifested by a decrease in the skin temperature of the digits of the hands and feet. The EDR sensors measure tonic or phasic changes in the electrical activity or conductivity of the skin (usually the hands) in response to anxiety. Fearful and anxious persons often have cold and clammy hands, which leads to a decrease in conductivity.

Biofeedback is used to treat anxiety and tension in conditions such as vascular and tension headaches, Raynaud's disease, and low back pain.

Relaxation

Practices for evoking the relaxation response are numerous. They are found in virtually every culture, and are credited with a generalized decrease in sympathetic nervous system activity and in musculoskeletal tension. According to Benson, four elements are integral to the various relaxation techniques: (1) a repetitive mental device, (2) a passive attitude, (3) decreased muscle tonus, and (4) a quiet environment. Benson developed a simple noncultural method that is commonly used for achieving relaxation. The instructions for this technique are as follows:

> Sit quietly in a comfortable position. Close your eyes. Deeply relax all your muscles, beginning at your feet and progressing up to your face. Keep them deeply relaxed.
>
> Breathe through your nose. Become aware of your breathing. As you breathe out, say the word "one" silently to yourself. Continue for 20 minutes. You may open your eyes to check the time, but do not use an alarm. When you are finished, sit quietly for several minutes, at first with closed eyes and later with open eyes.
>
> Do not worry about whether you are successful in achieving a deep level of relaxation. Maintain a positive attitude and permit relaxation to occur at its own pace. Expect distracting thoughts, ignore them, and continue repeating "one."
>
> Practice the technique once or twice daily, but not within two hours after a meal, since the digestive processes seem to interfere with elicitation of the anticipated changes.[26]

Progressive muscle relaxation, originally developed by Edmund Jacobson, is another method of relieving tension.[27] His procedure consisted of approximately 50 training sessions. Jacobson's methods have been modified by a number of therapists in an effort to increase their efficiency and practicality.[28,29] Progressive muscle relaxation involves the systematic contraction and relaxation of major muscle groups (typically, 15 groups are used initially). As the person learns to relax, the various muscle groups are combined. Eventually, the person learns to relax individual muscle groups without first contracting them.[30]

Imagery

Imagery is another technique that can be used to achieve relaxation. One method is scene visualization, in which the person is asked to sit back, close the eyes, and concentrate on a scene narrated by the therapist. Whenever possible all five senses are involved; the person is asked to see, feel, smell, hear, and taste aspects of the visual experience. Other types of imagery involve imaging the appearance of each of the major muscle groups and how they feel during tension.

In summary, stress is a normal part of everyday living. However, when the stress response is excessive or inappropriate, it can disrupt the body function and contribute to disease production. Nonpharmacologic methods used in the treatment of stress include biofeedback, relaxation, and imagery. Biofeedback involves the electronic monitoring of one or more physiologic responses with immediate feedback of the response to the person undergoing treatment. Relaxation involves physical and mental exercises to achieve mental relaxation and a decrease in muscle tension. Imagery uses scene visualization as a means of controlling the stress response.

■ Study Guide

☐ After you have studied this chapter, you should be able to meet the following objectives:

☐ State Selye's definition of stress.

☐ Define the term *stressor*.

☐ Cite two factors that influence the nature of the stress response.

☐ Compare specific and nonspecific stress responses.

☐ Explain the interaction of the nervous system structures in mediating the stress response.

☐ Describe the stress responses of the autonomic nervous system, the hypothalamus-pituitary-adrenal axis, the immune system, and the musculoskeletal system.

☐ Explain the purpose of adaptation.

☐ Describe the components of a simple control system.

☐ Describe the function of a negative feedback system.

☐ Cite Cannon's four features of homeostasis.

☐ List at least six factors that influence an individual's adaptive capacity.

☐ Relate experience and previous learning to the process of adaptation.

☐ Contrast anatomic and physiologic reserve.

☐ Describe the circadian rhythms for body temperature and cortisol.

☐ Relate the concept of entrainment to hunger.

☐ Relate the effect of social cues on the sleep-wakefulness cycle on third shift workers.

☐ Explain the methods used in biofeedback training.

☐ Describe the four factors that are involved in various relaxation techniques.

☐ Contrast relaxation exercises with the methods used in imagery.

■ References

1. Burchfield SR: The stress response: A new perspective. Psychosom Med 41:661, 1979
2. Hartmann F: An anthropological consideration of the stress response Contrib Nephrol 30:7, 1982
3. Selye H: The evolution of the stress concept. Am Sci 61:692, 1973

4. Mason JW: The re-evaluation of the concept of non-specificity in stress theory. J Psychiatr Res 7:323, 1971

5. Cohen F: Stress and bodily illness. Psychiatr Clin North Am 4, No. 2:269, 1981

6. Berne RM, Levy MN: Physiology. St. Louis, CV Mosby, 1983

7. Selye H: Stress Without Distress, p 6 New York, JB Lippincott, 1974

8. Dworkin SF: Psychosomatic concepts and dentistry: Some perspectives. J Peridontol 40:647, 1969

9. Solomon GF, Amkraut GF: Psychoneuroendocrinological effects on the immune response. Annu Rev Microbiol 35:155-184, 1981

10. Dubos R: Man Adapting, pp 256, 258, 261, 264 New Haven, Yale University Press, 1965

11. Cannon WB: The Wisdom of the Body, pp 299–300. New York: WW Norton, 1932

12. Guyton A: Textbook of Medical Physiology, 6th ed. Philadelphia, WB Saunders, 1980

13. Aschoff J: Circadian systems in man and their implications. Hosp Pract 11, No. 5:51, 1976

14. Halberg F: Implications of biological rhythms for clinical practice. Hosp Pract 12, No. 1:139, 1977

15. Wagner DR, Weitzman ED: Neuroendocrine secretion and biological rhythms in man. Psychiatr Clin North Am 3, No. 2:223, 1980

16. Wehr TA, Muscettola G, Goodwin FK et al: Phase advance of the circadian sleep-wake cycle as an antidepressant. Science 206:710, 1979

17. Arendt J, Marks V: Physiological changes underlying jet lag. Br Med J 284:144, 1982

18. Ortmeyer CF: Variations in mortality, morbidity, and health care by marital status. In Erhardt CE, Berlin JE (eds). Mortality and Morbidity in the United States. Cambridge, Harvard University Press, 1974

19. Gove WR: Sex, marital status, and mortality. Am J Soc 79:45, 1973

20. Greenblatt M, Becerra RM, Serafetinides EA: Social networks and mental health: An overview. Am J Psychiatr 139, No. 8:977, 1982

21. Berkman LF, Syme S: Social networks, host resistance, and morality: A nine-year follow-up study of Alameda County Residents. Am J Epidemiol 109:186, 1979

22. House JS, Robbins C, Metzner HL: The association of social relationships and activities with morality: Prospective evidence from the Tecumseh Community Health Study. Am J Epidemiol 116:123, 1982

23. Kaplan BH, Cassel J, Gore S: Social support and health. Med Care 15, No. 5 (Supplemental):48, 1977

24. Holmes TH, Rahe RH: The social readjustment rate scale. J Psychosom Res 11:213, 1967

25. Basmajian J: Biofeedback—Principles and Practice for Clinicians. Baltimore, Williams & Wilkins, 1979

26. Benson H: Systemic hypertension and the relaxation response. N Engl J Med 296, No. 20:1152, 1977

27. Jacobson E: Progressive Relaxation Chicago, University of Chicago Press, 1958

28. Wolpe J: The Practice of Behavior Therapy. New York, Pergamon, 1973

29. Nigl A, Fischer-Williams M: Treatment of musculo-ligamentous low back strain with electromyographic biofeedback and relaxation training. Psychosomatics 21:495, 1980

30. Fischer-Williams M, Nigl AF, Sovine DL: A Textbook of Biological Feedback. New York, Human Science Press, 1981

■ Additional References

Circadian rhythms

Bassler SF: The origins and development of biological rhythms. Nurs Clin North Am 11:575, 1976

Mann S, Millar Craig MW, Melville DI, et al. Physical activity and the circadian rhythm of blood pressure. Clin Sci 27:291s, 1979

Minors DS, Waterhouse JM: Circadian Rhythms and the Human. Boston, Wright PSG, 1981

Moore-Ede MC, Czeisler CA, Richardson GS: Circadian timekeeping in health and disease: Basic properties of circadian pacemakers. N Engl J Med 309:469, 1983

Moore-Ede MC, Czeisler CA, Richardson GS: Circadian timekeeping in health and disease: Clinical implications of circadian rhythmicity. N Engl J Med 309:530, 1983

Smolensky MH, Reinberg A: The chronotherapy of corticosteroids: Practical application of chronobiologic findings to nursing. Nurs Clin North Am 11:609, 1976

Stephens GJ: Periodicity in mood, affect, and instinctual behavior. Nurs Clin North Am 11:595, 1976

Surowiak JF: Circadian rhythms. Med Biol 56:117, 1978

Takahashi JS, Zatz M: Regulation of circadian rhythmicity. Science 217:1104, 1982

Tom CK: Nursing assessment of biological rhythms. Nurs Clin North Am 11:621, 1976

Weitzman ED: Biologic rhythms and hormone secretion patterns. Hosp Pract 11, No 8:79, 1976

Winfree AT: Circadian timing of sleepiness in man and woman. Am J Physiol 243:R193, 1982

Zucker I: Light, behavior, and biologic rhythms. Hosp Pract 11, No. 10:83, 1976

Stress

Brown GM, Seggie J: Neuroendocrine mechanisms and their implications for psychiatric research. Psychiatr Clin North Am 3:205, 1980

Davenport HW: Signs of anxiety, rage or distress. Physiologist 24:1, 1981

Donnelly GF: The simplest relaxation technique of all. RN 11:29, 1980

Everly GS, Rosenfeld R: The Nature and Treatment of the Stress Response. New York, Plenum, 1983

Haggerty RJ: Breaking the link between stress and illness in children. Postgrad Med 74:287, 1983

Haskett RF, Rose RM: Neuroendocrine disorders and psychopathology. Psychiatr Clin North Am 4:239, 1981

Rose RM: Endocrine responses to stressful psychological events. Psychiatr Clin North Am 3:251, 1980

Sachar EJ, Asnis G, Halbreich U, Nathan RS, Halpern F: Recent studies in the neuroendocrinology of major depressive disorders. Psychiatr Clin North Am 3:313, 1980

Selye H: Confusion and controversy in the stress field. J Human Stress 6:37, 1975

Stein M: A biophysical approach to immune function and medical disorders. Psychiatr Clin North Am 4:203, 1981

Strain GW: Nutrition, brain function and behavior. Psychiatr Clin North Am 4:253, 1981

Timmreck TC, Braza GF, Mitchell JH: Stress and aging. Geriatrics 6:113, 1980

Winogrod IR: Health, stress, and coping in the elderly. Wis Med J 81:27, 1982

Chapter 7

Infectious Processes

E. Ronald Wright

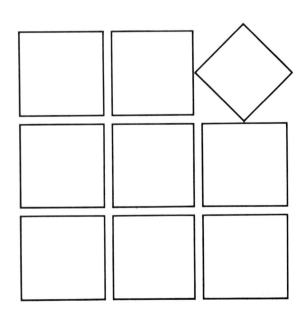

All the organisms on earth are constantly competing for the nutrients and space necessary for survival and replication. From the moment of birth until death, the human organism exists in constant contact with a myriad of life forms capable of utilizing the human body as an environment for their growth and propagation. Some of these organisms establish themselves in and on the body and are tolerated; in some cases they are encouraged at specific human body sites. These organisms make up what is termed the *normal flora* of the body. Although these organisms *infect* the body, they cause no damage because the body has developed an intricate system of excluding those organisms from potentially dangerous sites or destroying those organisms that stray from their tolerated sites. These mechanisms are discussed in Chapters 8 and 9. Some organisms, however, live at the expense of the *host* and produce damaging effects on the host cells and tissues. These organisms are classified as *parasites,* and their effects are termed *infectious disease.* This chapter will investigate the basis of the dynamic relationship that exists between these foreign invaders and the host organism.

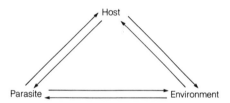

Figure 7-1 *The interactive host–parasite–environment triad. Each member of the triad exerts an effect on the other two members of the interaction.*

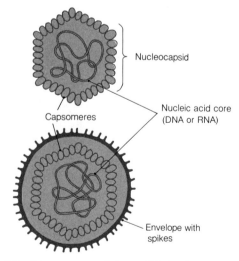

Figure 7-2 *The structure of viruses. The basic structure of a virus includes a protein coat surrounding an inner core of nucleic acid (either DNA or RNA). Some viruses may also be enclosed in a lipoprotein outer envelope.*

■ Infectious Disease

Infectious diseases are those diseases that produce body dysfunction because of the presence of another living agent in or on the human body. The key to this definition is the occurrence of some notable dysfunction. This dysfunction may be only a minor irritation, as in the case of the common cold, or it may be devastating and life threatening, as in spinal meningitis or rabies. The agents of infectious disease are found among the microbic groups of viruses, bacteria, mycoplasmas, chlamydiae, fungi, and protozoa.

Biologic Relationships of the Infectious Process

Not all infections by microorganisms lead to infectious disease. Figure 7-1 depicts the interactive, dynamic relationship that exists between microorganisms, the host (in this case the human body), and the environment. Each member of the triad influences the other two. The genetic and physiologic characteristics of the microorganisms interplay with the genetic and physiologic characteristics of the host and the environmental factors to determine the outcome of the interaction. Most interactions between the host and the microorganisms are inoffensive; the human body simply provides an environment for the microorganism and neither host nor parasite is harmed. This relationship is referred to as *commensalism* and the microorganism is called a *commensal.* Most microorganisms found on the skin, in the gastrointestinal tract, or in the urogenital tract fit this category. Some relationships are actually beneficial to both host and parasite; such a relationship is described as *mutualism.* For instance, some bacteria of the intestinal tract synthesize vitamin K for host use.

The state of *parasitism* exists when one member of the biologic partnership produces effects that are damaging to the host. Some microorganisms are so invasive or produce such toxic substances that they invariably cause pathobiologic effects in the normal host; these organisms are termed *pathogens.* It should be kept in mind, however, that the characteristics of the host play a significant role in determining whether or not a disease occurs. In most cases of infectious disease, there is an upset of the balance in favor of the replication and spread of the microorganism over the defense mechanisms of the host. The upset may occur as a result of an increase in the parasite's pathogenicity or a reduction in the resistance of the host.

Two other types of relationships between parasite and host are also encountered: (1) the *carrier state* and (2) *opportunistic pathogenicity.* In some cases, a host may be found to be harboring an overtly pathogenic organism without that organism producing any ill effects. For example, between 15% and 25% of the population carry the bacterium *Staphylococcus aureus* in their nasal tracts or on their skin and show no symptoms of disease. *S. aureus* is capable of causing a wide variety of pathologic effects ranging from boils to pneumonia, but it produces no ill effects in the carrier. This illustrates that more data than the presence of a certain pathogen in a sample are often needed to make a diagnosis of infectious disease. In other situations an organism known as an *opportunistic pathogen,* which is not normally considered to be a pathogen, may produce pathologic effects if the conditions are right. Such organisms are routinely controlled by the host's normal resistance mechanisms, but when the resistance of the host drops or there are dramatic shifts in normal physiology, such as in diabetes mellitus, opportunistic pathogens from the normal flora or from the environment may multiply and produce disease.

Infectious Disease Agents

Viruses

Viruses are the smallest obligate intracellular parasites. They are incapable of replication outside of another living cell. They have no cellular structure but rather consist of a protein coat (capsid) around a nucleic acid core of either RNA or DNA—never both, as is found in other living cells (Fig. 7-2). Some viruses also have an envelope of lipoprotein on the outside. Viruses must enter another living cell and usurp the biosynthetic machinery of the cell to replicate new viral particles. The steps in the viral replication process are depicted in Figure 7-3. In this case, the replication of the virus leads to the lysis of the host cell and its death (*e.g.,* poliomyelitis). Some other viruses do not lyse the host cell but are continuously released through the cell membrane to infect other cells (*e.g.,* influenza). Still other viruses enter the host cell, the nucleic acid becomes integrated into the host cell chromosome, and the viruses exist within the host cell for long periods of time without harming it. This type of virus, known as a *latent virus,* may then reappear and produce symptoms months or years later. Members of the *herpesvirus* group are the best example of this phenomenon. Herpesviruses include the viruses that cause fever blisters, genital infections, chickenpox and shingles, and cytomegalovirus infections. In each case, an initial infection is followed by a period of latency and a resurgence of the infection in the same form (fever blister) or a different form (shingles) months or years later.

Bacteria

Bacteria are unicellular life forms that exhibit a structure known as *prokaryotic* (lacking a *karyon,* or nucleus). The cell described in Chapter 1 is a *eukaryotic* (true nucleus) cell. The DNA of the eukaryotic cell is complexed with proteins, arrangd in chromosomes, and located in a

membrane-bound compartment known as a nucleus. Most of the cellular functions of the eukaryotic cell are compartmentalized into organelles within the cell, for purposes such as energy-derivation and protein synthesis. The prokaryotic bacterial cell differs dramatically in structure and function. Because of these differences between bacteria and animal cells in structure, enzymes, or function, it is sometimes possible to find agents (antibiotics) that selectively inhibit the function of the bacterium without doing damage to the animal cell. The structure of the bacterial cell is depicted in Figure 7-4.

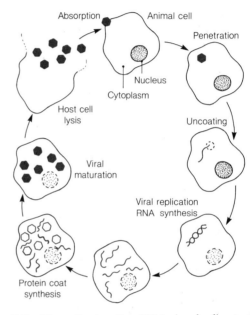

Figure 7-3 *The replication of an RNA virus leading to the lysis of the animal cell. This is the replication cycle of a cytolytic virus such as the poliovirus.*

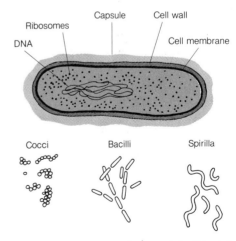

Figure 7-4 *The basic structure of a bacterial cell and the basic cell shapes found among bacteria that cause human infections.*

Bacteria are much smaller than animal cells. For purposes of comparison, refer to Figure 1-1; bacteria are about the size of the mitochondria within the cell pictured. Because of their small size and uniquely diverse metabolic capabilities, bacteria are found in virtually all inhabitable environments of the biosphere, including the human body. Some bacteria require oxygen *(aerobes)*, some require the absence of oxygen *(anaerobes)* and still others can adapt their metabolism to live in oxygen or in its absence *(facultative anaerobes)*. The varieties of bacteria are endless, and many are capable of living in the human body as commensals, as opportunistic pathogens, as overt pathogens in the carrier state, as *extracellular parasites*, or as *intracellular parasites*. Bacteria are capable of resisting many of the normal biologic defense mechanisms of the body because of the outer coverings of the *capsule* and *cell wall*. They have three basic cell shapes: spherical *(cocci)*, rod shaped *(bacilli)*, and spiral shaped *(spirilla)*. The cell shape is often used to identify bacteria. Another identifying characteristic used in classifying bacteria is the staining property of the bacteria. This property is based on the nature of the cell wall. The two most common staining procedures used to differentiate bacteria are the *Gram stain* and the *acid-fast stain*. If an organism stains pink with the Gram stain procedure it is said to be a *gram-negative* organism; if it stains purple, it is *gram-positive*. Organisms of the genus *Mycobacterium*, which includes the organisms that cause tuberculosis *(M. tuberculosis)* and leprosy *(M. leprae)*, stain red by the acid-fast stain and are said to be *acid-fast* organisms.

Mycoplasmas

Mycoplasmas are essentially bacterial cells that lack a cell wall. Because they do not have a cell wall, they may assume a variety of shapes, and compared with true bacteria, they have a severely restricted choice of environments in which they can live. They are difficult to isolate and identify. The lack of a cell wall makes them resistant to the antibiotics that kill bacteria by inhibiting cell wall synthesis, such as penicillins and cephalosporins. They are susceptible to other antibiotics, however. These microorganisms infect the surfaces and tissues of the respiratory, gastrointestinal, and urogenital tracts.

Rickettsiae and chlamydiae

Rickettsiae and chlamydiae are intracellular parasites. Their cellular structure and metabolism are similar to those of true bacteria, but they have adapted to an intracellular life that is dependent on the host cell's ability to provide nutrients and a suitable environment for their growth. The rickettsiae do not survive in the environment, and therefore they are transmitted from host to host through the bite of an arthropod vector. Their natural habitat seems to be the cells of arthropods such as

lice and ticks, and humans are only accidental hosts. Among these two groups, however, are found the causative agents for some highly dangerous diseases, such as typhus fever, Rocky Mountain spotted fever, and trachoma.

Fungi

The fungi are a diverse group of organisms, both structurally and in terms of the environments that they inhabit. The cells of the fungi are eukaryotic, and therefore their metabolism is more similar to human cell metabolism than that of bacteria. They do possess a protective cell wall, but it is different from that found in prokaryotic cells. Most fungi live as free-living cells in nature and are extremely important in the degradation and recycling of organic materials from plants and plant products. They can be divided into two basic groups, depending on cell structure: *yeasts*, which are ovoid, unicellular forms that reproduce by budding; and *molds*, which grow in long strands or filaments known as hyphae (Fig. 7-5). This division is entirely arbitrary, however, because some fungi that are pathogenic for humans can grow in either form. Such organisms are said to be *dimorphic*. The yeast form is often found in the tissues, and the mold form appears when the organism is grown in the laboratory.

Some fungal pathogens are restricted to the surfaces of the body because of their need for highly aerobic environment. These infections are referred to as *superficial mycoses* and include some commonly encountered diseases such as athlete's foot, vaginal yeast infections, and ringworm. Sometimes fungi spread into deeper tissues or throughout the body. These are called *systemic mycoses*. Examples of such infections are seen in histoplasmosis, coccidioidomycosis, and systemic candidiasis.

Protozoa

The protozoa are single-celled animals that normally exist as free-living organisms; however, a few can establish themselves in the human body. They are classified on the basis of their method of motility (cilia, ameboid movement, flagella) or lack of motility. The active, metabolizing forms of the cells are known as *trophozoites*. Most protozoan pathogens produce some type of resistant form, such as a *cyst*, to survive in the environment outside the host. Some protozoa have developed complicated life cycles involving alternating existences in the human host and the insect vector. Two diseases with worldwide distribution and enormous impact on human existence fit this description, malaria and trypanosomiasis (sleeping sickness).

Because both fungi and protozoa are eukaryotic, antibiotics that interfere with prokaryotic functions do not inhibit them. Because of the similarity in metabolic functions of eukaryotic pathogens and human host cells, the interference with the pathogen's activity by chemotherapeutic agents also produces adverse effects on host cells. This is the basis for the rather severe side-effects encountered with the use of some antifungal or antiprotozoan agents.

■ Host–Parasite Relationship

The presence or absence of infectious disease is based on the ever-changing relationship between host and parasite. Figure 7-6 is an attempt to illustrate this relationship. If the factors listed on the host side predominate, the relationship is tipped toward a healthy state, whereas an increase in the factors listed on the parasite side will push the relationship toward an expression of the symptoms of infectious disease. Chapters 8 and 9 will explore in greater detail the mechanisms associated with the host's resistance, and the factors contributing to the parasite's predominance and the resulting disease process will be explored in the remainder of this chapter.

Positive Effects of Normal Microbic Flora

In the balanced situation in which the organisms living in and on the human body are held in check by the normal host's biologic defense mechanisms, the microorganisms themselves play a significant role in maintaining that balance. Certain areas of the body are sterile, and finding organisms at such sites indicates an infectious disease.

Other areas are always colonized by a permanent resident (*endogenous*) microbic flora, which is often quite predictable in its composition (see Table 7-1). One of the primary functions of this resident population is protection against infection. This mechanism is termed *microbial antagonism,* and its importance is readily seen when patients receive extensive antibiotic therapy. When the endogenous flora of the upper respiratory tract is reduced by penicillin therapy, fungi such as the yeast *Candida albicans* may multiply on the mucous membranes of the mouth and upper respiratory tract to such a degree that serious disease results. The same phenomenon is observed when an antibiotic such as tetracycline upsets the normal microbic flora of the intestines and staphylococci gain predominance, leading to severe symptoms of gastrointestinal distress and inflammation. An upset of the normal flora may lead to a reduced supply of microbially contributed vitamins; therefore, extensive long-term antibiotic therapy may produce some degree of vitamin deficiency.

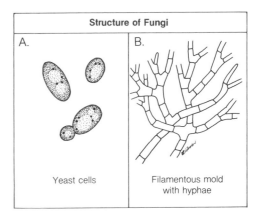

Figure 7-5 *The two shapes characteristic of fungi that infect humans.*

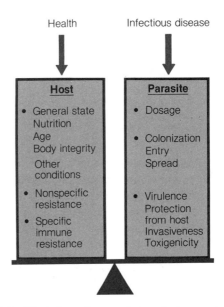

Figure 7-6 *The balance between factors: host-generated factors, which protect the host from infections, and the characteristics of the parasite, which contribute to the development of infectious disease.*

Factors Influencing the Host–Parasite Relationship

For an infectious disease to occur, a susceptible host must come into contact with sufficient numbers of the organism to establish an infection (*dosage*). The parasite must enter the host and gain access to a suitable site in the body. The infectious agent must multiply and spread. It must produce damaging effects on the host or initiate self-injuring responses from the host (*virulence*). Each of these events must occur and each event is influenced by the characteristics of both the host and the parasite.

Table 7-1   Distribution of Normal Microbic Flora

Region of Body	Sterile Areas	Nonsterile Areas	Organisms Commonly Found
Skin	None	All skin	*S. aureus, Bacillus, Corynebacterium, Mycobacterium, S. epidermidis, Streptococcus, transient environmental organisms*
Respiratory tract	Larynx, trachea, bronchi, bronchioles alveoli, sinuses	Nose, throat, mouth	*Staphylococcus, Candida, Streptococcus, Neisseria, Pneumococcus,* oral organisms
Gastrointestinal tract	Esophagus, stomach, upper small intestine	Esophagus and stomach (transiently), large intestine	Gram-negative rods, *Streptococcus, Bacteroides, Proteus, Clostridium, Lactobacillus*
Genitourinary tract	Cervix, uterus, fallopian tubes, ovaries, prostate, epididymis, testes, bladder, kidney	Exernal genitalia, anterior urethra, vagina	Skin organisms *Lactobacillus, Bacteroides*
Body fluids and cavities	Blood, pleural fluid, synovial fluid, spinal fluid, lymph	None	

Sources of the parasite

The sources of the pathogens are an important consideration in controlling infectious disease. These sources can be divided into *endogenous sources* (from organisms already present in or on the host) and *exogenous sources* (sources from the external environment).

In the hospitalized patient, one of the most common sources of infectious agents is the patient's own body. Endogenous infections usually occur when a normal flora organism is transferred from its normal habitat into an abnormal site. The organism may gain access to the new site because of the medical therapy. Thus, intestinal organisms may be introduced into the urinary tract during urinary catheterization or infect a wound following surgery. Upper respiratory tract organisms may descend the respiratory tract and cause pneumonia following intubation.

Exogenous sources of infection include *direct contact* with individuals harboring the infection. The person harboring the infection may or may not be showing the symptoms of the disease. There is little trouble in identifying the source if an individual has been exposed to an *active case* of the infection. This is the usual mode of contact with such diseases as chickenpox, whooping cough, tuberculosis, measles, herpes infections, and the common cold. It is more difficult to trace the source if direct contact has been with a *carrier* of the organism. The carrier harbors the organism without showing symptoms of the disease. Carriers can be classified into

groups: (1) *convalescent carriers,* who are recovering from an active case of the disease (typhoid, amebic dysentery, hepatitis); (2) *prodromal carriers,* who are carrying and spreading the organisms prior to the onset of the symptoms (chickenpox, influenza, common cold, infectious mononucleosis); and (3) *inapparent* or *subclinical carriers,* who have symptoms that are so slight that the presence of the disease goes completely unnoticed (gonorrhea, cytomegalovirus infections, staphylococcal infections, poliomyelitis, bacterial meningitis).

Other important sources of infectious agents include *soil, air, food, water,* and *animals.* Diseases that appear in both humans and animals are called *zoonoses,* for example, rabies, leishmaniasis, equine encephalitis, and bovine tuberculosis. Respiratory tract infections are usually encountered by the inhalation of *droplet nuclei* (small dried droplets of mucosal secretions) carrying the organism. Insects and arthropods such as mosquitoes (yellow fever, malaria, equine encephalitis), ticks (Rocky Mountain spotted fever), fleas (bubonic plague), and lice (typhus) all serve as *vectors* (carriers) of disease. Gastrointestinal tract diseases are most often acquired by ingestion of pathogen-contaminated food or water.

Dosage of the parasite

The number of parasites required to establish an infection varies from disease to disease and from host to host. Some diseases are established if only a few cells gain entrance, whereas others require contact with massive numbers of the agent. A small dosage of an extremely virulent organism might not produce disease in the normal host although a large dose would. If the host has been immunized against the agent, not even a massive dose will be infective. On the other hand, a small dose of an organism that is not especially virulent could develop into a devastating infection in the host who has been compromised by malnutrition, immunosuppression, or debilitation from some other disease or physiologic abnormality. Generally, however, the larger the dose of the pathogen, the more likely it is that an infectious disease will result.

Entry of the parasite into the host

To establish an infection, the parasite must gain access to a site in the human body that will support its growth. The surfaces of the human body present an array of defenses that must be breached or thwarted to gain such access. The epithelial tissues and mucous membranes present a formidable barrier to entrance, and few, if any, organisms can penetrate unbroken skin. The mucous membranes are protected by nonspecific substances and secreted antibodies of the immunoglobulin A (IgA) class (see Chap. 9), which are antimicrobial. The upward action of the mucous shield is ciliary movement, taking its entrapped organisms toward the mouth where the potential pathogens are swallowed and destroyed by the pH of the stomach, serving to protect the respiratory tract. The physical actions of salivation, the tearing and blinking of the eyes, and the movement of materials through and out of the intestine all provide protection to the host. The low pH of the stomach and vaginal secretions serve to inhibit the colonization of those sites by pathogens. It becomes extremely important, then, to maintain these physical and chemical barriers if infection is to be prevented. Adequate skin care and oral hygiene should not be considered simply niceties but rather as imperative for protection against infection.

Pathogens enter the body and gain access to the susceptible tissues by several routes:

1. *Breaks in the skin and mucous membranes.* Any break in the physical surface barriers is a significant site for the entrance of organisms. The break may be accidental (cuts, trauma, scratches), or it may be related to medical therapy (surgical incisions, catheterization, endoscopy) or damage to the tissues by another infection or physiologic trauma (lesions of chickenpox, bed sores, ischemic tissues).
2. *Alterations in tissue characteristics.* The tissue becomes more susceptible to invasion by pathogens when mucous membranes are allowed to dry out, when tissues become hypoxic, and when the nature of pH or normal secretions is altered.
3. *Direct contact between mucous membranes.* Some pathogens that infect the mucous membranes can be directly transmitted from an infected site to susceptible tissues. This is especially true of the infections classified as *sexually transmitted diseases*. Direct contact of the infected membranes with the uninfected membranes of the host occurs during intimate contact (kissing, genital–genital sex, oral–genital sex, or anal–genital sex).
4. *Inhalation.* The pathogens that produce respiratory tract infection (pneumonia, common cold, bronchitis, tuberculosis, influenza) and some infections of other sites (mumps, measles, chickenpox, smallpox) are most often inhaled.
5. *Ingestion.* The gastrointestinal tract becomes the point of entry for a number of infectious agents. Included among those diseases are cholera, viral gastroenteritis, traveler's diarrhea, typhoid fever, hepatitis, and poliomyelitis.

Multiplication and spread of the parasite

When the pathogen has gained access to the tissues, it does not immediately demonstrate untoward effects; rather the symptoms of the infectious process begin to appear only as the organism multiplies and spreads. In all cases, if the multiplication of the organism is prevented, there is no disease. Thus, it becomes a race between the ability of the bacterium, virus, or fungus to replicate and the ability of the host to attack and kill the pathogen.

The spread of the pathogen in the host depends on the nature of the invader and the ability of the host to isolate the infection. Some bacteria produce agents that facilitate their spread locally through the tissues (Table 7-2) by degrading the tissues or thwarting the defense mechanisms of the host. Other organisms reproduce so rapidly they simply overwhelm the host. The spread of the organism may occur by simple contiguous spread from the initial site of colonization to surrounding tissues. If the organism gains access to the lymphatic system or circulatory system, it can spread to distant sites. The finding of organisms in the blood is indicative of such a spread, which is referred to as a *viremia* (if viruses are found) or *bacteremia* (for bacteria). The agent may then invade other sites or tissues, establishing *secondary foci* of the infection. Spreading of organisms through the blood and lymph is cause for concern and indicates a less favorable prognosis. The host response to the pathogen (the inflammatory response) is designed to localize the injury and prevent its spread. Figure 7-7 illustrates the routes of spread in the human body.

Some microorganisms have characteristics that allow them to escape the primary cell-killing activity of phagocytosis during the inflammatory response. This can be accomplished by several different mechanisms. Some bacteria and yeast cells are surrounded by a *cap-

Table 7-2   Spreading and Invasive Factors of Bacteria

Factor	Genera Producing the Factor	Activity of Factor
Hyaluronidase	*Staphylococcus, Sreptococcus, Clostridium*	Degrades hyaluronic acid, a component of tissues
Coagulase	*Staphylococcus*	Clots blood, forming fibrin clots that protect the organism from phagocytosis
Hemolysin	Many bacterial genera but especially *Streptococcus, Staphylococcus,* and *Clostridium*	Lyses red blood cells
Collagenase	*Clostridium*	Digests collagen, a component of muscle and connective tissues
Fibrinolysin	*Streptococcus*	Digests fibrin clot
Leukocidin	*Staphylococcus*	Kills leukocytes
DNase	*Staphylococcus, Streptococcus*	Digests DNA, decreasing the viscosity of pus
Lecithinase	*Clostridium*	Destroys lecithin, a component of cell membranes

sule, which seems to protect the cell from recognition by the phagocyte and therefore interferes with ingestion. The importance of this mechanism is demonstrated by the observation that mutant strains of *Streptococcus pneumoniae* that have lost the ability to produce a capsule do not establish an infection, whereas encapsulated strains do. Other bacteria may be ingested by the phagocyte, but they escape degradation in the cell by resisting degradation or by producing agents *(leukocidins)* that kill the phagocyte before the parasite is destroyed. Still other bacteria are actually capable of living in the phagocyte, producing an *intracellular infection* of the cell.

Damage to the Host

The ability of the pathogen to cause host damage can be traced to one or a combination of three conditions created by the parasite: (1) direct damage produced by the multiplication and invasion of the pathogen, (2) elaboration of toxic substances, and (3) initiation of immunopathologic reactions.

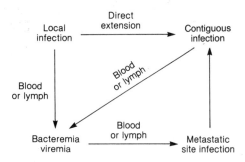

Figure 7-7   *The routes of spread of infections in the human body.*

Direct damage

The multiplication of viruses in cells leads to the loss of cell function or direct lysis (breakdown) of the cell. Cells can be rendered dysfunctional by the accumulation of viruses and viral products within the cell *(inclusion bodies)*. As these materials accumulate within the cell they interfere with normal cell metabolism and function. These inclusion bodies can be used to identify virally infected tissues and as a diagnostic tool. For example, the observation of Negri bodies in central nervous system cells provides a definitive diagnosis of rabies.

Viruses that lyse the infected cell lead to the immediate death of the cell and tissue necrosis. The severity of the disease then depends on the tissue destroyed. If the tissue is easily regenerated as in the case of epithelial tissue and cells lining the respiratory or intestinal tracts, little permanent damage is done *(e.g.,* chickenpox, common cold, influenza). If the tissue destroyed is not capable of regeneration, however, there is permanent damage *(e.g.,* paralytic poliomyelitis). The nonlysing viruses interfere with the normal cell function or alter the characteristics of the cell. These defects can produce changes ranging from inapparent infection to loss of function of the tissue infected.

Another cellular alteration of virally infected cells is the formation of *giant cells*. These abnormally large, multinucleated cells are produced by changes in the cell membranes of adjacent cells that allow the cells to fuse into *syncytial masses*. Syncytial tissues are sometimes observed in infections of measles, mumps, herpes, cytomegalovirus, and chickenpox viruses.

The role of virus infection in the development of cancer is well established but poorly understood. Certain viruses, termed *oncogenic viruses,* are capable of introducing into the host cell genetic information that alters the normal genetic expression of the cell so that the cell undergoes *transformation.* The mechanism by which this occurs has been the subject of extensive research. A unifying theory of carcinogenesis accounting for all of the diverse initiators of cancer (*e.g.,* chemicals, radiation, asbestos, toxins, viruses) is just now emerging; this is known as the *oncogene theory* (see Chap. 5). Oncogenic viruses seem to be viruses that have acquired one of the host cell *oncogenes* and incorporated it, probably accidentally, into the viral genome. In this way it becomes a carrier of genetic information that can cause the transformation of a normal cell to a *transformed,* or *cancer,* cell. Thus, by this mechanism the pathogen itself does not directly damage the host cells or tissues but rather creates conditions that are potentially devastating for the host.

The same type of situation is created by a viral agent that dramatically alters the host's immune response mechanisms, leading to a condition known as *acquired immune deficiency syndrome* (AIDS). Several pathogens can produce some degree of immunosuppression (among them tuberculosis, mumps, infectious mononucleosis) that renders the host more susceptible to secondary infections. However, in the case of AIDS, the effect of the agent is to directly alter the immune response mechanism in such a way that secondary infection (*Pneumocystis carinii pneumonia*) or malignant disease (*Kaposi's sarcoma*) are virtually ensured. Death from the secondary infection or malignancy may follow within one year of the appearance of the symptoms. The agent is probably a virus that is transmitted sexually and through blood and blood products. A human T-cell virus (lymphadenopathy-associated virus or human T-lymphotropic virus) has recently been implicated as a candidate for the causative agent of the condition.

Bacteria and fungi may release enzymes that degrade the surrounding intercellular matrix or directly lyse cells. These factors, known as *invasive factors,* allow the bacteria to spread and undermine the basic integrity of the tissues. Waste products produced during multiplication may accumulate and interfere with normal cell function. Fungi and protozoan parasites may directly lyse cells or compete for nutrients in their environment, thereby robbing cells of their normal supply of nutrients.

Toxins

Many pathogens produce *toxins,* but bacteria are especially important in this regard. Toxin production (*toxigenicity*) is the major factor determining the *virulence* (specific ability to cause disease) of many bacteria. The bacterial toxins can be divided into two general types: *exotoxins,* which are produced by the bacterial cell and released into the surrounding environment, and *endotoxins,* which are components of the cell itself, usually the cell wall material. The exotoxins cause direct effects on the cell structure and function (see Table 7-3), producing a variety of specific reactions such as blockage of nerve transmission, interference with the active transport of gut-lining cells, or lysis of red blood cells. The endotoxins, when present in sufficient amounts in the blood, exert their pathologic effects indirectly through the activation of plasma proteins, which mediate the inflammatory response. With the widespread activation of the

Table 7-3 Bacterial Exotoxins

Toxin	Toxin Producer	Action	Symptoms
Botulin	*Clostridium botulinum*	Produces neurotoxin	Double vision, difficulty in breathing and swallowing, death
Tetanus	*C. tetani*	Produces neurotoxin	Spasms, respiratory distress, death
Diphtheria	*Corynebacterium diphtheriae*	Inhibits protein synthesis	Heart damage, kidney damage, death
Staphylococcal enterotoxin	*S. aureus*	Induces vomiting	Vomiting
Erythrogenic toxin	*S. pyogenes*	Affects vasodilatation	Maculopapular rash
Exfoliatin	*S. aureus*	Induces intradermal separation	Exfoliation of skin
Choleragen	*V. cholera*	Produces water loss across gut wall	Massive diarrhea
Alpha toxin	*C. perfringens*	Splits lecithin	Hemolysis of RBCs
Anthrax	*B. anthracis*	Increases vascular permeability	Pulmonary edema, hemorrhage

complement system, kinin systems, and fibrin clot formation (see Chap. 8), progressive circulatory dysfunction occurs, which can lead to a generalized collapse known as *septic shock* (Chap. 21). This response is most often associated with a gram-negative bacteremia.

Viruses, pathogenic fungi, and protozoa are not noted for their production of toxic substances; however, some of the symptoms associated with diseases caused by these organisms are produced by the toxic effects of cellular materials released from host cells.

Immunopathologic effects

Often the symptoms that are associated with an infectious disease are not produced by the invading organisms but rather are the observable response of the body's resistance mechanisms to the presence of the organism in the host. For example, *Mycobacterium tuberculosis* is noted for being neither toxigenic nor especially invasive; however, it produces a devastating, relentlessly progressive disease in the body. The pathologic damage to the host does not come from what the bacterial cells are doing, but rather from the development of an immune response reaction known as delayed hypersensitivity (see Chap. 9), which is an allergic response. Some of the symptoms of viral infections, such as epithelial lesions and rashes, result from the immune response system's production of antibodies against viral antigens and the destruction of virally infected host cells by the cell-mediated immune response reaction. The same kinds of tissue-damaging effects are observed in rickettsial, fungal, and protozoan infections. In fact, during infection by organisms of these three groups, most of the observable tissue destruction is caused by the body's immune response reaction.

Other types of tissue-damaging effects mediated by the immune response mechanism are observed in the symptoms of *rheumatic fever* (Chap. 19) and *acute glomerulonephritis* (Chap. 29), which may follow infections of *Streptococcus pyogenes* (*e.g.,* strep throat, impetigo, cellulitis). Following an infection with certain strains of *S. pyogenes,* antibodies develop to antigens of the streptococcal cell. Those antibodies can combine with soluble streptococcal cell antigens in circulation, and the complexes then combine with complement. These complexes tend to accumulate on the basement membranes of capillaries in the renal glomeruli where they initiate an inflammatory reaction. The inflammatory reaction impairs the function of the glomeruli, producing the disease of acute glomerulonephritis. The clinical disease is not an infectious disease, as such, but rather represents an important clinical *sequela* of the primary infection.

Rheumatic fever is also a sequela of streptococcal infection. In this case, antibodies formed against certain components of the infectious agent *cross-react* with tissue antigens on the surface of myocardial (heart muscle) tissues. When the antibodies that are formed to protect against the infectious agent are carried by the circulation to the heart, they combine with the myocardial tissue antigen, bind and activate complement, and initiate an inflammatory reaction that produces the symptoms of *myocarditis.* Repeated inflammation and repair of the heart leads to damage of the heart valves through scar tissue formation and the chronic condition known as rheumatic heart disease.

■ Manifestations of Infectious Disease

The Course of Infectious Disease in the Host

Infectious diseases in the host follow different courses depending on the nature of the infecting organism and the ability of the host to respond to the presence of the infectious agent in the body. The different courses of infection are designated by the following terms: *primary acute infections, secondary acute infections, chronic infections, latent infections,* and *subclinical infections.*

Stages of infectious disease

Stages, or phases, can be recognized in the course of an infectious disease. Figure 7-8 depicts the stages of a *primary acute infection.* Although these stages are shown with lines drawn to differentiate them, there are no such clear-cut demarcations in the course of the disease in the human body. The figure plots the multiplication of the infectious agent in the body. The course of the clinical symptoms can be thought of as following the same development. The term *clinical horizon* is used to designate the appearance of definite clinically identifiable symptoms that might be associated with an infection (*e.g.,* fever, malaise, headache, rash, lesions). The line labeled *critical horizon* represents the apex of the dysfunction, system failure, or even death of the host. As will be discussed, the course (agent multiplication and degree of damage) is determined by the ability of the host to respond to the infection and destroy the infectious agent.

A *primary acute infection* is one that appears and runs its course over a short period of time, generally within a few days or weeks. Most infectious diseases fit this pattern (strep throat, the common cold, influenza, pneumonia). The outcomes of the infection in the host can be trivial (the common cold) or fatal (diphtheria). Trivial infections that normally run an uncomplicated course to resolution are also termed *self-limiting infections.* In these diseases, like the common cold, it is expected that the

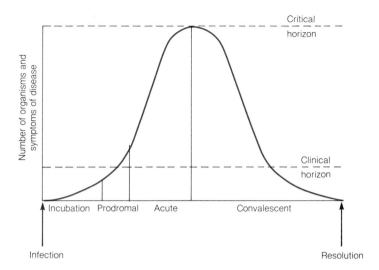

Figure 7-8 *The stages of a primary acute infection as they relate to numbers of infectious agents and severity of symptoms. The clinical horizon designates the appearance of observable symptoms of disease. The critical horizon represents the apex of dysfunction associated with the disease.*

body will respond and destroy the organism before it does significant damage.

The stages of a disease following the acute disease course are as follows:

1. *Infection*—the moment at which the pathogen enters the body.
2. *Incubation period*—the period of time between infection and the appearance of clinical symptoms of infection. For many diseases this is a very predictable period of time. In the case of chickenpox, the incubation period is usually around 12 to 14 days; for the common cold, it is 24 to 48 hours; for infectious hepatitis, it is 15 to 50 days (30 days is average). The length of the incubation period is affected by the dosage, the entry site, the virulence of the pathogen, and the immune state of the host. It is during this period that the pathogen is colonizing, multiplying, and spreading in the tissues of the host.
3. *Prodromal stage*—the period during which vague, nonspecific symptoms of infectious disease are experienced by the host. Classically, many infectious diseases begin with the same nondescript symptoms, including headache, low-grade fever, malaise, achiness, loss of appetite, and the feeling that one "is about to catch something." These symptoms are not characteristic of any specific disease. This period may take hours in a rapidly developing infection (common cold, influenza) or may persist for days in a disease with a slower progression (hepatitis, infectious mononucleosis).
4. *Acute stage*—the period of time from the appearance of symptoms specifically associated with the infection through the worsening of the condition. This is also referred to as the *active stage* of the infection. Symptoms now become correlated with the particular disease (rash, lesions, tissue damage, or dysfunction).

During this period the organism continues to multiply, releasing toxic substances and spreading.

5. *Convalescent stage*—the period of time marked by the destruction of the pathogen and the amelioration of symptoms. Once the host is able to halt the multiplication and spread of the pathogen, recovery from the disease progresses. Convalescent periods may vary in length depending on how severe the damage in the acute phase was and how quickly the host can repair the damage.
6. *Resolution*—the point at which the pathogen is no longer present in the body and repair is complete.

Figure 7-9 depicts the effects of the host's immune response and the action of antibiotic therapy on the course of a primary acute infection. Where the immune response curve intersects the line depicting the course of

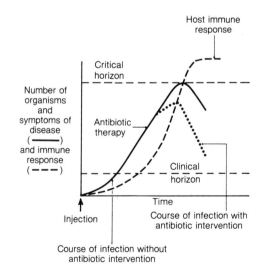

Figure 7-9 *Effects of host immune response and antibiotic therapy on the course of an infection.*

the infection, the body alters the course of infection. The more rapid and effective the host's response is, the shorter the course and the less severe the damage. If the host had already been primed to respond to the pathogen through immunization, the course of the infection would not even rise above the clinical horizon line and resolution would be early and complete. Figure 7-9 also illustrates the role of antibiotic therapy. With few exceptions, the role of an antibiotic is not to destroy the pathogen but rather to slow its multiplication and spread so that the body's own defense response can exert its effects and produce resolution. Notice that the slope of the line plotting the course of the infection is simply altered to intersect the host immune response line sooner. If the host were incapable of an immune response, the disease would continue to progress, but at a slower rate.

Variations in the course of infectious disease

Other infectious diseases may take a different course in the body. *Chronic infections* are diseases with a longer course. The initial stages of infection (incubation and prodromal periods) are the same as the primary acute infections, but the symptoms of the disease are protracted and may wax and wane depending on the state of the host. Such diseases as tuberculosis and chronic hepatitis fit this category. The course of the disease may actually drop below the clinical horizon as overt symptoms come and go. The key to these diseases is that there is no quick resolution to the infection. *Latent infections* such as herpesvirus infection or malaria have this lack of resolution in common with chronic infections; however, in latent infections the primary symptoms appear as in an acute infection and run their course. The symptoms disappear, but the organism persists in some type of cryptic form only to reemerge in an infectious form later. *Secondary acute infections* are those that follow a primary infection that has rendered the host susceptible to infection by another organism. For instance, a primary infection of a host with the influenza virus may be followed by a secondary bacterial pneumonia. Secondary infection of the chickenpox skin lesion with *Staphylococcus aureus* is also common. The *subclinical or inapparent infection* produces no observable symptoms in the host; therefore, it may be completely overlooked by the host. In some women gonorrheal or protozoan infections of the vagina produce only slight symptoms, which are easily overlooked. The significant problem of subclinical infections is that the unsuspecting host is a source of the infectious agent for others in the population.

Another group of diseases, designated *slow virus diseases,* depart from the normal pattern of viral disease in that the pathologic effects of their infection appear to proceed on a much longer time scale. Instead of the normal incubation period measured in days, or in some cases weeks, these diseases do not produce symptoms until months or years following infection. They are degenerative diseases of the central nervous system such as (1) *subacute sclerosing panencephalitis* (SSPE), which is caused by the measles virus, (2) *progressive multifocal leukoencephalopathy* (PML), caused by a papovavirus, (3) *kuru,* and (4) *Creutzfeldt-Jakob disease*. Each disease is marked by a slow, progressive involvement of more and more neurons of the central nervous system until the disease blocks normal CNS function and is fatal.

Systemic Manifestations of Infectious Disease

Depending on the nature and extent of an infection, the symptoms observed may be localized at one site or may become more generalized (systemic). Most of the systemic manifestations are the result of the nonspecific multisystem response that have been lumped under the descriptive term *inflammatory response* and are discussed in detail in Chapter 8. Infectious organisms are among the most common triggering mechanisms of inflammation, and because pathogens have the ability to multiply and spread, infections provide a persistent and ongoing source of injury to the tissues.

The classic systemic manifestations of infectious disease are *fever, leukocytosis* (or rarely *leukopenia*), *alteration of metabolic activity, cardiovascular changes, anemia,* and *malaise.*

Fever

The correlation of fever with disease has been recognized since ancient times, and although other etiologies of fever are common (trauma, immune reaction, neoplasia, tissue necrosis), when fever occurs infection is the first cause to be considered. Fever results from the chemical modification of the temperature set point in the hypothalamus mediated by the release of *endogenous pyrogens* from tissue cells, especially leukocytes. It should be noted that even though fever often accompanies infection, a large number of severe infections do not produce significant elevation of temperature. This is especially true of chronic diseases. Some diseases have specific fever patterns that can be discerned and may be of some diagnostic value.

Leukocyte response

Most acute infections caused by bacteria, fungi, and protozoa produce some degree of elevation of the total leukocyte count in the blood. This is the result of the release of substances into the circulation, which signals the mobilization of bone marrow stores of leukocytes and the acceleration of leukocyte synthesis in the bone marrow. When these stores are constantly called on, mature leukocytes begin to be depleted and less mature forms are placed in circulation. Among the leukocytes involved in inflammatory response, neutrophils make up the most important fraction (see Chap. 8). This increase is referred to as neutrophilia. As the demand for neutrophils in circulation continues to be signaled, the ability to supply mature neutrophils is soon outstripped, and immature neutrophils *(bands or stabs)* are released in an increasing proportion to the number of mature cells. In tabulating cell proportions, the column for reporting the number of immature cells has traditionally been to the left of the mature cell column, so that the slang term, *shift to the left,* is widely used to indicate the growing proportion of immature to mature cells in circulation.

Viral infections, chronic bacterial infections (tuberculosis, brucellosis, syphilis), and rickettsial infections all tend to be accompanied by an increase in the number of lymphocytes in the circulation. *Lymphocytosis,* an increase in lymphocytes, may also be a prominent feature during the convalescent phase of acute bacterial infections. In the case of whooping cough (pertussis), there is a drop in the neutrophil count *(neutropenia)* and a rise in the lymphocytes in the circulation. Table 7-4 summarizes some of the leukocyte manifestations associated with infectious diseases.

Metabolic alterations

Systemic alterations in metabolism and metabolic products can be detected during infection. Protein catabolism leading to a *negative nitrogen balance* (more protein being broken down than built up) is a common feature of both acute and chronic infections. The increase in overall metabolic demand and the lack of dietary protein replenishment is the underlying cause of this response. If this negative balance is maintained over long periods, a generalized wasting effect becomes apparent in the host. Alterations in the release and activity of the hormones controlling metabolism (corticosteroids, mineralocorticoids, growth hormone, insulin, and glucagon) lead to altered metabolism of protein and carbohydrates. Increased metabolism during fever results in increased caloric demand, disturbances of fluid and electrolyte balance, and increased respiratory rate to meet an elevated oxygen demand. If vomiting or diarrhea is present, dramatic dehydration of the host may be seen.

Cardiovascular changes

The flow, distribution, and composition of blood may be dramatically affected by the infectious process. With the elevation of body temperature, the *pulse rate* increases by approximately 10 beats/minute/degree Fahrenheit; however, in a few diseases (typhoid, mycoplasmal pneumonia, mumps, Colorado tick fever, and infectious hepatitis) the pulse rate slows. The dilation of peripheral capillary beds requires increased cardiac output to meet

Table 7-4 Leukocyte Responses to Infections

Leukocyte	Response	Associated Disease
Neutrophils	Neutrophilia	Most acute bacterial infections; many spirochete, rickettsial, viral, and protozoan systemic infections
	Neutropenia	Salmonellosis, brucellosis, pertussis, and some rickettsial, viral, and protozoan diseases
Lymphocytes	Lymphocytosis	Pertussis, tuberculosis, brucellosis, and syphilis; many rickettsial and viral infections; convalescent phase of some acute bacterial infections
Monocytes	Monocytosis	Tuberculosis, brucellosis, syphilis, and some rickettsial and protozoan infections
Eosinophils	Eosinophilia	Hypersensitivity reactions and some protozoan infections; scarlet fever

the increased volume. If the cardiac output cannot be maintained, the blood pressure falls and shock symptoms develop. The character of the blood may be altered by the appearance of *acute-phase proteins* (haptoglobin, fibrinogen, complement proteins, ceruloplasmin), whose synthesis by the liver is increased. Infection may also activate the enzymes of the coagulation cascade, which causes both thrombosis (clot formation) and consumption of the fibrin clot proteins, leading to bleeding. This condition is known as *disseminated intravascular coagulation* (DIC) (Chap. 12). In certain diseases (chronic infections and mycoplasmal infections) there may also be a pronounced *anemia* resulting from decreased red blood cell production in the bone marrow or increased destruction of cells by the spleen.

Malaise

Malaise is the generalized term used to describe the sick or bad feeling accompanying infection. There is no specific physiologic explanation for the condition. It may reflect the stresslike demands placed on the body by the altered metabolism of the host and the presence of abnormal levels of endogenous or exogenous toxic products.

■ Study Guide

After you have studied this chapter, you should be able to meet the following objectives:

☐ Define infection and infectious disease.

☐ Describe the basis of mutualism, commensalism, parasitism, carrier state, and opportunistic pathogenicity.

☐ List the groups of microorganisms that are responsible for infectious diseases.

☐ Describe the positive effects of the normal microbic flora.

☐ Describe the factors that influence the host—parasite relationship.

☐ Identify how parasites enter and spread in the human body.

☐ Describe the activities of parasites that damage the body.

☐ Describe the stages of an acute primary infection.

☐ Identify five types of infectious disease and give an example of each.

☐ Describe the systemic manifestations of infectious disease.

■ Additional References

Atkins E: Fever—New perspectives on an old phenomenon. N Engl J Med 308:958, 1983

Burnett M, White DO: Natural History of Infectious Disease. New York, Cambridge University Press, 1972

Dinarello CA, Wolff SM: Pathogenesis of fever in man. N Engl J Med 298:607, 1978

Holland JJ: Slow, inapparent and recurrent viruses. Sci Am 230:32, 1974

Karpas A: Viruses and leukemia. Am Sci 70:277, 1982

Land H, Parada LF, Weinberg RA: Cellular oncogenes and multistep carcinogenesis. Science 222:771, 1983

Lorian V: Significance of Medical Microbiology in the Care of Patients. Baltimore, Williams & Wilkins, 1977

McNeill WH: Plagues and People. Garden City, NY, Anchor Press/Doubleday, 1976

Mims CA: The Pathogenesis of Infectious Disease. New York, Academic Press, 1977

Reese PL, Dixon DM: Opportunistic mycoses. Am J Nurs 81:1160, 1981

Von Graevenitz A: The role of opportunistic bacteria in human disease. Annu Rev Microbiol 31:447, 1977

Wehrle PF, Top FH: Communicable and Infectious Diseases, 9th ed. St Louis, CV Mosby, 1981

Youmans GP, Patterson PY, Sommers HM: The Biologic and Clinical Basis of Infectious Disease, 2nd ed. Philadelphia, WB Saunders, 1980

Chapter 8

Inflammation and Repair

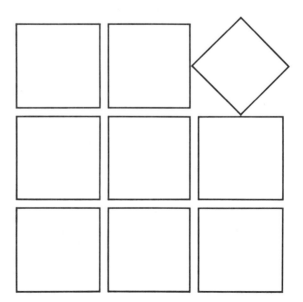

The ability of the body to sustain injury, resist attack by microbial agents, and repair damaged tissue is dependent on the inflammatory reaction, the immune response, tissue regeneration, and fibrous tissue replacement. This chapter focuses on the local manifestations of acute and chronic inflammation, the repair process, systemic signs of inflammation, and selected disease states that affect the inflammatory cells. Chapter 9 discusses the immune response.

Inflammation is the local reaction of vascularized tissue to injury.[1] Although the effects of inflammation are often viewed as undesirable because they are unpleasant and cause discomfort, the process is essentially a beneficial one that allows a person to live with the effects of everyday stress. Without the inflammatory response, wounds would not heal and minor infections would become overwhelming. On the other hand, inflammation also produces undesirable effects. The crippling effects of rheumatoid arthritis, for example, have their origin in the inflammatory response.

◼ The Inflammatory Response

The inflammatory response is closely intermeshed with wound healing and reparative processes. This process acts to neutralize or destroy the offending agent, restricts the tissue damage to the smallest possible area, alerts the individual to the impending threat of tissue injury, and prepares the injured area for healing. Wound healing and tissue repair begin during the active stages of inflammation and serve to repair the damage caused by the injurious agent.

The causes of inflammation are many and varied. Although it is quite common to equate inflammation with infection, it is important to recognize that almost all types of injury are capable of inciting the response and that only a small number of inflammatory responses are related to infections. The injurious agents that cause inflammation can arise from outside the body (*exogenous*) or from within the body (*endogenous*). Common causes of inflammation are trauma, surgery, infection, caustic chemicals, extremes of heat and cold, immune responses, and ischemic damage to body tissues.

Although the inflammatory response can be initiated by a wide variety of injurious agents, the sequence of physiologic events that follow is remarkably similar. Characteristic of the inflammatory response is that it involves *a sequence of specific physiologic behaviors that occur in response to injury by a nonspecific agent*. An acute inflammatory response will follow the same course, whether the injury is caused by a streptococcal infection or by tissue necrosis associated with myocardial infarction. The extent of the injury will vary and the site of inflammation will be different, but the tissue response and systemic manifestations will be similar. The body will, however, *use only those behaviors in the sequence that are needed to minimize tissue damage*. A small area of local swelling and redness may be sufficient to prevent injury from a mosquito bite, whereas other, more serious conditions, such as appendicitis, may incite leukocytosis, fever, and formation of an exudate.

Inflammation can be acute or chronic. Acute inflammation is the typical short-term response that is associated with all types of tissue injury. It involves hemodynamic changes, formation of an exudate, and the presence of granular leukocytes. Chronic inflammation follows a less uniform and more persistent pattern. It involves the presence of nongranular leukocytes and usually results in more extensive formation of scar tissue and deformities.

Inflammatory conditions are named by adding the suffix *itis* to the affected organ or system. For instance, neuritis refers to inflammation of a nerve, pericarditis to inflammation of the pericardium, and appendicitis to inflammation of the appendix. A further description of the inflammatory process might indicate whether the process was acute or chronic and what type of exudate was formed, for example, acute fibrinous pericarditis.

Acute Inflammation

The classic description of acute inflammation has been handed down through the ages. In the first century A.D., the Roman physician Celsus described the local reaction to injury in terms of what has come to be known as the cardinal signs of inflammation. These signs are *rubor* (redness), *tumor* (swelling), *calor* (heat), and *dolor* (pain). In the second century A.D., Galen added a fifth cardinal sign, *functio laesa* or "loss of function."

The manifestations of acute inflammation can be divided into two categories, *hemodynamic* and *white blood cell responses*. At the biochemical level, many of the responses that occur during acute inflammation are associated with the release of chemical mediators. Both the hemodynamic responses and white blood cell responses contribute to the *inflammatory exudates* that characterize the acute inflammatory response. Each of these aspects of acute inflammation is discussed separately.

Vascular response

The hemodynamic, or vascular, changes that occur with inflammation begin almost immediately following injury and are initiated by a momentary constriction of small vessels in the area. This momentary period of vasoconstriction is immediately followed by vasodilation of the arterioles and venules that supply the area. As a result, the area becomes congested and warm—the *redness* and *warmth* that are characteristic of acute inflammation.

bradykinin
prostaglandins

Accompanying this hyperemic response is an increase in capillary permeability that allows fluid to escape into the tissue and to cause *swelling*. *Pain* and *impaired function* occur as the result of tissue swelling and release of chemical mediators. The reader can simulate the hemodynamic responses that occur with acute inflammation by running the sharp edge of a fingernail along the inner aspect of the arm. The response has been termed the triple response.[2] Within seconds, the line becomes reddened. The second response is a red flare that develops on both sides of the line, which represents the hyperemic phase of the inflammatory response. Within several minutes, the line usually becomes slightly raised, because of swelling resulting from an increase in capillary permeability. The flare response that occurs with this type of stimulus is highly variable; some persons will have only a slight response while others will have an exaggerated one.

The hemodynamic changes that occur during the early stages of inflammation are beneficial in that they aid in controlling the effects of the injurious agent. During this stage, the exudation of fluid out of the capillary into the tissue spaces helps *dilute* the toxic and irritating agents. Sometime later, white blood cells accumulate in the area and leave the capillary as part of the exudate. As fluid moves out of the capillary, *stagnation* of flow and *clotting* of blood in the small capillaries that supply the inflamed area occur. This aids in *localizing* the effects of the injury.

Depending on the severity of injury, the hemodynamic changes that occur with the inflammatory reaction follow one of three patterns of response. The first is an immediate transient response that occurs with minor injury. The second is an immediate sustained response that occurs with more serious injury and continues for several days. With this response there is actual damage to the vessels in the area. The third type of response is a delayed response—the increase in capillary permeability is delayed for a period of 4 to 24 hours. A delayed response often accompanies radiation types of injuries, such as a sunburn.

Cellular response

The cellular stage of acute inflammation is marked by movement of white blood cells (leukocytes) into the area of injury. This stage includes (1) the margination or pavementing of white blood cells, (2) emigration of white blood cells, (3) chemotaxis, and (4) phagocytosis. A description of white blood cells precedes the discussion of cellular events that occur in acute inflammation.

Leukocytes. The leukocytes, or white blood cells, develop from the primordial stem cells that are located in the bone marrow and lymphoid tissue. The leukocytes are larger and less numerous than the red blood cells.

There are two types of white blood cells, granular and nongranular leukocytes. The different types of leukocytes are illustrated in Figure 8-1.

Granular leukocytes. The granular leukocytes are identifiable because of their cytoplasmic granules and are commonly referred to as granulocytes. In addition to their cytoplasmic granules, these white blood cells have distinctive multilobar nuclei (Fig. 8-1). The granulocytes are divided into three types (neutrophils, eosinophils, and basophils) according to the staining properties of the granules.

The *neutrophils*, which constitute 60% to 70% of the total number of white blood cells, have granules that are neutral and hence do not stain with either an acid or a basic dye. Because these white cells have nuclei that are divided into three to five lobes, they are often called *polymorphonuclear leukocytes (PMNs)*. The neutrophils are the first cells to arrive at the site of inflammation, usually appearing within 90 minutes of injury. Neutrophils increase greatly during the inflammatory process. When this happens, immature forms of neutrophils are released from the bone marrow. These immature cells are often called *bands* or *stabs* because of the horseshoe shape of their nuclei. The neutrophils have a life span of only about 10 hours and therefore must be constantly replaced if their numbers are to be adequate.

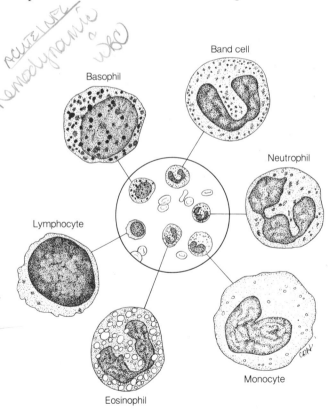

acute inflammation hemodynamic a WBC

Figure 8-1 *White blood cells that are involved in the inflammatory response.*

The cytoplasmic granules of the *eosinophils* stain red with the acid dye eosin. These leukocytes constitute 1% to 3% of the total number of white blood cells and increase during allergic reactions and parasitic infections. It is thought that they detoxify the agents or chemical mediators associated with allergic reactions and assist in terminating the response.

The granules of the *basophils* stain blue with a basic dye. These cells constitute only about 0.3% to 0.5% of the white blood cells. The granules in the basophils contain heparin and histamine and are similar to those of the mast cells. The basophils are thought to be involved in allergic and stress responses.

Nongranular leukocytes.   There are two groups of nongranular leukocytes, the monocytes and the lymphocytes. The *monocytes* are the second order of cells to arrive at the inflammation site and their arrival usually requires 5 hours or more. Within 48 hours, however, the monocytes are usually the predominant cell type in the inflamed area. Monocytes are the largest of the white blood cells and constitute about 3% to 8% of the total leukocyte count. The circulating life span of the monocyte is three to four times longer than that of the granulocytes, and these cells survive for a longer period of time in the tissues. The monocytes, which are phagocytic cells, are often referred to as *macrophages*. The monocytes engulf larger and greater quantities of foreign material than the neutrophils. These leukocytes play an important role in chronic inflammation and are also involved in the immune response. When the monocyte leaves the vascular system and enters the tissue spaces, it becomes known as a *histiocyte*. Histiocytes function as macrophages in the inflamed area. They can also proliferate to form a capsule, enclosing foreign material that cannot be digested.

The *lymphocytes* constitute 20% to 30% of the white blood cell count. There are two types of lymphocytes, B cells and T cells. The B cells form plasma cells and they are concerned with antibody formation. The T cells are concerned with cell-mediated immunity. Both types of lymphocytes play a major role in immunity and are discussed in Chapter 9.

Margination and pavementing of leukocytes.   During the early stages of the inflammatory response, fluid leaves the capillaries of the microcirculation causing blood viscosity to increase. As this occurs, the leukocytes begin to *marginate*, or move to the periphery of the blood vessel. As the process continues, the marginated leukocytes begin to adhere to the vessel lining in preparation for emigration from the vessel. The cobblestone appearance of the vessel lining due to margination of leukocytes has led to the term *pavementing*.

Emigration of leukocytes.   Emigration is a mechanism whereby the leukocytes extend *pseudopodia* (false feet), pass through the capillary walls by ameboid movement, and then migrate into the tissue spaces. The movement of red and white blood cells through the wall of the capillary is called *diapedesis*. Along with the emigration of leukocytes, there is also an escape of red cells from the capillary. The red cells may escape singly or in small jets at points where the capillaries have become distended.

Chemotaxis.   The leukocytes, after emigrating through the vessel wall, wander through the tissue space being guided by the presence of bacteria and cellular debris. The process by which leukocytes are attracted to bacteria and cellular debris is called *chemotaxis*. Chemotaxis can be positive or negative, meaning that it can act to either attract or repel the leukocytes. Many substances are capable of acting as chemotaxic agents, including infectious organisms, plasma-protein fractions (complement), and tissue debris.

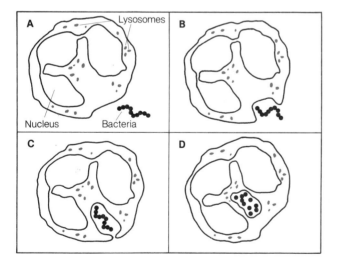

Figure 8-2 *Phagocytosis by a neutrophil. In A, a neutrophil that has emigrated from the capillary; in B, it is attracted to the bacteria through chemotaxis; and in C, it engulfs the bacteria. D shows the final stages of phagocytosis: the bacteria are degraded by the enzymes and digestive materials that are contained in the cytoplasmic granules of the neutrophil.*

Phagocytosis.   In the final stage of the cellular response, the neutrophils and monocytes engulf and degrade the bacteria and cellular debris in a process called *phagocytosis* (Fig. 8-2). The neutrophils are sometimes called *microphages* because they concentrate on the phagocytosis of bacteria and small particles. The monocytes, or *macrophages*, remove tissue debris and larger particles from the area of inflammation.

Leukocytosis. Leukocytosis refers to an increase in white blood cell numbers. Acute inflammatory conditions, particularly those of bacterial origin, are accompanied by marked increases in white blood cell numbers with a disproportionate increase seen in the neutrophilic count. A differential blood count measures both the total number of white blood cells and the percentage of each type of blood cell. Table 8-1 compares the normal white blood cell count with that sometimes seen in an acute infection.

The reticuloendothelial system. In addition to the mobile white cells that circulate in the bloodstream, there are nonmobile phagocytic cells that are widely scattered throughout the body. These cells are collectively referred to as the reticuloendothelial system. There are the Kupffer cells in the liver sinusoids, the alveolar macrophages, the microglia of the brain, and the macrophages located in the spleen, bone marrow, and lymphoid tissues. These cells ingest the debris of dead cells, bacteria, and inert foreign matter. The lymphoid organs (lymph nodes, spleen, and tonsils) are discussed in Chapter 9.

Inflammatory mediators

Although inflammation is precipitated by injury and cell death, its signs and symptoms are produced by chemical mediators such as histamine, the plasma proteases, prostaglandins, slow-reacting substance of anaphylaxis, and other neutrophil and lymphocyte factors. Other mediators have been identified, but their role in the inflammatory process is still unclear. The chemical mediators are stored in inactive form in various body cells such as neutrophils, basophils, mast cells, and platelets. The process of mediator activation requires a number of sequential steps that control the reaction and prevent the process from occurring by chance. If this were not true, most of us would be constantly covered with swollen and reddened areas over much of our bodies. Table 8-2 describes the prominent manifestations of inflammation and the chemical substances that mediate their occurrence.

Histamine. Histamine is widely distributed throughout the body. It can be found in platelets, basophils, and mast cells. Histamine causes dilatation of arterioles and enhanced permeability of capillaries and venules. It is the first mediator in the initial inflammatory response. Antihistamine drugs suppress this immediate transient response that is induced by mild injury.

Plasma proteases. The plasma proteases consist of the kinins, complement and its fractional components, and clotting factors. One of the kinins, bradykinin, causes increased capillary permeability and pain. The complement system consists of a number of component proteins and their cleavage products. These substances interact with the antigen-antibody complexes and mediate immunologic injury and inflammation (see Chap. 9). The clotting system is discussed in Chapter 12.

Prostaglandins. The prostaglandins, so named because they were first identified in the prostate gland, are ubiquitous tissue proteins composed of lipid-soluble acids derived from arachidonic acid, which is stored in cell membrane phospholipids. The synthesis of prostaglandins occurs in two stages: (1) arachidonic acid is liberated from the phospholipids of the cell membrane and (2) then converted to prostaglandins. This second stage requires the enzyme cyclo-oxygenase. Prostaglandins contribute to vasodilation, capillary permeability, and the pain and fever that accompany inflammation. There are a number of prostaglandins. The stable prostaglandins (PGE-1 and PGE-2) induce inflammation and potentiate the effects of histamine and other inflammatory mediators. The prostaglandin thromboxane A-2

Table 8-1 Example of a Normal White Blood Count (WBC) Compared with White Blood Count During an Acute Infection

	Normal	Acute Infection
Total WBC (cells per mm³)	5,000–10,000	16,000–18,000
Polymorphonuclear leukocytes (PMNs, %)	69	85
Stabs (% of PMNs)	—	12
Lymphocytes (%)	29	14
Monocytes (%)	2	1

Table 8-2 Signs of Inflammation and Corresponding Chemical Mediators

Inflammatory Response	Chemical Mediator
Swelling, redness, and tissue warmth (vasodilatation and capillary permeability)	Histamine Prostaglandins Bradykinin
Tissue damage	Neutrophil, macrophage, and lysosomal enzymes
Chemotaxis	Complement fractions
Pain	Prostaglandins Bradykinin
Fever	Prostaglandins Endogenous pyrogens
Leukocytosis	Leukocyte-stimulating factor

promotes platelet aggregation and vasoconstriction. Prostacycline (PGI-2) has the opposite effect. It relaxes vascular smooth muscle and inhibits platelet aggregation. Drugs such as aspirin and indomethacin (a nonsteroidal, anti-inflammatory drug) inhibit prostaglandin synthesis by suppressing cyclo-oxygenase activity. The glucocorticoid hormones secreted from the adrenal cortex (or given as a drug) are known to curtail the availability of arachidonic acid for prostaglandin production.[3] The glucocorticoid drugs have come to be known as anti-inflammatory drugs because of their ability to suppress the inflammatory response.

Leukotrienes.   The leukotrienes are a group of chemical mediators that are capable of inciting the inflammatory response. Their name was chosen because they were discovered on the leukocyte and they have a chemical triene structure. One of the leukotrienes, the slow-acting substance of anaphylaxis, causes slow and sustained constriction of the bronchioles and is an important inflammatory mediator in bronchial asthma and immediate hypersensitivity reactions (see Chap. 10). The leukotrienes have also been reported to have an effect on the permeability of the postcapillary venules; adhesion properties of the endothelial cells; extravasation of the white blood cells; and chemotaxis of polymorphonuclear cells, eosinophils, and monocytes.[4] Like the prostaglandins, the leukotrienes are formed from arachidonic acid but utilize the lipoxygenase pathway that involves the enzyme lipoxygenase. Thus, it now appears that prostaglandins and leukotrienes are part of a larger biologic control system based on arachidonic acid. Depending on the active enzymes in the stimulated cell, arachidonic acid can be converted to several biologically active compounds, which regulate various cellular responses to injury.

Neutrophil and lymphocyte products.   The neutrophils and lymphocytes contribute a number of mediators to the inflammatory process. The neutrophils release mediators that increase vascular permeability, act as a chemotactic factor for monocytes, and cause tissue damage. Much of the tissue damage done during the acute inflammatory process is caused by the lysosomal enzymes of the neutrophil. The lymphocytes release mediators called lymphokines. These mediators have numerous actions including chemotaxis of macrophages, neutrophils, and basophils.

Inflammatory exudates

Characteristically the acute inflammatory response involves production of exudates. These exudates can vary in terms of fluid, plasma protein, and cell content. Acute inflammation can produce serous, fibrinous, membranous, purulent, and hemorrhagic exudates. Inflammatory exudates are often composed of a combination of these types.

Serous exudate.   The initial exudate that enters the inflammatory site is largely plasma. Serous drainage is a watery exudate that is low in protein content. A blister contains serous fluid. A catarrhal inflammation is one that affects the mucous membranes and is associated with an increase in watery secretions and desquamation of the epithelial cells. Hay fever is an example of a catarrhal inflammatory response.

Fibrinous exudate.   Fibrinous exudates contain large amounts of fibrinogen and form a thick and sticky meshwork, much like the fibers of a blood clot. Fibrinous exudates are frequently encountered in the serous cavities of the body. Acute rheumatic fever often causes development of a fibrinous pericarditis. A fibrinous exudate must be removed through fibrinolytic activity of enzymes before healing can take place. Failure to remove the exudate leads to ingrowth of fibroblasts and subsequent development of scar tissue and adhesions. A fibrinous exudate may be beneficial in that it tends to glue the inflamed structures together thereby preventing the spread of infection. In appendicitis, for example, the initial formation of a fibrous exudate serves to localize the organisms in the region of the appendix and thus prevents the generalized spread of the infection to the peritoneal cavity.

Membranous exudate.   Membranous or pseudomembranous exudates develop on mucous membrane surfaces. The development of a membranous exudate occurs as necrotic cells become enmeshed in a fibropurulent exudate that coats the mucosal surface. *Diphtheria* was known for its ability to produce a membranous exudate on the surface of the trachea and major bronchi. *Thrush* is a monilial infection of the oral cavity that produces patches of membranous inflammation. *Membranous enterocolitis* is a severe membranous inflammatory condition of the bowel mucosa that is related to a disturbance in the normal bowel flora due to treatment with a variety of broad-spectrum antibiotics.

Purulent exudate.   A purulent (suppurative) exudate contains pus, which is composed of the remains of white blood cells, proteins, and tissue debris. Purulent infections are caused by a number of pyogenic or pus-forming bacteria. An *abscess* is a localized collection of pus. Abscesses may occur at the site of injury, or they may develop as the result of metastatic spread of infectious organisms and tissue debris through the bloodstream. An abscess is encapsulated in a so-called pyogenic membrane that consists of layers of fibrin, inflammatory cells, and granulation tissue. An abscess may need to be incised and the pus removed before healing can occur.

Cellulitis, or phlegmonous inflammation, is a subgroup of suppurative infections that involve massive necrosis of tissue along with production of purulent infiltrates. Instead of producing small localized collections of pus, certain pyogenic organisms (usually the streptococci) elaborate a large amount of spreading factor, the *hyaluronidases*, which break down the fibrin meshwork and other barriers designed to localize the infection.

Hemorrhagic exudate.   A hemorrhagic exudate occurs in situations in which severe tissue injury causes damage to blood vessels or when there is diapedesis of red blood cells from the capillaries. Often a hemorrhagic exudate accompanies other forms of exudate. A *serosanguineous* exudate describes a combination of serous and hemorrhagic exudates.

Resolution of acute inflammation

Acute inflammation can be resolved in one of three ways: (1) it can undergo resolution, with the injured area returning to normal or near-normal appearance and function; (2) it can progress, and suppurative processes may develop; or (3) it can proceed to the chronic phase. In the process of responding to injury, the body will use only those behaviors in the inflammatory sequence that are necessary to prevent or halt the destruction of tissue.

Chronic Inflammation

To this point, we have discussed acute inflammation associated with a self-limiting stimulus, such as a burn or infection, that is rapidly controlled by host defenses. Chronic inflammation, on the other hand, is self-perpetuating and may last for weeks, months, or even years. It may develop in the course of a recurrent or progressive acute inflammatory process or as the result of a low-grade smoldering response that fails to evoke an acute response. Characteristic of chronic inflammation is an infiltration by mononuclear cells (macrophages, lymphocytes, and plasma cells) rather than neutrophils, such as occurs in acute inflammation. Chronic inflammation also involves the proliferation of fibroblasts rather than exudates. As a result, the risk of scarring and deformity developing is usually considerably greater than in acute inflammation.

In contrast to agents that provoke sufficient initial tissue injury to evoke the acute inflammatory response, agents that evoke chronic inflammation are typically low-grade persistent irritants that are unable to penetrate deeply or spread rapidly. Among the causes of chronic inflammation are foreign bodies such as talc, silica, asbestos, and certain surgical suture materials. Many viruses provoke chronic inflammatory response, as do certain bacteria, fungi, and larger parasites of moderate to low virulence. Examples are the tubercle bacillus, the treponema of syphilis, and the actinomyces. The presence of injured or altered tissue, such as that surrounding a tumor or healing fracture, may also incite chronic inflammation. In many cases of chronic inflammation, such as sarcoidosis, the inciting agent is unknown. Little is known about the mediators of the chronic inflammatory response. Immunologic mechanisms are thought to play an important role in chronic inflammation.[5]

There are two patterns of chronic inflammation: (1) a nonspecific chronic inflammation and (2) granulomatous inflammation.

Nonspecific chronic inflammation

Nonspecific chronic inflammation involves a diffuse accumulation of macrophages and lymphocytes at the site of injury. Macrophages are accumulated from three sources: (1) continued recruitment of monocytes, the precursors of tissue macrophages, from the circulation in response to chemotaxic factors; (2) local proliferation of macrophages after they have left the bloodstream; (3) prolonged survival and immobilization of macrophages within the inflammatory site.[1] These mechanisms lead to fibroblast proliferation with subsequent scar formation that, in many cases, replaces normal supporting connective tissue elements or functional parenchymal tissue of the involved structure. For example, scar tissue resulting from chronic inflammation of the bowel causes narrowing of the bowel lumen, and in chronic glomerulonephritis there is a loss of functional nephrons.

Granulomatous inflammation

A granulomatous lesion is a form of chronic inflammation. A granuloma is typically a small, 1-mm to 2-mm lesion in which there is a massing of macrophages surrounded by lymphocytes. These modified macrophages resemble epithelial cells and are sometimes called *epithelioid cells*. Like other macrophages, the epithelioid cells that form a granuloma are derived from blood monocytes. Granulomatous inflammation is associated with foreign bodies such as splinters, sutures, silica, and talc particles, and with microorganisms such as those that cause tuberculosis, syphilis, sarcoidosis, deep fungal infections, and brucellosis. These types of agents have one thing in common—they are poorly digestible and are usually not easily controlled by other inflammatory mechanisms.

The epithelioid cells in granulomatous inflammation may either clump in a mass (granuloma) or coalesce, forming a large multinucleated giant cell that attempts to surround the foreign agent. Some giant cells may contain as many as 200 nuclei. A giant cell is usually surrounded by granuloma cells, and a dense membrane of connective tissue eventually encapsulates the lesion and isolates it. A tubercle is a granulomatous inflammatory response to the tubercle bacillus. Peculiar to the tuberculosis granuloma is the presence of a caseous (cheesy) necrotic center. In the past, surgical gloves were dusted with talc so they could be slipped on easily, but particles of talc frequently ended up in the surgical field and caused granulomatous lesions to develop. Surgical gloves are now dusted with an absorbable starch that does not cause this problem.

In summary, inflammation describes a local response to tissue injury and can present as an acute or chronic condition. Acute inflammation is the local response of tissue to a nonspecific form of injury. The classic signs of inflammation are redness, swelling, local heat, pain, and loss of function. Acute inflammation involves a hemodynamic phase in which blood flow and capillary permeability is increased and a cellular phase during which there is an increase in white cell movement in the area. Although acute inflammation is usually self-limiting, chronic inflammation is more prolonged and is usually caused by persistent irritants, most of which are insoluble and resistant to phagocytosis and other inflammatory mechanisms. Chronic inflammation usually involves the presence of lymphocytes, plasma cells, and macrophages.

■ Systemic Signs of Inflammation

Although inflammation is classically described as a local phenomenon, a number of systemic manifestations accompany its presence. Among the most commonly mentioned manifestations are leukocytosis (described earlier in the chapter), increased erythrocyte sedimentation rate (ESR), and fever.

Erythrocyte Sedimentation Rate

The ESR is a laboratory test that measures the speed at which the erythrocytes settle when an anticoagulant is added to the blood. In this test, the blood to which the anticoagulant has been added is placed in a long, narrow tube and the speed at which the cells settle is observed. Alterations in the plasma components that occur with inflammation are thought to increase the rate at which the red cells settle.

Fever

Fever may be caused by infections, tumors, infarction, tissue necrosis, hemolytic responses, hypersensitivity reactions, brain injury, dehydration, and metabolic disturbances. The role of fever in the inflammatory process is still unclear. It is possible that elevation of body temperature may decrease resistance of selected infectious agents to host defenses. It is also possible that the increased metabolism and blood flow associated with fever may enhance healing.

Body temperature is usually maintained within a range of 35.8°C to 37.4°C (98.6°F to 99.3°F). Within this range there are diurnal variations in body temperature; with the temperature reaching its highest point in late afternoon and evening, and its lowest point in the early-morning hours (Fig. 8-3). Fever can be defined as a rise in body temperature. It is an almost universal response to inflammation and infection. Fever is not a pathologic failure to maintain body temperature. On the contrary, when fever is present, the body retains the ability to regulate temperature very closely, but at a higher level than normal.

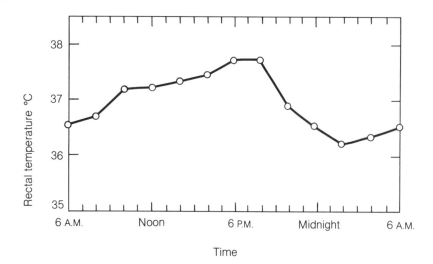

Figure 8-3 *Normal diurnal variations in body temperature.*

Regulation of body temperature

Body temperature is essentially the difference between body *heat production* and *loss of heat* from the body.

$$\text{Body temperature} =$$
$$\text{Body heat production} - \text{Body heat losses}$$

Heat production. The body's main source of heat production is metabolism. There is a 1-degree Fahrenheit increase in body temperature for every 7% increase in metabolism. The factors that influence body metabolism and heat production are (1) the metabolic rate of all the cells of the body, (2) the increased rate of muscle activity, including that caused by shivering, (3) the increased cell metabolism caused by the effect of thyroid hormones, (4) the increased cell metabolism caused by the effects of sympathetic nervous system stimulation, and (5) the increased cell metabolism caused by increased body temperature.[6] Much of the heat production takes place in the inner portions of the body (inner core); this heat is carried in the blood to the skin surface where it is dissipated into the surrounding environment.

Heat loss. Most of the body's heat losses occur at the skin surface as heat from the blood moves from the blood to the skin and from there into the environment. There are a number of arteriovenous (A-V) shunts, under the skin surface, that allow blood to move directly from the arterial to the venous system. These A-V shunts are much like the radiators in a heating system. When the shunts are open, body heat is freely dissipated to the skin and surrounding environment; and when the shunts are closed, heat is retained in the body. The opening and closing of these superficial vessels is regulated by the temperature control center in the hypothalamus.

There are four mechanisms that aid in dissipation of body heat from the skin surface: conduction, radiation, evaporation, and convection.

Conduction is the direct transfer of heat from one molecule to another. Blood carries or conducts heat from the inner core of the body to the skin surface. Normally only a small amount of body heat is lost through conduction to a cooler surface. Cooling blankets, or mattresses that are used for reducing fever, rely on conduction of heat from the skin to the cool surface of the mattress. Heat can also be conducted in the opposite direction—from the external environment to the body surface. For instance, body temperature may rise slightly after a hot bath.

Radiation is the transfer of heat through the air or a vacuum. Heat from the sun is carried by radiation. Heat loss by radiation varies with the temperature of the environment. It must be less than that of the body for loss of body heat to occur. Normally about 60% to 70% of body heat is dissipated by radiation.

Evaporation describes heat losses that occur as the result of energy used for vaporizing water on the skin surface. Sweating increases evaporative losses, and 0.58 calorie is lost from the body for each gram of water evaporated.[6]

Convection refers to heat transfer that occurs because of air currents. Normally there is a layer of heat that tends to remain near the body's surface; convection causes continual removal of this heat layer and replaces this air with that from the surrounding environment. The wind-chill factor that is often included in the weather report combines the effects of convection due to wind with the actual still-air temperature.

Body temperature is regulated by temperature-regulating centers in the hypothalamus. These centers integrate input from the various thermal receptors located throughout the body with output responses that either conserve body heat or increase its dissipation. The thermostatic centers in the hypothalamus are set so that the temperature of the body is regulated within the normal range of 35.8°C to 37.4°C. When body temperature begins to rise above the normal range, heat-dissipating behaviors are initiated; and when the temperature falls below that range, heat production is increased. Heat-conservation and production responses as well as heat dissipation behaviors are described in Table 8-3. Shivering increases metabolism through movement of the skeletal muscles. Release of epinephrine and norepinephrine acts at the cellular level to shift metabolism so that energy production (ATP) is reduced and heat production is increased. This may be one of the reasons that fever tends to produce feelings of weakness and fatigue. Thyroid hormone increases cellular metabolism, but this response usually requires several weeks to reach maximum effectiveness.

Pyrogens

Pyrogens are fever-producing substances. Leukocytes release endogenous pyrogens during inflammation. Pyrogens may also be released from other tissues. For example, in Hodgkin's disease the malignant cells reportedly produce endogenous pyrogens.[7] It is thought that pyrogens act directly on the hypothalamic temperature control center, increasing its set point so that body temperature is regulated within a new and higher range.

The reactions that occur as body temperature is increased during fever usually consist of four stages: a prodrome, a chill during which the temperature rises, a flush, and defervescence.[8] During the prodromal period, there are nonspecific complaints such as mild headache and fatigue, general malaise, and fleeting aches and pains. Vasoconstriction and piloerection usually precede the onset of shivering. At this point the skin is pale and covered with goose pimples. There is a feeling of being cold and an urgency to put on more clothing or covering

Table 8-3   Heat Loss and Heat Gain Responses Used in Regulation of Body Temperature

Heat Gain		Heat Loss	
Body response	*Mechanism of action*	*Body response*	*Mechanism of action*
Vasoconstriction of the superficial blood vessels	Restricts blood flow to the outer shell of the body, with the skin and subcutaneous tissues acting as insulation to prevent loss of core heat	Dilatation of the superficial blood vessels	Delivers blood containing core heat to the periphery where it is dissipated through: Radiation Conduction Convection
Piloerection (contraction of the piloerector muscles that surround the hairs on the skin)	Reduces the heat loss surface of the skin	Sweating	Increases heat loss through evaporation
Assumption of the "huddle" position with the extremities held close to the body	Reduces the heat los area of the body		
Shivering	Increases heat production by the muscles		
Increased production of epinephrine	Increases the heat production associated with metabolism		
Increased production of thyroid hormone	Is a long-term mechanism that increases metabolism and heat production		

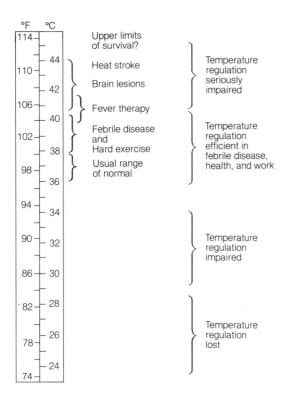

Figure 8-4 *Body temperatures under different conditions. (Dubois EF: Fever and the Regulation of Body Temperature. Springfield, IL, Charles C Thomas, 1948)*

and to curl up in a position that conserves body heat. This is followed by a generalized shaking chill; and even as the temperature rises, there is the uncomfortable sensation of being chilled. When the shivering has caused the body temperature to reach the new set point of the temperature control center, the shivering ceases and a sensation of warmth develops. At this point, cutaneous vasodilatation occurs and the skin becomes warm and flushed. The defervescence phase of the febrile response is marked by the initiation of sweating.

Harmful effects of fever

Fever can be damaging to body cells; delirium and convulsions often occur when the temperature reaches 40°C. Convulsions are more common in children than in adults. When the temperature goes above 41.1°C, damage to the internal structures of many cells results, including those in the brain. At this level of body temperature, regulation by the hypothalamic control center becomes impaired; and the body is no longer able to maintain the responses that increase heat loss (Fig.8-4).

Treatment of fever

The methods of fever treatment focus on (1) modification of the external environment as a means of increasing transfer of heat from the internal to the external environment, (2) support of the hypermetabolic state that accompanies fever, (3) protection of vulnerable body organs and systems, and (4) treatment of infection or the conditions causing the fever. Modification of the environment ensures that the environmental temperature facilitates the transfer of heat away from the body. Sponge baths (with cool water or an alcohol solution) can be used to increase evaporative heat losses. More profound cooling can be accomplished through the use of a cooling mattress, which facilitates the conduction of heat from the body into the coolant solution that circulates through the mattress. Adequate fluids and calories are needed to support the hypermetabolic state that is characteristic of fever. Additional fluids are needed for sweating and to replace insensible water losses from the lungs that occur with an increase in respiratory rate. Adequate vascular volume is needed for transport of heat to the skin surface. Antipyretic drugs, such as aspirin and acetaminophen, are used to protect vulnerable organs such as the brain from extreme elevations in temperature. These drugs act by resetting the thermostat of the hypothalamic temperature control center.

In summary, fever is a common systemic manifestation of inflammation. It is caused by pyrogens that are released from leukocytes. The pyrogens cause the temperature control center in the hypothalamus to be reset at a higher level. There are usually four stages that accompany fever. The first is the prodromal stage during which there are nonspecific complaints of discomfort. The second is the chill during which the body temperature is raised to the new setting of the temperature control center. When the temperature reaches the new setting, the third stage—flush—occurs. During this stage there is a feeling of warmth as the superficial blood vessels become dilated. The final stage of fever is the defervescence phase during which sweating occurs.

■ Tissue Healing and Repair

The degree to which body structures return to their normal state following injury is largely dependent on the body's ability to replace the parenchymal cells and to arrange them as they were originally. Repair can assume one of two forms: regeneration or fibrous scar-tissue replacement. Regeneration describes the process by which cells are replaced with cells of a similar type and function so that there is little evidence that injury has occurred. Healing by fibrous replacement, on the other hand, involves the substitution of a fibrous–connective tissue scar for the original tissue.

Regeneration

The ability to regenerate varies with tissue types. Body cells are divided into three types according to their ability to undergo regeneration: (1) labile, (2) stable, or (3) permanent cell types.

Labile cells are those that continue to regenerate throughout life. These cells include the surface epithelial cells of the skin and mucous membranes of the gastrointestinal tract. A constant daily turnover of cells occurs with these tissue types.

Stable cells are those that normally stop dividing when growth ceases. These cells are capable, however, of undergoing regeneration when confronted with an appropriate stimulus. In order for stable cells to regenerate and restore tissues to their original state, the underlying structural framework must be present. When this framework has been destroyed, the replacement of tissues will be haphazard. The reader will recall that epithelial tissue relies on the blood supply from the underlying connective tissues for nourishment. The hepatocytes of the liver are one form of stable cells, and the importance of the structural framework to regeneration is evidenced by two forms of liver disease. In viral hepatitis, for example, there is selective destruction of the parenchymal liver cells while the structural cells remain unharmed. Consequently, once the disease has subsided, the injured cells regenerate and liver function returns to normal. On the other hand, in cirrhosis of the liver, fibrous bands of tissue form and replace the normal structural framework of the liver, causing disordered replacement of liver cells and disturbance of liver function.

Permanent, or *fixed cells*, are those that cannot undergo mitotic division. The fixed cells include nerve cells, as well as skeletal and cardiac muscle cells. As will be discussed later, the nerve axon can regenerate under certain conditions in which the nerve cell body is uninjured.

Connective Tissue Repair

The sequence of events that occurs with laceration of the skin and underlying tissues is familiar to most readers. This type of injury is followed almost immediately by bleeding into the area and the development of a blood clot (Fig. 8-5). Within several hours, the clot loses fluid and becomes a hard, dehydrated scab that serves to protect the area. At about the same time, phagocytic white blood cells begin to enter the injured area and break down and remove the inflammatory debris. Shortly thereafter, cells called fibroblasts arrive and begin to build scar tissue by synthesizing collagen fibers and other proteins. Meanwhile, the epithelial cells at the margin of the wound begin to regenerate and move toward the center of the wound, forming a new surface layer that is similar to that destroyed by the injury. When healing is complete, the scab falls off. With the exception of the desiccated scab, repair of injury to internal structures follows a similar pattern.

The primary objective of the healing process is to fill the gap created by tissue destruction and to restore the

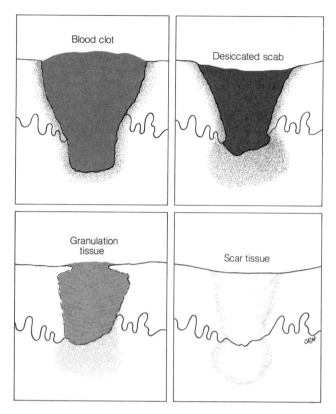

Figure 8-5 *Events that follow skin and subcutaneous tissue injury.*

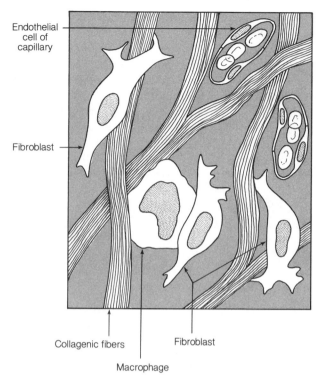

Figure 8-6 *Cells involved in the development of granulation tissue. Collagen fibers and vascular endothelial cells usually begin to enter the wound area around the third to sixth day following injury.*

structural continuity of the injured part. When regeneration cannot occur, healing by fibrous-tissue substitution provides the means for maintaining this continuity. Although scar tissue fills the gap created by tissue death, it does not repair the structure with functioning parenchymal cells.

Healing by fibrous substitution begins during the early stages of inflammation as macrophages invade the area and begin to digest the invading organisms and the cellular debris. The *fibroblasts* are connective-tissue cells that are responsible for the formation of *collagen* and other *intercellular elements* needed for wound healing.

As early as 24 hours following injury, fibroblasts and vascular endothelial cells begin to enter the area, and by the third to the fifth day proliferation of both fibroblasts and small blood vesssels occurs (Fig.8-6). As this happens, the area becomes filled with a specialized form of soft, pink granular tissue called *granulation tissue*. This tissue is edematous and bleeds easily because of the numerous, newly developed, fragile and leaky capillary buds. At times excessive granulation tissue, sometimes referred to as "proud flesh," may form. This excess granulation tissue protrudes from the wound and prevents reepithelization from taking place. Surgical removal or chemical cauterizaion of the defect allows healing to proceed.

As the process of scar-tissue development progresses, there is a further increase in extracellular collagen and a decrease in active fibroblastic function. The small blood vessels become thrombosed and degenerate. As this happens the collagen fibers begin to mature and shorten, and a dense devascularized scar is formed. *Wound contraction* contributes heavily to the healing of surface wounds. As a result, the scar that is formed is considerably smaller than the original wound. Cosmetically, this may be desirable because it reduces the size of the visible defect. On the other hand, contraction of scar tissue over joints and other body structures tends to limit movement and to cause deformities.

As a result of loss of elasticity, scar tissue that is stretched fails to return to its original length. Most wounds do not regain their original tensile strength once healing has occurred. They usually begin to increase in strength between 10 and 14 days following injury; after this they rapidly increase in strength and, by the end of 3 months, reach a plateau—at about 70% to 80% of their unwounded strength.[1]

Healing by first or second intention

Wounds can be divided into two types—those in which there is minimal tissue loss and that heal by first *intention* and those that have significant tissue loss and heal by *second intention* (Fig. 8-7). Both visible skin wounds and invisible wounds of the internal organs heal by either first or second intention. A sutured surgical incision is an example of healing by first intention (healing directly, without granulations). Visible wounds that heal by second intention are burns and decubitus ulcers. When healing by second intention occurs, granulation tissue proliferates into the injured area. The granulation tissue fills the defect and allows reepithelization to occur, beginning at the wound edges and continuing to the center, until the entire wound is covered. Healing by second intention is slower than healing by first intention and results in the formation of more scar tissue. A wound that might otherwise have healed by first intention may become infected and then heal by second intention.

Keloid formation

An abnormality in healing by scar tissue repair is *keloid* formation. Keloids involve excessive production of bulging tumorlike scar-tissue masses. The tendency to develop keloids is more common in blacks and seems to have a genetic basis.

Factors that affect wound healing

Many factors, both local and systemic, influence wound healing. Science has not found any way to hasten the normal process of wound repair, but there are many factors that impair healing.

Age. The rate of skin replacement slows with aging. Healing of open wounds and epithelization of skin takes longer in the elderly.

Nutrition. Adequate nutrition that includes essential amino acids, vitamins A and C, and zinc is essential for normal wound repairs. Cystine, an amino acid, is needed for synthesis of the mucopolysaccharides by the fibroblast. Vitamin C aids in collagen formation and capillary development. Zinc is thought to be an enzyme cofactor. In animal studies, zinc has been found to aid in reepithelization. It is of interest that although a zinc deficiency tends to impair healing, zinc therapy does not seem to improve healing.[9]

Infection. Infection tends to impair wound healing. Both wound contamination and host factors that increase susceptibility to infection predispose to wound infection. Increased susceptibility to infection is associated with conditions that lead to a deficiency in leukocytes or impaired leukocyte function. Neutrophils in the diabetic, for example, have diminished chemotaxic and phagocytic ability. This may explain why diabetics are highly vulnerable to bacterial wound invasion.

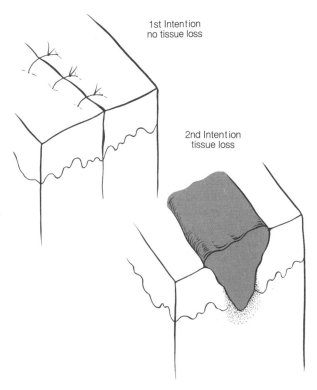

Figure 8-7 *Healing by first and second intention.*

Hormonal influences. The therapeutic administration of adrenal corticosteroids is known to influence the inflammatory process and to delay healing. These hormones decrease capillary permeability during the early stages of inflammation, impair the phagocytic property of the leukocytes, and inhibit fibroblast proliferation and function.

Blood supply. In order for healing to occur, wounds must have adequate blood flow to supply the necessary nutrients and to remove the resulting waste, local toxins, bacteria, and other debris. Impaired wound healing due to poor blood flow may occur as a result of wound conditions, such as swelling, or may be caused by preexisting conditions. Arterial disease and venous pathology are well-documented causes of impaired wound healing.

Wound separation. Approximation of the wound edges, that is, suturing of an incision type of wound, greatly enhances healing and prevents infection. Epithelization of a wound with closely approximated edges occurs within 1 to 2 days. Large gaping wounds tend to heal more slowly because it is often impossible to effect wound closure with these types of wounds.

Presence of foreign bodies. Foreign bodies tend to invite bacterial contamination and delay healing. Fragments of wood, steel, glass, and the like may have entered the wound at the site of injury and can be difficult to locate when the wound is treated. Sutures are also foreign bodies and, although needed for the closure of surgical wounds, they are an impediment to healing. This is why sutures are removed as soon as possible after surgery.

In summary, the ability of tissues to repair damage due to injury is dependent on the body's ability to replace the parenchymal cells and to organize them as they were originally. Regeneration describes the process by which tissue is replaced with cells of a similar type and function. Healing by regeneration is limited to tissue with cells that are able to divide and to replace the injured cells. Body cells are divided into types according to their ability to regenerate: (1) labile cells, such as the epithelial cells of the skin and gastrointestinal tract, which continue to regenerate throughout life; (2) stable cells, such as those in the liver, which normally do not divide but which are capable of regeneration when confronted with an appropriate stimulus; and (3) permanent or fixed cells, such as nerve cells, which are unable to regenerate. Scar-tissue repair involves the substitution of fibrous connective tissue for injured tissue that cannot be repaired by regeneration.

■ Study Guide

After you have studied this chapter, you should be able to meet the following objectives:

☐ Define inflammation.

☐ Explain why the inflammatory response is beneficial to the body.

☐ List at least five general causes of inflammation.

☐ Cite one universal characteristic of the inflammatory response.

☐ State the five cardinal signs of inflammation and describe the physiologic mechanisms involved in production of each of these signs.

☐ Describe the early hemodynamic changes that occur in acute inflammation.

☐ State the three patterns of the hemodynamic response that occur with an inflammatory reaction.

☐ Describe the four stages of the cellular phase of the acute inflammatory response.

☐ State the function of granular leukocytes.

☐ Define *diapedesis*.

☐ Relate chemotaxis to leukocytic activity.

☐ Describe the process of phagocytosis.

☐ List the components of the reticuloendothelial system.

☐ State one distinctive characteristic of chemical mediators.

☐ Contrast the five types of inflammatory exudates.

☐ Describe three patterns of resolution of acute inflammation.

☐ State the characteristics of chronic inflammation.

☐ State the purpose of the ESR.

☐ Relate heat production and heat loss to regulation of body temperature.

☐ Relate the sequence of events in fever.

☐ List five goals of fever treatment.

☐ Explain the action of aspirin and acetaminophen in terms of reducing the body temperature during fever.

☐ Explain the mechanism of fever reduction through the use of tepid sponge baths and a cooling mattress.

☐ Relate the sequence of events in soft tissue repair.

☐ Describe the process of scar tissue development.

☐ Define *first intention* and *second intention* in relation to wound healing.

☐ Relate the influence of local and systemic factors on wound healing.

■ References

1. Robbins SL, Cotran RS, Kumar V: Pathologic Basis of Disease, 3rd ed, pp 40, 62, 79. Philadelphia, WB Saunders, 1984
2. Lewis T: Blood Vessels of the Human Skin and Their Responses. London, Shaw, 1927
3. Claman HN: Glucocorticords I: Anti-inflammatory mechanisms. Hosp Pract 18, 7:123, 1983
4. Samuelsson B: Leukotrienes: Mediators of immediate hypersensitivity reactions and inflammation. Science 220:568, 1983
5. Houk JC: Inflammation: A quarter century of progress. J Invest Dermatol 67:124, 1976
6. Guyton A: Textbook of Medical Physiology, 6th ed, pp 887, 888. Philadelphia, WB Saunders, 1981
7. Badel P: Pyrogen release in vitro by lymphoid tissue in patients with Hodgkin's disease. Yale J Biol Med 47:101, 1974
8. Sodeman WA, Sodeman TM: Pathologic Physiology: Mechanisms of Disease, 6th ed, p 546. Philadelphia, WB Saunders, 1979
9. Neldner KH, Hambridge KM: Zinc therapy. N Engl J Med 292:879, 1975

■ Additional References

Inflammation and wound repair

Bornstein DL: Leukocytic pyrogen: A major mediator of the acute phase reaction. Ann NY Acad Sci 389:323, 1982

Bruno P: The nature of wound healing. Nurs Clin North Am 14, No 4:667, 1979

Bryant WM: Wound healing. Clin Symp 29, No 3:1, 1977

Gewurz H: Biology of C-reactive protein and the acute phase response. Hosp Pract 17, No 6:67, 1982

Gewurz H, Mold C, Siegel J, Fiedel B: C-reactive protein and the acute phase response. Ann Intern Med 27:345, 1982

Hotter A: Physiologic aspects and clinical implications of wound healing. Heart Lung 11:522, 1982

Jett MF, Lancaster LE: The inflammatory-immune response: The body's defense against invasion. Crit Care Nurs 5:64, 1983

Kushner I: The phenomenon of the acute phase response. Ann NY Acad Sci 389:39, 1982

McCarty M: Historical perspective on C-reactive protein. Ann NY Acad Sci 389:1, 1982

Montadon D, D'Andrian G, Gabbiani G: The mechanism of wound contraction and epithelialization. Clin Plast Surg 4, No 3:325, 1977

Peacock E Jr, Van Winkle W: Wound Repair, 2nd ed. Philadelphia, WB Saunders, 1976

Ryan GE, Majno G: Acute inflammation. Am J Pathol 86, No 1:185, 1977

Samuelsson B: Leukotrienes: Mediators of immediate hypersensitivity reactions and inflammation. Science 220, No 5:568, 1983

Weissman G, Smolen JE, Korchak HM: Release of inflammatory mediators from stimulated neutrophils. N Engl J Med 303, No 1:27, 1980

Fever

Bernheim HA, Block LH, Atkins E: Fever: Pathogenesis, pathophysiology, and purpose. Ann Intern Med 91:261, 1979

Castle M, Watkins J: Fever: Understanding the sinister sign. Nursing '78 9, No 2:26, 1978

Davis-Sharts J: Mechanisms and manifestations of fever. Am J Nurs 78, No 11:1874, 1978

Dinarello CA, Wolff SM: Pathogenesis of fever in man. N Engl J Med 298, No 11:607, 1978

Donaldson JF: Therapy of acute fever: A comparative approach. Hosp Pract 16, No 9:125, 1981

Done AK: Treatment of fever in 1982: A review. Am J Med 75, No 6:27, 1983

Chapter 9

The Immune Response

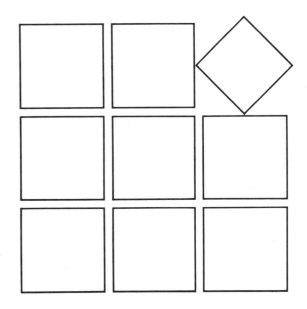

Immunology, the study of immune mechanisms, can be divided into four categories: immunity, serology, immunochemistry, and immunobiology.[1] Immunity is concerned with the prevention of infectious diseases and the growth of abnormal cells. Application of serologic procedures facilitates the diagnosis of diseases (rickettsial, viral, syphilitic, and others). Immunochemistry views immune mechanisms as complex chemical reactions between antigens, haptens, antibodies, and complement. At the molecular level, immunochemistry has advanced to the point of identifying the structure of the amino acid sequence of the immunoglobulins and other components of the immune response. Immunobiology encompasses a broader view of immunology: it proposes theories about how antibodies are formed, how hypersensitivity develops, and the origin of autoimmune disease. The discussion in this chapter focuses on the immune system and immune responses.

■ The Immune System

The immune system protects the body from destruction by foreign agents and microbial pathogens, degrades and removes damaged or dead cells, and exerts a surveillance function to prevent the development and growth of malignant cells. It is a complex network of specialized organs and cells. The immune system consists of the lymphoid organs (thymus, lymph nodes, spleen, and tonsils), all of the aggregates of lymphoid tissue occurring in nonlymphoid organs, and the immune cells (lymphocytes and macrophages). In many respects, its complexity parallels that of the nervous system. It is capable of distinguishing self from nonself, remembering previous experiences, and reacting accordingly.[2] Once an individual has the mumps, the immune system remembers the experience and protects against getting the disease again. Not only is the immune system capable of memory, it is also able to respond with diversity and specificity. It can recognize many millions of nonself molecules and produce specific molecules that match up with and counteract each of them.

The *immune response* describes the interaction between an antigen (immunogen*) and an antibody (immunoglobulin) or reactive T-lymphocyte. There are two types of immune responses—humoral and cell mediated. *Humoral immunity* is dependent on the pres-

---

*The terms antigen and immunogen are both used in describing a foreign substance that stimulates an immune response. Although the term antigen has been used for a number of years, the newer term immunogen is becoming more widely preferred. This text uses both terms interchangeably.

ence of circulating antibodies; *cell-mediated immunity* depends on lymphocytes that react directly with the antigen to cause its destruction.

Immunity

Immunity is a normal adaptive response. It involves the resistance to a disease resulting from immune mechanisms. Immunity can be either natural or acquired. *Natural immunity* is species specific. It is the reason that humans do not contract certain animal diseases, such as feline distemper. *Innate immunity* is the immunity one is born with. It is genetically controlled and involves natural immunity, heredity, race, and sex. *Acquired immunity* is that which an individual gains through active or passive means.

Active immunity

Active immunity is acquired through immunization or actually having had a disease. It is long-lived immunity that has been developed by the body's own immune system. Active immunity does not provide immediate protection on first exposure to a invading agent or vaccine; it takes a few days to weeks for the immune response to become sufficiently developed to contribute to the destruction of the pathogen. With subsequent exposure to the same agent, however, the immune system is usually able to react within minutes or hours.

Passive immunity

Passive immunity is temporary immunity that is transmitted or borrowed from another source. An infant receives passive immunity from its mother *in utero* and from antibodies that it receives from its mother's breast milk. Passive immunity can also be transferred through injection of antiserum, which contains the antibodies for a specific disease, or through the use of pooled gamma globulin, which contains antibodies for a number of diseases. Both antiserum and gamma globulin are obtained from blood plasma.

The Lymphoid Organs

The lymphoid system consists of central and peripheral lymphoid structures. The bone marrow, thymus, and bursa equivalent constitute the central lymphoid organs. The peripheral lymphoid structures consist of the lymph nodes, spleen, tonsils, intestinal lymphoid tissue, and aggregates of other lymphoid cells. The lymphoid organs are connected by networks of lymph channels and blood vessels. The effector units are the various immune cells that travel throughout the body and into and out of the lymphoid tissue.

Thymus

The thymus is an elongated, flat, bilobed structure located in the neck below the thyroid gland and extending into the upper part of the thorax behind the top of the sternum. The thymus is a fully developed organ at birth and weighs about 15 gm to 20 gm.[1] After birth, the thymus grows slowly, reaching a maximum size of about 40 gm at puberty. It then regresses in size, its lymphoid tissue being replaced by adipose tissue so that, in the adult, its substance is difficult to distinguish from the adipose tissue in which it is embedded. Nevertheless, some thymus tissue persists into old age.

The function of the thymus is central to the development of the immune system. During embryonic development, the thymus is the first organ to begin the manufacture of lymphocytes. There is evidence that precursor cells of some of the nonthymic lymphoid tissues (*e.g.*, lymph nodes and spleen) originate in the thymus and migrate at various times before and after birth to sites where they establish germinal centers for maintaining the body's immunologic defenses. Impaired thymus function has been associated with immunologic deficiency disorders. If the thymus is removed from certain animals at birth or is congenitally absent, as it is in certain

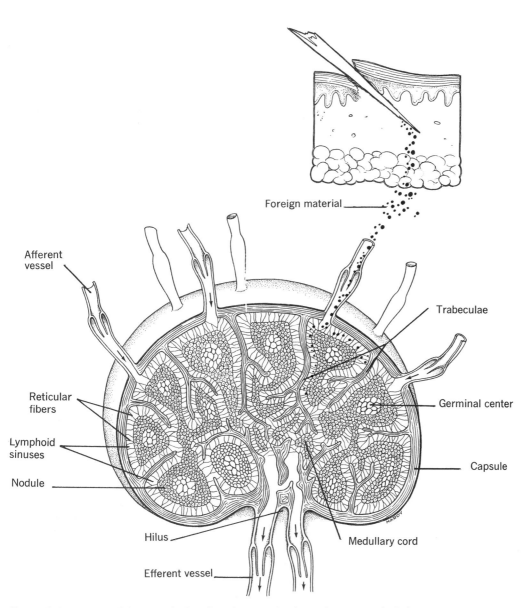

Figure 9-1 *Structural features of a lymph node. Bacteria that gain entry to the body are filtered out of the lymph as it flows through the node. (Chaffee EE, Lytle IM: Basic Physiology and Anatomy, 4th ed. Philadelphia, JB Lippincott, 1980)*

human conditions, there is a decrease of lymphocytes in the blood, a marked depletion or absence of T-lymphocytes, and an absence of thymus-dependent lymphocytes in the peripheral lymphoid tissues.[3]

In the adult, the thymus consists of many lobules, each containing a cortex and medulla. Lymphocytes produced in the cortex migrate to the medulla where they undergo further differentiation before they leave the thymus. Alterations in their surface antigens occur as these lymphocytes mature. Although the thymocytes are microscopically indistinguishable from lymphocytes in other tissues, they are antigenically distinguishable from the B lymphocyte by the unique surface antigens. For unknown reasons a substantial number of lymphocytes die in the thymus.

Maturation of the lymphocytes in the thymus takes about 2 to 3 days, after which the mature lymphocytes migrate from the thymus gland into the bloodstream. From the bloodstream they enter the inner cortex of the lymph nodes, the periarterial sheaths of the spleen, and other thymus-dependent regions of the peripheral lymphoid tissue.[3] In addition to lymphocytes that arise from resident cells within the thymus, certain hematopoietic cells from the bone marrow are capable of migrating to the thymus where they are somehow instructed to become mature lymphocytes. Before birth, the thymus is the major source of lymphocytes; in later life, the precursor cells migrate to the thymus.

Bursa equivalent

In fowls, the bursa of Fabricius is an organ, located near the hind part of the gut, in which the B-lymphocytes develop and mature. The location of the bursa equivalent in humans is not known. Current evidence suggests that the B-lymphocytes differentiate into B cells in the bone marrow and mature in the peripheral lymphoid structures.

Lymph nodes

The lymph nodes serve two functions: (1) they remove foreign materials from lymph before it enters the bloodstream and (2) they are centers for proliferation of immune cells. They are located along the lymph ducts, which lead from the tissues to the thoracic duct. Each lymph node processes lymph from a discrete, adjacent anatomic site. Many lymph nodes are situated in the axillae, groin, and along the great vessels of the neck, thorax, and abdomen (see Chap. 11, Fig. 11-3). A few are associated with the popliteal vessels and the vessels at the elbow.[4] A lymph node consists of an outer cortex and an inner medulla and is surrounded by a connective-tissue capsule (Fig. 9-1). Lymph enters the node through afferent channels that penetrate the capsule and then leaves through the deep indentation in the hilus. Because of the lymph nodes' spongelike structure, the mac-

rophages, lymphocytes, and granulocytes flow slowly through them. The reticular meshwork serves as a surface onto which macrophages attach and phagocytose antigens. The T-lymphocytes are more abundant in the medullary portion of the node and the B-lymphocytes in the cortex. The T-lymphocytes proliferate on antigenic stimulation and create germinal centers in the medullary region after stimulation. These centers contain macrophages, growing T-lymphocytes, and smaller adult cells. The cortical germinal centers contain mainly B-lymphocytes and appear to be concerned with antibody production.

Spleen

The spleen, which is roughly the size of a clenched fist, is located in the abdomen at the level of the 9th, 10th, and 11th ribs. The spleen is composed of red and white pulp. The red pulp is well supplied with arteries and is the area where senescent and injured red blood cells are destroyed. The white pulp contains concentrated areas of lymphocytes called periarterial lymphoid sheaths, which surround the central arterioles. Although T-lymphocytes are found in the spleen, it is primarily a B-lymphocyte–containing organ.

Other lymphoid tissues

The tonsils have a structure that is similar to the lymph thymus and lymph nodes. Like the thymus, the tonsils are rather large during childhood and regress in size with age. Other important collections of lymphoid tissue exist in the appendix and in Peyer's patches in the intestine.

Antigens

An antigen is any substance recognized as foreign (nonself) by the immune system. An antigen can be a virus, a bacterium, a fungus, or a parasite. Tissues or cells from another individual, unless it is an identical twin, can also act as antigens. Antigens have specific *antigenic determinant sites,* or *epitopes,* that interact with immune cells to induce the immune response. All antigens carry different epitopes, allowing the immune system to recognize the antigen as nonself and as different from other antigens. The number of antigenic determinant sites on a molecule is roughly proportional to its molecular weight, with one site existing for each 10,000 or so units of molecular weight.[1] A complete antigen has two or more sites. Large protein and polysaccharide molecules make good antigens because of their complex chemical structure and multiple antigenic determinant sites. Smaller molecules (those with a molecular weight of less than 10,000) usually make poor antigens. Some substances cannot act as antigens by themselves but have antigenic determinant sites and can combine with carrier substances and then act as antigens. These substances, which usually have a low molecular weight, are called haptens. House dust, animal danders, and plant pollens are haptens.

The site of access to the body may influence the antigenic strength of a substance. For example, the digestive enzymes often hydrolyze and destroy the antigenic quality of otherwise fully antigenic materials. When these same substances are given parenterally (injected), greater amounts of the antigen are available for interacting with the antigen-processing cells. The oral polio vaccine is one exception; when taken into the gastrointestinal tract, it invades the lining of the intestine and reproduces itself.[1]

Cells of the Immune System

At least three types of cells are involved in the immune response: the macrophage, the B-lymphocyte (B cell), and the T-lymphocyte (T cell). The macrophage processes the antigen and transfers the antigenic determinants to the lymphocytes. The T-lymphocytes are responsible for forming the sensitized lymphocytes that provide cellular immunity and the B-lymphocytes for forming the antibodies that provide humoral immunity.

Lymphocytes represent 20% to 30% of the leukocytes (Fig. 9-2). They begin their life in the bone marrow as lymphoblasts and travel in the blood to many organs, but are eventually imprinted in a series of critical events that occur in either the thymus or bursal equivalent tissue. Two types of lymphocytes, the T-lymphocytes and the B-lymphocytes, emerge as a result of the changes that occur in these two structures.

Both B-lymphocytes and T-lymphocytes manifest immunologic specificity, that is, they are programmed to respond to a specific antigen. Within the T-lymphocyte and B-lymphocyte populations are both effector cells and memory cells. Effector cells (activated lymphocytes and immunoglobulin-producing plasma cells of the B-cell population) are instrumental in the destruction of the antigen. *Memory cells* are formed following initial exposure to the antigen. They revert to an inactive state, but are able to rapidly increase the intensity of the immune response with subsequent exposure to the specific antigen of which they have a memory.

The functions of the B-lymphocytes and T-lymphocytes are not independent of each other. Only certain antigens will stimulate B cells. With most immune responses that elicit a humoral response, T-lymphocytes interact with B-lymphocytes, helping to stimulate them and regulating their differentiation.

T-lymphocytes

The *T-lymphocytes* are imprinted in the thymus and provide cell-mediated immunity. They are the smaller of the two types of lymphocytes and have a life span of years, much longer than the B-lymphocytes. Among the char-

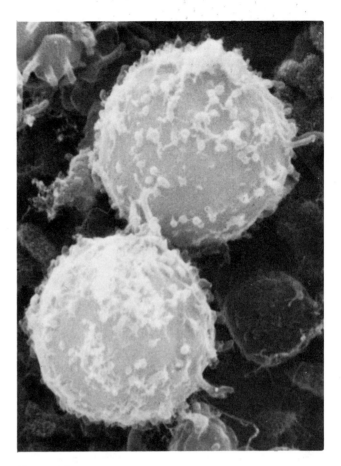

Figure 9-2 *A scanning micrograph of two lymphocytes. (Courtesy of Kenneth Siegesmund, Ph.D., Anatomy Department, Medical College of Wisconsin)*

acteristics shared by the T-lymphocytes is the presence of surface antigens (Thy 1, Lyt, and OKT antigens) that distinguish them from the B-lymphocytes. These antigens serve as useful markers for recognizing, identifying, and purifying T cells and their antigenic subsets. Other important surface markers are present on the T-lymphocyte including a receptor for sheep erythrocytes. When normal T-lymphocytes are incubated with sheep erythrocytes, they form rosettes, which can be visualized under the microscope. The reason for the spontaneous rosette formation is unknown, but humans, mice, and a few other species share this characteristic.[1]

B-lymphocytes

The second type of lymphocyte is called the *B-lymphocyte* because of its association with the bursa of Fabricius in fowls. The B cells are larger than the T cells and their life span is much shorter, only about 5 to 7 days. They can be identified by the presence of B antigen (now known as LyB antigen), immunoglobulins, and HLA antigens on their surface. The source of B-lymphocytes are the pre-B cells that originate from stem cells in the bone marrow.

The pre-B cells become immature B cells, which, on exposure to an antigen, develop into mature B cells. The pre-B cells are found in the bone marrow; the immature B cells are found in the bone marrow, the peripheral lymphoid tissues, and the blood; and the mature B-cells are found in the blood and the peripheral lymphoid tissues.

B-lymphocytes have the capacity to be transformed into *plasma cells* when exposed to an antigen. Antigen determinants that combine with corresponding antibody stimulate B-cell proliferation and differentiation into plasma cells that actively secrete antibodies. Several B-cell subsets are recognized, each forming a plasma cell specialized to produce only one type of immunoglobulin (IgA, IgD, IgE, IgG, or IgM). The immunoglobulins are discussed later.

Macrophages

It has been determined that the macrophages, the blood monocytes, and the tissue lymphocytes participate in the immune response by processing foreign substances and by presenting the antigen to the lymphocytes in a form that increases its immunogenicity (Fig. 9-3). In the process of phagocytosis, the macrophage ingests the foreign substance and digests it; then portions of the antigen move out through the cell membrane and become attached to receptors on the cell surface. The interaction between the modified antigen particles on the macrophage receptors and the lymphocyte stimulates lym-

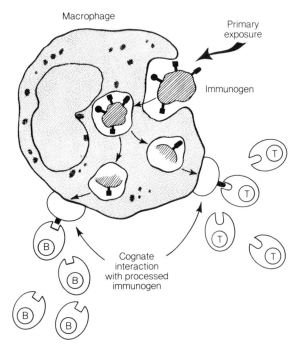

Figure 9-3 *The interaction between the immunogen (antigen), macrophage, and lymphocytes.*

phocyte differentiation and proliferation. These receptor-site interactions also appear to provide the stage for T-cell and B-cell interactions; they facilitate the helper role of the T-lymphocytes in terms of B-cell function. There is also evidence to suggest participation by the T-lymphocyte in humoral immunity, as well as evidence that the macrophage can act under T-cell influence to destroy bacteria and tumor cells. As will be discussed later, lymphokines that are produced by the effector T cells cause migration or activation of the macrophages.

In summary, the immune system protects the body against invasion by foreign agents and proliferation of abnormal and malignant cells. The immune system includes the lymphoid organs and the immune cells. An immune response involves an antigen, or substance that is recognized as foreign, and cells of the immune system. Antigens have antigenic determinant sites that the immune system uses to recognize the antigen as nonself and distinguish it from other antigens. Immunity is the resistance to a disease that the immune system provides. It can be acquired actively (through immunization or actually having a disease) or passively (by receiving antibodies or immune cells from another source).

■ Immune Mechanisms

Immune mechanisms are of two types: specific and nonspecific. *Specific immunologic responses* not only recognize self as distinct from nonself, but are also capable of distinguishing between antigens. They can be further divided into two types: humoral and cell-mediated immunity (Fig. 9-4). Humoral immunity is dependent on the presence of circulating antibodies that are formed by the B-lymphocytes. Cell-mediated immunity is effected by the T-lymphocytes that react directly with the antigen to cause its destruction. *Nonspecific immunologic* mechanisms such as the complement system, the activity of interferons, and the process of phagocytosis can distinguish between self and nonself but not between agents and pathogens.

Humoral Immunity

The B-lymphocytes, which form about 20% to 30% of the lymphocyte population, are capable of developing into plasma cells, which produce antibodies or immunoglobulins. Although the B cells produce large numbers of antibodies to a vast variety of antigens, each plasma cell produces only one type of antibody. It is implied that the B-cell antigen interaction results in an individual clone of plasma cells, which are committed to produce the antibody for that particular antigen. Some

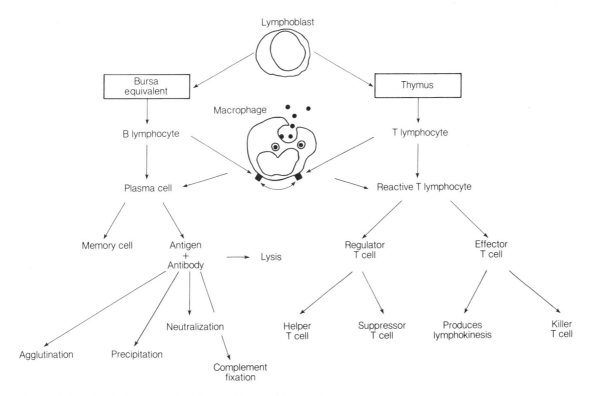

Figure 9-4 *The development of cellular and humoral immunity.*

cells in the clone are thought to produce antibodies, whereas others become memory cells.

The immunoglobulins are found in the globulin fraction of the plasma proteins. Only recently has the chemical structure of the immunoglobulins been identified (Fig. 9-5). Each of the immunoglobulins is composed of two heavy (H) chains and two light (L) chains. The amino acid sequence of each of the chains has a constant (C) region and a variable (V) region. The antigen reacts with the variable region. Each of the immunoglobulins has a different amino acid sequence in the variable region that provides it with the specificity needed to react with a single antigen. The heavy chains in each of the classes of immunoglobulins are antigenically distinctive, and it is this distinction that permits division of the immunoglobulins into classes through the use of immunoelectrophoresis.

The immunoglobulins have been divided into five classes—IgG, IgA, IgM, IgD, and IgE (Table 9-1). Each of these immunoglobulins is made by a different group of B-lymphocytes and each varies according to the nature of the antigen. IgG (gamma globulin) is the most abundant of the immunoglobulins. It circulates in body fluids and is the only immunoglobulin that crosses the placenta. IgG activates the complement system. IgA, the second most abundant of the immunoglobulins, is found in saliva, tears, and bronchial, gastrointestinal, prostatic,

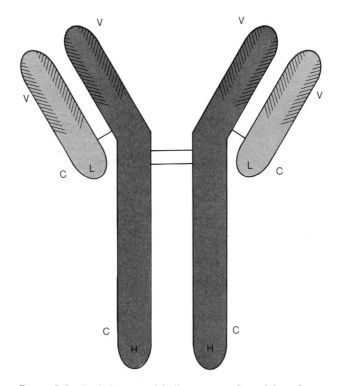

Figure 9-5 *Basic immunoglobulin structure formed from four polypeptide chains bound together. Light chains (L), heavy chains (H), constant amino acid region (C), and variable amino acid region (V). Antigens bind to the variable region of the immunoglobulin.*

Table 9-1   Classes of Immunoglobulins

Class	Percent of Total	Characteristics
IgG	75.0	Present in majority of B cells; contains antiviral, antitoxin, and antibacterial antibodies; only immunoglobulin that crosses the placenta; responsible for protection of newborn; activates complement and binds to macrophages
IgA	15.0	Predominant immunoglobulin in body secretions, such as saliva, nasal and respiratory secretions, breast milk; protects mucous membranes
IgM	10.0	Forms the natural antibodies such as those for ABO blood antigens; prominent in early immune responses; activates complement
IgD	0.2	Action is not known; may affect B-cell maturation
IgE	0.004	Binds to mast cells and basophils; involved in allergic and hypersensitivity reactions

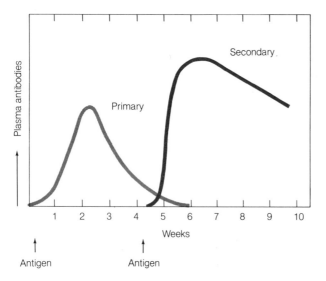

Figure 9-6   *Primary and secondary responses of the humoral immune system to the same antigen.*

and vaginal secretions. It is a secretory immunoglobulin and is considered to be a primary defense against local infections. The difference in protection afforded by the IgG and the IgA immunoglobulins can be illustrated using the two types of polio vaccine—Salk and Sabin. With some viral infections, such as poliovirus, systemic infection follows an initial mucosal phase during which the virus replicates in the mucosa of the portal of entry. In these infections, circulating IgG antibodies are important in preventing systemic disease. The Salk polio vaccine (killed virus administered by injection) prompts the production of systemic IgG antibodies and protects against the systemic effects of the virus. However, the Salk vaccine does not stimulate production of IgA secretory antibodies, and the organisms can grow in the gastrointestinal tract, resulting in establishment of a carrier state. With the oral Sabin polio vaccine, IgA secretory antibody production is induced and virus replication and subsequent mucosal penetration is prevented, as is systemic dissemination of the virus and development of the carrier state. IgM appears in response to most antigens early in the immune reaction. Like IgG, IgM activates the complement system. IgE is involved in allergic and hypersensitivity reactions. It binds to mast cells and causes the release of histamine and other mediators of allergic responses. The main function of IgD has not been determined.

Two types of responses occur in the development of humoral immunity (Fig. 9-6). A primary response occurs when the antigen is first introduced into the body. During this primary response, there is a latent period before the antibody can be detected in the serum. This latent period involves the recognition of the antigen by the antibody and the development of a clone of plasma cells that will produce the antibody. This period usually takes from 48 to 72 hours, after which the detectable antibody titer continues to rise for a period of 10 days to 2 weeks. Recovery from many infectious diseases occurs at about the time during the primary response when the antibody titer is reaching its peak. The secondary response occurs on second or subsequent exposures to the antigen. During the secondary response, the rise in antibody titer occurs sooner and reaches a higher level. There are two forms of plasma cells that develop during the primary response: one produces the antibody and the other becomes a memory cell that records the information needed for antibody production. During the secondary response, the memory cell recognizes the antigen and stimulates production of plasma cells, which produce the specific antibody. The booster immunization given for some infectious diseases, such as tetanus, makes use of the secondary response. For persons who have been previously immunized, administration of a booster shot causes an almost immediate rise in antibody titer to a level sufficient to prevent development of the disease.

Antigen–antibody reactions can take several forms. Combination of antigen with antibody can result in precipitation of the antigen–antibody complex; it can cause agglutination or clumping of cells; neutralization of bacterial toxins; lysis or destruction of the pathogen or cell membranes; adherence of the antigen to immunocytes or other structures; opsonization, which enhances phagocytosis; and complement fixation or activation. Some of these reactions, such as opsonization, occur because of complement fixation. Antigen–antibody reactions can be studied *in vitro* (in serum samples studied in the laboratory) or they can occur *in vivo* (in the body).

Cell-Mediated Immunity

In cell-mediated immunity, the action of the T-lymphocytes and the macrophages predominates. In addition to its protective effects, cell-mediated immunity is responsible for delayed hypersensitivity and transplant reactions. It is also thought to protect against tumor cell development.

The T-lymphocytes mature in the thymus and constitute about 70% to 80% of the lymphocytes. There are two populations of T cells: regulatory T cells and effector T cells. Regulatory cells act by either enhancing or suppressing the action of the B-lymphocytes. These cells are sometimes called the *T helper* cells or *T suppressor* cells. The effector cells synthesize and release immune mediators called lymphokines and cause the death of target cells by contact with cell-linked antigens. The type of effector T cell that causes cell death is called the *killer T cell*.

The *lymphokines* produced by the T cell are low-molecular-weight proteins that are capable of influencing other inflammatory cells, including the macrophage, the neutrophil, and the lymphocyte. The lymphokines also activate or suppress the macrophage. Lymphokines can act as chemotactic factors for neutrophils, eosinophils, and basophils and can cause histamine release from mast cells. Cytotoxic factor, or lymphotoxin, causes lysis of certain target cells.

Some subsets of effector T cells produce an intracellular RNA-type macromolecule called *transfer factor*. Its function is similar to that of RNA in that it provides the pattern for production of lymphokines. Immediately after a T cell responds to an antigen, it produces transfer factor. Transfer factor then converts other T-lymphocytes into lymphokine-producing cells. It has been shown that transfer factor can be used to transfer passive cell-mediated immunity from one animal to another. In humans, transfer factor has been used experimentally for treatment of resistant infections, such as mucocutaneous candidiasis and as an adjuvant therapy for certain types of cancer.

Cell-mediated immunity provides protection against viruses, cancer cells, and foreign tissue. Unlike humoral antibodies, which can be injected as an antiserum, cell-mediated immunity is not readily transferred from one individual to another.

The Complement System

The complement system is the primary mediator of the humoral immune response. The complement system, like the blood coagulation system, consists of a group of proteins that are normally present in the circulation as functionally inactive precursor components of the system. These proteins constitute 10% to 15% of the plasma–protein fraction. In order for a complement reaction to occur, each complement component must be activated in the proper sequence. There are two pathways for the activation of the complement system: the classic and the alternate pathways (Fig. 9-7).

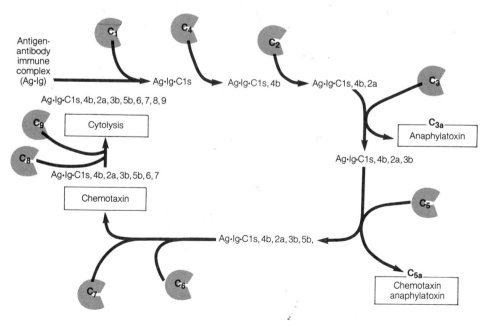

Figure 9-7 *Classic complement pathway and major biologic activities (in blocks). (Adapted from Barrett JT: Textbook of Immunology, 4th ed. St. Louis, CV Mosby, 1983)*

Table 9-2   Complement-Mediated Immune Responses

Response	Effect
Cytolysis	Destruction of cell membrane of body cells or pathogens
Adherence of immune cells	Adhesion of antigen–antibody complexes to the inert surfaces of cells or tissues such as the reticuloendothelial cells that line the blood vessels and have the capacity for phagocytosis
Chemotaxis	Chemical attraction of phagocytic cells to foreign agents
Anaphylaxis	Degranulation of mast cells with release of histamine and other inflammatory mediators
Opsonization	Modification of the antigen so that it can be easily digested by a phagocytic cell

The *classic complement pathway* is activated when target cells are able to evoke a complement-fixing antigen–antibody response (discussed in Chap. 10). Only immune responses involving IgG and IgM activate complement, and it is probable that complement is bound in all antigen–antibody reactions that involve these two classes of immunoglobulins. Portions of the complement system contribute to the chemotaxis, opsonization, immune adherence, anaphylatoxin formation, virus neutralization, and other responses associated with the immune response. Table 9-2 lists immune responses that occur as the result of complement fixation.

The *alternate (properdin) pathway* is activated by complex polysaccharides or enzymes. This system bypasses the first two steps of the classic complement pathway.

Phagocytosis

Phagocytosis is a nonspecific response in which injured cells and antigens are ingested by phagocytic cells. Phagocytosis is mainly the function of two types of cells: the neutrophils and the monocytes, or macrophages (described in Chap. 8). Phagocytosis involves four distinct but interrelated steps: (1) chemotaxis, (2) opsonization, (3) engulfment, and (4) intracellular killing. Although structurally different, both the neutrophils and the macrophages approach phagocytosis in a similar manner.

Chemotaxis involves the chemical attraction of phagocytic cells to foreign agent or pathogens. Granulocyte and macrophage chemotaxis can be stimulated by many factors, including fragments of the fifth complement factor, chemotaxic factors produced by lymphocytes, and compounds elaborated by bacteria. Defects in chemotaxis result in a decreased ability to respond to infections and overcome injury.

Opsonization renders pathogens more susceptible to ingestion by phagocytic cells. The virulence of many organisms, such as *Streptococcus pneumoniae, Klebsiella pneumoniae,* and *Haemophilus influenzae,* results from surface factors that inhibit attachment of the phagocytic cells. Opsonins provide binding sites for attachment of the phagocyte to the pathogen. Two opsonins are immunoglobulin (IgG) and the C_{3b} fragment of the complement system.

Engulfment occurs once the phagocyte recognizes the agent as foreign. Cytoplasm-filled extensions of the cell membrane surround and enclose the agent, forming a membrane-enclosed phagocytic vesicle, or *phagosome*. Interiorization occurs as the phagosome breaks away from the cell membrane and moves into the cell. Once inside the cell, the phagosome merges with a lysosome and lysosomal enzymes digest the agent.

Intracellular killing of pathogens is accomplished through a number of mechanisms in association with an acid pH environment, enzymes, and oxygen-dependent myeloperoxidases and peroxides. Neutrophils contain granules that participate in the destruction of the agent. Neutrophils are generally concerned with the phagocytosis of bacteria and organisms that rely on evading phagocytosis for survival.

The mononuclear phagocytic cells consist of blood monocytes and tissue macrophages. The blood monocytes ingest bacteria more slowly than the neutrophils and kill them less efficiently. Unlike the neutrophils, monocytes do not die when they leave the circulation but mature to become macrophages in the tissues, where they have a life span of many months or years. Macrophages are found in the lung (alveolar macrophages), liver (Kupffer's cells), spleen sinusoids, lymph nodes, peritoneum, central nervous system (microglial cells), and other areas. The term *reticuloendothelial system* is sometimes used to describe this distribution of phagocytic cells. One of the important functions of the macrophages is to phagocytize waste and foreign materials. For example, wornout red blood cells are removed by macrophages in the spleen; and in the lung, carbon and dust particles are ingested by the alveolar macrophages.

Several macrophages may fuse to form a giant cell that is large enough to enclose or wall off foreign material or debris too large to be incorporated into a single macrophage. Macrophages have several functions; they not only remove dead tissue and foreign materials, but they also release chemotaxic and other factors that participate in the inflammatory process, and they are important for antigen processing in the immune response.

Interferons

A discussion of the immune system would not be complete without mention of the interferons, which provide the body with protection from viruses and other intracellular pathogens. Interferons are a family of lymphokines that protect neighboring cells from invasion by intracellular parasites. This includes viruses, rickettsia, malarial parasites, and other intracellular organisms.[1] In addition, bacterial toxins, complex polysaccharides, and a number of other chemical substances are capable of inducing interferon production. Not all of these substances that induce interferon are antigenic. There are at least three types of interferon—α interferon (produced by T cells), β interferon (produced by fibroblasts), and γ interferon (produced by T cells). Interferon interacts at the gene level to inhibit the translation of messenger RNA, that regulate viral protein synthesis but not host protein synthesis. This antiviral activity can be transferred to neighboring cells without the continued presence of interferon. The actions of interferon are pathogen nonspecific, that is, they are effective against different types of viruses and intracellular parasites. They are, however, species specific. Animal interferons will not provide protection in humans. Of recent interest is the cell growth-regulating action of interferons. The ability of interferon to slow the growth of cancer cells has prompted investigation into its use in treatment of cancer (see Chap. 5).

Aging and the Immune Response

Aging is characterized by a declining ability to adapt to environmental stresses. One of the factors that is thought to contribute to this problem is a decline in immune responsiveness. This includes changes in both cell-mediated and antibody-mediated immune responses. Elderly persons tend to be more susceptible to infections; they have more evidence of autoimmune and immune complex disorders than younger persons, and they have a higher incidence of cancer.

The alterations in immune function that occur with advanced age are not fully understood. A decrease in the size of the thymus gland is thought to affect T-cell function. The size of the gland begins to decline shortly after sexual maturity, and by age 50 it has usually diminished to 15% or less of its maximum size.[5] There is also a progressive decrease in the absolute numbers of lympho-

Table 9-3　Major Human Histocompatibility Loci, 1977*

HLA-A	HLA-B		HLA-C	HLA-D	HLA-DR
HLA-A1	HLA-B5	HLA-Bw42	HLA-Cw1	HLA-Dw1	HLA-DRw1
HLA-A2	HLA-B7	HLA-Bw44	HLA-Cw2	HLA-Dw2	HLA-DRw2
HLA-A3	HLA-B8	HLA-Bw45	HLA-Cw3	HLA-Dw3	HLA-DRw3
HLA-A9	HLA-B12	HLA-Bw46	HLA-Cw4	HLA-Dw4	HLA-DRw4
HLA-A10	HLA-B13	HLA-Bw47	HLA-Cw5	HLA-Dw5	HLA-DRw5
HLA-A11	HLA-B14	HLA-Bw48	HLA-Cw6	HLA-Dw6	HLA-DRw6
HLA-Aw19	HLA-B15	HLA-Bw49		HLA-Dw7	HLA-DRw7
HLA-Aw23	HLA-Bw16	HLA-Bw50		HLA-Dw8	
HLA-Aw24	HLA-B17	HLA-Bw51		HLA-Dw9	
HLA-A25	HLA-B18	HLA-Bw52		HLA-Dw10	
HLA-A26	HLA-Bw21	HLA-Bw53		HLA-Dw11	
HLA-A28	HLA-Bw22	HLA-Bw54			
HLA-A29	HLA-B27				
HLA-Aw30	HLA-Bw35				
HLA-Aw31	HLA-B37				
HLA-AW32	HLA-Bw38				
HLA-Aw33	HLA-Bw39				
HLA-Aw34	HLA-B40				
HLA-Aw36	HLA-Bw41				
HLA-Aw43					
	HLA-Bw4				
	HLA-Bw6				

*The practice of applying "w" (workshop) prefixes is used to designate antigens that are only provisionally accepted by the International Histocompatibility Workshops. (Announcement: New Nomenclature for the HLA System. J Immunol 116, No 2:573, 1976)

(From Fudenberg HH et al: Basic and Clinical Immunology, 3rd ed. Copyright 1980 by Lange Medical Publications, Los Altos, California. Reproduced with permission.)

cytes, which begins during mid-life; by the sixth decade this number has decreased to 70% of the value seen in younger persons.[6] This mainly represents a decrease in T cells, especially helper T cells. As a result, delayed hypersensitivity responses, which are mediated by helper T cells, are diminished in the elderly. Likewise, there is impairment of antibody responses. This impairment is also thought to result from changes in the T-cell rather than the B-cell population. In addition to a decrease in helper T-cell function, there is evidence that suppressor functions of the immune system are altered as a result of the aging process. Impairment of suppressor function is thought to contribute to the increase in autoantibodies and autoimmune disorders in the elderly.

Histocompatibility Antigens

Histocompatibility refers to the sharing of transplantation genes. It has been found that all nucleated cells in the body contain surface antigens (histocompatibility antigens), which are genetically determined. In humans, these antigens are called the human leukocyte antigens (HLA) because they were first detected on the leukocyte. The histocompatability antigens are similar in many respects to the ABO antigens that are found on the red blood cell and that must be matched for transfusion purposes.

The histocompatibility antigens are inherited as part of the genetic makeup of an individual. Five closely linked gene loci—HLA-A, HLA-B, HLA-C, HLA-D, and HLA-DR—have been identified at the time this text is being written. These gene loci are located on the sixth chromosome. Each of the five loci is occupied by multiple alleles or genes that code the development of each cell surface antigen. There are at least 20 gene products or antigens for the A loci and 30 antigens for the B loci. Each of the antigens is numbered, HLA-A1, HLA-A2, and so on. Table 9-3 lists the major histocompatibility antigens.

Each individual receives a pair of genes, one from each parent. The pairs of genes that are inherited dictate a person's HLA type (Table 9-4). Because of the number of genes involved, the chances of common HLA types, such as persons with type A blood antigens, are unlikely.

The typing of histocompatibility antigens is important in tissue grafting and organ transplantation. The closer the matching of HLA types, the less the chance of organ or graft rejection.

It has been noted that specific HLA antigens are seen more frequently in persons with certain disease conditions (Table 9-5). For example, it has been observed that 90% of persons with ankylosing spondylitis have HLA-B27 antigen; whereas only 7% of a control group without the disease have the antigen. The mechanism responsible for the association of the HLA antigens with these diseases is not yet known.

Monoclonal Antibodies

Cell-surface antigens vary with cell type and degree of differentiation. The recent development of methods for producing monoclonal antibodies capable of recogniz-

Table 9-4   Genetic Transmission of HLA Antigens and Haplotypes

	A Antigens						B Antigens					
	1	*2*	*3*	*9*	*10*	*11*	*5*	*7*	*8*	*12*	*13*	*14*
Father	+	−	+	−	−	−	−	+	+	−	−	−
Mother	−	+	−	+	−	−	+	−	−	+	−	−
Children												
First	+	+	−	−	−	−	+	−	+	−	−	−
Second	+	−	−	+	−	−	−	−	+	+	−	−
Third	−	+	+	−	−	−	+	+	−	−	−	−
Fourth	−	+	+	−	−	−	+	+	−	−	−	−

Interpretation

	Phenotypes	*Haplotypes*
Father	A1, 3/ B7, 8	A1,B8/ A3, B7
Mother	A2, 9/ B5, 12	A2, B5/ A9, B12
Children		
First	A1, 2/ B5, 8	A1, B8/ A2, B5
Second	A1, 9/ B8, 12	A1, B8/ A9, B12
Third	A2, 3/ B5, 7	A3, B7/ A2, B5
Fourth	A2, 3/ B5, 7	A3, B7/ A2, B5

(From Barrett JT: Textbook of Immunology, 3rd ed, p 388. St Louis, CV Mosby, 1978)

Table 9-5 HLA and Disease Associations

Disease	HLA Antigen	Frequency In Patients (%)	In Controls (%)
Ankylosing spondylitis	B27	90	7
Reiter's disease	B27	76	6
Acute anterior uveitis	B27	55	8
Psoriasis	B13	18	4
	B17	29	8
	B16	15	5
Graves' disease	B8	47	21
Celiac disease (gluten-sensitive enteropathy)	D3	95	15
Dermatitis herpetiformis	B8	62	27
Myasthenia gravis	B8	52	24
Multiple sclerosis	D2	60	15
	B7	36	25
Acute lymphatic leukemia	A2	63	37
Hodgkin's disease	B5	25	16
	B1	39	32
	B8	26	22
Chronic hepatitis	B8	68	18
Ragweed hay fever Ra 5 sensitivity	B7	50	19
Allergen E sensitivity	Multiple (in family studies)		

(From Krupp MA, Chatton MJ (eds): Current Medical Diagnosis and Treatment. Copyright 1981 by Lange Medical Publications, Los Altos, California. Reproduced with permission.)

ing specific cell-surface antigens has revolutionized the study of immune cells. Monoclonal antibodies are produced in a laborious process that fuses a mouse spleen cell that has been activated by a specific cell-surface antigen with a malignant myeloma cell.[7,8] The fusion of the two cells results in single fused cell, or clone, capable of producing large amounts of a single antibody. The precision of the monoclonal antibody is such that it recognizes a single antigenic site, such as one of those located on the cell surface of hematopoietic or tumor cells. Monoclonal antibodies are used in dissecting cells of monocyte/macrophage and neutrophil lineage, in delineating between T-cells and B-cells, and in differentiating between subsets of helper and inducer T-cells. Of particular interest is the development of monoclonal antibodies that aid in the diagnosis and characterization of leukemia and other forms of cancer.

In summary, immune mechanisms can be classified into two types: specific and nonspecific. The immune response describes a specific interaction between an antigen and an antibody (humoral immunity) or an antigen and a reaction T-lymphocyte (cell-mediated immunity). It can distinguish between self and nonself and between different antigens. Nonspecific immune mechanisms include products of the complement system, phagocytosis, and interferon. These mechanisms can distinguish between self and nonself but not between pathogens. The effectiveness of the immune response decreases with aging. The HLA antigens are genetically determined antigens that are present on all nucleated cells. They are important in tissue grafting and organ transplantation. The recent development of methods of producing monoclonal antibodies capable of recognizing specific cell-surface antigens provides a means of differentiating among the different white blood cell types and an adjunct to diagnosis and characterization of hematologic and other cancers.

■ Study Guide

After you have studied this chapter, you should be able to meet the following objectives:

☐ Cite the functions of the immune system.

☐ Define the immune response.

☐ Describe the characteristics of an antigen.

☐ List the organs of the lymphoid system.

☐ Differentiate between passive and active immunity.

☐ Explain the origin of the T-lymphocyte and the B-lymphocyte.

☐ Cite the function of the plasma cell.

☐ Describe the function of the macrophage in terms of the immune response.

☐ Differentiate between specific and nonspecific immune mechanisms.

☐ Contrast humoral and cell-mediated immunity.

☐ List the five classes of immunoglobulins.

☐ Differentiate between primary and secondary immune responses.

☐ Differentiate between a regulatory T-lymphocyte and an effector T-lymphocyte.

☐ Cite the function of transfer factor in cell-mediated immunity.

☐ Relate the complement system to the immune response.

☐ Describe the four stages of phagocytosis.

☐ Describe the role of interferons in immunity.

☐ Characterize the changes in the immune response that occur in the elderly.

☐ Explain the origin of the histocompatibility antigens.

■ References

1. Barrett JT: Textbook of Immunology, 4th ed, pp 3, 40, 79, 87, 136, 215. Philadelphia, WB Saunders, 1983

2. National Institutes of Health: Understanding the Immune System, No. 84-529. Washington, DC, US Department of Health and Human Services, 1983

3. Smith LH, Their SO: Pathophysiology, p 167. Philadelphia, WB Saunders, 1981

4. Ham AW, Cormack DH: Histology, 8th ed, p 344. Philadelphia, JB Lippincott, 1979

5. Weksler ME: The senescence of the immune response. Hosp Pract 16, No. 10:55, 1981

6. Fundenberg HH, Sites DP, Caldwell JL, Well JV: Basic and Clinical Immunology, 3rd ed, p 328. Los Altos, CA, Lange Medical Publications, 1980

7. Diamond BA, Yelton DE, Scharff MD: Monoclonal antibodies. N Engl J Med 304:1344, 1981

8. Keller RH, Milson TJ, Janicek KM et al: Monoclonal antibodies: Clinical utility and the misunderstood epitope. Lab Med 15:795, 1984

Chapter 10

Alterations in the Immune Response

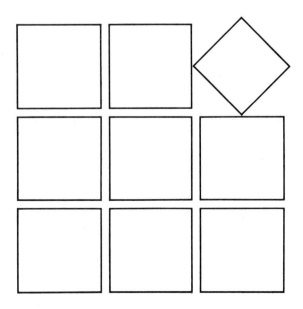

Although the immune response is a normal protective mechanism, it can cause disease when the response is deficient (immunodeficiency disease), inappropriate (allergy and hypersensitivity), or misdirected (autoimmune disease). Each of these alterations in the immune response are discussed in this chapter.

■ Immunodeficiency Disease

Immunodeficiency can be defined as an abnormality of the immune system that inhibits normal immune responsiveness. There are four major types of immune mechanisms that defend the body against assault by viral, bacterial, fungal, and other agents: (1) antibody-mediated (B-cell) immunity, (2) cell-mediated (T-cell) immunity, (3) complement factors, and (4) phagocytosis. The immunodeficiency state may be primary (hereditary or congenital) or secondary (acquired after birth), and it involves one or more of these immune mechanisms. Both primary and secondary deficiencies lead to the same spectrum of disease.[1] The severity and manifestations of the disorder depend on the type and degree of deficiency that is present.[2] The major categories of immunodeficiency are summarized in Table 10-1.

Antibody (B-Cell) Immunodeficiency

At birth a baby is partially protected by maternal IgG antibodies. During the first 4 to 5 months of life there is a gradual decline in serum IgG levels as these antibodies are destroyed; the IgG level reaches its lowest point at about 5 to 6 months. At about this time, the infant's immune system begins to function and the antibody level begins to rise, reaching adult levels when the infant is about 12 to 16 months of age. Some babies may, however, experience a delay in onset of gamma globulin production that could last until 2 to 3 years of age—*transient hypogammaglobulinemia.* These babies are particularly susceptible to bacterial and respiratory infections and to bronchitis. Usually, the condition is self-limiting and immunoglobulin production becomes normal sometime between the second and third year of life.

A much more serious disorder of immunoglobulin deficiency is a sex-linked inherited condition that is restricted to males and has an incidence of 1 in 100,000 live births.[3] This form of *X-linked hypogammaglobulinemia* was first described by Bruton in 1952 and is sometimes called Bruton's disease. It is thought that in these infants the bursa-equivalent stem cells fail to develop and as a result there is a deficiency in both B cells and plasma cells. Symptoms of the disorder usually begin to develop at about the time that maternal antibodies have been depleted (age 5 to 6 months). Children with this disorder are particularly prone to develop

severe recurrent episodes of pharyngitis, otitis media, skin infections, and respiratory tract infections from exposure to common pathogens. Diagnosis is based on demonstration of low levels of immunoglobulins in the serum. Treatment for the condition consists of injections of gamma globulin and treatment of the infections with antibiotics.

Common variable immunodeficiency (acquired hypogammaglobulinemia) consists of a group of clinical syndromes characterized by reduced levels of serum immunoglobulins, impaired ability to produce immunoglobulins following antigen exposure, and increased incidence of pyogenic (pus-forming) infections. The symptoms are similar to those of X-linked hypogammaglobulinemia but do not appear until later in life (usually between ages 15 and 35 years), and both males and females are affected equally. Affected individuals fail to produce significant levels of immunoglobulins secondary to a lack of plasma cells. Characteristically, there is a lack of germinal centers and plasma cells in the lymph nodes and spleen. These individuals have a high incidence of autoimmune disease and higher than normal incidence of abnormalities in T-cell immunity. A rheumatoidlike disorder develops in 30% of these individuals.[1] The cause of the disorder is unknown. Of interest is the greater than average incidence of autoimmune disease among first-degree relatives, which suggests a genetic basis. Treatment includes replacement therapy with human immune globulins.

A selective deficiency of IgA is the most common form of primary immunodeficiency state known. It occurs in 1 out of every 500 individuals and consists of a virtual lack of both serum and secretory IgA.[3] Most individuals with the disorder are asymptomatic, although some may have repeated respiratory infections, diarrhea, and increased incidence of asthma and other allergies. The disorder is thought to consist of a defect in the terminal stage of B-cell development. Patients with IgA deficiencies may experience an anaphylactic reaction when given a blood transfusion because the IgA in the donor blood is often recognized as a foreign agent.[4]

Cellular (T-Cell) Immunodeficiency

There are very few primary forms of T-cell deficiency. One such condition is a congenital failure of thymus gland development (*DiGeorge's syndrome*). The condition occurs as a defect associated with embryonic development of the third and fourth pharyngeal pouches. These embryonic structures are also involved in development of other parts of the head and neck, and babies born with this disorder also fail to develop the parathyroid gland and have congenital defects of the face and heart. Another condition, *Nezelof's syndrome*, is a genet-

Table 10-1   Immunodeficiency States*

Antibody (B-Cell) Immunodeficiency
Primary
  Transient hypogammaglobulinemia of infancy
  Common variable immunodeficiency
  X-linked hypogammaglobulinemia
  Selective deficiency of IgG, IgA, IgM
Secondary
  Decreased synthesis of immunoglobulins (lymphomas)
  Increased loss of immunoglobulins (nephrotic syndrome)
  Production of defective immunoglobulins (multiple myeloma)
Cellular (T-Cell) Immunodeficiency
Primary
  Congenital thymic aplasia (DiGeorge's syndrome)
  Abnormal T-cell production (Nezelof's syndrome)
Secondary
  Malignant disease (Hodgkin's disease and others)
  Transient suppression of T-cell production and function due to an acute
    viral infection such as measles.
  AIDS
Combined Antibody (B-Cell) and Cellular (T-Cell) Immunodeficiency
Primary
  Severe combined immunodeficiency (autosomal or sex-linked recessive)
  Wiskott–Aldrich syndrome (immunodeficiency, thrombocytopenia,
    and eczema)
  Immunodeficiency with ataxia and telangiectasia
Secondary
  X-radiation
  Immune suppressant and cytotoxic drugs
  Aging
Complement Abnormality
Primary
  Selective deficiency in a complement component
  Angioneurotic edema (complement 1 inactivator deficiency)
Secondary
  Acquired disorders in which complement is utilized
Phagocytic Dysfunction
Primary
  Chronic granulomatous disease
  Glucose-6-phosphate dehydrogenase deficiency
  Job's syndrome
Secondary
  Drug induced (*e.g.*, corticosteroid and immunosuppressive therapy)
  Diabetes

*Examples are not inclusive.

ically (autosomal recessive) determined disorder in which there is faulty development of the thymus gland and T-cell production, but lack of other developmental defects.

Temporary suppression of T-cell function has been reported following acute viral infections, such as measles. Viruses may actually damage the lymphocytes or mononuclear phagocytes, or they may inhibit their function. Some viruses have been found to damage cells in the thymus and thymus-dependent areas of the spleen and lymph nodes. Secondary forms of cellular immunodeficiency occur with some diseases of the lymphoid tissue, including Hodgkin's disease, a neoplastic disease of lymphoid tissue. Persons with Hodgkin's disease have impaired T-cell function and what is called *anergy*, or the failure to respond to a variety of skin antigens, including the tuberculin test. In terms of the protective function of the T cells, persons with Hodgkin's disease have a well-defined predisposition to develop tuberculosis, fungal and yeast infections, and herpes zoster varicella. The immunodeficiency observed with Hodgkin's disease and other neoplasms may be due to a number of factors including the effects of the tumor, depression of the immune system associated with irradiation and drugs used in treatment of cancer, and malnutrition.

Acquired immunodeficiency syndrome (AIDS)

The term *acquired immunodeficiency syndrome (AIDS)* is used to describe a diverse array of disorders, including opportunistic infections and Kaposi's sarcoma, that are predictive of defective cell-mediated immunity that cannot be attributed to a cause such as immunosuppressive therapy. The mortality due to the syndrome is as high as 80%.[5] The disease was initially seen in two groups of persons, male homosexuals and persons who abused intravenous drugs.[6-9] More recently, AIDS has been reported in persons with hemophilia who require treatment with factor VIII preparations, which are made from the plasma of multiple donors.[10] Cases have also been reported among native Haitians in both Haiti and the United States.[11]

The underlying problem in AIDS is a defective immune system that leaves the person unable to resist infections and, apparently, cancer. *Pneumocystis carinii* pneumonia, which accounts for 51% of all primary diagnoses, is the most common life-threatening opportunistic infection associated with AIDS.[8] Second is Kaposi's sarcoma, which accounts for 26% of all diagnoses.[8] Other opportunistic infections associated with AIDS are extensive mucosal candidas, cytomegalovirus pneumonia, herpes simplex virus infections, toxoplasmosis of the central nervous system, cryptococcal meningitis, avian tuberculosis, aspergillosis, nocardiosis, and prolonged varicella zoster.[7] Kaposi's sarcoma is a rare form of malignancy seldom seen in the United States.[12] The tumors usually begin in the skin and consist of pink to red lesions, progressing to slightly elevated plaques and nodules ranging in color from blue-purple to red-brown. Generalized lymphadenopathy follows, and finally there is spread to the gastrointestinal tract and lungs.

The clinical manifestations of AIDS are related to infections and other problems associated with the altered immune state. They include fatigue, fever, night sweats, weight loss, hepatomegaly, and splenomegaly. In the homosexual group, most of the cases have a history of multiple sexual partners, "recreational" drug use, and frequent sexually transmitted infections.[8]

The immune deficiency associated with AIDS is characterized by markedly impaired T-lymphocyte function without impairment of the humoral response. There is a reduction in helper T-lymphocytes and increased suppressor T-lymphocytes with an inverted helper/suppressor T-lymphocyte ratio.[13] There is also an abnormal response of T-lymphocytes to mitogen (a substance that stimulates mitosis) stimulation, a decreased natural killer-cell activity, and, paradoxically, hypergammaglobulinemia.[13]

Until recently, the cause of AIDS was unknown. Because most of the homosexual patients with AIDS appear to have been partially immunosuppressed before developing the disease, it had been suggested that the disorder might represent immune system exhaustion or an infectious process. Both homosexuals and drug users engage in practices that could have great impact on the immune system. Drug users have contact with numerous infections from sharing needles, and they are continually exposed to antigenic contaminants in "street" drugs. The earliest candidates proposed as agents of AIDS were the Epstein-Barr virus and cytomegalovirus, which are commonly found in the serum of AIDS patients and in individuals belonging to high-risk groups. Frequent exposure to the cytomegalovirus, which causes transient immunosuppression in the normal host, had been suggested.[6] It is now known that AIDS is caused by the human T-cell lymphotropic virus (HTLV) type III virus.[10] The antibody for the HTLV-III virus has been identified and is now available for screening of blood products and other testing purposes.

The mode of disease transmission appears to be through blood and body secretions. The most common forms of transmission are sexual contact, administration of contaminated blood products, use of contaminated needles by drug addicts, and from mother to fetus or newborn. It seems unlikely that the virus is transmitted through casual contacts with persons such as classmates or co-workers. Although the earliest reports of sexual transmission were confined largely to the homosexual population, reports of heterosexual transmission are becoming more common. Because of the seriousness of the disease, there is public concern about how to limit the sexual spread of the disease by persons known to be infected with the virus. Although much is known about the disease, many questions remain unanswered. For example, not all persons with the HTLV-III antibody develop AIDS, and it is not known what cofactors make an infected host more likely to develop the disease. Expression of the disease may depend on genetic and environmental factors.[9]

Combined Antibody (B-Cell) and Cellular (T-Cell) Immunodeficiency

A complete lack of both humoral and cellular immunity causes early susceptibility to infection. The deficiency state can be sex-linked or autosomal recessive. Infants with the disorder seldom survive beyond the first year of life because of poor resistance to infection unless confined to a sterile environment. Of recent interest was the boy from Houston, Texas, who was able to survive for more than 12 years in a sterile plastic bubble environment.[17] A histocompatible bone-marrow transplant is the treatment of choice.

There are several other combined forms of humoral and cellular immunodeficiency. These conditions are accompanied by other abnormalities. One of these is the Wiskott-Aldrich syndrome, which is accompanied by thrombocytopenia and eczema. Another is ataxia-telangiectasia, in which loss of muscle coordination and blood vessel dilatation are combined with deficits in IgA and IgE production and T-lymphocyte function.

Disorders of the Complement System

Complement plays a critical role in both specific and nonspecific immune responses. It is necessary for normal chemotaxis and killing of bacteria (Chap. 9). Alterations in the complement system can consist of a deficiency of one or more of its components or acquired disorders in which complement is involved in the pathogenesis of the condition.

There are several known abnormalities of the complement system. One of the better-known defects is a condition called *hereditary angioneurotic edema*, which is caused by a congenital deficiency of complement 1 inactivator. The uncontrolled activation of this component of the complement system leads to sporadic attacks of subcutaneous edema, which are associated with minor trauma to the affected part. In extensive reactions, edema of the face, neck, and joints may occur. Edema of the throat may make breathing difficult, and edema of the abdominal organs may produce intense abdominal pain.

Other deficiencies of the complement system have been described, and many are associated with recurrent infections. A decrease in complement levels has also been observed in a number of autoimmune disorders such as lupus erthymatosus, poststreptococcal glomerulonephritis, and autoimmune homolytic anemia. The reason for this deficiency is unknown. Many of the actions of complement are essential for phagocytosis and clearing the body of immune complexes. It has been suggested that a deficiency in classic complement components may lead to inadequate solubility and clearance of immune complexes.[18]

Disorders of Phagocytosis

Phagocytosis is an important defense mechanism in terms of removal of bacteria and foreign agents from the body. As with other alterations in immune function, defects in phagocytosis may occur as a primary genetic or congenital defect or secondary to drug therapy or disease states.

Primary disorders of phagocytosis are usually caused by enzyme deficiencies within the metabolic pathways used by the phagocytes for killing bacteria or destroying other agents. *Chronic granulomatous disease* is inherited as an X-linked disorder of phagocytosis. The metabolic pathways of both neutrophils and monocytes are abnormal, and susceptibility to organisms that usu-

ally are of low virulence such as *Staphylococcus epidermidis, Candida, and aspergillus* increases. The disorder usually becomes apparent during the first year of life. Manifestations include marked lymphadenopathy and heptatosplenomegaly associated with impaired phagocytic function of cells within these structures. Infections of the lymph nodes, skin, lungs, gastrointestinal tract, liver, and bone are common. Treatment includes use of antibiotics, and, in some cases, white cell infusions. *Job's syndrome* results in eczematoid skin lesions, otitis media, and chronic nasal discharge. It is thought to be a variant of chronic granulomatous disease. *Deficiency of leukocyte glucose-6-phosphate-dehydrogenase* is associated with a form of hemolytic anemia (Chap. 13). When this deficiency is present, there is impairment of glucose metabolism by the leukocytes, which are unable to destroy certain organisms.

Secondary disorders of phagocytosis can occur in a number of conditions. *Opsonins* are substances that alter an agent so that it can undergo phagocytosis. Antibodies and complement are the two main opsonins. Thus, deficiencies of either antibodies or complement cause impairment of phagocyte function. Immunosuppressive and corticosteroid drugs decrease the number of phagocytic cells and impair phagocytosis. Impaired phagocytic function is thought to contribute to the high incidence of infections that occur in persons with poorly controlled diabetes. The defect appears to involve a reduction in opsonic activity and a decrease in intracellular killing of organisms, probably related to altered metabolism of the phagocytes.[19]

In summary, immunodeficiency states describe an absolute or relative lack (or dysfunction) of immune cells or other factors, such as complement, which defend the body from invasion by foreign agents or the growth of malignant cells. There are four types of immunodeficiency states: (1) antibody (B-cell) immunodeficiency, (2) cellular (T-cell) immunodeficiency, (3) disorders of the complement system, and (4) impairment of phagocytosis. These immunodeficiency states can be primary (hereditary or congenital) or secondary (acquired after birth) and may involve one or more immune mechanisms. The severity of immunodeficiency states is dependent on the type and degree of deficiency that is present.

■ Allergy and Hypersensitivity

Allergy and hypersensitivity are immune responses in which the antigen is an environmental agent, food, or drug that is not intrinsically harmful. Gell and Coombs[20] have divided allergic responses into four categories:

I. *Type I* is an IgE-mediated response that causes release of histamine and slow-reacting substance of anaphylaxis (SRS-A) from mast cells. The types of reactions seen in this category are anaphylaxis and atopic allergies such as hay fever, asthma, and urticaria (hives).

II. *Type II* is an IgG- or IgM-mediated response. it is a cytotoxic reaction that most often involves complement, but this is not a requirement. Certain drug reactions fit into this category.

III. *Type III* is an IgG- or IgM-mediated antigen–antibody complex reaction. Serum sickness is a type III response.

IV. *Type IV* is a cell-mediated response in which sensitized T-lymphocytes react with an antigen to cause inflammation. Contact dermatitis is a type IV response; as is the tuberculin reaction.

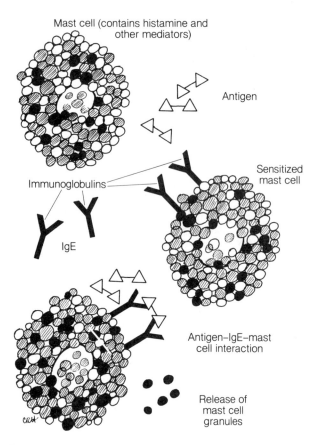

Mast cell (contains histamine and other mediators)

Antigen

Immunoglobulins

IgE

Sensitized mast cell

Antigen–IgE–mast cell interaction

Release of mast cell granules

Figure 10-1 *Type I immune response that involves an allergen (antigen), immunoglobulin (IgE), and mast cell. Exposure to the allergen causes sensitization of the mast cell with subsequent binding of the allergen, which causes release of mast cell granules containing inflammatory mediators such as histamine and SRS-A.*

Type I Allergic Responses

The term *atopy* is used to describe allergic conditions that have a familial predisposition. About 1 out of every 10 persons in the United States suffers from symptomatic allergies of this type.

Atopic immune responses result from immunoglobulin IgE activity. These immunoglobulins are sometimes called *reagins*. Reagins function only when they are attached to mast cells or basophils. Atopic reactions include anaphylaxis, seasonal pollen allergy (hay fever), allergic rhinitis, and atopic skin reactions. This discussion focuses on general concepts of atopy and seasonal pollen allergy, allergic rhinitis, food allergies, and atopic dermatitis. Anaphylactic shock is discussed in Chapter 21 and bronchial asthma in Chapter 23.

Mast cells (tissue cells) and basophils (blood cells) have granules that contain mediators involved in allergic reactions. In predisposed individuals, allergen stimulation causes IgE to bind to mast cells. On subsequent exposure, the allergen binds to the IgE on the sensitized mast cells, and this results in a series of reactions that culminate in the release of histamine and vasoactive substances from the mast cell (Fig. 10-1). There are four known mediators that are released from mast cells during an allergen-IgE-mediated response: (1) *histamine*, which causes increased vascular permeability; (2) *eosinophil chemotactic factor*, which attracts eosinophils; (3) *slow-reacting substance of anaphylaxis (SRS-A)*, which causes constriction of smooth muscle, such as bronchiole smooth muscle; and (4) *platelet-activating factor*, which causes platelet aggregation and lysis.

Seasonal pollen allergy and allergic rhinitis

Seasonal pollen allergy (hay fever) is associated with sneezing, itching, and watery drainage from the eyes and nose. The conjunctiva is usually reddened and swollen and there is often an accompanying irritation and itching of the pharynx and outer ear canal. The nasal mucosa is usually pale and boggy. Nasal polyps are grapelike cystic masses that are commonly associated with allergic rhinitis. Microscopic examination of a properly stained smear of nasal secretions usually demonstrates a large number of eosinophils, whereas neutrophils predominate in infectious rhinitis.

A person with hay fever may be allergic to one or more inhalants. Common inhalants that cause hay fever are pollens from ragweed, trees, grasses, weeds, and fungal spores. There is usually a season within each geographic location in the United States during which the common trees, grasses, and weeds pollinate. It is during these seasonal periods that persons with specific allergies are expected to have symptoms. In the Midwest, for example, ragweed season begins about August 15 and continues until after the first frost. Allergic rhinitis is usually a more perennial problem, caused by allergens such as house dust, animal danders, feathers, and fungal spores that are present the year round.

Diagnosis of seasonal pollen allergy and allergic rhinitis usually requires a careful history of food habits, exposure to inhalants, use of cosmetics and toiletries, presence of household pets, seasonal pattern of symptoms, and so forth. Skin tests provide a means for identifying the specific allergies. This is done by scratch or intradermal testing in which a small amount of a dilute solution of the antigen is applied to the skin; the area is then observed for edema and redness.

Treatment of hay fever and allergic rhinitis consists of avoiding the allergen when possible, treating the symptoms, and desensitizing for the antigen. When an individual responds to a single allergen, such as feathers in a bed pillow, it is often possible to eliminate the allergen. Antihistamine drugs usually provide symptomatic relief at the onset of the season, but their effectiveness often wanes as the season continues. Nasal decongestants of the sympathomimetic type are effective by themselves or with antihistamines. The anti-inflammatory steroid drugs are usually reserved for severe hay fever that cannot be controlled by other methods. Desensitization involves frequent (usually weekly) injections of the offending antigen(s). The antigens, which are given in increasing doses, stimulate production of high levels of IgG, which acts as a blocking antibody by combining with the antigen before it can combine with the cell-bound IgE antibodies.

Food allergies

Food allergies can occur at any age, although they are usually more common in children. They are usually type I allergic responses and frequently accompany other manifestations of atopic allergy. The reaction occurs when IgE antibodies in the intestinal mucosa react with the food allergen, causing release of mediators of the immune response. Systemic manifestations result from absorption of these mediators into the bloodstream. Allergens are usually food proteins or partially digested food products. Carbohydrates, fats, and food additives such as flavoring, preservatives, and food colorings are also potential allergens. Closely related foods can contain common or cross-reacting antigens. For example, some individuals may be allergic to all legumes (beans, peas, and peanuts). Some allergens are heat labile and are destroyed by cooking.[1] Diagnosis of food allergies is usually based on history rather than skin tests, which are often inaccurate. Avoidance of the food rather than desensitization is recommended.

Atopic dermatitis

Another form of type I hypersensitivity reaction is atopic dermatitis. The disorder is usually associated with a family history of atopy and a history of other allergies. Up to 70% of persons with atopic dermatitis have some type of allergic respiratory disorder and 70% have a family history of atopy.[21] This disorder typically appears in early childhood and either disappears or becomes less severe with age. Onset is in the first year of life in 60% of cases and within the first 5 years of life in 90%.[21] In infants the lesions are usually oozing, weeping, and eczematous. Consequently, the condition is often referred to as eczema in this age group. The lesions usually affect the forehead, cheeks, and extensor surfaces of the extremities in infants and small children. At later ages, the neck and anticubital and popliteal spaces are more commonly affected. The skin is dry, erythematous, and pruritic (itchy). This leads to excoriations, papules, and scaling. The disease usually improves spontaneously during the summer months.

The cause of atopic dermatitis is uncertain. IgE levels are elevated and histamine release seems important. It does not seem to be related to exposure to specific allergens, although food allergies may be demonstrated in children. Milk, wheat, eggs, corn, fish, and legumes are common food allergens. Recent studies suggest a partial defect in cell-mediated immunity.

Treatment includes the application of nonirritating lubricants to decrease the dryness of the skin. If a sensitivity to foods is noted, these foods are eliminated from the diet. Because foods have been implicated as a cause of eczema in infants, only one new solid food is usually added to an infant's diet at a time. Topical corticosteroid may be used to reduce the inflammatory response. The most common complication is secondary infection.

Type II Cytotoxic Reactions

In type II reactions IgM or IgG immunoglobulins react with cell-surface antigens to activate the complement system and produce direct damage to the cell surface (Fig. 10-2). The cytotoxic reactions include transfusion reactions, hemolytic disease of the newborn, autoimmune hemolytic anemia, and certain drug reactions in which antibodies are formed to react with the drug that is complexed to the red-cell antigens.

Type III Immune Complex Reactions

Type III reactions involve the complement-activating IgG and IgM immunoglobulins and the classic complement pathway. This type of reaction is characterized by the formation of an immune complex. These complexes

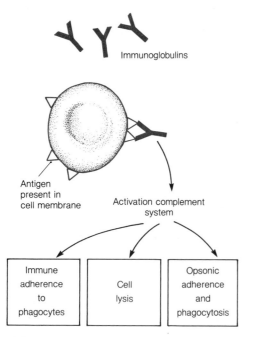

Figure 10-2 *Type II cytotoxic immune reactions that involve immunoglobulins (IgG and IgM) and cell-surface antigens with activation of the complement system.*

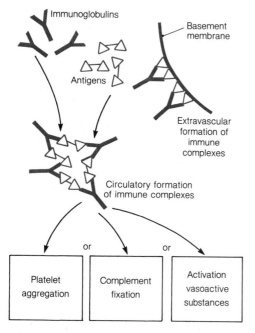

Figure 10-3 *Type III immune complex reactions that involve complement-activating IgG and IgM immunoglobulins with formation of blood-borne or extravascular immune complexes and their effects.*

become attached to walls of blood vessels where they cause tissue damage by activating the complement system. Two of the more common immune complex disorders are serum sickness and the Arthus reaction (see Fig. 10-3).

Serum sickness develops in about 50% of persons receiving bovine or horse antitoxin against tetanus, gas gangrene, and other infections.[22] Fortunately, antitoxin therapy is infrequently used today because most individuals have been actively immunized for tetanus and human antisera are available. At present the most common cause of serum sickness is an adverse reaction to drugs such as penicillin. The symptoms of serum sickness usually appear at about 7 to 10 days following exposure to the offending antigen. The signs and symptoms that occur at this time include urticaria, patchy or generalized rash, extensive edema (usually of the face, neck, and joints), and fever. In previously sensitized individuals, severe and even fatal forms of serum sickness may occur either immediately or within several days after the sensitizing drug or serum is administered.

The *Arthus reaction* is a local reaction to the immune complex. It consists of vasculitis and tissue necrosis at the site of antigen exposure. The reaction causes erythema and swelling, which begins within several hours, and progresses to form a central area of cellular necrosis. Usually the area dries and heals within a week. The Arthus reaction is involved in hypersensitivity pneumonitis and extrinsic alveolitis (Chap. 23). These disorders include farmer's lung, caused by breathing dust from moldy hay, pigeon breeder's disease, caused by exposure to pigeon droppings and danders, and humidifer lung from inhalation of fungal spores that grow in humidifiers. Allergic pneumonitis is characterized by a dry cough, shortness of breath, fever, and general malaise that appears about 6 to 8 hours after exposure to the antigen. The symptoms subside within a few days, but reappear with each subsequent exposure to the agent.

Type IV Cell-Mediated Hypersensitivity

Cell-mediated hypersensitivity reactions involve T-lymphocytes that have been sensitized to locally deposited antigens. The reaction is mediated by release of lymphokines, direct cytotoxicity, or both (Fig. 10-4). Cell-mediated immunity is also called delayed hypersensitivity, compared with immediate hypersensitivity, which is caused by immunoglobulins such as IgE. Two of the more common types of cell-mediated immunity are the tuberculin test and contact dermatitis.

The *tuberculin test*, in which a purified component of the tubercle bacillus is injected intradermally, produces a delayed type of hypersensitivity reaction. In a

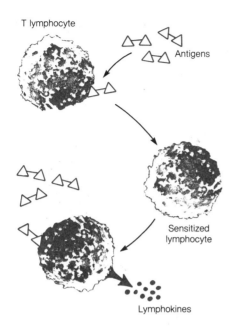

T lymphocyte

Antigens

Sensitized
lymphocyte

Lymphokines

Figure 10-4 *Type IV immune response that involves an antigen, sensitized T-lymphocyte, and lymphokines. Exposure to the antigen causes sensitization of the lymphocyte with release of lymphokines on subsequent exposures.*

previously sensitized individual, there is redness and swelling at the site of injection as the sensitized T-type lymphocytes interact with the tuberculin antigen. The reaction usually develops gradually over a period of 48 to 72 hours. As a point of clarification, it is important to recognize that the tuberculin test merely indicates that an individual has been sensitized to the tuberculosis bacillus through a previous exposure—it does not mean that the person has the disease.

Contact dermatitis is an acute or chronic dermatitis that results from direct contact with different chemical agents or other irritants, such as cosmetics, hair dyes, metals, and drugs applied to the skin. Two of the best known types of contact dermatitis are due to poison ivy and poison oak. When the sap from these plants comes in contact with the skin, neoantigens are formed, and sensitization to these new antigens develops. Contact dermatitis lesions usually consist of erythematous macules, papules, and vesicles (blisters). The affected area often becomes swollen and warm, with exudation, crusting, and development of a secondary infection. The location of the lesions often provides a clue as to the nature of the antigen causing the disorder.

In summary, hypersensitivity and allergic reactions are immune responses in which the antigen is an environmental agent, food, or drug usually considered harmless. There are four basic types of hypersensitivity responses: (1) a type I response that is mediated by the IgE immu-

noglobulins and includes anaphylactic shock, hay fever, and bronchial asthma; (2) type II cytotoxic reactions that are caused by IgG- or IgM-activated complement and include hemolytic responses due to blood transfusion reactions; (3) type III hypersensitivity reactions in which IgG or IgM reacts with an antigen to form an immune complex that causes local tissue injury; and (4) type IV cell-mediated responses in which sensitized T-lymphocytes react with an antigen to cause inflammation and tissue injury.

■ Transplant Rejection

In transplant rejection the body recognizes the histocompatibility (HLA) antigens of the donor as foreign. In organ transplantation (*e.g.*, kidney transplant) immunosuppressive therapy is used to lessen the chance of rejection. Rejection usually involves both cell-mediated and humoral immunity and is a complex process. There are three basic patterns of transplant rejection: hyperacute, acute, and chronic.

A hyperacute response occurs almost immediately following the transplant; in kidney transplants, it can often be noted at the time of surgery. As soon as blood flow from the recipient to the donor kidney has been established, the kidney, instead of becoming pink and viable-looking, becomes cyanotic, mottled, and flaccid in appearance. Sometimes the onset of the reaction is not so sudden, but develops over a period of hours or several days. The hyperacute transplant rejection is caused by the presence of existing recipient antibodies to the graft that act at the level of the vascular epithelium to incite an Arthus type of reaction. These antibodies have usually developed in response to previous blood transfusions, pregnancies in which the mother develops antibodies to fetal antigens that have been inherited from the father, or infections with HLA crossreacting bacteria or viruses.

Acute rejection is seen in the first months following transplant. In the patient with a kidney transplant, acute rejection is evidenced by signs of renal failure. Acute rejection often involves both humoral and cell-mediated immune responses.

Chronic rejection occurs over a period of months following transplant and is largely caused by cell-mediated immune responses. In renal transplant patients this rejection pattern causes a gradual rise in serum creatinine over a period of 4 to 6 months.[23]

■ Autoimmune Disease

Inherent in the normal immune response is the ability of the immune system to recognize body cells as self and to distinguish them from nonself. There is a normal immunologic tolerance that prevents damage to body tissues by the immune response. In autoimmune disease, self-antigens or abnormal immune cells that incite the immune response develop. Autoimmunity can involve abnormal or excessive activity of T cells, B cells, or the complement system.

Probable Mechanisms

There are at least five probable mechanisms to explain the development of autoimmune disease. The *first* is based on the hidden antigen theory in which it is postulated that the contact of developing lymphocyte clones, with their respective antigens during fetal or early postfetal life, leads to destruction of the corresponding clones. It is also possible that circulating self-antigens, which are present throughout life, continually destroy their corresponding clones of lymphocytes before they can develop into immunocompetent cells. If this is true, autoimmune disease can develop if cells that have been hidden from the immune system during lymphocyte development were released. For example, trauma to the testes, with release of sperm into the tissues and circulation, has resulted in the development of sperm antibodies.[24] *Second*, it is possible that body cells or tissues are *altered* by chemical, physical, or biologic means so that they become self-antigens. It has been suggested that certain drugs can combine with body cells, converting them into autoantigens. Autoimmune anemia associated with such drugs as the antihypertensive medication alpha-methyldopa may result from the drug's effect on the red-cell surface.[23] A *third* potential is that similarities exist between exogenous antigens and self-antigens, which allows for *cross-reactions* to occur. For example, evidence suggests that in rheumatic fever, the antibody formed to the streptococcus cross-reacts with tissues found in the heart. *Fourth*, it is possible that *mutations* or alterations in the function of the immune cells develop and that these lead to inappropriate immune responses. For example, loss of T-cell suppressor function or B-cell activity and production of immunoglobulins to self-antigens have been suggested as contributing to autoimmune diseases such as systemic lupus erythematosus. A *fifth* possibility is that inherited immune genes that are linked to the *histocompatibility antigens* may predispose to altered immune responses and rejection of one's own tissues.

Autoimmune diseases can affect almost any cell or tissue in the body. There are known autoimmune disorders of blood cells and various body tissues, and disorders that affect multiple organs and systems. Table 10-2 describes some of the probable autoimmune diseases. Lupus erythematosus is presented in this chapter as an example of an autoimmune disease. A discussion of many of the other autoimmune disorders is included in other sections of the book.

Systemic Lupus Erythematosus

Systemic lupus erythematosus (SLE) is a chronic autoimmune disease that affects multiple body systems. Recent studies indicate that the prevalence of the disease is about 1 in 2000.[25] The disease is seen most frequently in the 20- to 40-year-old age group, with about 85% of the affected persons being women. Blacks are affected more frequently than whites. There is a strong familial predisposition for development of the disease.

A lupuslike reaction that is indistinguishable both clinically and in the laboratory from spontaneously occurring SLE can also develop from the continual use of a number of drugs, especially the antihypertensive drug hydralazine and the antiarrhythmic drug procainamide. Drug-induced reactions usually disappear once the drug has been discontinued.

One of the first cellular changes to develop in SLE of immunologic origin is the presence of *LE cells* in the blood. The LE cells are neutrophils that contain a large LE body that has been engulfed. This LE body originates from the nucleus of certain white blood cells that have undergone nuclear changes and have been stripped of their cytoplasm by other phagocytic leukocytes. The LE factor responsible for this reaction has been identified as an antideoxyribonucleoprotein (anti-DNA) antibody of the IgG type. The relationship between the LE factor found in the serum and the development of the body changes that occur with SLE is still obscure, particularly because the LE cells are found in only about 75% to 80% of persons with SLE and in about 15% of persons with other collagen diseases such as rheumatoid arthritis and scleroderma.[1]

The disease affects many organs and body systems, including the skin, joints, kidneys, and serosal surfaces. Its course may vary from a mild episodic disorder to a rapidly fatal illness.

The *skin* lesions include the classic "butterfly" rash that extends over the nose and cheeks—the sign of the red wolf for which the disease is named. There is extreme sensitivity to sunlight, and the rash appears in areas of the body that are exposed to sunlight. Depending on the course of the disease, the rash may resolve without problems or it may progress to form scars, hypo- or hyperpigmentation, or discoid lesions. A *polyarthritis* occurs in about 90% of persons with SLE; it can affect any of the joints and is often the first manifestation of the disease. The arthritis seldom causes deformities, and erosive lesions usually are not observed on x-ray films. Involvement of the *serous cavities* can lead to pleural and pericardial effusion and pleurisy. *Renal* involvement is a common and serious complication of SLE. The most severe type of renal lesion observed in SLE is proliferative glomerulonephritis, which may be associated with nephrosis and renal failure. It is probably due to

Table 10-2 Probable Autoimmune Diseases

Disorder	Probable Antigens
Systemic	
Systemic lupus erythematosus	Numerous nuclear and cellular components
Rheumatoid arthritis	IgG
Dermatomyositis	Nuclear antigens, myosin (?)
Scleroderma	Nuclear antigens, IgG
Sjögren's syndrome	salivary gland, thyroid, nuclear antigens
Mixed connective-tissue disease	Ribonucleoprotein
Blood	
Autoimmune hemolytic anemia	Erythrocyte antigens
Idiopathic thrombocytopenic purpura	Platelet surface antigens
Neutropenia and lymphopenia	Surface antigens
Other Organs	
Hashimoto's thyroiditis	Thyroglobulin
Thyrotoxicosis	Cell surface TSH receptors
Goodpasture's syndrome	Kidney and lung basement membranes
Pernicious anemia	Parietal cell antigens, intrinsic factor
Myasthenia gravis	Acetylcholine receptors, muscle
Primary biliary cirrhosis	Mitochondria, bile duct cells
Chronic active hepatitis	Liver cells, virally infected
Ulcerative colitis	Colonic mucosal cells
Autoimmune adrenalitis	Adrenal cells
Juvenile autoimmune diabetes	Islet-cell antigens
Premature gonadal failure	Cells of the ovary and testes
Sympathetic ophthalmia	Uvea
Temporal arteritis	Blood-vessel antigens
Acute idiopathic polyneuritis	Peripheral nerve myelin
Insulin-resistant diabetes	Insulin receptors

(From Robbins SL, Cotran RS: Pathologic Basis of disease, p. 293, Philadelphia, WB Saunders, 1979)

immune-complex deposition in the glomerular basement membrane. Among the other manifestations of SLE are neurologic disorders such as severe depression, psychosis, and convulsions. Ocular disturbances may also occur, including conjunctivitis. The disease is often called the great imitator because it affects so many body systems and can imitate so many different disease conditions.

In summary, autoimmune disease represents a disordered immune response in which the body recognizes its own tissues as foreign. Autoimmune disorders can involve the T cells, B cells, or the complement system and can affect any of the body cells and tissues. Among the theories that have been used to explain the origin of autoimmunity are the (1) hidden antigen theory, which suggests that autoimmunity develops as a result of release of substances that were sequestered from the immune system during the fetal or early postfetal period when the developing lymphocyte clones for autoantigens were being destroyed by their corresponding antigens; (2) development of an altered body antigen that comes about by chemical, physical, or biologic means; (3) occurrence of a cross-reaction in which an exogenous antigen and a body tissue or cell type share antigenic properties; (4) establishment of a mutation of immune cells that leads to an inappropriate immune response; and (5) influence of the HLA antigens in rejection of a person's own tissues.

■ Study Guide

After you have studied this chapter, you should be able to meet the following objectives:

☐ List the most important categories of immunodeficiency disorders, and state one example of each category.

☐ List populations at risk for developing AIDS.

☐ State the immune mechanism that is impaired in AIDS.

☐ Describe the effect of impaired immune function in AIDS.

□ Explain the pathogenesis of type I allergic responses.

□ List the possible causes of serum sickness.

□ Define the Arthus reaction.

□ Explain the pathogenesis of type IV cell-mediated hypersensitivity.

□ Describe the three patterns of transplant rejection.

□ Describe three or more postulated mechanisms underlying autoimmune disease.

□ State the significance of the LE factor in systemic lupus erythematosus.

■ References

1. Fundenberg HH, Stites DP, Caldwell JL, Wells JV: Basic and Clinical Immunology, pp 409, 445, 529. Los Altos, CA, Lange Medical Publications, 1980

2. Wedgewood RJ, Rosen FS, Paul NW (eds): Primary immunodeficiency disease: Report of the International Workshop held September 12-16, 1982 at Rosario Resort, Orcas Island, Washington. Birth Defects 19:345, 1983

3. Baradana EJ: A conceptual approach to immunodeficiency. Med Clin North Am 65, No 5:959, 1981

4. Sodeman WA, Sodeman TM: Pathologic Physiology: Mechanisms of Disease, p 125. Philadelphia, WB Saunders, 1979

5. Hallansbee SE, Busch DF, Wofsy CB et al: An outbreak of *Pneumocystis carinii* pneumonia in homosexual man. Ann Intern Med 96:705, 1982

6. Curran JW, Evatt BL, Lawrence DN: Acquired immune deficiency syndrome: The past as a prologue. Ann Intern Med 98:401, 1983

7. Marx J: New disease baffles medical community. Science 217:618, 1982

8. Aledort LM: AIDS: An update. Hosp Pract 18, No 9:159, 1983

9. Curran JW: AIDS—Two years later. N Engl J Med 309:610, 1983

10. Davis KC, Horsburgh CR, Ute H et al: Acquired immunodeficiency syndrome in a patient with hemophilia. Ann Intern Med 98:284, 1983

11. Pitchenik AE, Fischl MA, Dickson GM et al: Opportunistic infections and Kaposi's sarcoma among Haitians: Evidence of a new acquired immunodeficiency state. Ann Intern Med 98:277, 1983

12. Friedman-Kien AE, Laubenstein LJ, Rubinstein P: Disseminated Kaposi's sarcoma in homosexual men. Ann Intern Med 96:693, 1982

13. Kornfeld H, Stouwe RA, Lange M: T-lymphocyte subpopulations in homosexual men. N Engl J Med 307:729, 1982

14. Check WA: Preventing AIDS transmission: Should blood donors be screened? JAMA 249:567, 1983

15. Prevention of acquired immune deficiency syndrome (AIDS): Report of inter-agency recommendations. JAMA 249:1544, 1983

16. Marx J: Health officials seeks ways to halt AIDS. Science 219:272, 1983

17. Plastic bubble remains boy's home. JAMA 237:521, 1977

18. Smith LH, Their SO: Pathophysiology, p 234. Philadelphia, WB Saunders, 1981

19. Rayfield EJ, Ault MJ, Keutsch GT et al: Infection and diabetes: The case for glucose control. Am J Med 72:439, 1982

20. Gell RGH, Coombs RRA, Lachman PJ(eds): Clinical Aspects of Immunology, 3rd ed. Oxford, Blackwell Scientific, 1975

21. Hanifin JM: Atopic dermatitis. Postgrad Med 74, No 3:188, 1983

22. Barrett JT: Textbook of Immunology, 4th ed, pp 380, 424. St Louis, CV Mosby, 1983

23. Robbins SL, Cotran RS, Kumar V: Pathologic Basis of Disease, 3rd ed, pp 174, 179. Philadelphia, WB Saunders, 1984

24. Heckman A, Rumke P: Autoimmunity and isoimmunity against spermatozoa. In Miescher PA, Miller-Eberhard HJ (eds): Textbook of Immunopathology, Vol II, 2nd ed, p 947. New York, Grune & Stratton, 1976

25. Shearn MA, Engleman EP: Arthritis and allied rheumatic disorders. In Krupp MA, Marcus A, Chatton MJ (eds): Current Medical Diagnosis and Treatment, p 505. Los Altos, CA, Lange Medical Publications, 1984

■ Additional References

Becker MJ, Drucker I, Farkas R et al: Monocyte-mediated regulation of cellular immunity in humans: Loss of suppressor activity with ageing. Clin Exp Immunol 45:439, 1981

Benacerraf Baruj: Suppressor T cells and suppressor factor. Hosp Pract 13, No 4:65, 1978

Bridgewater SC, Voignier RR, Smith CS: Allergies in children: Recognition. Am J Nurs 78, No 4:613, 1978

Colten HR, Alper CA, Rosen FS: Genetics and biosynthesis of complement proteins. N Engl J Med 304:653, 1981

Czernicki J, Rzetelski B, Offierska M: Suppressor cells function in healthy persons. Acta Physiol 32:461, 1981

Dharan M: The immune system: Immunoglobulin abnormalities. Am J Nurs 76, No 10:1626, 1976

Donley DL: The immune system: Nursing the patient who is immunosuppressed. Am J Nurs 76, No 10:1619, 1976

Fauci AS (moderator): Activation and regulation of human immune responses: Implications in normal and disease states (NIH Conference). Ann Intern Med 99:61, 1983

Fruth R: Anaphylaxis and drug reactions: Guidelines for detection and care. Heart Lung 9, No 4:662, 1980

Groenwald SL: Physiology of the immune system. Heart Lung 9, No 4:645, 1980

Goodwin JS, Searles RP, Tung SK: Immunological responses of a healthy elderly population. Clin Exp Immunol 48:403, 1982

Hanson JM, Rumjanek VM, Morley J: Mediators of cellular immune reactions. Pharmacol Ther 17:165, 1982

Herberman RB: Natural killer cells. Hosp Pract 17, No 4:93, 1982

Hirschhorn R: Metabolic defects and immunodeficiency disorders. N Engl J Med 308:714, 1983

Ishizaka K: Structure and biologic activity of immunoglobulin E. Hosp Pract 12, No 1:57, 1977

Jett MF, Lancaster LE: The inflammatory-immune response: The body's defense against invasion. Crit Care Nurs 5:64, 1983

Jones JV: Plasmapheresis: Current research and success. Heart Lung 9:671, 1980

Lane HC, Masur H, Edgar LC et al: Abnormalities of B-cell activation and immunoregulation in patients with the acquired immunodeficiency syndrome. N Engl J Med 309:453, 1983

Lind M: The immunologic assessment: A nursing focus. Heart Lung 9, No 4:658, 1980

Lippman SM, Arnett FC, Conley CL et al: Genetic factors predisposing to autoimmune diseases. Am J Med 73:827, 1982

McAdams CW: Interferon the penicillin of the future? Am J Nurs 80:714, 1980

McLeod BC: Immunologic factors in reactions to blood transfusions. Heart Lung 9, No 4:675, 1980

Nysather JO, Katz EE, Lenth JL: The immune system: Its development and functions. Am J Nurs 76, No 10:1614, 1976

Rana AN, Luskin A: Immunosuppression, autoimmunity, and hypersensitivity. Heart Lung 9, No 4:651, 1980

Rosen FS, Cooper MD, Wedgwood RJ: The primary immunodeficiencies. N Engl J Med 311:300, 1984

Sasazuki T, McDevitt HO: The association between genes in the major histocompatibility complex and disease susceptibility. Annu Rev Med 28:425, 1977

Schaller JG, Hansen JA: HLA relationships to disease. Hosp Pract 16, No 5:41, 1981

Schoenfeld Y, Schwartz RS: Immunologic and genetic factors in autoimmune disease. N Engl J Med 311:1019, 1984

Schumak KH: Therapeutic plasma exchange. N Engl J Med 310:762, 1984

Shahinpour N: The patient with systemic lupus erythematosus: Prototype of autoimmunity. Heart Lung 9, No 4:682, 1980

Torbett MP, Ervin JC: The patient with systemic lupus erythematosus. Am J Nurs 77:1299, 1977

Unanue ER: The macrophage as a regulator of lymphocyte function. Hosp Pract 14, No 11:61, 1979

Voignier RR, Bridgewater SC: Allergies in children: Testing and treating. Am J Nurs 78:617, 1978

Weksler ME: Senescence of the immune system. Med Clin North Am 67:263, 1983

Weksler ME: The senescence of the immune system. Hosp Pract 16, No 10:53, 1981

Chapter 11

White Blood Cell and Lymphoproliferative Disorders

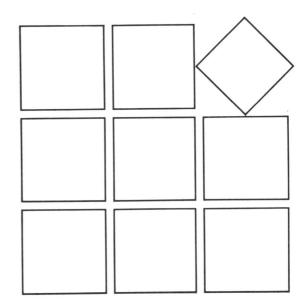

The white blood cells and lymphoid system serve to protect the body against invasion by foreign agents. The functions of the leukocytes and lymphoid system in terms of inflammation and immunity were discussed in Chapters 8, 9, and 10. In this chapter neutropenia and lymphoproliferative disorders are discussed.

■ Lymphoreticular System

The lymphoreticular system includes the white blood cells, their precursors, and their derivatives. It includes the *myeloid,* or bone marrow, tissue in which the white blood cells are formed and the *lymphoid tissues* of the lymph nodes, thymus, spleen, tonsils, and adenoids. Aggregates of lymphoid tissue are also found in the lungs and gastrointestinal tract.

White Blood Cells

White blood cells have their origin in the bone marrow as pluripotential stem cells (Fig. 11-1). These stem cells are capable of providing progenitors for both lymphopoiesis and hemopoiesis (processes by which mature lymph and blood cells are made). Several levels of differentiation lead to the development of committed unipotential cells that are the progenitor cells for each of the blood cell types. These committed cells develop into the precursors of blood cells such as the myeloblast from which the granulocytes develop. The myeloblasts differentiate into promyelocytes and then myelocytes. At this point it should be emphasized that immature, or blast, forms of blood cells do not normally appear in the peripheral circulation. Generally, a cell is not called a myelocyte until it has at least 12 granules.[1] The myelocytes mature to become metamyelocytes (Greek *meta,* "beyond"), at which point they lose their capacity for mitosis. Subsequent development of the neutrophil involves reduction in size with transformation from an indented to an oval to a horseshoe-shaped nucleus (band cell), and then to a mature cell with a segmented nucleus. At this point the neutrophil enters the bloodstream (Fig. 11-2). Neutrophil development (from stem cell to mature neutrophil) requires about 2 weeks.

After release from the marrow, the neutrophils spend only a short time (4 to 8 hours) in the circulation before moving into the tissues. Their survival in the tissues is short (about 5 days). They die either in discharging their function or of senescence. The pool of circulating neutrophils (those that appear in the blood count) are in rapid equilibrium with a similar-sized pool of cells marginating along the walls of small blood vessels.[2] Epinephrine, exercise, and corticosteroid drug therapy can cause rapid increases in the circulating neutrophil count by shifting cells from the marginating to

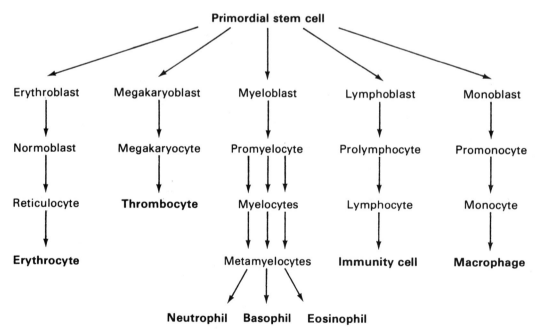

Figure 11-1 *Diagrammatic summary illustrating orderly development of erythrocytes, thrombocytes, and leukocytes from a primary cell, or forefather, called a primordial stem cell. (Chaffee EE, Lytle IM: Basic Physiology and Anatomy, 4th ed. Philadelphia, JB Lippincott, 1980)*

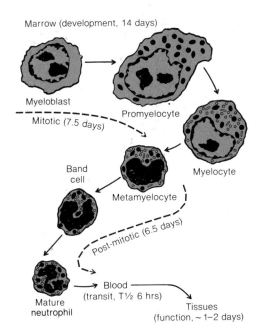

Figure II-2 *The development of neutrophil (PMNs) leukocytes. Azurophile granules (lysosomes) are represented in black, and specific neutrophilic granules are depicted as circles. A description of the stages is given in the text. (Adapted from Bainton DF, Ullyot JL, Farquhar MG: J Exp Med 134:907, 1971, by copyright permission of The Rockefeller University Press)*

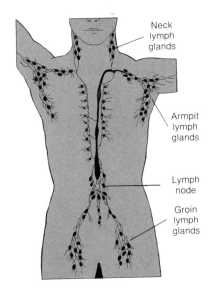

Figure II-3 *Location of some of the lymph nodes in the human body. (What You Need to Know About Hodgkin's Disease. Washington, DC, Department of Health and Human Services, July 1981)*

the circulating pool. Endotoxins have the opposite effect, producing a transient decrease in neutrophils.

The T-lymphocytes and B-lymphocytes develop in the lymphatic tissue (thymus gland and bursa equivalent) from committed stem cells that originated in the bone marrow.

Lymphoid Tissues

Lymphoid tissues make up the body's lymphatic system, which consists of the lymphatic vessels, the lymph nodes, the spleen, and the thymus. Lymph is body fluid that originates as excess fluid from the capillaries (Chap. 27). It is returned to the vascular compartment and right heart through lymphatic vessels.

Lymph nodes are situated along the course of the lymphatic channels and serve to filter the lymph before it is returned to the circulation (Fig. 11-3). Lymph enters a lymph node through afferent lymphatic channels, percolates through a labyrinthine system of minute channels lined with endothelial and phagocytic cells, and then emerges through efferent lymphatic vessels. A number of efferent vessels join to form collecting trunks. Each collecting trunk drains a definite area of the body. By filtering bacteria and other particulate matter, the lymph nodes serve a secondary line of defense even when clinical disease is not present. In the event of malignant neo-

plasm development, cancer cells are filtered and retained by the lymph nodes for a period of time before being disseminated to other parts of the body. Because of their contribution to the development of the immune system, the lymph nodes are relatively large at birth and undergo progressive atrophy throughout life.

■ Disorders of White Blood Cells

Leukopenia

Normally, the number of white blood cells in the peripheral circulation ranges from 5000 to 10,000 per mm^3 of blood. The term *leukopenia* describes an absolute decrease in white blood cell numbers. The disorder may affect any of the specific types of white blood cells, but most often it affects the neutrophils. Lymphopenia, when it occurs, is usually associated with specific clinical conditions such as Hodgkin's disease or corticosteroid therapy.

Agranulocytosis

Agranulocytosis refers specifically to a decrease in the granulocytes, mainly the neutrophils. It is usually defined as a circulating neutrophil count of below 1500 per mm^3. It can occur because (1) granulocyte production (granulopoiesis) fails to keep pace with granulocyte turnover or (2) accelerated destruction removes neutrophils from the circulating blood. Impairment of granulocytosis occurs in conditions such as cancer chemotherapy, irradiation, and aplastic anemia, which interfere with the formation of all blood cells. Overgrowth of neoplastic cells in nonmyelocytic leukemia and lymphoma may crowd out the granulopoietic precursors. Because of the very short life span of the neutrophil (less than a day in the peripheral blood), agranulocytosis occurs rapidly when there is impairment of granulopoiesis. Under these conditions, granulocytopenia is usually accompanied by thrombocytopenia (platelet deficiency).

Accelerated removal of neutrophils from the circulation may occur in a number of conditions. Infections drain neutrophils from the blood faster than they can be replaced. Autoimmune disorders or idiosyncratic drug reactions may cause increased and premature destruction of neutrophils. In splenomegaly, neutrophils may be trapped in the spleen along with other blood cells. In Felty's syndrome (a variant of rheumatoid arthritis) there is increased destruction of neutrophils in the spleen.

The most common cause of agranulocytosis is drug-related depression or destruction of neutrophils. Implicated drugs include chemotherapeutic drugs used in the treatment of cancer (alkalating agents, antimetabolites, and others) and chloramphenicol (an antibiotic), which cause predictable dose-dependent depression of bone-marrow function. The term *idiosyncratic* is used to describe drug reactions that are different from the usual effects obtained in the majority of persons and that cannot be explained in terms of allergy. A number of drugs such as phenothiazine tranquilizers, propylthiouracil (used in treatment of hyperthyroidism), phenylbutazone (used in the treatment of arthritis), and many other drugs may cause idiosyncratic depression of bone-marrow function. Some drugs, such as hydantoinates and primidone (used in the treatment of epilepsy) can cause intramedullary destruction of granulocytes and thereby impair production. In addition, many idiosyncratic cases of drug-induced neutropenia are thought to be caused by immunologic mechanisms, with the drug or its metabolites acting as an antigen (or hapten) to incite production of antibodies reactive against the neutrophils. It is known that neutrophils possess not only HLA antigens but other antigens specific to a given leukocyte line. Antibodies to these specific antigens have been identified in some cases of drug-induced neutropenia.[3] The causes of agranulocytosis are summarized in Table 11-1.

Because the neutrophil is essential to the cellular phase of inflammation, infections are common in per-

Table 11-1 Causes of Agranulocytopenia

Cause	Mechanism
Accelerated removal, *e.g.,* inflammation and infection	Removal of neutrophils from the circulation exceeds production
Drug-induced granulotcytopenia	
Defective production	
Cytotoxic drugs used in cancer therapy and chloramphenicol	Predictable damage to precursor cells, usually dose dependent
Phenothiazine, thiouracil, phenylbutazone, and others	Idiosyncratic depression of bone-marrow function
Hydantoinates, primidone, others	Intramedullary destruction of granulocytes
Immune destruction	Immunologic mechanisms with cytoloysis or leukoagglutination
Aminopyrine, others	
Periodic or cyclic neutropenia (occurs during infancy and later)	Unknown
Neoplasms involving bone marrow, e.g., leukemias and lymphomas	Overgrowth of neoplastic cells, which crowd out granulopoietic precursors
Idiopathic neutropenia that occurs in the absence of other disease or provoking influence	Autoimmune reaction
Felty's syndrome	Intrasplenic destruction of neutrophils

sons with agranulocytosis, and extreme caution is needed to protect them from exposure to infectious organisms. Infections that might go unnoticed in a person with a normal neutrophil count may prove fatal in a person with agranulocytosis.

The symptoms of agranulocytosis usually stem from severe infections that are characteristic of the disorder. These infections commonly occur with organisms that colonize the skin and gastrointestinal tract. Initially there is malaise, chills, and fever, followed by extreme weakness and fatigability. The white blood cell count is often reduced to 1000 cells per mm.[3] Ulcerative necrotizing lesions of the mouth are common in agranulocytosis. Ulcerations of the skin, vagina, and gastrointestinal tract may also occur.

Treatment with antibiotics provides a means of controlling infections in those situations in which the destruction of neutrophils can be controlled or recovery of granulopoietic function of the bone marrow is possible. The prognosis is variable and depends on the cause.

In summary, one of the major disorders of the white blood cells is agranulocytosis, with marked reduction of the circulating neutrophils. Agranulocytosis can occur as the result of defective production or accelerated removal of neutrophils from the circulation. Severe agranulocytosis can occur in lymphoproliferative diseases, in which neoplastic cells crowd out granulocyte precursor cells, and during radiation therapy or treatment with cytotoxic drugs, which destroy granulocyte precursor cells. Because the neutrophil is essential to the cellular stage of inflammation, severe and often life-threatening infections are common in persons with agranulocytosis.

■ Lymphoproliferative Disorders

The term *lymphoproliferative* is used to describe a number of localized and systemic disorders of the cells of the lymphoreticular system. The discussion in this section focuses on infectious mononucleosis, the leukemias, lymphomas, and plasma cell dyscrasias.

Infectious Mononucleosis

Infectious mononucleosis is, for the most part, a benign lymphoproliferative syndrome caused by the Epstein–Barr virus (EBV), one of the herpesviruses. The highest incidence is in adolescents and young adults. The disease tends to be seen more frequently in the upper socioeconomic classes of developed countries. This is probably because the disease, which is relatively asymptomatic when it occurs during childhood, confers complete immunity to the virus. In upper socioeconomic families,

exposure to the virus may be delayed until late adolescence or early adulthood. In such individuals, the mode of infection, size of the viral pool, and physiologic and immunologic condition of the host may determine whether the infection will occur or not.

The mode of transmission of the virus is unclear. Infectious mononucleosis has been called the "kissing disease," and evidence suggests that virally contaminated saliva is one of the main modes of transfer. The incubation period is 20 to 30 days or longer.

The disease is characterized by fever, generalized lymphadenopathy, sore throat, and the appearance in the blood of atypical lymphocytes. In the course of infection, the EBV invades the B-lymphocytes of oropharyngeal lymphoid tissues.[3] A replication of the virus ensues, with the subsequent death of the B-lymphocytes and release of the virus into the blood, causing the febrile reaction and specific immunologic responses. Concurrent with the febrile response, viral neutralizing antibodies appear and the virus disappears from the blood. However, some EBV-transformed B-lymphocytes remain in the circulation with the genome of the virus integrated into their genetic structure. The presence of virus-determined antigens on the surface of these B-lymphocytes is recognized by killer T cells and stimulates their multiplication. These killer T cells are the atypical lymphocytes seen in the blood of persons with infectious mononucleosis. The stimulation of the T-lymphocytes throughout the body is responsible for the lymphadenopathy and hepatosplenomegaly.

The signs and symptoms of infectious mononucleosis are usually insidious in onset, with a prodromal period of 1 to 2 weeks during which there is fever, fatigue, general malaise, and anorexia. Occasionally, the onset is abrupt with a high fever. Lymphadenopathy is present in 90% of cases, with symmetrically enlarged and often tender lymph nodes.[4] Splenomegaly or hepatomegaly occurs in about 50% of cases. Splenomegaly occasionally leads to the rupture of the spleen. This is associated with severe abdominal pain. Fewer than 1% of cases, usually in the adult age group, develop symptoms referable to the central nervous system. These symptoms can include cranial nerve palsies, encephalitis, meningitis, transverse myelitis, and the Guillain–Barré syndrome. Occasionally, severe toxic pharyngotonsillitis may cause airway obstruction. Most cases of infectious mononucleosis recover without incident. Usually the acute phase of the illness lasts for 2 to 3 weeks, after which recovery occurs rapidly. However, some degree of debility and lethargy may persist for 2 to 3 months.

The peripheral blood usually shows an increase in leukocytes, with a white blood cell count between 12,000 and 18,000, 95% of which are lymphocytes. The rise in white blood cells begins during the first week, rises even higher during the second week of the infection, and then returns to normal around the fourth week. Although leukocytosis is common, leukopenia may be seen in some persons during the first 3 days of the illness. Atypical lymphocytes are frequent, constituting over 20% of the total lymphocyte count. A number of circulating immunoglobulins, including heteroantibodies (sheep red cell agglutinins), are found in persons with infectious mononucleosis. These antibodies are typically not absorbed by guinea pig kidneys but are absorbed by beef erythrocytes, a means used to differentiate the antibodies due to the EBV virus from other disorders that produce antibodies that react with sheep red blood cells.[5]

The treatment of infectious mononucleosis is usually symptomatic and supportive. It includes bed rest and analgesic agents such as aspirin to control fever, headache, and sore throat. In cases of severe pharyngotonsillitis, corticosteroid drugs are given to reduce inflammation.

Leukemias

The leukemias are malignant neoplasms of white blood cells and their precursors. The term *leukemia (white blood)* was first used by Virchow to describe a reversal of the usual ratio of red to white blood cells. Because the leukemias involve blood cells, they are disseminated throughout the body from their earliest recognizable stages. They are characterized by (1) diffuse replacement of bone marrow with leukemic cells, (2) appearance of abnormal immature white blood cells in the peripheral circulation, and (3) widespread infiltration of the liver, spleen, lymph nodes, and other tissues throughout the body.[3]

Leukemias strike 25,000 persons in the United States each year and cause 17,000 deaths annually.[6] The disease strikes more children than any other form of cancer and is the leading cause of death in children ages 3 to 14 years. Although leukemia is commonly thought of as childhood disease, it affects more adults than children (22,000 adults per year compared with 2500 children).[6]

Classification

There are several types of leukemias. The leukemias are usually classified according to the predominant cell type and whether the condition is acute or chronic. Thus, a rudimentary classification system divides leukemia into four types: acute lymphocytic (lymphoblastic) leukemia (ALL), chronic lymphocytic leukemia (CLL), acute myelocytic (myeloblastic) leukemia (AML), and chronic myelocytic leukemia (CML). There are a number of subgroups within each of these types, and variants of these subgroups continue to be identified. In myelocytic

types of leukemia, any of the cell lines (erythroid, granulocytic, monocytic, and megakaryocytic) may be involved. Acute leukemias are rapidly fatal when untreated (usually 2 to 4 months from the time of diagnosis) and are characterized by the appearance of poorly differentiated cells.[3] Chronic types of leukemia are characterized by more mature cells that permit longer survival even when left untreated (2 to 6 years in many cases).

About 90% of all cases of leukemia are caused by neoplastic transformation of two types of leukocytes—the lymphocytes (lymphocytic leukemia) and the granulocytes (granulocytic leukemia).[7] Acute lymphocytic leukemia (ALL) is the most common form of leukemia in children. Acute granulocytic leukemia is most common in young adults and chronic leukemia (granulocytic or lymphocytic) is generally seen after age 40.

Causes

The causes of leukemia are unknown. There is an unusually high incidence of leukemia among persons exposed to high levels of radiation. The number of cases of leukemia in the most heavily exposed survivors of the atomic blasts at Hiroshima and Nagasaki during the 20-year period from 1950 to 1970 was nearly 30 times the expected rate.[8] There is also an increased incidence of leukemia associated with exposure to benzene and use of antitumor drugs and chloramphenicol.[9,10] There are hints of genetic predisposition. It is known that persons with Down's syndrome have a higher incidence of leukemia, and leukemia has been seen in a significant number of twins. There are chromosomal changes in many forms of leukemia. For example, the Philadelphia chromosome (translocation from chromosome 22 to 9) is evident in approximately 90% of persons with chronic myelogenous leukemia.[3] Interest in the role of viruses as etiologic agents in leukemia is also increasing. Leukemia viruses have been identified in a number of animal species.

Clinical manifestations

Leukemic cells are an immature and mobile type of white blood cell. In Chapter 5 it was explained that differentiation of a cell line determines its structure, function, and life span. Because leukemic cells are immature and poorly differentiated, they are capable of an increased rate of proliferation and a prolonged life span. They are also unable to perform the functions of mature leukocytes, that is, they are ineffective as phagocytes or immune cells. Because they are rapidly proliferating, leukemic cells tend to crowd out the normal bone-marrow cells, including the erythroblasts (red blood cells) and the megakaryocytes (platelets). Being mobile, they are able to travel throughout the circulatory system, cross the blood–brain barrier, and infiltrate many body organs.

Acute leukemias. Acute leukemias have sudden and stormy onsets with signs and symptoms related to depression of bone-marrow function (Table 11-2). Generalized lymphadenopathy, splenomegaly, and hepatomegaly due to infiltration by leukemic cells are characteristic of ALL but are not usually predominant in acute myelocytic leukemia (AML).[3] Both forms are characterized by anemia, depression of platelet count, and blast-form peripheral leukocytes. Signs of central nervous system and bone involvement occur in ALL and to a lesser degree in AML. Hyperuricemia occurs as the result of increased proliferation and metabolic alterations of the leukemic cells.

Chronic leukemias. Chronic leukemias have a more insidious onset than acute leukemias and may be discovered during a routine medical examination. Symptoms, which include low-grade fever, night sweats, and weight loss, are usually related to hypermetabolism of the leukemic cells. Anemia causes weakness, easy fatigability, and exertional dyspnea. Hepatomegaly, splenomegaly, and lymphadenopathy often cause a feeling of abdominal fullness and discomfort. Generalized lymphadenopathy is more common in chronic lymphocytic leukemia (CLL), whereas marked splenomegaly is more characteristic of chronic myelogenous leukemia (CML). Bleeding manifestations result from thrombocytopenia. As a generalized disorder of the lymphocytes, CLL is often accompanied by impaired humoral and cell-mediated immunity. This tends to lead to hemolytic anemia and increased vulnerability to infection.

Treatment

The treatment of leukemia varies with the type. The goal of treatment is to effect a remission. Chemotherapy is by far the most effective initial method of treatment. In certain patients, especially children with ALL, x-ray therapy of the central nervous system is used during chemotherapy. In some medical centers, the use of combination chemotherapy (multiple anticancer drugs) has produced an up to 75% 5-year-survival rate in children with ALL.[6] It is hoped that these children have been cured. In some cases a bone marrow transplant may be indicated.

Lymphomas

There are two types of lymphomas: Hodgkin's disease and non-Hodgkin's lymphomas. The most common of these two types is Hodgkin's disease.

Hodgkin's disease

Hodgkin's disease is a malignant neoplasm of the lymphatic structures, named after an English physician, Thomas Hodgkin, who first described the disease in

Table 11-2   Clinical Manifestations of Leukemia and Their Pathologic Basis*

Clinical Manifestations	Pathologic Basis
Symptoms of Bone-Marrow Depression	
Malaise, easy fatigability	Anemia
Fever	Infection or increased metabolism by neoplastic cells
Bleeding	Decreased thrombocytes
Petechiae	
Ecchymosis	
Gingival bleeding	
Epistaxis	
Bone pain and tenderness on palpation	Subperiosteal bone infiltration, bone-marrow expansion, and bone resorption
Headache, nausea, vomiting, papilledema, cranial nerve palsies, seizures, coma	Leukemic infiltration of central nervous system
Abdominal discomfort	Generalized lymphadenopathy, hepatomegaly, splenomegaly due to leukemic cell infiltration
Increased Vulnerability to Infections	Immaturity of the white cells and ineffective phagocytic and immune function.
Hematologic Abnormalities	
Anemia	Physical and metabolic encroachment of leukemic cells on red blood cell and thrombocyte precursors
Thrombocytopenia	
Hyperuricemia and other Metabolic Disorders	Abnormal proliferation and metabolism of leukemic cells

* The manifestations will vary with the type of leukemia.

1832. This disease constitutes 40% of malignant lymphomas. There were an estimated 6900 new cases of Hodgkin's disease in 1985, resulting in 1500 deaths.[6] About 50% of the cases occur in persons between the ages of 20 and 40 years.[11] Recent reports suggest that, in contrast with patients with many types of cancer, the majority of cases of Hodgkin's disease can be cured with appropriate therapy if diagnosed early. In 60% to 90% of persons with localized Hodgkin's disease there is the possibility of a definitive "cure" (normal life expectancy for age, 10 or more years after treatment).[11]

Hodgkin's disease is characterized by painless and progressive enlargement of lymphoid tissue, usually a single node or group of nodes. It is believed to originate within one area of the lymphatic system and, if unchecked, it will spread throughout the lymphatic network. Splenic enlargement usually occurs early in the course of the disease. The malignant proliferating cells may invade almost any area of the body and may produce a wide variety of symptoms. Low-grade fever, night sweats, unexplained weight loss, fatigue, pruritus, and anemia are indicative of disease spread. In its advanced stages, the liver, lungs, digestive tract, and occasionally the central nervous system may be affected.

As the disease progresses, the rapid proliferation of abnormal lymphocytes leads to an immunologic defect, particularly in cell-mediated responses, rendering the person more susceptible to bacterial, viral, fungal, and protozoal infections. Neutrophilic leukocytosis and mild normocytic normochromic anemia are common. Eosinophilia may also occur. Leukopenia is usually a late manifestation. Hypergammaglobulinemia is common during the early stages of the disease, whereas hypogammaglobulinemia may develop in advanced disease.

Lymph node biopsy is used to diagnose the disease. Characteristic of Hodgkin's disease is the presence of a distinctive giant tumor cell known as the Reed–Sternberg (RS) cell, which can be detected on microscopic examination. Computerized tomography (CT) scans of the abdomen are commonly used in screening for involvement of abdominal and pelvic lymph nodes. Radiologic visualization of the abdominal and pelvic lymph structures can be achieved through the use of lymphangiography. A staging laparotomy, in which the abdominal and pelvic lymph nodes are biopsied, is usually done when involvement of these nodes is suspected. Because the spleen is a frequent site of extralymphatic spread, it is often removed during a staging laparotomy.

The cause of Hodgkin's disease is unknown. There is a long-standing suspicion that the disease may begin as an inflammatory reaction to an infectious agent. This belief is supported by epidemiologic data that include the clustering of the disease among family members and among students who have attended the same school. There also seems to be an association between the presence of the disease and a deficient immune state. As with other forms of cancer, it is likely that no single agent is responsible for the development of Hodgkin's disease.

Non-Hodgkin's lymphomas

The non-Hodgkin's lymphomas are a group of neoplastic disorders of the lymphoid tissue. There are about 15,000 new cases of non-Hodgkin's lymphoma each year in the United States and about 13,200 deaths.[11]

The non-Hodgkin's lymphomas are divided into three main groups according to the type of cell that is involved: lymphocytic lymphoma (or lymphosarcoma), histiocytic lymphoma (or reticulum cell sarcoma), and mixed cell lymphoma.

A viral etiology is suspected in at least some of the lymphomas. Cell cultures and immunologic studies of

one type of lymphoma, Burkitt's lymphoma, found in some parts of Africa has implicated the Epstein–Barr herpeslike virus without proving a causal relationship.[12] There is also a reported increase in lymphomas in persons treated with chronic immunosuppressive therapy and in other immune deficiency states.

The signs and symptoms of non-Hodgkin's lymphoma are similar to those of Hodgkin's disease except for the early involvement of the oropharyngeal lymphoid tissue, skin, gastrointestinal tract, and bone marrow. Leukemic transformation with high peripheral lymphocyte counts occurs in about 13% of persons with non-Hodgkin's lymphoma. There is increased susceptibility to bacterial, viral, and fungal infections associated with hypogammaglobulinemia and poor humoral antibody response, rather than impaired cellular immunity as seen in Hodgkin's disease.

As with Hodgkin's disease, a lymph node biopsy is used to confirm the diagnosis. Treatment is dependent on the stage of the disease. It may include surgical resection of the diseased tissue, combination chemotherapy, and irradiation.

Multiple Myeloma

Multiple myeloma is a plasma cell cancer of the osseous tissue that, in the course of its dissemination, may involve other nonosseous sites. It is characterized by the uncontrolled proliferation of an abnormal clone of plasma cells, usually of the IgG or IgA type. In 1985 there were an estimated 9900 new cases of the disease in the United States.[6] Over 90% of the cases occur in persons over age 40.[11]

In multiple myeloma, plasma cells that are seldom found in healthy bone marrow proliferate and erode into the hard bone, predisposing to pathologic fractures and hypercalcemia due to bone dissolution. Bone pain, concentrated in the back, is often one of the first symptoms to occur in this form of cancer. Bone destruction also impairs the production of erythrocytes and leukocytes and predisposes to anemia and recurrent infections. There is often weight loss and a feeling of weakness. In some forms of the disease, there is an unbalanced synthesis of light and dark chains for the immunoglobulins, resulting in an excess of light chains. Proteinuria develops as these light chains, called *Bence Jones proteins,* are excreted in the urine. The most effective treatment for multiple myeloma is chemotherapy.

In summary, lymphoproliferative disorders affect the cells of the lymphoreticular system, including the lymphocytes and plasma cells. Infectious mononucleosis is a benign lymphoproliferative disorder caused by the Epstein–Barr virus. Malignant lymphoproliferative disorders include the leukemias, Hodgkin's disease, non-Hodgkin's lymphomas, and multiple myeloma. Leukemias are classified according to the cell type (lymphocytic, myelocytic [myelogenous], or monocytic) and whether the disease is acute or chronic. Acute lymphocytic leukemia occurs most often in children. In adults, acute granulocytic and chronic lymphocytic leukemias are most common. Because leukemic cells are immature and poorly differentiated, they proliferate rapidly and crowd out precursors of other blood cells (thrombocytes, granulocytes, and erythrocytes) and they are unable to perform the functions of mature leukocytes. Hodgkin's disease is a malignant neoplasm of the lymphatic structures. It usually begins in a single lymph node or group of lymph nodes and, if unchecked, it invades the spleen and other lymphatic structures. Multiple myeloma results in the uncontrolled proliferation of plasma cells, usually a single clone of IgG- or IgA-producing cells.

■ Study Guide

After you have studied this chapter, you should be able to meet the following objectives:

☐ List the cells and tissues of the lymphoreticular system.

☐ Describe the production and life span of the granulocytes.

☐ Define leukopenia.

☐ Cite two general causes of granulocytosis.

☐ Describe three mechanisms of drug-induced granulocytosis.

☐ Describe the mechanism of symptom production in agranulocytosis.

☐ Describe the pathogenesis of infectious mononucleosis.

☐ List the six major types of leukemia.

☐ State the characteristics of leukemia.

☐ Explain the manifestations of leukemia in terms of altered cell differentiation.

☐ State the major treatment modalities used in leukemia.

☐ Discuss the prognosis associated with different types of leukemia.

☐ Describe the signs and symptoms of Hodgkin's disease.

☐ Discuss the prognosis of Hodgkin's disease in relation to the stage of the disease.

☐ Cite the major treatment modalities used in Hodgkin's disease.

☐ Describe the lymphoproliferative disorder that occurs with multiple myeloma.

☐ Explain the origin of the Bence Jones protein that appears in the urine in multiple myeloma.

■ References

1. Ham AW, Cormack DH: Histology, 8th ed, p 314. Philadelphia, JB Lippincott, 1979
2. Smith LH, Their SO: Pathophysiology, p 421–428. Philadelphia, WB Saunders, 1981
3. Robbins SL, Cotran RS: Pathologic Basis of Disease, 2nd ed, pp 445, 746, 779, 780, 781, 788. Philadelphia, WB Saunders, 1979
4. Henle W et al: Epstein-Barr virus specific diagnostic test in infectious mononucleosis. Hum Pathol 5:551, 1974
5. Lai PK: Infectious mononucleosis: Recognition and management. Hosp Pract 12, No 8:47, 1977
6. American Cancer Society: Cancer Facts and Figures 1985, pp 8, 12. New York, 1985
7. American Cancer Society: Facts on Leukemia. New York, American Cancer Society, 1978
8. Jablon S, Kato H: Studies of the mortality of A-bomb survivors. Radiat Res 50:658, 1972
9. Pederson-Bjergaard J, Larsen SO: Incidence of acute non-lymphocytic leukemia, preleukemia and acute myeloproliferative syndrome up to 10 years after treatment for Hodgkin's disease. N Engl J Med 307:964, 1982
10. Boise JD, Greene MH, Killen JY et al: Leukemia and preleukemia after adjuvant treatment of gastrointestinal cancer with Semustine. N Engl J Med 309:107, 1983
11. Rubin P (ed): Clinical Oncology, 6th ed, pp 346, 354, 355, 361. New York, American Cancer Society, 1983
12. Ziegler JL: Burkitt's lymphoma. N Engl J Med 305, No 13:735, 1981

■ Additional References

Arlin ZA, Bayard D, Clarkson BD: The treatment of acute nonlymphoblastic leukemia in adults. Adv Intern Med 28:303, 1983

Berard CV, Greene MH, Jaffee ES: A multidisciplinary approach to non-Hodgkin's lymphomas. Ann Intern Med 94:218, 1981

Cassileth PA: Adult acute leukemia. Med Clin North Am 68, No 3:675, 1984

Chessels JM: Acute lymphoblastic leukemia. Semin Hematol 19:155, 1982

DeVita V, Hubbard SM, Molloy JH: The cure of Hodgkin's disease with drugs. Adv Intern Med 28:277, 1983

Ersek MT: The adult leukemia patient in the intensive care unit. Heart Lung 13:183, 1984

Feely AM, Houlihan NG, Ern M: The treatment of leukemia. Cancer Nurs 4:233, 1982

Gaynor ER, Ultmann JE: Non-Hodgkin's lymphoma: Management strategies. N Engl J Med 311:1506, 1984

Haller DG: Non-Hodgkin's lymphoma. Med Clin North Am 68, No 3:741, 1984

Houlihan NG: Leukemia: A hematologic review. Cancer Nurs 4:61, 1981

Jacobs AD, Gale RP: Recent advances in biology and treatment of acute lymphoblastic leukemia in adults. N Engl J Med 311:1219, 1984

Kamani N, August CS: Bone marrow transplantations: Problems and prospects. Med Clin North Am 68:657, 1984

Koeffler HP, Golde DW: Chronic myelogenous leukemia— New concepts. N Engl J Med 304:1269, 1981

Niederman JC: Infectious mononucleosis: Observations on transmission. Yale J Biol Med 55:259, 1982

Oken MM: Multiple myeloma. Med Clin North Am 68:757, 1984

Portlock CS: Hodgkin's disease. Med Clin North Am 68, No 3:729, 1984

Poweles R, McElwain T: Introduction to leukemia and lymphoma. Semin Hematol 19:152, 1982

Rai KR, Sawitsky A, Kandasamy J et al: Chronic lymphocytic leukemia. Med Clin North Am 68, No 3:697, 1984

Rappeport JM: Sowing hematopoietic seeds. N Engl J Med 309:1385, 1983

Snugden B: Epstein-Barr virus: A human pathogen inducing lymphoproliferation in vivo and in vitro. Rev Infect Dis 4:1048, 1982

Spiers ASD: Chronic granulocytic leukemia. Med Clin North Am 68, No 3:713, 1984

Wessler RM: Care of the hospitalized adult patient with leukemia. Nurs Clin North Am 17, No 4:649, 1982

Chapter 12

Alterations in Hemostasis and Blood Coagulation

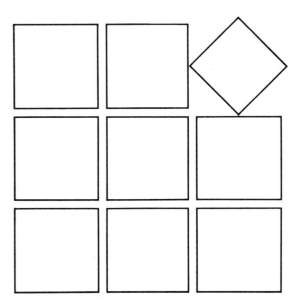

The term *hemostasis* refers to the stoppage of blood flow. Hemostasis is designed to maintain the integrity of the vascular system and to prevent blood from leaving its channels. Disorders of hemostasis fall into two main categories: (1) the inappropriate formation of clots within the vascular system and (2) the failure of blood to clot in response to an appropriate stimulus.

■ Mechanisms Associated with Hemostasis

Hemostasis is generally divided into five stages: (1) vessel spasm, (2) formation of the platelet plug, (3) blood coagulation or development of an insoluble fibrin clot, (4) clot retraction, and (5) clot dissolution. These steps are summarized in Table 12-1.

Vessel Spasm

Vessel spasm is the first of the stages involved in the formation of a blood clot; it is caused by local and neural reflex mechanisms. Vessel spasm constricts the vessel and reduces blood flow. It is a transient event that usually lasts less than a minute.

Formation of the Platelet Plug

Platelets, or thrombocytes, are large fragments from the cytoplasm of bone stem cells called the megakaryocytes. They are enclosed in a membrane but have no nucleus. They have a life span of only 5 to 9 days. Platelet production is controlled by a substance called thrombopoietin. The source of thrombopoietin is unknown, but it appears that its production and release is regulated by the number of platelets in the circulation. The newly formed platelets that are released from the bone marrow spend 24 to 36 hours in the spleen before they are released into the blood.

The platelet plug is the second line of defense, which is initiated as platelets come into contact with the vessel

---

Table 12-1 Steps in Hemostasis

Vessel spasm
Formation of the platelet plug
   Platelet adherence to the vessel wall
   Platelet aggregation to form the platelet plug
Blood coagulation
   Activation of the intrinsic or extrinsic coagulation pathway
   Conversion of prothrombin to thrombin
   Conversion of fibrinogen to fibrin
Clot retraction
Clot dissolution (fibrinolysis)

---

wall. As the platelets adhere to the subendothelial layer of the vessel wall, they become "sticky." This allows them to interact with other platelets and to form an aggregate—a process called platelet aggregation. A platelet plug usually forms within seconds of vessel injury. At least two plasma factors are needed for platelet adhesiveness and aggregation to occur: fibrinogen and von Willebrand's factor, a protein with a structure similar to factor VIII. Persons with von Willebrand's disease are deficient in von Willebrand's factor and have bleeding problems.

During the third stage of hemostasis, the unstable platelet plug is cemented together with fibrin strands. When vessel injury is slight, the platelet plug may be all that is needed to close the defect; and when this happens, the formation of the fibrin clot is not needed. In addition to sealing vascular breaks, platelets play an almost continuous role in maintaining normal vascular integrity. Persons with thrombocytopenia have decreased capillary resistance and develop small skin hemorrhages, which result from the slightest trauma or change in blood pressure.

Blood Coagulation

Blood coagulation is the third stage of hemostasis. This is the process by which fibrin strands form and create a meshwork that cements blood components together (Fig. 12-1). Blood coagulation occurs as a result of activation of either the intrinsic or extrinsic coagulation pathways (Fig. 12-2). The intrinsic pathway, which is a relatively slow process, occurs in the vascular system; the extrinsic pathway, which is a much faster process, occurs in the tissues. The terminal steps in both pathways are the same, consisting of the interaction between thrombin and the plasma protein fibrinogen. A final interaction for both pathways converts fibrinogen to fibrin, the material that forms the structural matrix of the clot. Both pathways are needed for normal hemostasis. Bleeding, however, when it occurs because of defects in the extrinsic system, is usually not as severe as that which results from defects in the intrinsic pathway. Both systems are activated when blood passes out of the vascular system. The intrinsic system is activated as blood comes in contact with the injured vessel wall and the extrinsic system when blood is exposed to tissue extracts.

The purpose of the coagulation process is to form an insoluble fibrin clot. This process may involve as many as 30 different substances that either promote clotting (procoagulation factors) or inhibit it (anticoagulation factors). The procoagulation factors are identified by Roman numerals (Table 12-2). The decision to use Roman numerals resulted from the discovery that two factors were identified by the same name. It is easy to see how this could happen with the various names that

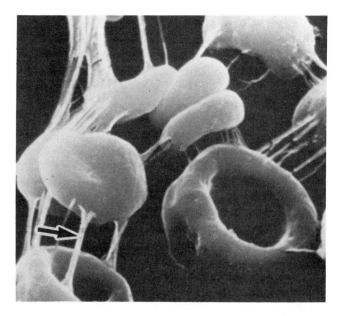

Figure 12-1 *Scanning electron micrograph of a blood clot at a magnification of 5000. The fibrous bridges (indicated by the arrow) that form a meshwork between red blood cells are fibrin fibers. (Chaffee EE, Lytle IM: Basic Physiology and Anatomy, 4th ed. Philadelphia, JB Lippincott, 1980)*

appear in Table 12-2. There is no factor VI, because that number was originally assigned to what is now known to be the activated form of factor V.

Each of the procoagulation factors performs a specific step in the coagulation process. The action of one coagulation factor is usually designed to activate the next factor in the sequence (cascade effect). Some sources

Table 12-2   Coagulation Factors

Factor I	Fibrinogen
Factor II	Prothrombin
Factor III	Tissue thromboplastin
Factor IV	Calcium
Factor V	Proaccelerin, labile factor, A-C globulin
Factor VII	Proconvertin, serum prothrombin conversion accelerator (SPCA)
Factor VIII	Antihemophilic factor (AHF)
Factor IX	Plasma thromboplastin component (PTC), antihemophilic factor B (AH-B), Christmas factor
Factor X	Stuart factor, Stuart–Prower factor
Factor XI	Plasma thromboplastin antecedent (PTA)
Factor XII	Hageman factor
Factor XIII	Fibrin stabilizing factor

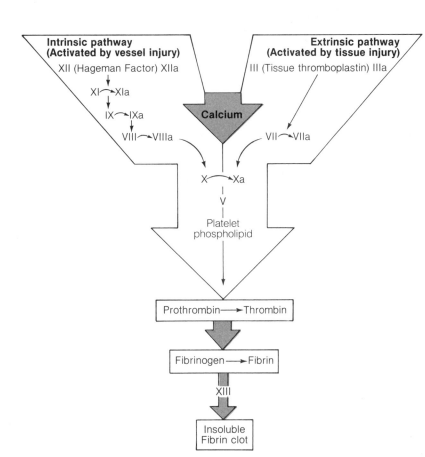

Figure 12-2 *The intrinsic and extrinsic coagulation pathways. The terminal steps in both pathways are the same. Calcium, factors X and V, and platelet phospholipids combine to form prothrombin activator, which then converts prothrombin to thrombin. This interaction, in turn, causes conversion of fibrinogen into the fibrin strands that create the insoluble blood clot.*

identify the activated form of the factor by inserting the subscript *a* after the factor number (factor Va). Because most of the inactive procoagulation factors are present in the blood at all times, the multistep coagulation process ensures that a massive episode of intravascular clotting does not occur by chance. It also means that abnormalities of the clotting process will occur when one or more of the factors are deficient or when conditions lead to inappropriate activation of any of the steps.

Calcium (factor IV) is required in all but the first two steps of the clotting process. Fortunately, the living body almost always has sufficient calcium to interact in the clotting process. The inactivation of the calcium ion is used to prevent blood that has been removed from the body from clotting. The addition of a citrate-phosphate-dextrose solution to blood stored for transfusion purposes prevents clotting by combining with the calcium ions. Both oxalate and citrate are often added to blood samples used for analysis in the clinical laboratory.

Clot Retraction

Clot retraction occurs immediately once the clot has formed. Clot retraction, which requires large numbers of platelets, contributes to homostasis by pulling the edges of the broken vessel together.

Clot Dissolution (Fibrinolysis)

The dissolution of a blood clot begins shortly after its formation; this allows blood flow to be reestablished and allows tissue repair to take place. The process by which a blood clot dissolves is called fibrinolysis. As with clot formation, clot dissolution requires a sequence of steps (Fig. 12-3).

Plasminogen, the proenzyme for the fibrolytic process, is normally present in the blood in its inactive form. It is converted to its active form, *plasmin*, by plasminogen activators formed in the tissues, plasma, urine, or blood clot. The plasmin formed from plasminogen digests the fibrin strands of the clot as well as other proteins. It also digests certain clotting factors such as fibrinogen, factor V, and factor VIII. Circulating plasmins are inactivated by *antiplasmins*, which are normally present in the circulation in concentrations ten times those of plasmins. This high level of antiplasmins protects the blood clotting factors.

The plasma-activating factor is released from the endothelial cells by a number of stimuli, including the action of vasoactive drugs, elevated body temperature, and exercise. Plasma activator is unstable and is rapidly inactivated by substances in the blood and by the liver. For this reason, chronic liver disease may cause altered fibrinolytic activity. The tissue activation factor does not normally enter the blood unless there is extensive tissue damage, such as that caused by burns. The urine-activating factor, urinokinase, is thought to be produced by the kidney and probably assists in maintaining the patency of the renal tract.

In summary, hemostasis is designed to maintain the integrity of the vascular compartment. The process is divided into five phases: (1) vessel spasm, which constricts the size of the vessel and reduces blood flow, (2) platelet adherence and formation of the platelet plug, (3) formation of the fibrin clot, which cements the platelet plug together, (4) clot retraction, which pulls the edges of the injured vessel together, and (5) clot dissolution, which involves the action of fibrinolysins that dissolve the clot and allow blood flow to be reestablished and healing of tissues to take place. The process of blood coagulation requires the stepwise activation of coagulation factors, which ensures that the process is not activated by chance.

■ Disorders of Hemostasis and Blood Coagulation

Blood clotting is normal when it seals a blood vessel thereby preventing blood loss and hemorrhage. It is abnormal when it causes inappropriate blood clotting or

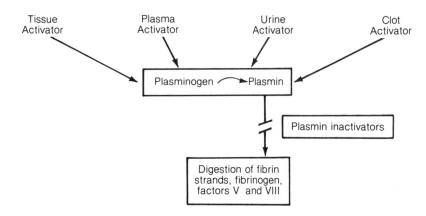

Figure 12-3 *The steps in the fibrinolytic sequence. Fibrinolysis can be initiated by tissue, plasma, urine, or clot-activating factors.*

when clotting is insufficient to stop the flow of blood from the vascular compartment. Clotting disorders, discussed in the following sections, have been divided into two groups: (1) the hypercoagulability states and (2) bleeding diatheses (disorders).

Hypercoagulability States

All of the components or factors necessary to trigger the intrinsic coagulation pathway are present in the blood at all times. There are two general forms of hypercoagulability states: (1) conditions that create hyperreactivity of the platelet system and (2) conditions that cause accelerated activity of the coagulation system. Current evidence suggests that hyperreactivity of the platelet system results in arterial thrombosis and that increased activity of the clotting system causes venous thrombosis and its sequelae.[1] Table 12-3 summarizes conditions commonly associated with hypercoagulability states.

Hyperreactivity of platelet function

The causes of increased platelet function tend to be twofold: (1) disturbances in flow and changes in the vessel wall and (2) increased sensitivity of platelets to factors that cause adhesiveness and aggregation. Atherosclerotic plaques disturb flow and render the inner lining of the arterial wall more susceptible to platelet adherence. There is now considerable evidence that disturbed flow and platelet function contribute to the development of atherosclerosis as well as arterial thrombosis. It appears that platelets adhering to the vessel wall may release factors that are damaging to the underlying vessel and thereby contribute to the development and progression of atherosclerosis. Diabetes mellitus not only increases the incidence of atherosclerosis but also appears to increase platelet adherence and aggregation. Smoking and elevated levels of blood lipids and cholesterol also appear to cause increased platelet sensitivity to factors that cause platelet adherence and aggregation.

Increased clotting activity

Factors that increase the activation of the coagulation system are (1) stasis of flow and (2) alterations in the coagulation components of the blood (either an increase in procoagulation factors or a decrease in anticoagulation factors). Venous thrombosis usually begins in regions of slow and disturbed flow. Venous thrombosis is a common event in the immobilized and postsurgical patient. Heart failure also contributes to venous congestion and thrombosis. Blood coagulation factors have been found to be increased in women using oral contraceptive agents. The incidence of stroke, thromboemboli, and myocardial infarction is greater among women who use oral contraceptives than among those who do not. Clotting factors are also increased during normal

Table 12-3   Conditions Associated with Hypercoagulability States

Hyperreactivity of Platelets
- Atherosclerosis
- Diabetes mellitus
- Smoking
- Elevated blood lipids and cholesterol
- Increased platelet levels

Accelerated Activity of the Clotting System
- Pregnancy and the puerperium
- Use of oral contraceptives
- Postsurgical state
- Immobility
- Congestive heart failure
- Malignant diseases

pregnancy; and these changes, along with limited activity during the puerperium, predispose to venous thrombosis. A third condition that predisposes to hypercoagulability is malignant disease. Many tumor cells are thought to release procoagulation factors, which, along with the increased immobility and sepsis seen in patients with malignant disease, contribute to the increased incidence of thrombosis in these patients.

Bleeding Disorders

As with the hypercoagulability states, bleeding disorders or impairment of blood coagulation can result from defects in any of the factors that contribute to hemostasis. This includes defects in platelets and coagulation factors.

Impairment of platelet function

Platelet function can be impaired because of a decrease in the number of circulating platelets or because of impaired platelet function.

Platelets are produced by cells in the bone marrow and are then stored in the spleen before being released into the circulation. Consequently, a decrease in the number of circulating platelets can result from either a decrease in platelet production by the bone marrow or an increased pooling of platelets in the spleen. Replacement of bone marrow by malignant cells, such as occurs in leukemia, impairs the bone marrow's ability to produce platelets. Radiation and drugs such as those used in the treatment of cancer often depress bone marrow function and cause reduced platelet production (thrombocytopenia). On the other hand, there may be normal production of platelets but excessive pooling of platelets in the spleen. Normally the spleen sequesters about 30% to 40% of the platelets. When the spleen is enlarged (splenomegaly), however, as many as 80% of the platelets can be sequestered in the spleen.

Another cause of thrombocytopenia is the abnormal destruction of platelets that is thought to result from an autoimmune response in which the body produces antibodies against its own platelets. Often the cause of platelet destruction cannot be determined, in which case it is referred to as idiopathic thrombocytopenia. In acute disseminated intravascular clotting, discussed later, excessive platelet consumption leads to a deficiency.

Failure of platelet adherence and aggregation is seen in a number of conditions. Aspirin, which impairs platelet function by inhibiting platelet aggregation, is one of the most common causes of this impairment. The effect of aspirin on platelet aggregation lasts for the life of the platelet—usually about 7 to 8 days. In a study in which maternal ingestion of aspirin occurred within 5 days of delivery, six of ten mothers and nine of ten infants had bleeding tendencies.[2] The recent interest in aspirin's effect on hemostasis has been not so much in its ability to

---

Table 12-4 Drugs That May Predispose to Bleeding

Interference with Platelet Production or Function
Acetazolamide
Alcohol
Antihistamines
Antimetabolite and anticancer drugs
Aspirin and salicylates
Chloramphenicol
Clofibrate
Colchicine
Dextran
Dipyridamole
Diuretics (furosemide, ethacrynic acid, and the thiazide diuretics)
Lidocaine
Nonsteroidal anti-inflammatory drugs
Penicillins
Phenylbutazone
Propranolol
Quinine derivatives (quinidine and hydroxychloroquine)
Sulfonamides
Theophylline
Tricyclic antidepressants
Vitamin E
Interference with Coagulation Factors
Anabolic steroids
Coumadin
Heparin
Thyroid preparations
Decrease in Vitamin K Levels
Antibiotics
Clofibrate

(From Hansten P (ed): Drug Interactions, 4th ed. Philadelphia, Lea & Febiger, 1979; Koda-Kimble MA (ed): Applied Therapeutics for Clinical Pharmacists, 2nd ed, p 260. San Francisco, Applied Therapeutics, 1978; Packman MA, Mustard JF: Clinical pharmacology of platelets. Blood 50, No 4:1977)

---

cause bleeding as its ability to prevent blood clotting. Table 12-4 describes other drugs that impair platelet function.

The depletion of platelets must be relatively severe (10,000-20,000 per mm^3 compared with the normal values of 150,000-200,000 per mm^3) before hemorrhagic tendencies become evident. Bleeding that results from platelet deficiencies is usually spontaneous and affects the small vessels of the skin and mucous membranes. Bleeding of the intracranial vessels is also a danger with severe platelet depletion.

Coagulation defects

Impairment of blood coagulation can result from deficiencies in one or more of the known clotting factors. Deficiencies can arise because of deficient synthesis, production of inactive factors, or increased consumption of the clotting factors.

Impaired synthesis. Coagulation factors V, VII, IX, X, and XIII, prothrombin, fibrinogen, and probably factors XI and XII are synthesized in the liver. Factor VIII is synthesized in the endothelial cells.

Of the coagulation factors synthesized in the liver, factors VII, IX, and X, and prothrombin require the presence of vitamin K for normal activity. In liver disease synthesis of the entire clotting factor is reduced. In vitamin K deficiency, the liver produces the clotting factor but in an inactive form. Vitamin K is a fat-soluble vitamin that is being continuously synthesized by intestinal bacteria. This means that a deficiency in vitamin K is not likely to occur unless intestinal synthesis is interrupted or absorption of the vitamin is impaired. Vitamin K deficiency can occur in the newborn infant prior to establishment of the intestinal flora and can also occur as a result of treatment with broad-spectrum antibiotics that cause destruction of intestinal flora. Because vitamin K is a fat-soluble vitamin, its absorption requires bile salts. A vitamin K deficiency, therefore, may result from impaired fat absorption due to liver or gallbladder disease.

Hereditary defects. Hereditary defects usually affect one factor and have been reported for each of the clotting factors. The three most common defects occur in (1) factor VIII (classic hemophilia), (2) factor IX (Christmas disease or hemophilia B), and (3) factor XI (hemophilia C). Factor VIII defects account for about 80% of the total cases of hemophilia and Christmas disease for about 15%. The other 5% are due to defects in factor XI. Hemophilia is a sex-linked recessive disorder that primarily affects males. Although it is a hereditary disorder, there is no family history of the disorder in about one-third of newly diagnosed cases, suggesting that it has arisen as a new mutation.[3] Factor VIII is produced by the endothelial cells, and until recently it was thought that persons with hemophilia failed to produce factor VIII (or XI). It has been shown that the factor is present but in an inactive form. An individual with normal coagulation function possesses about 50% to 150% procoagulation activity for most of the coagulation factors. In hemophilia, this amount is only 1% to 20%, with 5% to 20% in mild hemophilia, 1% to 5% in moderate hemophilia, and 1% or less in severe forms of hemophilia.[3] In mild or moderate forms of the disease, bleeding usually does not occur unless there is a local lesion or trauma. The disorder may not be detected in childhood. On the other hand, in severe hemophilia, bleeding is usually present in childhood (it may be noted at the time of circumcision) and tends to be both spontaneous and severe. Spontaneous hemorrhage into the joint is damaging and is a frequent cause of disability.

Prevention of bleeding is of primary concern in persons with hemophilia. Contact sports and physically hazardous occupations should be avoided. Preparations containing concentrated clotting factors obtained from the plasma of multiple donors are available and are used to prevent and control bleeding. Cryoprecipitate consists of specific clotting factors that have been separated from plasma by cooling. Preparations of clotting factors are produced by pooling and processing cryoprecipitated clotting factors from 2500 to 22,500 individuals.[4] Receiving plasma or plasma products from multiple donors exposes hemophiliacs to hepatitis and acquired immune deficiency disease (AIDS).[5] AIDS is discussed in Chapter 10.

Abnormal consumption. Acute disseminated intravascular clotting (DIC) is a paradox in the hemostatis sequence in which blood coagulation, clot dissolution, and bleeding all take place at the same time. The condition begins with activation of the coagulation system with formation of microemboli and is accompanied by consumption of specific clotting factors, aggregation, and loss of platelets and activation of the fibrinolytic mechanisms responsible for clot dissolution.

Disseminated intravascular clotting is not a primary disorder; it occurs as a complication in a variety of disease conditions. The coagulation process can be initiated by activation of either the extrinsic coagulation pathway, through liberation of tissue factors, or the intrinsic pathway, through extensive endothelial damage or stasis of blood. Among the clinical conditions known to incite DIC are massive trauma, burns, sepsis, shock, meningococcemia, and malignant disease. About 50% of individuals with DIC are patients with obstetrical complications. Table 12-5 summarizes the conditions that have been associated with DIC.

Secondary activation of the fibrinolytic system is localized at the sites of intravascular clotting. Breakdown of the fibrin, however, leads to release of products that prevent conversion of fibrinogen to fibrin and thus to further bleeding problems.

Although the coagulation and formation of microemboli initiate the events that occur in DIC, its acute manifestations are usually more directly related to the bleeding problems that occur. The bleeding may be present as petechiae, purpura, or severe hemorrhage. Uncontrolled postpartum bleeding may indicate DIC. Microemboli may cause tissue hypoxia and damage to organ structures. The kidney is usually the most severely damaged organ, but there may also be damage to the heart, lungs, and brain. A form of hemolytic anemia may develop as red cells become damaged when they pass through vessels partially blocked by thrombus.

The treatment for DIC is directed toward the primary disease, correcting the bleeding, and preventing further activation of clotting mechanisms. Heparin may be given to decrease blood coagulation, thereby interrupting the process that leads to consumption of coagulation factors and secondary activation of the fibrolytic system. It is usually given as a continuous intravenous infusion that can be interrupted promptly if bleeding is accentuated. Fresh coagulation factors in the form of fresh whole blood, platelets, cryoprecipitate, or plasma

---

Table 12-5 Conditions That Have Been Associated with Disseminated Intravascular Clotting (DIC)

Obstetric Conditions
Abruptio placenta
Dead fetus syndrome
Preeclampsia and eclampsia
Amniotic fluid embolism
Malignancies
Metastatic cancer
Leukemia
Infections
Acute bacterial infection, *e.g.,* meningococcal meningitis
Acute viral infections
Rickettsial infections, *e.g.,* Rocky Mountain spotted fever
Parasitic infections, *e.g.,* malaria
Shock
Septic shock
Severe hypovolemic shock
Trauma or Surgery
Burns
Massive trauma
Surgery involving exracorporeal circulation
Snake bite
Heat stroke
Hematologic Conditions
Blood transfusion reactions

may be used in case of uncontrolled hemorrhage. E-aminocaproic acid, which is a powerful antifibrolytic agent, may be used when hemorrhage is severe.[6]

Vascular disorders

Vascular disorders cause easy bruising and spontaneous bleeding from small blood vessels. These disorders occur because of structurally weak vessels or vessels that have been damaged by inflammation or immune responses. Among the vascular disorders that cause bleeding are hemorrhagic telangiectasia (an uncommon autosomal dominant trait in which there are dilatations of capillaries and arterioles), vitamin C deficiency (scurvy), and Cushing's disease. Vascular defects also occur in the course of DIC as a result of the presence of the microthrombi.

Vascular disorders are characterized by easy bruising and spontaneous appearance of petechiae and purpura of the skin and mucous membranes. In persons with bleeding disorders due to vascular defects, the platelet count and other tests for coagulation defects are normal.

Effects of Drugs on Hemostasis

A number of drugs serve to either enhance or impair hemostasis. Oral contraceptives and the corticosteroid drugs are associated with an increase in coagulation factors. Drugs that impair platelet production or function and those that interfere with coagulation are summarized in Table 12-4. Two drugs are commonly used as anticoagulant agents—heparin and coumadin.

Coumadin

The anticoagulant drug coumadin acts by decreasing prothrombin and other procoagulation factors that require vitamin K for biologic activity. Coumadin acts at the level of the liver and competes with vitamin K during the synthesis of the vitamin K-dependent coagulation factors. Because the relationship between vitamin K and coumadin is competitive, vitamin K is used as the antidote for coumadin overdose.

Heparin

Heparin is an anticoagulant that is found in many body cells. It is formed in large quantities in mast cells located in the pericapillary connective tissues and in the basophilic cells of the blood. Pharmacologic preparations of heparin are extracted from animal tissues. Heparin acts at several steps in the coagulation process to inhibit blood clotting. It interferes with the prothrombin activator in the intrinsic pathway and inhibits the action of thrombin on fibrinogen. Heparin also acts directly to inactivate thrombin and to increase its removal through increased absorption of fibrin.

Fibrinolytic enzymes

A number of fibrinolytic enzymes have been purified to treat thrombi and emboli. Two of the plasminogen activators that are used are streptokinase and urinokinase. Streptokinase, a protein elaborated by certain β-hemolytic streptococci, may be used in the treatment of coronary artery occlusion (Chap. 19) or acute arterial or venous occlusion (Chap. 15). The enzyme combines with plasminogen to form plasmin and activate the fibrinolytic pathway. Normal urine contains urinokinase that is elaborated and excreted by the kidneys. Like streptokinase, it can be used for the dissolution of thrombi and emboli.

In summary, there are two types of disorders of hemostasis and blood clotting: (1) the hypercoagulability states and (2) bleeding disorders. Hypercoagulability causes excessive clotting and contributes to thrombus formation. It results from conditions that cause hyperreactivity of platelets or accelerated activity of the clotting system. Bleeding disorders result from impaired formation of the platelet plug that seals the vessels or from defects in the coagulation process. The formation of the platelet plug is impaired when the number of platelets is deficient (because of inadequate production, excessive pooling in the spleen, or excessive destruction) or adherence or aggregation is defective (because of aspirin and other drug effects). Deficiencies of clotting factors can arise because of inadequate synthesis (resulting from liver disease or vitamin K deficiency), production of inactive factors (from hemophilia), or increased consumption (from DIC).

■ Study Guide

After you have studied this chapter, you should be able to meet the following objectives:

- [ ] State the five stages of hemostasis.
- [ ] Describe the formation of the platelet plug.
- [ ] State the purpose of coagulation.
- [ ] State the function of clot retraction.
- [ ] Trace the process of fibrinolysis.
- [ ] Compare normal and abnormal clotting.
- [ ] State the causes of platelet hyperreactivity.
- [ ] State two conditions that contribute to increased clotting activity.
- [ ] State two causes of impaired platelet function.
- [ ] Describe the role of vitamin K in coagulation.

☐ State three common defects of coagulation factors and the distribution of each.

☐ Describe the physiologic basis of acute disseminated intravascular clotting.

☐ Describe the effect of vascular disorders on hemostasis.

☐ State the mechanism by which coumadin and heparin inhibit coagulation.

■ References

1. Arkin CF, Hartman AS: The hypercoagulability states. CRC Crit Rev Clin Lab Sci 10:397, 1979
2. Stuart MJ, Gross MJ, Elrad H et al: Effects of acetyllsalicylic-acid ingestion on maternal or neonatal hemostasis. N Engl J Med 307:909, 1982
3. Lazerson J: Prophylactic infusion therapy in hemophilia. Hosp Pract 14, No 5:49, 1979
4. Curran JW, Evatt BL, Lawrence DN: Acquired immune deficiency syndrome: The past as prologue. Ann Intern Med 98:401, 1983
5. Lederman MM, Ratnoff OD, Scillina JJ et al: Impaired cell-mediated immunity in patients with classic hemophilia. N Engl J Med 308:79, 1983
6. Merskey C: DIC: Identification and management. Hosp Pract 17, No 12:83, 1982

■ Additional References

Arkin CF, Hartman AS: The hypercoagulability states. Crit Rev Clin Lab Sci 10, No 4:397, 1979

Bennett JS: Blood coagulation and coagulation tests. Med Clin North Am 68:557, 1984

Bosl GJ, Edson JR: Intravascular coagulation. Minn Med 62, No 7:544, 1979

Chamberlain SL: Low-dose heparin therapy. Am J Nurs 80, No 6:1115, 1980

Chart IS, Sanderson JH: General aspects of the blood coagulation system. Pharmacol Ther 5, No 1-3:220, 1979

Dressler D: Understanding and treating hemophilia. Nursing '80 10, No 8:72, 1980

Franco LM: Acute disseminated intravascular coagulation. Cardio-Vasc Nurs 15, No 5:22, 1979

Green D: Role of the von Willenbrand factor in atherogenesis. Artery 5, No 3:262, 1979

Gill FM: Congenital bleeding disorders: Hemophilia and von Willebrand's disease. Med Clin North Am 68:601, 1984

Hand J: Keeping anticoagulants under control. RN 42, No 4:25, 1979

Harrington WJ, Ahn YN, Byrnes JJ et al: Treatment of idiopathic thrombocytopenic purpura. Hosp Pract 18, No 9:205, 1983

Kouts J, Howard M, Firkin BG: Factor VIII physiology and pathology in man. Prog Hematol 11:115, 1979

Marcus AJ: Aspirin as an antithrombotic medication. N Engl J Med 309:1515, 1983

Mielke CH: Influence of aspirin on platelets and the bleeding time. Am J Med 72:72, 1983

Salzman EW: Aspirin to prevent arterial thrombosis. N Engl J Med 307:113, 1982

Sharma GV, Cella G, Parisi AF, Sasahara AA: Thrombolytic therapy. N Engl J Med 306:1268, 1982

Shattil SJ, Bennett JS: Platelets and their membranes in hemostasis: Physiology and pathophysiology. Ann Intern Med 94:108, 1980

Schafer AI: Bleeding disorders: Finding the cause. Hosp Pract 19, No 11:88K, 1984

Stuart MJ, Gross SJ, Elrad H, Graeber JE: Effects of acetyllsalicylic-acid ingestion on maternal and neonatal hemostasis. N Engl J Med 307:909, 1982

Vargaftic BB, Conrad J, Samama M: Blood coagulation and platelet function. Pharmacol Ther 5:225, 1979

Wall RT: The endothelium and thrombosis. Annu Rev Med 31:361, 1980

Wessler S, Gitel SN: Warfarin: From bedside to bench. N Engl J Med 311:645, 1984

Zalamas J, Simon C: Anticoagulants: Accepted treatment and current trends. Nurs Drug Alert 3:105, 1979

Unit III

Alterations in Oxygenation of Tissues

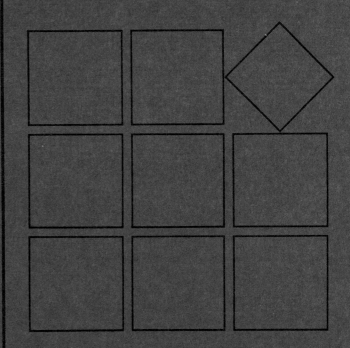

Chapter 13

The Red Blood Cell and Alterations in Oxygen Transport

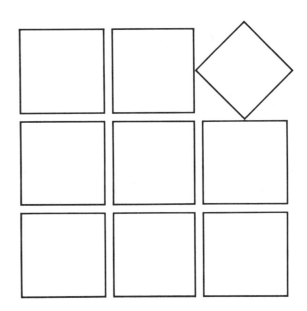

Although the lungs provide the means for gas exchange between the external and internal environment, it is the hemoglobin in the red blood cells that transports oxygen to the tissues. The red blood cells also function as carriers of carbon dioxide and participate in acid–base balance. The function of the red blood cells, in terms of oxygen transport, is discussed in Chapter 22 and acid–base balance is covered in Chapter 26. This chapter presents a discussion of the red blood cell, anemia, and polycythemia.

■ The Red Blood Cell

The red blood cell (erythrocyte) is a concave, spherical disk (Fig. 13-1). This shape serves to increase the surface area available for diffusion of oxygen and allows the cell to change in volume and shape without rupturing its membrane. The biconcave form presents the plasma with a surface 20 to 30 times greater than if the red blood cell were an absolute sphere. The erythrocytes, 500 to 1000 times more numerous than other blood cells, are the most common type of blood cell.

The function of the red blood cell, facilitated by the hemoglobin molecule, is to transport oxygen to the tissues. In addition, hemoglobin binds some carbon dioxide and carries it from the tissues to the lungs. The hemoglobin molecule is composed of two pairs of struc-

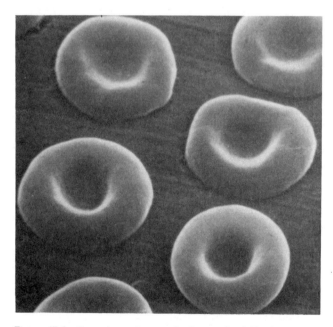

Figure 13-1 *Scanning micrograph of normal red blood cells (× 5000). The normal concave disk appearance of these cells is apparent. (Courtesy of STEM Laboratories and Fischer Scientific Company)*

turally different polypeptide chains. Each of the four polypeptide chains is attached to a heme unit, which, in turn, surrounds an atom of iron that binds oxygen. The rate at which hemoglobin is synthesized in anemia depends on the availability of iron for heme synthesis. Lack of iron results in relatively small amounts of hemoglobin in the red blood cells.

There are two types of normal hemoglobin: adult hemoglobin (HbA) and fetal hemoglobin (HbF). *Adult hemoglobin consists of a pair of α chains and a pair of β chains. Fetal hemoglobin is the predominant hemoglobin in the fetus from the third through the ninth month of gestation. It has a pair of γ chains substituted for the β* chains. Because of this chain substitution, fetal hemoglobin has a high affinity for oxygen. This facilitates the transfer of oxygen across the placenta. Fetal hemoglobin is replaced soon after birth with adult hemoglobin.

Red Cell Production and Regulation

Erythropoiesis is the production of red blood cells. After birth, the red cells are produced in the red bone marrow. Until the age of 5 years, almost all bones produce red cells to meet growth needs. Following this period, bone marrow activity gradually declines; after age 20, red cell production takes place mainly in the membranous bones of the vertebrae, sternum, ribs, and pelvis. With this lessened activity, the red bone marrow is replaced with fatty yellow bone marrow.

The red cells derive from the erythroblasts, which are continuously being formed from the primordial stem cells in the bone marrow. In developing into a mature red cell, the primordial stem cell moves through a series of stages—*erythroblast* to *normoblast* to *reticulocyte* and finally to *erythrocyte* (Fig. 13-2). Hemoglobin synthesis begins at the erythroblast stage and continues until the cell becomes an erythrocyte. During its transformation from normoblast to reticulocyte, the red blood cell loses its nucleus. Normally, the period from stem cell to emergence of the reticulocyte in the circulation takes about a week. Maturation of reticulocyte to erythrocyte takes about 24 to 48 hours, and during this process the red cell loses its mitochondria and ribosomes along with its ability to produce hemoglobin and engage in oxidative metabolism. Most maturing red cells enter the blood as reticulocytes. Normally about 1% of the red blood cells are generated from bone marrow each day, and therefore the reticulocyte count serves as an index of the erythropoietic activity of the bone marrow.

The red cell relies on glucose and the glycolytic pathway for its metabolic needs. It relies on the enzyme-mediated anaerobic metabolism of glucose for the generation of the adenosine triphosphate (ATP) needed for normal membrane function and ion transport. Depletion of glucose or the functional deficiency of one of the glycolytic enzymes leads to the premature death of the red blood cell. Another essential enzyme pathway in the red cell is needed to maintain hemoglobin in the reduced state and prevent the formation of methemoglobin when oxygen becomes attached to the iron atom of the heme unit. The enzyme glucose 6-phosphate dehydrogenase (G6PD) is essential to the function of this pathway. A deficiency of this eynzyme can lead to denaturing of hemoglobin with hemolysis of the red blood cell.

Erythropoiesis is governed, for the most part, by tissue oxygen needs. *Hypoxia* is the main *stimulus* for red cell production. Hypoxia does not, however, act directly on the bone marrow. Instead, red cell production by the bone marrow is regulated by *erythropoietin,* sometimes called the erythropoietic factor. Erythropoietin, a glycoprotein with a molecular weight of 39,000 to 70,000, is released in response to hypoxia, although the precise mechanism of its formation is unclear. It is known that erythropoietin levels are lower in persons with impaired kidney function and in those who have had a kidney removed. It is thought that the kidney, when exposed to hypoxia, releases an enzyme—renal erythropoietic factor—that converts a circulating plasma protein into erythropoietin.

Erythropoietin takes several days to effect release of red blood cells from the bone marrow, and only after 5 or more days does red blood cell production reach maximum. Because red blood cells are released into the blood as reticulocytes, the percentage of these cells in relation to the total red blood cell count is higher when there is a marked increase in red blood cell production. In some severe anemias, for example, the reticulocytes may account for as much as 30% to 50% of the total.[1] In some situations, red cell production is so accelerated that numerous normoblasts appear in the blood.

Red Blood Cell Destruction

Mature red blood cells have a life span of about 4 months or 120 days. As the red blood cell ages, a number of changes occur. The metabolic activities within the cell decrease; enzyme activity falls off; and ATP, potassium, and membrane lipids decrease. Normally the rate of red cell destruction (1% per day) is equal to red cell production, but in some conditions, such as hemolytic anemia, the cell's life span may be shorter.

Destruction of red blood cells is accomplished by a group of large phagocytic cells found in the spleen, liver, bone marrow, and lymph nodes. These phagocytic cells ingest and destroy the erythrocytes in a series of enzymatic reactions during which the amino acids from the globulin chains and iron from the heme units are salvaged and reutilized. The bulk of the heme unit is

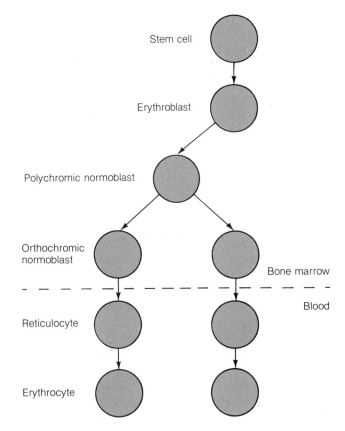

Figure 13-2 *Red blood cell development.*

converted to bilirubin (the pigment of bile), which is insoluble in plasma and attaches to the plasma proteins for transport. Bilirubin is removed from the blood by the liver and conjugated with glucuronide to render it water soluble so that it can be excreted in the bile. The plasma-insoluble form of bilirubin is referred to as unconjugated bilirubin and the water-soluble form as conjugated bilirubin. Serum levels of conjugated and unconjugated bilirubin can be measured in the laboratory using the Van der Bergh test, which is described in Chapter 43.

If the rate of bilirubin production is excessive and the ability to conjugate and excrete bilirubin is deficient, excess unconjugated bilirubin will accumulate in the blood. This not only results in a yellow discoloration of the skin (jaundice), but because unconjugated bilirubin is lipid soluble it can cross neuronal cell membranes. In infants this can cause bilirubin encephalopathy. Such damage may be subtle and may not be apparent for several years, or it may cause a severe neurologic condition called *kernicterus,* which can cause visual–motor defects, deafness, cerebral palsy, mental retardation, and even death. Hyperbilirubinemia is most apt to occur in sick and immature infants, but it can occur in normal newborns as well. The condition affects 50% of newborns but only 10% require treatment.[2] Unconjugated bilirubin cannot cross the cell membrane as long as it remains bound to albumin or other plasma proteins. Many factors combine to raise serum bilirubin levels in the newborn, including hypoalbuminemia (common in the newborn), acidosis, sepsis, hypoxia, hemolytic disease of the newborn (to be discussed), dehydration, and certain drugs that compete for bilirubin-binding sites on albumin.

Two types of treatment are used for hyperbilirubinemia in the newborn: exchange transfusions and phototherapy. Bilirubin is photolabile. Under visible light in the absorption range of 450 nm to 500 nm, bilirubin is broken down to a less lipid-soluble form that is readily excreted by the liver. Whole body radiation can be used. Phototherapy units, consisting of banks of eight to ten fluorescent lamps placed about 2 feet above the skin surface of the infant, are generally used.

When red blood cell destruction takes place in the vascular circulation, as in hemolytic anemia, the hemoglobin remains in the plasma. The plasma contains a hemoglobin-binding protein called haptoglobin. Other plasma proteins, such as albumin, may also bind hemoglobin. With extensive intravascular destruction of red blood cells, hemoglobin levels may exceed the hemoglobin-binding capacity of haptoglobin. When this happens, free hemoglobin appears in the blood (hemoglobinemia) and is excreted in the urine (hemoglobinuria). Because this can occur in hemolytic transfusion reactions, urine samples are tested for free hemoglobin following a transfusion reaction.

Laboratory Tests

The red cells can be studied by means of a sample of blood (Table 13-1). In the laboratory, modern automated blood cell counters are used to provide rapid and accurate measurements of red cell content and cell indices.

The *red blood cell count (RBC)* measures the *total number* of RBCs in a cubic millimeter of blood. The *percentage of reticulocytes* (normally about 1%) provides an index of the rate of red cell production. The *hemoglobin* (grams per 100 ml of blood) measures the *hemoglobin content* of the blood. The major components of the blood are the red cell mass and plasma volume. The *hematocrit* measures the volume of red cell mass in 100 ml of plasma volume. To determine the hematocrit, a sample of blood is placed in a glass tube, which is then centrifuged to separate the cells and the plasma. The hematocrit may be deceptive, since it varies with the quantity of extracellular fluid present, rising with dehydration and falling with overexpansion of the extracellular fluid volume.

The word *corpuscle* means "little body." The *mean corpuscular volume (MCV)* reflects the *volume* or *size* of the red cells. The MCV falls in microcytic anemia and rises in macrocytic anemia. The *mean corpuscular hemoglobin concentration (MCHC)* is the *concentration of hemoglobin* in each cell, and it decreases in hypochromic anemia. A stained red cell study gives information about the size, color, and shape of the red blood cells. They may be normocytic (of normal size), microcytic (of small size), or macrocytic (of large size); normochromic (of normal color) or hypochromic (of decreased color).

Bone marrow function in blood cell production is studied by means of the *bone marrow smear,* in which the marrow is aspirated with a short, rigid sharp-pointed needle equipped with a stylet.

In summary, the red blood cell provides the means for transport of oxygen from the lungs to the tissues. The red cells develop from stem cells in the bone marrow and are released into the blood as reticulocytes, where they become mature erythrocytes. The life span of a red cell is about 120 days. Red cell destruction normally occurs in the spleen, liver, bone marrow, and lymph nodes. In the process of destruction the heme portion of the hemo-

Table 13-1   Standard Laboratory Values for Red Blood Cells

Test	Normal Values	Significance
Red blood cell count (RBC)		
Men	4.2 to 5.4 million/mm³	Number of red cells in the blood
Women	3.6 to 5 million/mm³	
Reticulocytes	1.0% to 1.5% of total RBC	Rate of red cell production
Hemoglobin (Hb)		
Men	14 to 16.5 gm/100 ml	Hemoglobin content of the blood
Women	12 to 15 gm/100 ml	
Hematocrit (HCT)		
Men	40 to 50/100 ml	Volume of cells in 100 ml of blood
Women	37 to 47/100 ml	
Mean corpuscular volume (MCV)	85 to 100 cu U	Size of the red cell
Mean corpuscular hemoglobin concentration (MCHC)	31 to 35 gm/100 ml	Concentration of hemoglobin in the red cell

globin molecule is converted to bilirubin. Bilirubin, which is insoluble in plasma, attaches to plasma proteins for transport in the blood. It is removed from the blood by the liver and conjugated to a water-soluble form so that it can be excreted in the bile.

Anemia

Anemia is a condition in which an abnormally low number of circulating red blood cells, abnormally low hemoglobin, or both occur. There may be (1) excessive loss (bleeding) or destruction (hemolysis) of red blood cells or (2) deficient red cell production because of a lack of iron or other nutritional elements or bone marrow failure (aplastic anemia).

Manifestations

Anemia is not a disease but rather an indication of some disease process or alteration in body function. The manifestations of anemia can be grouped into three categories: (1) impaired oxygen transport, (2) alterations in red cell structure, and (3) signs and symptoms associated with the pathologic process causing the anemia. The manifestations of anemia also depend on its severity and the rapidity of its development. With rapid blood loss circulatory shock and circulatory collapse may occur. On the other hand, the body tends to adapt to slowly developing anemia, and the loss of red cell mass may be considerable without any signs and symptoms.

Anemia interferes with oxygen transport to the tissues and, unlike respiratory failure, causes hypoxia but not hypercarbia. Decreased oxygen transport can give rise to fatigue, syncope, dyspnea, angina, and organ dysfunction. There is tachycardia, especially with slight exertion, as the body tries to compensate with an increase in cardiac output. A flow-type systolic heart murmur, resulting from changes in blood viscosity, may develop. Ventricular hypertrophy may develop in severe and chronic anemia.

Oxygenated hemoglobin provides the red pigment for blood. Lack of red blood cells in the superficial vessels causes pallor of the skin, mucous membranes, conjunctiva, skin folds, and nail beds. Jaundice (due to increased bilirubin in the blood) often accompanies the pallor in hemolytic anemia. In aplastic anemia there may be petechiae and purpura associated with thrombocytopenia.

Blood Loss Anemia

With anemia due to bleeding, iron and other components of the erythrocyte are lost from the body. Blood loss may be acute or chronic. In the acute form, there is a risk of hypovolemia and shock rather than anemia (Chap. 21). The red cells are normal in size and color. A fall in the red blood cell count, hematocrit, and hemoglobin results from hemodilution caused by movement of fluid into the vascular compartment. The hypoxia resulting from blood loss stimulates red cell production by the bone marrow. If the bleeding is controlled and sufficient iron stores are available, the red cell concentration returns to normal within 3 to 4 weeks. Chronic blood loss does not affect the blood volume but instead leads to iron-deficiency anemia (discussed later). Red blood cells are produced with too little hemoglobin, giving rise to microcytic hypochromic anemia.

Hemolytic Anemias

Hemolytic anemia is characterized by the premature destruction of red cells with retention in the body of iron and the other products of red cell destruction. Virtually all types of hemolytic anemia are characterized by normocytic and normochromic red cells. Because of the shortened life span of the red cell, the bone marrow is usually hyperactive, resulting in increased numbers of reticulocytes in the circulating blood. As with other types of anemias there is easy fatigability, dyspnea, and other signs of impaired oxygen transport. In addition, mild jaundice is often present. In hemolytic anemia, red cell breakdown can occur within the vascular compartment or it can result from phagocytosis by the reticuloendothelial system. Intravascular hemolysis is manifest by hemoglobinemia and hemoglobinuria.

Hemolytic anemias result from a wide variety of causes. These disorders can be either intrinsic or extrinsic to the red cell. The intrinsic disorders include defects of the red cell membrane, the various hemoglobinopathies, and inherited enzyme defects that cause hemolytic anemia. There are also acquired forms of hemolytic anemia caused by agents extrinsic to the red cell, such as drugs, bacterial and other toxins, antibodies, and trauma.[3] Although all of these disorders cause premature and accelerated destruction of red cells, they cannot all be treated in the same way. Some respond to splenectomy and others to the adrenocorticosteroid hormones, whereas still others do not resolve until the primary disorder is corrected.

Inherited disorders of the red cell membrane

Hereditary spherocytosis, which is inherited as an autosomal dominant trait, is the most common inherited disorder of the red cell membrane. The disorder leads to gradual loss of the membrane surface during the life span of the red blood cell, resulting in a tight sphere instead of a concave disk. While the spherical cell retains its ability to transport oxygen, its shape renders it susceptible to destruction as it passes through the venous sinuses of the splenic circulation.

An aplastic crisis may occur in any of the congenital hemolytic anemias that are manifest in childhood. In the face of a shortened life span, a sudden disruption of red cell production (in most cases caused by a viral infection) causes a rapid drop in hematocrit and hemoglobin levels and a worsening of the anemia that may be life threatening.

The disorder is usually treated with splenectomy to reduce the red cell destruction. In children, this is usually not done until after age 4 to 5 years to avoid the risk of infectious complications, including septicemia.[3]

Hemoglobinopathies

Abnormalities in hemoglobin structure can lead to accelerated red cell destruction. Two main types of hemoglobinopathies can cause red cell hemolysis: (1) the abnormal substitution of an amino acid in the hemoglobin molecule as in sickle cell anemia and (2) defective synthesis of one of the polypeptide chains that form the globin portion of hemoglobin, as in the thalassemias.

Sickle cell anemia.   Sickle cell anemia, affecting approximately 50,000 Americans is largely a disease of blacks. About one out of every ten black Americans is estimated to carry the trait.[4] In sickle cell anemia, there is a defect of the β-chain of the hemoglobin molecule, with an abnormal substitution of a single amino acid. Sickle hemoglobin (HbS) is transmitted by recessive inheritance and can present as either sickle cell trait (heterozygote) or sickle cell disease (homozygote). In the heterozygote only about 40% of the hemoglobin is HgS, whereas in the homozygote almost all of the hemoglobin is HbS. Sickle cell trait is not a mild form of sickle cell anemia, although in severe hypoxia, persons with sickle cell trait may experience some sickling.

In the homozygote, the HbS becomes sickled when deoxygenated. These deformed red blood cells obstruct blood flow in the microcirculation. In order for sickling to occur, one HbS molecule must interact with another. Thus, the person with sickle cell trait who has 60% HbA has little tendency to sickle except in hypoxia. Fetal hemoglobin does not interact with HbS, and therefore the child with sickle cell anemia does not usually begin to experience the effects of the sickling until sometime after 4 to 6 months of age when the fetal hemoglobin has been replaced by HbS.

Factors that precipitate sickling are exertion, infection, other illnesses, hypoxia, acidosis, dehydration, or even such trivial incidents as reduced oxygen tension induced by sleep. Hardly an organ is spared in sickle cell anemia. Affected persons develop severe anemia, painful crises, organ damage, and chronic hyperbilirubinemia. A painful crisis results from vessel occlusion and can appear suddenly in almost any part of the body. The common sites are the abdomen, the chest, and the joints. Infarctions due to sluggish blood flow may cause chronic damage to the liver, spleen, heart, kidney, and other organs. The hyperbilirubinemia resulting from the breakdown products of hemoglobin often leads to production of pigment stones in the gallbladder.

At present, there is no known cure or therapeutic regimen that prevents the problems associated with sickle cell anemia, and treatment is largely supportive. There is an emphasis on avoiding situations that precipitate sickling episodes, such as infections, cold exposure, severe physical exertion, acidosis, and dehydration. Genetic counseling may be of value in family planning.

Thalassemias.   In contrast to sickle cell anemia, which involves a single amino acid on the beta chain of the hemoglobin molecule, the thalassemias are the result of absent or defective synthesis of either the α- or β-chains of Hb.[5] The β-thalassemias represent a defect in β-chain synthesis and the α-thalassemias a defect in α-chain synthesis. The defect is inherited as a mendelian trait, and a person may be heterozygous for the trait and have a mild form of the disease or be homozygous and have the full-blown disease. Like sickle cell anemia, the thalassemias occur with high frequency in certain populations. They are most prevalent in Mediterranean populations (*e.g.,* southern Italy and Greece) and in Asian populations (*e.g.,* Thailand, China, and the Philippines). The β-thalassemias, sometimes called *Cooley's anemia* or *Mediterranean anemia,* are most common in Mediterranean populations, and the α-thalassemias are most common among Asians. Both α- and β-thalassemias are common in Africans and American blacks.

Two factors contribute to the anemia that occurs in thalassemia: reduced hemoglobin synthesis and an imbalance in globin chain production. In both α- and β-thalassemia, defective globin chain production leads to deficient hemoglobin production and the development of a hypochromic microcytic anemia. Because only one type of globin chain (either the α chain or the β chain) is affected in the thalassemias, the unaffected type of chain is unable to find a complementary chain for binding. The unpaired chains accumulate in the red cell, contributing to red cell destruction and anemia.

The clinical manifestations of β-thalassemias are based on the severity of the anemia. The presence of one normal gene in heterozygous persons usually results in sufficient normal hemoglobin synthesis to prevent severe anemia. Persons who are homozygous for the trait have very severe transfusion-dependent anemia. The unpaired synthesis of α-chains leads to the precipitation of insoluble aggregates or inclusion bodies (Heinz bodies) within the bone marrow red cell precursors.[6] These inclusion bodies impair DNA synthesis and cause damage to the red cell membrane. Severely affected red cell precursors are destroyed in the bone marrow, and those that escape intramedullary death are at increased risk of destruction in the spleen. Severe growth retardation is present in children with the disorder. With transfusions, survival to the second or third decade is possible.[6] An increased stimulus for hematopoiesis causes bone marrow expansion and increased iron absorption, and splenomegaly and hepatomegaly result from increased red cell destruction. Bone marrow expansion leads to thinning of the cortical bone, with new bone formation on the external aspect. Changes are evident on the maxilla and frontal bones of the face. The long bones, ribs, and vertebrae may become vulnerable to fracture. Excess iron stores, which accumulate secondary to increased dietary absorption and intake from repeated transfusions, become deposited in the myocardium, liver, and pancreas to induce organ injury.

Synthesis of the α-globin chains of hemoglobin is controlled by two pairs of (four) genes; hence the severity of α-thalassemia shows great variations. Silent carriers have deletion of a single α-globin gene. As with β-thalassemia, anemia results from defective hemoglobin production and the accumulation of unpaired globin chains, in this case the β-chains. The most severe form of α-thalassemia occurs in infants in whom all four α-globin genes are deleted. Such a defect results in a hemoglobin molecule (Hb Barts) that is formed exclusively from the α-chains of fetal hemoglobin. Hb Barts, which has an extremely high oxygen affinity, is unable to release oxygen in the tissues. Affected infants suffer from severe hypoxia and are either stillborn or die shortly after birth. Deletion of three of the four α-chain genes leads to unstable aggregates of β-chains called *hemoglobin H* (HbH). The β-chains are more soluble than the α-chains; therefore, their accumulation tends to be less toxic to the red cells, so that senescent rather than precursor red cells are affected. Persons with HbH usually have only mild to moderate hemolytic anemia, and manifestations of ineffective erythropoiesis (bone marrow expansion and iron overload) are absent.

Inherited enzyme defects

The most common inherited enzyme defect resulting in hemolytic anemia is a deficiency of G6PD. The disorder causes direct oxidation of hemoglobin to methemoglobin and denaturing of the hemoglobin molecule to form what are called *Heinz bodies*. Hemolysis usually occurs as the damaged red blood cells move through the narrow vessels of the spleen. The gene determining this enzyme is located on the X chromosome, and the defect is expressed only in males and homozygous females.

There are a number of genetic variants of this disorder. The African variant has been found in 10% of American blacks.[6] A deficiency of G6PD is thought to protect against malaria, and this may be one of the reasons that the genetic trait has persisted. In blacks, the defect is mildly expressed and is not associated with chronic hemolytic anemia unless exposed to oxidant drugs or chemicals. Numerous oxidant drugs may trigger a hemolytic crisis, principally the antimalarial drugs (primaquine phosphate and Atabrine), the sulfonamides, nitrofurantoin, aspirin, and phenacetin, among others. A more severe deficiency of G6PD is found in peoples of Mediterranean descent (Sardinians, Sephardic Jews, Arabs, and others). In some of these persons chronic hemolysis occurs in the absence of exposure to oxidants. The disorder can be diagnosed through the use of a G6PD assay or screening test.

Acquired hemolytic anemias

A number of acquired factors, exogenous to the red blood cell, produce hemolysis. These include various drugs, chemicals, toxins, venoms, and infections such as malaria. Antibodies that cause premature destruction of red cells may develop. Hemolytic anemia may also be caused by mechanical factors such as prosthetic heart valves, vasculitis, severe burns, and other conditions that directly injure the red cell. In all types of drug-related hemolytic anemia, discontinuance of the drug results in the eventual disappearance of the antibody.

The antibodies that cause red cell destruction fall into two categories: warm-reacting antibodies of the IgG type, which are maximally active at 37°C, and cold-reacting antibodies of the IgM type, which are optimally active at or near 4°C.

The warm antibodies cause no morphologic or metabolic alteration in the red cell. Instead, they react with antigens on the red cell membrane, causing destructive changes that lead to spherocytosis, with subsequent phagocytic destruction in the spleen or reticuloendothelial system. They lack specificity for the ABO antigens but may react with the Rh antigens. The hemolytic reactions associated with the warm-reacting antibodies have varied etiologies; they are often related to malignancies of the lymphoproliferative system (chronic lymphocytic leukemia and lymphoma) or collagen diseases (systemic lupus erythematosus). Treatment with the antihypertensive drug alpha-methyldopa produces an antibody that closely resembles the warm-reacting antibodies found in nondrug hemolytic anemias. The diagnosis of warm-reacting antibody hemolytic anemia is made through use of the Coombs' test.

The *Coombs' test* detects the presence of immune globulins on the surface of the red cell. A *direct Coombs' test* detects the antibody on red blood cells. In this test red cells, which have been washed free of serum, are mixed with Coombs' antiserum. The red cells will agglutinate if the specific immune globulins or other proteins attach to the red cell membrane. The direct Coombs' test is positive in autoimmune hemolytic anemia, erythroblastosis fetalis (Rh disease of the newborn), transfusion reactions, and following exposure to certain drugs such as large doses of penicillin, cephalothin, and the antihypertensive drug alpha-methyldopa. The *indirect Coombs' test* detects the presence of antibody in the serum and is positive in the presence of specific antibodies resulting from previous transfusions or pregnancy.

The cold-reacting antibodies activate complement. Chronic hemolytic anemia due to cold-reacting antibodies occurs with lymphoproliferative disorders and as an idiopathic disorder of unknown etiology. The hemolytic process occurs in distal body parts where the temperature may fall below 30°C. Vascular obstruction by red cells results in pallor, cyanosis of the body parts exposed to cold temperatures, and Raynaud's phenomenon (Chap. 15). Hemolytic anemia develops in only a few persons. In contrast to hemolytic anemia caused by warm-reacting antibodies, the direct Coombs' test is only weakly positive with hemolytic conditions caused by cold-reacting antibodies.

Hemolytic disease of the newborn

Erythroblastosis fetalis, or hemolytic disease of the newborn, occurs in Rh-positive infants of Rh-negative mothers who have been sensitized by previous pregnancies in which the infants are Rh positive or by blood transfusions of Rh-positive blood. The Rh-negative mother usually becomes sensitized during the first few days following delivery. During this time the antigens from the placental site are released into the maternal circulation. Because the development of the antibodies requires several weeks, the first Rh-positive infant of an Rh-negative mother is usually not affected. Infants with Rh-negative blood have no antigens on their red cells to react with the maternal antibodies and are also not affected.

Once an Rh-negative mother has been sensitized, the Rh antibodies from her blood are transferred to the baby through the placental circulation. These antibodies react with the red cell antigens of the Rh-positive infant, causing agglutination and hemolysis. This leads to severe anemia with compensatory hyperplasia and enlargement of the blood-forming organs, including the spleen and liver, in the fetus. Liver function may be impaired, with decreased production of albumin and development of a generalized edema called *hydrops fetalis*. Blood levels of unconjugated *bilirubin* in the blood are abnormally high due to red cell hemolysis, and with these elevated levels there is danger that the bilirubin will precipitate in neuronal tissue and cause destructive changes; this condition is called *kernicterus*.

Not all babies born to Rh-negative mothers are Rh-positive, and those that are Rh-negative are not likely to develop erythroblastosis. If, for example, the father carries a complex of both Rh-positive and Rh-negative genes, there is a chance that the baby will be Rh-negative.

Three recent advances have served to decrease the threat to babies born to Rh-negative mothers: (1) prevention of sensitization, (2) intrauterine transfusion to the affected fetus, and (3) exchange transfusion. Injection of *Rh immune globulin* (gamma globulin containing Rh antibody) prevents sensitization in Rh-negative mothers who have given birth to Rh-positive infants if administered within 72 hours of delivery. The Rh immune globulin must be given after each delivery (or abortion) of an Rh-positive infant to prevent sensitization—once sensitization has developed, the immune globulin is of no known value. In the past, about 20% of erythroblastotic fetuses died *in utero*. It is now possible to increase their chances of survival by studying the amniotic fluid to determine whether intrauterine blood transfusions are necessary. If the specimen of amniotic fluid indicates that the fetus is erythroblastotic, the intrauterine transfusions will be given. Exchange transfusions are given after birth. In this technique, 10 ml to 20 ml of the infant's blood is removed and replaced with an equal amount of type O, unsensitized Rh-negative blood. This procedure is repeated until twice the blood volume of the infant has been exchanged. The purpose of the exchange transfusion is to prevent hyperbilirubinemia with consequent damage to the brain.

Nutritional Anemias

A true nutritional anemia must meet two criteria: (1) deficiency or lack of a nutrient alone must produce the anemia and (2) providing the nutrient must correct the anemia.[7] The common types of nutritional anemias are iron-deficiency and megaloblastic anemia due to vitamin B_{12} or folic acid deficiencies.

Iron-deficiency anemia

Iron is an integral constituent of the heme in the hemoglobin molecule, and its deficiency leads to a decrease in hemoglobin synthesis. In iron-deficiency anemia there is a decrease in serum iron. The red cells are decreased in number and are microcytic, hypochromic, and often malformed (poikilocytosis). Membrane changes may predispose to hemolysis causing further loss of red cells.

Body iron is repeatedly reused. When red cells

become senescent and are broken down, their iron is released and reused in the production of new red cells. The normal diet contains about 12 mg to 15 mg iron of which normally only 5% to 10% is absorbed. In iron deficiency, the absorption increases. Normally, less than 1 mg iron is lost from the body daily. About 30% of body iron is stored in the bone marrow, the spleen, muscle, and other organs; the remainder is present in the form of hemoglobin.

In the adult, a blood loss of 2 ml to 4 ml per day is the usual reason for an iron deficiency.[8] This blood loss may be due to gastrointestinal bleeding, such as occurs with peptic ulcer, intestinal polyps, hemorrhoids, or malignancy. Excessive aspirin intake may cause undetected gastrointestinal bleeding. In women, blood is lost during menstruation. Each milliliter of blood contains 0.5 mg iron, and the average menstrual flow is about 44 ml, with a loss of 22 mg of iron.[8] Although cessation of menstruation spares iron loss in the pregnant woman, iron requirements increase at this time; the expansion of the mother's blood volume requires about 480 mg of additional iron, and the growing fetus requires about 390 mg.[8]

A child's growth places extra demands on the body: blood volume increases, with a greater need for iron. Iron requirements are proportionally higher in infancy (3 to 24 months) than at any other age, though childhood and adolescence also bring increased requirements.

In infancy the two main causes of iron-deficiency anemia are low iron levels at birth (due to maternal deficiency) and a diet consisting mainly of cow's milk, which is low in absorbable iron. The peak increase in iron deficiency during adolescence stems from increased body requirements resulting from growth spurts at the same time dietary intake may be inadequate.

The signs and symptoms of iron-deficiency anemia are related to the cause and impairment of oxygen transport and lack of hemoglobin. Depending on its severity, fatigability, palpitations, dyspnea, angina, and tachycardia may occur. Late signs are waxy pallor, brittle hair and nails, smooth tongue, and sores in the corners of the mouth. A poorly understood symptom sometimes seen is pica, the bizarre compulsive eating of ice or dirt. Also there may be extreme dysphagia.

The treatment of iron-deficiency anemia is directed toward controlling chronic blood loss, increasing dietary intake of iron, and administering supplemental iron. Parenteral iron may be given if oral forms are not tolerated. Special care is required when administering an iron preparation (Imferon) intramuscularly; it must be injected deeply by pulling the skin to one side before inserting the needle (Z track) to prevent leakage with skin discoloration.

Megaloblastic anemias

Megaloblastic anemias are characterized by a mean corpuscular volume above 100 with increase in red cell size due to abnormalities of maturation in the bone marrow. There may be a vitamin B_{12} deficiency (pernicious anemia) or a folic acid deficiency. (One form of megaloblastic anemia, unresponsive to either vitamin B_{12} or folic acid therapy, is not discussed here.) Because megaloblastic anemias develop slowly, there are often few symptoms until the anemia is far advanced.

Pernicious anemia. Vitamin B_{12} *(cyanocobalamin)* is an essential nutrient required for synthesis of DNA; when it is deficient, failure of nuclear maturation and cell division occurs, especially of the rapidly proliferating red cells. Moreover, when B_{12} is deficient, the red cells that are produced are abnormally large, have flimsy membranes, and are oval rather than the normal biconcave disk shape. The resulting condition is called pernicious anemia. These odd-shaped cells have a short life span that can be measured in weeks rather than months. Pernicious anemia is also accompanied by neurologic changes in which degeneration of the dorsal and lateral columns of the spinal cord causes symmetrical paresthesias of the feet and fingers, which eventually progress to spastic ataxia.

Absorption of vitamin B_{12} in the intestine requires the presence of *intrinsic factor*, which is produced by the gastric mucosa. Intrinsic factor binds to vitamin B_{12} in food and protects it from the enzymatic actions of the gut. As discussed in Chapter 42, production of intrinsic factor is impaired in chronic gastritis (in which atrophic changes occur in the gastric mucosa) and following total removal of the stomach. Treatment consists of intramuscular injections of vitamin B_{12}.

Folic acid deficiency anemia. *Folic acid* is also required for red cell maturation, and its deficiency produces the same type of red cell changes that occur in pernicious anemia. Folic acid deficiency does not, however, induce the neurologic manifestations that are seen in pernicious anemia. Folic acid is readily absorbed from the intestine. It is found in vegetables (particularly the green leafy types), fruits, cereals, and meats. However, much of the vitamin is lost in cooking. The most common cause of a folic acid deficiency is malnutrition, especially in association with alcoholism; it is also seen with malabsorption syndromes such as sprue. Pregnancy increases the need for folic acid five- to tenfold, so a deficiency can occur at this time. Poor dietary habits, anorexia, and nausea are other reasons for a folic acid deficiency during pregnancy. Several groups of drugs may also contribute to a deficiency. Primidone, phenytoin, and phenobarbital (drugs used to treat seizure disorders) and triamterene (a diuretic) predispose to a deficiency by interfering with its absorption. Methotrexate (a folic acid analog used in treatment of cancer) impairs the action of folic acid by blocking its conversion to the active form.

Bone Marrow Depression (Aplastic Anemia)

Bone marrow depression or failure usually is an outcome of stem cell dysfunction with failure to produce blood cells. True red cell aplasia (failure to develop) can occur, but is rare. More commonly the bone marrow fails to produce leukocytes and thrombocytes, as well as erythrocytes.

With aplastic anemia, there is failure to replace the senescent red cells that are destroyed and leave the circulation, although the cells that remain are of normal size and color. At the same time, because the leukocytes, particularly the neutrophils, and the thrombocytes have a short life span, a deficiency of these cells usually is apparent before the anemia becomes severe.

Aplastic anemia can occur at any age. It may be insidious in onset, or it may strike with suddenness and great severity. Weakness, fatigability, and pallor are present. Thrombocytopenia (decrease in the number of platelets) develops and leads to purpura; and the decrease in neutrophils increases susceptibility to infection.

Among the causes of bone marrow depression are exposure to radiation, infections, and chemical agents that are toxic to bone marrow. The best-documented of the identified toxic agents are benzene, the antibiotic chloramphenicol, and the alkylating agents and antimetabolites used in the treatment of cancer (Chap. 5). Bone marrow depression due to exposure to a chemical agent may sometimes be an idiosyncratic reaction, that is, it affects only certain susceptible persons. Such reactions are often severe and sometimes irreversible and fatal. Although aplastic anemia can develop in the course of many infections, it is seen most often in viral hepatitis and military tuberculosis. In two-thirds of the cases there is no known cause, and these are termed *idiopathic aplastic anemia.*[6]

The treatment of aplastic anemia includes avoidance of the offending agent and prevention of infection and trauma. Deficient blood cells may be replaced by transfusions. Transplantation of bone marrow is a relatively recent procedure and may be tried in selected cases. In radiation and many drug-induced aplastic anemias, bone marrow function gradually recovers once the offending agent has been discontinued.

In summary, anemia describes a condition in which a decrease in red cell mass occurs. It is not a disease but a manifestation of some disease process or alteration in body function. It is generally caused by excess loss of red cells (blood loss or hemolytic anemias) or by impaired production (nutritional and aplastic anemias). The manifestations of anemia include those associated with (1) impaired oxygen transport, (2) alterations in red blood cell structure, and (3) signs and symptoms of the underlying process causing the anemia.

■ Polycythemia

Polycythemia is an abnormally high total red blood cell mass. It is categorized as relative, primary, or secondary. In *relative polycythemia* the hematocrit rises because of a loss of blood volume without a corresponding decrease in red cells. *Polycythemia vera (primary polycythemia)* is a proliferative disease of the bone marrow characterized by an absolute increase in total red blood cell mass and volume. It is seen most commonly in men aged 40 to 60 years. *Secondary polycythemia* results from an increase in the level of erythropoietin. This elevation is related to living at high altitudes and to chronic heart and lung disease, both of which cause hypoxia. Smoking more than one and a half packs of cigarettes daily may also cause secondary polycythemia.

In polycythemia vera, signs and symptoms are those related to increased blood viscosity and hypermetabolism—increase in red cell count, hemoglobin, and hematocrit. The increased blood volume gives rise to hypertension. There may be complaints of headache, inability to concentrate, and some difficulty in hearing. There is a plethoric appearance, or dusky redness—even cyanosis—particularly of the lips, fingernails, and mucous membranes. Because of the concentration of blood cells, the person may experience itching and pain in the fingers or toes, and the hypermetabolism may induce night sweats and weight loss. With the elevated blood viscosity and stagnation of blood flow, thrombosis and hemorrhage are possible.

Relative polycythemia is corrected by increasing the vascular fluid volume. Treatment of secondary polycythemia focuses on relieving the hypoxia. For example, the use of continuous low-flow oxygen therapy is a means of correcting the severe hypoxia that occurs in some persons with chronic obstructive lung disease. This form of treatment is thought to relieve the pulmonary hypertension and polycythemia and delay the onset of cor pulmonale. The goal in primary polycythemia is a reduction in blood viscosity. This can be done by phlebotomy (withdrawal of blood) or chemotherapy or radiation to suppress bone marrow function.

In summary, polycythemia describes a condition in which there is an increase in red blood cell mass. It may be relative in type, with red cell mass increased due to a loss of vascular fluid; primary, with proliferative changes in the bone marrow; or secondary, with elevation of erythropoietin levels due to hypoxia.

■ Transfusion Therapy

Transfusion therapy provides the means for (1) replacing deficient red cell mass in the blood and thereby improving oxygen transport and (2) volume replacement. It consists of the transfusion of whole blood or one of its components. In modern blood banking, only the needed components are administered rather than whole blood.[6] In this way a single unit of blood can supply components for more than one person, and there is less risk to recipients because they are not being exposed to antigens or other foreign substances contained in the unneeded portion of the blood. This discussion focuses on the administration of whole blood or the red cell component. Plasma or its components (platelets, granulocytes, albumin, clotting factors) may be administered separately. Table 13-2 describes the red cell components that are used for transfusion.

Blood transfusions must be carefully typed (ABO and Rh type) and carefully cross-matched before they are administered. Failure to do so may cause a fatal blood transfusion reaction. In cross-matching, cells and serum from donor and recipient are selectively combined and observed for agglutination following direct mixing, addition of a high-protein solution to promote agglutination, and addition of Coombs' reagent following thorough washing of the red cells (direct Coombs).

ABO Types

There are four major ABO blood types as determined by the presence or absence of two types of red cell antigens (A and B). Persons who have no red cell antigens are classified as having type O blood, those with A antigens as having type A blood, those with B antigens as having type B blood, and those with AB antigens as having type AB blood (Table 13-3). The ABO blood types are genetically determined. The type O gene is apparently functionless in production of a red cell antigen. Each of the other genes is expressed by the presence of a strong antigen on the red blood cell. Six genotypes and four blood types stem from the four gene types.

Table 13-2   Red Blood Cell Components Used in Transfusion Therapy

Component	Preparation	Advantages
Whole blood	Drawn from the donor. Anticoagulants are added, usually acid-citrate-dextrose or citrate-phosphate-dextrose. Stored at 1°C 5°C until used or expiration date is reached.	Useful in blood loss. Does not require additional preparation except for typing and to cross-matching. Contains both red cells and colloids that are in the plasma.
Packed red cells	Red cells are separated from the plasma of whole blood	Can replace whole blood transfusion when red cells are needed. Minimizes exposure to potentially dangerous materials in the plasma such as potassium, various allergens, and free hemoglobin. Also reduces the danger of volume overload.
Buffy coat–poor red cells	The buffy coat is the white layer that lies above the red cells when whole blood is centrifuged. It is removed in addition to the plasma.	Removes the leukocytes and platelet antigens and reduces the risk of nonhemolytic febrile reactions.
Washed red cells	Packed red cells are washed by special centrifuge method using normal saline.	Futher lessens the antigens in sensitized persons. Cost is high and the cells must be used within 24 hours to avoid bacterial contamination.
Frozen red cells	Red cells are mixed with glycerol to prevent ice crystals from forming and rupturing the cell membrane. Cells must be washed before they have been thawed in preparation for administration.	Lessens the risk of febrile reactions and decreases the sensitization to the HLA antigens on the lymphocytes. Eliminates hepatitis risk. Used in kidney transplant recipients and other high-risk individuals. Costly and takes too long to prepare for use in emergency transfusions.

(Data obtained from Reich PR: Blood Groups II: Pathology and Transfusion Therapy. In Beck WS: Hematology, 2nd ed, pp 317–334. Cambridge, MIT Press, 1977)

Table 13-3   ABO System for Blood Typing

Genotype	Red Cell Antigens	Blood Type	Serum Antibodies
OO	None	O	AB
AO	A	A	B
AA	A	A	B
BO	B	B	A
BB	B	B	A
AB	AB	AB	None

Normally, the body does not develop antibodies to its own tissues or blood cells. When an ABO antigen is not present on the red cell, antibodies develop in the plasma. Thus, persons with type A antigens on their red cells develop type B antibodies in their serum; persons with type B antigens develop type A antibodies in their serum; and persons with type O blood develop both type A and type B antibodies. The ABO antibodies are usually not present at birth but begin to develop 2 to 8 months following birth and reach maximum at about 8 to 10 years of age.[11]

Rh Types

Blood to be transfused must also be typed for Rh type. The Rh type is coded by a triple-gene complex: Cc, Dd, and Ee. The Rh (positive) factors—C, D, and E—are inherited as dominant mendelian traits so that if either of the two chromosomes carrying these genes contains one or more of these dominant genes, the antigen will be present on the red cell. For blood to be Rh negative (lacking the red cell Rh antigens), it is necessary that none of the dominant (C, D, or E) genes be present. Unlike serum antibodies for the ABO blood types that develop spontaneously after birth, development of the Rh antibodies requires exposure to one or more of the Rh factors or their protein products. This means that transfusion of Rh-positive blood into a person with Rh-negative blood who has never been exposed to the Rh-positive factor will have no immediate consequences, because it takes several weeks to build antibodies. After several weeks a reaction might occur, but it is usually mild. If, however, subsequent transfusions of Rh-positive blood are given to the person who has now become sensitized, there may be a severe immediate reaction.

Blood Transfusion Reactions

The seriousness of blood transfusion reactions prompts the need for extreme caution when blood is administered. Care should be taken to ensure proper identification of the recipient and transfusion source. Once the transfusion has been started, careful observation for signs of a transfusion reaction is imperative.

The most critical transfusion reaction is that between the antibody of the recipient's serum and the antigen on the donor's red cells. The signs and symptoms of such a reaction include sensation of heat along the vein where the blood is being infused, flushing of the face, urticaria, headache, pain in the lumbar area, chills and fever, constricting pain in the chest, cramping pain in the abdomen, nausea and vomiting, tachycardia, hypotension, and dyspnea. The transfusion should be stopped immediately should any of these signs occur. Access to the vein should be maintained, since it may be necessary to administer intravenous medications. The blood must be saved for studies to determine the cause of the reaction. One of the complications of a blood transfusion reaction is oliguria and renal shutdown. The urine should be examined for hemoglobin, urobilinogen, and red blood cells.

In summary, transfusion therapy provides the means for replacement of red blood cells and other blood components. Red blood cells contain surface antigens and antibodies. There are four major ABO blood types determined by the presence of two red cell antigens (A and B). There are also Rh antigens. Blood contains antibodies to the antigens that are not present in the blood. Both recipient and donor blood must be carefully typed and cross-matched to prevent blood transfusion reactions, which can prove fatal.

■ Study Guide

After you have studied this chapter, you should be able to meet the following objectives:

☐ Trace the development of a red blood cell from erythroblast to erythrocyte.

☐ Describe the formation, transport, and elimination of bilirubin.

☐ Explain the function of the enzyme G6PD in the red blood cell.

☐ Describe the manifestations of anemia and their mechanisms.

☐ Explain the difference between intravascular and extravascular hemolysis.

☐ Cite the factors that predispose to hyper-bilirubinemia in the infant.

☐ Explain the action of phototherapy in the treatment of hyperbilirubinemia in the newborn.

☐ Describe the pathogenesis of hemolytic disease of the newborn.

- ☐ Compare conjugated and unconjugated bilirubin in terms of production of encephalopathy in the neonate.
- ☐ Compare the hemoglobinopathies associated with sickle cell anemia and thalassemia.
- ☐ Explain the cause of sickling in sickle cell anemia.
- ☐ Cite the criteria for nutritional anemia.
- ☐ Cite common cause of iron-deficiency anemia in infancy and adolescence.
- ☐ Describe the relationship between vitamin B_{12} deficiency and megaloblastic anemia.
- ☐ List three causes of bone marrow depression.
- ☐ Compare characteristics of the red blood cells in acute blood loss, hereditary spherocytosis, sickle cell anemia, iron-deficiency anemia, and aplastic anemia.
- ☐ Compare polycythemia vera and secondary polycythemia.
- ☐ Differentiate between red cell antigens and antibodies in persons with type A, B, AB, and O blood.
- ☐ Explain the determination of the Rh factor.
- ☐ List signs and symptoms of a blood transfusion reaction.

■ References

1. Guyton A: Textbook of Medical Physiology, 6th ed, pp 59, 85. Philadelphia, WB Saunders, 1981
2. Sisson RC: Molecular basis of hyperbilirubinemia and phototherapy. J Invest Dermatol, 77:158, 1981
3. Forget BG: Hemolytic anemias: Congenital and acquired. Hosp Pract 15, No 4:67, 1980
4. Proceedings of the First National Sickle Cell Education Symposium, p 6. Department of Health, Education and Welfare, 1976
5. Lin-Fu JS: Cooley's Anemia. (DHHS Publication No(HSA) 81-5125). US Department of Health Services, Rockville, MD, 1981
6. Robbins SL, Cotran R, Kumar V: Pathologic Basis of Disease, 3rd ed, pp 625, 639. Philadelphia, WB Saunders, 1984
7. Herbert V: The nutritional anemias. Hosp Pract 15, No 3: 65, 1980
8. Beck WS: Hematology, 2nd ed, pp 288, 129, 322. Cambridge, MIT Press, 1977

■ Additional References

Adamson JW: Hemoglobin—From F to A, and back. N Engl J Med 310:917, 1984
Alavi JB: Sickle cell anemia: Pathophysiology and treatment. Med Clin North Am 68:545, 1984
Axelson JA, LoBuglio AF: Immune hemolytic anemia. Med Clin North Am 64 (No 4):597, 1980
Brewer GJ: Inherited erythrocyte metabolic and membrane disorders. Med Clin North Am 64 (No 4):579, 1980
Camitta BM, Storb R, Thomas ED: Aplastic anemia: Part 1 and 2. N Engl J Med 306:645,712, 1982
Cook JD: Clinical evaluation of iron deficiency. Semin Hematol 19:6, 1982
Crosby WH: Red cell mass: Its precursors and its perturbations. Hosp Pract 15, No 2:71—81, 1980
Dallman PR: Manifestations of iron deficiency. Semin Hematol 19:19, 1982
Erythropoietin and the regulation of erythropoiesis. N Engl J Med 308:520, 1983
Goldstein M: The aplastic anemias. Hosp Pract 15, No 5:85—96, 1980
Green R, Kuhl W, Jacobson R et al: Masking of macrocytes by α-thalassemia in blacks with pernicious anemia. N Engl J Med 307:1322, 1982
Halberg L: Iron nutrition and food iron fortification. Semin Hematol 19:31, 1982
Hamilton E: Intrauterine transfusion for Rh disease: A status report. Hosp Pract 13 (No 8):113—124, 1978
Huebers H, Finch CA: Clinical aspects of iron deficiency. Semin Hematol 19:3, 1982
Katz AJ: Transfusion therapy: Its role in the anemias. Hosp Pract 15, No 6:77—84, 1980
Kellermeyer RW: General principles of evaluation and therapy of anemias. Med Clin North Am 68:533, 1984
McFee JG: Iron metabolism and iron deficiency during pregnancy. Clin Obstet Gynecol 22 (No 4):788—808, 1979
Nimeh N, Bishop RC: Disorders of iron metabolism. Med Clin North Am 64 (No 4):631—644, 1980
Peschle C: Erythropoiesis. Annu Rev Med 31:303, 1980
Scott RB: Reflections on the current status of the national sickle cell disease program in the United States. J Natl Med Assoc 71(No 7):679—681, 1979
Shohet SB, Ness PM: Hemolytic anemias: Failure of the red cell membrane. Med Clin North Am 60 (No 5):913—932, 1976
Silver BJ, Zuckerman KS: Aplastic anemia: Recent advances in pathogenesis and treatment. Med Clin North Am 64 (No 4):607—629, 1980
Spaet TH: Anemia is a symptom. Hosp Pract 17, No 2:17, 1980
Steinberg MH, Hebbel RP: Clinical diversity of sickle cell anemia: Genetic and cellular modulation of disease severity. Am J Hematol 14:405, 1983
Trubowitz S: The management of sickle cell anemia. Med Clin North Am 60 (No 5):933—944, 1976

Chapter 14

The Circulatory System and Control of Blood Flow

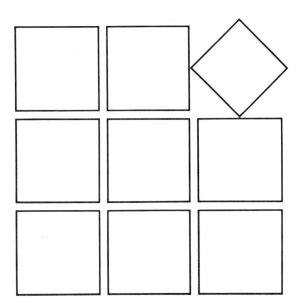

The circulatory system, which consists of the heart and blood vessels, has only one main function—transport. It delivers oxygen and nutrients needed for metabolic processes to the tissues, carries waste products from cellular metabolism to the kidneys and other excretory organs for elimination, and circulates electrolytes and hormones needed to regulate body function. Temperature regulation relies on the circulatory system for transport of core heat to the periphery, where it can be dissipated into the external environment. In addition, the circulatory system plays a vital role in the transport of various immune substances that contribute to the body's defense mechanisms. The purpose of this chapter is to discuss the functional components of the circulatory system and the control of blood flow. Control of blood pressure is discussed in Chapter 16 and control of cardiac function in Chapter 18.

Functional Organization of the Circulatory System

Systemic and Pulmonary Circulations

The circulatory system can be divided into two parts: the systemic and the pulmonary circulations. The systemic circulation supplies all of the body's tissues except the lungs, which are supplied by the pulmonary circulation.

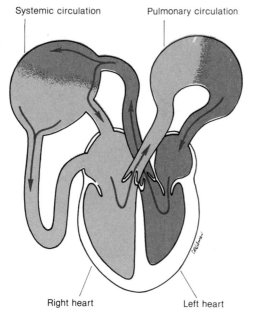

Figure 14-1 *Systemic and pulmonary circulations. The right side of the heart pumps blood to the lungs and the left side of the heart pumps blood to the systemic circulation.*

The systemic circulation is often referred to as the *peripheral circulation*. Because it must pump blood to distant parts of the body, often against gravity, the systemic circulation functions as a high-pressure system (mean arterial pressure approximately 90 mm Hg to 100 mm Hg). The pulmonary circulation along with the blood that is in the heart is often called the *central circulation*. The pulmonary circulation provides a gas exchange function; its location is the chest in close proximity to the heart, which propels blood through it. In contrast to the systemic circulation, the pulmonary circulation functions as a low-pressure system (mean arterial pressure is approximately 12 mm Hg).

Each division of the circulation has a pump, an arterial system, capillaries, and a venous system. The heart is the pump that propels blood through both divisions. It is divided into a right heart, which delivers blood to the pulmonary circulation, and a left heart, which delivers blood to the systemic circulation (Fig. 14-1). Each side of the heart is further divided into two chambers, an atrium and a ventricle. The ventricles are the main pumping chambers of the heart. The atria act as collection chambers for venous blood returning to the heart and as axillary pumps for the ventricles. In each system the arteries and arterioles serve as a distribution system, the capillaries as an exchange system, and the veins and venules as a collection system.

The circulation of blood through the heart and blood vessels will function effectively only as long as that flow is unidirectional and if the outputs of the right and left hearts are equal. Unidirectional flow through the heart is ensured by the heart valves. The distribution of pressure and volumes throughout the circulatory system requires that both sides of the heart pump equal amounts of blood. If the output of the left heart were to fall below that of the right heart, blood would accumulate in the pulmonary circulation. If the right side of the heart pumped less than the left, blood would accumulate in the systemic circulation.

Pressure and Volume Distribution

The systemic circulation contains about 83% of the total blood volume, the pulmonary circulation 8%, and the heart 8%. Of the blood in the heart and systemic circulation, 4% is in the left heart, 16% in the arteries and arterioles, 4% in the capillaries, 64% in the veins and venules, and 4% in the right heart (Fig. 14-2)[2]. The pulmonary blood volume (about 450 ml in the adult) can vary from as low as 50% of normal to as high as 200% of normal.[1] Increases in intrathoracic pressure (e.g., that involved in blowing a trumpet) can cause a shift from the pulmonary to the systemic circulation of as much as 250 ml of blood. Hemorrhage or loss of blood

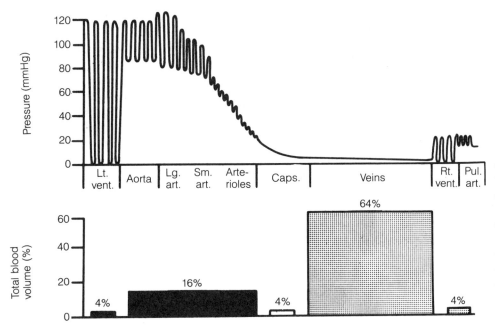

Figure 14-2 Pressure and volume distribution in the systemic circulation. The graphs illustrate the inverse relationship between internal pressure and volume in different portions of the circulatory system. (Smith JJ, Kampine JP: Circulatory Physiology: The Essentials, 2nd ed. Baltimore, Williams & Wilkins, 1984)

volume produces a shift in blood from the pulmonary to the systemic circulation. With mitral valve stenosis and left heart failure, blood flow between the veins and the arteries of the systemic circulation is impaired, causing an increase in pulmonary blood volume. Because the volume of the systemic circulation is about seven times that of the pulmonary circulation, a shift of blood from one system to the other has a much greater effect in the pulmonary than in the systemic circulation.

Blood moves from the arterial to the venous side of the circulation along a pressure gradient. The pressure distribution of the systemic circulation is opposite that of volume distribution (Fig. 14-2). The pressure in the arterial side of the circulation, which contains only about one-sixth of the blood, is greater than that in the venous side, which contains about two-thirds of the blood. Mean arterial pressure (in a young adult) is about 90 mm Hg and vena caval pressure is about 6 mm Hg. It is this difference in pressure (about 84 mm Hg) that provides the driving force for flow of blood in the systemic circulation. The pulmonary circulation has similar arterial-venous pressure differences, albeit of a lesser magnitude, that facilitate blood flow.

Pressure Pulses

The intermittent pumping action of the ventricles produces a pressure pulse that serves as a driving force for the circulation. In the systemic circulation, the pressure pulse has its origin in the rapid ejection of blood from the left ventricle into the aorta at the onset of systole. This rapid ejection of blood creates an impulse that is transmitted from molecule to molecule throughout the entire length of the vessel. These pressure pulses are what is felt when assessing a peripheral pulse, and they produce the Korotkoff sounds that are heard during blood pressure measurement. This impulse, or pressure wave, is transmitted through the aortic blood column at a velocity of 4 m to 6 m per second, which is about 20 times faster than the actual flow of blood. These pressure waves are similar to those created by splashing water in a basin or tub.

As the pressure wave moves out through the aorta into the arteries, it is reflected backward and thus collides with the next advancing pressure wave (Fig. 14-3). Just as the waves created by splashing water in a tub increase in amplitude as they hit the edge of the tub and reverse their direction of flow, the pressure pulse increases as it moves to the peripheral arteries; therefore, the pulse pressure in the femoral artery, for example, is usually greater than that in the aorta. With peripheral arterial disease, resistance to transmission of the pressure wave increases and a delay occurs in the transmission of the reflected wave, so that the pulse decreases in amplitude.

Following its initial amplification, the pressure pulse becomes smaller and smaller as it moves through the smaller arteries and arterioles, until it disappears entirely in the capillaries. This damping of the pressure pulse is caused by the resistance and distensibility characteristics of these vessels. The increased resistance of these small vessels impedes the flow that carries the pressure waves. Their distensibility is great enough, however, that any small change in flow does not cause a pressure change. Although the pressure pulses are not usually

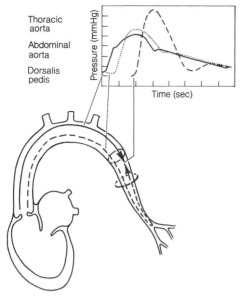

Figure 14-3 *Amplification of the arterial pressure wave as it moves forward in the peripheral arteries. This amplification occurs as a forward-moving pressure wave merges with a backward-moving reflected pressure wave.*

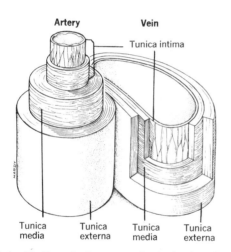

Figure 14-4 *Medium-sized artery and vein showing the relative thickness of the three layers. (Chaffee EE, Lytle IM: Basic Physiology and Anatomy, 4th ed. Philadelphia, JB Lippincott, 1980)*

transmitted to the capillaries, there are situations in which this does occur. For example, injury to a finger or other area of the body often results in a throbbing sensation. In this case, extreme dilatation of the capillaries in the injured area produce a reduction in the damping of the pressure pulse. Capillary pulsations also occur in conditions that cause exaggeration of aortic pressure pulses, such as aortic regurgitation or patent ductus arteriosus (Chap. 19).

In summary, the circulatory system is designed to deliver nutrients and remove waste products for body tissues. The heart pumps blood throughout the system. The blood vessels serve as tubes through which blood flows; the arterial system carries fluids from the heart to the tissues and the veins carry them back to the heart. The circulatory system can be divided into two parts: the systemic and the pulmonary circulations. The systemic circulation, which is served by the left heart, supplies all of the tissues except the lungs, which are served by the right heart and the pulmonary circulation. Blood moves throughout the circulation along a pressure gradient, moving from the high-pressure arterial system to the low-pressure venous system.

■ Blood Vessel Structure

All of the blood vessels, except the capillaries, have walls composed of three layers (Fig 14-4). The *tunica externa*, or *tunica adventitia*, is the outermost covering of the vessel. This layer is composed of fibrous and connective tissue that serves to support the vessel. The *tunica media*, or *middle layer*, is largely a smooth muscle that constricts and relaxes in order to control the diameter of the vessel. The *unica intima*, or *inner layer*, has an elastic layer that joins the media and a thin layer of epithelial cells that lie adjacent to the blood. The epithelial layer provides a smooth and slippery inner surface for the vessel. This smooth inner lining, as long as it remains intact, prevents blood clotting.

Arteries and Arterioles

The layers of the vessel vary with the vessel's function. Arteries are thick-walled vessels with large amounts of elastic fibers. The elasticity of these vessels allows them to stretch during cardiac systole and recoil during diastole. The arterioles, which are predominantly smooth muscle, serve as resistance vessels for the circulatory system. Sympathetic vasoconstrictor tone enables these vessels to constrict or to relax as needed to maintain blood pressure. The mean arterial pressure in the large arteries of the systemic circulation is normally about 90 mm Hg to 100 mm Hg; in the small arteries, 60 mm Hg to 90 mm Hg, and in the arterioles, 40 mm Hg to 60 mm Hg.

Veins and Venules

The veins and venules are thin-walled, distensible, and collapsible vessels. The structure of the veins allows these vessels to act as a reservoir, or blood storage system. The venous system is a low-pressure system that relies on changes in intra-abdominal pressure and the action of muscle pumps to assist in the movement of blood back to the heart. Their pressure ranges from about 10 mm Hg at the end of the venules to about 0 mm Hg at the entrance of the vena cavae into the heart. The peripheral veins have valves that prevent the retrograde, or backward, flow of blood and aid in the return of blood to the heart (Fig. 14-5).

Capillaries

The capillaries are microscopic single-thickness vessels that connect the arterial and venous segments of the circulatory system. In the systemic circulation, the intra-capillary pressure is about 25 mm Hg at the arterial end and about 10 mm Hg at the venous end. Exchange of gases, nutrients, and waste materials occurs through the thin permeable walls of the capillaries.

In summary, the walls of all blood vessels, except the capillaries, are composed of three layers: the tunica externa, tunica media, and tunica intima. The layers of the vessel vary with its function. Arteries are thick-walled vessels with large amounts of elastic fibers. The walls of the arterioles, which control blood pressure, have large amounts of smooth muscle. Veins are thin-walled, distensible, and collapsible vessels. Capillaries are single-thickness vessels designed for the exchange of gases, nutrients, and waste materials.

■ Principles of Blood Flow

Blood flow is brought about by a pressure difference between the various parts of the circulatory system (Fig. 14-6). This pressure difference provides the force that overcomes the resistance to blood flow. Blood pressure is measured in millimeters of mercury (mm Hg) and blood flow in milliliters (ml).

Pressure, Resistance, and Flow

Resistance refers to the forces that blood must overcome as it moves through a vessel. In the vascular system, resistance is affected by the *length of the vessel*, its *radius*, and the *viscosity of the blood*. It is related directly to the length of the vessel and inversely to its radius. The longer the vessel, the greater the overall resistance that the blood must overcome as it moves through the vessel. Because the length of most vessels does not change, we shall not be concerned with that relationship in this discussion. A more important consideration is the radius of the vessel. Resistance to flow is inversely related to the fourth power of the radius. The larger the radius of a vessel, the less the

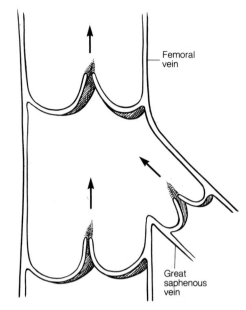

Figure 14-5 *Drawing of the venous valves located at the junction of the great saphenous and the common femoral veins. Arrows indicate direction of blood flow.*

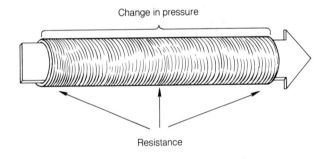

$$\text{Flow Q} = \frac{\text{Change in pressure} \times \pi \text{ radius}^4}{8 \times \text{length} \times \text{viscosity}}$$

Figure 14-6 *The factors that affect blood flow (Poiseuille's law). Increasing the pressure difference between the two ends of the vessel or enlarging the diameter of the vessel causes the flow to increase. Increasing the length or the viscosity of the fluid causes the flow to decrease. Flow diminishes as resistance increases. Resistance is directly proportional to blood viscosity and the length of the tube and inversely proportional to the fourth power of the radius.*

resistance and the greater the flow. For example, the rate of flow is 16 times greater in a vessel with a radius of 2 cm than in one with a radius of 1 cm. Thus, even small changes in a vessel's diameter can produce marked changes in blood flow. The reader is asked to consider the consequences of a 25%, 50%, and 75% narrowing of a coronary artery in terms of blood flow to the myocardium.

The term *viscosity* refers to the ease with which molecules of fluid slide over each other when the fluid is moving. Water flows more rapidly through a tube than syrup because the water molecules slide over each other more easily. As a general rule, the viscosity of a fluid is related to its thickness. The more particles of solute that are present in a liquid, the greater the interaction and frictional forces that develop between the molecules. Blood cells contribute to the viscosity of blood.

Resistance cannot be measured directly in the vascular system. Instead, it is calculated from measurements of blood flow and the pressure difference between the ends of the vessel.

$$\text{resistance} = \text{flow} \times \text{pressure difference between vessel ends}$$

Total peripheral resistance refers to the total resistance encountered by blood as it flows through the systemic circulation. It considers the entire systemic circulation as a single tube that begins at the aorta and ends in the right atrium. The pressure difference between these two points (about 100 mm Hg) is the mean arterial pressure (about 100 mm Hg) minus right atrial pressure (about 0 mm Hg). The cardiac output (about 100 ml/sec at rest) is the flow through the system. Thus, the total peripheral resistance is 100/100 or 1 peripheral resistance unit (PRU). The total resistance in the pulmonary circulation is only about 0.12 PRU. In this case, the blood flow is the same as in the systemic circulation, but the pressure difference between the pulmonary artery (mean pressure about 16 mm Hg) and the left atrium (about 4 mm Hg) is much less.

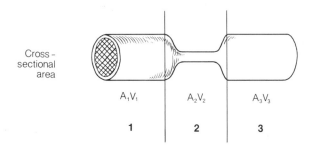

Figure 14-7 *Effect of cross-sectional area on velocity of flow. In section 1, velocity is low because of an increase in cross-sectional area. In section 2, velocity is increased because of a decrease in cross-sectional area. In section 3, velocity is low again.*

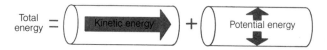

Figure 14-8 *Total energy in the vascular system is spent either in moving blood forward (kinetic energy) or in stretching the vessel wall (potential energy).*

Velocity and Cross-Sectional Area

In the circulatory system, *velocity* refers to the speed with which blood moves through a vessel. Flow is determined by the vessel's cross-sectional area and velocity of flow (Fig. 14-7). A decrease in its cross-sectional area, assuming that flow remains constant, will cause the velocity of flow to increase. Conversely, an increase in the cross-sectional area of the vessel will result in a decrease in the velocity of flow.

The total energy in a system can be divided into two types: potential and kinetic. *Potential energy* is energy that can be stored and that has the potential for later use. *Kinetic energy* involves motion. Both types of energy contribute to the flow and pressure of blood in the vascular system (Fig. 14-8). Potential energy is associated with the stretching of blood vessel walls and the exertion pressure against the side of the vessel. It is converted to active energy when the vessel wall rebounds after being stretched. Kinetic energy involves the velocity or forward movement of blood. The total energy of a system, including the vascular system, can be described in terms of the sum of the kinetic and potential energies (total energy equals kinetic energy plus potential energy). If the total energy in a fluid system remains constant, changes in velocity must be accompanied by changes in pressure. In Figure 14-7, it can be seen that the velocity of flow associated with the kinetic portion of the total energy will be decreased in sections 1 and 3 of the tube. The lateral pressure associated with the storing of potential energy (tension on the vessel wall) will be high in these two segments. In section 2, the kinetic energy (velocity) is great, whereas the lateral pressure is low. Similar changes can occur in circulatory disorders that cause changes in vessel or heart valve diameter.

Laminar and Turbulent Flow

Laminar or *streamlined flow* is smooth flow in which the blood components are layered so that the plasma is adjacent to the smooth, slippery surface of the blood vessel and the cellular components, including the platelets, are in the center of the bloodstream (Fig. 14-9). This arrangement reduces friction by allowing the blood layers to slide smoothly over each other.

Structural changes in the vessel wall often disrupt flow and produce turbulence (Fig. 14-9). Turbulence means that blood flows crosswise as well as lengthwise along a vessel in a manner similar to the eddy currents seen in a rapidly flowing river at a point of obstruction. The tendency for turbulence to occur increases in direct proportion to the velocity of flow. Atherosclerotic narrowing of a vessel increases the velocity of flow leading to turbulent flow, which can often be heard through a stethoscope. An audible murmur in a blood vessel is referred to as a bruit. Turbulent flow also predisposes to clot formation as platelets and other coagulation factors come in contact with the endothelial lining of the vessel.

Wall Tension, Intraluminal Pressure, and Radius

The relationship between wall tension, pressure, and the radius of a vessel or sphere was described more than 200 years ago by the French astronomer and mathematician *Pierre de Laplace.*[3] This relationship, which is expressed by the formula Pressure (P) = Tension (T)/radius (R), has come to be known as Laplace's law (Fig. 14-10). Among other things, it explains why soap bubbles and balloons burst. Laplace's law states that the tension in the wall of a sphere is equal to the product of its radius and its intraluminal pressure. In general, Laplace's law applies only to a sphere with an infinitely thin wall.[3] Wall tension is also inversely related to wall thickness—the thicker the wall, the less the tension and the thinner the wall, the greater the tension. As shall be seen in Chapter 15, the principles related to wall thickness, wall tension, radius, and intraluminal pressure contribute to the progress and often to the eventual rupture of aneurysms.

The law of Laplace can also be applied to the pressure required to maintain the patency of small blood vessels. Providing that the thickness of a vessel wall and its tension remain constant, it takes more pressure to keep a vessel open as its diameter decreases in size. This is analogous to blowing up a balloon. When the balloon is small it takes more effort to inflate the balloon than it does when the balloon is larger. The critical closing pressure refers to the pressure at which blood vessels close to the point where blood can no longer flow through them. In circulatory shock, for example, many of the small vessels collapse as blood pressure drops to the point where it can no longer overcome the tension in the vessels' walls.

In summary, blood flow is controlled by many of the same mechanisms that control fluid flow in other systems. It is influenced by vessel length, vessel radius, the viscosity of the blood, the pressure difference between the two ends, cross-sectional area, and wall tension. The rate of flow is directly related to pressure difference between the two ends of the vessel and inversely related to vessel length, vessel radius, and blood viscosity. The cross-sectional area of a vessel influences the velocity of flow; as the cross-sectional area decreases, the velocity is increased, and vice versa. The relationship between wall tension, pressure, and radius is described by the law of Laplace, which states that wall tension becomes greater as the radius increases.

■ Control of Blood Flow

Microcirculation

The entire circulatory system is designed to supply body tissues with sufficient blood flow to meet their metabolic needs. The capillaries, where exchange of nutrients and metabolites occur, are single-layer vessels located

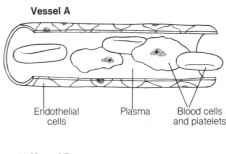

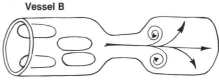

Figure 14-9 *Laminar flow in blood vessels. Vessel A illustrates laminar flow in which the plasma layer is adjacent to the vessel endothelial layer and blood cells are in the center of the bloodstream. Vessel B depicts the presence of turbulent flow. The axial location of the platelets and other blood cells is disturbed.*

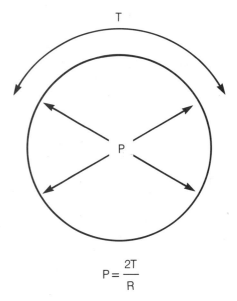

Figure 14-10 *Law of Laplace (for a sphere P = 2T R, and for a tube P = T R), where P = the pressure needed to distend an elastic sphere or tube; T = the tension in the wall of the sphere or tube; and R = the radius of the sphere or tube.*

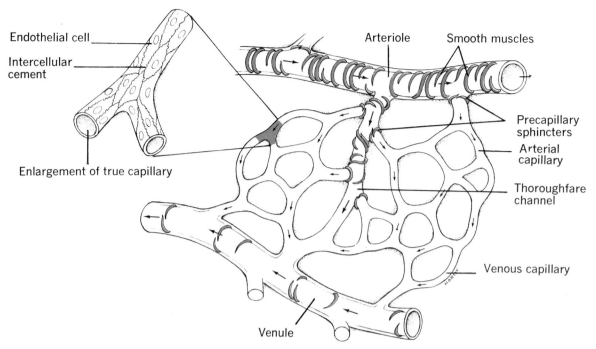

Figure 14-11 *A capillary bed. Precapillary sphincters are relaxed, thus permitting the flow of blood through the capillary network. A greatly magnified portion of capillary wall is shown in the inset* (upper left). *(Chaffee EE, Lytle IM: Basic Physiology and Anatomy, 4th ed. Philadelphia, JB Lippincott, 1980)*

between an arteriole and a venule (Fig. 14-11). Metarterioles serve as thoroughfare vessels that link the arterioles and venules. The capillaries, venules, and metarterioles are collectively referred to as the *microcirculation*. Blood flow through capillary channels designed for exchange of gases and nutrients is called *nutritional flow*. Precapillary sphincters control blood flow through the nutritional channels of the microcirculation, and when all of the precapillary sphincters are closed, blood flows directly from an arteriole into a venule. Blood flow that bypasses the nutrient channels of the capillary bed is called *nonnutrient flow*. In some capillary beds, such as those that supply the skin, another type of bypass channel called an arteriovenous (AV)shunt, which directly connects an arteriole with a venule, carries nonnutrient blood flow. The AV shunts in the capillaries of the skin are important in temperature regulation.

The control of blood flow through the microcirculation performs two functions: (1) it provides for the tissue exchange of gases, nutrients, and metabolites and (2) it controls the total peripheral resistance of the circulatory system. The total cardiac output travels through the microcirculation; therefore, the size of the vessels, particularly the arterioles, determines the total peripheral resistance and, as will be discussed later, the arterial blood pressure. If, for example, all of the arterioles were to open fully, the total peripheral

resistance, and thus the blood pressure, would fall catastrophically. These two somewhat conflicting functions require a degree of independent control over arteriole resistance and flow in the capillaries of the microcirculation. The nervous system controls the peripheral resistance by regulating the smooth muscle tone of the arterioles, and local factors control the precapillary sphincters, which regulate flow through the nutrient channels of the capillary bed.

Local control of blood flow

Local control is governed largely by the nutritional needs of the tissue. For example, blood flow to organs such as the heart, brain, and kidney remains relatively constant although blood pressure may vary over a range of 60 mm Hg to 180 mm Hg (Fig. 14-12). The ability of the tissues to regulate their own blood flow is called *autoregulation*. Autoregulation of blood flow is controlled by local tissue factors, such as oxygen lack or accumulation of tissue metabolites. It involves the selective opening and closing of capillary channels. Local control is particularly important in tissues such as skeletal muscle, which has varying blood flow requirements according to the level of activity.

Autocoids. *Autocoids* are vasoactive substances that are formed in the tissues from cell constituents and aid in autoregulation of blood flow.[4] The most important of these are histamine, serotonin (5-hydroxytryptamine), the kinins, and the prostaglandins. *Histamine* increases blood flow. Most blood vessels contain histamine in mast cells and nonmast cell stores; when these tissues are injured, histamine is released. In certain tissues, such as skeletal muscle, the activity of the mast cells is mediated by the sympathetic nervous system; that is when sympathetic control is withdrawn, the mast cells release histamine. This mechanism augments with withdrawal of vasoconstrictor activity. *Serotonin* is liberated from aggregating platelets during the clotting process; it causes vasoconstriction and plays a major role in control of bleeding. Serotonin is found in brain and lung tissues, and there is some speculation that it may be involved in the vascular spasm associated with some allergic pulmonary reactions and migraine headaches. The *kinins* (*kallidins* and *bradykinin*) are liberated from the globulin kininogen, which is present in body fluids. The kinins cause relaxation of arteriole smooth muscle, increase capillary permeability, and constrict the venules. In exocrine glands, the formation of kinins contributes to the vasodilatation that is needed for glandular secretion. Prostaglandins are synthesized from constituents (the long-chain fatty acid, arachidonic acid) of the cell membrane. Tissue injury incites the release of arachidonic acid from the cell membrane, which initiates prostaglandin synthesis. There are several prostaglandins (E_2, F_2, and D_2) that are subgrouped according to their solubility; some produce vasoconsriction and some produce vasodilatation. As a general rule of thumb, those in the E group are vasodilators and those in the F group are vasoconstrictors.[4] The adrenal glucocorticoid hormones can produce an anti-inflammatory response by blocking the release of arachidonic acid, and thus preventing prostaglandin synthesis.

Hyperemia. An increase in local blood flow is called *hyperemia*. When the blood supply to an area has been occluded and then restored, local blood flow through the tissues increases within seconds to restore the metabolic equilibrium of the tissues. This increased flow is called *reactive hyperemia*. The transient redness seen after leaning an arm on a hard surface is an example of reactive hyperemia. The ability of tissues to increase blood flow in situations of increased activity, such as exercising, is called *functional hyperemia*. Local control mechanisms rely on a continuous flow from the main arteries and, therefore, the blood flow through capillary channels cannot increase when these arteries are narrowed. For example, if a major coronary artery becomes occluded, the opening of capillary channels supplied by that vessel cannot restore blood flow.

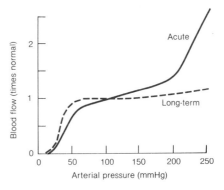

Figure 14-12 *Effect on blood flow through a muscle of increasing arterial pressure. The solid curve shows the effect if pressure is raised over a period of a few minutes. The dashed curve shows the effect if the arterial pressure is raised slowly over a period of many weeks. (Guyton A: Medical Physiology, 6th ed. Philadelphia, WB Saunders, 1981)*

Neural Control of Blood Flow

The neural control centers for regulation of cardiovascular function are located in the reticular formation of the lower pons and medulla of the brain. The area of the reticular formation in the brain that controls vasomotor function is called the *vasomotor center*. The sympathetic nervous system serves as the final common pathway for controlling the smooth muscle tone of the blood vessels. Most of the sympathetic preganglionic fibers that control vessel function travel in the intermediolateral column of the spinal cord and exit with the ventral nerves; they then synapse with postganglionic fibers in the paravertebral ganglia. The sympathetic neurons that supply the blood vessels maintain them in a state of tonic activity, so that even under resting conditions the blood vessels are partially constricted. Vessel constriction and relaxation is accomplished by altering this basal input. Both vasodilator and vasoconstrictor fibers control the smooth muscle tone in blood vessels. Increasing sympathetic activity causes constriction of some vessels, such as those of the skin, the gastrointestinal tract, and the kidney. Skeletal muscle is innervated by both vasoconstrictor and vasodilator fibers. The response of the sympathetic *vasoconstrictor* fibers is mediated by *norepinephrine* and *epinephrine*, and the *vasodilator fibers* are mediated by *acetylcholine*. These vasodilator fibers are referred to as *cholinergic fibers*. Although the parasympathetic nervous system contributes to the regulation of heart function, it has little, if any, control over the blood vessels.

Collateral Circulation

Collateral circulation is a mechanism for the long-term regulation of local blood flow. In the heart and other vital structures, anastomotic channels exist between some of the smaller arteries. These channels permit perfusion of an area by more than one artery. When one artery becomes occluded, these anastomotic channels increase in size, allowing blood from a patent artery to perfuse the area supplied by the occluded vessel. For example, persons with extensive obstruction of a coronary blood vessel may rely on collateral circulation to meet the oxygen needs of the myocardial tissue normally supplied by that vessel. As with other long-term compensatory mechanisms, the recruitment of collateral circulation is most efficient when obstruction to flow is gradual rather than sudden.

In summary, mechanisms that control blood flow are designed to ensure the delivery of blood to the tissues. Local control is governed largely by the needs of the tissues and is regulated by local tissue factors such as lack of oxygen or the accumulation of metabolites. Hyperemia is a local increase in blood flow that occurs following a temporary occlusion of blood flow. It is a compensatory mechanism that serves to decrease the oxygen debt of the deprived tissues. The vasomotor center of the reticular formation of the lower pons and medulla provides for neural control of blood flow via the sympathetic nervous system. Collateral circulation is a mechanism for long-term regulation of local blood flow involving the development of collateral vessels.

- ☐ Compare laminar and streamlined flow in terms of the development of turbulent flow in the vascular system.
- ☐ Define the term microcirculation.
- ☐ State the difference between nutrient and non-nutrient blood flow.
- ☐ Describe the regulation of blood flow in terms of local, neural, and humoral components.
- ☐ Define the term hyperemia.

■ References

1. Guyton A: Textbook of Medical Physiology, 6th ed, p 291. Philadelphia, WB Saunders, 1981
2. Smith JJ, Kampine JP: Circulatory Physiology, 2nd ed, p 10. Baltimore, Williams & Wilkins, 1984
3. Johansen K: Aneurysms. Sci Am 247, No. 1:110, 1982
4. Shepard JT, VanHoutte PM: The Human Cardiovascular System, p 101, 103. New York, Raven Press, 1979

■ Study Guide

After you have studied this chapter, you should be able to meet the following objectives:

- ☐ Describe the organization of the circulatory system.
- ☐ Compare the distribution of blood flow and blood pressure in the systemic and pulmonary circulations.
- ☐ Describe the origin of the pressure pulse.
- ☐ Compare the structure of arteries, arterioles, veins, and capillaries.
- ☐ Define the term *resistance* as it relates to blood flow.
- ☐ Explain how vessel radius, vessel length, blood viscosity, and blood pressure affect blood flow.
- ☐ Relate the cross-sectional area to pressure and the velocity of flow in a blood vessel.
- ☐ Relate kinetic energy and potential energy to lateral wall pressure and the velocity of blood flow in a vessel.
- ☐ Use the law of Laplace to explain the effect of radius size on the pressure and wall tension in a vessel.

Chapter 15

Alterations in Blood Flow

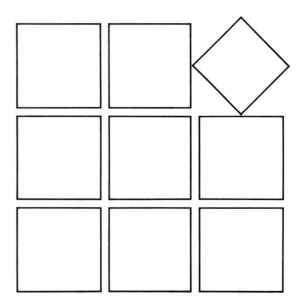

Interruption of blood flow in either the arterial or the venous system interferes with the delivery of oxygen and nutrients to the tissues. Alterations in arterial flow produce ischemia, or the temporary holding back of blood from the tissues. Venous obstruction, on the other hand, causes congestion and edema. This chapter is organized into four sections: (1) the mechanisms of vessel obstruction, (2) the disorders of the arterial circulation, (3) alterations of the venous circulation, and (4) pressure sores caused by the localized interruption of blood flow.

■ Mechanisms of Vessel Obstruction

Occlusion of flow within a vessel can result from (1) thrombus formation, (2) emboli, (3) compression, (4) vasospasm, or (5) structural defects in the vessel (Fig. 15-1). Each of these mechanisms is discussed briefly in preparation for the discussion on specific alterations in arterial and venous flow.

Thrombus Formation

A thrombus is a blood clot. Blood clotting is a homeostatic mechanism intended to seal off blood vessels, to prevent bleeding, and to maintain the continuity of the

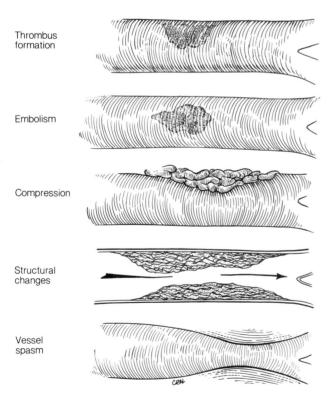

Thrombus formation

Embolism

Compression

Structural changes

Vessel spasm

Figure 15-1 Conditions that cause disruption of blood flow.

vascular system. A thrombus can develop in either the arterial or the venous system and obstruct flow. Alterations in hemostasis are discussed in Chapter 12.

Embolus

An embolus is a foreign mass that is transported in the bloodstream. Although an embolus moves freely in the larger blood vessels, it becomes lodged and obstructs flow once it reaches a smaller vessel. An embolus can be a dislodged thrombus or can consist of air, fat, tumor cells, or other materials. Approximately 95% of venous emboli have their origin in the veins of the legs. These emboli move through the venous system, into the right heart, and then into the pulmonary circulation where they can become lodged and obstruct blood flow. Arterial emboli commonly have their origin in the heart itself and can travel to the brain, spleen, kidney, or vessels and the lower extremity before they become lodged and obstruct flow.

Compression

The lumen of a blood vessel can be occluded by external forces. The external pressure of a tourniquet, for example, is intended to compress blood vessels and interrupt blood flow. Likewise, casts and circular dressings predispose to vessel compression, particularly when swelling occurs after these devices have been applied. Tumors may encroach on blood vessels as they grow. Blood vessels may be compressed between bony structures such as the sacrum and the supporting surfaces of a chair or bed.

Vasospasm

Vasospasm may result from locally or neurally mediated reflexes. Exposure to cold causes severe vasoconstriction in many of the superficial blood vessels. Fortunately, local control mechanisms produce brief periods of vasodilatation designed to maintain tissue oxygen needs. Those who have spent time on the ski slopes, or elsewhere in the cold, may have noticed the intermittent redness of their companions' noses during these periods of vasodilatation. In certain disease states, vasospasm from exposure to cold or other stimuli is excessive and may lead to ischemia and tissue injury.

Structural Defects

Structural changes in blood vessels can take many forms. Defects in venous valves may impair blood flow in the venous system, causing varicose veins. Arteriosclerosis causes rigidity and narrowing of the arterioles. Aneurysms are dilatations in arteries that appear at points where the vessel wall has been weakened.

In summary, interruption of flow in either the arterial or the venous system interferes with the flow of oxygen and nutrients to the tissues. Occlusion of flow can result from (1) the presence of a thrombus, (2) emboli, (3) vessel compression, (4) vasospasm, or (5) structural changes within the vessel.

■ Alterations in Arterial Flow

Pathology of the arterial system affects body function through impaired blood flow. The discussion in this section focuses on arteriosclerosis, aneurysms, acute arterial occlusion, peripheral vascular diseases—Raynaud's syndrome and Buerger's disease—and assessment of arterial flow.

Vascular disease is a relatively silent disorder. To be more explicit, the diseased vessel itself seldom gives rise to symptoms that warn of its presence. Rather, signs and symptoms arise because of ischemia in the body part that is served by the vessel. The pain associated with coronary heart disease (angina pectoris) and the intermittent claudication (pain and weakness in the leg occurring with exercise and relieved by rest) provide evidence of impaired blood flow. Unfortunately, arterial disease is usually far advanced by the time these symptoms occur.

Arteriosclerosis: Atherosclerosis

Arteriosclerosis is a general term that literally means *hardening of the arteries*. The term describes several conditions. One form of arteriosclerosis, Mönckeberg's medial sclerosis, affects the media of medium-sized arteries and is characterized by a hyaline thickening of the arterioles and small blood vessels. This form of arteriosclerosis increases vessel rigidity but does not encroach on the lumen of the vessel and obstruct blood flow. This chapter addresses the most common form of arteriosclerosis—atherosclerosis, which does encroach on the vessel lumen.

Atherosclerosis affects the large and medium-sized arteries—the aorta and its branches, the coronaries, and the large vessels that supply the brain (Fig. 15-2). In 1981, complications of atherosclerosis (heart attack, aneurysms, stroke, and peripheral vascular disease) caused 873,000 deaths—almost half of all deaths in the United States.[1] In that same year, atherosclerosis cost an estimated $39 billion in health care expenditures and lost productivity. The bright side of this grim picture is the recent decline in death rates from coronary heart disease. In 1978 alone, there were 114,000 fewer deaths among people ages 35 to 74 years than would have been expected had the rate not declined from its high level in the 1960s.[1] This decline probably reflects new and improved methods of medical treatment as well as improved health care practices resulting from an increased public awareness of the factors that predispose to development of the disorder.

Atherosclerosis begins as an insidious process, and clinical manifestations of the disease often do not become evident for 20 to 40 years or longer. Fibrous plaques often begin to appear in the arteries of Americans in their twenties. Among 300 American soldiers (average age 22 years) killed during the Korean war, 77% were found to have gross evidence of atherosclerosis.[2]

Atherosclerosic lesions are characterized by (1) the accumulation of intracellular and extracellular lipids, (2) proliferation of smooth muscle cells, and (3) formation of large amounts of scar tissue and connective tissue proteins.[3] The lesions begin as a gray to pearly white elevated thickening of the vessel intima with a core of extracellular lipid (mainly cholesterol, which is usually complexed to proteins) covered by a fibrous cap of connective tissue and smooth muscle. Later lesions contain hemorrhage, ulceration, and scar tissue deposits. As the lesions increase in size, they encroach on the lumen of the artery and eventually may either occlude the vessel or predispose to thrombus formation, causing reduction of blood flow (Fig. 15-3). Because blood flow is related to the fourth power of the radius (Chap. 14), reduction in blood flow becomes more severe as the disease progresses.

Mechanisms of development

The cause of atherosclerosis is largely unknown. In the past decade three important hypothesized causes have been investigated: vessel injury, the manner in which vascular cells respond to lipoproteins and metabolize cholesterol (lipid infiltration hypothesis), and the manner in which vascular cells multiply (monoclonal hypothesis).

Vessel wall injury. The normal intact endothelial layer of blood vessels acts as a selective barrier that protects the subendothelial layers from interacting with platelets and other blood components. A current hypothesis of atheroma formation is that injury to the arterial endothelium is the initiating factor that permits platelets, cholesterol, and other blood components to come in contact with and stimulate abnormal proliferation of muscle cells and connective tissue in the vessel wall (Fig. 15-4). Platelets contain a potent smooth-muscle mitogenic factor (a substance that induces cell mitosis and cell transformation). According to current theory, this factor is released from platelets when they aggregate over a denuded area of the vessel wall. Recent evidence suggests that the low-density lipoproteins (LDL) act as the cofactors necessary for growth and proliferation of the smooth muscle cells but

Affected site

Cerebral vessels

Carotid arteries

Aorta

Coronary arteries

Renal arteries

Iliac arteries

Femoral arteries

Tibial arteries

Complication

Stroke
Transient ischemic attacks
Chronic ischemic brain disease

Stroke
Ischemic attacks

Aneurysm

Heart attack
Angina

Hypertension

Peripheral vascular disease

Peripheral vascular disease

Peripheral vascular disease

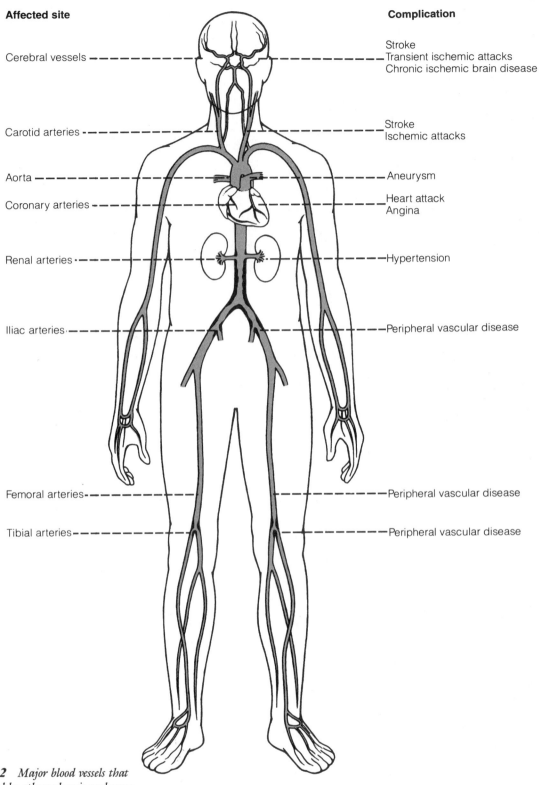

Figure 15-2 *Major blood vessels that are affected by atherosclerosis and some complications of the process. (Report of the 1977 Working Group to Review the Report by the National Heart and Lung Institute Task Force on Arteriosclerosis: Arteriosclerosis. DHEW Publication No NIH 78-1526)*

are not able to stimulate the process by themselves.[4] A number of factors are regarded as possible injurious agents of the vessel endothelium, including products associated with smoking, immune mechanisms, and mechanical stress associated with hypertension.

Cholesterol and the lipoproteins. The association between high serum levels of cholesterol and the development of atherosclerosis has been appreciated for a number of years.

Cholesterol is an important constituent of cell membranes and is also used by some cells in the synthesis of steroid hormones. Although most cells can synthesize their own cholesterol, they prefer to remove it from the plasma. Because lipids are insoluble in plasma, they are encapsulated by certain fat-carrying proteins—the lipoproteins—for transportation in the blood. There are five classes of lipoproteins: (1) chylomicrons, (2) very low density lipoproteins (VLDL), (3) intermediate-den-

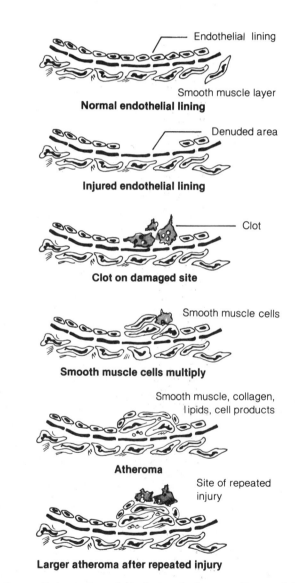

Normal endothelial lining

Injured endothelial lining

Clot on damaged site

Smooth muscle cells multiply

Atheroma

Larger atheroma after repeated injury

Figure 15-3 *Evolution of occlusion in an atherosclerotic vessel. (Report of the 1981 Working Group to Review the Report by the National Heart and Lung Institute Task Force on Arteriosclerosis: Arteriosclerosis. DHEW Publication No NIH 1526)*

Figure 15-4 *A theory for evolution of atheroma. (Report of the 1977 Working Group to Review the Report by the National Heart and Lung Institute Task Force on Arteriosclerosis: Arteriosclerosis. DHEW Publication No NIH 78-1526)*

sity lipoproteins (IDL), (4) low-density lipoproteins, and (5) high-density lipoproteins (HDL). The naming of these proteins is based on ultracentrifugation, by which the proteins are separated according to their density and rate of flotation. The greater the ratio of lipids to protein, the lower the density. Accordingly, the LDL carry large amounts of lipid compared with the HDL. The LDL and HDL are the major carriers of cholesterol. About two-thirds of plasma cholesterol is carried by the LDL, therefore, its measurement provides a good estimate of blood cholesterol in most people. The chylomicrons and VLDR are the major triglyceride-carriers.

The lipoproteins are synthesized in two types of cells, the mucosal cells of the small intestine and the parenchymal cells of the liver. The chylomicrons are synthesized by the intestinal cells and are involved in the transport of fats absorbed from the gastrointestinal tract. The liver synthesizes and secretes VLDL and HDL. LDL are derived mainly from the catabolism of VLDL, and the IDL are thought to be an intermediate in this pathway.

The entry of LDL-bound cholesterol into vascular smooth muscle cells occurs through receptor-mediated and nonreceptor mechanisms. Arterial vascular smooth muscle cells have been shown to possess highly specific LDL surface receptors. The uptake of LDL-bound cholesterol is preceded by receptor binding, followed by the formation of a pinocytotic vesicle that carries the LDL into the cell. Once inside the cell, the protein from the pinocytotic vesicle is digested by enzymes in the lysosomes and the free cholesterol is liberated (Fig. 15-5). When the needs of the cell have been met, excess cholesterol is stored in the cytoplasm as a cholesterol ester. These cholesterol esters, when present in excess amounts, form the typical fat-filled cell seen in atherosclerotic lesions. Normally the intracellular concentration of cholesterol is regulated by three important negative feedback mechanisms: (1) saturation of the limited number of receptors on the cell surface, (2) inhibition of new receptor formation due to the presence of the free cholesterol liberated from LDL, and (3) inhibition of intracellular synthesis of cholesterol by increased intracellular levels of free cholesterol.

There is also a nonreceptor pathway for cholesterol entry into cells. This system is not regulated by negative feedback control; rather, the cellular uptake of cholesterol by this pathway is strictly related to the concentra-

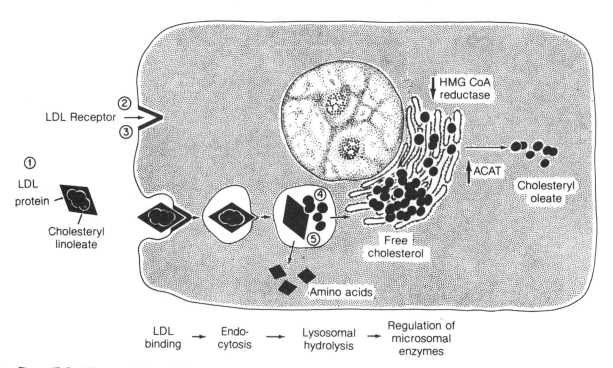

Figure 15-5 *The metabolism of cholesterol. This figure illustrates the entry of low-density lipoproteins into the cell after interaction with cell receptors. The cholesterol esters are then broken down, and the cholesterol that is released inhibits the synthesis of new cholesterol and increases the rate of esterification of cholesterol. States of hypercholesterolemia can occur when the receptors for lipoproteins are reduced. (Brown MS, Goldstein JL: N Engl J Med 294:1387, 1976. Reprinted by permission of the New England Journal of Medicine)*

tion of LDL in the plasma. With excess entry of LDL, the ability of the lysosomes to degrade the cholesterol esters can be exceeded, causing accumulation within the cell.

Cholesterol is not metabolized in peripheral tissues such as vascular smooth muscle, and amounts that are not used in synthesis of cell membranes would accumulate if no mechanism were available for its removal. It is now believed that the HDL serve as carriers that remove cholesterol from the peripheral tissues and transport it back to the liver for catabolism and excretion.[5] The HDL are also believed to inhibit cellular uptake of LDL. These two mechanisms could help to explain the protective effect that the HDL have been observed to provide in relation to the risk of coronary heart disease.

The mechanisms by which hypercholesterolemia contributes to the development of atherosclerosis is still unknown. A number of factors are likely involved. For example, the normal LDL receptor is deficient or defective in the genetic disorder known as familial hypercholesterolemia. This results in decreased catabolism of LDL and increased circulating cholesterol levels.[6] Myocardial infarction may develop before age 20 in individuals with this disorder. A number of other genetic defects that affect the LDL receptor pathway have been identified. In one variant, there is a lack of receptors; in another, receptors are defective. Genetic defects in the handling of cholesterol within the cell may also cause its accumulation.

Monoclonal hypothesis. The monoclonal hypothesis suggests that atherosclerotic lesions begin as a mutation in the proliferation of a single cell line, similar to the development of a benign neoplasm.[7] Such a transformation could result from a number of agents such as hydrocarbons produced by cigarette smoking or potentially mitogenic metabolites of fat-rich diets.

Risk factors

Although the exact cause and mechanisms of atherosclerosis are unclear, epidemiologic studies have identified predisposing risk factors, which are listed in Table 15-1. Some of these risk factors can be changed and others cannot.

Major risk factors that cannot be changed. Risk factors such as heredity, sex, race, and age cannot be changed. It appears that the tendency to develop atherosclerosis runs in families. A number of genetically determined alterations in lipoprotein and cholesterol metabolism have been identified, and it seems likely that others will be identified in the future. Black Americans have a greater incidence of hypertension (a contributing factor in the development of atherosclerosis) than whites. The incidence of atherosclerosis increases with age. Men are at greater risk of developing coronary heart disease than women; even though the death rate of women increases after menopause, it never reaches that of men.

Major risk factors that can be changed. The major risk factors that can be changed include cigarette smoking, high blood pressure, blood cholesterol levels, and diabetes. Risk factors such as high blood pressure, diabetes, and high blood cholesterol levels can often be controlled with the aid of a physician. The responsibility for changing other risk factors such as smoking rests entirely with the individual.

High cholesterol and LDL levels. The mechanism linking hypercholesterolemia to atherosclerosis has been described. Recent epidemiologic evidence suggest that the potentially serious effects of these substances depend not so much on the level of serum lipoproteins as on the type of lipoproteins that are present. High levels of LDL are linked with the development of atherosclerosis, whereas, high levels of HDL appear to provide some protection against the disorder. It has been observed that HDL levels are increased in individuals who engage in regular exercise and in persons who consume a moderate amount of alcohol. Smoking and diabetes, themselves risk factors for atherosclerosis, are associated with high levels of LDL and low levels of HDL.

Diabetes. Atherosclerosis is a common complication of diabetes mellitus. In persons with type II diabetes mellitus, the atherosclerotic changes may be well advanced at the time the diabetes is diagnosed. The cause

Table 15-1 Risk Factors of Atherosclerosis

Major Risk Factors That Cannot Be Changed	Major Risk Factors That Can Be Changed	Contributing Factors
Heredity	Cigarette smoking	Obesity
Sex	High blood pressure	Lack of Exercise
Race	Blood cholesterol levels	Stress
Age	Diabetes	

(From Heart Facts 1984. Dallas, American Heart Association, 1984)

of accelerated atherosclerosis development in diabetes is unclear. It is probably related to alterations in fat and carbohydrate metabolism.

Blood pressure.   Blood pressure levels are closely correlated with coronary heart disease. The risk of coronary artery disease in men 30 to 59 years of age with a diastolic pressure above 105 mm Hg is reported to be almost four times greater than it is when the diastolic pressure is less than 85 mm Hg.[8] Hypertension increases the risk of atherosclerosis more markedly when associated with other risk factors, such as diabetes mellitus and cigarette smoking.

Cigarette smoking.   Cigarette smoking is closely linked with coronary heart disease and sudden death. The risk of death from coronary heart disease is about 60 to 70 times greater for smokers than for nonsmokers.[9] The greatest effects of smoking are noted in younger men and women, particularly those below the age of 55. The effects are directly related to the number of cigarettes smoked.

Contributing factors.   The association between coronary heart disease and contributing risk factors is not as convincing as it is for the established risk factors. These factors often are linked with the established or other risk factors. For example, obesity and physical inactivity are often observed in the same individual. Furthermore, both of these situations are reported to bring about alterations in lipid levels. Likewise, smoking patterns, blood pressure levels, and other risk factors are closely associated with stress and personality patterns.

Prevention

At the present time there is no known cure for atherosclerosis; efforts are directed at ways of preventing it and halting its progression. As was mentioned earlier, the presence of atherosclerotic changes in young soldiers killed in the Korean War suggests that the process starts at an early age. It therefore seems apparent that prevention, in terms of sound nutrition and diagnosis and treatment of hypertension, cannot be delayed until the middle years when symptoms of atherosclerosis begin to manifest themselves. As the late cardiologist Dr. Paul Dudley White so aptly stressed, prevention of atherosclerosis needs to begin at the time of conception based on wise and prudent health practices of the expectant mother and then continued after birth by the wise and careful parenting efforts of both father and mother.*

* From a speech given by Dr. Paul Dudley White, which the author was privileged to attend.

Arterial Aneurysms

An aneurysm is an abnormal localized vessel dilatation caused by weakness of the arterial wall. Aneurysms can assume several forms and may be classified according to their etiology, location, and anatomic features (Fig. 15-6). A *berry aneurysm* consists of a small, spherical dilatation of the vessel, rarely exceeding 1 cm to 1.5 cm in diameter.[10] They are usually found in the circle of Willis in the cerebral circulation. A *fusiform aneurysm* involves the entire circumference of the vessels and is characterized by a gradual and progressive dilatation of the vessel. These aneurysms, which vary in diameter (up to 20 cm) and length, may involve the entire ascending and transverse portions of the thoracic aorta or may extend over large segments of the abdominal aorta. A *saccular aneurysm* extends over part of the circumference of the vessel and appears saclike. They can vary in size up to 15 cm to 20 cm but are frequently about 5 cm to 10 cm in diameter.[10] In a *dissecting aneurysm,* vessel dilatation occurs because of the accumulated blood within the layers of the vessel wall. This occurs when blood enters the wall of the artery, dissecting its layers to create a blood-filled cavity.

The weakness that leads to aneurysm formation may be due to several factors, including congenital defects, trauma, infections, and arteriosclerosis. Once initiated, the size of the aneurysm tends to progress because the tension on the vessel wall increases in accordance with Laplace's law (Chap. 14). Untreated, the aneurysm may burst because of internal pressure. Even an unruptured aneurysm can cause damage by exerting pressure on adjacent structures and interrupting blood flow.

Aortic aneurysms

Aortic aneurysms may involve any part of the aorta: the ascending aorta, aortic arch, descending aorta, or thoracic-abdominal aorta. Multiple aneurysms may be present. Aortic aneurysms were, until recently, caused largely by tertiary syphilis. Now, with better control of syphilis, atherosclerosis has become the leading cause of aneurysmal development. Atherosclerotic aneurysms are most common in men over 50 years of age.

Aortic aneurysms may or may not cause symptoms. The first evidence of an aneurysm may be associated with vessel rupture. With aneurysms of the thoracic aorta, substernal, back, and neck pain may occur. There may also be dyspnea, stridor, or a brassy cough due to pressure on the trachea. Hoarseness may result from pressure on the recurrent laryngeal nerve, and there may be difficulty swallowing because of pressure on the esophagus. The aneurysm can compress the superior vena cava causing distention of neck veins and edema of the face and neck. It may also cause enlargement of the aorta in the

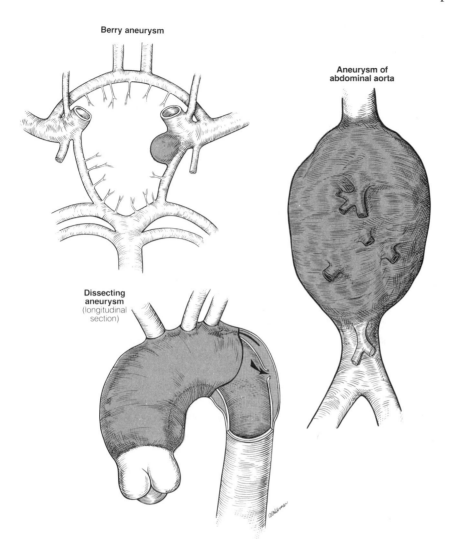

Berry aneurysm

Aneurysm of
abdominal aorta

Dissecting
aneurysm
(longitudinal
section)

Figure 15-6 *Three forms of aneurysms—berry aneurysm in the circle of Willis, fusiform-type aneurysm of the abdominal aorta, and a dissecting aortic aneurysm.*

areas of the aortic valve to the point of preventing complete valve closure and causing aortic regurgitation.

Aneurysms of the abdominal aorta are usually below the level of the renal artery. Because an aneurysm is of arterial origin, a pulsating mass may provide the first evidence of the disorder. This mass may be discovered during a routine physical examination, or the affected person may complain of its presence. Calcification, which frequently exists on the wall of the aneurysm, may be detected during an abdominal x-ray examination. Pain may be present, varying from mild midabdominal or lumbar discomfort to severe abdominal and back pain. The aneurysm may extend to and impinge on the renal, iliac, or mesenteric arteries. Stasis of blood favors thrombus formation along the wall of the vessel, and peripheral emboli may develop causing symptomatic arterial insufficiency. With both thoracic and abdominal aneurysms the most dreaded complication is rupture.

Arteriography, using a radiopaque dye to render the aneurysm visible on x-ray, may be used in diagnosis.

Recently, two noninvasive diagnostic techniques have come into use—ultrasound and computerized axial tomography (CAT scanning). Surgical repair, in which the involved section of the aorta is replaced with a synthetic graft of woven dacron, is frequently the treatment of choice. Hypertension, if present, should be controlled.

Dissecting aneurysms

A dissecting aneurysm is an acute, life-threatening condition. It involves hemorrhage into the vessel wall with longitudinal tearing (dissection) of the vessel wall to form a blood-filled channel. Unlike syphilitic or atherosclerotic aneurysms, dissecting aneurysms often occur without evidence of previous vessel dilatation.

Dissecting aneurysms are caused by conditions that weaken or cause necrosis of the medial layer of the aorta. They are seen most often in the 40- to 60-year-old age group and are more common in men than in women. There is a history of hypertension in 94% of cases.[10]

Dissecting aneurysms are also associated with connective tissue diseases such as Marfan's syndrome and during pregnancy because of histochemical changes in the aorta that occur during this time.

Approximately 75% of dissections have their origin in the ascending aorta. Dissection is usually bidirectional, moving proximally toward the heart and distally into the descending aorta. When the ascending aorta is involved, expansion of the vessel wall may impair closure of the aortic valve. Although the length of the dissection varies, it is possible for the abdominal aorta to be involved, with, finally, progression into the renal, iliac, or femoral arteries.

A major symptom of a dissecting aneurysm is the abrupt appearance of excruciating pain described as tearing or ripping. The location of the pain may point to the site of dissection. Pain associated with dissection of the ascending aorta is frequently located in the anterior chest; whereas pain associated with dissection of the descending aorta is often located in the back. In the early stages, blood pressure is often moderately or markedly elevated. Later, both the blood pressure and the pulse become unobtainable in one or both arms as the dissection disrupts arterial flow to the arms.

Mortality due to dissecting aneurysm is high. Within the first 48 hours, 50% of all untreated patients die, and 90% die within 6 weeks.[11] Treatment may be medical or surgical. Surgical treatment consists of resection of the involved segment of the aorta and replacement with a prosthetic graft. Medical treatment involves control of hypertension and drugs to lessen the force of systolic blood ejection from the heart.

Acute Arterial Occlusion

Acute arterial occlusion usually results from a thrombus or an embolus. Trauma or arterial spasm due to arterial cannulation is another cause.

The signs and symptoms of acute arterial occlusion depend on the artery involved and the adequacy of the collateral circulation. Emboli tend to lodge in bifurcations of the major arteries, including the aorta and iliac and the femoral and popliteal arteries. Occlusion in an extremity causes sudden onset of acute pain with numbness, tingling, weakness, pallor, and coldness. These changes are rapidly followed by cyanosis, mottling, and loss of sensory, reflex, and motor function. Pulses are absent below the level of the occlusion.

Treatment of acute arterial occlusion is aimed at restoring blood flow. Antifibrolytic therapy (streptokinase) may be used in an attempt to dissolve the clot.[12] Anticoagulant therapy (heparin) is usually given to prevent extension of the embolus. An embolectomy—surgical removal of the embolus—may be indicated. It is important that application of heat and cold be avoided and that the extremity be protected from hard surfaces and overlying bedclothes.

Peripheral Arterial Disease

The peripheral arterial circulation is usually described as arterial circulation outside the heart. For our purposes, we will consider the peripheral circulation as that outside the pulmonary and cerebral circulation. Arteriosclerosis, discussed earlier, is a major cause of peripheral vascular disorders. Two other conditions, Raynaud's phenomenon and thromboangiitis obliterans (Buerger's disease) will serve as prototypes of peripheral arterial disease.

Raynaud's syndrome

Raynaud's syndrome is a functional disorder caused by intense vasospasm of the arteries and arterioles in the fingers and, less often, in the toes. Raynaud's syndrome is divided into two types: Raynaud's disease, which occurs without demonstrable cause, and Raynaud's phenomenon, which occurs secondary to some other disease condition. Raynaud's disease is seen most frequently in otherwise healthy young women; it is often precipitated by exposure to cold or by strong emotions. Raynaud's phenomenon is associated with occupational trauma such as that caused by use of heavy vibrating tools, neurologic disorders, and chronic arterial occlusive disorders. It is often the first symptom of collagen diseases. In 70% of persons with scleroderma, it is the first symptom, and it is the presenting problem in 8% to 16% of lupus erythematosus cases.[13]

In Raynaud's disease or phenomenon, ischemia due to vasospasm causes changes in skin color that progress from pallor to cyanosis, a sensation of cold, and changes in sensory perception such as numbness or tingling. The color changes are usually first noted in the tips of the fingers, later moving into one or more of the distal phalanges. Following the ischemic episode, there is a period of hyperemia with intense rubor, throbbing, and paresthesias. The period of hyperemia is followed by a return to normal color. If Raynaud's disease begins asymmetrically (does not affect both hands in the same manner) it usually becomes symmetrical within 4 to 6 months.[13] During the attack there may be slight swelling. With repeated episodes of ischemia, the nails may become brittle, and the skin over the tips of the affected fingers thickened. Nutritional impairment of these structures may give rise to nutritional arthritis. Ulceration and superficial gangrene of the fingers, although infrequent, may occur.

In primary Raynaud's disease, the anatomy of the blood vessels appears normal and the cause of the vasospasm is unknown. It appears that local circulatory control mechanisms such as the prostaglandins may be involved. Raynaud's phenomenon is usually characterized by anatomic abnormalities of the vessels.

Treatment measures are directed toward eliminating factors that cause vasospasm and protecting the digits from trauma during an ischemic episode. Abstinence from smoking and protection from cold are first priorities. Avoidance of emotional stress is another important factor in controlling the disorder because anxiety and stress may precipitate a vascular spasm in predisposed individuals. Treatment with vasodilator drugs may be indicated, particularly if episodes are frequent, because frequency tends to encourage the potential from thrombosis and gangrene. The calcium-channel—blocking drugs that exert a vasodilator effect on vascular smooth muscle are currently being tested. Intravenous infusion of prostaglandin E seems to be beneficial during an acute attack of vasospasm, and its effects may last for several weeks. The McIntyre maneuver, which is used by skiers to warm their hands, has been shown to be helpful in the early stages of the vasospastic attack.[14] To do this maneuver, the person assumes standing position and briskly swings the hands downward and behind the body and then upward and in front of the body at a rate of about 180 times per minute. The centrifugal force of this maneuver moves blood into the fingers. Biofeedback training may be helpful in persons with Raynaud's disease but does not seem to be as effective in those with Raynaud's phenomenon.[15] Sympathectomy may be indicated if the attacks become severe, particularly if trophic changes have developed and medical treatment is ineffective.

Thromboangiitis obliterans (Buerger's disease)

Thromboangiitis obliterans is, as the name implies, an inflammatory arterial disorder that causes thrombus formation. The disorder affects the medium-sized arteries, usually the plantar and digital vessels in the foot and in the lower leg. Arteries in the arm and hand may also be affected. Although primarily an arterial disorder, the inflammatory process often extends to involve adjacent veins and nerves. The cause of Buerger's disease is unknown. It is a disease of men between 25 and 40 years of age who are heavy cigarette smokers.

Pain is the predominant symptom. During the early stages of the disease, there is intermittent claudication of the calf muscles and the arch of the foot. In severe cases, pain is present even when the person is at rest. The impaired circulation increases sensitivity to cold. The peripheral pulses are diminished or absent, and there are changes in the color of the extremity. In moderately advanced cases, the extremity becomes cyanotic when the person assumes a dependent position, and the digits may turn reddish blue in color even when in a nondependent position. With lack of blood flow, the skin assumes a thin, shiny look, and hair growth and skin nutrition suffer. Chronic ischemia brings thick malformed nails. If the disease continues to progress, tissues will eventually ulcerate, and gangrenous changes will arise that may necessitate amputation.

In the treatment program for thromboangiitis obliterans, it is mandatory that the person stop smoking cigarettes. Other treatment measures are of secondary importance and focus on methods for producing vasodilatation and for preventing tissue injury. Sympathectomy may be done to alleviate the vasospastic manifestations of the disease. Buerger's exercises take advantage of the gravitational effects of position change to improve blood flow to the affected part. The exercises consist of a cycle of approximately 2-minute positional changes: horizontal, legs elevated 45°, legs in a dependent position, and then horizontal again. The exercises are usually repeated five times and are done three times a day. Patients are usually instructed to wiggle their toes while exercising.

Assessment of Arterial Flow

There are a number of methods for assessing arterial flow and detecting arterial disease. These include monitoring of arterial pulses, angiography, Doppler ultrasound flow studies, impedance plethysmography, and thermography.

The volume of the peripheral pulses and capillary refill time are useful indirect methods for assessing peripheral perfusion.

Peripheral arterial pulses are palpated over vessels in the head, neck, and extremities. In situations associated with potential vessel spasm or thrombus formation, it may be necessary only to check for the presence of pulses. In many situations, however, the pulse volume provides useful information about vascular volume and the condition of the arterial circulation. Pulse volume can be graded on a scale of 0 to +4.

0— Pulse is not palpable.

+1— Pulse is thready, weak, and difficult to palpate; it may fade in and out and is easily obliterated with pressure.

+2— Pulse is difficult to palpate and may be obliterated with pressure, so light palpation is required. Once located, however, it is stronger than +1.

+3— Pulse is easily palpable, does not fade in and out, and is not easily obliterated by pressure. This pulse is considered to have normal volume.

+4— Pulse is strong, bounding, hyperactive, easily palpated, and not obliterated with pressure. In some cases, such as aortic regurgitation, it may be considered pathologic.[16]

Arterial auscultation is used to listen to the flow of blood with a stethoscope. A *bruit* is an audible murmur that can be heard over a peripheral artery. It is caused by turbulent blood flow and is suggestive of obstructive arterial disease.

Capillary refill time is an indicator of the efficiency of the microcirculation. It is measured by depressing the nailbed of a finger or toe until the underlying skin blanches. The refill time is normal if the capillary vessels refill within 3 seconds following release of the pressure.[16]

Angiography involves the injection of a radiopaque dye into the vascular system to allow visualization of the blood vessels on x-ray.

Ultrasonic Doppler flow studies use reflected ultrasound waves, which are transmitted back to the skin surface where they are sensed by an appropriate transducer. With moving objects such as blood cells, the frequency of the reflected sound is shifted in relation to the transmitted signal. This frequency shift is used in determining both the velocity and direction of blood flow.

Impedance plethysmography estimates blood flow in a limb or digit using measurements of resistance (impedance) changes that occur as the fluid volume of the limb changes due to the pulsatile nature of arterial blood flow. With this method four electrodes are placed in a row along the limb. A high-frequency AC voltage of very low amplitude is transmitted across the skin by the two outer electrodes, while the two inner electrodes monitor the changes in electrical resistance that occur because of changes in blood flow.

The temperature of the skin is determined by many factors, including arterial blood flow. One of the observations in atherosclerotic and acute arterial occlusion is that the affected area is colder than normal. Skin temperature may be measured with a skin thermometer. Infrared *thermography* uses an infrared camera to map the skin temperature of an area.

In summary, there are two types of arterial disorders: (1) diseases such as atherosclerosis and peripheral arterial diseases that obstruct blood flow and (2) disorders such as aneurysms that weaken the vessel wall. Atherosclerosis, which is a leading cause of death in the United States, affects large and medium-sized arteries such as the coronary and cerebral arteries. It has an insidious onset and its lesions are usually far advanced before symptoms appear. Although the mechanisms of atherosclerosis are uncertain, risk factors associated with its development have been identified. These include (1) factors such as heredity, race, sex, and age, which cannot be controlled; (2) factors such as smoking, high blood pressure, high serum cholesterol levels, and diabetes, which can be controlled; and (3) other contributing factors such as obesity, lack of exercise, and stress. Aneurysms are abnormal vessel dilatations of an artery. The weakness that leads to aneurysm formation can be caused by several factors including congenital defects in vessel structure, trauma, infections, and atherosclerosis. Peripheral arterial diseases affect blood vessels outside the heart and thorax. They include Raynaud's phenomenon, caused by vessel spasm and thromboangiitis obliterans (Buerger's disease), which is characterized by an inflammatory process that involves medium-sized arteries and adjacent veins and nerves of the lower extremities.

■ Alterations in Venous Flow

Veins are low-pressure, thin-walled vessels that rely on the ancillary action of skeletal muscle pumps and changes in abdominal and intrathoracic pressure to return blood to the heart. Unlike the arterial system, the venous system is equipped with valves that prevent retrograde flow of blood. Although its structure enables the venous system to serve as a storage area for blood, it also renders the system susceptible to problems related to stasis and venous insufficiency. This section focuses on two common problems of the venous system: varicose veins and venous thrombosis. Pulmonary embolism, a complication of deep vein thrombosis, is discussed in Chapter 23.

Varicose Veins

Varicose, or dilated, tortuous veins of the lower extremities, are common and often lead to secondary problems of venous insufficiency. Estimates suggest that 10% of the adult population is affected by varicose veins and another 40% or 50% have slight asymptomatic varicosities.[17] Customarily, varicose veins are described as being primary or secondary. Primary varicosities originate in the superficial saphenous veins, and secondary varicose veins result from impaired flow in the deep venous channels.

A brief review of the anatomy of the venous system of the legs explains why varicosities may develop. The venous system in the legs might well be described as being composed of two venous channels: the superficial (saphenous and its tributaries) veins and the deep venous channels (Fig. 15-7). Perforating or communicating veins connect these two systems. Blood from the skin and subcutaneous tissues in the leg collects in the superficial veins and is then transported across the commu-

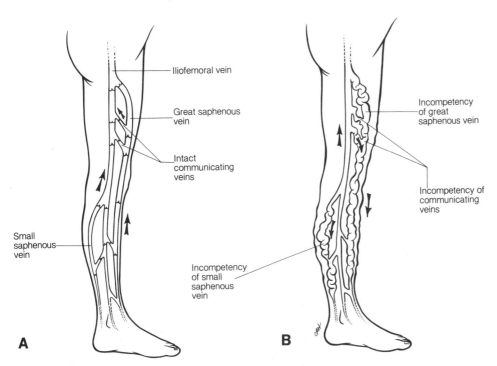

Figure 15-7 *The superficial and deep venous channels of the leg. View A represents normal venous structures and flow patterns. View B illustrates varicosities in the superficial venous system that are the result of incompetent valves in the communicating veins. The arrows in both views indicate the direction of blood flow. (Modified from Abramson DI: Vascular Disorders of the Extremities, 2nd ed. New York, Harper & Row, 1974)*

nicating veins into the deeper venous channels for return to the heart. When a person walks, the action of the muscle pumps produces an increase in flow in the deep channels and facilitates movement of blood from the superficial to the deep veins.

Valves present in the veins prevent the retrograde flow of blood and play an important role in the function of the venous system. Although these valves are irregularly located along the length of the veins, they are almost always found at junctions where the communicating veins merge with the larger deep veins and where two veins meet. The number of venous valves differs somewhat from one individual to another as does the structural competence, factors that may help to explain the familial predisposition to development of varicose veins.

Causes
Varicose veins result from prolonged dilatation and stretching of the vascular wall as a result of increased venous pressure. One of the most important factors in the elevation of venous pressure is the hydrostatic effect associated with the standing position. When a person is in the erect position, the full weight of the venous columns of blood is transmitted to the leg veins. The effects

of gravity are compounded in persons who stand for long periods of time without using their leg muscles to assist in pumping blood back to the heart. Because there are no valves in the inferior vena cava or common iliac veins, blood in the abdominal veins must be supported by the valves located in the external iliac or femoral veins. When intra-abdominal pressure increases, as it does during pregnancy, or when the valves in these two veins are absent or defective, the stress on the saphenofemoral junction is increased. The high incidence of varicose veins in women who have been pregnant also suggests a hormonal effect on venous smooth muscle leading to venous dilatation and valvular incompetence.

Prolonged exposure to increases in pressure causes the venous valves to become incompetent so they no longer close properly. When this happens, blood regurgitates into the superficial veins. Furthermore, once varicose veins have developed, the venous structures become deformed, promoting further dilatation.

Another consideration is that the superficial veins have only subcutaneous fat and superficial fascia for support, whereas the deep venous channels are supported by muscle, bone, and connective tissue. Therefore, obesity tends to increase the risk for varicose veins.

Normally, about 80% to 90% of venous blood from the lower extremities is transported through the deep channels. The development of secondary varicose veins becomes inevitable when flow in these channels is impaired or blocked. Among the causes of secondary varicose veins are thrombophlebitis, congenital or acquired arteriovenous fistulas, congenital venous malformations, and pressure on the abdominal veins due to pregnancy or a tumor.

Venous insufficiency

Signs and symptoms associated with varicose veins vary. Most women complain of their unsightly appearance. In addition to their cosmetic effects, varicose veins tend to impair venous emptying giving rise to a condition known as venous insufficiency. This often causes a sensation of progressive heaviness and, with prolonged standing, aching legs. In contrast to the ischemia due to arterial insufficiency, venous insufficiency tends to lead to tissue congestion, edema, and eventual impairment of tissue nutrition. The edema is exacerbated by long periods of standing. In its advanced form, impairment of tissue nutrition causes stasis dermatitis and the development of stasis or varicose ulcers. Stasis dermatitis is characterized by the presence of thin, shiny bluish brown, irregularly pigmented desquamative skin that lacks the support of the underlying subcutaneous tissues. Minor injury leads to relatively painless ulcerations that are difficult to heal. The lower part of the leg is particularly prone to develop stasis dermatitis and varicose ulcers.

Diagnosis and treatment

Several procedures are used to assess the extent of venous involvement associated with varicose veins. One of these, the Trendelenburg test, involves the use of a tourniquet in the following manner. A tourniquet is applied to the affected leg while it is elevated and the veins are empty. The person then assumes the standing position, and the tourniquet is removed. If the superficial veins are involved, the veins distend quickly. To assess the deep channels, the tourniquet is applied while the person is standing and the veins are filled. The person then lies down and the affected leg is elevated. Emptying of the superficial veins indicates that the deep channels are patent. The Doppler ultrasonic flow probe may also be used to assess the flow in the large vessels. Angiographic studies employing a radiopaque contrast medium are also used to assess venous function.

Ideally, measures should be taken to prevent the development and progression of varicose veins. Once the venous channels have been repeatedly stretched and the valves rendered incompetent, little can be done to restore normal venous tone and function. These measures center on avoiding any activities that involve prolonged elevation of venous pressure.

Treatment measures for varicose veins focus on improving venous flow and preventing tissue injury, such as avoiding prolonged standing and providing for frequent leg elevation. When properly fitted, elastic support stockings compress the superficial veins and thus prevent distention. These stockings should be applied before the standing position is assumed at a time when the leg veins are empty. Surgical treatment consists of removing the varicosities and the incompetent perforating veins, but it is limited to persons with patent, deep venous channels. Sclerotherapy, which is usually done on small residual varicosities, is another treatment measure; it involves injection of a sclerosing agent into the collapsed superficial veins in order to produce fibrosis of the vessel lumen.

Venous Thrombosis

In thrombophlebitis there is inflammation of a vein with subsequent thrombus formation, while in phlebothrombosis thrombus formation is followed by inflammation. In phlebothrombosis, the clot is less firmly attached to the vessel wall than is the case in thrombophlebitis, so that embolization is a greater risk. From a clinical standpoint, it is often difficult to determine which came first—the inflammation or the clot. Therefore, this discussion treats thrombophlebitis and phlebothrombosis as one and the same.

In 1846, Virchow described the triad that has come to be associated with thrombosis: (1) stasis of blood, (2) increased blood coagulability, and (3) vessel-wall injury.[18] It is thought that two of the three factors must be present for thrombi to form. Thrombi can develop in either the superficial or the deep veins (DVT). Thrombus formation in deep veins is a precursor to venous insufficiency and embolus formation.

A number of factors may be present that promote venous thrombosis (Table 15-2). Immobilization, trauma, and surgery are definite risk factors, as are aging, heart failure, hypercoagulability states, and a previous history of venous disorders. The patient immobilized by a hip fracture or joint replacement is particularly vulnerable to DVT. Persons in the older age groups (over 40 years) are more susceptible than younger people. Although there is no single explanation for it, factors known to promote venous stasis, such as heart failure, venous pathology, and cancer occur more frequently in older individuals. Hypercoagulability is in itself a homeostatic mechanism that is invoked in conditions of stress or injury. It may be that thrombi form as a result of changes in clotting factors or in the fibrinolytic system (see Chap. 12). When body fluid is lost because of injury or disease, the resulting hemoconcentration will cause the clotting factors to become more concentrated. Certain malignancies are associated with increased clotting tendencies, and although the reason for this is largely unknown, substances that promote blood coagulation may be released from the tissues due to the cancerous growth. In congestive heart failure and shock, there is impaired circulation with stasis of coagulation factors.

What part oral contraceptive agents play in promoting blood coagulation and, as a consequence, a predisposition to venous thrombosis and pulmonary embolism is controversial. Certainly, if other risk factors are present, both the risk and benefits of oral contraceptives need to be carefully weighed.

Signs and symptoms

The most common signs of thrombophlebitis are those related to the inflammatory process: pain, swelling, deep muscle tenderness, and fever. Generally, the pain is described as localized, deep, aching, and throbbing and is exacerbated by walking. A positive Homans' sign— pain in the popliteal area when the foot is forcefully dorsiflexed—suggests thrombophlebitis. Swelling of the leg usually occurs soon after the onset of pain. How much swelling there is depends on the extent to which venous flow is impaired. Fever, general malaise, and an elevated white blood cell count and sedimentation rate are accompanying signs of inflammation.

Phlebothrombosis differs from thrombophlebitis in that the early signs of inflammation are often absent. Frequently, a positive Homans' sign or manifestations of pulmonary embolism are the only evidence that thrombosis has occurred.

Diagnosis and treatment

The risk of pulmonary embolism emphasizes the need for early detection and treatment of thrombophlebitis. Several tests are useful for this purpose: radioactive fibrinogen (I^{125}), Doppler ultrasonic flowmeter studies, and impedance plethysmography. At present, the most reliable test appears to be the intravenous injection of radioactive fibrinogen, which becomes incorporated into any developing thrombus. The thrombus is then detected by a scintillation counter, which records the radioactivity at selected points in the extremity.

These three methods provide means for frequent assessment of venous flow or fibrinogen accumulation and are useful in monitoring persons at risk for developing venous thrombosis.

Venography, in which a contrast medium is injected into a vein and x-ray studies are done, is another diagnostic procedure, but it is not done routinely.

Whenever possible, venous thrombosis should be prevented, in preference to being treated. Early ambula-

Table 15-2 Risk Factors Associated with Venous Thrombosis

Aging
Anesthesia and surgury
Circulatory failure
   Congestive heart failure
   Shock
Dehydration
Hematologic disorders
   Polycythemia
   Disorders of blood clotting
   Disorders of fibrinolytic activity
Malignancy
Massive trauma or infection
Obesity
Reproductive processes
   Pregnancy
   Parturition
   Oral contraceptive therapy
Venous disorders
   Venous insufficiency
   Vascular trauma
   Venous obstruction

tion following childbirth and surgery is one measure that decreases the risk of thrombus formation. Exercising the legs and wearing support stockings also improve venous flow. A further precautionary measure is to avoid assuming body positions that favor venous pooling. For example, in the hospitalized patient, if both the head and knees of the hospital bed are raised, blood will tend to pool in the pelvic veins. Long unbroken auto and plane trips also promote venous pooling and thrombus formation.

In both thrombophlebitis and phlebothrombosis, bed rest with elevation of the affected extremity is prescribed. In one study, contrast medium remained in the soleus veins, on the average, for 10 minutes in supine patients whose legs were in horizontal position.[19] This may explain why postoperative thrombi frequently originate in the soleus vein. A 20° elevation of the legs will prevent stasis.[20] It is important that the entire lower extremity or extremities be carefully extended to avoid acute flexion of the knee or hip. Heat is often applied to the leg to relieve vasospasm and to aid in the resolution of the inflammatory process. Measures are also taken to prevent the bed coverings from resting on the leg because this increases discomfort.

Two anticoagulants, warfarin and heparin, are used both to treat and to prevent thrombophlebitis. *Treatment* is usually initiated with either continuous or periodic intravenous heparin infusions. This is followed by *prophylactic* therapy with either subcutaneous minidose heparin injections or oral warfarin sodium to prevent further thrombus formation. Minidose heparin is usually injected into the subcutaneous tissue of the lower abdomen or laterally above the iliac crest.[21,22] Prophylactic therapy is usually continued for 6 to 10 weeks following uncomplicated DVT and for up to 6 months following pulmonary embolism. The mechanisms of action of the anticoagulant drugs are discussed in Chapter 12. Antifibrolytic therapy (streptokinase) may be used in an attempt to dissolve the clot.

In summary, the storage function of the venous system renders it susceptible to venous insufficiency, stasis, and thrombus formation. Varicose veins occur with prolonged distention and stretching of the superficial veins due to venous insufficiency. Varicosities can arise because of defects in the superficial veins (primary varicose veins) or because of impaired blood flow in the deep venous channels (secondary varicose veins). Venous thrombosis, thrombophlebitis, and pulmonary embolism are associated with three factors: vessel injury, stasis of venous flow, and hypercoagulability states.

■ Impairment of Local Blood Flow: Pressure Sores

Pressure sores are ischemic lesions of the skin and underlying structures caused by external pressure, which impairs the flow of blood and lymph. *Decubitus* comes from the Latin term meaning "lying down"; pressure sores are often referred to as decubitus ulcers or bedsores. However, a pressure sore may result from pressure exerted in either the seated or supine positions. It is most likely to develop over a bony prominence, but it may occur on any part of the body that is subjected to external pressure, friction, or shearing forces.

Sources of Tissue Injury

Shearing forces

Shearing forces are caused by the sliding of one tissue layer over another with stretching and angulation of blood vessels causing injury and thrombosis. Clinically, injury due to shearing forces commonly occurs when the head of the bed is elevated, causing the torso to slide down thus transmitting pressure to the sacrum and deep fascia; at the same time, friction and perspiration cause the sacral skin to remain fixed to the bed. Another source of shearing forces is pulling rather than lifting a patient up in bed. In this case the skin remains fixed to the sheet while the fascia and muscles are pulled upward.

Pressure

External pressure that exceeds capillary pressure interrupts the blood flow in the capillary beds. When this pressure is greater than the pressure in the arterioles, it also interrupts the flow in these vessels. The average blood pressure of the normal skin capillaries is about 25 mm Hg. A pressure exceeding 50 mm Hg applied to the skin over a bony prominence is sufficient to interrupt the blood flow and cause ischemia.[23] Approximately 7 pounds of pressure per square inch of tissue surface is sufficient to shut off blood flow.[24] Great pressure distributed over a small area will cause more rapid breakdown of tissue than a small amount distributed over a larger area. If this pressure is applied constantly for 2 hours, oxygen deprivation coupled with an accumulation of metabolic end products leads to irreversible tissue damage. Altering the distribution of pressure from one skin area to another prevents tissue damage. If a man weighing 70 kg with a total surface area of 1.8 m² were in the supine position, with pressure evenly distributed, the pressure at any given point would be 5.7 mm Hg.[25] Normally, pressure on the skin and underlying tissues is continually shifted to prevent ischemia. During the night, for example, frequent turning prevents ischemic injury of tissues overlying the bony prominences that support the weight of the body; the same is true for sitting for any length of time. The movements needed to shift the body weight are made unconsciously, and only when movement is restricted do we become aware of discomfort. Pressure ulcers occur most commonly with conditions, such as spinal cord injury, in which normal sensation and movement to effect redistribution of body weight are impaired.

Whether a person is sitting or lying down, the weight of the body is borne by tissues covering the bony prominences. Ninety-six percent of pressure sores are located on the lower part of the body, most often over the sacrum, the coccygeal areas, the ischial tuberosities, and the greater trochanter.[25] Pressure over a bony area is transmitted from the surface to the underlying dense bone; all the underlying tissue is compressed with the greatest pressure at the surface of the bone and dissipating in conelike fashion toward the surface of the skin (Fig. 15-8). The skin lesion is often just the tip of the iceberg; extensive underlying tissue damage is often present when a small superficial skin lesion is first noted.

Grading of Pressure Sores

Pressure sores can be graded according to four categories developed by Shea.[26] Grade 1 lesions are characterized by a hardened, warm, reddish brown swelling. These lesions are essentially reversible and will resolve in 5 to 10

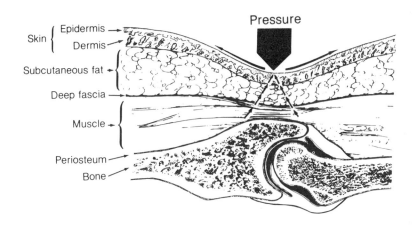

Figure 15-8 *Pressure over a bony prominence compresses all intervening soft tissue, with a resulting wide, three-dimensional pressure gradient that causes varying degrees of ischemia and damage. (Shea JD: Pressure sores: Classification and management. Clin Orthop, 112:90, 1975)*

days if treated by relieving of pressure and taking measures to prevent bacterial contamination. Grade 2 lesions involve all of the soft tissue, with development of a shallow, full-thickness skin ulcer with pigmented edges that blend into a broad area that is warm, swollen and hardened, and reddish brown in color. Grade 2 ulcers are also reversible; they take longer to heal than grade 1 ulcers, however, and require treatment directed toward further breakdown. Grade 3 pressure sores extend through the skin into the subcutaneous fat with extensive undermining; they are frequently infected and foul smelling. There may be profound loss of fluid and protein from these open draining wounds. Although grade 3 pressure sores will heal by second intention, the resulting scar tissue is thin and subject to easy breakdown. A grade 4 ulcer includes penetration of the deep fascia with involvement of muscle and bone. Dislocation, resulting from septic joints and osteomyelitis, may occur. Septicemia is a frequent cause of death in persons with grade 4 pressure ulcers.[27]

Prevention and Treatment

Prevention of pressure ulcers is preferable to treatment. In 1978 it was estimated that the cost of treating a pressure ulcer ranged from $6000 for less severe ulcers to $17,500 for severe ulcers requiring extensive care and convalescent time, not to mention the discomfort and other problems arising from their occurrence.[23] Risk factors that have been identified as contributing to the development of pressure sores are unconsciousness, dehydration, paralysis, restricted mobility, circulatory impairment, and emaciation. The elderly are particularly prone to develop pressure sores; in one institution, 76% of the pressure ulcers that occurred during two 6-month periods of time were in persons over 70 years of age.[28] Identifying patients who are at risk for development of decubitus ulcers allows health care facilities to focus

prevention measures on this group, and this has been shown to reduce the incidence of pressure sores.[28,29]

Prevention includes frequent position change, meticulous skin care, and careful and frequent observation to detect early signs of skin breakdown. Bed linens should be kept clean, dry, and wrinkle free. A natural or synthetic sheepskin that is soft and resilient, does not wrinkle, and distributes weight evenly may be used. Usually a synthetic sheepskin that is easily laundered is used. Special pads and mattresses that distribute weight more evenly may be used. Such items as silicone-filled pads, egg-crate cushions, turning frames, flotation pads, and other devices minimize contact pressure. Adequate exposure of the skin to air is necessary to avoid the buildup of heat and perspiration. A bed cradle may be used to keep bedclothes away from the skin. Care should be taken to maintain the individual at a position of 30° to 40° to minimize slipping and shearing forces from sliding against the sheets. It is also important that the person be lifted and not dragged across the sheet. A lifting sheet works well for this purpose. Elevation of the ankles and heels off the sheets with foam pads can reduce skin breakdown in these areas of the body.

Casts, braces, and splints can exert extreme pressure on underlying tissues, and persons with these devices require special attention to avoid skin breakdown.

Prevention of dehydration improves the circulation, reduces the concentration of urine, minimizing skin irritation in incontinent patients, and reduce urinary problems contributing to incontinence. Maintenance of adequate nutrition is important. Anemia and malnutrition contribute to tissue breakdown and delay healing once tissue injury has occurred.

Once skin breakdown has occurred, special treatment measures are needed to prevent further ischemic damage, reduce bacterial contamination and infection, and promote healing. Frequent cleansing and irrigation with sterile water, normal saline, or other cleansing agents are done to remove drainage and any other contamination that has occurred.

Numerous topical agents have been used as adjuvants in the treatment of pressure sores. Some of the more widely used are enzyme preparations, such as fibrinolysin and desoxyribonuclease (Elase) and Sutilains ointment (Travase), which are used to assist in debridement of the ulcer. A preparation of trypsin, balsam of Peru, and castor oil (Granulex) may also be used for this purpose. Dextranomer (Debrisan) is a long-chain polysaccharide that is used to absorb the products of collagen and tissue breakdown and contaminating bacteria and allows the wound to heal without crusting.

Op-site is a self-adhesive transparent dressing that seals in the body's own defenses against invasion—leukocytes, plasma, and fibrin.[30] It promotes natural healing without the usual formation of a dry crust over the wound. Although Op-site is nonporous and prevents the escape of fluid, it is permeable to air and water vapor and prevents the growth of anaerobic bacteria.

In summary, pressure sores are caused by ischemia of the skin and underlying tissues. They are caused by external pressure, which disrupts blood flow, or by shearing forces, which cause stretching and injury to blood vessels. Pressure sores are divided into four grades: grade 1 lesions, which are reversible and are characterized by hardened, warm, reddish brown swelling; grade 2 lesions, which involve all the soft tissue with development of a shallow, full-thickness skin ulcer; grade 3 lesions, which extend through the skin into the subcutaneous fat with extensive undermining and are frequently infected; grade 4 lesions, which penetrate the deep fascia and involve bone and muscle. Prevention of pressure sores is accomplished through frequent change of position, careful skin care, adequate nutrition and hydration, and use of special pads and mattresses that aid in the distribution of weight.

■ Study Guide

After you have studied this chapter, you should be able to meet the following objectives:

☐ List five mechanisms of blood vessel obstruction.

☐ Describe vessel changes that occur in atherosclerosis.

☐ Use the principles of blood flow from Chapter 14 to explain why atherosclerosis is usually a silent disease until extensive vessel occlusion has occurred.

☐ Cite three current theories used to explain the pathogenesis of atherosclerosis.

☐ State the three categories of risk factors for atherosclerosis.

☐ State the function of the lipoproteins in terms of cholesterol transport and metabolism.

☐ Distinguish between berry aneurysms, aortic aneurysms, and dissecting aneurysms.

☐ Relate the law of Laplace to wall tension in an aneurysm.

☐ List the signs and symptoms associated with thoracic and abdominal aneurysms.

☐ State the signs and symptoms of acute arterial occlusion.

☐ State a method for describing gradations in pulse volume.

☐ Explain the pathology involved in Raynaud's syndrome.

☐ Explain why pain is the predominant symptom of thromboangiitis obliterans.

☐ Describe the effect of gravity on the venous system.

☐ State the signs and symptoms of venous insufficiency.

☐ Describe the pathology involved in venous thrombosis.

☐ Cite two causes of pressure sores.

☐ Explain how shearing forces contribute to ischemic skin damage.

☐ Explain why pressure sores are most apt to develop over bony prominences.

☐ List four measures that contribute to the prevention of pressure sores.

■ References

1. Report of the 1981 Working Group to Review the Report by the National Heart and Lung Institute Task Force on Arteriosclerosis. Ateriosclerosis, p 37, 1983

2. Enos WF, Beyer JC, Holmes RF: Pathogenesis of coronary artery disease in American soldiers killed in Korea. JAMA 158:912, 1955

3. Campbell GR, Chambley-Campbell VH: Invited review: The cellular pathobiology of atherosclerosis. Pathology 13:424, 1981

4. Smith LH, Thier SO: Pathophysiology. p 1163, Philadelphia, WB Saunders, 1981

5. Steinberg D: Research related to underlying mechanisms in atherosclerosis. Circulation 60:1562, 1979

6. Wittels EW, Gotto AM: Atherogenic mechanisms. In Froelich ED (ed): Patholphysiology, 3rd ed, p 114. Philadelphia, JB Lippincott, 1984

7. Benditt EP: Implications of the monoclonal character of human atherosclerotic plaques. Am J Pathol 86:693, 1977

8. McIntosh HD, Stamler J, Jackson D: Introduction to risk factors in coronary artery disease. Heart Lung 7:126, 1978

9. Report of the 1977 Working Group to Review the Report of the National Heart and Lung Institute Task Force on Arteriosclerosis. Arteriosclerosis, p 20, 1977

10. Robbins SL, Cotran RS, Kumar V: Pathologic Basis of Disease, 3rd ed, pp 529, 529, 532. Philadelphia, WB Saunders, 1984

11. Webb RW, Bunswick RA: Management of acute dissection of the aorta. Heart Lung 9:284, 1980

12. Berni GA, Bandyk DF, Zierler RE et al: Streptokinase treatment in acute arterial occlusion. Ann Surg 198:185, 1983

13. Lipsmeyer EA: Raynaud's syndrome. J Arkansas Med Soc 79:63, 1982

14. McIntyre DR: A maneuver to reverse Raynaud's vasospasm. JAMA 240:2760, 1978

15. Gordon RS: From National Institutes of Health. Biofeedback for patients with Raynaud's disease. JAMA 242:509, 1979

16. Miller KM: Assessing peripheral perfusion. Am J Nurs 78:1673, 1978

17. Lofgren KA: Varicose veins: Their symptoms, complications and management. Postgrad Med 65, No 6:131, 1979

18. Virchow R: Weinere untersuchungen uber dic verstropfung der lungenrarterie und ihre folgen. Beitr Exp Pathol Physiol 2:21, 1846

19. Nicolaides AN, Kakkar VV, Renney JTG: Soleal sinuses and stasis. Br J Surg 58:307, 1971

20. Nicolaides AN, Gordon-Smith I: The prevention of deep venous thrombosis. In Hobbs JT (ed): The Treatment of Venous Disorders, A Comprehensive Review of Current Practice in the Management of Varicose Veins and Postthrombotic Syndrome. Philadelphia, JB Lippincott, 1977

21. Caprini JA, Zoellner JL, Weisman M: Heparin therapy—Part II. Cardiovasc Nurs 13, No 4:17, 1977

22. Chamberlain SL: Low-dose heparin therapy. Am J Nurs 80:1115, 1980

23. Terry C, Silverstein P (eds): Management of Dermal Ulcers. Deerfield, IL, Travenol Laboratories, 1981

24. Beland I, Passos JY: Clinical Nursing, 4th ed, p 1112. New York, Macmillan, 1981

25. Reuler JB, Cooney TG: The pressure sore: Pathophysiology and principles of management. Ann Intern Med 94:661, 1981

26. Shea JD: Pressure sores. Clin Orthop 12:89, 1975

27. Galpin JE, Chow AW, Bayer AS et al: Sepsis associated with decubitus ulcers. Am J Med 61:346, 1976

28. Anderson KE, Korning SA: Medical aspects of decubitus ulcer. Int J Dermatol 5:265, 1982

29. Ameis A, Chiarcossi A, Jimenez J: Management of pressure sores. Postgrad Med 67, No 2:177, 1980

30. Ahmed MC: Op-site for decubitus care. Am J Nurs 82:61, 1982

■ Additional References

Atherosclerosis and arterial pathology

Barboriak JJ, Menahan LA: Alcohol, lipoproteins and coronary heart disease. Heart Lung 8, No 4:736, 1979

Barnes RW: Axioms on acute arterial occlusion in an extremity. Hosp Med 14, No 6:34, 1978

Barnes RW: Diagnosing vascular disease with noninvasive tests. Consultant 17:56, 1978

Bernstein EF, Fronek A: Current status of noninvasive tests in the diagnosis of peripheral arterial disease. Surg Clin North Am 62, No 3:473, 1982

Bjorkerud S: Mechanisms of atherosclerosis. Pathobiol Annu 9:277, 1979

Brown MS, Goldstein JL: Familial hypercholesterolemia: A genetic defect in the low-density lipoprotein receptor. N Engl J Med 294, No 25:1386, 1976

Cohen I: Role of endothelial injury and platelets in atherogenesis. Artery 5, No 3:237, 1979

deWolfe VG: Intermittent claudication and after. Emerg Med 11:204, 1979

Dillon P, Seasholtz J: Oral contraceptives and myocardial infarction. Cardiovasc Nurs 15, No 2:5, 1979

Fagan-Dubin L: Atherosclerosis: A major cause of peripheral vascular disease. Nurs Clin North Am 12, No 1:101, 1977

Farrell PA, Barboriak J: The time course of alterations of plasma lipid and lipoprotein concentrations during eight weeks of endurance training. Atherosclerosis 37:231, 1980

Friedman SA: Guide to diagnosis of peripheral arterial disease. Hosp Med 15, No 1:87, 1979

Garrison RJ et al: Cigarette smoking and HDL cholesterol—The Framingham offspring study. Atherosclerosis 30:17, 1978

Harker L, Ross R: Pathogenesis of arterial vascular disease. Semin Thromb Hemost 5, No 4:274, 1979

Hertzer NR: Abdominal aortic aneurysm: Guide to diagnosis and management. Hosp Med 15, No 3:65, 1979

Hoffman GS: Raynaud's disease and phenomenon. Am Fam Physician 21, No 1:91, 1980

Johansen K: Aneurysms. Sci Am 247, No 1:101, 1982

Lee K: Aneurysm precautions: A physiologic basis for minimizing rebleeding. Heart Lung 9, No 2:336, 1980

Lees RS, Lees AM: High-density lipoproteins and the risk of atherosclerosis. N Engl J Med 306, No 25:1546, 1982

Lees RS, Myers GS: Noninvasive diagnosis of arterial disease. Adv Intern Med 27:475, 1982

Levy RI: Current status of the cholesterol controversy. Am J Med 72:1, 1983

Morriss NS: Dissecting aortic aneurysms. J Emerg Nurs 5:10, 1979

Roenigk HH Jr: Leg ulcers in the elderly. Geriatrics 34:21, 1979

Samuel P, McNamara DJ, Shapiro J: The role of diet in the etiology and treatment of atherosclerosis. Annu Rev Med 34:179, 1983

Sanderson CJ et al: Acute aortic dissection: An historical review. J R Coll Surg Edinb 27, No 4:195, 1982

Sexton DL: The patient with peripheral arterial occlusive disease. Nurs Clin North Am 12:89, 1977

Shionoya S et al: Pattern of arterial occlusion in Buerger's disease. Angiology 31:375, 1982

Spittell JA Jr: Diagnosis and treatment of occlusive peripheral arterial disease. Geriatrics 37, No 1:57, 1982

Spittell JA Jr: Occlusive peripheral arterial disease: Guidelines for office management. Postgrad Med 71, No 2:137, 1982

Stadel BV: Oral contraceptives and cardiovascular disease. Part
     1 and Part 2. N Engl J Med 305:612, 672, 1981
Taggart E: The physical assessment of the patient with arterial
     disease. Nurs Clin North Am 12, No 1:109, 1977
Thomas WA, Kim DN: Biology of disease: Atherosclerosis as a
     hyperplastic and/or neoplastic process. Lab Invest 48, No
     3:245, 1983
Weksler BB, Nachman RL: Platelets and atherosclerosis. Am J
     Med 71, No 3:331, 1981

Venous pathology

Barnes RW: Current status of noninvasive tests in the diagnosis
     of venous disease. Surg Clin N Am 62, No 3, 1982
Bennison J: The support of the venous circulation. Angiology
     32:442, 1982
Bloomberg AE: Stripping varicose veins. NY J Med :184,
     1982
Kakkar VV: Deep vein thrombosis: Detection and prevention.
     Circulation 51:8, 1975
Summer DS: Venous dynamics—Varicosities. Clin Obstet
     Gynecol 24, No 3, 1981

Chapter 16

Control of Arterial Blood Pressure

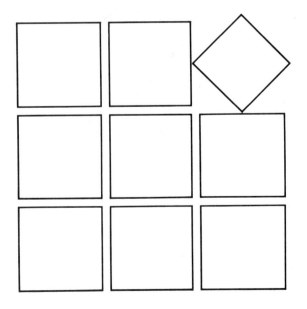

The arterial blood pressure is the driving force for blood in the circulatory system. Although blood pressure varies from moment to moment, it is perhaps the most controlled variable in the circulatory system. In Chapter 14, the blood vessels and local control of blood flow were discussed. To function effectively, mechanisms that control local blood flow (Chap. 14) must be accompanied by an adequate perfusion pressure. The focus of this chapter is on the systemic arterial blood pressure and its regulation, pulmonary arterial pressure, and blood pressure measurement. A discussion of the autonomic nervous system is included to assist the reader in understanding the regulation of blood pressure and the medications used in the treatment of hypertension.

■ Arterial Pressure Pulses

The arterial pressure reflects the intermittent ejection of blood from the left ventricle into the aorta. It rises as the left ventricle contracts and falls as it relaxes, giving rise to what is termed a pressure pulse or pressure wave. This pressure pulse is responsible for the Korotkoff sounds heard when blood pressure is measured using a blood pressure cuff. The ejection of blood from the right ventricle into the pulmonary artery also produces pressure

pulses similar to, albeit of lesser magnitude than, those of the systemic arterial system. The contour of the arterial pressure tracing shown in Figure 16-1 is typical of the pressure changes that occur in the large arteries of the systemic circulation. There is a rapid rise in the pulse contour during left ventricular contraction (systole), followed by a slower rise in peak pressure. The end of systole is marked by a brief downward deflection and formation of the dicrotic notch, which results from the reversal of the blood flow when ventricular pressure decreases below that in the aorta. The sudden closure of the aortic valve and subsequent rebound of blood from it cause a brief rise in pressure immediately following the notch. As the blood flows into the peripheral vessels during ventricular relaxation (diastole), the pressure falls rapidly at first and then declines slowly as the driving force decreases.

The maintenance of blood pressure during ventricular diastole results from the elastic properties of the aorta. If the amount of blood that was ejected from the heart were the same as that which flowed out of the arteries into the arterioles, the volume of blood in the arteries would remain constant and there would be no change in the pressure pulse. This, however, is not the case. Instead, the elastic walls of the aorta stretch during systole in a manner that prevents systolic pressure from rising excessively, and during diastole they recoil to augment the pumping action of the heart. Only about one-third of the ejected blood leaves the aorta during ventricular systole. The remainder distends the elastic walls of the aorta. During diastole, the stretched aortic walls rebound, providing the force that continues to drive blood through the arteries to maintain the diastolic blood pressure. The elastic properties of the aortic walls and their ability to store energy as a means of maintaining diastolic blood pressure are similar to the elastic properties of a rubber band and its ability to store energy when it is stretched.

In a healthy young adult, the pressure at the height of the pressure pulse (systolic blood pressure) is about 120 mm Hg and about 80 mm Hg at the lowest pressure (diastolic pressure). The pulse pressure (about 40 mm Hg) is the difference between the systolic and diastolic pressures. It reflects the magnitude of the pressure pulse. The mean arterial pressure represents the average pressure in the arterial system during both ventricular contraction and relaxation (about 90 mm Hg–100 mm Hg) and is depicted by the shaded areas under the pressure tracing in Figure 16-1.

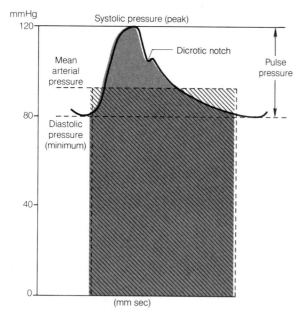

Figure 16-1 *Intra-arterial pressure tracing made from the brachial artery. Pulse pressure is the difference between systolic and diastolic pressures. The shaded area under the pressure tracing represents the mean arterial pressure, which can be calculated by using the formula: mean arterial pressure = diastolic pressure + pulse pressure.*
                                        3

In summary, the alternating contraction and relaxation of the heart produces a pressure pulse that moves the blood through the circulatory system. The elastic walls of the aorta stretch during systole and recoil during diastole to maintain the diastolic blood pressure. It is the pressure pulse that is responsible for the Korotkoff sounds heard when blood pressure is measured using a blood pressure cuff, and it is this impulse that is felt when the pulse is taken.

Blood Pressure Measurement

Clinically, arterial blood pressure is usually monitored by an *indirect method* using a sphygmomanometer with an *inflatable rubber bladder* connected to a *mercury manometer* or an *aneroid gauge* by means of rubber tubing (Fig. 16-2). Blood pressure is measured in *millimeters of mercury* (mm Hg).

In the measurement of blood pressure, the uninflated cuff is wrapped around an extremity, usually the upper arm, and the rubber bladder is placed superficial to the brachial artery. The cuff is then inflated to the point at which its pressure exceeds that of the artery, thus occluding blood flow. The cuff is then slowly deflated until the pressure in the vessel once again exceeds the pressure in the cuff. At this point, a small amount of blood is forced through the partially obstructed artery and, by placing a stethoscope over the artery distal to the cuff, one can audibly monitor the tapping sounds that are produced as a result.

Blood pressure is recorded in terms of both systolic and diastolic pressure, for example, 120/70 mm Hg. The *systolic pressure* reflects the initial tapping sound heard as the blood is first forced through the artery. *Diastolic pressure* reflects the point at which the sounds are no longer heard; it measures the point at which arterial pressure is sufficient to prevent vessel compression by the cuff, that is, when the vessel pressure just exceeds the cuff pressure (Fig. 16-2). The auscultatory sounds, or tapping sounds heard during blood pressure measurement, are often referred to as the Korotkoff sounds after the Russian physician who first described them. Both phases IV and V have been used to describe diastolic pressures. It has been suggested that phase IV is the best indicator of diastolic pressure.[1] When there is a marked difference between phases IV and V, it is suggested that both pressures be recorded (*e.g.*, 142/85/70). (See Chart 16-1.)

Accuracy of blood pressure measurement requires that the equipment be properly calibrated, the correct cuff size be used, the arm be properly positioned, and the cuff be inflated and deflated correctly. The room should be free of distracting noises, and the blood pressure gauge should be at eye level. The appropriate cuff size is essential for accurate blood pressure measurement—too large a cuff is apt to give low readings whereas an inappropriately small cuff may give too high a reading. In

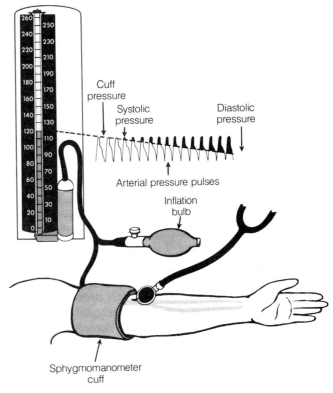

Figure 16-2   *Indirect method for measuring blood pressure. When the sphygmomanometer cuff pressure is above arterial pressure, no auscultatory sounds can be heard. As the cuff is deflated and the arterial pressure becomes greater than the cuff pressure, the blood spurts into the artery below the cuff, producing vibrations that can be heard through the stethoscope. The pressure at which the auscultatory sounds are first heard is called the systolic pressure. As the cuff is deflated, the sounds increase in intensity, then suddenly become muffled, and finally disappear. This represents phases IV and V of the Korotkoff sounds.*

Chart 16-1   *Korotkoff Sounds*

Phase I: That period marked by the first tapping sounds, which gradually increase in intensity.

Phase II: The period during which a murmur or swishing sound is heard.

Phase III: The period during which sounds are crisper and greater in intensity.

Phase IV: The period marked by distinct, abrupt muffling or by a soft blowing sound.

Phase V: The point at which sounds disappear.

---

adults, the bladder of the cuff should completely encircle the upper arm (or leg) and should be 20% wider than the diameter of the limb.[1a] The arm being used should be positioned so that the artery is at the level of the heart. Deflation should be slow enough so that accurate measurements can be obtained (2 mm Hg/beat).

Blood pressure can also be measured intra-arterially. Intra-arterial measurement requires the insertion of a catheter into a peripheral artery. The arterial catheter is connected to a pressure transducer that converts pressure into an electronic signal that can be measured and recorded (see Fig. 16-1).

Blood Pressure Measurement in Children

There are special methods for obtaining blood pressure measurements in infants and small children. Either the Doppler (ultrasonic) or the flush method is recommended for infants and children under 1 year of age. In the *Doppler method,* blood movement through the artery is interpreted audibly by a special transducer contained in the cuff. Although this method provides accurate measurement of systolic pressure, its reliability for diastolic pressures has not been established. The *flush technique* is done in the following manner: (1) a cuff of appropriate size is placed around the infant's upper arm; (2) the entire arm is elevated; (3) an elastic bandage is wrapped around the arm (from the level of the hand to the cuff), forcing blood into the upper arm; (4) at the point at which the hand becomes pale, the cuff is rapidly inflated and the elastic bandage removed; (5) the cuff is slowly deflated as with the auscultatory method. The mean arterial pressure coincides with the first evidence of a flush; as with the auscultatory method, this is the point at which blood is able to move through the partially occluded vessel.

When the auscultatory method is used for children or adolescents, it is recommended that phase IV Korotkoff sounds be used as an indicator of diastolic pressure; this is because heart sounds are often audible throughout deflation of the cuff.

In summary, blood pressure can be measured either directly or indirectly. Direct measurement requires the insertion of a catheter into an artery. Clinical measurement of blood pressure is usually done by the indirect method using a blood pressure cuff and either the auscultatory or Doppler method. Special methods of measurement are required for infants and small children.

■ Determinants of Blood Pressure

Arterial blood pressure is determined by the cardiac output (heart rate × stroke volume) and the total peripheral resistance and can be expressed as the product of the two.

$$\text{blood pressure} = \text{cardiac output} \times \text{total peripheral resistance}$$

The body maintains its blood pressure by adjusting the cardiac output to compensate for changes in total peripheral resistance, and it changes the total peripheral resistance to compensate for changes in cardiac output.

Systolic Blood Pressure

During systole the ejection of blood into the aorta raises the aortic and arterial pressures (Fig. 16-3). The extent to which the systolic pressure rises is determined by the amount of blood that is ejected into the aorta; the velocity of ejection; and the distensibility, or elasticity, of the aorta. For example, systolic pressure rises with the rapid ejection of a large stroke volume from the heart. This rise in pressure is accentuated when the aorta becomes stiffened, contributing to the rise in systolic blood pressure that is sometimes seen in elderly persons with arteriosclerosis of the aorta.

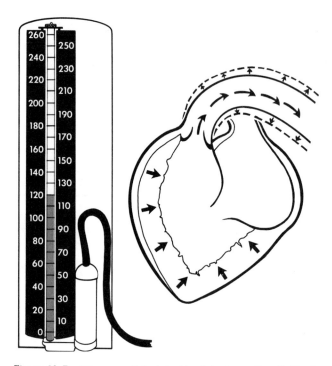

Figure 16-3 *Diagram of the left side of the heart. Systolic blood pressure results from ejection of blood into the aorta during systole; it reflects the stroke volume, the distensibility of the aorta, and the velocity with which the blood is ejected.*

Diastolic Blood Pressure

As discussed previously, diastolic pressure is maintained by the elastic recoil properties of the aorta (Fig. 16-4). The level of the diastolic blood pressure is determined largely by the condition of the arteries and their ability to accept the runoff of blood from the aorta during diastole. The vasoconstriction of the arterioles during shock increases the resistance to movement of blood out of the aorta and large arteries and serves to maintain the diastolic pressure. In atherosclerosis the arteries may become rigid and unable to stretch adequately to accept the diastolic runoff of blood from the aorta, resulting in an elevation of diastolic pressure.

Pulse Pressure

The pulse pressure (systolic pressure − diastolic pressure) is an important component of blood pressure. Because diastolic pressure remains relatively constant, the pulse pressure is usually considered to be a good indicator of stroke volume. In hypovolemic shock, for example, there is usually a marked decrease in pulse pressure. This reflects an increase in total peripheral resistance, which serves to maintain the diastolic pressure, whereas systolic pressure declines because of a decrease in stroke volume.

Mean Arterial Blood Pressure

The mean arterial blood pressure represents the average blood pressure in the systemic circulation. It is the mean arterial pressure that determines tissue blood flow. It can be estimated by adding one-third of the pulse pressure to the diastolic pressure (diastolic blood pressure + pulse pressure/3). Hemodynamic monitoring equipment in intensive care or coronary care units can usually compute mean arterial pressure automatically. Because it is a good indicator of tissue perfusion, the mean arterial pressure is often monitored along with systolic and diastolic blood pressures in critically ill patients.

In summary, blood pressure is determined by the cardiac output and the total peripheral resistance. Systolic pressure occurs at the height of the pulse pressure and diastolic pressure at the lowest point. The pulse pressure is the difference between these two pressures. The mean arterial pressure reflects the average pressure throughout the cardiac cycle. It can be estimated by adding one-third of the pulse pressure to the diastolic pressure. Systolic pressure is determined primarily by the characteristics of the stroke volume, whereas diastolic pressure is determined largely by the condition of the arteries and their ability to accept runoff from the aorta.

■ Control of Blood Pressure

Although each tissue bed is able to regulate its own blood flow, it is necessary for the arterial pressure to remain relatively constant as blood shifts from one area of the body to another. The mechanisms for regulating blood pressure are so efficient that the mean arterial pressure (in the young adult) is normally regulated within a narrow range of 90 mm Hg to 100 mm Hg. The method by which the arterial blood pressure is regulated depends on whether short-term or long-term adaptation is needed.

Short-Term Regulation of Blood Pressure

Short-term adjustments (those occurring over minutes or hours) are intended to correct temporary imbalances in blood pressure, such as those caused by postural change, exercise, or hemorrhage. They involve neural and hormonal mechanisms, the most rapid of which are the neural mechanisms.

Autonomic nervous system

The neural control centers for regulation of cardiovascular function are located in the reticular formation of the lower pons and medulla of the brain where the

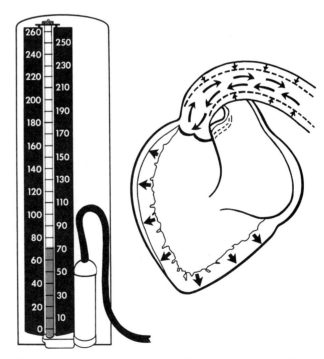

Figure 16-4 *Diagram of the left side of the heart. Diastolic blood pressure represents the pressure in the arterial system during diastole; it is largely determined by the ability of the arterial system to accept the runoff of blood that is ejected into the aorta during systole.*

integration and modulation of autonomic nervous system responses occur. The area of the reticular formation in the brain that controls vasomotor function is referred to as the *vasomotor center.*

The heart is innervated by both the parasympathetic and the sympathetic nervous systems. Increased parasympathetic activity by means of the vagus nerve causes a slowing of heart rate. The sympathetic nervous system influences both the heart rate and cardiac contractility, with increased sympathetic activity producing an increase in both heart rate and cardiac contractility.

Vascular smooth muscle is innervated by the sympathetic nervous system, and even under resting conditions the blood vessels are partially constricted. Vessel constriction and relaxation is accomplished by altering this basal tone. The parasympathetic nervous system has little, if any, control over the blood vessels.

Autonomic neurotransmitters.   The transmission of impulses in the autonomic nervous system occurs in the same manner as transmission in other neurons (Chap. 44). There are self-propagating action potentials, transmission of impulses across synapses and other tissue junctions through neurohumoral transmitters.

The main neurotransmitters of the autonomic nervous system are acetylcholine and the catecholamines: epinephrine and norepinephrine. Acetylcholine is released at all of the autonomic ganglia and at parasympathetic nerve endings. It is also released at sympathetic nerve endings that innervate the sweat glands and at cholinergic vasodilator fibers found in skeletal muscle. Norepinephrine is released at most sympathetic nerve endings. The adrenal medulla, which is an extension of the sympathetic nervous system, produces epinephrine along with small fractions of norepinephrine. Because norepinephrine is sometimes called noradrenalin and epinephrine adrenalin, sympathetic neurons are called *adrenergic neurons.* Dopamine, which is an intermediate compound in the synthesis of norepinephrine, also acts as a neuromediator. It has a vasodilator effect on renal, splanchnic, and coronary blood vessels and is sometimes used in the treatment of shock (Chap. 21).

The catecholamines are synthesized in the axoplasm of sympathetic terminal nerve endings from the amino acid tyrosine (Fig. 16-5). About 80% of the norepinephrine released during an action potential is removed from the synaptic area by an active reuptake process. This process not only terminates the action of the neuromediator but also allows it to be reused by the neuron. The remainder of the released catecholamines either diffuse into the surrounding tissue fluids or are degraded by two special enzymes: catechol-O-methyltransferase (COMT) and monoamine oxidase (MAO). Some drugs, such as the tricyclic antidepressants, are thought to increase the level of catecholamines at the site of nerve endings in the brain by blocking the reuptake process. Others, such as the MAO inhibitors, decrease the enzymatic degradation of the neuromediators and thus increase their levels. The catecholamines that are produced and released from sympathetic nerve endings are referred to as *endogenous neuromediators.* Sympathetic nerve endings can also be activated by *exogenous* forms of these neuromediators, which reach the nerve endings through the bloodstream after being injected into the body or being administered by mouth. These drugs mimic the action of the neuromediators and are said to have a *sympathomimetic* action.

Adrenergic receptors.   The responses of organs to neurotransmitters are mediated by interaction with special structures in the cell membrane called *receptors.* The receptors in sympathetic neurons are called *adrenergic receptors.* The use of pharmacologic agents that selectively stimulate or block the actions of the sympathetic nervous system has facilitated the classification of adrenergic receptors into alpha (α) and beta (β) receptors. The actions of α-adrenergic responses and β-adrenergic responses are defined in terms of their responsiveness to norepinphrine, epinephrine, and the artificially synthesized catecholamine isoproterenol. The α receptors are most sensitive to the actions of norepinephrine, and an α-adrenergic action is defined by a decreasing response to the sequence norepinephrine, isoproterenol, and epi-

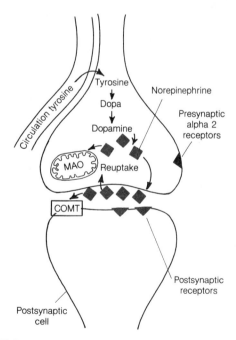

Figure 16-5 *Synthesis, reuptake, and metabolism of norepinephrine. Presynaptic alpha$_2$ receptors control norepinephrine release in the central nervous system.*

nephrine and the selective blocking of these effects by specific blocking agents. The β-adrenergic actions are characterized by a decreasing response to the sequence isoproterenol, epinephrine, and norepinephrine.[2] The beta-adrenergic actions can be eliminated by specific beta-blocking drugs such as propranolol.

In vascular smooth muscle, excitation of α receptors causes vasoconstriction, and excitation of β receptors causes vasodilatation. Both endogenously and exogenously administered norepinephrine produces marked vasoconstriction of the blood vessels in the skin, kidneys, and splanchnic circulation that are supplied with α receptors. Beta receptors are most prevalent in the heart, in blood vessels of skeletal muscle, and in the bronchioles. Blood vessels in skeletal muscle have both α and β receptors. In these vessels, high levels of norepinephrine produce vasoconstriction, and low levels produce vasodilatation. It is thought that β receptor activity predominates when norepinephrine levels are low.[2] In vessels with few receptors such as those that supply the brain and heart, norepinephrine has little effect.

Alpha-adrenergic receptors have been further subdivided into α_1 and α_2 receptors and β-adrenergic receptors into β_1 and β_2 receptors. Beta$_1$ receptors are found primarily in the heart and can be selectively blocked by β_1 receptor blockers. Beta$_2$ receptors are found in the bronchioles and in other sites that have beta-mediated functions. Alpha$_1$ receptors are found primarily in postsynaptic effector sites and appear to mediate the vasoconstrictor responses to norepinephrine. Alpha$_2$ receptors are mainly presynaptically located and can inhibit the release of norepinephrine from sympathetic nerve terminals. Alpha$_2$ receptors are abundant in the central nervous system and thought to influence the central control of blood pressure. Table 16-1 summarizes α and β receptor–mediated actions in the cardiovascular system.

Table 16-1   Responses of Cardiovascular Structures to Sympathetic Nerve Impulses

Effector Organs	Receptor Type*	Response
Heart		
SA node	β_1	Increase in heart rate
Atria	β_1	Increase in contractility and conduction velocity
AV node	β_1	Increase in automaticity and conduction velocity
Bundle of His and Purkinje system	β_1	Increase in automaticity and conduction velocity
Ventricles	β_1	Increase in contractility, conduction velocity, automaticity, and rate of idioventricular (ectopic) pacemakers
Arterioles		
Coronary	α	Constriction
	β_2	Dilatation (dilatation predominates because of metabolic autoregulatory mechanisms)
Skin and mucosa	α	Constriction
Skeletal muscle	α	Constriction
	β_2	Dilatation (vasodilatation predominates)†
Cerebral	α	Slight constriction
Pulmonary	α	Constriction
	β_2	Dilatation (dilatation predominates because of metabolic autoregulatory mechanisms)†
Abdominal organs	α	Constriction
	β_2	Dilatation (β receptor vasodilatation predominates in blood vessels of the liver and α receptor vasoconstriction predominates in blood vessels of other viscera)†
Kidney	α	Constriction
	β_2	Dilatation (α receptor vasoconstriction predominates)†
Salivary glands	α	Constriction
Veins (systemic)	α, β_2	Constriction, dilatation

*α indicates receptors found in postsynaptic receptor sites, which are mainly α_1.
†Indicates the normal physiologic range of catecholamine release.
(Developed from information in Goodman LS, Gilman A: The Pharmacological Basis of Therapeutics, 6th ed., pp 60–61. New York, Macmillan, 1980)

Neural control mechanisms

Neural mechanisms that control blood pressure include intrinsic circulatory reflexes, extrinsic reflexes, and higher center influences.[3] The intrinsic reflexes are located within the circulatory system and are essential to the short-term regulation of blood pressure. They include the baroreceptors and the chemoreceptors. The extrinsic reflexes are found outside the circulation and exert their effects through the somatic neural pathways. They include blood pressure changes observed with pain, cold, and isometric handgrip exercise. The brain pathways for these reflexes are unknown, and their responses are less consistent than the intrinsic pathways. Higher center influences include the central nervous system (CNS) ischemic response. The hypothalamus plays a key role in determining the sympathetic nervous system responses that accompany swings in mood and emotion.

Baroreceptors.   The baroreceptors are pressure-sensitive receptors located in the walls of blood vessels and the heart. The carotid and aortic baroreceptors are located in strategic positions between the heart and the brain (Fig. 16-6). The baroreceptors respond to a change in the stretch of the vessel wall by sending impulses to cardiovascular centers in the brain to effect appropriate changes in heart action and vascular smooth muscle tone. For example, a fall in blood pressure on moving from the lying to the standing position produces a decrease in the stretch of the aortic and carotid baroreceptors with a resultant increase in heart rate and vasoconstriction. The rapidity with which the baroreflex response occurs is such that a change in heart rate can often be observed within one or two heartbeats. The vasoconstrictor response may take several seconds to occur.

The carotid and aortic baroreceptors are often referred to as the high-pressure baroreceptors because they are located in the arterial side of the circulation. There are also low-pressure baroreceptors, which are located in the right atria and pulmonary artery (the low pressure side of the circulation). As with other neural receptors, the baroreceptors adapt to prolonged changes in blood pressure and are probably of little importance in the long-term regulation of blood pressure.

Chemoreceptors.   The chemoreceptors are sensitive to changes in the oxygen, the carbon dioxide, and the hydrogen ion content of the blood. The arterial chemoreceptors are located in the carotid bodies, which lie in the bifurcation of the two common carotids and in the aortic bodies of the aorta (Fig. 16-6). Because of their location, these chemoreceptors are always in close contact with the arterial blood. Although the main function of the chemoreceptors is to regulate ventilation, they also communicate with the vasomotor center and can induce widespread vasoconstriction. Whenever the arterial pressure drops below a critical level, the chemoreceptors are stimulated because of a diminished oxygen supply and a buildup of carbon dioxide and hydrogen ions. As we shall see in Chapter 23, persons with hypoxemia due to chronic lung disease may develop both systemic and pulmonary hypertension.

Central nervous system responses.   It is not surprising that the central nervous system, which plays an essential role in regulating vasomotor tone and blood pressure, would have a mechanism for controlling the blood flow to the cardiovascular centers that control circulatory function. When the blood flow to the brain has been sufficiently interrupted to cause ischemia of the vasomotor center, these vasomotor neurons become strongly excited, causing massive vasoconstriction as a means of raising the blood pressure to levels as high as the heart can pump against. This response is called the CNS ischemic response and it can raise the blood pressure to levels as high as 270 mm Hg for as long as 10 minutes.[4] The CNS ischemic response is a last-ditch stand to

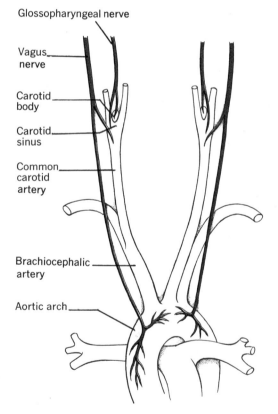

Glossopharyngeal nerve

Vagus nerve

Carotid body

Carotid sinus

Common carotid artery

Brachiocephalic artery

Aortic arch

Figure 16-6   *Location and innervation of the aortic arch and carotid sinus baroreceptors and the carotid body chemoreceptors. (Chaffee EE, Lytle IM: Basic Physiology and Anatomy, 4th ed. Philadelphia, JB Lippincott, 1980)*

preserve the blood flow to vital brain centers; it does not become activated until blood pressure has fallen to at least 50 mm Hg and it is most effective in the range of 15 mm Hg to 20 mm Hg. If the cerebral circulation is not reestablished within 3 to 10 minutes, the neurons of the vasomotor center cease to function, so that the tonic impulses to the blood vessels stop and the blood pressure falls precipitously.

The Cushing reflex is a special type of CNS reflex resulting from an increase in intracranial pressure. When the intracranial pressure rises to levels that equal intra-arterial pressure, blood vessels to the vasomotor center become compressed, initiating the CNS ischemic response. The purpose of this reflex is to produce a rise in arterial pressure to levels above intracranial pressure so that the blood flow to the vasomotor center can be reestablished.

Hormonal control mechanisms

In addition to the previously discussed neural control mechanisms, there are at least four hormonal mechanisms that contribute to the regulation of blood pressure: (1) the circulating catecholamines, epinephrine and norepinephrine, (2) the renin–angiotensin mechanism, (3) vasopressin (antidiuretic hormone), and (4) the kallikrein–kinin system.

Circulating catecholamines.   Stimulation of the sympathetic nervous system results in the release of norepinephrine and epinephrine from the adrenal gland as well as the direct stimulation of the heart and blood vessels. These neuromediators circulate in the blood for several minutes before they are inactivated and serve to prolong the effects of direct neural stimulation. They also reach areas of the circulation, such as the metarterioles, that are not directly innervated by the sympathetic nervous system but respond to the catecholamines.

Renin–angiotensin mechanism.   The renin–angiotensin mechanism regulates blood pressure through vasoconstriction and changes in body fluid volume (Fig. 16-7). Renin is an enzyme produced by the kidneys; the main stimulus for its release is a decrease in the renal blood flow. Renin combines with a circulating plasma protein, angiotensinogen, to form angiotensin I. Angiotensin I is then activated in the small vessels of the lung by a converting enzyme to form angiotensin II. Although angiotensin II is inactivated within minutes, it is one of the most potent vasoconstrictors known. Angiotensin II also has a direct effect on the kidney to decrease the elimination of salt and water, and it stimulates an increase in the release of aldosterone from the adrenal cortex to provide more long-term regulation of salt and water metabolism.

Renal kallikrein–kinin system.   Recent investigations have revealed that the renal kallikrein–kinin system may influence the regulation of blood pressure. This system involves the release of renal prostaglandins. The kinins and prostaglandins share the ability to effect salt diuresis (natriuresis) and vasodilation of the renal blood vessels.

Vasopressin.   Vasopressin, or antidiuretic hormone (ADH), is released from the posterior pituitary gland in response to decreases in blood volume and blood pressure. Its release is also mediated by the osmolality of the blood. The antidiuretic actions of vasopressin are discussed in Chapter 25. Vasopressin has a direct vasoconstrictor effect on blood vessels, particularly those of the splanchnic circulation. For this reason, the hormone may be administered when gastrointestinal hemorrhage occurs. Recent research suggests that vasopressin plays a major role in restoring blood pressure following acute blood loss.[4]

Long-Term Regulation of Blood Pressure

Both neural and hormonal regulation of blood pressure are short-term mechanisms that act rapidly to restore blood pressure. Short-term mechanisms are capable of completely correcting changes in blood pressure that occur during the performance of normal, everyday activities such as physical exercise and changes in posture. These mechanisms are also responsible for the

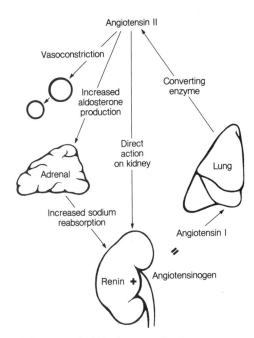

Figure 16-7 *Control of blood pressure by the renin–angiotensin–aldosterone mechanism.*

maintenance of blood pressure at survival levels during acute life-threatening situations. They are, however, ineffective in the long-term regulation of blood pressure; the day-by-day, week-by-week, and month-by-month regulation of blood pressure is vested in what Guyton terms the "renal–body fluid pressure control system."[4]

In the renal–body fluid system for the long-term regulation of blood pressure, the kidneys respond to a change in arterial pressure by either increasing or decreasing salt and water excretion. For example, an increase in arterial pressure greatly increases the rate at which both water (pressure diuresis) and sodium (pressure natriuresis) are excreted by the kidney. Figure 16-8 illustrates the control of blood pressure by renal output mechanisms. The only point on the graph at which the intake and output are balanced is at point A. At point B, where intake has increased almost fourfold, the blood pressure has increased to only 106 mm Hg, demonstrating that the kidney adjusts the output of urine to balance the input. The function of the kidney in regulating body fluids is discussed in Chapter 28.

The only way to change the long-term regulation of blood pressure using the concept of the renal–body fluid control system is to change either the pressure range of the renal output curve or the net rate of intake. For example, kidney disease, which impairs salt and water excretion, results in a shift of the curve to the right so that points A and B occur at a higher arterial pressure. It is important to consider that the renal mechanisms will control the blood volume at a level required to attain the blood pressure needed to balance the intake and output. In some situations such as hot weather, which produces vasodilatation, more volume is required to attain this balance.

It is often difficult to imagine how small a change in body fluid is needed to cause a marked change in blood pressure. For example, a 2% (about 500 ml) chronic increase in body fluid is sufficient to increase the cardiac output by 5%, the total peripheral resistance by 25% to 30%, and the blood pressure by 30% to 57%.[4] This example demonstrates how treatment measures that decrease body fluid levels can effect a reduction in blood pressure in some persons with hypertension. On the

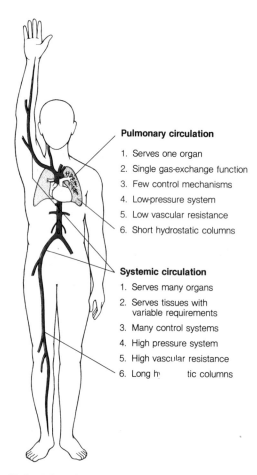

Figure 16-9 *The pulmonary and systemic circulations. There are marked differences in the systemic and pulmonary circulations that are related to the structure, function, and location of these two vascular beds. (Adapted from Rushmer RF: Structure and Function of the Cardiovascular System, 2nd ed. Philadelphia, WB Saunders, 1976)*

Pulmonary circulation

1. Serves one organ
2. Single gas-exchange function
3. Few control mechanisms
4. Low-pressure system
5. Low vascular resistance
6. Short hydrostatic columns

Systemic circulation

1. Serves many organs
2. Serves tissues with variable requirements
3. Many control systems
4. High pressure system
5. High vascular resistance
6. Long hydrostatic columns

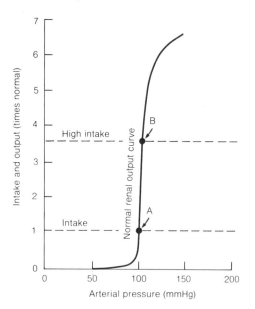

Figure 16-8 *Graphic representation of long-term regulation of blood pressure based on the renal–body fluid mechanism for pressure control. The steep part of the curve is the normal urinary output curve and indicates that a 3.5 times normal intake will only increase arterial pressure from a level of 100 mm Hg to 106 mm Hg. (Guyton A: Medical Physiology, 6th ed. Philadelphia, WB Saunders, 1981)*

other hand, it is difficult to understand how a large volume of fluid can be acutely infused into a patient without causing a marked elevation in blood pressure unless one remembers that neural reflexes such as vasodilatation and other short-term mechanisms prevent significant changes in blood pressure for short periods of time.

Pulmonary Blood Pressure

Systemic and pulmonary blood pressures vary in magnitude and function (Fig. 16-9).

To this point, the discussion has focused on blood pressure in the systemic circulation, which controls the blood flow to all parts of the body except the lungs, which are supplied by the pulmonary circulation. The pulmonary circulation is controlled in much the same manner as the systemic circulation. In this system, the right heart serves to pump blood through the lungs. The pressure in the pulmonary circulation is much lower than in the systemic circulation (22/8 mm Hg compared with 120/70 mm Hg). The pulse pressure in the pulmonary circulation is maintained at two-thirds that of the systemic circulation. The low-resistance, low-pressure characteristics of the pulmonary circulation are consistent with the close proximity of the lungs to the heart and with the single gas exchange function of the lungs. Unlike the systemic circulation, sympathetic activity has little effect on blood pressures in the pulmonary vessels.

In summary, short-term and long-term mechanisms for blood pressure control normally maintain the mean arterial blood pressure within a very narrow range of 90 mm Hg to 100 mm Hg. Short-term mechanisms occur over minutes or hours and are intended to correct temporary imbalances in blood pressure, such as those caused by postural changes, exercise, or hemorrhage. They involve neural mechanisms (autonomic nervous system responses) and hormonal mechanisms (the circulating catecholamines, the renin–angiotensin mechanism, the antidiuretic hormone, and the kallikrein–kinin system). Long-term control mechanisms affect the day-by-day, week-by-week, and month-by-month regulation of blood pressure and involve the excretion of salt and water by the kidneys (the renal–body fluid pressure control system).

The low-resistance, low-pressure characteristics of the pulmonary circulation are consistent with the close proximity of the lungs to the heart and with the single gas exchange function of the lungs. Pulmonary arterial pressure, although much lower than systemic arterial pressure, is controlled in much the same manner as systemic blood pressure.

Study Guide

After you have studied this chapter, you should be able to meet the following objectives:

☐ State the physiologic origin of the arterial pressure pulse.

☐ Compare the methods of blood pressure measurement in the adult and the small child or infant.

☐ Define systolic, diastolic, pulse, and mean arterial pressures.

☐ State the determinants of systolic, diastolic, pulse, and mean arterial blood pressures.

☐ Describe the autonomic nervous system control of blood pressure.

☐ Describe the synthesis, release, and reuptake of norepinephrine.

☐ Compare the alpha- and beta-adrenergic receptors in terms of their effect on vascular smooth muscle.

☐ Construct a diagram illustrating the neural pathways involved in the baroreflex control of the heart rate.

☐ Trace the physiology of the renin–angiotensin–aldosterone mechanism.

☐ State the effect of ADH on blood pressure regulation.

☐ Describe the effect of salt and water intake on the long-term regulation of blood pressure.

☐ Compare the characteristics of blood pressure in the systemic and pulmonary circulations.

References

1. Kirkendall WM, Burton AC, Epstein FH et al: Recommendations on Human Blood Pressure Determination by Sphygmomanometers, p 14. New York, American Heart Association, 1967

1a. Lancour J: How to avoid pitfalls in measuring blood pressure. Am J Nurs 76:773, 1976

2. Schmitt RF, Thews G: Human Physiology, p 115, 116. New York, Springer-Verlag, 1983

3. Smith JJ, Kampine JP: Circulatory Physiology, p 161. Baltimore, Williams & Wilkins, 1983

4. Guyton A: Textbook of Medical Physiology, 6th ed, pp 253, 257, 259, 260. Philadelphia, WB Saunders, 1981

Chapter 17

Alterations in Blood Pressure: Hypertension and Orthostatic Hypotension

Darlene Gene Thornhill

Carol Mattson Porth

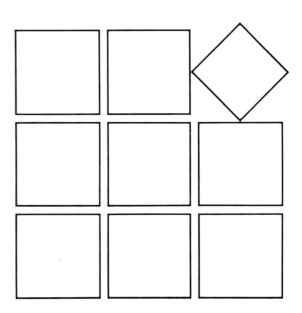

Under ordinary conditions there are moment-by-moment variations in blood pressure related to normal activities of daily living such as change in position, exercise, and emotional stress. Normally, however, blood pressure is regulated at levels sufficient to ensure adequate tissue perfusion but within a range low enough not to cause vessel damage. This chapter discusses two alterations in blood pressure regulation: hypertension and orthostatic hypotension.

■ Hypertension

Hypertension, or high blood pressure, is probably the most common of all cardiovascular disorders. More than 60 million persons in the United States have an elevated blood pressure (140/90 mm Hg or greater) or have reported being told by a physician that they have high blood pressure. The prevalence of hypertension increases with age, and the rate among black Americans is higher than among white Americans.[1] It occurs in all geographic areas of the country and affects individuals from low-, middle-, and upper-income groups. Hypertension is credited with causing 31,800 deaths annually; it takes its toll mainly through vascular complications that lead to stroke, coronary heart disease, and chronic renal failure.[2]

Hypertension is commonly divided into the categories of primary and secondary hypertension. In primary hypertension, often called essential hypertension, the chronic elevation in blood pressure occurs without evidence of other disease. In secondary hypertension, the elevation of blood pressure accompanies some other disorder, such as kidney disease. Malignant hypertension, as the name implies, is an accelerated form of hypertension. The discussion that follows focuses on these forms of hypertension, hypertension in children and the elderly, and the complications and treatment of hypertension.

The 1984 report of the Joint National Committee on Detection, Evaluation, and Treatment of High Blood Pressure of the National Institutes of Health has recommended criteria for the diagnosis of high blood pressure in those individuals aged 18 years and older.[3] The diagnosis of hypertension is made if the diastolic blood pressure measurement is 90 mm Hg or higher or the systolic blood pressure measurement is 140 mm Hg or higher when at least two blood pressure measurements are averaged on two or more successive visits. High blood pressure may be further categorized into high normal blood pressure, mild hypertension, moderate hypertension, severe hypertension, borderline isolated systolic hypertension, and isolated systolic hypertension (Table 17-1). The report emphasizes that obtaining one elevated blood pressure reading should not constitute the diagnosis of hypertension. Blood pressure measurements should be taken when the individual is relaxed and not after a stressful situation such as climbing stairs. A mercury manometer with the appropriately sized cuff or an aneroid manometer that is accurately calibrated should be utilized for blood pressure measurements. At least two measurements should be made at each visit in the same arm while the individual is seated. The diastolic pressure is recorded at the disappearance of sound, or phase V of the Korotkoff sounds.[3]

Primary, or Essential, Hypertension

Unlike secondary hypertension, which has a specific cause in each individual, essential or primary hypertension does not have a singular cause. It is a disorder of blood pressure regulation and has numerous physiologic causes, associated risk factors, and treatments.[4] Approximately 90% to 95% of those individuals with high blood pressure have essential hypertension.

Mechanisms of blood pressure elevation
A number of factors are suspected of contributing to long-term elevation of blood pressure that is characteristic of essential hypertension. These factors include hemodynamic mechanisms, neural mechanisms, and humoral and renal mechanisms. As with other disease conditions, it is improbable that a single cause is responsible for the development of essential hypertension or, for that matter, that the condition is a single disease.

Table 17-1 Classification of Blood Pressure (BP)

BP Range, mm Hg	Category*
Diastolic	
<85	Normal blood pressure
85–89	High normal blood pressure
90–104	Mild hypertension
105–114	Moderate hypertension
>115	Severe hypertension
Systolic (diastolic BP < 90)	
<140	Normal BP
140–159	Borderline isolated systolic hypertension
>160	Isolated systolic hypertension

*A classification of borderline isolated systolic hypertension (systolic BP = 140 mm Hg to 159 mm Hg) or isolated systolic hypertension (systolic BP > 160 mm Hg) takes precedence over a classification of high normal BP (diastolic BP = 85 mm Hg to 89 mm Hg) when both occur in the same person. A classification of high normal BP (diastolic BP, 85 mm Hg to 89 mm Hg) takes precedence over a classification of normal BP (systolic BP ≤ 140 mm Hg) when both occur in the same person.
(From The 1984 Report of the Joint Committee on Detection, Evaluation, and Treatment of High Blood Pressure. Arch Intern Med 144:1045, 1984)

Hemodynamic mechanisms. Arterial blood pressure reflects the interaction of two factors, cardiac output and total peripheral resistance. The question whether the hypertensive state is initiated by an increase in cardiac output or total peripheral resistance remains unanswered. Some investigators believe that an expanded blood volume and increased cardiac output precede a state of sustained hypertension.[5] According to these investigators, the enlarged cardiac output in turn produces an increase in total peripheral resistance that remains after adaptive renal mechanisms (salt and water elimination) have returned the cardiac output to normal. Other investigators believe that an increase in arterial and venular smooth muscle tone constitutes the initiating event in the development of hypertension.[6]

Neural mechanisms. Most of the hemodynamic alterations associated with essential hypertension (increased cardiac output, increased total peripheral resistance, and renin release by the kidney) can be explained in terms of an exaggerated influence of the sympathetic nervous system. The impulses that control sympathetic outflow to the heart and blood vessels are generated from various centers in the central nervous system. Currently, central nervous system mechanisms are only beginning to be understood. For example, central alpha-adrenergic receptors (see Chap. 16) are now known to inhibit the sympathetic outflow from the brain. Several of the antihypertensive medications exert their effect at this level. At present it is not known if the neural mechanisms that contribute to the development of hypertension are caused by a defect in the sympthetic nervous system or if the mechanism is reinforced or exaggerated by other factors such as sodium.

Renal and humoral mechanisms. Renal mechanisms and humoral (blood-borne) substances are known to play an essential role in the regulation of blood pressure. Normally, renal excretion of sodium and water are regulated so that the blood pressure remains within a normal range. As it rises because of increased sodium and water, there is an automatic increase in the elimination of water (diuresis) and sodium (natriuresis) by the kidney until the blood pressure returns to normal.[5] One feature of this system is that it can be altered by other factors, such as neural mechanisms (*e.g.*, sympathetic or renal nerve stimulation) and humoral influences (*e.g.*, angiotensin, aldosterone, and other adrenocorticosteroid hormones).[7] For example, secondary hypertension occurs in some forms of kidney disease resulting from increased renin levels and in primary aldosteronism due to increased production of aldosterone by the adrenal gland. Although plasma renin levels are usually normal in essential hypertension, about 25% of those with essen-

tial hypertension have what has been determined to be low renin levels. Interestingly, patients with low renin levels have normal aldosterone levels, which suggests that there is a defect in the renin-angiotensin-aldosterone feedback mechanism. Low-renin hypertensives tend to have fewer vascular complications and a better response to diuretic therapy.[8]

Of recent interest are reports of a natriuretic hormone that may affect blood pressure control. The hormone is thought to inhibit sodium transport out of cells in exchange for potassium. In the kidney, inhibition of sodium-potassium transport causes increased sodium excretion. In vascular smooth muscle it results in a net uptake of calcium and, in turn, increased vascular tone. In sympathetic neurons, the inhibition of sodium transport enhances norepinephrine release and inhibits its uptake. It is thought that some individuals who are prone to develop hypertension have a congenital or acquired defect in sodium excretion by the kidney and that excess sodium ingestion in these individuals stimulates increased secretion of the natriuretic factor as a compensatory mechanism. In these individuals, hypertension develops as a side-effect of the natriuretic hormone and its action on vascular smooth muscle and the sympathetic nervous system.[9-11]

Risk factors

Although the cause or causes of essential hypertension are largely unknown, several risk factors have been implicated as contributing to its development. These contributing factors include (1) family history, (2) advancing age, (3) race, (4) high salt intake, (5) and other life-style factors such as obesity and alcohol consumption (Chart 17-1).

Family history. The inclusion of inheritance as a contributing factor in the development of hypertension is supported by the fact that hypertension is seen most frequently among persons with a family history of hypertension. Current studies suggest that in persons with a

---

Chart 17-1   Risk Factors Associated with Development of Essential Hypertension

Family history of hypertension
Advancing age
Race
High salt intake or exaggerated response to sodium
Environmental factors
  Obesity
  Stress
  Alcohol consumption

positive family history the risk for developing essential hypertension is approximately twice that of persons with a negative family history. The inherited predisposition does not seem to rely on other risk factors, but when they are present the risk is apparently additive. This is particularly true of obesity. When obesity and a genetic predisposition are both present, the risk of developing hypertension becomes three to four times higher.[12] The pattern of inheritance is unclear, that is, it is not known whether a single gene or multiple genes are involved. Whatever the explanation, the high incidence of hypertension among close family members seems significant enough to be presented as a case for recommending that persons from so-called high-risk families be encouraged to participate in hypertensive screening programs. This recommendation should include the children from such families. It is recommended that all children 3 years and older, particularly those with a family history of hypertension, should have their blood pressure checked annually.[13]

Advancing age.   Maturation and growth are known to cause predictable increases in blood pressure. For example, in the newborn, arterial blood pressure is normally only about 50 mm Hg systolic and 40 mm Hg diastolic. Sequentially, blood pressure increases with physical growth from a value of 78 mm Hg systolic at 10 days of age to 120 mm Hg at the end of adolescence. Blood pressure usually continues to undergo a slow rate of increase during the adult years. The relationship between the aging process and hypertension is commonly accepted. The author can recall many older persons describing the normal range of blood pressure as being "100 plus your age." While this definition is not entirely correct, it is quite possible that the cardiovascular and autonomic nervous system changes that are part of the normal aging process do, in fact, contribute to the increased blood pressures observed in older persons. It must be remembered that individuals tend to age differently; this factor undoubtedly accounts for some of the great variations in blood pressure among elderly persons. However, the finding of isolated systolic hypertension is common in the elderly population and will be discussed later in this chapter.

Race.   Hypertension is not only more prevalent in blacks than in whites, it is also more severe. The mortality risk for hypertensive blacks is approximately two to three times that of the white population. There is a greater prevalence of diastolic hypertension among young black men than among young white men.[12,14] The reasons for this are largely unknown. It has been proposed that many blacks have a diet that is high in salt and low in potassium and that they may have difficulty excreting sodium.[15] It may also be that stress associated with social and economic problems contributes to the development of hypertension in blacks.

Salt.   Increased salt intake has long been suspected as an etiologic factor in the development of hypertension. The relationship between body levels of sodium and hypertension is based, at least partially, on the finding of a decreased incidence of hypertension among primitive, unacculturated people from widely differing parts of the world.[16,17] For example, among the Yanomamo Indians of northern Brazil, who excrete only about 1 mEq of sodium per day, the average blood pressure in men 40 to 49 years of age is 107/67 mm Hg and 98/62 mm Hg in women of the same age.[18] From childhood through adult life, acculturated societies consume 10 gm to 20 gm of salt daily. Drinking water may be another source of increased sodium intake; in some cities there is considerable sodium in the water supply. Of recent interest is the relationship between the feeding practices of infants who are exposed to high salt intake at a very early age and the development of hypertension. Findings from one study indicate that on a weight basis, infants consumed more sodium (through prepared formula and baby foods) than older children.[19]

Just how increased salt intake contributes to the development of hypertension is still unclear. Evidence to support individual and group susceptibility to the hypertensive effects of sodium comes from observations made from the development of a strain of spontaneously hypertensive rats. These rats develop hypertension earlier than other strains, and their hypertension is more severe when extra salt is added to their diet. It may be that salt causes an elevation in blood volume, increases the sensitivity of cardiovascular or renal mechanisms to adrenergic influences, or exerts its effects through some other mechanism such as the renin-angiotensin-aldosterone mechanism. Interestingly, it has been observed that excessive salt intake does not cause hypertension in all persons, nor does the reduction in salt intake reduce blood pressure in all hypertensives. This probably means that some people are more susceptible than others to the effects of increased sodium intake. The impact of long-term nationwide restriction of sodium consumption is not known, for example, it could create problems in persons who respond poorly to volume-depleting stresses in the absence of readily available salt in their diet.[20] Identification of persons at risk who would specifically benefit from salt reduction would facilitate hypertension management.

More recently, it has been proposed that it may be the ratio of sodium to potassium intake, rather than sodium intake alone, that influences blood pressure.[15] A high-potassium diet does not alter blood pressure in individuals with normal blood pressure but tends to lower blood pressure in hypertensive individuals.[21-23] It has been suggested that food preparation today involves not only the addition of salt but the leaching out of potassium as a result of modern cooking methods in which cooking water is discarded.

The interrelationship of high blood pressure, calcium, and magnesium levels is also being investigated. Studies suggest that reduced consumption of calcium and magnesium is associated with an increased risk of developing hypertension and cardiovascular disease.[24]

Obesity. Excessive weight is commonly observed in association with hypertension. In a large nationwide screening program of more than a million persons, it was found that the frequency of hypertension in overweight persons 20 to 39 years of age was double that of persons of normal weight and triple that of underweight persons.[25] The exact manner in which obesity contributes to the development of hypertension is largely unknown, although it may be that mechanisms responsible for elevating blood pressure in the overweight person are related to the metabolic needs of the excess adipose tissue, along with the increased demands on the cardiovascular system to provide adequate blood flow through the enlarged body mass. It is also quite possible that the dietary habits of the overweight person include the ingestion of excessive amounts of salt along with increased caloric intake. Hyperinsulinemia (excess insulin in the blood), which reduces sodium excretion and causes neuroendocrine disturbances such as abnormalities of the sympathetic nervous system, may also contribute to the development of hypertension in obese individuals.[26] Whatever the cause, it is known that weight loss is effective in reducing blood pressure in a significant number of obese hypertensive individuals. It is important to emphasize, however, that any beneficial effects of weight reduction will probably be determined by the duration and severity of the hypertension and its residual damaging effects on the circulatory system.

Stress. Physical and emotional stress undoubtedly conributes to transient alterations in blood pressure. Studies in which arterial blood pressure was continually monitored on a 24-hour basis as individuals performed their normal activities showed marked fluctuations in pressure associated with normal life stresses—increasing during periods of physical discomfort and family crisis and declining during rest and sleep.[27] As with other risk factors, the role of stress-related episodes of transient hypertension in producing the chronically elevated pressures seen in essential hypertension is still speculative. It may be that vascular smooth muscle hypertrophies with increased activity in a manner similar to that of skeletal muscle or that the central integrative pathways in the brain become adapted to the frequent stress-related input.

Psychologic techniques involving biofeedback, relaxation, and transcendental meditation have emerged as methods to control alterations in blood pressure. It is still too early to tell whether these techniques will offer information about the role of stress in the production of hypertension or will prove useful in its treatment.

Alcohol consumption. A study of close to 84,000 persons with known drinking habits at the Oakland-San Francisco Kaiser-Permanente Medical Care Program revealed an interesting relationship between alcohol consumption and blood pressure;[28] regular consumption of three or more alcoholic drinks per day increases the risk of hypertension. Systolic blood pressures were more markedly affected in persons with increased alcohol consumption than the diastolic pressures. The interaction between alcohol abuse, changes in blood pressure, and deranged mineral metabolism are complex. The loss of one mineral may affect the metabolism of several others, and a hemodynamic effect may stimulate a hormonal effect.[29,30] Vasoconstrictor hormones, renin, aldosterone, and catecholamines rise after acute alcohol intake and during withdrawal. Only recently has the link between alcohol consumption and hypertension come to light, and it is expected that further studies will shed more light on this relationship.

High blood pressure in children

The incidence of high blood pressure in children is not known. One reason for this uncertainty is that blood pressure measurement in children has been a neglected part of the physical examination. According to one survey, only 5% of children in three large outpatient clinics had their blood pressures measured during a physical examination.[31] Although there has been some change in these figures, the extent of change is not known. Lauer (1975) found a 1.2% incidence of high blood pressure in children ages 6 to 9 and a 12.2% incidence in adolescents of 14 to 18 years.[32] Secondary causes of high blood pressure are more common in children and are usually related to some other health problem such as kidney disease. There is a greater incidence of essential hypertension among adolescents; probably as much as 25% of adolescent hypertension can be labeled essential.[33] The risk factors associated with essential hypertension are similar to those in the adult—a family history of hypertension, increased salt intake, and obesity.

The National Heart, Lung, and Blood Institute (NHLBI) convened a task force to review the situation, consult with experts in the field, and develop recommendations for evaluation and treatment of high blood pressure in children.[34] The task force developed a grid of blood pressures for children ages 2 to 18 years (Fig. 17-1), based on readings obtained from more than 11,000 normal children. It recommended that the term "high normal blood pressure" be used to describe an otherwise healthy child with a single systolic and diastolic pressure reading above the 95th percentile; it was also recommended that these children be reexamined. The term "sustained elevated blood pressure" was suggested to describe those children whose reading is above the 95th percentile on four separate consecutive occasions. The original "Report of the Task Force on Blood Pressure Control in Children" was published in 1977.[34] A revised report is scheduled for publication in 1985. The new nomograms will incorporate the child's height and weight along with age in providing blood pressure ranges.[35] The reader is referred to these reports and to other readings for further discussion.

Hypertension in the elderly

Isolated systolic hypertension (systolic pressure greater than 160 mm Hg and diastolic pressure less than 90 mm Hg) is considered an abnormal clinical finding in old age.[36] It is found in approximately 25% to 30% of men and women over age 75.[37] For years this form of hypertension was considered innocuous and was not treated. The results of the Framingham study have shown, however, that there is approximately a twofold to fivefold increase in death from cardiovascular disease associated with isolated systolic hypertension.[36a] Appropriate treatment methods for this form of hypertension are currently being investigated.

Data from the Framingham study also indicate that hypertension, whether systolic or diastolic, is a risk factor for cardiovascular morbidity and mortality in older as well as younger persons.[37] Stroke is two to three times more common in elderly hypertensives than with age-matched normotensive subjects.[38,39] Hypertension may also be an etiologic factor in senile dementia when it is due primarily to vascular disease.[36]

The aging processes that tend to increase blood pressure are stiffness of the arteries, decreased baroreceptor sensitivity, increased peripheral resistance, and decreased renal blood flow. Normally, other aging processes such as an increased volume capacity of the aorta, decrease in blood volume, and a decrease in cardiac output tend to counteract the rise in pressure.[39] The disproportionate rise in systolic pressure that is observed in some elderly persons is explained by the increased rigidity of the aorta and peripheral arteries that accompanies the aging process; this is caused by a loss of elastic fibers in the media; increase in the amount of collagen, calcium deposition in the media, and atheroma formation in the intima.[40,41] Normally the elastic properties of the aorta allow it to stretch during systole as a means of buffering the rise in pressure that occurs as blood is ejected from the heart. Then, during diastole the recoil of the elastin fibers serves to transmit the stored pressure to the peripheral arterioles as a means of maintaining the diastolic blood pressure. As the aorta loses its elasticity

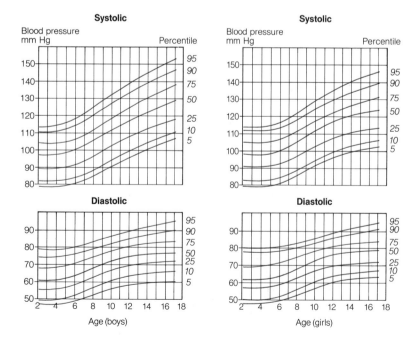

Figure 17-1 Percentiles of blood pressure measurement in boys and girls (right arm, seated). (High Blood Pressure Information Center, 120/80, NIH, Bethesda, MD)

and becomes more rigid with aging, the pressure generated during ventricular systole is transmitted to the peripheral arteries practically unchanged.

Blood pressure measurement methods require special considerations in the elderly. The indirect measurement of blood pressure (using a blood pressure cuff and the Korotkoff sounds) has been reported to give falsely elevated readings of diastolic pressure as much as 15 mm Hg to 30 mm Hg higher than direct intra-arterial measurements.[42] On the other hand, in elderly persons with hypertension, a silent interval, called the auscultatory gap, may occur between the end of the first and beginning of the third phases of the Korotkoff's sounds, providing the potential for underestimating the systolic pressure, sometimes by as much as 50 mm Hg.[41] Since the gap occurs only with auscultation, it is recommended that a preliminary determination of systolic blood pressure be made by palpation and the cuff then be inflated above this value for the auscultatory measurement of blood pressure. It is also recommended that the cuff be deflated slowly to avoid missing the first Korotkoff's sounds.

There is often a transient fall in blood pressure during the first 2 to 3 minutes of standing, after which reflex-mediated increases in heart rate and total peripheral resistance (vascular constriction) normally return the blood pressure to normal values. Because these reflexes are often less responsive in the elderly and may be impaired by hypertensive medications, it has been recommended that blood pressure be recorded 2 to 5 minutes after assumption of the standing position as well as in the supine and seated positions. This should be done not only during pretreatment examinations but during follow-up examinations once treatment has been instituted. This is done to detect the complication of postural hypotension that can occur with some medications.[36]

Signs and symptoms

Essential hypertension is frequently asymptomatic, and diagnosis is often made by chance during screening procedures or when an individual seeks medical care for other purposes. Although headache is often considered to be an early symptom of hypertension, it is present only in a small number of hypertensives at the time of diagnosis. When present, the headache associated with hypertension is believed to be due to intense vasodilatation. It occurs most frequently on awakening and is usually felt in the back of the head or neck. A common early symptom of long-term hypertension is nocturia, which indicates that the kidney is losing its ability to concentrate urine. Epistaxis (nosebleeds), tinnitus (ringing in the ears), and vertigo (dizziness), although often claimed to be characteristic of hypertension, have been found to be no more frequent among persons with recognized hypertension than among those with normal blood pressures.

Other commonly associated signs and symptoms are probably related to the complications of hypertension—the long-term effects of blood pressure elevation on other organ systems in the body, such as the kidneys, eyes, heart, and blood vessels.

Aside from elevated blood pressure measurements, there are few diagnostic tests that are useful in detecting and diagnosing essential hypertension. In this respect, the increased availability of hypertensive screening clinics provides a means for early detection. The reader is reminded that blood pressure varies in response to stress, time of day, and other factors; therefore, a diagnosis of essential hypertension is never based on a single blood pressure reading. Contributing factors such as a family history of hypertension or the presence of obesity often assist in confirming the diagnosis. Laboratory tests, x-ray films, and other diagnostic tests are usually done to rule out secondary hypertension or associated complications.

Effects

The complications and mortality associated with primary and secondary hypertension can be explained as the increased wear and tear on the heart and blood vessels.

The increase in the work load of the left ventricle as it pumps against the elevated pressures in the systemic circulation is directly related to the degree and duration of the hypertension. This increased work is the stimulus for ventricular muscle hypertrophy and it increases the heart's need for oxygen. If the increased work demands exceed the heart's compensatory efforts, heart failure occurs because the heart can no longer pump effectively. Heart failure is discussed in Chapter 20. The individual who develops coronary artery disease along with hypertension is at especially high risk, because the heart's oxygen transport facilities are impaired in the presence of increased oxygen needs. Surprisingly, many individuals seem to tolerate elevated levels of blood pressure for many years before its detrimental effects on cardiac function are detected. The hypertrophied left ventricle is usually visible on an x-ray film and shows a characteristic left axis deviation on the electrocardiogram.

Arteries and arterioles throughout the body experience the effects of the mechanical stress associated with hypertension. Again, it is the severity and duration of the increase that largely determine the extent of vascular changes. In general, hypertension has been implicated in accelerating the development of atherosclerosis, which causes a narrowing of the vessel lumen, and in weakening the vessels. Also, there is greater risk of aortic aneurysm, coronary heart disease, renal complications, retinopathy, and cerebral vascular disease.

Secondary Hypertension

Only 5% to 10% of hypertensive cases are currently classified as secondary hypertension—that is, hypertension due to another disease condition. In secondary hypertension, as with other alterations in physiologic function, the presence of an elevation in blood pressure may be a homeostatic response that is recruited in an effort to maintain body function at least partially; or the elevated pressure may be due to an actual alteration in body structures that control or affect blood pressure. The disease states that most frequently give rise to secondary hypertension are (1) kidney disease, (2) vascular disorders, (3) alterations in endocrine function and hormone levels, and (4) acute brain lesions. To avoid duplication in descriptions, the mechanisms associated with elevations of blood pressure in these disorders are discussed briefly, and a more detailed discussion of specific disease disorders is reserved for other sections of the book.

Renal disease

With the dominant role that the kidney assumes in blood pressure regulation, it is not surprising that the largest single cause of secondary hypertension is renal disease (for further discussion of hypertension in renal disease see Chapter 30). By controlling salt and water levels, the kidney is probably involved in virtually all types of hypertension. In renal disease, salt and water retention undoubtedly plays a major role in elevated blood pressure. Also implicated in the development of renal hypertension is an imbalance between the vasoconstrictor and vasodepressor substances produced by the kidney.

The classic Goldblatt kidney experiments of the 1930s showed that renal ischemia contributes to the development of hypertension through the renin-angiotensin-aldosterone mechanism. In these experiments hypertension occurred regularly in animals in which one renal artery was constricted to produce renal ischemia. These experiments revealed that the ischemic kidney secretes large amounts of renin; this secretion leads to formation of angiotensin II and an aldosterone-mediated increase in salt and water retention by the nonischemic kidney. There is also evidence that the kidneys produce one or more vasodepressor substances. The most likely candidate for this action is a member of the prostaglandin family, although other substances such as kallikrein, a neutral lipid from the medulla of the kidney, and bradykinin have also been suggested. The data are inconclusive, but continuing research will probably bring further insight.

Vascular disorders

Arteriosclerosis.   As mentioned earlier in this chapter, hypertension itself predisposes to vascular disorders and vascular pathology tends to produce or perpetuate hypertension. The effects of arteriosclerosis on blood pressure are generally interpreted as changes in total peripheral resistance. In arteriosclerosis of the aorta and large arteries, the rigid vessel walls resist the runoff of blood ejected from the heart during systole, so the blood pressure rises and remains elevated during diastole. When renal blood vessels are affected, additional renal mechanisms contribute to the blood pressure elevation. The exaggerated vascular changes seen in malignant hypertension are discussed later in this chapter.

Coarctation of the aorta.   An unusual form of hypertension occurs in coarctation of the aorta (adult form) in which there is a narrowing of that vessel as it exits from the heart, most commonly beyond the subclavian arteries (see Chap. 19). In the infantile form, the narrowing occurs proximal to the ductus arteriosus, in which case heart failure and other problems are present. As a result, many affected babies die within their first year of life. In the adult form of coarctation there is often an increase in cardiac output that results from renal compensatory mechanisms. The ejection of a large stroke volume into a narrowed aorta with limited ability to accept the runoff results in an increase in systolic blood pressure and blood flow to the upper part of the body. Blood pressure in the lower extremities may be normal, although it is frequently low. For this reason, blood pressures in the legs may be assessed as a screening method for this disorder. The pulse pressure in the legs is almost always narrowed and the femoral pulses are weak. Because the aortic capacity is diminished, there is usually a marked increase in systolic pressure (measured in the arms) during exercise when both stroke volume and heart rate are exaggerated.

Alterations in endocrine function

Secondary hypertension due to endocrine disorders is rare; when it does occur it is usually of adrenal origin and involves either the adrenal medullary or cortical tissue.

Pheochromocytoma.   A *pheochromocytoma* is a tumor of chromaffin tissue usually found in the adrenal medulla; but it may also arise in other sites where there is chromaffin tissue, such as the sympathetic ganglia. Like adrenal medullary cells, the tumor cells of a pheochromocytoma produce and secrete the catecholamines epinephrine and norepinephrine. Thus, the hypertension results from the massive release of these catecholamines. Often their release is paroxysmal rather than continuous, causing periodic episodes of hypertension, tachycardia, sweating, anxiety, and other signs of excessive sympathetic activity. Several tests are available to differentiate this type of hypertension from other types.

Currently the most commonly used diagnostic measure is the determination of urinary catecholamines and their metabolites, including vanillylmandelic acid (VMA).

Elevated levels of adrenocortical hormones.   Increased levels of *adrenal cortical hormones* can also give rise to hypertension. Both primary hyperaldosteronism (excess production of aldosterone by the adrenal cortex) and excess levels of glucocorticoids (Cushing's disease or syndrome) tend to raise the blood pressure (see Chap. 38). These hormones facilitate salt and water retention by the kidney; the hypertension that accompanies excessive levels of either hormone is probably related to this factor. It has been observed that in primary hyperaldosteronism a salt-restricted diet often brings the blood pressure down. Because aldosterone acts on the distal renal tubule to promote sodium exchange for the potassium lost in the urine, persons with hyperaldosteronism usually have decreased potassium levels. The drug spironolactone is an aldosterone antagonist and is therefore used in the medical management of patients with an excess of this hormone; the drug increases sodium excretion and potassium retention.

Pregnancy and contraceptive medications.   About 1 out of every 15 pregnancies is accompanied by hypertension resulting from preeclampsia, eclampsia, or other forms of hypertension. The triad of hypertension (blood pressures above 140/90 on at least two occasions, 6 or more hours apart), or a rise in systolic pressure of at least 30 mm Hg or in diastolic pressure of at least 15 mm Hg over previously known blood pressures, proteinuria (300 mg/liter in 24 hours), and edema (weight gain in excess of 2 lb/week) developing after the 20th week of pregnancy is a classic finding in preeclampsia. Eclampsia is an exaggerated form of preeclampsia that has progressed to include convulsions and possibly coma.

Preeclampsia, or toxemia of pregnancy, is seen most frequently in young teenage primigravidae (first pregnancy), in diabetics, in pregnant women with multiple fetuses, and in women with hydatidiform moles. Preeclampsia disappears spontaneously within about 48 hours after the pregnancy is terminated. No specific causes of preeclampsia or the hypertension that symbolizes its presence have been established. It is known that renin levels are reduced in preeclampsia and that plasma levels of aldosterone and desoxycorticosterone fall considerably, although not back to the prepregnant state. The observed decrease in both renin and aldosterone has prompted questions about the advisability of routine salt restriction and frequent use of diuretics during pregnancy. For a more thorough discussion of toxemias of pregnancy, the reader is referred to an appropriate text.

Oral contraceptives are known to cause hypertension. Why this is true is largely unknown, although it has been suggested that increased sodium retention, plasma volume, and weight gain, along with changes in the level and action of renin, angiotensin, and aldosterone may play a part. The fact that the various contraceptive drugs contain different amounts and combinations of estrogen and progestational agents may contribute to the varying incidence of hypertension among pill users. Fortunately, the hypertension associated with contraceptives usually disappears once the drugs have been discontinued. Reduction to normal may require as much as 6 months. However, in some women the blood pressure may not return to normal, and it may be that they are among that portion of the population that was at risk for developing hypertension.

Brain lesions.   The hypertension associated with brain lesions is usually of short duration and should be considered a protective homeostatic mechanism. It is mentioned here because it tells us quite a bit about intracranial pressure and cerebral blood flow. The brain and other cerebral structures are located within the rigid confines of the skull with no room for expansion, and any increase in intracranial pressure tends to compress the blood vessels that supply the brain. Because adequate blood flow is essential to life, it is not surprising that brain lesions that increase intracranial pressure and impede cerebral blood flow trigger a vasoconstrictor response (the Cushing reaction) designed to elevate blood pressure as a way to restore blood flow to the brain. This flow is reestablished when the arterial pressure increases to a level higher than the increase in the intracranial pressure that caused the compression of the vessels. Should the intracranial pressure rise to the point that the blood supply to the vasomotor center becomes inadequate, vasoconstrictor tone is lost, and the blood pressure begins to fall.

Treatment

In *secondary hypertension*, efforts are made to correct or control the disease condition that is the cause of the hypertension. Antihypertensive medications and other treatment measures supplement the treatment of the underlying disease.

For some individuals, restriction of dietary sodium, weight loss, and efforts to reduce stress factors may be sufficient to control the blood pressure in *essential hypertension*. When changes in life-style are ineffective or inappropriate, antihypertensive medications are often prescribed. The medications fall into three categories: (1) diuretics, (2) sympathetic inhibitors, and (3) vasodilators (Table 17-2).

Table 17-2 Actions and Side-Effects of Antihypertensive Drugs†

Drug	Actions	Frequent Side-Effects (greater than 5%)*
Sympathetic Inhibitors		
Rauwolfia alkaloids (reserpine)	Acts centrally and peripherally; causes depletion of catecholamines	Nasal congestion, drowsiness, sedation, *depression,* increased appetite, and weight gain*
Methyldopa (Aldomet)	Reduces the level of neurotransmitter in the central and peripheral nervous system	Fatigue, drowsiness, and sedation; postural and exercise dizziness; dry mouth and headache; may cause abnormal liver function tests and positive direct Coombs' test*
Prazosin Hydrochloride (Minipres)	Smooth muscle relaxant; alpha-adrenergic blocker which acts directly on peripheral arterioles	Dizziness, postural hypotension, syncope, weakness, palpitations, drowsiness, lack of energy, weakness, nausea, and vomiting; patients usually started on low initial dose to avoid severe syncope*
Clonidine (Catapres)	Diminishes sympathetic outflow from the brain	Dry mouth, drowsiness, sedation, fatigue, dizziness, and vertigo; dry mouth and constipation; *sudden discontinuance of the drug may result in hypertensive crisis*
Guanabenz (Wytensin)	Diminishes sympathetic outflow from the brain	Drowsiness, sedation, dizziness, weakness, dry mouth, headache; *sudden discontinuance of the drug may lead to hypertensive crisis.*
Propranolol (Inderal)	Adrenergic beta receptor blocking drug (central and peripheral); reduces cardiac output and renin release	Nausea, anorexia, fatigue, dizziness, lightheadedness, bradycardia; blocks beta receptors on bronchioles and can cause bronchospasm in predisposed persons; may intensify hypoglycemia in diabetics on insulin or oral agents*
Guanethidine (Ismelin)	Postganglionic sympathetic blocking agent	Orthostatic hypotension, bradycardia, diarrhea, muscular weakness and fatigue, nasal stuffiness, edema, weight gain, headaches, inhibition of ejaculation, impotence, elevation of BUN and creatinine*
Vasodilators		
Hydralazine hydrochloride (Apresoline)	Reduces the total peripheral resistance by relaxing smooth muscle in the arterioles	Headache, nausea, vomiting, tachycardia, palpitations, dizziness, weakness, lethargy, and postural hypotension*
Minoxidil (Loniten)	Smooth muscle relaxant; action most pronounced at level of arterioles	Fluid retention, angina, tachycardia, hair growth (hypertrichosis) of face and extremities*
Converting Enzyme Inhibitors		
Captopril (Capoten)	Inhibits conversion of angiotensin I to angiotensin II and breakdown of the vasodilators bradykinin and prostaglandins	Rash, flushing, taste impairment, hypotension

*(Based on data from McMahon FG: Management of Essential Hypertension. Mount Kisco, Futura Publishing, 1978)
†The actions of diuretic drugs are given in Chapter 25, Table 25-1.

Diuretics, such as the thiazides, spironolactone, triamterene, and amiloride, produce a decrease in vascular volume that helps reduce blood pressure. Of the four, the thiazides appear to have a direct blood pressure lowering effect that is separate from their diuretic action.

Sympathetic inhibitors act at various levels of the sympathetic nervous system. They decrease sympathetic outflow from the brain; they decrease the level of sympathetic neuromediators that are available; or they block transmission of impulses at the sympathetic ganglia or peripheral nerve endings. Inhibition of sympathetic activity often affects functions other than those related to blood pressure; it also tends to enhance parasympathetic nervous system activity. Thus, a number of the side-effects of these drugs are related to the altered autonomic responses they induce—either decreased sympathetic or increased parasympathetic function.

Vasodilator drugs promote a decrease in the total peripheral resistance by causing relaxation of vascular smooth muscle, particularly the arterioles. These drugs often stimulate tachycardia as a result of the decreased filling of the vascular compartment.

Several drugs are under investigation for use in the treatment of hypertension, including new beta-adrenergic blocking drugs and enzyme inhibitors, which prevent conversion of angiotensin I to angiotensin II. Captopril is one of the converting enzyme inhibitors that has recently been released for use.[43]

Calcium-channel blocking drugs (slow channel blocking agents or calcium antagonists) have been approved by the FDA for use in the treatment of hypertension. These drugs inhibit the movement of calcium ions into myocardial and smooth muscle cells. They probably reduce blood pressure by several mechanisms, including a reduction in cardiac output or reduction of smooth muscle tone in the venous or the arterial systems.[44] Some calcium blockers have a direct myocardial effect that reduces the cardiac output through a decrease in cardiac contractility and fall in heart rate. Other drugs influence venous tone and reduce the cardiac output through a decrease in venous return. Still others influence arterial vascular smooth muscle by either inhibiting calcium transport across the membrane channels or inhibiting the vascular response to norepinephrine or angiotensin.

There are at least three factors that the physician usually considers when prescribing drugs to control hypertension: (1) the drug is not highly toxic and causes minimal side-effects, (2) the cost of the drug is not prohibitive, and (3) the procedure for taking the medication is compatible with the patient's life-style, that is, he or she may take antihypertensive drugs once a day but may refuse (or forget) to comply with a plan that requires taking medications more frequently. More than one drug may be prescribed to take advantage of drug synergism; that is, each of the drugs enhances the action of the others so that none needs to be prescribed in high doses.

The Joint National Committee on Detection, Evaluation, and Treatment of High Blood Pressure[3] has recommended a stepwise approach to the treatment of hypertension. Step 1 involves the initiation of a thiazide-type diuretic or a beta blocker. If blood pressure control is not achieved, step 2 is initiated. Either a small dose of an adrenergic-inhibiting medication or a small dose of a diuretic is added to the initial medication dependent on the drug that was used for step 1 therapy. If the blood pressure remains elevated, a step 3 medication (vasodilator) is added to the other two medications that were prescribed in steps 1 and 2. When necessary, guanethidine is added as a step 4 drug to achieve blood pressure control. The purpose of the stepped care approach is to achieve blood pressure control with the least amount of medication and the fewest side-effects for the least cost. The specific drugs recommended for each step are not cited in this discussion because newer drugs undoubtedly will become available, which may or may not fit the stepwise approach.[3]

Malignant Hypertension

Five to 10% of persons with essential and secondary hypertension develop an accelerated and potentially fatal form of the disease—malignant hypertension. This is usually a disease of younger persons, particularly young black men, women with toxemias of pregnancy, and persons with renal and collagen diseases.

Malignant hypertension is characterized by marked elevations in blood pressure with diastolic values above 120 mm Hg, encephalopathy, renal disorders, vascular changes, and retinopathy. There may be intense arterial spasm of the cerebral arteries with hypertensive encephalopathy. Cerebral vasoconstriction is probably an exaggerated homeostatic response designed to protect the brain from excesses of blood pressure and flow. The regulatory mechanisms are often insufficient to protect the capillaries, and cerebral edema frequently develops. As it advances, papilledema (swelling of the optic nerve at its point of entrance into the eye) ensues, giving evidence of the effects of pressure on the optic nerve and retinal vessels. There may be headache, restlessness, confusion, stupor, motor and sensory deficits, and visual disturbances. In severe cases convulsions and coma follow.

Prolonged and severe exposure to exaggerated levels of blood pressure in malignant hypertension injures the walls of the arterioles, and intravascular coagulation and fragmentation of red blood cells may occur. The renal blood vessels are particularly vulnerable to hypertensive damage. In fact, renal damage due to vascular changes is probably the most important prognostic determinant in malignant hypertension. Elevated levels of blood urea nitrogen and serum creatinine, metabolic acidosis, hypocalcemia, and proteinuria provide evidence of renal impairment.

The complications associated with hypertensive crisis demand immediate and rigorous medical treatment. With proper therapy, the death rate from this cause can be markedly reduced, as can further episodes. Two drugs to treat hypertensive emergencies are mentioned here, although others also may be required to bring the blood pressure down to a safe level. These two drugs—diazoxide, which causes arteriolar dilatation, and sodium nitroprusside, a vasodilator that also affects the venous system—are administered intravenously.

In summary, hypertension is a chronic health problem that presently affects about one out of every five Americans. It may present as a primary disorder or may be a symptom of some other disease. The incidence of hypertension increases with age, is seen more frequently in men than women, and is more prevalent among blacks. It is also linked to a family history of the disorder, obesity, and increased salt intake. Because hypertension is often silent, hypertension screening programs provide an effective means of early detection. The importance of screening lies in the fact that hypertension can usually be controlled and its complications prevented or minimized with appropriate treatment measures.

■ Orthostatic Hypotension

The term *orthostatic hypotension* refers to a fall in both systolic and diastolic blood pressure on standing. In the absence of normal baroreflex function, blood pools in the lower part of the body when the standing position is assumed, cardiac output falls, and blood flow to the brain is inadequate. Dizziness, fainting, or both may then occur.

When the upright position is assumed, there is usually a momentary shift in blood to the lower part of the body with an accompanying fall in central blood volume and arterial pressure. Normally, this fall in blood pressure is transient, lasting through several cardiac cycles. This is because the baroreceptors located in the thorax and carotid sinus area sense the fall in blood pressure and initiate reflex constriction of the veins and arterioles as well as an increase in heart rate that brings blood pressure back to normal. Within a few minutes of standing, blood levels of ADH and sympathetic neuromediators increase as a secondary means of ensuring maintenance of normal blood pressure in the standing position. Muscle movement in the lower extremities also aids venous return to the heart by pumping blood out of the legs.

In persons with healthy blood vessels and normal autonomic function, cerebral blood flow is usually not reduced in the upright position unless arterial pressure falls below 70 mm Hg. The strategic location of the arterial baroreceptors between the heart and brain is designed to ensure that the arterial pressure is maintained within a range sufficient to prevent a reduction in cerebral blood flow.

Causes

In orthostatic hypotension, the mean arterial and pulse pressure are decreased by at least 30 mm Hg to 35 mm Hg after 10 minutes of standing.[45] It has been reported to occur with (1) increased age, (2) decreased blood volume, (3) defective autonomic function, (4) severe varicose veins, and (5) immobility or impaired function of the skeletal muscle pumps.

Aging
Weakness and dizziness on standing are common complaints of the elderly. It has been reported that about 10% of persons over the age of 65 have a fall in systolic pressure of 20 mm Hg or more on assumption of the upright position.[46] Since cerebral blood flow is primarily dependent on systolic pressure, patients with impaired cerebral circulation may experience symptoms of weakness, ataxia, dizziness, and syncope when their arterial pressure falls even slightly. This may happen in older persons who are immobilized for brief periods of time or whose blood volume is decreased due to inadequate fluid intake or overzealous use of diuretics.

Fluid deficit
Orthostatic hypotension is often an early sign of fluid deficit. When blood volume is decreased, the vascular compartment is only partially filled; although cardiac output may be adequate when a person is in the recumbent position, it often decreases to the point of causing weakness and fainting when the person assumes the standing position. Common causes of orthostatic hypotension related to hypovolemia are (1) excessive use of diuretics, (2) excessive diaphoresis, (3) loss of gastrointestinal fluids through vomiting and diarrhea, and (4) loss of fluid volume associated with prolonged bed rest.

Autonomic dysfunction
The sympathetic nervous system plays an essential role in adjustment to the upright position. Sympathetic stimulation increases heart rate and cardiac conractility and causes constriction of peripheral veins and arterioles. Orthostatic hypotension caused by altered autonomic function is common in peripheral neuropathies associated with diabetes mellitus, following injury or disease of the spinal cord, or as the result of a cerebral vascular accident in which sympathetic outflow from the brain stem is disrupted. Another cause of autonomically mediated orthostatic hypotension is the use of drugs that interfere with sympathetic activity (Table 17-3).

Bed rest
With prolonged bed rest there is a reduction in plasma volume, a decrease in venous tone, failure of peripheral vasoconstriction, and weakness of the skeletal muscles of

Table 17-3 Drugs Known to Cause Orthostatic Hypotension*

Drug Groups	Specific Drugs	Mechanism of Action
Antihypertensive drugs	Pentolinium (Ansolysen) Trimetapahn (Arfonad)	Blocks transmission of sympathetic impulses at the autonomic ganglia
	Guanethidine (Ismelin)	Blocks sympathetic impulses at the postganglionic sites
	Methyldopa (Aldomet) Clonidin (Catapres)	Decreases sympathetic outflow from the central nervous system
	Hydralazine (Apresoline) Prazosin (Minipres) Minoxidil (Loniten)	Direct vasodilator action
Antiparkinson drugs	Levodopa preparation Amantadine (Symmetrel)	Vasodilatation due to beta-adrenergic stimulation or alpha blockade of the peripheral vascular system
Antipsychotic drugs	Chlorpromazine (Thorazine) Thiethylperazine (Torecan) Thioridazine (Mellaril)	Loss of reflex vasoconstriction due to blocking of alpha receptors; these drugs also impair sympathetic outflow from the brain
Calcium channel blockers	Diltiazem (Cardizem) Nifedipine (Procardia) Verapamil (Calan, Isoptin)	Direct vasodilator action
Tricyclic and related antidepressant drugs	Amitriptyline (Elavil, Endep, Amitid, Amtril, others) Amoxapine (Asendin) Desipramine (Norepramine, Pertofrane) Doxepin (Adapin, Sinequan) Imipramine (Tofranil, Imavate, others) Nortriptyline (Aventyl, Pamelor) Maprotiline (Ludiomil) Traxodone (Desyrel)	Blocks norepinephrine uptake in central adrenergic neurons, with a resultant increase in stimulation of central alpha-adrenergic receptors, causing a decrease in peripheral sympathetic nervous system activity
Vasodilator drugs	Nitrates (nitroglycerin and long-acting nitrates)	Direct vasodilator action

*This list is not intended to be inclusive; it encompasses some of the widely prescribed drugs.

the veins, which help return blood to the heart. Orthostatic intolerance is a recognized problem of space flight—a potential risk upon reentry into the earth's gravitational field. Physical deconditioning follows even short periods of bed rest. After 3 to 4 days, the blood volume is decreased. Loss of vascular and skeletal muscle tone is less predictable but probably becomes maximal after about 2 weeks of bed rest.

Idiopathic orthostatic hypotension

Idiopathic orthostatic hypotension is unrelated to drug therapy or pathologic conditions. It may be of two types: (1) idiopathic orthostatic hypotension not accompanied by other signs of neurologic deficits and (2) idiopathic hypotension accompanied by multiple neurologic deficits (Shy-Drager syndrome). The Shy-Drager syndrome is characterized by upper motor neuron damage with uncoordinated movements, urinary incontinence, constipation, and other signs of neurologic pathology.

Diagnosis and Treatment

Orthostatic hypotension can be assessed with the blood pressure cuff. A reading should be made when the patient is supine, immediately upon assumption of the seated or upright position, and at 2- to 3-minute intervals for a period of 10 to 15 minutes. It is strongly recommended that a second person be available when blood pressure is measured in the standing position, to prevent injury should the patient become faint. A tilt table can also be used for the purpose. With a tilt table, the patient is recumbent, while the table is tilted so that the patient is in a head-up position.

Treatment of orthostatic hypotension is usually directed toward alleviating the cause or, if this is not possible, toward helping the patient cope. Correcting the fluid deficit and trying a different antihypertensive medication are examples of measures designed to correct the cause. Measures designed to help the patients cope are (1) gradual ambulation, that is, sitting on the edge of the bed for several minutes before standing, to allow the circulatory system to adjust, (2) avoidance of situations that encourage excessive vasodilatation (such as drinking alcohol or exercising vigorously in a warm environment), and (3) avoidance of excess diuresis (use of diuretics), diaphoresis, or loss of body fluids. Tight-fitting elastic support hose or an abdominal support garment may help prevent pooling of blood in the lower extremities and abdomen.

In summary, orthostatic hypotension refers to an abnormal fall in both systolic and diastolic blood pressures that occurs on assumption of the upright position. Among the factors that contribute to its occurrence are (1) advanced age, (2) decreased blood volume, (3) defective function of the autonomic nervous system, (4) severe varicose veins, and (5) the effects of immobility.

■ Study Guide

After you have studied this chapter, you should be able to meet the following objectives:

☐ Cite the current definition of hypertension as cited by the Joint National Committee on Detection, Evaluation, and Treatment of Hypertension.

☐ Define systolic hypertension.

☐ Describe the possible influence of age, race, family history, and environment on essential hypertension.

☐ State the postulated roles of obesity, stress, and salt intake in hypertension.

☐ Cite the criteria for diagnosis of hypertension in children.

☐ Describe consideration for blood pressure measurement in the elderly.

☐ Differentiate essential, or primary, hypertension from secondary hypertension.

☐ Relate renal disease to the occurrence of hypertension.

☐ Describe the relationship between arteriosclerosis and blood pressure.

☐ State the role of aortic coarctation in the development of hypertension.

☐ Explain the role of catecholamines in the development of hypertension.

☐ State the parameters used to determine the presence of preeclampsia.

☐ Explain why the vasoconstrictor response is protective in brain lesions.

☐ Describe the effects of malignant hypertension on the vascular system.

☐ List the advantages of the stepped care approach to treatment of hypertension.

☐ List the three categories of drugs used to treat hypertension and the chief characteristics of each.

☐ Cite a definition for orthostatic hypotension.

☐ Describe the pathologic changes that culminate in orthostatic hypotension.

☐ State why older persons are more likely than younger ones to experience orthostatic hypotension.

☐ State the relationship between orthostatic hypotension and fluid deficit.

☐ Describe the mechanisms of drug action that may induce orthostatic hypotension.

☐ Describe treatment measures in orthostatic hypotension.

■ References

1. Rowlands M, Roberts J: Blood pressure levels in persons 6-74 years: United States 1967-1980, Advancedata. National Center for Health Statistics No 84, US Dept of Health and Human Services, Public Health Service, October 8, 1982

2. Heart Facts 1984. Dallas, American Heart Association, 1982

3. The 1984 Report of the Joint National Committee on Detection, Evaluation, and Treatment of High Blood Pressure. Arch Intern Med 144:1045, 1984

4. Gross F, Guyton AC, Lever AF et al: Cardiac output and volume in hypertension. Clin Sci 57:59s, 1979

5. Guyton AC, Hall JE, Lohmeier TE et al: The ninth JAF Stevenson memorial lecture: The many roles of the kidney in arterial pressure control and hypertension. Can J Physiol Pharmacol 59:513, 1981

6. Frohlich ED: Mechanisms contributing to hypertension. Ann Intern Med 98 (Pt 2): 709, 1983

7. Genst J: Volume hormones and hypertension. Ann Intern Med 98 (pt 2): 744, 1983

8. Kaplan NM: Clinical Hypertension, 2nd ed, p 299. Baltimore, Williams & Wilkins, 1978

9. New natriuretic hormone, Key to essential hypertension? Hosp Pract 19, No 9:39, 1983

10. Blaustein MP, Hamlyn JM: Role of natriuretic factor in essential hypertension: An hypothesis. Ann Intern Med 98 (Pt 2): 785, 1983

11. Haddy FJ: Sodium-potassium pump in low-renin hypertension. Ann Intern Med 98 (Pt 2): 781, 1983

12. Stamler J, Stamler R, Riedinger WF et al: Hypertension screening in 1 million Americans. JAMA 235, 21:2299, 1976

13. Recommendations of the Task Force on Blood Pressure Control in Children. Pediatrics 59, No 5 (Suppl): 797, 1977

14. Itskovitz HF, Kochar MS, Anderson AJ et al: Patterns of blood pressure in Milwaukee. JAMA 238, 8:864, 1977

15. Langford HG: Hypertension in blacks. Cardiovasc Clin 9, 1:323, 1978

16. Berglund G: The role of salt in hypertension. Acta Med Scand (Suppl) 672:117, 1983

17. Hunt JC: Sodium intake and hypertension: A cause for concern. Ann Intern Med 98 (Pt 2): 724, 1983

18. Oliver WJ, Cohen EL, Neel JV: Blood pressure, sodium intake, and sodium related hormones in the Yanomamo Indians, a "no-salt" culture. Circulation 52, 1:146, 1975

19. Berensen GS, Voors AW, Frank GC et al: Studies of blood pressure and dietary sodium intake in children in semirural southern United States: The Bogalusa Heart Study. In Fregly MJ, Kare MR (eds): The Role of Salt in Cardiovascular Hypertension, pp 49-62. New York, Academic Press, 1982

20. Laragh JH, Pecker MS: Dietary sodium and essential hypertension: Some myths, hopes, and truths. Ann Intern Med 98 (Pt 2): 735, 1983

21. Meneely GR, Battarbee HD: High sodium-low potassium environment and hypertension. Am J Cardiol 38:768, 1976

22. Lanford HG: Dietary potassium and hypertension: Epidemiologic data. Ann Intern Med 98 (Pt 2): 770, 1983

23. Fregly MJ: Estimates of sodium and potassium intake. Ann Intern Med 98 (Pt 2): 792, 1983

24. McCarron DA: Calcium and magnesium in human hypertension. Ann Intern Med 98 (Pt 2): 800, 1983

25. Stamler R, Stamler J, Riedlinger WR: Weight and blood pressure. JAMA 240, 15:1607, 1978

26. Dustan HP: Mechanisms of hypertension associated with obesity. Ann Intern Med 98 (Pt 2): 860, 1983

27. Bevan AT, Hanour AJ, Stott FH: Direct arterial pressure recording in unrestricted man. Clin Sci 36:329, 1969

28. Klatsky AL, Freidman GD, Siegelaub AB: Alcohol consumption and blood pressure. N Engl J Med 296, 21:1194, 1977

29. Beevers DB, Bannan LT, Saunders JB: Alcohol and hypertension. Contrib Nephrol 30:92, 1982

30. Kaysen G, Noth RH: The effects of alcohol on blood pressure and electrolytes. Med Clin North Amer 68, No 1:221, 1984

31. Pazdral PT, Lieberman HM, Pazdral WE et al: Awareness of pediatric hypertension: Measuring blood pressure. JAMA 235, 21:2320, 1976

32. Lauer RM, Connor WE, Leaverton PS et al: Coronary heart disease risk factors in school children: The Muskatine Study. J Pediatr 86:696, 1975

33. Adelman RD: Elevated blood pressures in infants and children. J Fam Pract 6, 2:360, 1978

34. National Heart, Lung and Blood Institute: Report of the Task Force on Blood Pressure Control in Children. Pediatrics 59:797, 1977

35. Personal communication, Michael Horan, MD. Hypertension and Kidney Branch National Heart, Blood, and Lung Institute. National Institute of Health, Bethesda, MD, 1984

36. Statement on hypertension in the elderly. US Department of Health and Human Services, Revised April 1980

36a. Kannel WB, Dawber TR, McGee DL: Perspectives on systolic hypertension: The Framington study. Circulation 61:1179, 1980

37. Kannel WB, Gordon T: Evaluation of cardiovascular risk in the elderly: The Framingham Study. Bull NY Acad Med 54:573, 1978

38. Ostfeld AM, Shekelle RB, Klawans H et al: Epidemiology of stroke in an elderly welfare population. Am J Public Health 64:450, 1974

39. Shekelle RB, Ostfeld AM, Klawans HI Jr: Hypertension and risk of stroke in an elderly population. Stroke 5:71, 1974

40. Kohn RR: Heart and cardiovascular system. In Finch CE, Hayflick L: (eds) Handbook of the Biology of Aging, pp 300-301. New York, Van Nostrand Reinhold, 1977

41. Niarchos AP, Laragh JH: Hypertension in the elderly: Pathophysiology. Mod Concepts Cardiovasc Dis 9:49, 1980

42. Spence JD, Sibbald WJ, Cape RD: Psydeohypertension in the elderly. Clin Sci 55:399s, 1978

43. Swartz Sl, Williams GH: Angiotensin-converting enzyme inhibition and prostaglandins. Am J Cardiol 49:1405, 1982

44. Cohn JN: Calcium, vascular smooth muscle, and calcium entry blockers in hypertension. Ann Internal Med 98 (Pt 2): 806, 1983

45. Ziegler MG, Lake CR, Kopin IJ: The sympathetic nervous-system deficit in primary orthostatic hypotension. N Engl J Med 296, 6:293, 1977

46. Johnson RH et al: Effect of posture on blood pressure in elderly patients. Lancet 731, 1965

◼ Additional References

Hypertension

Agras S: Relaxation therapy and hypertension. Hosp Pract 17:129, 1983

Bear RA, Erenrich N: Essential hypertension and pregnancy. Can Med Assoc J 118, No 8:936, 1978

Beauchamp GK, Bertino M, Engelman K: Modification of salt taste. Ann Intern Med 98:763, 1983

Bravo EL, Gifford RW: Pheochromocytoma: Diagnosis, localization, and management. N Engl J Med 311, No 20:1298, 1984

Chobanian AV: Pathophysiologic considerations in the treatment of the elderly hypertensive patient. Am J Cardiol 52:49D, 1983

Daniels L, Kochar MS: Monitoring and facilitating adherence to hypertension therapeutic regimens. Cardio-Vasc Nurs 16, No 2:7, 1980

Davidman M, Opsahl J: Mechanisms of elevated blood pressure in human essential hypertension. Med Clin North Am 68, No 2:301, 1984

Ferris TF: The kidney and hypertension. Arch Intern Med 142:1889, 1982

Franklin SS: Geriatric hypertension. Med Clin North Am 67, No 2:395-417, 1983

Friedman GD, Klatsky AL, Siegelaub AB: Alcohol intake and hypertension. Ann Intern Med 98:846, 1983

Frishman WH: Atenolol and Timolol: Two new systemic-adrenoceptor antagonists. N Engl J Med 306, No 24:1456, 1982

Frishman WH: Pindolol: A new-adrenoceptor antagonist with partial agonist activity. N Engl J Med 308, No 16:940, 1983

Gifford RW et al: The dilemma of "mild" hypertension. JAMA 250, No 23:3171, 1983

Gillum RF et al: Nonpharmacologic therapy of hypertension: The independent effects of weight reduction and sodium restriction in overweight borderline hypertensive patients. Am Heart J 106, No 1:128, 1983

Green KG: The role of hypertension and downward changes of blood pressure in the genesis of coronary atherosclerosis and acute myocardial ischemic attacks. Am Heart J 103, No 4:579, 1982

Harburg E et al: Skin color, ethnicity, and blood pressure I: Detroit blacks. Am J Public Health 68, No 12:1177, 1978

Hartshorn JC: What to do when the patient's in hypertensive crisis. Nursing '80 10, No 7:37, 1980

Havlik RJ et al: Weight and hypertension. Ann Intern Med 98:855, 1983

Jones MB: Hypertensive disorders of pregnancy. J Obstet Gynecol Neonatal Nurs 8, No 2:92, 1979

Kannel WB, Sorlie P, Gordon T: Labile hypertension: A faulty concept: The Framingham study. Circulation 61, No 6:1183, 1980

Kaplan NM: Hypertension: Prevalence, risks, and effect of therapy. Ann Intern Med 98:705, 1983

Kaplan NM: Renal dysfunction in essential hypertension. N Engl J Med 309, No 17:1052, 1983

Lieberman E: Hypertension in childhood and adolescence. Clin Symp 30, No 3:3, 1978

Luft FC et al: Estimation of dietary sodium intake in children. Pediatrics 73, No 3:318, 1984

Marcinek MB: Hypertension: What it does to the body. Am J Nurs 80, No 2:928, 1980

Messerli FH: Essential hypertension in the elderly: Haemodynamics, intravascular volume, plasma renin activity, and circulating catecholamine levels. Lancet 2 (8357):983, 1983

Perloff D, Sokolow M, Cowan R: The prognostic value of ambulatory blood pressures. JAMA 249, No 20:2792, 1983

Reisin E et al: Effect of weight loss without salt restriction on the reduction of blood pressure in overweight hypertensive patients. N Engl J Med 298, No 1:1, 1978

Stamler R et al: Family (parental) history and prevalence of hypertension. JAMA 241, No 1:43, 1979

Tarazi RC: Pathophysiology of essential hypertension: Role of the autonomic nervous system. Am J Med 72:2-8, 1983

Thurnau GR et al: The development of a profile scoring system for early identification and severity assessment of pregnancy-induced hypertension. Am J Obstet Gynecol 146, No 4:406-416, 1983

Tunbridge RDG, Donnai P: Pregnancy-associated hypertension, a comparison of its prediction by "roll-over test" and plasma noradrenaline measurement in 100 primigravidae. Br J Obstet Gynaecol 90:1027-1032, 1983

Vardan S et al: Systolic hypertension in the elderly: Hemodynamic response to long-term Thiazide diuretic therapy and its side effects. JAMA 250, No 20:2807-2813, 1983

Vidt DG, Bravo EL, Fouad FM: Captopril. N Engl J Med 306, No 4:214-220, 1982

Orthostatic hypotension

Adelman EM: When the patient's blood pressure falls: What does it mean? What do you do? Nursing '80 10, No 2:26, 1980

Hickler RB: Orthostatic hypotension and syncope. N Engl J Med 296, No 6:336, 1977

Johnson RH, Smith AC, Spalding JMK et al: Effect of posture on blood pressure in elderly patients. Lancet:731, 1965

Mooss AN, Sketch MH: Orthostatic hypotension: Evaluation and therapy. Hosp Med 15, No 12:16, 1979

Moss AJ, Glaser W, Topol E: Atrial tachypacing in the treatment of a patient with primary orthostatic hypotension. N Engl J Med 302, No 26:1456, 1980

Myers MG, Kearns P, Shedletsky R et al: Postural hypotension and mental function in the elderly. Can Med Assoc J 119:1061, 1978

Chapter 18

Control of Cardiac Function

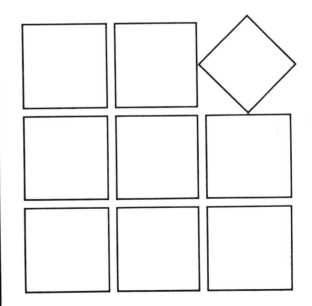

The heart is a four-chambered muscular pump about the size of a man's fist that beats an average of 70 times a minute, 24 hours a day, 365 days a year for a lifetime. In one day this pump moves over 1800 gallons of blood throughout the body, and the work performed by the heart over a lifetime would lift 30 tons to a height of 30,000 feet. In this chapter, the embryonic development of the heart, its overall structure and function, and diagnostic methods for assessing cardiac function are discussed.

■ Functional Anatomy of the Heart

The heart is located between the lungs, in the mediastinal space of the intrathoracic cavity, within a loose-fitting sac called the pericardium. It is suspended by the great vessels, with its broader side (base) facing upward and its tip (apex) pointing downward, forward, and to the left. The heart is positioned obliquely, so that the right heart is almost fully in front of the left heart with only a small portion of the lateral left ventricle on the frontal plane of the heart (Fig. 18-1). The impact of the heart's contraction is felt against the chest wall at a point between the fifth and sixth ribs, a little below the nipple and about 3 inches to the left of the midline. This is called the point of maximum impulse (PMI).

The heart is divided longitudinally into a right and a left pump, each composed of two muscular chambers: a thin-walled atrium, which serves as a reservoir for blood coming into the heart, and a thick-walled ventricle, which pumps blood out of the heart. The two halves of the heart are separated by the interatrial and interventricular septa.

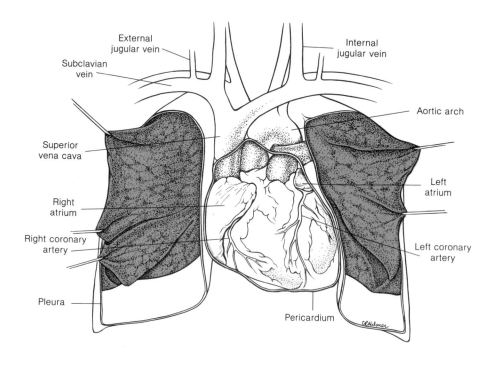

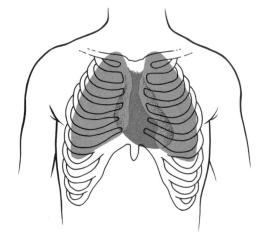

Figure 18-1 (Top) *Anterior view of the heart and great vessels;* (bottom) *position of the heart in relation to the skeletal structures of the chest cage.*

The right heart delivers blood to the lungs where the blood is oxygenated and carbon dioxide is removed. Because of the close proximity of the lungs to the heart and the low resistance to flow in the pulmonary circulation, the right heart operates as a low-pressure pump (pulmonary artery pressure is about 22/8 mm Hg).

In contrast to the right heart, which functions as a low-pressure pump, the left heart must pump blood throughout the entire systemic circulation. Because of the distance the blood must travel and the resistance to blood flow, this side must operate as a high-pressure system (systemic arterial blood pressure is approximately 120/70 mm Hg). The increased thickness of the left ventricular wall results from the additional work that this ventricle is required to perform.

Although the right and the left heart function under different pressure requirements, both must pump the same amount of blood over a period of time. This concept has a particular meaning in relation to both right-sided and left-sided heart failure (Chap. 20).

Embryonic Development of the Heart

The heart is the first functioning organ in the embryo; its first pulsative movements begin during the third week following conception. This early development of the heart is essential for the rapidly growing embryo, because the embryo soon outgrows its ability to meet its nutritional and elimination needs through diffusion alone.

The developing heart begins to function as a single tubular structure and then rapidly undergoes a series of synchronized folding and positional changes as both it and the embryo continue to grow and develop (Fig. 18-2). As it changes externally, the tubular embryonic heart also changes internally, partitioning into two parts, a right and a left heart.

The atrial and ventricular septa divide the tubular heart into separate right and left hearts. The development of a closed ventricular septum is usually completed by the end of the seventh week. The formation of a closed atrial septum is more complex and closure does not occur until after birth. During the formation of the atrial septum, an opening called the foramen ovale develops to establish a communicating channel between the two upper chambers of the heart. This opening allows blood from the umbilical vein to pass directly into the left heart, bypassing the lungs (Fig. 18-3). As the lungs expand following birth, the pulmonary and systemic circulations separate into two systems and the foramen ovale closes.

Separation of the heart occurs as the tissue bundles, called the *endocardial cushions,* begin to form in the midportion of the dorsal and ventral walls and grow inward. As the endocardial cushions enlarge, they meet and fuse

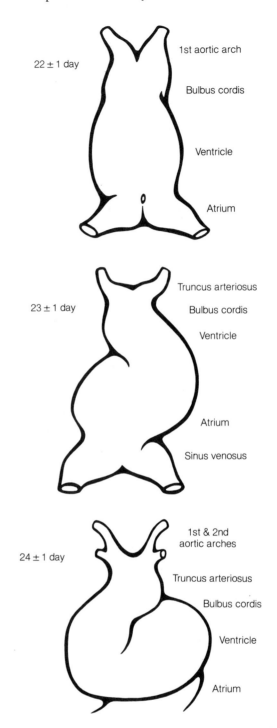

Figure 18-2 *Ventral views of the developing heart (20–25 days). (Adapted from Moore KL: The Developing Human, 2nd ed. Philadelphia, WB Saunders, 1977)*

to form a right and left atrioventricular channel (Fig. 18-4). It is in these channels that the mitral and tricuspid valves develop.

To complete the transformation into a four-chambered heart, provision must be made for separating the

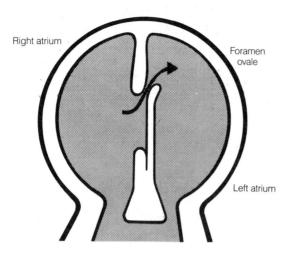

Figure 18-3 *The foramen ovale. (Adapted from Moore KL: The Developing Human, 2nd ed. Philadelphia, WB Saunders, 1977)*

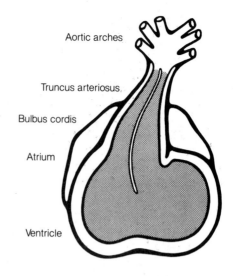

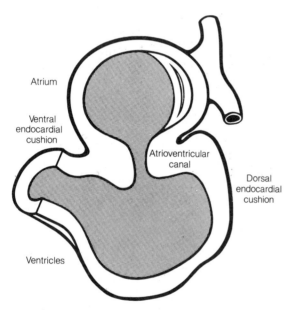

Figure 18-4 *Development of the endocardial cushions. (Adapted from Moore KL: The Developing Human, 2nd ed. Philadelphia, WB Saunders, 1977)*

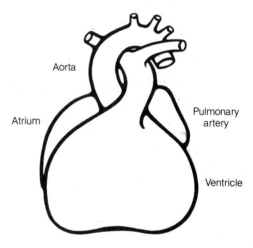

Figure 18-5 *Separation and twisting of the truncus arteriosus to form the pulmonary artery and aorta. (Adapted from Moore KL: The Developing Human, 2nd ed. Philadelphia, WB Saunders, 1977)*

blood pumped from the right heart, which is to be diverted into the pulmonary circulation, from the blood pumped from the left heart, which is to be pumped to the systemic circulation. This separation of blood flow is accomplished by developmental changes in the outlet channels of the tubular heart, the bulbus cordis and the truncus arteriosus, which undergo spiral twisting and vertical partitioning (Fig. 18-5). In the process of forming a separate pulmonary trunk and aorta, the ductus arteriosus arises to allow the blood entering the pulmon-

ary trunk to be shunted into the aorta as a way of bypassing the lungs. Like the foramen ovale, the ductus arteriosus usually closes shortly after birth.

Structures of the Heart

The wall of the heart is composed of an outer epicardium, which lines the pericardial cavity, a fibrous skeleton, the myocardium or muscle layer, and the smooth endocardium, which lines the chambers of the heart.

Pericardium

The pericardium forms a fibrous covering around the heart, holding it in a fixed position in the thorax. It provides both physical protection and a barrier to infec-

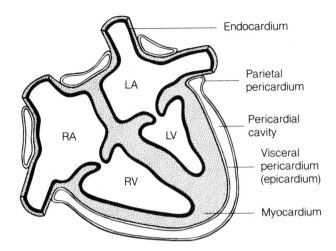

Figure 18-6   *The layers of the heart showing the visceral pericardium, the pericardial cavity, and the parietal pericardium.*

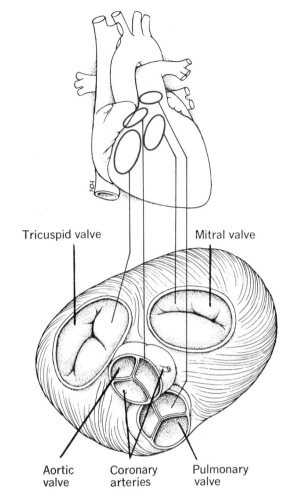

Figure 18-7   *Fibrous skeleton of the heart, which forms the four interconnecting valve rings and support for attachment of the valves and insertion of cardiac muscle. (Chaffee EE, Lytle IM: Basic Physiology and Anatomy, 4th ed. Philadelphia, JB Lippincott, 1980)*

tion. The pericardium consists of a tough outer fibrous layer and an inner serous layer. The outer layer is attached to the great vessels that enter and leave the heart, the sternum, and the diaphragm. The fibrous pericardium is highly resistive to distention; it prevents acute dilatation of the heart chambers and exerts a restraining effect on the left ventricle. The serous layer consists of a visceral layer and a parietal layer. The visceral layer, also known as the epicardium, covers the entire heart and great vessels and then folds over to form the parietal layer that lines the fibrous pericardium (Fig. 18-6). Between the visceral and parietal layers is the pericardial cavity, a potential space containing 5 ml to 30 ml of serous fluid that acts as a lubricant to minimize friction as the heart contracts and relaxes.

Fibrous skeleton

An important structural feature of the heart is its fibrous skeleton, which consists of four interconnecting valve rings and surrounding connective tissue. It separates the atria and ventricles and forms a rigid support for attachment of the valves and insertion of the cardiac muscle (Fig. 18-7). The top of the valve rings are attached to the muscle masses of the atria, pulmonary trunks, and aorta. The bottoms are attached to the ventricular walls.

Myocardium

The myocardium, the muscular portion of the heart, includes the atrial and ventricular muscle fibers (which contract in a manner similar to skeletal muscle) and the specialized muscle fibers of the conduction system (which contract only slightly). Cardiac muscle cells have properties somewhere between those of skeletal and smooth muscle. They are small striated and branched

cells with interconnecting fibers (Fig. 18-8). The cell membranes of the interconnecting fibers fuse to form tight junctions, or intercalated disks, which are low-resistance pathways for the passage of ions and electrical currents from one cardiac cell to another. The myocardium therefore behaves as a single unit, or syncytium, rather than as a group of isolated units, as does skeletal muscle. When one myocardial cell becomes excited, the impulse travels rapidly to all of the other cells.

Endocardium

The endocardium is a thin, three-layered membrane that lines the heart. The innermost layer consists of smooth endothelial cells supported by a thin layer of connective tissue. The endothelial lining of the endocardium is continuous with the lining of the blood vessels that enter

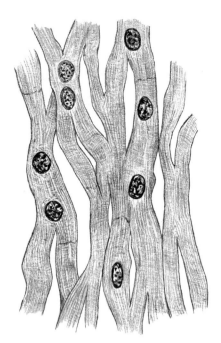

Figure 18-8　*Cardiac muscle. Branching fibers, centrally placed nuclei, and intercalated disks can be seen. (Chaffee EE, Lytle IM. Basic Physiology and Anatomy, 4th ed. Philadelphia, JB Lippincott, 1980)*

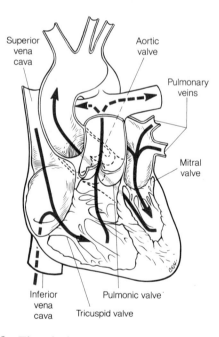

Figure 18-9　*The valvular structures of the heart. The atrioventricular valves are in an open position and the semilunar valves are closed. There are no valves to control the flow of blood at the inflow channels (vena cava and pulmonary veins) to the heart.*

and leave the heart. The middle layer consists of dense connective tissue with elastic fibers. The outer layer, composed of irregularly arranged connective tissue cells, contains blood vessels and branches of the conduction system and is continuous with the myocardium.

Heart valves

In order for the heart to function effectively, blood must move forward through its chambers. This directional control is provided by the heart's two atrioventricular (tricuspid and mitral) and two semilunar (aortic and pulmonic) valves (Fig. 18-9).

The atrioventricular (AV) valves control the flow of blood between the atria and the ventricles. The thin edges of the AV valves form cusps, two on the left (bicuspid) side of the heart and three on the right (tricuspid) side. The bicuspid valve is also known as the mitral valve. The atrioventricular valves are supported by the papillary muscles, which project from the wall of the ventricles, and the chordae tendineae, which attach to the valve. Contraction of the papillary muscles at the onset of systole ensures closure by producing tension on the leaflets of the AV valves before the full force of ventricular contraction pushes against them. The chordae tendineae are cordlike structures that support the AV valves and prevent them from turning inside out and everting into the atria during systole.

The aortic valve controls the flow of blood into the aorta; the pulmonic valve controls blood flow into the pulmonary artery. The aortic and pulmonic valves are often referred to as the semilunar valves because their flaps are shaped like half-moons. Both the pulmonic and aortic valves have three leaflets shaped like little teacups. These cuplike structures collect the retrograde, or backward, flow of blood that occurs toward the end of systole, enhancing closure. For the development of a perfect seal along the free edges of the semilunar valves, each valve cusp must have a triangular shape when it is closed, which is caused by a nodular thickening at the apex of each leaflet (Fig. 18-10). The openings for the coronary arteries are located in the aorta just above the aortic valve.

There are no valves at the atrial sites (venae cavae and pulmonary veins) where blood enters the heart. This means that excess blood will be pushed back into the veins when the atria become distended. For example, the jugular veins often become prominent in severe right-sided heart failure when they normally should be flat or collapsed. Likewise, the pulmonary venous system becomes congested when outflow from the left atrium is impeded.

In summary, the heart is a four-chambered muscular pump that lies in the pericardial sac within the mediastinal space of the intrathoracic cavity. The embryonic development of the heart occurs during weeks 3 to 8 following conception. During this time, development of the atrial and ventricular septa divides the embryonic tubular heart into a right heart and a left heart. The endocardial cushions develop to form the AV valves, which separate the atria and ventricles. The wall of the heart is composed of an outer epicardium, which lines the pericardial cavity; a fibrous skeleton; the myocardium, or muscle layer; and the smooth endocardium that lines the heart. The right heart pumps blood to the pulmonary circulation and the left heart pumps blood to the systemic circulation. The four heart valves control the direction of blood flow as it moves through the heart. The AV valves control the flow of blood between the atria and ventricles; the pulmonic valve controls the flow of blood from the right ventricle into the pulmonary artery; and the aortic valve controls the flow of blood from the left ventricle into the aorta. There are no valves at the atrial sites (venae cavae and pulmonary veins) where blood enters the heart; blood flows into the heart along a pressure gradient.

■ Conduction System and Electrical Activity of the Heart

Heart muscle differs from skeletal muscle in its ability to generate and rapidly conduct its own action potentials (electrical impulses). This unique rhythmic property allows the heart to continue beating independently of the nervous system.

In certain areas of the heart, the myocardium has been modified to form the specialized cells of the conduction system. Although most myocardial cells are capable of initiating and conducting impulses, it is the heart's conduction system that maintains its pumping efficiency. Specialized pacemaker cells *generate* impulses at a faster rate than other types of heart tissue, and the conduction tissue *transmits* impulses at a faster rate than other types of heart tissue. It is because of these properties that the conduction system is able to control the rhythm of the heart.

Each cardiac contraction is initiated by an impulse that originates in the sinoatrial (SA) node, which is located in the posterior wall of the right atrium near the entrance to the superior vena cava. The SA node is called the *pacemaker* of the heart because it has the fastest inherent firing rate in the conduction system. Impulses from the SA node travel through the atria to the atrioventricular (AV) node (Fig. 18-11). There are at least four intra-atrial pathways, including Bachmann's bundle, that connect the SA and AV nodes.[1]

The heart has essentially two separate conduction systems—one controls atrial activity and the other con-

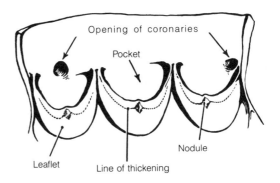

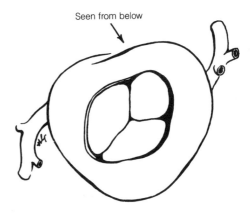

Figure 18-10   (Top) *The three leaflets of the aortic valve as they appear when the aorta is cut open and spread out flat. Note that the openings of the coronary arteries are located just above this valve.* (Bottom) *The appearance of the aortic valve in its closed position, as seen from below. (Ham H, Cormack DH: Histology, 8th ed. Philadelphia, JB Lippincott, 1979)*

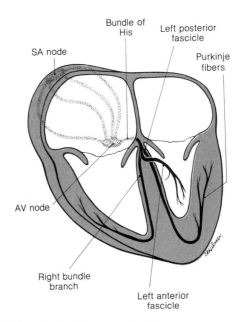

Figure 18-11   *Conduction system of the heart.*

trols ventricular activity. These two systems are connected by the AV node. Within the AV node, atrial fibers connect with the very small junctional fibers of the node itself. The velocity of conduction through these fibers is very slow (about 1/25th that of normal cardiac muscle), which greatly delays transmission of the impulse into the AV node.[2] A further delay occurs as the impulse travels through the AV node into the transitional fibers and finally into the bundle of His (also called the AV bundle). The delay in transmission of impulses through the AV node is important in that it allows the atria to empty before the ventricle contracts. Because the AV node provides the only connection between the two conduction systems, the atria and the ventricles will beat independently of each other if the transmission of impulses through the AV node is blocked.

The Purkinje system, which supplies the ventricles, has large fibers that allow for rapid conduction and almost simultaneous excitation of the entire right and left ventricles. This rapid rate of conduction throughout the Purkinje system is necessary for the rapid and efficient ejection of blood from the heart. The Purkinje fibers originate in the AV node and then form the bundle of His, which extends through the fibrous tissue between the valves of the heart and into the ventricular system. The bundle of His divides almost immediately into right and left bundle branches as it reaches the interventricular septum. The bundle branches move through the subendocardial tissues toward the papillary muscles and then subdivide into the Purkinje fibers that branch out and supply the outer walls of the ventricle. The left bundle branch fans out as it enters the septal area and divides further into two segments: the left posterior and left anterior fascicles.

Cardiac Muscle Contraction

Cardiac muscle, like skeletal muscle, is composed of sarcomeres containing myosin and actin filaments (see discussion of muscle tissue in Chap. 1).

Calcium ions are of particular importance in the regulation of cardiac muscle contraction. During an action potential, calcium is released from the sarcoplasmic reticulum and the transverse (T) tubules; these ions diffuse into the area of the actin and myosin filaments where they provide the signal for the contraction process to begin. Muscular relaxation results from cessation of the calcium influx, its removal from the actin–myosin sites, and its energy-dependent reuptake from the cytoplasm into the sarcoplasmic reticulum and other storage sites. Compared with skeletal muscle cells, cardiac muscle cells are smaller, have less-well-defined sarcoplasmic reticulum, and have a shorter distance from the cell membrane to the myofibrils. Because of this,

cardiac muscle relies more heavily than skeletal muscle on extracellular calcium ions for participation in the contractile process. The entry of extracellular calcium into myocardial cells is facilitated by two important mechanisms that have been identified. Calcium enters the cell through the cell membrane, particularly during the plateau of the action potential. Calcium for cardiac muscle contraction also enters by means of the nonenergy-dependent sodium–calcium exchange, in which two internal calcium ions are exchanged for one external sodium ion. Because of the normally low concentration of sodium within the cell, this mechanism is usually not an important source of calcium for cardiac contraction, but it may become important in conditions such as heart failure. Drugs such as digitalis, which block the sodium pump, increase the contractile properties of cardiac muscle by making more calcium available through this exchange system.

Action Potentials

The action potential of a cardiac muscle is divided into five phases: phase 0 is depolarization, which is characterized by the rapid upstroke of the action potential; phase 1 is the brief period of repolarization; phase 2 is the plateau, which lasts for 0.1 second to 0.2 second; phase 3 is the period of repolarization; and phase 4 is the resting membrane potential (Fig. 18-12). The plateau, or phase 2, of the action potential contributes to the unique electrical properties of cardiac muscle. It causes the action potential of cardiac muscle to last 20 to 50 times longer in skeletal muscle and causes a corresponding increased period of contraction.[1]

The electrical activity of the myocardial cell depends on changes in the permeability of the cell membrane to cations, primarily sodium, potassium, and calcium. There are two types of membrane channels through which ions flow during the depolarization phase of the action potential: the fast and slow channels. During phase 0 the membrane permeability to sodium increases rapidly, resulting in the fast inward movement of current through the fast channels. With phase 1, immediately following this rapid increase in sodium permeability, an abrupt decrease in sodium permeability occurs. If the sodium permeability remained low and potassium permeability increased to its resting level, the cell would rapidly repolarize. This is not the case. Instead, when the membrane has become partially depolarized, a second slow inward current develops and continues throughout the plateau of phase 2. The slow channels, which are much more permeable to calcium than sodium, are sometimes called the calcium channels. During the phase-3 repolarization period, there is a sharp rise in the membrane permeability to potassium as the slow inward movement of sodium and calcium is inactivated. The rapid outward movement of the potassium ions during this phase facilitates the reestablishment of the resting membrane potential. Phase 4 corresponds to diastole; it is the period during which the membrane is impermeable to sodium.

Action potentials from the contracting cells of the atria and ventricles, the specialized intracardiac conduction system, and the distal portion of the AV node depend on both the fast and slow channels. There are, however, two main types of action potentials in the heart (Fig. 18-12). One type, the so-called fast response, occurs in the normal myocardial cells of the atria and ventricles and in the conducting fibers (interatrial conduction fibers and Purkinje fibers) of these chambers. The amplitude and rapid rise of phase 1 is important to the conduction velocity of the fast response. The other type, the so-called slow response, is found in the SA node, which is the natural pacemaker of the heart and the conduction fibers of the AV node. The hallmark of these pacemaker cells is a spontaneous phase-4 depolarization. The rise in the membrane potential during phase 4 reflects the slow inward flow of current through the slow channels until the threshold for firing is reached. The rate of pacemaker cell discharge varies with the resting membrane potential and the slope of phase-4 depolarization. The catecholamines (epinephrine and norepinephrine) increase the heart rate by increasing the slope of phase 4. Acetylcholine, which is released during vagal stimulation of the heart, decreases the slope of phase 4.

The fast response of atrial and ventricular muscle can be converted to a slow pacemaker response under cetain conditions. For example, such conversions may occur spontaneously in persons with severe coronary artery disease, in areas of the heart in which blood supply has been severely curtailed. Impulses generated by these cells can lead to ectopic beats and serious arrhythmias.

Refractory Period of the Heart

The pumping action of the heart requires alternating contraction and relaxation. Following an action potential, there is a refractory period during which the membrane is resistant to a second stimulus. During the absolute refractory period, the membrane is completely insensitive to stimulation. This period is followed by the relative refractory period during which a more intense stimulus is needed to initiate an action potential. In skeletal muscle the refractory period is very short compared with the duration of the contraction, so that a second contraction can be initiated before the first is over. This results in a summated tetanized contraction. In cardiac muscle, the absolute refractory period is almost as long as the contraction, and a second contraction

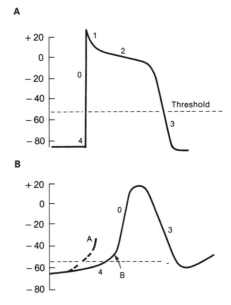

Figure 18-12 *Action of cardiac muscle and pacemaker cells. (A) Fast action potential that occurs in myocardial cells of atria and ventricular muscle. The phases are identified by numbers: phase 4, resting membrane potential; phase 0, depolarization; phase 1, brief period of repolarization; phase 2, plateau; and phase 3, repolarization. (B) Slow response, SA and AV nodes. The slow response is characterized by a slow, spontaneous rise in the phase 4 membrane potential to threshold levels; it has a lesser amplitude and shorter duration than the fast response. Increased automaticity (A) occurs when rate of phase 4 depolarization is increased.*

cannot be stimulated until the first is over. The longer length of the absolute refractory period of cardiac muscle is important in maintaining the alternating contraction and relaxation that is essential to the pumping action of the heart and to the prevention of fatal arrhythmias.

In summary, the rhythmic contraction and relaxation of the heart relies on the specialized cells of the heart's conduction system. Specialized cells in the SA node have the fastest inherent rate of impulse generation and act as the pacemaker of the heart. Impulses from the SA node travel through the atrial to the AV node, and then to the AV bundle and the ventricular Purkinje system. The AV node provides the only connection between the atrial and ventricular conduction systems. The atria and ventricles are independent of each other when AV node conduction is blocked.

The action potential of cardiac muscle is divided into five phases: phase 0 represents depolarization and is characterized by the rapid upstroke of the action potential; phase 1 is characterized by a brief period of repolarization; phase 2 consists of a plateau, which prolongs the duration of the action potential; phase 3 represents repolarization; and phase 4 is the resting membrane potential. The calcium ions contribute to the unique electrical properties of the heart and help in cardiac muscle contraction. Calcium ions enter the cardiac cells through special channels called the slow channels or calcium channels. Drugs that selectively block the calcium channels are used in the treatment of heart disease.

■ The Cardiac Cycle

The cardiac cycle can be divided into two parts: systole, the period during which the ventricles are contracting and blood is being ejected from the heart, and diastole, the period during which the ventricles are relaxed and the heart is filling with blood. During diastole the ventricles normally increase their volume to about 120 ml (called the end-diastolic volume), and at the end of systole about 50 ml of blood remains in the ventricles (end-systolic volume). The difference between the end-diastolic volume and the end-systolic volume is the stroke volume. There are simultaneous changes in left atrial pressure, left ventriclar pressure, aortic pressure, ventricular volume, electrocardiogram (ECG), and phonocardiogram during the cardiac cycle (Fig. 18-13).

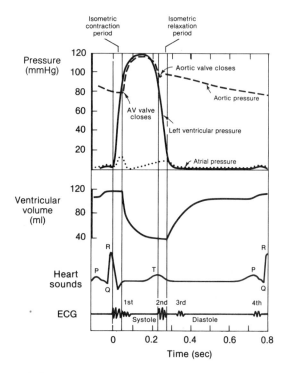

Figure 18-13 *Events in the cardiac cycle, showing changes in aortic pressure, left ventricular pressure, atrial pressure, left ventricular volume, heart sounds, and the electrocardiogram.*

Ventricular Systole and Diastole

During ventricular systole, the ventricles are contracting and blood is leaving the heart. The electrical activity, recorded on the ECG, precedes the mechanical events of the cardiac cycle. As the wave of depolarization (the QRS complex on the ECG) passes through the ventricles, it triggers a contraction. As the ventricles begin to contract, the AV valves close giving rise to the first heart sound. Following the closure of the AV valves, there is an additional 0.02 second to 0.03 second during which contraction is occurring in the ventricles, but the volume remains the same because both sets of valves are closed and no blood is leaving the heart. This period of the cardiac cycle is called isovolumic or isometric contraction. The ventricular pressures rise precipitately during isometric contraction until left ventricular pressure is slightly above aortic pressure (and right ventricular pressure is above pulmonary artery pressure). At this point, the semilunar valves open and blood is ejected from the heart. About 60% of the stroke volume is ejected during the first quarter of systole and the remaining 40% is ejected during the next two-quarters of systole. Little blood is ejected from the heart during the last quarter of systole although the ventricle remains contracted. At the end of systole, there is a sudden fall in intraventricular pressures due to the relaxation of the ventricles. As this occurs, blood from the large arteries flows back toward the ventricles causing the aortic and pulmonic valves to snap shut; an event that is marked by the second heart sound. The T wave on the ECG occurs during the last half of systole and represents repolarization of the ventricles.

The movement of blood into the aorta at the onset of systole causes the elastic fibers in the walls of the vessel to stretch and the pressure to rise. During the last quarter of systole, the arterial pressure begins to fall as blood flows out of the aorta into the peripheral vessels. At the end of ejection, the left ventricle begins to relax and its pressure falls below that in the aorta, at which point the aortic valve closes. The incisura, or notch, in the aortic pressure tracing represents closure of the aortic valve. Recoil of the elastic fibers in the aorta that were stretched during systole serve to maintain arterial blood pressure during the diastolic phase of the cardiac cycle.

Following the closure of the semilunar valves, the ventricles continue to relax for another 0.03 second to 0.04 second (the period of isovolumic relaxation), during which time the ventricular pressure becomes less than the atrial pressure. At this time, the AV valves open and the blood that has been accumulating in the atria during systole flows into the ventricles. Most of ventricular filling occurs during the first third of diastole, or the rapid filling period. During the middle third of diastole, inflow into the ventricles is almost at a standstill.

The last third of diastole is marked by the atrial contraction, which gives an additional thrust to ventricular filling. When audible, the third heart sound is heard during the rapid filling period of diastole as blood flows into a distended or noncompliant ventricle. The fourth heart sound occurs during the last third of diastole.

Atrial Systole and Diastole

Atrial contraction occurs during the last third of diastole. It is preceded by the P wave on the ECG, which represents depolarization of the atria. There are three main atrial pressure waves that occur during the cardiac cycle. The *a* wave is caused by atrial contraction. The *c* wave occurs as the ventricles begin to contract, and their increased pressure causes the AV valves to bulge into the atria. The *v* wave results from a slow buildup of blood in the atria toward the end of systole when the AV valves are still closed. The atrial pressure waves are transmitted to the internal jugular veins as pulsations. These pulsations can be observed visually and may be used to assess cardiac function. For example, exaggerated *a* waves occur when the right atrium has difficulty emptying into the right ventricle.

Although the main function of the atria is to store blood as it enters the heart, these chambers also act as primer pumps that aid in ventricular filling. This function becomes more important during periods of increased activity, when the diastolic filling time is decreased, or when heart disease impairs ventricular filling. In these two situations, the cardiac output would fall drastically were it not for the action of the atria. It has been estimated that atrial contraction can contribute as much as 30% to cardiac reserve during periods of stress, while having little or no effect on cardiac output during rest.

In summary, the cardiac cycle is divided into two parts: systole, during which the ventricles contract and blood is ejected from the heart, and diastole, during which the ventricles are relaxed and blood is filling the heart. The stroke volume (about 70 ml) represents the difference between the end-diastolic volume (about 120 ml) and the end-systolic volume (about 50 ml). The electrical activity of the heart, as represented on the electrocardiogram, precedes the mechanical events of the cardiac cycle. The heart sounds signal the closing of the heart valves during the cardiac cycle. Atrial contraction occurs during the last third of diastole. Although the main function of the atria is to store blood as it enters the heart, atrial contractions act to increase cardiac output during periods of increased activity when the filling time is reduced or in disease conditions in which ventricular filling is impaired.

■ Regulation of Cardiac Performance

The efficiency of the heart as a pump is often measured in terms of cardiac output. Cardiac output is the product of the stroke volume and the heart rate:

$$\text{cardiac output} = \text{stroke volume} \times \text{heart rate}$$

The cardiac output varies with body size and the metabolic needs of the tissues. It increases with physical activity and decreases during rest and sleep. The normal average cardiac output in an adult ranges from 3.5 liters to 8.0 liters/minute. In the trained athlete this value can increase to levels as high as 35 liters/minute. The *cardiac reserve* refers to the maximum percentage of increase in cardiac output that can be achieved above the normal resting level. The normal young adult has a cardiac reserve of about 400%.[2]

Factors Affecting Cardiac Output

The heart's ability to increase its output according to body needs is mainly dependent on four factors: (1) the preload or ventricular filling, (2) the afterload or resistance to ejection of blood from the heart, (3) cardiac contractility, and (4) the heart rate.

Preload

The volume achieved during diastolic filling of the ventricles is referred to as the preload because it is work imposed on the heart before the contraction begins. The preload varies with venous return to the heart, which in turn is determined by the right atrial pressure and mean systemic pressure. It contributes to the force of ventricular contraction by means of the Frank–Starling mechanism.

Right atrial and systemic filling pressures. During diastole, the ventricles fill with venous blood that has been returned to the atria. Venous return to the right atrium is determined by the right atrial and mean systemic filling pressures. The mean systemic filling pressure refers to the degree of filling of the systemic circulation. It is the force that moves blood back to the heart. Venous return is greatest when the right atrial pressure is low and the mean systemic filling pressure is high. Because the heart is in the thoracic cavity, the right atrial pressure reflects the intrathoracic pressure. Therefore, venous return is increased during inspiration when the intrathoracic and right atrial pressures are decreased and it is decreased during expiration when the intrathoracic and right atrial pressures are increased.

Starling's law of the heart. The anatomic arrangement of the myocardial fibers is such that the tension or force of contraction is greatest if the muscle is stretched just before it begins to contract. The maximum force of contraction is achieved when an increase in diastolic filling (preload) causes the muscle fibers to be stretched about two and one-half times their normal resting length. When the muscle fibers are stretched to this degree, the actin and myosin filaments are optimally approximated. The increased force of contraction that accompanies an increase in diastolic filling is referred to as the Frank–Starling mechanism or Starling's law of the heart. The Frank–Starling mechanism allows the heart to adjust its pumping ability to accommodate various levels of venous return. The Frank–Starling mechanism can be graphically represented by the Starling curve (Fig. 18-14).

Afterload

The afterload is the force, or resistance, against which the heart must pump to eject blood. It is the work that is presented to the heart after the contraction has commenced. The arterial blood pressure is the main source of afterload strain on the heart. The afterload of the left ventricle is increased with narrowing (stenosis) of the aortic valve and the afterload of the right ventricle is increased when stenosis of the pulmonic valve is present. In the late stages of aortic stenosis, the left ventricle may need to generate systolic pressures up to 300 mm Hg in order to move blood through the diseased valve.[3]

Cardiac contractility

Cardiac contractility refers to the ability of the heart to change its force of contraction without changing its resting (diastolic) length. The contractile state of the myocardial muscle is determined by biochemical and biophysical properties that govern the actin and myosin interactions within the myocardial cells. An *inotropic* influence is one that modifies the contractile state of the myocardium. For instance, hypoxia exerts a negative inotropic effect by decreasing cardiac contractility, whereas sympathetic stimulation produces a positive inotropic effect by increasing it.

Heart rate

The heart rate increases the cardiac output by increasing the frequency with which blood is ejected from the heart. As the heart rate increases, however, the time spent in diastole is reduced, and there is less time for the filling of the ventricles before the onset of systole. At a heart rate of 75 beats/minute, one cardiac cycle lasts 0.8 second, of which about 0.3 second is spent in systole and about 0.5 second in diastole. As the heart rate increases, the time spent in systole remains about the same while that spent in diastole decreases. This leads to a decrease in stroke volume; and at high heart rates, it may actually cause a decrease in cardiac output. In fact, one of the dangers of ventricular tachycardia is a reduction in cardiac output because the heart does not have time to fill adequately.

Autonomic Control of Cardiac Function

The autonomic nervous system modifies the activity of the conduction system and the contractile properties of the heart. The parasympathetic outflow to the heart originates from the vagal nucleus in the medulla. The axons of these neurons pass to the heart in the cardiac branches of the vagal nerve. Sympathetic outflow to the heart and blood vessels arises from neurons located in the reticular formation of the brain stem. The axons of these neurons descend in the intermediolateral columns of the spinal cord. The central sympathetic outflow is eventually transmitted to the heart by means of cell bodies in the paravertebral ganglia and their postganglionic axons. Synaptic transmission in the parasympathetic nervous system is mediated by acetylcholine (cholinergic). Sympathetic control of cardiac function is mediated by the catecholamines. The autonomic control of cardiac function is mediated by a number of sensors that are located throughout the circulatory system. For example, the baroreceptors, which are located in the aortic arch and carotid sinus, monitor blood pressure and effect changes in the heart rate through the autonomic nervous system (Chap. 16). There are also atrial and ventricular receptors that respond to distention and other stimuli.

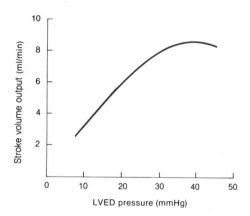

Figure 18-14 *The Starling ventricular function curve. An increase in left end-diastolic pressure (volume) produces an increase in stroke volume by means of the Frank–Starling mechanism. The maximum force of contraction and increased stroke volume are achieved when diastolic filling causes the muscle fibers to be stretched about two and one-half times their resting length.*

Parasympathetic control of cardiac function

The parasympathetic nervous system has two effects on heart action: it slows the rate of impulse generation in the SA node and it slows transmission of impulses through the AV node. As a consequence, the heart rate is slowed. Normally, the parasympathetic nervous system is tonically active and has a constraining effect on the heart rate. Strong vagal stimulation can actually stop impulse formation in the SA node or block transmission in the AV node. When this happens, there is a delay of about 10 seconds to 15 seconds, after which a ventricular pacemaker takes over, causing the ventricles to begin beating at a rate of 15 to 40 beats/minute. The drug atropine, which has an anticholinergic action, blocks vagal stimulation to the heart and causes the heart rate to increase.

Sympathetic control of cardiac function

Cardiac sympathetic fibers are widely distributed to the SA and AV nodes as well as the myocardium. Stimulation of these fibers activates beta$_1$-adrenergic receptors and causes an increase in both the heart rate and the velocity and force of cardiac contraction. These receptors respond to both neural stimulation and endogenous or exogenous sympathetic neuromediators in the blood. Adrenergic beta-blocking drugs are used to inhibit the effect of sympathetic stimulation on the heart.

Autonomic response to circulatory stresses

The response of the cardiovascular system to the stresses of everyday living is mediated largely through the autonomic nervous system. These stresses include postural stress, the Valsalva maneuver, and face immersion.

Postural stress. During movement from the supine to the standing position, about 20% of the blood in the heart and lungs is displaced into the legs.[3] The venous filling of the heart is decreased, and consequently, the cardiac output decreases. The body compensates for this decrease in cardiac output through autonomically mediated increases in heart rate and total peripheral resistance. These responses prevent the blood pressure from falling when the standing position is assumed. With prolonged standing, an increase in plasma volume and the action of the skeletal muscle pumps aid in the return of blood to the heart. Decreased tolerance of the upright position causes orthostatic hypotension, which is discussed in Chapter 17.

Valsalva maneuver. The Valsalva maneuver, which involves forced expiration against a closed glottis, incites a sequence of rapid changes in preload and afterload stresses along with autonomically mediated changes in the heart rate and total peripheral resistance.[4] The Valsalva maneuver is a normal accompaniment of many everyday activities. It is used in coughing, lifting, pushing, vomiting, and straining at stool. The pushing that occurs during the final stages of childbirth makes extensive use of the maneuver. The rise in intrathoracic pressure (often to levels of 40 mm Hg or greater) during the strain of the Valsalva maneuver causes a decrease in venous return to the heart, with a resultant decrease in stroke volume output from the heart, a decrease in systolic and pulse pressures, and a baroreflex-mediated increase in the heart rate and the total peripheral resistance. Following the release of the strain, venous return is suddenly reestablished; both stroke volume and arterial blood pressure undergo marked, but transient, elevations. The sudden rise in arterial pressure that occurs at a time when reflex vasoconstriction is still present gives rise to a vagal slowing of the heart rate that normally lasts for several beats. The Valsalva maneuver may be used as a method of testing circulatory reflexes, because the increase in heart rate and total peripheral resistance that occurs during the Valsalva strain, as well as the bradycardia that follows its release, is mediated through the baroreceptors and the autonomic nervous system.

Face immersion (diving reflex). The diving reflex is a potent protective mechanism against asphyxia in birds and submerged vertebrates; it allows for gross redistribution of the circulation in order to ensure the oxygenation of the brain and the heart. The diving response has three main features: (1) apnea, (2) an intense vagal slowing of heart rate, and (3) a powerful peripheral vasoconstriction. Except for the coronary and cerebral blood vessels, there is massive vasoconstriction to the extent that the circulation becomes, in effect, a heart–brain circuit.[5] Because of the severe vasoconstriction, arterial pressure remains relatively unchanged. The reflex enables the duck to remain submerged for 15 minutes, the sea lion for 30 minutes, and the whale for 2 hours.[5]

In humans, application of cold water to the face produces a similar reduction in the heart rate and the skin and muscle blood flow. The slowing of the heart rate is greater with ice water than cool water, and an even lesser slowing of heart rate can be produced by dry cold. Because of the powerful vagal effects, pathologic arrhythmias such as premature ventricular contractions can occur after only 30 seconds of diving.[5] Immersion of the face in ice water may be used clinically to terminate supraventricular paroxysmal tachycardia. Because the reflex is potent in the newborn, it may protect against asphyxia during the birth process. It has also been credited with increasing the survival of children who have accidentally fallen into cold water and remained submerged for longer periods of time than are normally associated with survival.

In summary, the efficiency of the heart as a pump is often measured in terms of cardiac output (the product of stroke volume and heart rate). The heart's ability to increase its output according to body needs is dependent on: (1) the preload, or filling of the ventricles (end-diastolic volume), (2) the afterload, or resistance to ejection of blood from the heart, (3) cardiac contractility, which is determined by the interaction of the actin and the myosin filaments of cardiac muscle fibers, and (4) the heart rate, which determines the frequency with which blood is ejected from the heart. The maximum force of cardiac contraction is greatest when an increase in preload stretches muscle fibers of the heart to approximately two and one-half times their resting length (Frank–Starling mechanism). The autonomic nervous system contributes to the regulation of cardiac output by altering the heart rate, cardiac contractility, the preload, and the afterload. Activation of the parasympathetic nervous system slows the heart rate. The sympathetic nervous system innervates the conduction system of the heart, the arterioles, and the veins; its stimulation produces an increase in heart rate and cardiac contractility, in preload (venous constriction), and in afterload (arterial vasoconstriction). The autonomic nervous system plays a major role in regulatory circulatory responses to everyday activities such as postural stress, the Valsalva maneuver, and exposure to cold.

■ Coronary Circulation

The blood supply for the heart is provided by the coronary arteries, which arise in the aorta just distal to the aortic valve. There are two coronary arteries: the right coronary artery, which mainly supplies the right ventricle and atrium, and the left coronary artery, which divides near its origin to form the left circumflex artery and the anterior descending artery. The left coronary artery mainly supplies the left ventricle and atrium. After passage through the arteries and capillary beds, most of the venous blood from the myocardium returns to the right atrium through the coronary sinus; some blood returns to the right atrium by way of the anterior coronary veins. There are also vascular channels that communicate directly between the vessels of the myocardium and the chambers of the heart; these are the arteriosinusoidal, the arterioluminal, and the thebesian vessels.

Regulation of Coronary Blood Flow

Blood flow in the coronary arteries is regulated by the metabolic and oxygen needs of the heart muscle. The mechanisms for controlling the coronary blood flow have not yet been fully determined. Numerous agents, generally referred to as metabolites, have been suggested as mediators of coronary artery vasodilatation observed during increased cardiac work.[1] Among the substances implicated are carbon dioxide, reduced oxygen tension, lactic acid, hydrogen ions, histamine, potassium ions, increased osmolality, and adenine nucleotides. These substances are released from myocardial cells when there is an increased need for oxygen delivery.

The sympathetic nervous system also plays a role in regulating coronary blood flow. Both alpha receptors, which cause vessel constriction, and beta receptors, which produce vessel dilatation, are known to exist in the coronary vessels. There is also evidence that prostaglandins (prostaglandin I_2) play a role in the modulation of coronary artery tone; and aspirin, which suppresses prostaglandin synthesis, has been reported to increase coronary artery spasm when given in large doses to patients with variant angina.[6]

Contraction of myocardial muscle fibers affects the flow of blood through the coronary arteries. During systole, the contraction of myocardial muscle compresses the coronary arteries and causes a reduction in blood flow. Because of the high pressure that the left ventricle must generate, the decrease in flow is greatest in the arteries that supply this chamber. It has been estimated that about 70% of blood flow through the coronaries occurs during diastole. This is particularly significant in tachycardia when the increase in heart rate causes an increase in oxygen consumption, while the time spent in diastole is markedly reduced. An increase in heart rate probably has little effect on oxygen delivery in the normal heart because the process of autoregulation causes the coronary arteries to dilate. On the other hand, rigid atherosclerotic vessels probably have a limited capacity for dilatation, in which case an increase in heart rate may impair oxygen delivery to the myocardium.

Metabolic Needs of the Myocardium

The energy expended for myocardial contraction requires constant utilization of oxygen and other nutrients (fatty acids, glucose, and ketones). Although muscles can store limited supplies of nutrients, they are unable to store oxygen. Oxygen must, instead, be supplied continuously for metabolic processes to continue. The oxygen supply for the heart is derived from the blood that flows through the coronary arteries. Under normal conditions, the heart extracts and uses about 60% to 80% of the oxygen from the blood flowing through the coronary arteries, compared with the 25% to 30% that is extracted by skeletal muscles. Because there is little oxygen reserve in the blood, the coronary arteries must increase their flow to meet the metabolic needs of the myocardium during periods of increased activity. The normal resting blood flow through the coronary arteries averages about 225 ml/min.[1] During strenous exercise, coronary blood flow must increase four- to fivefold to meet the energy requirements of the heart.

Normally, the heart uses fats as a fuel source; about 70% of the heart's energy supply is derived from fatty acids, which must be metabolized by aerobic mechanisms.[1] Under conditions of oxygen deprivation, the heart must convert to the anaerobic metabolism of glucose, with subsequent production of lactic acid, to meet its energy needs. Lactic acid is thought to be the source of pain stimulation during myocardial ischemia.

Determinants of Oxygen Consumption

The oxygen needs of the heart are determined by the tension that the heart must generate to pump blood, the stroke volume that is ejected, the contractile state of the heart, and the heart rate.

Oxygen consumption and the need for oxygen delivery by the coronary arteries are determined largely by the tension that the heart muscle must generate during contraction to eject blood into the aorta (left ventricle) and pulmonary artery (right ventricle) and the length of time that this tension must be maintained (tension × time). When the heart is dilated at the onset of systole, it must use additional energy just to overcome the wall tension and decrease its size before it can generate the tension needed to eject blood. When some cardiac muscle fibers are damaged, others must take up the load. They do this by increasing their length so that the heart dilates and the wall tension is increased (see Chap. 15, law of Laplace). The oxygen consumption is therefore greater for the same work load.

The stroke work is the effort the heart expends to pump blood. Work is generally defined as force multiplied by distance, for example, the work required to carry a heavy box up a flight of stairs is equal to the weight of the box times the height of the stairs. The main (external) work of the heart is determined by the amount of blood (like the weight of the box) that is pumped with each beat and the pressure (distance) that the ventricle must develop to move the blood into the aorta or pulmonary artery.

$$stroke\ work = stroke\ volume \times mean\ arterial\ blood\ pressure$$

The stroke work of the left ventricle pumping against a mean systemic pressure of 85 mm Hg is going to be greater than the stroke work of the right ventricle pumping against a mean pulmonary artery pressure of 15 mm Hg. Stroke work is increased in the presence of hypertension and valvular disorders, which reduce the size of the valve opening through which blood must be pumped.

The contractile state of the heart refers to its ability to change its force of contraction without a change in end-diastolic volume, the heart rate, or arterial pressure. Oxygen consumed during the contractile state is used to produce and maintain the interactions between the actin and myosin filaments of the myocardial fibers. The cardiac glycosides (digitalis drugs) increase the myocardial contractility, allowing the heart to increase its stroke volume without an increase in metabolic demands. The catecholamines increase cardiac contractility, but they also increase the metabolic requirements of the myocardium.

The heart rate increases the myocardial oxygen requirements by increasing the frequency with which the heart goes through the processes that require oxygen consumption.

In summary, the blood supply for the heart is provided by the coronary arteries, which arise in the aorta just distal to the aortic valve. Coronary blood flow is regulated by the metabolic and oxygen needs of the heart muscle. Contraction of myocardial muscle fibers compresses the coronary arteries so that blood flow is greatest during diastole. Under normal conditions the heart extracts 60% to 80% of the oxygen from the blood flowing through the coronary arteries, compared with the 25% to 30% that is extracted by skeletal muscle. Because the blood that flows through the coronary arteries contains little reserve oxygen, the coronary arteries must increase their flow during periods of increased activity. The oxygen needs of the heart are determined by the tension that the heart must generate to pump blood, the stroke volume that is ejected, and the heart rate.

■ Diagnostic Methods

There are a number of methods for assessing the function of the heart and its structures. Among those used in assessing cardiac function are interpretation of heart sounds, electrocardiography, echocardiography, nuclear imaging, exercise stress testing, cardiac catheterization, and hemodynamic monitoring (central venous pressure, pulmonary capillary wedge pressure, and cardiac output measurement). Each of these methods is described briefly.

Heart Sounds

Closure of the heart valves produces vibrations of the surrounding heart tissues and blood that can be detected as the audible "lub dup" sounds heard with a stethoscope during cardiac auscultation. There are four heart sounds. The first and second are heard normally in all healthy individuals. The third and fourth heart sounds are not usually heard and may or may not indicate pathology.

The first and second heart sounds represent closure of the AV and the semilunar valves, respectively. The first heart sound (lub), which has a lower pitch and lasts longer (about 0.14 second) than the second sound, marks the onset of systole and the closure of the AV valves. The second heart sound (dup) occurs with the closure of the semilunar valves; it is shorter (0.10 second) and has a higher pitch than the first heart sound. The second heart sound is a composite sound resulting from the closure of both the aortic and the pulmonic valves. Normally, the aortic valve closes slightly before the pulmonic valve, causing a separation of the two components of the second heart sound. During expiration, aortic valve closure precedes pulmonic valve closure by 0.02 second to 0.04 second; during inspiration this difference is increased to 0.04 second to 0.06 second. This is because during inspiration there is an increase in venous return to the right heart, and as a result it takes longer for the right ventricle to empty and for the pulmonic valve to close. At the same time, less blood is returning to the left ventricle, causing the aortic valve to close slightly earlier. An audible widening of the second heart sound that occurs with inspiration is a normal finding. It is often referred to as a physiologic splitting and can be heard only in the left second intercostal space.

The third heart sound is low pitched and occurs during rapid filling of the ventricles early in diastole, about 0.12 second after the second heart sound. It is usually only heard in young individuals or in persons with heart failure. The fourth heart sound is produced by atrial contraction during the last third of diastole; it is audible only in conditions in which resistance to ventricular filling occurs during late diastole. The heart sounds and their relationship to the cardiac cycle are illustrated in Figure 18-13.

The loudness of the first and second heart sounds depends on the rate of change in pressure across the valve.[2] At high heart rates, intraventricular pressures rise rapidly, whereas atrial pressures remain relatively low. As a result, the first heart sound is intensified. The same principle occurs during exercise when the force of ventricular contraction is increased. Conversely, the intensity of the first heart sound is decreased when ventricular contractions are sluggish as a result of a weakened heart muscle. The loudness of the second heart sound is related to the rate of decrease in ventricular pressure at the end of systole. In persons with hypertension, the second heart sound is accentuated because ventricular pressure is high at the time the aortic valve closes, and therefore the rate at which ventricular pressure falls is accelerated.

Heart murmurs are caused by abnormal vibrations produced by turbulent blood flow. In the heart, turbulence occurs when the velocity of blood flow is increased, the valve diameter is decreased, or the viscosity of the blood is decreased. For example, very high velocities of flow may be reached when blood is ejected through a narrowed, or stenotic, heart valve. Severe anemia may reduce blood viscosity to the point at which turbulence occurs.

Auscultation to detect murmurs or abnormalities of the heart sounds is a valuable diagnostic procedure. Although auscultation of the heart does not involve the use of expensive equipment, it does require a trained ear and a thorough understanding of the physiologic events associated with valvular function and the cardiac cycle.

A permanent recording of the heart sounds can be obtained through use of a phonocardiograph. This is obtained by placing a high fidelity microphone on the chest wall over the heart while a recording is being made. Usually, an electrocardiographic tracing is recorded simultaneously for timing purposes.

Electrocardiography

The electrocardiogram (ECG) is a recording of the electrical activity of the heart. The electrical currents that are generated by the heart spread through the body to the skin, where they can be sensed by appropriately placed electrodes, amplified, and then recorded on an oscilloscope or chart recorder. The horizontal axis of the ECG measures time (seconds), and the vertical axis measures the amplitude of the impulse (millivolts). Each heavy vertical black line represents 0.2 second and each thin black line 0.04 second (Fig. 18-15). On the horizontal axis, each heavy horizontal line represents 0.05 mV. The connections of the ECG are such that an upright deflection indicates a positive potential, and a downward deflection indicates a negative potential.

The deflection points of an ECG are designated by the letters P, Q, R, S, and T. The P wave represents SA node and atrial depolarization; the QRS complex (beginning of the Q wave to the end of the S wave)

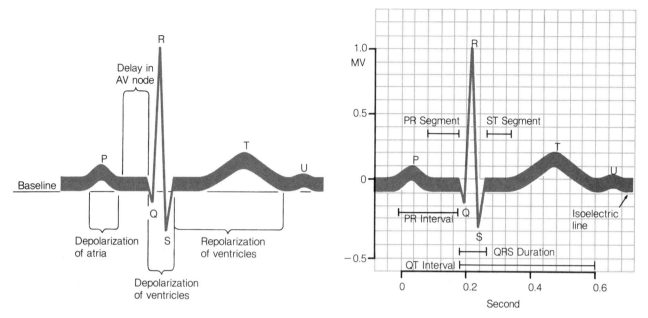

Figure 18-15 *Diagram of the electrocardiogram (lead II) and representative depolarization and repolarization of the atria and ventricle. The P wave represents atrial depolarization, the QRS complex ventricular depolarization, and the T wave ventricular repolarization. Atrial repolarization occurs during ventricular depolarization and is hidden under the QRS complex.*

represents ventricular depolarization; and the T wave represents ventricular repolarization. Atrial repolarization occurs during ventricular depolarization and is hidden in the QRS complex.

The process of impulse generation in the heart and other excitable tissue involves the movement or flow of electrically charged ions at the level of the cell membrane. The ECG records three types of electrical events: the resting membrane potential, depolarization, and repolarization. During the resting state the membrane is impermeable to the flow of charge and the inside is negative in relation to the outside (Fig. 18-16). The electrical potential (difference in charge) between the two electrodes is zero. Depolarization occurs when the cell is stimulated and the cell membrane becomes selectively permeable to a current-carrying ion such as sodium. During the process of depolarization, the membrane potential is reversed so that the inside becomes positive in relation to the outside. Repolarization involves the reestablishment of the resting membrane potential. During repolarization, potassium moves back into the cell as sodium is pumped out of the cell, and the membrane again becomes negative on the inside in relation to the outside.

The shape of the recorder tracing is determined by the direction in which the impulse spreads through the heart muscle in relation to electrode placement. A depolarization wave that moves toward the recording electrode will register as a positive, or upward, deflection. Conversely, if the impulse moves away from the recording electrode, the deflection will be downward, or negative. When there is no difference in charge between the two electrodes, the potential is zero and a straight line is recorded at the baseline of the chart. If the direction of current flow is perpendicular to the recording electrode, the recorder will also register zero because the electrode cannot detect the direction of current flow. The electrocardiograph recorder is much like a camera in that it can record different views of the electrical activity of the heart depending on where the recording electrode is placed.

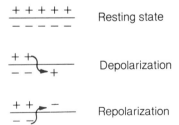

Figure 18-16 *The flow of charge during impulse generation in excitable tissue. During the resting state, opposite charges are separated by the cell membrane. Depolarization represents the flow of charge across the membrane and repolarization of the return of the membrane potential to its resting state.*

Unlike laboratory experiments, which record from a single nerve or muscle fiber, the ECG records the sum of all the electrical activity of the heart. A force that has both magnitude and direction is referred to as a vector. The electrical vector of the heart, which can be measured using the ECG, designates all of the electromotive forces of the heart: it has magnitude, direction, and polarity. A vector can be represented by an arrow in which the length of the shaft represents the magnitude of the force and the tip of the arrow represents the direction of the force. The mean QRS vector can be estimated from the standard leads of the ECG and is used in describing the size and position of the heart.

Conventionally, 12 leads are recorded for a diagnostic ECG, each viewing the electrical forces of the heart from a different position on the body's surface. The electrodes are attached to the four extremities or representative areas on the body (near the shoulders and lower chest or abdomen). The electrical potential recorded from any one extremity should be the same no matter where the electrode is placed on the extremity.[7] Chest electrodes are moved to different positions on the chest. The right limb lead is used as a ground electrode. Additional electrodes may be applied to other areas of the body, such as the back, when indicated.

Bipolar limb leads

The three standard, or bipolar, limb leads record the potential difference between two electrodes (the indifferent [−] electrode and the recording [+] electrode). Lead I records the difference in potential between the left and right arms, with the right arm negative in relation to the left arm (Fig. 18-17). Lead II records the potential

difference between the right arm, which is negative and the left leg, which is positive. Lead III records the potential between the left arm (negative) and the left leg (positive). The relationship between the three leads is expressed algebraically by Einthoven's equation: lead II = lead I + lead III. This equation is based on Kirchoff's law, which states that the algebraic sum of all the potential differences in a closed circuit is equal to zero. The equation is used to obtain the mean electrical vector for the heart.

Augmented unipolar limb leads

The augmented unipolar limb leads measure impulses from the heart without being influenced by an indifferent electrode as in the bipolar limb leads. Lead aVr records the potential from the right arm, aVl the potential from the left arm, and aVf the potential from the left leg (foot). This results in amplification of the recording signal of about 50%.[3] Instead of lead II = lead I + lead III, lead aVf equals the total electrical vector from the heart as recorded from the foot. Likewise, aVl equals the total electrical vector from the heart, as recorded from the left arm, and aVr the total vector, as recorded from the right arm.

Unipolar chest leads

Usually six unipolar chest leads are recorded with an electrode that can be moved to specific areas of the chest. As with the unipolar limb leads, the chest leads record the potential from the heart without being influenced by an indifferent electrode.

Vectorcardiography

A vectorcardiogram is a three-dimensional ECG. It displays a vector loop of impulses on the frontal (right to left and head to toe), saggital (front to back and head to toe), or horizontal (front to back and left to right) planes of the body. Whereas an electrocardiographic lead records in one single axis, a vectorcardiograph records the same electrical event simultaneously in two perpendicular axes.

Echocardiography

Echocardiography uses ultrasound to record an image of heart structures. An ultrasound signal has a frequency greater than 20,000 Hz (cycles per second) and is inaudible to the human ear. Echocardiography uses ultrasound signals in the range of 2 million Hz to 5 million Hz. The ultrasound signal is reflected (echos) whenever tissue resistance to the transmission of the sound beam changes. It is possible to image the internal structures of the heart, because the chest wall, the blood, and the different heart structures all reflect ultrasound differently.

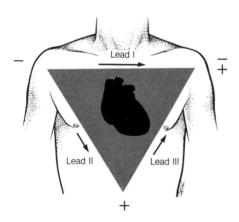

Figure 18-17 *Einthoven's triangle, illustrating the connections of the bipolar limb leads. The heart is the center of the triangle. Lead I records the potential difference between the left arm and the right arm. Lead II records the potential difference between the right arm and the left leg. Lead III registers the difference between the left arm and left leg.*

The echocardiograph transducer, which is placed on the chest, serves as both transmitter for the ultrasound waves and receiver for the echos reflected back from the heart structures. The transducer emits pulses of microwaves, each lasting 1 μsec (1 millionth of a second) at a rate of 1000 times/second, the remaining 99.9% of the time is used in receiving the echo. When the echo reaches the transducer, it is converted to an electronic signal and recorded. The ultrasound signal travels through different tissues at variable speeds depending on the density. The time that has elapsed between the emission of the signal and the return of the echo is automatically converted into a measurement of distance from the chest wall. In this manner, an echocardiograph can record a dynamic, or moving, image of the heart, with the depth of the structures on the vertical axis and time on the horizontal axis. An ECG is recorded simultaneously for timing purposes (M-mode echo). A second and more recent method (two-dimensional, or 2D, echo) permits examination of larger areas of the heart in multiple planes (Fig. 18-18).

The echocardiogram is useful for determining ventricular dimensions and valve movements, obtaining data on the movement of the left ventricular wall and septum, estimating diastolic and systolic volumes, and viewing the motion of individual segments of the left ventricular wall during systole and diastole. It can also be used for studying valvular disease (Fig. 18-18) and detecting pericardial effusion.

Nuclear Imaging

Nuclear cardiology techniques involve the use of radionuclides (radioactive substances) and are essentially noninvasive. Three types of nuclear cardiology tests are commonly used: infarct imaging, myocardial perfusion imaging, and ventriculography. With all three types of tests a scintillation camera is used to record the radiation that is emitted from the radionuclide.

Acute infarct imaging uses an agent (*e.g.*, technetium pyrophosphate) that is taken up by the cells in the infarcted zone. With this method the radionuclide becomes concentrated in the damaged myocardium, allowing its visualization as a hot spot, or positive area, of increased uptake of the radionuclide.

Myocardial perfusion imaging uses agents that are extracted from the blood and taken up by functioning myocardial cells. Thallium-201, an analog of potassium, is usually used for this purpose. The physical half-life of thallium-201 is 72 hours. Thallium-201 is distributed to the myocardium in proportion to the magnitude of blood flow. Following injection, an external detection device describes the distribution of the radioactive material. An ischemic area appears as a "cold spot" that lacks radioactive uptake. Thallium-201 can be used to assess myocardial blood flow during both rest and exercise.

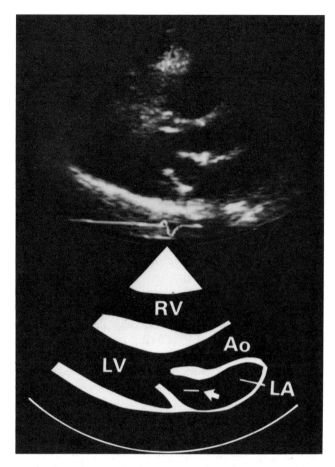

Figure 18-18 *A two-dimensional echocardiogram. Parasternal long-axis view of a patient with a Hancock porcine mitral valve prosthesis. (RV = right ventricle; LV = left ventricle; Ao = aorta; LA = left atrium; arrow points to the valve leaflets.) (Courtesy of LS Wann, M.D., Zablocki Veterans Administration Medical Center, Wood, Wisconsin)*

Radionuclide ventriculography provides actual visualization of ventricular structures during systole and diastole and provides a means for evaluating ventricular function during rest and exercise. A radioisotope such as technetium-labeled albumin, which does leave the capillaries but remains in the blood and is not bound to the myocardium, is used for this type of imaging. This type of nuclear imaging can be used to determine right and left ventricular volumes, ejection fractions, regional wall motion, and cardiac contractility. This method is also useful in the diagnosis of intracardiac shunts.

Radionuclide ventriculography can be performed using first-pass techniques in which the initial transit of the radioactive material is used in evaluating cardiovascular function. With this technique the radionuclide bolus can be localized as it passes through the cardiac chambers, making it possible to visualize one side of the heart at a time. A second technique, called multiple image gated acquisition (MUGA), produces computerized composite images of the heart that have been accumulated over hundreds of cardiac cycles. The distribution of these images is regulated by a gating signal from the ECG that controls the scintillation camera so that repeated images are taken during a designated portion of the cardiac cycle. This allows for calculation of left ventricular end-diastolic volumes, left ventricular end-systolic volumes, and left ventricular ejection fractions.

Exercise Stress Testing

Exercise stress testing is a means of observing cardiac function under stress. Three types of tests are utilized: the step test, the bicycle ergometer, and the treadmill. The treadmill is used most frequently in the United States. Many people are not accustomed to riding bicycles, and the usefulness of the step test is limited because it requires considerable motivation on the part of the patient and it also produces greater distortion of the ECG than the other tests. During treadmill testing, the person walks or runs on a moving belt. The level of physical activity, or work load, that the person performs can be gradually increased by changing the speed and the incline of the belt; this is usually done in stages. The ECG is monitored continuously during the test, and the blood pressure is taken at predetermined intervals. It is also possible to monitor oxygen consumption, although a person is assumed to have reached the limit for oxygen uptake at the point of exhaustion. Usually the person being tested continues to exercise, completing successive stages of the test, until exhaustion or a predetermined heart rate is reached. The maximal heart rate is determined by age. Tables of heart rate by age are available; but as a general rule, the maximal heart rate can be determined by subtracting age from 220, for example, the target heart rate for a 30-year-old would be 190 beats/minute. The person may be asked to continue until the maximum heart rate is achieved or until a percentage (*i.e.*, 85% to 90%) of the maximal rate is reached.

The presence of chest pain, severe shortness of breath, arrhythmias, S-T segment changes on the ECG, or a decrease in blood pressure is suggestive of coronary heart disease, and the test is usually terminated if these signs appear.

Metabolic equivalents (METs), which are multiples of the basal metabolic rate, are commonly used to express the work load at various stages of the exercise protocols. A MET is equivalent to the energy expended in resting in a supine position, sitting, standing, eating, or having an ordinary conversation. Walking at 4 miles per hour (mph), cycling at 11 mph, playing tennis (singles), digging a garden, or doing heavy carpentry requires 5 to 6 METs. Running 6 mph requires 10 METs, and running

10 mph requires 17 METs. Physically trained individuals can achieve work loads beyond 16 METs. Healthy sedentary individuals, however, seldom exercise beyond 10 or 11 METs; and in persons with coronary heart disease work loads of 8 METs are usually sufficient to produce angina.

Cardiac Catheterization

Cardiac catheterization involves the passage of flexible catheters into the great vessels and chambers of the heart. In right heart catheterization, the catheters are inserted into a peripheral vein (usually the basilic or femoral) and then advanced into the right heart. The left heart catheter is inserted retrograde through a peripheral artery (usually the brachial or femoral) into the aorta and left heart. The cardiac catheterization laboratory, where the procedure is done, is equipped for viewing and recording fluoroscopic images of the heart and vessels in the chest and for measuring pressures within the heart and great vessels. There is also equipment for cardiac output studies and for obtaining samples of blood for blood gas analysis. Angiographic studies are made by injecting a contrast medium into the heart, so that an outline of the moving structures can be visualized and filmed. Coronary arteriography involves the injection of a contrast medium into the coronary arteries, this permits visualization of lesions within these vessels.

Hemodynamic Monitoring

Central venous pressure
Central venous pressure reflects the amount of blood returning to the heart and the ability of the heart to pump the blood forward into the arterial system. Measurements of central venous pressure can be obtained by means of a catheter inserted into the superior vena cava through a peripheral vein. This pressure is decreased in hypovolemia and increased in heart failure. The changes that occur in central venous pressure over time are usually more significant than the absolute numerical values obtained during a single reading.

Pulmonary capillary wedge pressure
Pulmonary capillary wedge pressure (PCWP) is obtained by means of a flow-directed, balloon-tipped Swan–Ganz catheter. This catheter is introduced through a peripheral vein and is then advanced into the superior vena cava. The balloon is inflated with air once the catheter is in the thorax; it then floats through the right heart and pulmonary artery until it becomes wedged in one of the small pulmonary arteries (Fig. 18-19). Once the catheter is in place, the balloon is inflated *only* when

the PCWP is being measured, to prevent necrosis of pulmonary tissue. With the balloon inflated, the catheter monitors pulmonary capillary pressures in direct communication with pressures from the left atrium. The pulmonary capillary pressures provide a means of assessing the pumping ability of the left heart.

One type of Swan–Ganz catheter is equipped with a thermistor probe to obtain *thermodilution measurements of cardiac output*. In this method, a known amount of iced solution of a known temperature is injected into the right atrium through an opening in the catheter, and the temperature of the blood is measured downstream in the pulmonary artery by means of a thermistor probe located at the end of that catheter. A microcomputer calculates blood flow (and cardiac output) by the difference between the temperatures recorded from the two sites.

Cardiac output measurement

Cardiac output is the amount of blood ejected from the heart per unit time (stroke volume × heart rate) and is reported in milliliters per minute. There are three commonly used methods for measuring cardiac output: (1) the Fick method, (2) the dye-dilution method, and (3) thermodilution. All of these methods are based on the indicator–dilution technique and rely on the principle that the total uptake or release of a substance by an organ is the product of blood flow to the organ and the arteriovenous concentration difference of a substance.

The Fick method uses oxygen as the substance that is released into the blood; the cardiac output is determined by measuring the oxygen content of the expired air and subtracting it from the oxygen content of room air, making adjustments for barometric pressure. The difference between the two oxygen concentrations is then divided by the arteriovenous oxygen difference (the difference between the oxygen content of the pulmonary artery blood and that of the left ventricular, or systemic, arterial blood). This method uses both arterial and venous blood samples and requires that the patient be in a constant or steady state and able to cooperate in collecting the expired air sample.

With the dye-dilution method for cardiac output determination, a dye such as indocyanine green or Evans blue is released into the blood. A predetermined amount of the dye is injected into the venous system while arterial blood is steadily withdrawn through a densitometer, which uses a light beam and photocell to measure the concentration of the dye. Through use of the densitometer, a timed concentration curve is recorded as the dye passes through one circulation of the body and the cardiac output is calculated from the area under the curve. This method of cardiac output determination is usually used during cardiac catheterization, because it

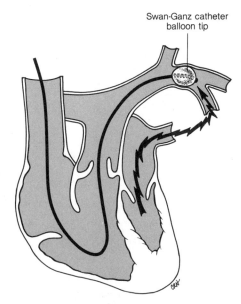

Figure 18-19 *Swan–Ganz balloon tip catheter positioned in a pulmonary capillary. The pulmonary capillary wedge pressure, which reflects the left ventricular diastolic pressure, is measured with the balloon inflated.*

requires placement of both central venous and arterial catheters.

In summary, a number of diagnostic measures are used in assessing cardiac function, including interpretation of heart sounds, electrocardiography, echocardiography, nuclear imaging, exercise stress testing, cardiac catheterization, and hemodynamic monitoring. Closure of the heart valves produces vibrations that can be detected with cardiac auscultation. Heart sounds provide information about the function of the heart valves and abnormal vibrations of the ventricles that occur in heart failure (S_3). Electrocardiography is used to assess the function of the heart's conduction system. Echocardiography uses ultrasound to construct an image of heart structures during different phases of the cardiac cycle. Nuclear imaging techniques employ radionuclides in studying cardiac function. Three types of nuclear cardiology test are currently used: infarct imaging, myocardial perfusion imaging, and first-pass or MUGA ventriculography. Exercise stress testing utilizes the step test, bicycle ergometer, or treadmill as a means of observing cardiac function under stress. Cardiac catheterization involves the passage of flexible catheters into the great vessels and chambers of the heart as a means of studying heart pressures, obtaining cardiac output measurements, viewing fluoroscopic images of the heart and great vessels, and performing angiographic studies of the coronary arteries. Hemodynamic monitoring includes methods for measuring central venous pressure, pulmonary capillary wedge pressure, and cardiac output.

■ Study Guide

After you have studied this chapter, you should be able to meet the following objectives:

☐ Describe how the ventricular wall thickness and the pressure generated by the right and left ventricles are related.

☐ Describe the sequential development of the embryonic heart.

☐ State the function of the pericardium.

☐ Cite the function of the valvular structures of the heart.

☐ State the function of the intercalated disks in cardiac muscle.

☐ Trace an impulse that is generated in the SA node through the conduction system of the heart.

☐ Relate systolic and diastolic changes in the left ventricular pressure and volume to changes in the ECG and phonocardiogram.

☐ Define the terms preload and afterload.

☐ Explain the effects that increased and decreased venous return to the heart have on cardiac output using Starling's law of the heart.

☐ Describe the permeability characteristics of cells in the ventricular conduction system to sodium, potassium, and calcium ions during the five phases of an action potential.

☐ Explain the importance of the plateau and length of the refractory period in cardiac muscle.

☐ State the formula for calculating the cardiac output.

☐ Define cardiac reserve.

☐ Explain the effect of the Valsalva maneuver on venous return, heart rate, and blood pressure.

☐ Cite the distribution of sympathetic and parasympathetic nervous system innervation and their effects on heart rate and cardiac contractility.

☐ Describe the determinants of oxygen consumption by the myocardium.

☐ Compare the amount of oxygen that is normally extracted from blood flowing through the skeletal and coronary circulations and relate it to the mechanisms for increasing oxygen delivery.

☐ Explain the relationship between the loudness of the first heart sound and the heart rate.

☐ State the difference between a 12-lead electrocardiogram and a vectorcardiogram.

☐ Cite the information that can be obtained from an echocardiogram.

☐ State the difference between infarct nuclear imaging, myocardial perfusion imaging, and radionuclide ventriculography.

☐ Explain the purpose of a treadmill exercise stress test.

☐ State the definition of a metabolic equivalent (MET).

☐ Describe the measurement of pulmonary capillary wedge pressure.

■ References

1. Berne RM, Levy MN: Physiology, pp 457, 442, 601. St Louis, CV Mosby, 1983
2. Guyton A: Textbook of Medical Physiology, 6th ed, pp 167, 317, 298, 302, 322, 335. Philadelphia, WB Saunders, 1981
3. Shepard JT, Van Houtte PM: The Human Cardiovascular System, pp 238, 158. New York, Raven Press, 1979
4. Porth CJM, Bamrah VS, Tristani FE, Smith JJ: The Valsalva: Mechanisms and clinical implications. Heart Lung 13:507, 1984
5. Smith JJ, Kampine JP: Circulatory Physiology, 2nd ed, pp 255–256, Baltimore, Williams & Wilkins, 1984
6. Miwa K, Kambara H, Kawai C: Effect of aspirin in large doses on variant angina. Am Heart J 105:351, 1983
7. Goldman MJ: Clinical Electrocardiography, p 3. Los Altos, Lange Medical Publications, 1984

Chapter 19

Alterations in Cardiac Function

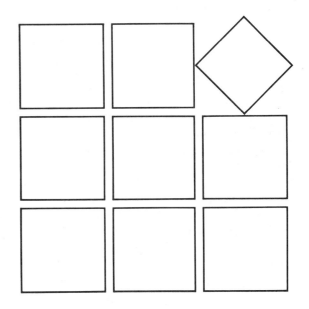

The latest estimates indicate that more than 42 million persons in the United States have some form of cardiovascular disease. About 50% of all deaths, 989,610 in 1981, result from cardiovascular disease.[1] Heart attack is the nation's number one killer; it is responsible for more than one-third of all deaths and is the predominant cause of early disability in the American labor force. Eight out of every 1000 children are born with congenital heart defects and 100,000 children and 1,750,000 adults are affected with rheumatic fever. In 1981, heart and blood vessel diseases cost the nation an average of 46.2 billion dollars. In an attempt to focus on common heart problems that affect persons of all age groups, this chapter has been organized into seven sections: (1) disorders of the pericardium, (2) coronary heart disease, (3) arrhythmias and disorders of the conduction system, (4) disorders of the endocardium, (5) valvular heart disease, (6) cardiomyopathies, and (7) congenital heart defects.

■ Disorders of the Pericardium

The pericardium isolates the heart from the other thoracic structures, maintains its position in the thorax, and prevents it from overfilling. The two layers of the pericardium are separated by a thin layer of serous fluid, which serves to prevent frictional forces from developing as the inner visceral layer, or epicardium, comes in contact with the outer parietal layer of the fibrous pericardium. The mechanisms that control the movement of fluid between the capillaries and the pericardial space are the same as those that control fluid movement between the capillaries and the interstitial spaces of other body tissues (see Chap. 26). Normally, the pericardial sac contains 30 ml to 50 ml of clear straw-colored fluid.[2] Conditions, such as kidney disease and heart failure, that produce edema in other structures of the body may also produce an accumulation of fluid in the pericardial sac. This is often called *pericardial effusion*. In hydropericardium, the excess pericardial fluid is a serous transudate with a low specific gravity. Although a liter or more of transudates may accumulate, volumes of over 500 ml are uncommon.

The pericardium is subject to many of the pathologic processes such as inflammation, neoplastic disease, and congenital disorders that affect other structures of the body (Table 19-1). Pericardial disease is usually associated with or occurs secondary to another disease, either within the heart or in the surrounding structures.[2] The discussion in this chapter focuses on the pathologic processes associated with acute inflammation of the pericardium (pericarditis), pericardial effusion, cardiac tamponade, and constrictive pericarditis.

Table 19-1 Classification of Disorders of the Pericardium

Inflammation

Acute inflammatory pericarditis
1. Infectious
    Viral (echo, coxsackie and others)
    Bacterial (tuberculosis, staphylococcus, streptococcus, etc.)
    Fungal
2. Immune and collagen disorders
    Rheumatic fever
    Rheumatoid arthritis
    Systemic lupus erythematosus
3. Metabolic disorders
    Uremia and dialysis
    Myxedema
4. Ischemia and tissue injury
    Myocardial infarction
    Cardiac surgery
    Chest trauma
5. Physical and chemical agents
    Radiation therapy
    Untoward reactions to drugs, such as hydralazine, procainamide, and anticoagulants
Chronic inflammatory pericarditis
    Can be associated with most of the agents causing an acute inflammatory response

Neoplastic Disease
1. Primary
2. Secondary (carcinoma of the lung or breast, lymphoma, etc.)

Congenital Disorders
1. Complete or partial absence of the pericardium
2. Congenital pericardial cysts

Types of Pericardial Disorders

Acute pericarditis

Acute pericarditis is characterized by inflammation of the pericardium, often with the development of an exudate. It can result from a number of diverse causes. In many cases the same cause may persist over time and produce a recurrent subacute, or chronic, disease.[3]

Acute pericarditis can be classified according to etiology (infections, trauma, or rheumatic fever) or the nature of the exudate (fibrinous, purulent, hemorrhagic). Like other inflammatory conditions, acute pericarditis is often associated with increased capillary permeability. The capillaries that supply the serous pericardium become permeable, allowing plasma proteins, including fibrinogen, to leave the capillaries and enter the pericardial space. This results in an exudate that varies in type and amount depending on the causative agent. The most common type of exudate in acute pericarditis is fibrinous or serofibrinous (serous fluid mixed with fibrinous exudate). If the exudate contains red cells it is hemorrhagic, and if it contains pus cells it is purulent. Acute pericarditis is frequently associated with a fibrous exudate, which has been described as having a shaggy bread-and-butter appearance because it resembles the surfaces of a bread and butter sandwich that has been pulled apart. Acute fibrinous pericarditis may heal by resolution or progress to organization of the fibrin strands with deposition of scar tissue and formation of adhesions between the layers of the serous pericardium.

Perhaps the most common form of acute pericarditis is what has been termed *idiopathic* pericarditis. The disorder is commonly attributed to a viral agent or an immune response. It is seen most commonly in men 20 to 50 years of age and is often preceded by a prodromal phase during which fever, malaise, and other flulike symptoms are present. The condition usually lasts for several weeks, during which precordial pain, friction rub, and electrocardiographic (ECG) changes are present. Although the acute symptoms may subside shortly, easy fatigability often continues for several months.

Other causes of acute pericarditis are infections, rheumatic fever, myocardial infarction, the postpericardiotomy syndrome, posttraumatic pericarditis, metabolic disorders, physical and chemical agents, and pericarditis associated with connective tissue diseases. With the increased use of open-heart surgery in the treatment of various heart disorders, the postpericardiotomy syndrome has become a commonly recognized form of pericarditis. Although this type of pericarditis is thought to be due to an inflammatory response resulting from the presence of blood in the pericardium, it has been suggested that a viral agent, possibly arising from the multiple transfusions required during this type of surgery, may also play a role. Among the connective tissue diseases that cause acute pericarditis are rheumatic fever and systemic lupus erythematosus. Pericarditis has been noted in up to 90% of persons with systemic lupus erythematosus.[3] It may be the first sign of the disease and may precede the onset of other manifestations by months. In childhood the most common cause is rheumatic fever. Among the metabolic disorders that cause pericarditis are myxedema and uremia. Pericarditis with effusion is a common complication in persons being maintained on hemodialysis for the treatment of renal failure.

Manifestations of acute pericarditis. The manifestations of acute pericarditis include a triad of chest pain, friction rub, and ECG changes. The clinical findings and other manifestations may vary according to the etiologic agent. Leukocytosis and elevation in sedimentation rate are common.

Nearly all persons with acute pericarditis have chest pain. The pain is usually abrupt in onset, occurs in the precordial area, and is described as sharp. It may radiate to the neck, back, abdomen, or side. It is usually worse with deep breathing, coughing, swallowing, and positional changes. Often the patient will seek relief by sitting up and leaning forward. Only a small portion of the pericardium, the outer layer of the lower parietal pericardium below the fifth and sixth intercostal spaces, is sensitive to pain. This means that pericardial pain probably results from inflammation of the surrounding structures, particularly the pleura. Pain is more common when considerable effusion of fluid is present in the pericardial sac, probably because of the increased stretching of the lower parietal pericardium.

A pericardial friction rub, which is heard when a stethoscope is placed on the chest, results from movement between the inflamed pericardial surfaces. The sound associated with a friction rub has been described as leathery or close to the ear. It is usually heard best when the patient is leaning forward in the seated position and the diaphragm of the stethoscope is placed firmly along the left sternal border over the xiphoid process or near the lower border of the sternum. There are usually three components to the pericardial friction rub: the first occurs during atrial contraction, the second during the rapid filling phase of diastole, and the third during ventricular systole.[4] The two diastolic components of the friction rub may become merged to produce what has been termed a to-and-fro rub. In some patients, only a systolic rub is present. The friction rub associated with acute pericarditis usually lasts from 7 to 10 days.

Four stages of ECG changes occur during acute pericarditis:

Stage one: There is an acute elevation of the S-T segment.
Stage two: The S-T segment becomes isoelectric.
Stage three: The T wave becomes inverted.
Stage four: The ECG returns to normal.[5]

The S-T segment changes begin within hours to days following the onset of acute pericarditis. Serial ECGs are useful in differentiating between myocardial infarction in which the S-T segment does not return to the isoelectric line, before the T wave inversion occurs, and acute pericarditis, in which T wave inversion occurs after the S-T segment has returned to normal. The reader is referred to a specialty text for a more complete description of these ECG changes.

Pericardial effusion

Pericardial effusion refers to the presence of exudate in the pericardial cavity. The amount of exudate, the rapidity with which it accumulates, and the elasticity of the pericardium will determine the effect that the effusion has on cardiac function. Small pericardial effusions may produce no symptoms or abnormal clinical findings. Even a large effusion that develops slowly may cause few, if any, symptoms providing the pericardium is able to stretch and avoid compressing the heart. On the other hand, a sudden accumulation of 200 ml may raise intracardiac pressure to levels that seriously limit the venous return to the heart. Signs of cardiac compression may also occur with relatively small accumulations of fluid when the pericardium has become thickened by scar tissue or neoplastic infiltrations.

Cardiac tamponade. Cardiac tamponade is defined as cardiac compression due to excess fluid or blood in the pericardial sac. It can occur as the result of trauma, effusion, cardiac rupture, or dissecting aneurysm. The seriousness of the condition results from restriction in

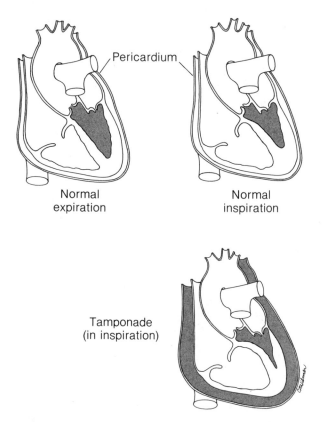

Figure 19-1 *Effect of respiration and cardiac tamponade on ventricular filling and cardiac output. During inspiration venous flow into the right heart increases, causing the interventricular septum to bulge into the left ventricle. This produces a decrease in left ventricular volume, with a subsequent decrease in stroke volume output. In cardiac tamponade, the fluid in the pericardial sac produces further compression of the left ventricle, causing an exaggeration of the normal inspiratory decrease in stroke volume and systolic blood pressure.*

ventricular filling with a subsequent critical reduction in stroke volume and depends on the amount of fluid that is present and the rate at which it accumulates. A rapid accumulation of fluid results in an increase in central venous pressure, a decrease in venous return to the heart, distention of the jugular veins, a decrease in cardiac output despite an increase in heart rate, a decrease in systolic blood pressure, and signs of circulatory shock.

Pulsus paradoxus refers to an exaggeration of the normal inspiratory decrease in systolic blood pressure and is a clinical indicator of cardiac tamponade. Pulsus paradoxus is easiest to detect when the blood pressure cuff is inflated to a value above the systolic pressure and then deflated slowly at a rate of 2 mm Hg/sec until the first Korotkoff sound is detected with expiration. Following the notation of this pressure, the cuff is deflated until the Korotkoff sounds can be heard throughout the respiratory cycle. A difference greater than 10 mm Hg between the two readings is indicative of pulsus paradoxus. In cardiac tamponade, this implies a large reduction in ventricular volume. Inspiration normally accelerates venous flow, increasing right atrial and ventricular filling; this causes the interventricular septum to bulge to the left, producing internal compression of the left ventricle. In cardiac tamponade, the left ventricle is compressed from within by movement of the interventricular septum and from without by fluid in the pericardium (Fig. 19-1). With pulsus paradoxus, left ventricular output can decrease within a beat of the beginning of inspiration.

Chronic pericarditis with effusion. Chronic pericarditis with effusion is characterized by an increase in inflammatory exudate that continues beyond the anticipated period of time. In some cases the exudate will persist for several years. In most cases of chronic pericarditis no specific pathogen can be identified. The process is commonly associated with other forms of heart disease, such as rheumatic fever, congenital heart lesions, or hypertensive heart disease. Systemic diseases such as lupus erthymatosus, rheumatoid arthritis, scleroderma, and myxedema are also causes of chronic pericarditis, as are metabolic disturbances associated with acute and chronic renal failure. Unlike those of acute pericarditis, the signs and symptoms of chronic pericarditis are often minimal; many times the disease is detected for the first time on routine chest film. As the condition progresses, the fluid may accumulate and compress the adjacent cardiac structures and impair cardiac filling.

Constrictive pericarditis

In constrictive pericarditis, scar tissue develops between the visceral and parietal layers of the serous pericardium. In time the scar tissue contracts and interferes with cardiac filling, at which point cardiac output and cardiac reserve become fixed. Ascites is a prominent early finding, often occurring without signs of accompanying peripheral edema. The jugular veins are also distended. Kussmaul's sign is an inspiratory distention of the jugular veins due to the inability of the right atrium, encased in its rigid pericardium, to accommodate the increase in venous return that occurs with inspiration.

Diagnosis and Treatment

Various diagnostic tests are used to confirm the presence of pericardial disease. These measures include auscultation, chest x-ray, electrocardiography, echocardiography, and cardiac catheterization with angiographic studies. Aspiration and laboratory analysis of the pericardial fluid may be used to identify the causative agent.

Treatment is dependent on the etiology. When infection is present, antibiotics specific for the causative agent are usually prescribed. Anti-inflammatory drugs may be given to minimize the inflammatory response and the accompanying undesirable effects. Pericardiocentesis, the removal of fluid from the pericardial sac, may be a life-saving measure in severe cardiac tamponade. Surgical treatment may be required in traumatic lesions of the heart or in constrictive pericarditis in which cardiac filling is severely impaired.

In summary, disorders of the pericardium include acute pericarditis, pericardial effusion, cardiac tamponade, and constrictive pericarditis. Acute pericarditis is characterized by chest pain, ECG changes, and a friction rub. Among the causes of acute pericarditis are infections, uremia, rheumatic fever, connective tissue diseases, and myocardial infarction. Pericardial effusion refers to the presence of an exudate in the pericardial cavity and can be either acute or chronic. Pericardial effusion can increase intracardiac pressure, compress the heart, and interfere with venous return to the heart. The amount of exudate, the rapidity with which it accumulates, and the elasticity of the pericardium determine the effect that the effusion has on cardiac function. Cardiac tamponade is a life-threatening cardiac compression resulting from excess fluid in the pericardial sac. In constrictive pericarditis, scar tissue develops between the visceral and parietal layers of the serous pericardium. In time, the scar tissue contracts and interferes with cardiac filling.

◼ Coronary Heart Disease

The major cause of death in the United States is coronary heart disease, which accounts for two-thirds of all cardiovascular deaths. In 1981 it caused 559,000 deaths;

4,600,000 persons alive today have a history of heart attack or angina pectoris or both.[1]

In most of the cases, coronary heart disease is due to atherosclerosis. Epidemiologic studies have identified three treatable risk factors: hypertension, elevated blood cholesterol, and cigarette smoking. A number of additional contributing factors in the development of coronary heart disease such as obesity, diabetes, physical inactivity, male sex, and certain personality types have been implicated. Coronary heart disease is often a silent disorder; most men and women over 50 years of age probably have moderately far advanced coronary atherosclerosis although most of them have no symptoms of heart disease.[6]

No simple screening tests exist at present to detect coronary artery disease. Disease of the coronary vessels can cause angina, myocardial infarction, cardiac arrhythmias, conduction defects, heart failure, and sudden death; diagnostic tests are usually done when symptoms are present and are often used to determine severity and localize the areas of involvement.

Coronary Arteries and Distribution of Blood Flow

There are two main coronary arteries, the right and left, which arise from the coronary sinus just above the aortic valve (Fig. 19-2). The *left coronary artery* divides almost immediately into the anterior descending and circumflex branches. The *left anterior descending artery* passes down through the groove between the two ventricles, giving off *diagonal branches* that supply the left ventricle and *perforating branches* that supply the anterior portion of the intraventricular septum and the anterior papillary muscle of the left ventricle. The *circumflex branch* of the left coronary artery passes to the left and moves posteriorly in the groove that separates the left atrium and ventricle, giving off branches that supply the left lateral wall of the left ventricle. The *right coronary artery* lies in the right atrioventricular groove, and its branches supply the right ventricle. The right coronary artery usually moves to the back of the heart where it forms the *posterior descending artery*, which supplies the posterior portion of the heart (the intraventricular septum, atrioventricular node, and posterior papillary muscle). The sinoatrial node is also usually supplied by the right coronary artery. In about 10% of the population, the left circumflex rather than the right coronary artery moves posteriorly to form the posterior descending artery. The term *dominant* designates the main coronary artery that extends to form the posterior descending artery. Dominant left circulation tells us that the posterior descending artery is a branch of the left circumflex, and dominant right circulation tells us

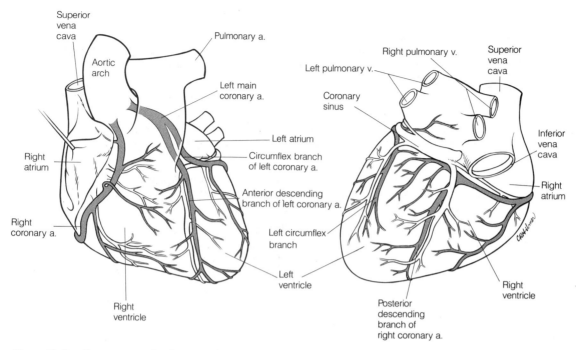

Figure 19-2 *Coronary arteries that arise from the aorta and some of the coronary veins.*

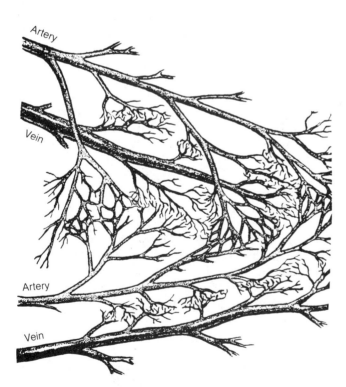

Figure 19-3 *Anastomoses of the smaller coronary arterial vessels. (Guyton AC: Textbook of Medical Physiology, 6th ed. Philadelphia, WB Saunders, 1981)*

that the posterior descending artery is a branch of the right coronary artery.

The large coronary arteries lie on the surface of the heart, with smaller intramuscular branches coming off and penetrating the myocardium. Although there are no connections between the large coronary arteries, there are anastomotic channels that join the small arteries (Fig. 19-3). With gradual occlusion of the larger vessels, the smaller collateral vessels increase in size and provide alternative channels for blood flow. One of the reasons that coronary disease does not produce symptoms until it is far advanced is that the collateral channels develop at the same time the atherosclerotic changes are occurring.

Coronary heart disease can affect one or all of the coronary arteries (1-, 2-, or 3-vessel disease) and can be diffuse or localized to one area of a single vessel. Usually 75% or more of the vessel lumen must be occluded before there is significant reduction in coronary blood flow.

Angina Pectoris

Angina pectoris is a choking paroxysmal pain associated with transient myocardial ischemia. The pain of angina is assumed to occur when the myocardial need for oxygen exceeds the ability of the coronary vessels to supply adequate blood flow to meet the need. Angina may be caused by atherosclerotic lesions of the coronary arteries, by vasospasm of these vessels, or by a combination of these two conditions. Angina associated with atherosclerotic disease of the coronaries is commonly referred to as classic angina; when it is due to spasm of the coronaries it is called variant angina. Unstable angina includes features of both classic and variant angina. In rare instances, other factors that increase the work load of the heart, such as severe aortic stenosis or anemia, may cause angina.

Pain is a classic manifestation of angina. Typically, the pain is described as constricting, squeezing, or suffocating. The pain is usually steady, increasing in intensity only at the onset and end of the attack. The pain of angina is usually located in the precordial or substernal area; it is similar to myocardial infarction in that it may radiate to the left shoulder, jaw, arm, or other areas of the chest. In some persons, the arm or shoulder pain may be confused with arthritis; in others, the epigastric pain is thought to result from indigestion (Fig. 19-4). The duration of anginal pain is brief—seldom does it last more than 5 minutes.

Electrocardiographic changes are not always present in angina, particularly if the recording is made while the person is resting or at a time when pain is not present. Exercise and pain may cause S-T segment displacement. Exercise stress testing is useful in differentiating angina from other forms of chest pain.

Types of angina

Classic angina.   Classic angina, sometimes called exertional angina, is associated with atherosclerotic disease of the coronary arteries and occurs when the metabolic needs of the myocardium exceed the ability of the occluded coronary arteries to deliver adequate blood flow. Despite the fact that the overwhelming majority of persons with angina have atherosclerotic heart disease, angina does not develop in a considerable number of persons with advanced coronary atherosclerosis. This is probably because of their sedentary life-style, the development of adequate collateral circulation, or the inability of these persons to perceive the pain. In many instances, myocardial infarction occurs without a prior history of angina. Pain is usually precipitated by situations such as physical exertion, exposure to cold, and emotional stress, that increase the work demands of the heart. Of particular diagnostic significance is the fact that the pain is relieved by rest or the administration of nitroglycerin; this is not true of other forms of chest pain.

Variant angina.   The syndrome of variant angina was first described by Prinzmetal and associates in 1959 and is sometimes referred to as Prinzmetal's angina.[7] Evidence suggests that variant angina is caused by spasms of the coronary arteries. In most instances, the spasms

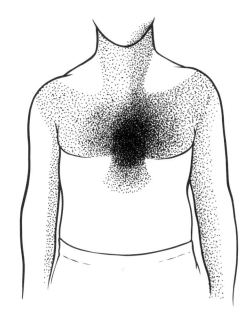

Figure 19-4   *Areas of pain due to angina. (Adapted from Heart Facts 1984. American Heart Association, 1984)*

occur in the presence of coronary artery stenosis; however, variant angina has been shown to occur in the absence of visible disease. Unlike the classic form of angina that occurs with exertion or stress, variant angina usually occurs during rest or with minimal exercise and is frequently nocturnal. It may be associated with REM sleep. It commonly follows a cyclic or regular pattern of occurrence (*e.g.,* it happens at the same time each day). Arrhythmias are often present when the pain is severe and the individual suffering the attack is often aware of their presence. Electrocardiographic changes are significant if recorded during the attack. Typically the S-T segment is elevated on the same lead during each attack, suggesting the involvement of a single vessel. A provocative test that may be performed to confirm the diagnosis of variant angina is the administration of ergonovine or another agent that produces coronary vasospasm. This test is done during angiographic studies performed in the cardiac catheterization laboratory. The mechanism of coronary vasospasm is uncertain. It has been suggested that it may result from hyperactive sympathetic nervous system responses, from a defect in the handling of calcium in vascular smooth muscle, or from a reduced production of prostaglandin I_2. In one clinical study of four patients with variant angina, the administration of aspirin (4 gm/day) markedly increased the frequency of anginal attacks.[8] As in classic angina, nitroglycerin is usually effective in relieving the attack of variant angina. The calcium-channel blocking drugs have proved extraordinarily effective in treating variant angina.

Unstable angina. Unstable angina is an accelerated form of angina in which the pain is characterized by a changing pattern. It begins to appear more frequently, is more severe, lasts longer, and may appear at rest. Ischemic ECG changes occur with the pain. Unstable angina is usually associated with obstructive coronary artery disease, but at present it is uncertain whether or not coronary artery vasospasm plays an important role in its progression. Unstable angina is sometimes called preinfarction angina because of its propensity for accelerating to myocardial infarction. Individuals with unstable angina are commonly admitted to the coronary care unit of a hospital for stabilization and treatment. Cardiac catheterization followed by transluminal angioplasty or bypass surgery may be needed.

Diagnosis and treatment

Diagnosis of angina is usually based on history, ECG findings, response to the administration of nitroglycerin, and the results of exercise stress testing. Cardiac catheterization and nuclear imaging may be used in describing the location and extent of the disease. These diagnostic methods are described in Chapter 18.

Measures for the treatment of angina are usually directed toward reducing the work demands of the heart, since in classic and unstable angina the diseased coronary vessels are probably maximally dilated and carrying as much blood as they are capable of carrying. Treatment measures directed at decreasing preload and afterload stress include the selective pacing of physical activities, stress reduction, avoidance of cold, weight reduction if obesity is present, use of nitroglycerin and long-acting nitrates, beta-blocking drugs, and a new group of drugs called calcium antagonists. Immediate cessation of activity is often sufficient to abort an anginal attack. Sitting down or standing quietly is often preferable to lying down, since these positions tend to decrease preload by producing pooling of blood in the lower extremities. Sudden exposure to cold tends to increase vasoconstriction and afterload stress; thus, patients with angina are usually cautioned against drinking cold liquids and breathing extremely cold air. Anxiety often precipitates angina because it causes an increase in both heart rate and blood pressure.

Nitroglycerin. *Nitroglycerin* (glycerol trinitrate) provides prompt relief from anginal pain. It is a vasodilating drug that causes the relaxation of both venous and arterial vessels. Venous dilatation reduces venous return to the heart, thereby emptying the heart and decreasing the amount of blood that the heart must pump. With this decrease the tension on the wall of the ventricle is reduced, and less pressure is needed to pump blood. Nitroglycerin also relaxes the arterioles, reducing the

pressure against which the left heart must pump. Nitroglycerin must be given *sublingually*, because it is rapidly destroyed in the liver once it has been absorbed. Absorption is rapid, and relief of pain usually begins in 30 seconds. Nitroglycerin is available in ointment and adhesive patch forms for topical application. Ointment has a duration of action of 4 to 6 hours. The adhesive patches have a longer duration of action (24 hours). Although they are more costly than the ointment, they tend to increase compliance in many individuals.

Beta-adrenergic blocking drugs. The beta-adrenergic blocking drugs act as antagonists that block stimuli mediated by the beta receptors of the sympathetic nervous system. There are two types of beta receptors: beta $(\beta)_1$ and β_2 receptors. β_1 receptors are found in the heart and β_2 receptors are found in other parts of the body. At present there are six beta-blocking drugs approved by the Food and Drug Administration (FDA); these are propranolol, nadolol, timolol, pindolol, atenolol, and metaprolol; of these drugs atenolol and metaprolol are cardioselective in low doses (preferentially block β_1 receptors), whereas the other four drugs block both β_1 and β_2 receptors and are nonselective in their actions. Blockade of beta receptors in the heart reduces the heart rate, cardiac contractility, and myocardial oxygen consumption.

Calcium-channel blocking drugs. The calcium-channel blocking drugs, sometimes called calcium antagonists, are currently approved for the treatment of angina pectoris and cardiac arrhythmias; they are being investigated for treating cardiomyopathy and hypertension. At present the three drugs that are most used in the United States are diltiazem, nifedipine, and verapamil. Although these three drugs have different chemical structures, they are effective in blocking a number of calcium-dependent functions; that is, they block the function of the calcium channels or enter the cell and substitute for calcium at intracellular receptor sites.[9]

Free intracellular calcium serves to link many membrane-initiated events with cellular responses, such as muscle contraction and action potential generation. Vascular smooth muscle lacks the sarcoplasmic reticulum and other structures that are necessary for intracellular storage of calcium; it relies on the influx of calcium from the extracellular fluid into the cell to initiate and sustain contraction. In cardiac muscle, the slow inward calcium current contributes to the plateau of the action potential and to cardiac contractility. The slow calcium current is particularly important in the pacemaker activity of the SA node and the conduction properties of the AV node. The therapeutic effect of the calcium antagonists results from coronary and peripheral artery dilatation and decreased myocardial metabolism associated with the decrease in myocardial contractility. In patients with variant angina, nifedipine has proven to have a 82% to 94% good to excellent response; diltiazem, 85% to 91%; and verapamil, 61% to 86%.[10] In clinical doses, verapamil and diltiazem depress the SA and AV nodes. The extent of slowing is dependent on the dose, the route of administration, and the concomitant use of other drugs. Verapamil may be administered intravenously for the termination of paroxysmal supraventricular tachycardia. Nifedipine, in the usual clinical doses, has no direct effect on AV node conduction.

Percutaneous transluminal coronary angioplasty. Percutaneous transluminal coronary angioplasty (PTCA) involves the dilatation of a stenotic coronary vessel. The procedure is similar to that for coronary angiography. With this procedure, a double lumen balloon dilatation catheter is introduced percutaneously into the femoral or brachial artery and then advanced under fluoroscopic control to the coronary ostium. It is then directed into the affected coronary artery and advanced until the balloon segment is within the stenotic area of the vessel. Once in place, the balloon is inflated for 3 seconds to 5 seconds using a pressure-controlled pump. The inflation may be repeated several times if needed. The mechanism for reduction of stenosis is not completely understood. It has been suggested that compression of the lipids and loose connective tissue within the atheromatous lesion may occur or that splitting and separation of the smooth muscle fibers may produce a controlled injury to the vessel that serves to increase the outer diameter of the vessel.[11] If the dilatation is successful, the patient is monitored for 6 to 8 hours and then discharged in 1 to 2 days. Selection criteria for this treatment include demonstrated evidence of myocardial ischemia; disease limited to one vessel, or at most coronary artery disease in which only one vessel has a major obstruction; and suitable candidacy for coronary bypass surgery, should it be needed. At this time, use of the procedure in multiple vessel disease is investigational. Some persons with previous coronary bypass surgery who have developed stenosis of the vein graft may be considered suitable candidates for the procedure.[11]

Coronary bypass surgery. The surgical treatment of angina—aortocoronary bypass surgery—has gained popularity, particularly in patients who have significant coronary artery disease. In this surgical procedure, revascularization of the myocardium is effected by placing a saphenous vein graft between the aorta and the affected coronary artery distal to the site of the occlusion or by using the internal mammary artery as a means of revascularizing the left anterior descending artery or its

branches. Figure 19-5 illustrates the placement of a saphenous vein graft and a mammary artery graft. Although it cannot be documented that this surgery significantly alters the progress of disease, it does relieve pain, so that patients may have a more productive life. In one study, 60% of patients who had bypass surgery for angina showed marked improvement or were pain free 1 year later, compared with 16% who had corresponding relief when treated medically.[12] In another study, which viewed patients' employment patterns following bypass surgery, 90% of men under age 55, 68% of men 55 to 59, and 44% of men over age 60 were still employed 4 years later.[13]

Myocardial Infarction

Myocardial infarction is the ischemic death of myocardial tissue associated with the obstruction of a coronary vessel. There are three views on the origin of the obstruction. One is that the obstruction is caused by thrombosis. Another view is that the occlusion is caused by hemor-

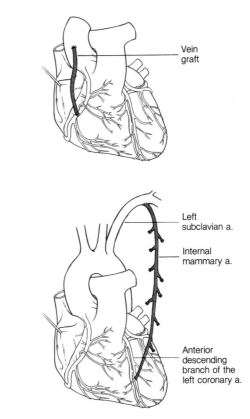

Vein graft

Left subclavian a.

Internal mammary a.

Anterior descending branch of the left coronary a.

Figure 19-5 *Coronary artery revascularization.* (Top) *Saphenous vein bypass graft. The vein segment is sutured to the ascending aorta and the right coronary artery at a point distal to the occluding lesion.* (Bottom) *Mammary artery bypass. The mammary artery is anastomosed to the anterior descending left coronary artery, bypassing the obstructing lesion.*

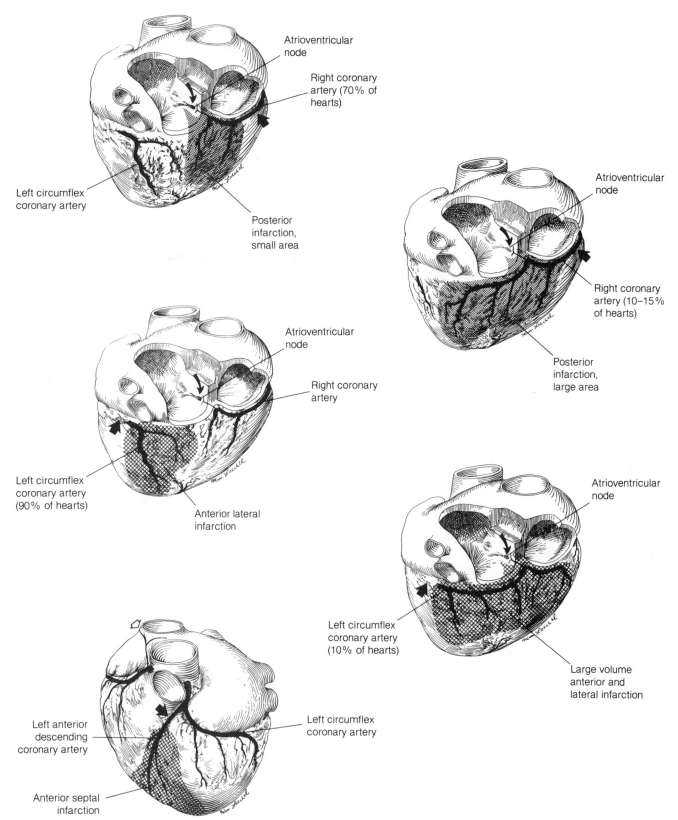

Figure 19-6 *Anatomy and distribution of the coronary arteries and the topography of infarction. Shaded areas represent extent of infarction. Arrows point to affected arteries. Percentages relate to persons with described involvement of right, left circumflex, or left anterior descending coronary artery. (James TN: Arrhythmias and conduction disturbances in acute myocardial infarction. Am Heart J 64(3):416, 1962)*

rhage in an atherosclerotic plaque. According to the third view, the ischemia is precipitated by a sudden increase in oxygen demand by the myocardium or by spasm of a diseased vessel.

Recently, it has been suggested that thrombosis follows, rather than precedes, the ischemic event. This opinion is supported by necropsy data in which complete occlusion with thrombosis was not demonstrated in a large percentage of patients dying from myocardial infarction.[14] The frequency of thrombosis increases with the duration of survival and the size of the infarct. It is quite possible that the event responsible for the infarct—vessel spasm or excessive myocardial oxygen requirements—may also predispose to thrombus formation in the vessel supplying the area. Even though thrombosis may not be the initiating event in myocardial infarction, almost all patients dying of myocardial infarction have been found to have severe coronary atherosclerosis.[2]

An infarct may involve the endocardium, myocardium, epicardium, or a combination of these. An *intramural* infarct is one that is contained within the myocardium whereas a *transmural* infarct involves all three layers. Most infarcts are transmural, involving the free wall of the left ventricle and the intraventricular septum. The increased vulnerability of the left ventricle is probably related to its increased work demands. According to Robbins,[2] about 30% to 40% of infarcts affect the right coronary artery, 40% to 50% the left anterior descending artery, and the remaining 15% to 20% the left circumflex artery. This distribution is depicted in Figure 19-6.

Although gross tissue changes are not apparent for hours following myocardial infarction (Table 19-2), it has been reported that the ischemic area ceases to function within a matter of minutes and that irreversible damage to cells occurs in about 40 minutes. There is also evidence to suggest that an area of injury and ischemic zone borders the necrotic area (Fig. 19-7). There is reason to believe that the fate of the remaining viable cells in the area of injury and ischemic zone is not determined until sometime after the onset of infarction.[15] Recently, there has been considerable concern for salvaging the ischemic area and thereby reducing the size of the infarct. Measures said to reduce infarct size are (1) decreasing the myocardial oxygen consumption and (2) increasing the oxygen availability. Because *sympathetic activity* increases the *metabolic activity of the myocardium* and myocardial oxygen consumption, beta-adrenergic blocking drugs may be used to reduce sympathetic stimulation of the heart following infarction. A second means of decreasing oxygen consumption is the use of vasodilator drugs, such as nitroglycerin, nitroprusside, and hydralazine, because they decrease venous return (reduce preload) and the arterial pressure against which the left ventricle must pump (afterload). Oxygen is administered to make it

Table 19-2 Tissue Changes Following Myocardial Infarction

Time Following Onset	Gross Tissue Changes
6–12 hours	No gross changes
18–24 hours	Pale to gray-brown Slight pallor of area
2–4 days	Necrosis of area is apparent. Area is yellow-brown in center and hyperemic around the edges
4–10 days	Area becomes soft; fatty changes in the center are well developed Hemorrhagic areas are present in the infarcted area. Rupture of the heart, when it occurs, happens during this period
10 days or more	Fibrotic (scar) tissue replacement and revascularization commences
6 weeks	Scar tissue replacement of necrotic tissue is usually complete, depends on size of infarct

(Developed from data in Robbins SL, Cotran R, Kumar V: Pathologic Basis of Disease, 3rd ed, pp 559–560. Philadelphia, WB Saunders, 1984)

readily available to the ischemic myocardium. Of interest is the possibility of augmenting the production of ATP by the myocardial cells through the anaerobic pathway in an effort to supply needed energy. Efforts in this area have focused on the use of glucose-insulin-potassium infusions, antilipolytic agents, and lipid-free albumin solutions.

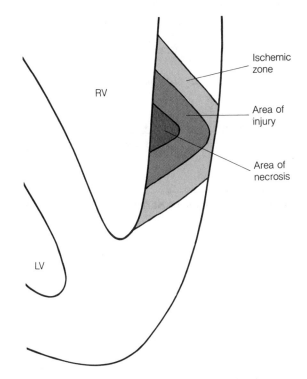

Figure 19-7 *Tissue damage after myocardial infarction.*

Signs and symptoms

The signs and symptoms of myocardial infarction can be categorized into four groups: (1) pain and autonomic responses associated with the ischemic event, (2) weakness and signs related to impaired myocardial function, (3) arrhythmias and electrocardiographic changes associated with ischemia and death of myocardial cells, and (4) signs of inflammation and elevated serum enzyme levels indicative of tissue death.

Pain.   The onset of infarction is usually abrupt, with pain as the significant symptom. Typically, the pain is severe and crushing, often described as being constrictive, suffocating, or like "someone sitting on my chest." The pain is usually substernal, radiating to the left arm, neck, or jaw, although it may be experienced in other areas of the chest. Unlike that of angina, the pain associated with infarction is more prolonged and is not relieved by rest or nitroglycerin, and narcotics are frequently required.

Manifestations of circulatory dysfunction.   There may be a sensation of *epigastric distress*; nausea and vomiting may occur. These symptoms are thought to be related to the severity of the pain and to vagal stimulation. This epigastric distress may be mistaken for indigestion and the patient may seek relief with the use of antacids or other home remedies, which only delays getting medical attention. Frequently, there are complaints of *fatigue and weakness*, especially of the arms and legs. Pain and sympathetic stimulation combine to give rise to *tachycardia, anxiety, restlessness,* and *feelings of impending doom.* The *skin* is often *pale, cool,* and *moist.* The impaired myocardial function may lead to hypotension and shock.

Electrocardiographic changes.   Electrocardiographic changes may not be present immediately following the onset of symptoms, except as arrhythmias. Typical changes associated with the death of myocardial tissue include prolongation of the Q wave, S-T segment eleva-

tion, and T wave inversion. The ECG changes are variable and complex, and interested readers and those intending to work in the coronary care unit are referred to specialty texts for full discussion.

Serum enzymes.   Cell death causes inflammation and the release of intracellular enzymes. Fever and leukocytosis usually develop within about 24 hours and continue for 3 to 7 days. The sedimentation rate rises on the second and third days and remains elevated for 1 to 3 weeks. Enzymes released include creatine phosphokinase (CPK), lactic dehydrogenase (LDH), and glutamine-oxaloacetic transaminase (GOT). As indicated in Table 19-3, these enzymes become elevated at different times after infarction and provide useful diagnostic information. The enzyme CPK (MB band), which is one of three isoenzymes of CPK, has been found to be a more reliable indicator of myocardial infarction than other enzymes (singly or in combination) or the electrocardiogram.[16]

Complications

The stages of recovery are closely related to the size of the infarct and the changes that have taken place within the infarcted area. Fibrous tissue lacks the contractile, elastic, and conductive properties of normal myocardial cells; hence, the residual effects as well as complications are determined essentially by the extent and location of injury.

Sudden death.   Sudden death is death occurring within an hour after the onset of symptoms, and it is usually attributed to fatal arrhythmias, which may occur without evidence of infarction. Sulfinpyrazone, a drug that inhibits platelet aggregation, has been reported to decrease the incidence of sudden death.[17] At this writing, the benefits of the drug are investigational. Should its effectiveness be established, it will then be necessary to develop a means of identifying persons at risk, because many of those who die suddenly have had no history of heart disease.

Table 19-3   Elevation of Serum Enzymes Postmyocardial Infarction

Enzyme	Time Postinfarction		
	Exceeds Normal Value	Reaches Peak Value	Returns to Normal
CPK (Creatine phosphokinase)*	4–8 hours	24 hours	3–4 days
GOT (Glutamine oxaloacetic transaminase)	8–12 hours	24–48 hours	4–7 days
LDH (Lactic dehydrogenase)†	12–24 hours	3–6 days	8–14 days

*There are three isoenzymes of CPK; myocardial cells possess the isoenzyme MB.

†There are five isoenzymes of LDH; myocardial cells have both LDH_1 and LDH_2. Normally the ratio of LDH_1 to LDH_2 is less than 1; following myocardial infarction, this ratio is reversed.

Heart failure and cardiogenic shock. Both heart failure and cardiogenic shock are dreaded complications of myocardial infarction. They are discussed in Chapters 20 and 21.

Pericarditis and Dressler's syndrome. Pericarditis may complicate the course of acute myocardial infarction. It usually appears on the second or third day postinfarction. At this time, the patient experiences a new type of pain, which is sharp and stabbing in nature and aggravated with deep inspiration and positional changes. A pericardial rub may or may not be heard in all patients who have postinfarction pericarditis, and often it is transitory, usually resolving uneventfully. Dressler's syndrome describes signs and symptoms associated with pericarditis, pleurisy, and pneumonitis: fever, chest pain, dyspnea, and abnormal laboratory (elevated white blood cell count and sedimentation rate) and ECG findings. The symptoms may arise between 1 day and several weeks following infarction and are thought to represent a hypersensitivity response to tissue necrosis.

Thromboemboli. Thromboemboli are a potential complication, arising either as venous thrombi or, occasionally, as a clot from the wall of the ventricle. Immobility and impaired cardiac function contribute to the stasis of blood in the venous system. Elastic stockings, along with active and passive leg exercises, are usually included in the postinfarction treatment plan as a means of preventing thrombus formation. If a clot is detected on the wall of the ventricle (usually by echocardiography), treatment with anticoagulants is used.

Rupture of heart structures. The acute postmyocardial infarction period can be complicated by rupture of the myocardium, the intraventricular septum, or a papillary muscle. Myocardial rupture is usually fatal, occurring at the time when the injured ventricular tissue is soft and weak, about the seventh to the tenth day. Necrosis of the septal wall or papillary muscle may also lead to the rupture of either of these structures with a worsening of ventricular performance. Surgical repair is usually indicated, but whenever possible, it is delayed until the heart has had time to recover from the initial infarction. Vasodilator therapy and the aortic balloon counterpulsation pump may provide supportive assistance during this period.

Ventricular aneurysm. Scar tissue does not have the characteristics of normal myocardial tissue. When a large section of ventricular muscle is replaced by scar tissue, that section does not contract with the rest of the ventricle; instead there is outpouching—aneurysm—of the ventricle during systole, which diminishes myocardial pumping efficiency (Fig. 19-8). This increases the work of the left ventricle and predisposes to heart failure. The ischemia in the surrounding area predisposes to the development of arrhythmias; and within the aneurysm, stasis of blood can lead to thrombus formation. Surgical resection is often corrective.

Diagnosis and treatment

Diagnosis of myocardial infarction is based on the presence of prolonged chest pain and other signs of distress, changes in heart rate and blood pressure, ECG changes, and elevation of cardiac enzymes. Diagnostic methods such as nuclear imaging may be used to confirm the diagnosis and the extent of the injury.

The treatment of myocardial infarction has changed drastically in the past two decades. Patients are ambulated earlier, leave the hospital sooner, and are encouraged to return to an active and productive life; this contrasts with the requirements of prolonged activity restriction and limited return to work that were imposed in the past. The current treatment methods focus on detection and early treatment of arrhythmias and other types of acute cardiac dysfunction, relief of pain and provision for rest of the heart to minimize the size of the infarcted area, and rehabilitation and exercise. In selected cases, streptokinase may be used to dissolve the clot during the immediate postinfarction period.

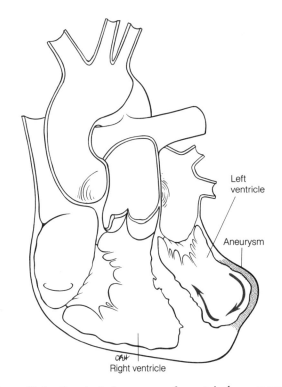

Left ventricle

Aneurysm

Right ventricle

Figure 19-8 *Paradoxical movement of a ventricular aneurysm during systole.*

Prevention of arrhythmias and acute complications.
The immediate postinfarction care focuses on the early detection and treatment of arrhythmias, cardiac failure, and cardiogenic shock. The danger of potentially fatal arrhythmias soon after infarction usually warrants continual electrocardiographic monitoring. The continual or frequent monitoring of other hemodynamic measurements such as blood pressure and pulmonary capillary wedge pressure may also be indicated. The coronary care unit ensures access to constant supervision, monitoring, and emergency treatment if required.

Rest and pain relief.   Protecting the oxygen supply of the heart and decreasing the myocardial oxygen consumption as much as possible are additional concerns during the early treatment of myocardial infarction. Patients with myocardial infarction are usually maintained on bed rest for at least 48 hours, although the use of the bedside commode for elimination purposes may be allowed. This is followed by a gradual increase in activity depending on the severity of the infarct and the presence of complications. The severe pain of myocardial infarction gives rise to anxiety, with recruitment of autonomic responses, and these increase the work demands on the heart. Morphine and meperidine (Demerol) are often given intravenously because they have a rapid onset of action, and the intravenous route does not elevate cardiac enzyme levels. A second early treatment measure involves the administration of oxygen to augment the oxygen content of the inspired air and increase the oxygen saturation of the hemoglobin. Arterial oxygen levels may fall precipitously following myocardial infarction, and oxygen administration maintains the oxygen content of the blood perfusing the coronary circulation. Modifying the diet to include foods that are low in salt and easy to digest is another treatment measure. Stool softeners are often prescribed to prevent constipation and straining on defecation.

Streptokinase.   Intracoronary artery infusion of streptokinase, an enzyme that dissolves blood clots, has recently been introduced as a treatment for patients in whom myocardial infarctions are caused by intracoronary thrombi. The treatment requires 20 to 40 minutes to reestablish the blood flow; to be effective, the treatment must be done within 3 to 4 hours following the onset of acute myocardial infarction while the heart tissue that is supplied by the affected vessel can still be salvaged. The procedure is carried out during cardiac catheterization using angiographic studies.

Rehabilitation and exercise.   An exercise program has become an integral part of the rehabilitation program for most cardiac patients. It includes such activities as walking, swimming, and bicycling. These exercises cause changes in muscle length and rhythmic contractions of muscle groups. The exercise program is usually individually designed to meet the patient's physical and psychologic needs. The goal of the exercise program is to increase the maximal oxygen uptake by the tissues, so that these patients will be able to perform more work at a lower heart rate and blood pressure.

In summary, coronary heart disease is usually due to atherosclerosis. It is frequently a silent disorder, and symptoms do not occur until the disease is far advanced. Angina pectoris is a choking paroxysmal chest pain that occurs when there is a disparity between the metabolic needs of the myocardium and the amount of blood that the coronary arteries can deliver. There are three types of angina. Classic angina is associated with atherosclerosis of the coronary arteries, in which pain is precipitated by increased work demands on the heart and is relieved by rest; variant angina is due to spasms of the coronary arteries; and unstable angina is an accelerated form of angina in which the pain occurs more frequently, is more severe, and lasts longer. Myocardial infarction refers to the ischemic death of myocardial tissue associated with obstructed blood flow in the coronary arteries. The infarct can involve the endocardium, myocardium, pericardium, or a combination of all three layers. The complications of myocardial infarction include potentially fatal arrhythmias, heart failure, cardiogenic shock, pericarditis, thromboemboli, rupture of cardiac structures, and ventricular aneurysms.

■ Arrhythmias and Conduction Disorders

The specialized cells in the conduction system manifest four inherent properties: (1) automaticity, (2) excitability, (3) conductivity, and (4) refractoriness (see Chap. 18). The term *arrhythmia* refers to an alteration in cardiac rhythm.* An alteration in any of these properties may produce arrhythmias or conduction defects. There are many causes of altered cardiac rhythms, including congenital defects of the conduction system, degenerative changes, ischemia and myocardial infarction, fluid and electrolyte imbalances, and the effects of drug ingestion. Arrhythmias are not necessarily patholologic; they can occur in the healthy as well as the diseased heart. Disturbances in cardiac rhythms exert their harmful effects by interfering with the heart's pumping ability. Rapid heart rates reduce the diastolic filling time, causing a subsequent decrease in the stroke volume output and in

---

*The term *dysrhythmia* is also used to describe disorders of cardiac rhythm.

coronary perfusion while increasing the myocardial oxygen needs. Abnormally slow heart rates may impair the blood flow to vital organs such as the brain.

Mechanisms of Arrhythmias and Conduction Disorders

Automaticity is the ability of certain cells of the conduction system to spontaneously initiate an impulse or action potential. The SA node has an inherent discharge rate of 60 to 100 times a minute; normally it acts as the pacemaker of the heart because it reaches the threshold for excitation before other parts of the conduction system have recovered sufficiently to be depolarized. If the sinus node fires more slowly, or if the SA node conduction is blocked, another site that is capable of automaticity will take over as pacemaker. Other regions that are capable of automaticity include the atrial fibers that have plateau-type action potentials, the AV node, the bundle of His, and the bundle-branch Purkinje fibers. These pacemakers generally have a slower rate of discharge. The AV node has an inherent firing rate of 40 to 60 times per minute, and the Purkinje system 30 to 40 times per minute. Even though the SA node is functioning properly, other cardiac cells can assume accelerated properties of automaticity and begin to initiate impulses when they are injured, oxygen-deprived, or exposed to certain chemicals or drugs.

An *ectopic pacemaker* is an excitable focus outside the normally functioning SA node. These pacemakers can reside in other parts of the conduction system or in muscle cells of the atria or ventricles. A premature contraction occurs when an ectopic pacemaker initiates a beat. In general, premature contractions do not follow the normal conduction pathways, they are not coupled with normal mechanical events, and they often render the heart refractory or incapable of responding to the next normal impulse arising in the SA node. Premature contractions occur without incident in persons with healthy hearts in response to sympathetic stimulation or to stimulants such as caffeine. In the diseased heart, the premature contraction may lead to more serious arrhythmias.

Excitability describes the ability of a cell to respond to an impulse and generate an action potential. Myocardial cells that have been injured or replaced by scar tissue do not possess normal excitability. For example, cells within the ischemic zone become depolarized during the acute phase of myocardial ischemia. These ischemic cells remain electrically coupled to the adjacent nonischemic area, and thus current from the ischemic zone can induce reexcitation of cells in the nonischemic zone.

Conductivity is the ability to conduct impulses, and *refractoriness* is the inability to respond to an incoming stimulus. The refractory period of cardiac muscle is the interval in the repolarization period during which an excitable cell has not recovered sufficiently to be reexcited. Disturbances in either conductivity or refractoriness predispose to arrhythmias.

An important condition in the development of arrhythmias is the phenomenon of reentry. Reentry occurs when an impulse reexcites an area through which it previously traveled, disrupting the normal conduction sequence. For reentry to occur, there must be a unidirectional, or one-way, block in one limb of a conduction pathway (Fig 19-9). When this occurs, the impulse is conducted through the unaffected limb of the pathway and then reenters the affected limb from the reverse direction; if sufficient time has elapsed for the refractory period in the reentered area to have ended, a self-perpetuating "circus-type" movement can be initiated. The functional components of a reentry circuit can be large and include an entire specialized conduction system or it can be microscopic; it can include myocardial tissue, AV nodal cells, or junctional cells.

Types of Arrhythmias

Sinus arrhythmias
The normal rhythm of the heart with the sinus node in command is regular and ranges from 60 to 100 beats/minute. On the electrocardiogram a P wave may be observed to precede every QRS complex.

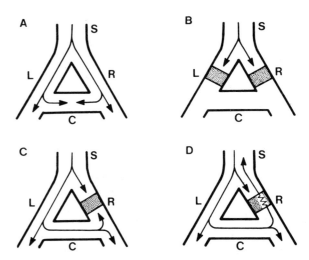

Figure 19-9 *The role of unidirectional block in reentry. An excitation wave traveling down a single bundle (S) of fibers continues down the left (L) and right (R) branches. The depolarization wave enters the connecting branch (C) from both ends and is extinguished at the zone of collision, (B). The wave is blocked in the L and R branches. (C) Bidirectional block exists in Branch R. (D) Unidirectional block exists in branch R. The antegrade impulse is blocked, but the retrograde impulse is conducted through and reenters bundle S. (From: Berne RM, Levy MN: Physiology. St. Louis, CV Mosby, 1983)*

Alterations in the function of the SA node lead to a change in the rate and regularity of the heartbeat. *Sinus bradycardia* describes a slow heart rate (less than 60 beats/minute). In sinus bradycardia, a P wave precedes each QRS; this confirms that the impulse is originating in the SA node rather than in a part of the conduction system that has a slower heart rate. Vagal stimulation decreases the firing rate of the SA node and conduction through the AV node to cause a decrease in the heart rate. A slow resting rate of 50 to 60 beats/minute may be normal in a well-trained athlete who maintains a large stroke volume. *Sinus tachycardia* refers to a rapid heart rate (100 to 160 beats/minute) that has its origin in the SA node (a P wave precedes every QRS complex). Sympathetic stimulation or withdrawal of vagal tone incites an increase in heart rate. Sinus tachycardia is normal during fever, exercise, and in situations that incite sympathetic stimulation. *Sinus arrhythmia* is a condition in which the heart rate speeds up and then slows down in an irregular, but cyclic, pattern; it is often associated with respiration and alterations in autonomic control. It is common and normal in young people. *Sinus arrest* refers to failure of the SA node to discharge and results in an irregular pulse. An escape rhythm develops as another pacemaker takes over. Sinus arrest may result in prolonged periods of asystole and often predisposes to other arrhythmias. Causes of sinus arrest include disease of the SA node, digitalis toxicity, and excess vagal tone. The *sick sinus syndrome* is a term that describes a condition of periods of bradycardia alternating with tachycardia. The bradycardia is caused by disease of the sinus node (or other intra-atrial conduction pathways) and the tachycardia, by paroxysmal atrial or junctional arrhythmias.

Arrhythmias originating in the atria

The impulse from the SA node passes through the conductive pathways in the atria to the AV node. An *atrial premature contraction* can originate in the atrial conduction pathways or in atrial muscle cells. This contraction is transmitted to the ventricle as well as back to the SA node. The retrograde transmission to the SA node often interrupts the timing of the next sinus beat so that a pause occurs between the two normally conducted beats. *Atrial flutter* describes an atrial rate of 160 to 350 beats/minute. There is a delay in conduction through the AV node, and the ventricles respond to every second, third, or fourth beat (*e.g.,* when conduction from the atria to the ventricles is 3:1, an atrial flutter rate of 225 will result in a ventricular rate of only 75). *Atrial fibrillation* describes an atrial rate in excess of 350, usually 450 to 600 beats/minute. Here, conduction through the AV node is totally disorganized, the peripheral pulse is grossly irregular, and a pulse deficit can be observed. The pulse deficit is the difference between the apical and peripheral pulses. In atrial fibrillation, the rate may be such that there is not sufficient stroke output to be felt at the wrist, causing a difference between the apical heartbeat and peripheral pulses. Atrial fibrillation can occur as the result of left atrial distention due to mitral stenosis. It is the most common atrial arrhythmia in the elderly. Atrial fibrillation predisposes to thrombus formation in the atria, with subsequent risk of formation of systemic emboli. Figure 19-10 illustrates the electrocardiographic changes that occur with atrial arrhythmias.

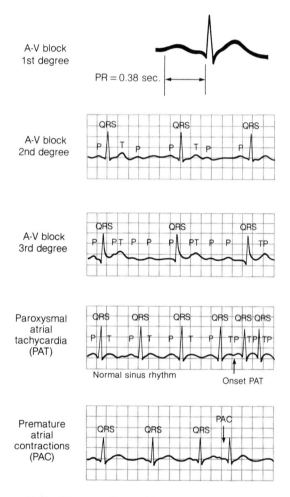

Figure 19-10 *Electrocardiographic (ECG) changes that occur with alterations in AV node conduction and atrial arrhythmias. The top tracing shows the prolongation of the PR interval, which is characteristic of first-degree AV block. The second tracing illustrates second-degree AV block, in which the conduction of one or more P waves is blocked. In third-degree AV block, complete block in conduction of impulses through the AV node occurs, and the atria and ventricles each develop their own rate of impulse generation (middle tracing). The fourth tracing illustrates paroxysmal atrial tachycardia (PAT), preceded by a normal sinus rhythm. The fifth tracing illustrates a premature atrial contraction (PAC) followed by normal QRS complex.*

During rest and moderate activity, ventricular filling is not dependent on atrial contraction. Atrial contraction contributes only about 25% to 30% of cardiac reserve; therefore, atrial arrhythmias may go unnoticed unless they are transmitted to the ventricle. In persons with marginal cardiac output, however, the loss of atrial function may result in a sufficient decrease in cardiac output to produce symptoms.

Alterations in AV Conduction

The AV node provides the only connection for transmission of impulses between the atrial and the ventricular conduction systems. Junctional fibers in the AV node have high resistance characteristics, which cause a delay in the transmission of impulses from the atria to the ventricles; this allows for filling of the ventricles and protects them from abnormally rapid rates that arise in the atria. Conduction defects are most commonly due to fibrosis or scar tissue in fibers of the conduction system. Conduction defects of the AV node can also occur as the result of digitalis toxicity.

Heart block occurs when conduction through the AV node is delayed or interrupted. It may occur in the AV nodal fibers or in the AV bundle (bundle of His), which is continuous with the Purkinje conduction system that supplies the ventricles. The P-R interval on the ECG corresponds with the time that it takes for the cardiac impulse to travel from the SA node to the ventricular pathways; the normal range is 0.12 second to 0.20 second. A *first-degree heart block* occurs when conduction through the AV pathway is delayed and the P-R interval is longer than 0.20 second (Fig. 19-10). In *second-degree block*, one or more of the atrial impulses are blocked. There are two types of second-degree block: the *Mobitz type I*, or *Wenckebach phenomenon*, describes a progressive increase in the P-R interval until the point at which one P wave is totally blocked; the *Mobitz type II block* describes the situation in which there is a sudden block in one or more atrial impulses without an antecedent prolongation of the P-R interval. In a Mobitz type II block, the ventricular rate is irregular and reflects the degree of block; this type of block is significant because it often precedes complete heart block. *Third-degree,* or *complete,* heart block occurs when the conduction link between the atria and ventricles is completely lost; the atria continue to beat at a normal rate and the ventricles develop their own rate, which is normally slow (30 to 40 beats/minute). Complete heart block causes a decrease in cardiac output with possible periods of syncope (called a Stokes-Adams attack). Patients with complete heart block usually require a pacemaker.

The AV node can act as a pacemaker in the event that the SA node fails to initiate an impulse. Junctional fibers in the AV node or bundle can also serve as ectopic pacemakers, producing *premature junctional contractions*.

Disorders of ventricular conduction

The junctional fibers in the AV node join with the bundle of His, which divides to form the right and left bundle branches; they then branch to form the Purkinje fibers, which supply the walls of the ventricles (Chap. 18, Fig. 18-10). On leaving the junctional fibers, the cardiac impulse travels through the AV bundle, moves down the right and left bundle branches that lie beneath the endocardium on either side of the septum, and then spreads out through the walls of the ventricles. Interruption of impulse conduction through the bundle branches does not usually cause alterations in the rhythm of the heartbeat; this is because the impulse is usually conducted along an alternate or detour pathway. It does, however, take longer for the impulse to be transmitted through the Purkinje system when there is a conduction defect; this produces changes in the QRS complex of the ECG and causes the QRS complex to be wider than the normal 0.08 second to 0.12 second. The left bundle branch is divided into two parts called fascicles. A hemiblock refers to involvement of one of the fascicles of the left bundle branch.

Ventricular arrhythmias

Arrhythmias arising in the ventricles are usually considered more serious than those arising in the atria because they afford the potential for interfering with the pumping action of the heart. A *premature ventricular contraction* (PVC) is caused by a ventricular ectopic pacemaker. Following a PVC, the ventricle is usually not able to repolarize sufficiently to respond to the next impulse that arises in the SA node; this causes the "compensatory pause," which occurs while the ventricle waits to reestablish its previous rhythm (Fig. 19-11). With a PVC, the diastolic volume is usually insufficient for ejection of blood into the arterial system; this causes a skipped beat. In the absence of heart disease, PVCs are usually not of great clinical significance. They can also occur in digitalis toxicity and in myocardial ischemia and infarction. A special type of PVC is called ventricular bigeminy. Here the PVCs occur in such a way each normal beat is followed by or paired with a PVC. It is often an indication of digitalis toxicity or heart disease. The occurrence of frequent PVCs in the diseased heart predisposes to other more serious arrhythmias, including ventricular tachycardia and fibrillation. *Ventricular tachycardia* describes a ventricular rate of 160 to 250 beats/minute; it is dangerous because it causes a reduction in the diastolic filling time to the point at which the cardiac output is severely diminished or nonexistent (Fig. 19-12). Ven-

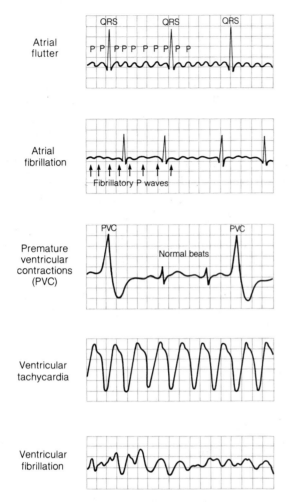

Figure 19-11 *Electrocardiographic (ECG) tracings of atrial and ventricular arrhythmias. On the top is a tracing of atrial flutter, characterized by the presence of atrial flutter (P) waves occurring at a rate of 160 to 350 beats per minute. The ventricular rate remains regular because of the conduction of every sixth atrial contraction. In atrial fibrillation (second tracing) there is an atrial rate of in excess of 350 beats per minute; the P waves are no longer distinct and the ventricular rate becomes irregular. Premature ventricular contractions (PVCs) originate from an ectopic focus in the ventricles, causing a distortion of the QRS complex (third tracing). Because the ventricle usually cannot repolarize sufficiently to respond to the next impulse that arises in the SA node, a PVC is followed by a compensatory pause. Ventricular tachycardia is characterized by a rapid ventricular rate of 160 to 250 beats per minute and the absence of P waves (fourth tracing). In ventricular fibrillation, which is illustrated in the bottom tracing, there are no regular or effective ventricular contractions and the ECG tracing is totally disorganized.*

tricular tachycardia requires prompt correction because it leads to compromised coronary perfusion and predisposes to fibrillation. *Ventricular fibrillation* is a fatal arrhythmia, unless it is immediately treated with cardiopulmonary resuscitation and defibrillation. During

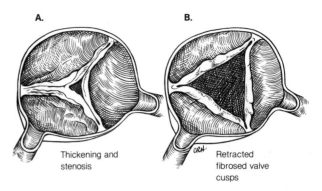

Figure 19-12 *Disease of the aortic valve as viewed from the aorta; (A) Stenosis of the valve opening and (B) an incompetent or regurgitant valve that is unable to close completely.*

ventricular fibrillation, the ventricle quivers but does not contract; with the cessation of cardiac output no pulse is palpable or audible (Fig. 19-11).

Diagnosis and Treatment

Diagnosis of conduction defects and cardiac arrhythmias is usually made on the basis of the elctrocardiograph tracing.

The treatment of arrhythmias is directed toward controlling the arrhythmia and correcting the cause and preventing more serious or fatal arrhythmias. Correction may involve simply adjusting an electrolyte disturbance or withholding a medication such as digitalis. Preventing more serious arrhythmias often involves drug therapy. Antiarrhythmic drugs act by modifying disordered formation and conduction of impulses that induce cardiac muscle contraction. These drugs are currently classified into four groups (Table 19-4).[18] The cardiac glycosides are also used in the management of arrhythmias such as atrial tachycardia, flutter, and fibrillation.

Correction of the conduction defect can also involve the use of an electronic pacemaker or cardioversion when ventricular defibrillation occurs. A *pacemaker* is an electronic device that delivers an electrical stimulus to the heart, and it may be a temporary or a permanent measure. Temporary pacing involves the passage of a venous catheter with electrodes at its tip. The catheter is advanced under fluoroscopic or electrocardiographic control into the right atrium or ventricle, where it is wedged against the endocardium. Permanent pacing requires insertion of pacemaker electrodes attached directly into the epicardium, or the transvenous insertion into the apex of the right ventricle, where the electrode comes in contact with the endocardium. Defibrillation or DC cardioversion (400 watt-seconds) is the only reliable method for treating ventricular fibrillation. The current from the defibrillator interrupts the disorganized impulses, allowing the SA node to regain control of the heartbeat.

In summary, disorders of cardiac rhythm arise as the result of disturbances in impulse generation or conduction of impulses in the heart. Cardiac arrhythmias are not necessarily pathologic—they occur in healthy as well as diseased hearts. Sinus arrhythmias have their origin in the SA node. They include sinus bradycardia (heart rate less than 60 beats/minute); sinus tachycardia (heart rate 100 to 160 beats/minute); sinus arrhythmia, in which the heart rate speeds up and slows down; sinus arrest, in which there are prolonged periods of asystole; and the sick sinus syndrome, a condition characterized by periods of bradycardia alternating with tachycardia. Atrial arrhythmias arise from alterations in impulse generation that occur within the conduction pathways or muscle of the atria. They include atrial premature contractions, atrial flutter (atrial depolarization rate of 160 to 350 beats/minute), and atrial fibrillation (atrial depolarization rate in excess of 350 beats/minute). Arial arrhythmias often go unnoticed unless they are transmitted to the ventricles. Alterations in the conduction of impulses through the AV node lead to disturbances in the transmission of impulses from the atria to the ventricles. There can be a delay in transmission (first-degree heart block), failure to conduct one or more impulses (second-degree heart block), or complete failure to conduct impulses between the atria and ventricles (third-degree heart block). Conduction disorders of the bundle of His, called bundle branch blocks, cause a widening of and changes in the configuration of the QRS complex of the ECG. Because of their potential for interfering with the pumping action of the heart, arrhythmias arising in the ventricles are usually considered more serious than those arising in the atria. Premature ventricular contraction (PVC) is caused by a ventricular ectopic pacemaker. Ventricular tachycardia is characterized by a ventricular rate of 160 to 250 beats/minute. Ventricular fibrillation (ventricular rate in excess of 350 beats/minute) is a fatal arrhythmia unless it is successfully treated with defibrillation.

■ Disorders of the Endocardium

The endocardium has a smooth surface that interfaces with blood moving through the heart. The endocardium covers the septum, the papillary muscles, the latticework of muscular columns called the trabeculae carneae, and the valvular structures. The smoothness of this layer is an essential characteristic in preventing platelet aggregation and clot formation. This section discusses two diseases of the endocardium, rheumatic fever and endocarditis.

Table 19-4 Antiarrhythmic Drugs and Mechanisms of Action

Drug	Dominant Mechanisms of Action[*]
Class I	
Lidocaine (Xylocaine)	Change the rate of action potential depolarization by depressing the fast inward sodium channels. Lengthen the effective refractory period of the action potential. Depress the spontaneous depolarization by delaying the return of excitability.
Tocainide (Tonocard)	
Procainamide (Pronestyl)	
Disopyramide (Norpace)	
Phenytoin (Dilantin)	
Quinidine	
Class II	
Atenolol (Tenormin)	Beta-adrenergic receptor blocking agents. Inhibit effects of sympathetic nervous system activity on the heart.
Metoprolol (Lopressor)	
Nadolol (Corgard)	
Propanolol (Inderal)	
Pindolol (Visken)	
Timolol (Blocadren, Timoptic)	
Class III	
Bretylium (Bretylol)	Alter repolarization, producing a prolongation of the action potential.
Class IV	
Diltiazem (Cardizem)	Block the slow channels in the myocardium. Prolong the effective and functional refractory periods of the AV node.
Nifedipine (Procardia)	
Verapamil (Celan, Isoptin)	

*Actions cited are the dominant actions of the drug group. Many of the individual drugs have other actions that influence their basic antiarrhythmic properties.

Rheumatic Fever

Rheumatic fever is an important disease because of its potential for causing chronic heart problems. It currently affects 2,010,000 adults and children in the United States. Although it is generally a preventable disease, the death rate from rheumatic fever in 1981 was 7700.[1] Rheumatic fever is more prevalent in groups subjected to poor nutrition, crowded living conditions, and inadequate health care.

Age plays an important role in the epidemiology of rheumatic fever. It is most prevalent in school-age children. The incidence of acute rheumatic fever peaks between ages 6 and 16 years.[2] However, one-fifth of all first attacks occur in adults.[2]

Etiology and manifestations

Rheumatic fever is associated with infection due to group A beta-hemolytic streptococcus and usually follows an inciting pharyngeal infection by 1 to 4 weeks. It is of particular significance that rheumatic fever and its cardiac complications can be prevented by antibiotic treatment of the initial streptococcal infection.

The pathogenesis of the disease is unclear, and why only 3% of persons with uncomplicated streptococcal infections develop rheumatic fever remains to be answered. The time frame for development of symptoms in relation to the sore throat, as well as the presence of antibodies to the streptococcus organism, strongly suggests an immunologic origin. Like other immunologic phenomena, rheumatic fever requires an initial sensitizing exposure to the offending (streptococcus) agent, and the risk of recurrence is high following each subsequent exposure. Rheumatic fever can present as an acute, recurrent, or chronic disorder.

The acute stage includes a history of an initiating streptococcal infection and subsequent involvement of the mesenchymal connective tissue of the heart, blood vessels, joints, and subcutaneous tissues. Common to all is the presence of a lesion called the *Aschoff body*. The Aschoff body is a localized area of tissue necrosis containing fibrinoid material. The recurrent phase usually involves extension of the cardiac effects of the disease. The chronic problems are associated with valvular defects due to the disease.

The child with rheumatic fever usually has had a history of sore throat, headache, fever, abdominal pain, nausea and vomiting, swollen glands (usually at the angle of the jaw), and other signs of a streptococcal infection. Throat cultures taken at the time of the acute infection are positive for streptococcus. The sedimentation rate, C-reactive protein, and white blood cell count are usually elevated at the time that heart or joint manifestations begin to appear. A high or rising antistreptolysin O titer is also suggestive of rheumatic fever. Streptolysin O is a hemolytic factor produced by most strains of group A beta-hemolytic streptococci; antistreptolysin O (ASO) is an antibody against the hemolytic factor produced by the streptococci. Other signs and symptoms associated with an acute episode of rheumatic fever are related to the structures involved in the disease process.

Rheumatic fever can affect any of the three layers of the heart: pericardium, myocardium, and endocardium. Usually all three layers are involved. Rheumatic pericarditis causes the production of a fibrinous or serofibrinous exudate. For the most part myocardial changes are reversible and produce minimal changes in cardiac function. It is the involvement of the endocardium and valvular structures that produces the permanent and disabling effects of the disease. Although any of the four valves can be involved, it is the mitral and aortic valves that are affected most often. During the acute inflammatory stage of the disease, the valvular structures become reddened and swollen; small vegetative lesions develop on the valve leaflets. Gradually, the acute inflammatory changes proceed to fibrous scar tissue development, which tends to contract and cause deformity of the valve leaflets and shortening of the chordae tendineae. In some cases, the edges or commissures of the leaflets fuse together as healing occurs.

The manifestations of rheumatic carditis include a heart murmur in a child without a previous history of rheumatic fever, change in the character of a murmur in a person with a previous history of the disease, cardiomegaly or enlargement of the heart, friction rub or other signs of pericarditis, and congestive heart failure in a child without discernible cause (Jones Criteria, American Heart Association).[1]

Polyarthritis, although not a cause of permanent disability, is the most common finding in rheumatic fever. The inflammatory process affects the synovial membrane of the joint, causing swelling, heat, redness, pain, tenderness, and limitation of motion. The arthritis is almost always migratory, affecting one joint and then moving to another. The joints most frequently affected are the larger ones, particularly the knees, ankles, elbows, and wrists.

The *skin lesions* seen in rheumatic fever are of two types, subcutaneous nodules and erythema marginatum. The *subcutaneous nodules* range in size from 1 cm to 4 cm; they are hard, painless, and freely movable, and usually overlie the extensor muscles of the wrist, elbow, ankle, and knee joints. *Erythema marginatum* lesions are maplike macular areas, seen most commonly on the trunk or inner aspects of the upper arm and thigh. Skin lesions are present only in about 10% of patients who have rheumatic fever; they are transitory and disappear during the course of the disease.

Chorea (Sydenham's chorea), sometimes called St. Vitus' dance, is the major central nervous system manifestation. It is seen most frequently in girls. Typically, there is an insidious onset of irritability and other behavior problems. The child is often fidgety, cries easily, begins to walk clumsily, and tends to drop things. The choreic movements are spontaneous, rapid, purposeless jerking movements, which tend to interfere with voluntary activities. Facial grimaces are common and even speech may be affected. Fortunately, the chorea is self-limiting, usually running its course within a matter of weeks or months.

Recurrent nosebleeds (epistaxis) are thought to be a subclinical manifestation of rheumatic fever.

Diagnosis and treatment

The diagnosis of rheumatic fever is based on clinical and laboratory findings. The Jones Criteria for guidance in diagnosis of rheumatic fever were initially proposed in 1955 and revised in 1966 by a committee of the American Heart Association. The criteria were developed because no single laboratory test, sign, or symptom is pathognomonic of the disease, although several combinations of them are diagnostic. The criteria group the signs and symptoms into major and minor categories.

Chart 19-1   *Jones Criteria (Revised) for Guidance in Diagnosis of Rheumatic Fever*[*]

Major Manifestations	**Minor Manifestations**
Carditis	History of previous rheumatic
Polyarthritis	fever or rheumatic heart
Chorea	disease
Erythema marginatum	Arthralgia
Subcutaneous nodules	Fever
	Laboratory findings
	Acute phase reactants
	Erythrocyte sedimentation
	rate, C-reactive protein,
	leukocytosis
	Prolonged P–R interval on
	ECG

Supporting evidence of streptococcal infection

Increased titer of antistreptolysin
   antibodies, ASO (antistreptolysin O),
   others
Positive throat culture for group A
   streptococcus
Recent scarlet fever

[*]The presence of two major criteria, or of one major and two minor criteria, indicates a high probability of acute rheumatic fever, if supported by evidence of preceding group A streptococcal infection.
(Reprinted with permission. American Heart Association, 1982)

The presence of two major signs or one major and two minor signs indicates a high probability of the presence of rheumatic fever, if supported by a history of a preceding group A streptococcal infection. The revised criteria are summarized in Chart 19-1.

Treatment is designed to control the acute inflammatory process and to prevent cardiac complications and recurrence of the disease. During the acute phase, prevention of residual cardiac effects is of primary concern. Administration of antibiotics and anti-inflammatory drugs and selective restriction of physical activities are usually carried out during the acute stage of illness. Secondary prevention involves the prophylactic use of penicillin (or another antibiotic in penicillin-sensitive patients) for a period of at least 5 years to prevent recurrence. Penicillin is also the antibiotic of choice for treating the acute illness. Salicylates and corticosteroids are also widely used.

Secondary prevention and compliance with a plan for prophylactic administration of penicillin require that the patient and the family understand the rationale for such measures as well as the measures themselves. Patients also need to be instructed to report possible streptococcal infections to their physician. They should be instructed to inform their dentist about them so that they can be adequately protected during dental procedures that might traumatize the oral mucosa.

Bacterial Endocarditis

Etiology and manifestations

The significance of bacterial endocarditis lies in its tendency to develop in persons with a damaged heart. It can be caused by almost any pathogen, the most common being *Streptococcus viridans*. Staphylococci, gram-negative bacteria, and fungi have also been isolated as causes of endocarditis.

Two predisposing factors contribute to the development of endocarditis—a *damaged endocardial surface* and a *portal of entry* by which the organism gains access to the bloodstream. The presence of valvular disease, rheumatic heart disease, or congenital heart defects provides an environment conducive to bacterial growth. The second factor, bacteremia, may emerge in the course of seemingly minor health problems, such as an upper respiratory tract infection, a skin lesion, or a dental procedure. Simple gum massage or an innocuous oral lesion may afford the pathogenic bacteria access to the bloodstream. Bacterial endocarditis is reported to be a significant potential disease in narcotic addicts who "mainline." And it is a potential complication in patients with intravascular catheters that remain in place for long periods of time.

The vegetative lesion characteristic of bacterial endocarditis consists of a collection of pathogens and cellular debris enmeshed in the fibrin strands of clotted blood. These lesions may be singular or multiple, may reach a size of several centimeters, and are usually found loosely attached to the free edges of the valve surface. The loose organization of the lesion permits the organisms to disseminate, and fragments are carried by the blood to give rise to small hemorrhages, abscesses, and infarcted areas in other parts of the body—kidneys, spleen, brain, and joints.

Bacterial endocarditis may occur in an acute or subacute form. *Acute bacterial endocarditis* is thought to affect primarily persons with normal hearts, whereas *subacute bacterial endocarditis* (SBE) is seen most frequently in patients with damaged hearts. The signs and symptoms include fever, change in the character of an existing heart murmur, and evidence of embolic distribution of the vegetative lesions. In the acute form, the fever is usually spiking and accompanied by chills. In the subacute form, the fever is usually low grade and of gradual onset and is frequently accompanied by other systemic signs of inflammation such as anorexia, malaise, and lethargy. Small petechial hemorrhages frequently result when emboli lodge in the small vessels of the skin, nailbeds, and mucous membranes.

Diagnosis and treatment

The blood culture is the most significant diagnostic aid in bacterial endocarditis. Usually a series of three to six cultures are obtained during a 36- to 48-hour period to ensure adequate sampling.

The focus of treatment is toward identifying and destroying the causative organism, minimizing the residual cardiac effects, and treating the pathology induced by the emboli. The blood cultures usually identify the organism so its sensitivity to antibiotics can be assessed. An appropriate antibiotic is prescribed to eradicate the pathogen. This active treatment stands in contrast to preantibiotic days when bacterial endocarditis often was fatal. Of even greater importance is prevention in persons known to be at risk. Prevention can be largely accomplished through prophylactic administration of an antibiotic prior to dental and other procedures that may cause bacteremia.

In summary, the endocardium lines the heart and covers the valvular structure; it provides a smooth surface that interfaces with the blood. Rheumatic fever, which is associated with an antecedent group A streptococcal infection, is an important cause of heart disease. Its most serious and disabling effects result from involvement of the heart valves. Because there is no single laboratory test, sign, or symptom that is pathognomonic of acute

rheumatic fever, the Jones Criteria are used to establish the diagnosis during the acute stage of the disease. Bacterial endocarditis involves the invasion of the endocardium by pathogens that produce vegetative lesions of the endocardial surface. The loose organization of these lesions permits the organisms and fragments of the lesions to be disseminated throughout the systemic circulation. It can be caused by a number of organisms. Two predisposing factors contribute to the development of endocarditis: (1) a damaged endocardium and (2) a portal of entry through which the organisms gain access to the bloodstream.

■ Valvular Disease

Dysfunction of the heart valves can result from a number of disorders, including congenital defects, trauma, ischemic damage, degenerative changes, and inflammation. Rheumatic endocarditis is the most common cause. Its inflammatory changes cause scar tissue to form on the valve leaflets and the chordae tendineae with a subsequent shortening of the chordae and deformation of the valve structure. Two types of mechanical disruptions may occur in valvular disease: (1) narrowing or stenosis of the valve opening or (2) failure of a valve to close completely (Fig. 19-12). Although any of the four heart valves can become diseased, the most commonly affected are the mitral and aortic valves.

Hemodynamic Manifestations

Valvular disease can be either stenotic (failure to open completely) or regurgitant (failure to close completely), but often there is a combination of both stenotic and regurgitant effects. The influence of valvular disease on cardiac function is related to alterations in blood flow and increased work demands on the heart.

Stenosis causes a decrease in flow through the valve, with an increased work demand on the heart chamber in front of the diseased valve. In mitral stenosis, for example, the left atrium becomes distended and the work output required of this chamber is increased. As the condition advances, blood return from the lungs is impeded, and the pulmonary circulation becomes congested. Blood flow through a normal valve can increase to five to seven times the resting value; consequently, valvular stenosis must be severe before it causes life-threatening problems.[19] The first evidence of symptoms usually is noted during exercise.

An incompetent (regurgitant) valve permits blood flow to continue while the valve is closed, flowing into the left ventricle during diastole when the aortic valve is affected, and into the left atrium during systole when the mitral valve is diseased. With an incompetent valve, the work demands of both the heart chamber in front and that in back of the affected valve are increased. In mitral regurgitation, the left atrium is presented with an increased volume and the left ventricle with a bidirectional flow pattern such that blood is propelled into both the left atrium and the aorta during systole.

Types of Valvular Disorders

Aortic valve defects

The orifices of the coronary arteries are strategically located in the aorta, just distal to the aortic valve leaflets (Fig. 19-13). In aortic stenosis, the velocity of flow through the narrowed valve orifice is increased at the expense of the lateral pressure needed to perfuse the coronary arteries. In aortic regurgitation, failure of aortic valve closure during diastole causes diastolic pressure to fall; this decreases the pressure needed to perfuse the coronary arteries.

Aortic valve stenosis. *Aortic stenosis* causes resistance to ejection of blood into the aorta, so the work demands on the left ventricle are increased and the volume of blood ejected into the systemic circulation decreases. The most common causes of aortic stenosis are rheumatic fever and congenital heart defects. In the elderly, it may be related to degenerative atherosclerotic changes of the valve leaflets.

Obstruction to aortic outflow causes a decrease in stroke volume, in which systolic blood pressure is reduced and pulse pressure is narrow. Thus, it takes a longer time for the heart to eject blood; the heart rate is often slow and the pulse of low amplitude. Resistance to flow through the aortic valve gives rise to an auscultatory murmur in systole.

The onset of signs and symptoms is dependent to a large extent on the person's activity level; in one who leads a sedentary life, the disease may be far advanced before symptoms are noted. Exertional dyspnea is a common presenting symptom. It is characterized by vertigo and syncope when the stroke volume falls to levels insufficient for cerebral needs. Also, the combination of increased work demands on the hypertrophied left ventricle and decreased perfusion of the coronary vessels may cause angina.

Aortic valve regurgitation. An *incompetent aortic valve* allows blood to return to the left ventricle during diastole. This defect may result from conditions that cause scarring of the valve leaflets or from enlargement of the valve orifice to the extent that the valve leaflets no

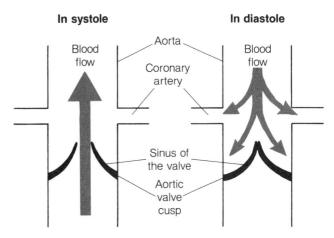

Figure 19-13 *Location of the orifices for the coronary arteries and the direction of flow during systole and diastole.*

longer meet. Rheumatic fever ranks first on the list of causes of aortic regurgitation.

A widening of the pulse pressure is characteristic of aortic regurgitation, so that the systolic pressure is frequently increased and the diastolic pressure decreased. Widening of the pulse pressure has two underlying mechanisms: first, there is an increase in the stroke volume as the left ventricle must eject blood entering from the lungs, as well as the blood that has leaked back across the aortic valve into the ventricle during diastole; second, because the aortic valve fails to close completely, diastolic pressure cannot be maintained. The left ventricle hypertrophies because of the increased volume load on this chamber. Turbulence of flow across the aortic valve during diastole produces a high-pitched or blowing type of murmur.

The large stroke volume and rapid runoff of blood from the aorta produce characteristic changes in the peripheral pulses: prominent carotid pulsations in the neck, throbbing peripheral pulses, and a left ventricular impulse that causes the chest to move with each beat. The term *waterhammer* pulse is often used to describe the hyperkinetic peripheral pulse found in persons with aortic regurgitation.

Symptoms of aortic regurgitation are those associated with heart failure: exertional dyspnea, dizziness, pulmonary edema, and orthopnea. Angina follows the impaired coronary perfusion due to a low diastolic pressure and the increased work demands on the left ventricle. Patients with significant aortic regurgitation complain of throbbing of the chest due to the hyperdynamic left ventricle.

Mitral valve defects

The mitral valve controls the directional flow of blood between the left atrium and the left ventricle. The cusps of the atrioventricular valves are thinner than those of the semilunar valves; they are anchored to the papillary muscles by the chordae tendineae. During much of systole, the mitral valve is subjected to the high pressure that is generated by the left ventricle as it pumps blood into the systemic circulation and the chordae tendineae prevent the eversion of the valve leaflets into the left atrium.

Mitral valve stenosis.   Mitral valve stenosis is characterized by fibrous replacement of valvular tissue, along with stiffness and fusion of valve commissures. Involvement of the chordae tendineae causes shortening, which pulls the valvular structures more deeply into the ventricles. As the impediment to flow through the valve increases, the left atrial pressure rises and eventually dilatation of this heart chamber occurs; eventually the increased left atrial pressure is transmitted to the pulmonary venous system, causing pulmonary congestion. The rate of flow across the valve is dependent on the size of the valve orifice, the driving pressure (atrial minus ventricular pressure), and the time available for flow during diastole. As the condition progresses, symptoms of decreased cardiac output occur during extreme exertion or other situations that cause tachycardia and thereby reduce diastolic filling time. In the late stages of the disease, pulmonary vascular resistance increases with the development of pulmonary hypertension; this increases the arterial pressure against which the right heart must pump and eventually leads to failure of this side of the heart.

The signs and symptoms of mitral valve stenosis depend on the severity of the obstruction and are generally related to (1) elevation in left atrial pressure and pulmonary congestion, (2) decreased cardiac output due to impaired left ventricular filling, and (3) left atrial enlargement with development of atrial arrhythmias and mural thrombi. The symptoms are those of pulmonary congestion, including nocturnal paroxysmal dyspnea and orthopnea. Premature atrial beats, paroxysmal atrial tachycardia, and atrial fibrillation may occur as a result of distention of the left atria. Together, the fibrillation and distention predispose to mural thrombus formation, from which systemic emboli may form. Palpitations, chest pain, weakness, and fatigue are common complaints. The murmur of mitral valve stenosis is found during diastole when blood is flowing through the constricted valve orifice; it is characteristically a low-pitched rumbling murmur, best heard at the apex of the heart. The first heart sound is often accentuated and somewhat delayed because of the increased left atrial pressure; an opening snap often precedes the diastolic murmur as a result of the elevation in left atrial pressure.

Mitral valve regurgitation.   In addition to rheumatic fever, the causes of mitral regurgitation are rupture of the chordae tendineae, which is commonly caused by bacterial endocarditis, papillary muscle dysfunction, or rupture due to coronary heart disease, and secondary stretching of the valve structures due to dilatation of the left ventricle. With mitral valve insufficiency, blood from the left ventricle is forced back into the left atrium during systole; this blood is then returned to the left ventricle during diastole. With chronic regurgitation, dilatation of the left ventricle occurs as a result of the increased volume and muscle mass needed to eject a much larger stroke volume (the forward stroke volume that is ejected into the aorta and the regurgitant stroke volume that is ejected into the left atrium). As the disorder progresses, left ventricular function becomes impaired and the left atrial pressure increases with the subsequent development of pulmonary hypertension. The increased volume work associated with mitral regurgitation is relatively well tolerated and persons with the disorder often remain asymptomatic for 10 to 20 years despite severe regurgitation. A characteristic feature of mitral valve regurgitation is an enlarged left ventricle and a pansystolic (throughout systole) murmur.

Mitral valve prolapse.   Mitral valve prolapse, sometimes referred to as the floppy mitral valve syndrome, has been reported to be present in 6% to 21% of otherwise healthy persons.[20,21] The disorder is seen three times more frequently in men than women and may have a familial basis. Although the cause of the disorder is unknown, it has been associated with Marfan's syndrome, osteogenesis imperfecta, and other connective tissue disorders, as well as scoliosis and coronary heart disease.

Pathologic findings in mitral valve prolapse include a myxedematous (mucinous) degeneration of the spongiosum, which lies between the collagen and elastic tissue covering the atrial aspect of the valve and the thick layer of connective tissue that provides the main support for the valve, causing a redundancy of valve tissue and ballooning of the valve leaflets into the left atrium during systole when the ventricular pressure is high. It has also been suggested that certain forms of the disorder may arise from disorders of the myocardium that result in abnormal movement of the ventricular wall or papillary muscle; this places undue stress on the mitral valve. In epidemiologic survey studies, the majority of persons with the disorder were unaware that they had it. The most commonly encountered symptoms in the clinical setting are chest pain, weakness, dyspnea, fatigue, anxiety, palpitations, and lightheadedness. The chest pain differs from angina in that it is often prolonged, ill defined, and not associated with exercise or exertion. The pain has been attributed to ischemia resulting from traction of the prolapsing valve leaflets. It has recently been suggested that the anxiety, palpitations, and arrhythmias that accompany the disorder may be due to the abnormal function of the autonomic nervous system.[22] Rare cases of sudden death have been reported in persons with mitral valve prolapse, mainly in persons with a family history of similar occurrences.

The disorder is characterized by a spectrum of auscultatory findings ranging from a silent form to one or more midsystolic clicks followed by a late systolic murmur.[23] A variety of abnormal electrocardiographic changes can occur. Arrhythmias may be brought out by exercise stress testing or 24-hour ECG monitoring. Echocardiographic studies have become a method for the diagnosis of mitral valve prolapse, and the availability of this technique has undoubtedly contributed to increased recognition of the problem, particularly in its asymptomatic form.

The treatment of mitral valve prolapse focuses on the relief of symptoms and the prevention of complications. The beta-adrenergic blocking drugs have proved useful in treating the chest discomfort and arrhythmias that occur in the symptomatic form of the disease. Infective endocarditis is an uncommon complication in patients with a murmur; antibiotic prophylaxis is usually recommended before dental treatments or surgery.

Diagnosis and Treatment

Valvular defects are usually detected through cardiac auscultation. Diagnosis is aided by the use of the phonocardiogram, echocardiogram, and catheterization. The phonocardiogram, obtained by placing a microphone on the chest wall, provides a graphic recording of heart sounds. Simultaneous ECG recordings are usually made to provide reference points for use in interpreting the phonocardiogram.

The treatment of valvular defects consists of (1) medical management of heart failure and associated problems and (2) surgical intervention to either repair or replace the defective valve. Mitral commissurotomy is the surgical enlargement of a stenotic valve. It may be performed as either an open or a closed procedure. The open procedure requires extracorporeal circulation (cardiopulmonary bypass) but has the advantage of affording the surgeon direct visualization of the operative site. Valvular replacement, either with a prosthetic device or a homograft, is usually reserved for severe disease. Unfortunately, the ideal substitute valve has not yet been invented, and consequently, valve replacement is usually reserved for patients with severe disease.

In summary, dysfunction of the heart valves can result from a number of disorders, including congenital defects, trauma, ischemic heart disease, degenerative changes, and inflammation. Rheumatic endocarditis is a common cause. Valvular heart disease produces its effects through disturbances in the blood flow. A stenotic valvular defect is one that causes a decrease in blood flow through a valve, resulting in impaired emptying and increased work demands on the heart chamber in front of the diseased valve. A regurgitant valvular defect permits the blood flow to continue when the valve is closed; it increases the work demands of the chamber in front and in back of the affected valve. Valvular heart disorders produce blood flow turbulence and are often detected through cardiac auscultation.

◼ Cardiomyopathies

The cardiomyopathies are a group of disorders that affect the heart muscle. They can develop as either primary or secondary disorders. The primary cardiomyopathies, which are discussed in this chapter, are heart muscle diseases of unknown cause. Secondary cardiomyopathies are conditions in which the cardiac abnormality is due to another cardiovascular disease, such as myocardial infarction. In the United States, an estimated 1% of cardiac deaths can be attributed to primary cardiomyopathies. The onset of the primary cardiomyopathies is often silent and the symptoms do not occur until the disease is well advanced. The diagnosis is suspected when a young, previously healthy normotensive individual develops cardiomegaly and heart failure.

Types of Cardiomyopathies

The International Society and Federation of Cardiology/World Health Organization has categorized the primary cardiomyopathies into three groups: (1) congested, (2) hypertrophic, and (3) constrictive cardiomyopathies (Fig. 19-14).[24]

Dilated cardiomyopathies

The dilated, or congestive, cardiomyopathies are recognized by the dilatation of the heart chambers (often all four) and the impaired pumping function of the ventricles, with increases in both end-systolic and end-diastolic volumes of the heart. There is a profound reduction in the left ventricular ejection fraction (the ratio of stroke volume to end-diastolic volume) to 40% or less, compared with a normal value of about 67%. Microscopically, there is evidence of scarring and atrophy of myocardial cells. The ventricular wall is usually thickened and mural thrombi are common, most often in the left ventricle but also in the right ventricle or in either atrium.

The cause of congestive cardiomyopathy is unknown. The disease itself is probably the result of several factors acting in concert in a susceptible person, with alcohol, viral infections, the puerperium, and other causes acting as risk factors. In one study 20% of persons with the disorder had a history of excessive alcohol con-

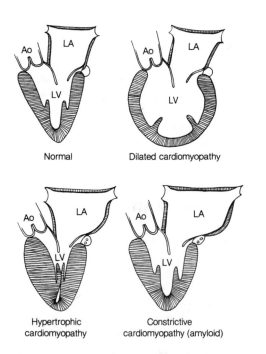

Figure 19-14 *The various types of cardiomyopathies compared to the normal heart. (Roberts WC, Ferrans VJ: Pathologic anatomy of the cardiomyopathies. Hum Pathol 6:289, 1975)*

sumption, 20% had had a severe influenzalike syndrome within 60 days of the appearance of the cardiac manifestations, and another 8% had a previous history of rheumatic fever without valvular involvement.[25]

There is considerable evidence that acute alcohol consumption reduces cardiac contractility and can produce arrhythmias and conduction disorders. In the heart, the presence of alcohol or its metabolite acetaldehyde interferes with a number of cellular functions that involve the transport and binding of calcium. With chronic alcohol consumption, the toxic effects of alcohol on the myocardium can persist after the alcohol has been metabolized. Although it is rare, congestive cardiomyopathy can also develop during the peripartum period.

Most cases of peripartal cardiomyopathy have their onset 1 to 6 weeks after delivery, but a few women begin to develop symptoms during the last month of pregnancy.[26] The incidence of peripartal cardiomyopathy is significantly higher in women over 30 years of age, in a third or subsequent pregnancy, and in the presence of twins or toxemia.[27] The cause of the condition is unknown.

There are two possible outcomes of peripartal cardiomyopathy. In approximately half of the cases, the heart returns to normal within 6 months and the chances for long-term survival are good. In these women, heart failure returns only during subsequent pregnancies. In

the other half of the cases, the cardiomegaly persists, and the prognosis is poor and death is very probable if another pregnancy occurs.[26]

In congestive cardiomyopathy, heart failure occurs because impairment of left ventricular ejection requires that the left ventricle dilate (Starling mechanism) to compensate for the fall in stroke volume that would otherwise occur. Dilatation of the heart and pump failure may be present for years before symptoms are noted. However, once symptoms have developed, the course of the disorder is distinguished by a propensity for the development of heart failure, embolism, and a poor prognosis. In a 13-year Mayo Clinic study of 104 patients with a diagnosis of congestive cardiomyopathy, 77% had an accelerated death rate, two-thirds of the deaths occurring within the first 2 years of diagnosis.[25] The most striking symptoms are those of heart failure, dyspnea on exertion, orthopnea, weakness, fatigue, and peripheral edema. On physical examination, tachycardia, an enlarged apical beat with the presence of both a third and fourth heart sound, and a murmur associated with regurgitation of one or both atrioventricular valves are frequently found. The systolic blood pressure is either normal or low, and the peripheral pulses are often of low amplitude. Pulsus alternans, in which the pulse regularly alternates between weaker and stronger, may be present.

Treatment. The treatment of congestive cardiomyopathy is directed toward relieving the symptoms of heart failure. Abstinence from alcohol is imperative in those individuals with a history of excessive consumption. In selected patients, heart transplantation may be an alternative, although the emotional, financial, and other costs must be carefully considered in view of the limited long-term survival of transplant recipients.

Hypertrophic cardiomyopathy

Hypertrophic cardiomyopathy is characterized by a small left ventricular volume with hypertrophy of ventricular muscle mass. Although the hypertrophy may be symmetrical, the involvement of the ventricular septum is often disproportionate in some patients, producing obstruction of the left ventricular outflow channel. Synonyms for this disorder include idiopathic hypertrophic subaortic stenosis (IHSS) and asymmetric septal hypertrophy (ASH).

A distinctive finding in hypertrophic cardiomyopathy is the microscopic presence of myofibril disarray. Instead of the normal parallel arrangement of myofibrils, the myofibrils branch off at random angles, sometimes at right angles to an adjacent fiber with which they may connect. Small bundles of fibers may course haphazardly through normally arranged muscle fibers.[2] It is thought that the presence of these disordered fibers may produce abnormal movements of the ventricles with uncoordinated contraction and impaired relaxation.[28]

The cause of hypertrophic cardiomyopathy is unknown. Often it is of familial origin, the disorder being inherited as an autosomal dominant trait.

The manifestations of hypertrophic cardiomyopathy are variable; for reasons that are unclear, some persons with the disorder remain asymptomatic whereas others become incapacitated. Symptomatic hypertrophic cardiomyopathy is commonly a disease of young adulthood. The most common symptom is dyspnea associated with an elevation in left ventricular diastolic pressure resulting from impaired ventricular filling and increased wall stiffness secondary to ventricular hypertrophy.[29] Because of the obstruction to outflow from the left ventricle, the systolic pressure difference between the left ventricle and the aorta increases. Chest pain, fatigue, and syncope are also common and become worse during exertion. Arrhythmias, both atrial and ventricular, may occur. Sudden death can occur and is especially common in certain families.

Treatment. The treatment of hypertrophic cardiomyopathy includes medical and surgical management. The goal of medical management is to relieve the symptoms by lessening the pressure difference between the left ventricle and the aorta, thereby improving cardiac output. Beta-adrenergic receptor blocking drugs may be used in persons with chest pain, arrhythmias, or dyspnea. These drugs reduce the heart rate and myocardial contractility, allowing more time for ventricular filling and reduction of ventricular stiffness. Recent use of the calcium-channel blocking drug verapamil has proved useful in relieving the symptoms of dyspnea, chest pain, and syncope.[30] Increased calcium uptake and increased intracellular calcium content are associated with an increased contractile state, a characteristic finding in persons with hypertrophic cardiomyopathy. Surgical treatment may be used if severe symptoms persist despite medical treatment. It involves incision of the septum (myotomy) with or without the removal of part of the tissue (myectomy) and it is accompanied by all of the risks of open-heart surgery.

Restrictive cardiomyopathies

Of the three categories of cardiomyopathies, the restrictive type is the least common in the Western countries. With this form of cardiomyopathy ventricular filling due to excessive rigidity of the ventricular walls is restricted, while the contractive properties of the heart remain relatively normal. The most common causes of restrictive cardiomyopathy are endocardial fibroelastosis and infiltrations, such as amyloidosis. Although the cause of fibroelastosis is unknown, about one-third of the cases are associated with congenital heart defects. The extent of the manifestations is dependent on the extent of the involvement. When there are only focal lesions, there may be few effects and normal longevity. On the other hand, when the lesions are diffuse, cardiac decompensation and death may result. The manifestations of restrictive cardiomyopathy resemble those of constrictive pericarditis.

In summary, the cardiomyopathies represent a disorder of the heart muscle. Cardiomyopathies may present as primary or secondary disorders. Secondary cardiomyopathies are conditions in which damage to the cardiac muscle occurs as the result of another disease process, such as myocardial infarction. There are three main types of primary cardiomyopathies: (1) dilated or congestive cardiomyopathy, in which fibrosis and atrophy of myocardial cells with dilatation of all four heart chambers occur; (2) hypertrophic cardiomyopathy, which is characterized by a disproportionate involvement of the ventricular septum, causing obstruction of the left ventricular outflow channel, and a disarray in the organization of myocardial fibers and ventricular hypertrophy; and (3) restrictive cardiomyopathy, in which there is excessive rigidity of the ventricular wall. The cause of the primary cardiomyopathies is largely unknown. The disease is suspected when a young, previously healthy individual develops cardiomegaly and heart failure.

■ Congenital Heart Disease

Normal development of the heart requires a precise and orderly sequence of differentiation and growth. Congenital heart defects can arise at any stage of development, with structural abnormalities reflecting growth that was occurring at the time the disturbance arose. Table 19-5 is designed to assist the reader in understanding the embryonic origin of specific defects.

Approximately 8 out of every 1000 babies are born with a congenital heart defect. About one-third of these have a severe defect that would cause death within the first year if it were not corrected. This section of the chapter is designed to provide an overview of congenital heart defects, including the hemodynamic changes that accompany congenital heart disorders and the more common defects. Depending on the type of defect that is present, children with congenital heart disease will experience varying signs and symptoms associated with altered heart action, heart failure, and difficulty in supplying the peripheral tissues with oxygen and other nutrients.

Table 19-5 Classification of Congenital Heart Defects According to Site of Embryonic Origin

Stage of Embryonic Development	Defect
Development of the atrial septum	Atrial septal defect of septum secondum
	Atrial septal defect of septum primum
Development of the ventricular septum	Ventricular septal defect of muscular septum
	Ventricular septal defect of membranous septum
Development of the endocardial cushions	Ebstein's anomaly of the tricuspid valve
	Abnormalities of the tricuspid and mitral valve
	Defect in ostium primum
	Defect in membranous portion of the ventricular septum
Spiraling and partitioning of the truncus arteriosus and bulbus cordis	Transposition of the great vessels
	Persistent truncus
	Tetralogy of Fallot
	Pulmonary stenosis
	Pulmonary outflow obstruction
Development of the aortic arches	Coarctation of the aorta
	Patent ductus arteriosus

Causes of Congenital Heart Defects

Development of the heart and major blood vessels is usually completed by the end of the eighth week of gestation. Included in this brief span of time is the critical period between weeks 3 and 8 with its complex changes in cardiac development. Congenital heart defects have been attributed to environmental, genetic, and chromosomal causes.

Maternal rubella during this critical period of fetal development is associated with an increased incidence of heart defects; in one study, congenital heart disease was identified in 52% of babies who were born with congenital rubella during the 1964-65 New York City epidemic.[31] Also, it appears that other viruses, some drugs, and radiation can cause congenital heart defects.

Chromosomal and genetic factors are thought to account for about 5% of congenital heart defects. Characteristic of these influences is the number of cardiac lesions observed in children born with Down's syndrome (trisomy of chromosome 21). The familial clustering of a number of congenital heart defects suggests that these defects are polygenic in origin. The 3% risk of polygenic recurrence that occurs with the presence of one affected child increases substantially as a second and third child are found to have similar defects.

Although both environmental and genetic influences have been cited as causes of congenital heart disease, the cause is often unknown, and it has been postulated that perhaps genetic and environmental factors interact and contribute to the defect.

Hemodynamic Changes

Congenital heart defects produce their major effects through (1) the shunting or mixing of arterial and venous blood and (2) the alterations in pulmonary blood flow and production of pulmonary hypertension.

Shunting of blood
Shunting of blood refers to the diverting of blood flow from one system to the other—from the arterial to the venous or the venous to the arterial system. The shunting of blood in congenital heart defects usually originates with the presence of an *abnormal opening* between the right and left circulations and the presence of a *pressure difference* that facilitates flow.

In atrial defects, blood usually moves from the left atrium into the right atrium because of the higher pressure in the left heart. In a more complicated pressure-flow situation, such as a ventricular septal defect accompanied by obstruction of the pulmonary outflow channel, pressure builds up in the right ventricle to the extent that it may exceed left ventricular pressure; in this case, blood is pushed from the right side of the heart to the left side. The presence of a right-to-left shunt results in unoxygenated blood being ejected into the systemic circulation, causing cyanosis. In the left-to-right shunt, blood intended for ejection into the systemic circulation is recirculated through the right heart and back through the lungs; the increased volume distends the right heart and pulmonary circulation and increases the work load placed on the right ventricle. Children with a septal defect that causes left-to-right shunting usually have an enlarged right heart and pulmonary blood vessels.

Changes in blood flow and pressure
Many of the complications of congenital heart disorders result from their effect on the pulmonary circulation, which may be exposed to either an increase or a decrease in blood flow.

In contrast to the arterioles in the systemic circulation, the mature pulmonary arterioles are thin-walled vessels, so they can accommodate various levels of stroke volume from the right heart. The maturation process that produces thinning of the smooth muscle layer in these vessels is delayed until after birth. In many forms of congenital heart disease, increased pulmonary blood flow during the early neonatal period results in delay or impairment of maturation. If vascular disease is allowed to progress, pulmonary vascular resistance increases and pulmonary hypertension develops. How damaging this blood flow will be to the maturing pulmonary vessels depends on the time of onset and the extent of the increased flow. In many instances, the volume overload occurs after the pulmonary vessels have already developed their low-resistance properties.

In situations in which the shunting of systemic blood flow into the pulmonary circulation threatens permanent injury to the pulmonary vessels, a surgical procedure may be done in an attempt to reduce the flow by increasing resistance to outflow from the right ventricle. This procedure, called pulmonary banding, consists of placing a constrictive band around the main pulmonary artery. The banding technique is often used as a temporary measure to alleviate the symptoms and protect the pulmonary vessels in anticipation of later surgical repair of the defect.

There are also defects that decrease pulmonary blood flow, producing inadequate oxygenation of blood. The affected child often experiences fatigue, exertional dyspnea, impaired growth, and even syncope.

Types of Congenital Heart Defects

Atrial septal defects

Atrial septal defects are more common in girls than in boys. Embryologically, division of the atria is facilitated by the development of two separate septa, which lie side by side; the septum primum is formed first and the septum secondum develops later. Neither septum completely separates the atria, and an oblique opening, the foramen ovale, allows blood to flow from the right atria into the left heart as a means of bypassing the uninflated lungs. The septum primum acts as a one-way valve to prevent the backward flow of blood. At birth, the lungs expand, umbilical blood flow is interrupted, and left atrial pressure rises, pushing the septum primum against the septum secondum. The continued contact of septum primum with septum secondum induces permanent closure of the foramen ovale, which is usually completely closed by the second or third month of extrauterine life.

Atrial septal defect occurs with the aberrant development of the septum primum or septum secondum or, more frequently, because the foramen ovale fails to close. The affected child often is asymptomatic because the defect is so small. In the case of an isolated septal defect that is large enough to allow shunting, the flow of blood will usually be from the left to the right side of the heart (remember that the pressure in the left heart is greater than that in the right); when this happens, there is an increase in the volume of the right heart and pulmonary artery (Fig. 19-15, A). This increased blood volume that

must be ejected from the right heart prolongs closure of the pulmonic valve and produces a separation, or fixed splitting, of the aortic and pulmonic components of the second heart sound.

Ventricular septal defects

Ventricular septal defects are the most common form of congenital heart defect; in 20% of all patients with congenital heart disease a ventricular defect is the only abnormality, and males are affected more frequently than females. These defects vary in size and can be located in almost any part of the structure, the site being determined by the embryologic event that was occurring at the time that growth was interrupted. The ventricular septum originates from two sources: the intraventricular groove of the folded tubular heart gives rise to the muscular part of the septum, and the endocardial cushions fuse to separate the atria and extend to form the membranous portion of the septum. The upper membranous portion of the septum is the last area to close and it is here that most defects occur.

A ventricular septal defect may be the only cardiac defect or may be one of multiple cardiac anomalies. Many defects of medium or small size in the muscular septum close spontaneously.

As with atrial septal defects, the alterations in cardiac function related to openings in the ventricular septum depend on the presence of other heart defects and their size and location. The shunting of blood across the defect is determined largely by the pressures within the two ventricles. Flow is usually left to right because of the higher pressure in the left ventricle (Fig. 19-15, B). In situations in which an obstruction to pulmonary outflow accompanies a ventricular defect, right ventricular pressure may exceed left ventricular pressure, and then the flow will be from right to left. Depending on the size of the opening, the signs and symptoms may range from the presence of an asymptomatic systolic murmur to frank congestive heart failure. Often, ventricular septal defects are a component of a defect of greater complexity, such as tetralogy of Fallot.

Tetralogy of Fallot

As the name implies, tetralogy of Fallot consists of four associated congenital heart defects: (1) ventricular septal defects involving the membranous septum and the anterior portion of the muscular septum; (2) dextroposition or shifting to the right of the aorta, so that it overrides the right ventricle and is in communication with the septal defect; (3) obstruction or narrowing of the pulmonary outflow channel, including a pulmonic valve stenosis, a decrease in the size of the pulmonary trunk, or

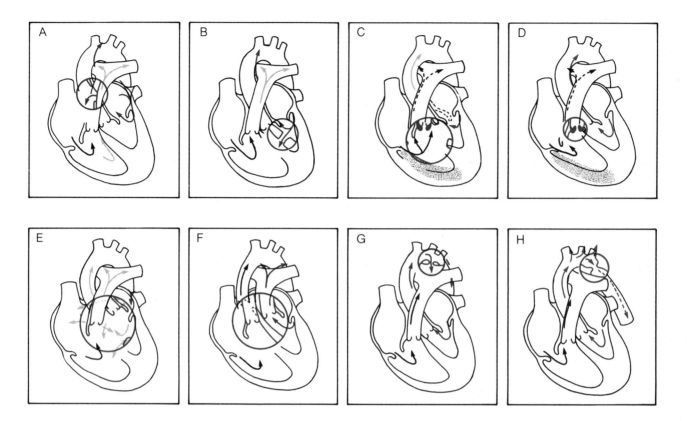

Figure 19-15 *Congenital heart defects. (A) Atrial septal defect. Blood is shunted from left to right. (B) Ventricular septal defect. Blood is usually shunted from left to right. (C) Tetralogy of Fallot. This involves a ventricular septal defect, dextroposition of the aorta, right ventricular outflow obstruction, and right ventricular hypertrophy. (D) Pulmonary stenosis, with decreased pulmonary blood flow and right ventricular hypertrophy. (E) Endocardial cushion defects. Blood flows between the chambers of the heart. (F) Transposition of the great vessels. The pulmonary artery is attached to the left side of the heart and the aorta to the right side. (G) Patent ductus arteriosus. The high pressure blood of the aorta is shunted back to the pulmonary artery. (H) Postductal coarctation of the aorta.*

both; and (4) hypertrophy of the right ventricle due to the increased work required to pump blood through the obstructed pulmonary channels (Fig. 19-15, C).

Most children with tetralogy of Fallot display varying degrees of cyanosis—hence the term *blue babies*. The cyanosis develops as the result of decreased pulmonary blood flow and because the right-to-left shunt causes mixing of unoxygenated blood with the oxygenated blood being ejected into the peripheral circulation. Because of the decreased availability of oxygen, these children have limited exercise tolerance. As a means of coping with this exercise intolerance, the child often is observed to spontaneously assume the squatting position, though just how the squatting effects an increase in blood oxygen levels is still conjectural. Some authorities suggest that the position increases blood flow to the brain and other vital organs by temporarily reducing blood flow to the lower extremities, while others suggest

that the compression of vessels in the lower extremities may incite a vasoconstrictor response that serves to elevate blood pressure.

Pulmonary stenosis

Pulmonary stenosis may occur as an isolated valvular lesion or in conjunction with more complex defects, such as tetralogy of Fallot. In isolated valvular defects, the pulmonary cusps may be absent or malformed or may remain fused at their commissural edges; often, all three abnormalities are present. Pulmonic valvular defects usually cause some impairment of pulmonary blood flow and increase the work load imposed on the right heart (Fig. 19-15, D). In infants with severe defects causing marked impairment of pulmonary blood flow, the ductus arteriosus may provide the vital accessory route for perfusing the lungs during early postnatal life. Medical treatment efforts designed to maintain the patency of the ductus in affected infants are discussed later in this chapter in the section on patent ductus arteriosus. If pulmonary stenosis is extreme, increased pressures in the right heart may delay closure of the foramen ovale.

Endocardial cushion defects

Children with Down's syndrome have a high incidence of endocardial cushion defects, with estimates indicating that as many as 50% of such children have some form of endocardial cushion defect. The endocardial cushions form the atrioventricular canals, the upper part of the ventricular septum, and the lower part of the atrial septum. Considering the embryologic contributions of the endocardial cushions to heart development, it is easy to see why the defect can cause so many different types of problems. In its most severe form, the defect involves both the atrial and ventricular septa and the tricuspid and mitral valves. When growth is halted at a later stage of development, there may be an ostium primum defect and a cleft in the mitral valve. Any single defect or combination of endocardial defects is possible (Fig. 19-15, E).

Ebstein's anomaly is a defect in endocardial cushion development characterized by displacement of tricuspid valvular tissue into the ventricle. The displaced tricuspid leaflets are attached either directly to the right ventricular endocardial surface or to shortened or malformed chordae tendineae.

Transposition of the great vessels

In transposition of the great vessels, the aorta originates in the right ventricle and the pulmonary trunk in the left. The structural defect present in this anomaly suggests that during embryonic partitioning of the aorta and pulmonary trunk there was failure in the spiral movement of the bulbus cordis and truncus arteriosus (Fig. 19-15, F). In infants born with this defect, survival is dependent on communication between the right and left heart, either in the form of a septal defect or as a patent ductus arteriosus. A procedure called a balloon atrial septostomy may be done to increase the blood flow between the two sides of the heart. This is done by inserting a balloon-tipped catheter into the heart through the vena cava, then passing the catheter through the foramen ovale into the left atrium. The balloon is then inflated and as it is brought back through the foramen ovale, the opening is enlarged.

A surgical procedure, the Mustard operation, in which the atrial septum is removed and a new wall is created so that blood is directed into the proper outflow channels, corrects the defect.

Patent ductus arteriosus

In fetal life, the ductus arteriosus is the vital link by which blood from the right heart bypasses the lungs and enters the systemic circulation (Fig. 19-15, G). Following birth this passage is no longer needed, and it usually closes during the first 24 to 72 hours. The physiologic stimulus and mechanisms associated with permanent closure of the ductus are not entirely known, but the fact that infant hypoxia predisposes to a delayed closure suggests that arterial oxygen levels play a role. As is true of other heart and circulatory defects, patency of the ductus arteriosus may be present in various forms; the opening may be small, medium-sized, or large.

The function of the ductus arteriosus in providing a right-to-left shunt in prenatal life has prompted the surgical creation of an aortic-pulmonary shunt as a means of improving pulmonary blood flow in children with severe pulmonary outflow disorders. Recent research has focused on the role of type E prostaglandins in maintaining the patency of the ductus; several researchers have found that, by injecting prostaglandin E into the umbilical vein of infants who require a ductal shunt, closure has been delayed or prevented.[32] Other research suggests that inhibiting prostaglandin activity with drugs such as aspirin and indomethacin has prompted closure of the ductus.[33,34]

Coarctation of the aorta

Coarctation of the aorta can be described as a localized narrowing of the aorta, either proximal to (preductal) or distal to the ductus (postductal). (See Fig. 19-15, H.)

In *preductal* coarctation, the ductus remains open and shunts blood from the pulmonary artery, through the ductus arteriosus, into the aorta. It is frequently seen with other cardiac anomalies and carries a high mortality. Because of the position of the defect, blood flow throughout the systemic circulation is reduced, and the affected infant develops heart failure at an early age due to the increased work load imposed on the left ventricle.

In *postductal* coarctation, symptoms often do not arise until late adolescence or adult life. In these persons, the narrowing of the aorta distal to the subclavian artery and proximal to the descending aorta creates disparity between the pulses and blood pressure of the upper and lower extremities (Chap. 17).

Manifestations and Treatment

Congenital heart defects present with numerous signs and symptoms. Some defects, such as patent ductus arteriosus and small ventricular septal defects, often close spontaneously, and in other less severe defects, there are no signs and symptoms. Often, the disorder is discovered during a routine health examination. Pulmonary congestion, cardiac failure, and decreased peripheral perfusion are the chief concerns in children with more severe defects. Such defects often cause problems shortly after birth or in early infancy. The child often exhibits cyanosis, respiratory difficulty, and fatigability, and is likely to have difficulty with feeding and failure to thrive. A generalized cyanosis that persists more than 3 hours following birth is suggestive of congenital heart disease.

One technique for evaluating the infant consists of administering 100% oxygen for 10 minutes. If the infant "pinks up," the cyanosis is probably due to respiratory problems. Because infant cyanosis may appear as a duskiness, it is important to assess the color of the mucous membranes, fingernails, toenails, tongue, and lips. Pulmonary congestion in the infant causes an increase in respiratory rate, orthopnea, grunting, wheezing, coughing, and rales. The baby whose peripheral perfusion is markedly decreased may appear to be in a shocklike state. The manifestations and treatment of heart failure in the infant and small child are similar in many ways to those in the adult (Chap. 20), but the infant's small size and limited physical reserve make them more serious and treatment more difficult. The treatment plan usually includes supportive therapy designed to help the infant compensate for the limitations in cardiac reserve and to prevent complications. Surgical intervention is often required in severe defects, and it may be done in the early weeks of life or, conditions permitting, may be delayed until the child is older. The reader is referred to a pediatric textbook for a complete description of treatment.

In summary, congenital heart defects affect about 8 out of every 1000 neonates. The fetal heart develops during weeks 3 to 8 following conception, and it is during this period that defects in its development arise. The defect reflects the stage of development at the time when the causative event occurred. A number of factors are thought to contribute to the development of congenital heart defects, including genetic and chromosomal influences, viruses, and environmental agents such as drugs and radiation. Often the cause of the defect is unknown. The defect may produce no effects or it may markedly affect cardiac function. Infants with severe congenital heart defects often suffer from pulmonary congestion, heart failure, and decreased peripheral perfusion.

■ Study Guide

After you have studied this chapter, you should be able to meet the following objectives:

☐ List at least five causes of pericarditis.

☐ Compare the manifestations of acute pericarditis with those of chronic pericarditis with effusion.

☐ State the mechanisms associated with pulsus paradoxus.

☐ State the characteristics of constrictive pericarditis.

☐ Relate the term *tamponade* to its manifestations in cardiac tamponade.

☐ Describe the anatomy of the right and the left coronary arteries.

☐ State the significance of atherosclerosis in the occurrence of coronary heart disease.

☐ State the physiologic cause of angina.

☐ Distinguish unstable angina from variant angina.

☐ State the overall goal in treatment of angina and its rationale.

☐ Describe the difference between sites of action of β_1- and β_2- adrenergic blocking drugs.

☐ Describe the action of calcium-channel blocking drugs as they relate to the relief of angina.

☐ State the relationship between thrombosis and myocardial infarction.

☐ List the chief signs and symptoms by which the health professional can recognize myocardial infarction.

☐ State four or more possible complications of myocardial infarction and the manifestations of each.

☐ Describe the immediate postinfarction and later postinfarction treatment measures that the professional health care team should follow.

☐ State the anatomic changes created with aortocoronary bypass surgery and the mammary artery revascularization procedure.

☐ Relate the action of streptokinase in the treatment of myocardial infarction.

☐ Describe the sequence of events by which the conduction system controls cardiac rhythm and pumping action.

☐ Compare sinus arrhythmia with atrial arrhythmia.

☐ Describe the characteristics of first-, second-, and third-degree heart block.

☐ State the potential complications associated with premature ventricular contractions.

☐ State the major manifestations of acute rheumatic fever.

☐ State the probable sequence of events in rheumatic fever.

☐ State the predisposing factors in bacterial endocarditis and the significance of each.

☐ Distinguish between the role of infectious organisms in the production of rheumatic fever and of bacterial endocarditis.

☐ Relate the pathologic changes that occur with bacterial endocarditis to production of signs and symptoms of the disease.

☐ Relate the presence of valvular disease to cardiac function.

☐ State the differences in blood flow and cardiac function that occur with a stenotic and regurgitant heart valve.

☐ Compare the hemodynamic derangements that occur with aortic stenosis and aortic regurgitation.

☐ Describe the clinical findings in mitral valve defects.

☐ Discuss the epidemiology of mitral valve prolapse.

☐ Compare the heart changes that occur with dilated, hypertrophic, and constrictive cardiomyopathies.

☐ Relate the occurrence of Down's syndrome to congenital heart defects.

☐ State the effect of altered pulmonary blood flow on congenital heart disease.

☐ Compare the features of atrial septal defects with those of ventricular septal defects.

☐ Explain why the phrase "blue baby" is used to describe a baby with tetralogy of Fallot.

☐ State the effect of congenital pulmonary stenosis on pulmonary blood flow.

☐ Explain the significance of endocardial cushion defects.

☐ Describe the anatomical situation in transposition of the great vessels.

☐ Explain the function of the ductus arteriosus in fetal life.

☐ Describe the effect on blood flow of preductal and postductal coarctation of the aorta.

■ References

1. Facts 1984. Dallas, American Heart Association, 1982
2. Robbins SL, Cotran RS, Kumar V: Pathologic Basis of Disease, 3rd ed, pp 602, 556, 553, 559, 571, 598. Philadelphia, WB Saunders, 1984
3. Spodick DH: Acute pericarditis and pericardial effusion: Guide to diagnosis and management. Hosp Med 15, No. 5:72, 1979
4. Spodick D: Acoustic phenomena in pericardial disease. Am Heart J 81:114, 1971
5. Spodick D: The normal and diseased pericardium: Current concepts of pericardial physiology, diagnosis, and treatment. J Am Coll Cardiol 1:240, 1983
6. Arteriosclerosis. Report of the 1977 Working Group to Review the Report of the National Heart and Lung Institute Task Force on Arteriosclerosis. Washington, DC, US Department of Health, Education and Welfare, p 14, 1977
7. Prinzmetal M, Kennamer R, Merliss R et al: A variant form of angina pectoris. Am J Med 27:375, 1959
8. Miwa K, Kambara H, Kawai C: Effect of aspirin in large doses on attacks of variant angina. Am Heart J 106:351, 1982
9. Braunwald E: Mechanisms of calcium-channel-blocking agents. N Engl J Med 307:1618, 1982
10. Zelis R, Flaim SF: Calcium-blocking drugs for angina pectoris. Annu Rev Med 33:465, 1982
11. Block PC, Baughman KL, Pasternak RC et al: Transluminal angioplasty: Correlation of morphologic and angiographic findings in an experimental model. Circulation 61:778, 1980
12. Peduzzi P, Haltgren H: Effect of medical vs. surgical treatment on symptoms of stable angina pectoris. Circulation 60:888, 1979
13. Anderson AJ, Barboriak JJ, Hoffman RG et al: Retention or resumption of employment after aortocoronary bypass operation. JAMA 246:543, 1980
14. Robbins SL: Cardiac pathology—A look at the last five years. Hum Pathol 5:9, 1974
15. Hillis LD, Braunwald E: Myocardial ischemia. N Engl J Med 296:1034, 1977
16. Grande P, Christiansen C, Peterson A et al: Optimal diagnosis in acute myocardial infarction. Circulation 61:723, 1980
17. The Anturane Reinfarction Trial Research Group Sulfinpyrazone in the prevention of sudden death after myocardial infarction. N Engl J Med 302:250, 1980
18. Singh BN, Nademanee K: New agents in antiarrhythmia therapy. Primary Cardiol 8, No 2:16, 1982
19. Sololow M, McIlroy MB: Clinical Cardiology, p 351. Los Altos, Lange Medical Publications, 1977
20. Markiewicz W, Stoner J, Londone E et al: Mitral valve prolapse in one hundred presumably healthy young females. Circulation 53:464, 1976
21. Procacci PM, Savran SV, Schreiter SL, Bryson AL: Prevalence of clinical mitral-valve prolapse in 1169 young women. N Engl J Med 294:1086, 1976
22. Gaffney FA, Karlson ES, Campbell W et al: Autonomic dysfunction in women with mitral valve prolapse syndrome. Circulation 59:894, 1979
23. Jerasaty RM: Mitral valve prolapse-click syndrome. Prog Cardiovasc Dis 15:623, 1973
24. Report of the WHO/ISFC Task Force on the Definition and Classification of the Cardiomyopathies. Br Heart J 44:672, 1980
25. Fuster V, Gersh BJ, Giuliani ER et al: The natural history of dilated cardiomyopathy. Am J Cardiol 47:525, 1981
26. Johnson AR, Palacios I: Dilated cardiomyopathies of the adult. N Engl J Med 307:1051, 1982
27. Demakis JG, Shahbudin H, Rahimtoola MB et al: Natural course of peripartum cardiomyopathy. Circulation 44:1053, 1971
28. Bohachick P, Rongaus AM: Hypertrophic cardiomyopathy. Am J Nurs 84:320, 1984

29. Braunwald, E (ed): Heart Disease: A Textbook of Cardiovascular Medicine, Vol 2, p 1451. Philadelphia, WB Saunders, 1980

30. Chatterjee D, Raff G, Anderson D, Parmley WW: Hypertrophic cardiomyopathy—Therapy with slow channel inhibiting agents. Prog Cardiovasc Dis 25:193, 1982

31. Engle MA, Adams F, Betson C et al: Primary prevention of congenital heart disease. Circulation 41:A26, June 1970

32. Rudolph AM, Heymann MA: Medical treatment of ductus arteriosus. Hosp Pract 12, No 2:57, 1977

33. Heymann MA, Rudolph AM, Silverman NH: Closure of the ductus arteriosus in premature infants by inhibition of prostaglandin synthesis. N Engl J Med 295, No 10:530, 1976

34. Smith ME: Nonsurgical closure of patent ductus arteriosus in preterm infants. Heart Lung 8, No 2:308, 1979

■ Additional References

Bacterial endocarditis and rheumatic fever

DiSciascio G, Taranta A: Rheumatic fever in children. Am Heart J 99, No 5:635, 1980

Kaplan EL et al: Prevention of bacterial endocarditis. Circulation 56, A139, 1977

Pankey GA: The prevention and treatment of bacterial endocarditis. Am Heart J 98, No 1:102, 1979

Cardiomyopathies

Altman GB: Alcoholic cardiomyopathy. Cardio-Vasc Nurs 17:25, 1981

Bohachick P, Rongaus AM: Hypertrophic cardiomyopathy. Am J Nurs 3:320, 1984

Bulkley NH: The cardiomyopathies. Hosp Pract 6:59, 1984

James TN: Myocarditis and cardiomyopathy. N Engl J Med 308:39, 1983

Nishimura RA, Giuliani ER, Brandenburg RO: Hypertrophic cardiomyopathy. Cardio VascRev Rep 4:931, 1983

Olsen EG: The pathology of cardiomyopathies: A critical analysis. Am Heart J 98:385, 1979

Cardiovascular drugs

Braunwald E, Muller JE, Kloner RA, Maroko PR: Role of beta-adrenergic blockade in the therapy of patients with myocardial infarction. Am J Med 74:113, 1983

Calcium-blocker therapy for unstable angina pectoris. N Engl J Med 306:926, 1982

Conti RC, Feldman RL, Pepine CJ, Hill JA, Conti JB: Effect of glyceryl trinitrate on coronary and systemic hemodynamics in man. Am J Med 105:28, 1983

Kennedy GT: Slow channel calcium blockers in the treatment of chronic stable angina. Cardio-Vasc Nurs 20:1, 1984

Lapinski ML: Cardiovascular drugs and the elderly population. Heart Lung 11:430, 1982

O'Rourke RA: New drugs for the treatment of angina pectoris. Med Times 111:85, 1983

Rossi LP, Antman EM: Calcium channel blockers. Am J Nurs 83:382, 1983

Conduction defects

Duke DM: Intraventricular conduction blocks. Crit Care Nurs 3:30, 1982

Heger JJ, Fisch C: Axioms on cardiac arrhythmias. Hosp Med 15, No 1:20, 1979

Roffman JA, Fieldman A: Ventricular conduction defects: Significance and prognosis. Heart Lung 9, No 1:111, 1980

Selzer A: Atrial fibrillation revisited. N Engl J Med 306:1044, 1982

Spear JF, Moore EN: Mechanisms of cardiac arrhythmias. Annu Rev Physiol 44:485, 1982

Standford JL, Felmer JM, Arenberg D: Antiarrhythmic drug therapy. Am J Nurs 80, No 7:1288, 1980

Congenital heart defects

Hoffman JI, Rudolph AM, Heymann MA: Pulmonary vascular disease with congenital heart lesions: Pathologic features and causes. Circulation 64:873, 1981

Modrcin MA, Schott J: An update of congestive heart failure in infants. Issues Comp Pediatr Nurs 3:5, 1979

Nadas AS: Heart disease in children. Hosp Pract 12, No 1:103, 1977

Nadas AS: Indomethacin and the patent ductus arteriosus. N Engl J Med 305:97, 1981

Nadas AS: Update on congenital heart disease. Med Clin North Am 31, No 1:153, 1984

Rudolph AM, Heymann MA: Medical treatment of ductus arteriosus. Hosp Pract 12, No 2:57, 1977

Sacksteder S: Embryology and fetal circulation. Am J Nurs 78, No 2:262, 1978

Sacksteder S, Gildea H, Dassy C: Common congenital cardiac defects. Am J Nurs 78, No 2:266, 1978

Shor VZ: Congenital cardiac defects. Am J Nurs 78, No 2:256, 1978

Smith ME: Nonsurgical closure of patent ductus arteriosus in preterm infants. Heart Lung 8, No 2:308, 1979

Exercise testing and rehabilitation

Dehn M: Rehabilitation of the cardiac patient: The effects of exercise. Am J Nurs 80, No 3:435, 1980

Fletcher GF: Exercise and exercise testing—A symposium. Heart Lung 13:5, 1984

Johnston BL: Exercise testing for patients after myocardial infarction and coronary bypass surgery: Emphasis on predischarge phase. Heart Lung 13:18, 1984

Merril S, Froelicher VF: Exercise testing. Cardio-Vasc Nurs 13, No 6:23, 1977

Sivarajan ES, Halpenny CJ: Exercise testing. Am J Nurs 79, No 12:1262, 1979

Winslow EH, Weber TM: Rehabilitation of the cardiac patient. Progressive exercise to combat the hazards of bed rest. Am J Nurs 80, No 3:440, 1980

Diseases of the myocardium

Alexander JK, Fred HL, Wright KE, Turell DJ, Jackson RA, Jackson D: Exercise and coronary artery disease. Heart Lung 7, No 1, 1978

Arcebal AG, Lemberg L: Angina pectoris in the absence of coronary artery disease. Heart Lung 9, No 4:728, 1980

Braunwald E: Treatment of the patient after myocardial infarction. N Engl J Med 302, No 5:290, 1980

Cain RS, Ferguson R, Tillisch JH: Variant angina: A nursing approach. Heart Lung 8, No 6:1122, 1979

Come PC: Coronary arterial spasm. J Fam Pract 14:119, 1982

Devny AM: Rehabilitation of the cardiac patient: Bridging the gap between in-hospital and outpatient care. Am J Nurs 80, No 3:446, 1980

Epstein SE, Palmeri ST, Patterson RE: Evaluations of patients after acute myocardial infarction. N Engl J Med 307:1487, 1982

Foster SB, Canty KA: Pump failure following myocardial infarction: An overview. Heart Lung 9, No 2:293, 1980

Fuchs RM, Becker LC: Pathogenesis of angina pectoris. Arch Intern Med 142:1685, 1982

Fuller EO: The effect of antianginal drugs on myocardial oxygen consumption. Am J Nurs 80, No 2:250, 1980

Grande P, Hansen BF, Christiansen C, Naestoft J: Acute myocardial infarct size estimated by CK-MB determinations: Clinical accuracy and prognostic relevance utilizing a practical modification of the isoenzyme approach. Am Heart J 101:582, 1981

Gronim SS: Helping the client with unstable angina. Am J Nurs 78, No 10:1677, 1978

Hirsh AT: Postmyocardial infarction syndrome. Am J Nurs 79, No 7:1240, 1979

Kannel WB, Sorlie P, McNamara PM: Prognosis after initial myocardial infarction: The Framingham study. Am J Cardiol No 44:53, 1979

Maseri A, Chierchia S: Coronary artery spasm: Demonstration, definition, diagnosis, and consequences. Prog CardioVasc Dis 25:169, 1982

McCarthy CL: Percutaneous transluminal coronary angioplasty: Therapeutic intervention in the cardiac catheterization laboratory. Heart Lung 11:499, 1982

Miller D, Waters DD, Warnica W, Szlachcic J, Kreeft J, Theroux P: Is variant angina the coronary manifestation of a generalized vasospastic disorder? N Engl J Med 304:763, 1981

Mirvis DM: Management of acute myocardial infarction. Adv Intern Med 28:1, 1983

Pitt B: Prognosis after acute myocardial infarction. N Engl J Med 305:1147, 1981

Scheer E: Enzymatic changes and myocardial infarction: A nursing update. Cardio-Vasc Nurs 14, No 2:5, 1978

Schroeder JS, Lamb I, Hu M: Do patients in whom myocardial infarction has been ruled out have a better prognosis after hospitalization than those surviving infarction? N Engl J Med 303, No 1:1, 1980

Schuster EH, Bulkley BH: Early post-infarction angina. N Engl J Med 305:1101, 1981

Spann JF: Changing concepts of pathophysiology, prognosis, and therapy in acute myocardial infarction. Am J Med 74:877, 1983

Vaughan P: Bedside assessment of the myocardial infarction patient. Crit Care Nurs 4:60, 1984

Vaughan P: Complications of myocardial infarction. Crit Care Nurs 3:44, 1982

Wenger NK: Early ambulation physical activity: Myocardial infarction and coronary artery bypass surgery. Heart Lung 13:14, 1984

Diseases of the pericardium

Buselmeier TJ, Davin TD, Simmons RL, Najarian JS, Kjellstrand CM: Treatment of intractable uremic pericardial effusion. J Am Med A 240:1358, 1978

Domby WR, Whitcomb MF: Pleural effusion as a manifestation of Dressler's syndrome in the distant post infarction period. Am Heart J 96, No 2:243, 1978

Hirschmann JV: Pericardial constriction. Am Heart J 96, No 1:110, 1978

Spodick DH: Acute pericarditis and pericardial effusion: Guide to diagnosis and management. Hosp Med 15:72, May 1979

Zeluff GW, Eknoyan G, Jackson D: Pericarditis in renal failure. Heart Lung 8, No 6:1139, 1979

Valvular heart disease

Jeresaty RM: Mitral valve prolapse-click syndrome: Etiology, clinical findings, and therapy. CardioVasc Med 3:597, 1978

Savage DD, Garrison RJ, Devereux RB et al: Mitral valve prolapse in the general population. I. The Framingham study. Prog Cardiol 106:571, 1983

Gaasch WH: Management of aortic valve disease. Hosp Pract 9:133, 1982

Chapter 20

Heart Failure

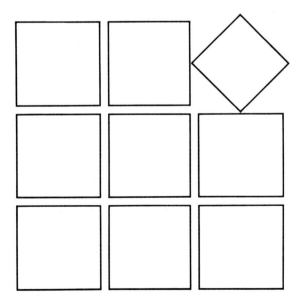

Heart failure is a major health problem in the United States. In 1980, 401,000 patients were discharged from the hospital with a diagnosis of heart failure. As many as 50% of those discharged died within 12 months of diagnosis.[1] Although heart failure affects all age groups, 75% of persons with heart failure are over age 60.[2]

Heart failure is not a specific disease, but rather the inability of the heart to pump blood commensurate with the metabolic needs of body tissues. It may result either from a diseased heart that is unable to pump blood or from excessive demands placed on a normal heart, as in the case of thyrotoxicosis. Heart failure may present as an acute or chronic disorder. In persons with asymptomatic heart disease, heart failure may be precipitated by an unrelated illness or stress. The discussion in this chapter focuses on congestive heart failure and acute pulmonary edema.

Primary disorders of the heart such as coronary heart disease, valvular heart disease, and cardiomyopathies clearly account for most cases of heart failure. Of the various types of primary heart disease, most involve abnormalities of the contractile properties of the left ventricle. A normal ventricle ejects about two-thirds of the blood that is present in the ventricle at the end of diastole (ejection fraction). In heart failure, the ejection fraction declines progressively with increasing degrees of myocardial dysfunction. In very severe forms of heart failure, the ejection fraction may be as low as 20% to

25%.[3] The resultant increased residual volume leads to cardiac dilatation and a rise in diastolic filling pressure. This leads to a passive congestion of organs proximal to the failing ventricle (the lungs when it is the left ventricle, and the liver and extremities when it is the right). Cardiac dilatation also increases the tension in the wall of the ventricle, and as a result more work is needed to eject blood from the heart (see law of Laplace, Chap. 14).

■ Compensatory Mechanisms

The heart has the amazing capacity to adjust its activity to meet the varying needs of the body—during sleep its output declines, and during exercise it increases markedly. This ability to increase output during increased activity is called the *cardiac reserve*. For example, competitive swimmers and long-distance runners have large cardiac reserves. During exercise the cardiac output of these athletes rapidly increases to as much as five to six times the normal level. In sharp contrast with the healthy athlete, persons with heart failure often use their cardiac reserve even at rest. For them, even such simple activities as climbing a flight of stairs may cause shortness of breath because they have exceeded their cardiac reserve.

Cardiac reserve is maintained mainly through three processes: (1) the Frank-Starling mechanism, (2) increased sympathetic nervous system activity, and (3) myocardial hypertrophy. The diseased as well as the healthy heart employs these mechanisms. In many forms of heart disease, early decreases in cardiac function go unnoticed because these compensatory mechanisms maintain the cardiac output. Unfortunately, the mechanisms were not intended for long-term use, and in severe and prolonged heart failure, the compensatory mechanisms themselves begin to cause problems (Fig. 20-1).

The Frank-Starling Mechanism

As was discussed in Chapter 18, the Frank-Starling mechanism produces an increase in stroke volume by means of an increase in ventricular end-diastolic volume. The increased volume leads to increased filling and stretching of the myocardial fibers during diastole and a resultant increase in the force of the next contraction (Fig. 20-2). In heart failure, the increase in ventricular end-diastolic volume results from an increase in vascular volume, which yields a subsequent increase in venous return to the heart.

Several mechanisms contribute to fluid retention in heart failure. Normally, the kidneys receive about 25% of the cardiac output. With heart failure and the sympathetic-mediated vasoconstriction of the renal blood vessels that accompanies a decrease in cardiac output,

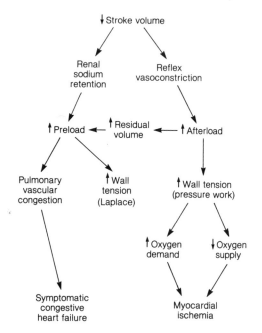

Figure 20-1 *Sequence of responses after reduction in cardiac pump performance due to heart failure. (From Ross G: Pathophysiology of the Heart. New York, Masson Publishing, 1982. Reproduced with permission)*

this amount may be decreased to as low as 8% to 10%; the result is an increase in sodium and water retention by means of the renin-angiotensin-aldosterone mechanism.[3] A second mechanism involves the metabolism in the liver of aldosterone, which stimulates the retention of sodium and water by the kidneys. In heart failure, passive congestion of the liver leads to decreased destruction of aldosterone, and thus to sodium and water retention. Finally, there is evidence of abnormal secretion of antidiuretic hormone in heart failure, which may contribute to water retention.

Cardiac output may be normal at rest in persons with heart failure due to increased ventricular end-diastolic volume and the Frank-Starling mechanism. This mechanism becomes ineffective, however, when the heart becomes overfilled and the muscle fibers overstretched. With the deterioration of myocardial contractility, the ventricular function curve depicted in Figure 20-1 flattens out, so that with any given increase in cardiac output, such as occurs with increased physical activity, there is a greater rise in left ventricular end-diastolic volume and pressure, with an elevation of pulmonary capillary pressure and development of dyspnea.[4] Overfilling of the ventricle also results in an increase in wall tension to maintain the same pressure as a smaller ventricle (law of Laplace, Chap. 14). Because the increased wall tension increases myocardial oxygen requirements, it contributes to the impairment of cardiac function.

Sympathetic Stimulation

The importance of the sympathetic nervous system in the control of cardiac function is well established. Sympathetic stimulation increases both heart rate and cardiac contractility. Although sympathetic activity does not appear to contribute to the intrinsic contractile state of the heart, it augments contractility during periods of stress. Persons with heart failure have been shown to have increased concentration of plasma norepinephrine at rest and during exercise, compared with persons without heart failure.[5] In addition, 24-hour urine norepinephrine levels were markedly increased in persons with heart failure, which indicates increased activity of the sympathetic nervous system, including the adrenal medulla.[6] There is evidence that in cardiac failure the sympathetic receptors in the heart remain functional and able to respond to norepinephrine. The failing heart, however, is unable to synthesize the neuromediator and must depend on increased catecholamines in the blood.

Increased sympathetic activity also causes vasoconstriction and a compensatory redistribution of cardiac output. Blood from the skin, kidneys, and gastrointestinal tract is diverted to the more critical cerebral and coronary circulations. This general increase in sympathetic tone produces an increase in vascular resistance and the afterload against which the heart must pump.

Myocardial Hypertrophy

Myocardial hypertrophy is a long-term compensatory mechanism. Cardiac muscle, like skeletal muscle, responds to an increase in work demands by undergoing hypertrophy. Heart diseases that increase resistance to the ejection of blood from the ventricles are the greatest stimulus for hypertrophy; for example, the left ventricle may increase in size to six times normal in severe aortic stenosis. If portions of the heart muscle are damaged and replaced with scar tissue, the undamaged part of the myocardium often hypertrophies as a means of improving the pumping capacity of the ventricle. However, myocardial hypertrophy is no longer beneficial when the oxygen requirements of the increased muscle mass exceed the ability of the coronary vessels to bring blood to the area.

In summary, heart failure is characterized by the impaired pumping ability of the heart and represents the outcome of many forms of heart disease or other conditions that place excessive demands on the heart. The cardiac reserve represents the heart's ability to increase its output according to the needs of the body. Three compensatory mechanisms contribute to the cardiac reserve: the Frank-Starling mechanism, the activity of the sympathetic nervous system, and myocardial hypertrophy. In many forms of heart disease, early decreases in cardiac

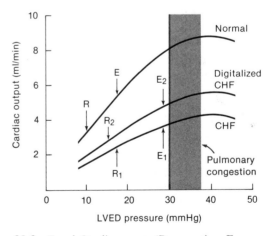

Figure 20-2 *Frank-Starling curves (R = resting; E = exercise; LVED = left ventricular end-diastolic pressure; CHF = congestive heart failure; CI = cardiac index.) (From Iseri LT, Benvenuti DJ: Pathogenesis and management of congestive heart failure—revisited. Am Heart J, 105, No 2: 346, 1983)*

function go unnoticed because of these compensatory mechanisms. As heart failure progresses, however, the compensatory mechanisms may contribute to the production of signs and symptoms and a worsening of cardiac function.

■ Congestive Heart Failure

Heart failure occurs when the heart fails to pump sufficient blood to meet the metabolic needs of body tissues. In congestive heart failure, fluid accumulates in body tissues along with a decrease in cardiac output. Table 20-1 lists the causes of heart failure.

When the heart fails as a pump, there may be two direct effects on the circulation: backward or forward failure. *Backward failure* refers to signs and symptoms that arise from inadequate emptying, which allows blood to accumulate in vessels or heart chambers located behind the failing ventricles (in the lungs when there is failure of the left ventricle and in the systemic circulation when there is failure of the right ventricle), resulting in congestion of the pulmonary and venous systemic circulations. *Forward failure* results in impaired output of blood into the vessels emerging from the heart. Heart failure may also be classified according to the side of the heart (right or left) that is affected. Although the initial event that leads to heart failure may be primarily right-sided or left-sided in origin, long-term heart failure usually involves both sides. It is easier, however, to understand the physiologic mechanisms associated with heart failure when right- and left-sided failure are discussed separately.

Right-Sided Failure

The right side of the heart moves deoxygenated blood from the systemic circulation into the pulmonary circulation. Right-sided heart failure is characterized by an accumulation or damming back of blood in the systemic venous system. This causes an increase in right atrial and peripheral venous pressures, with subsequent development of edema in the peripheral tissues and congestion of the abdominal organs. Fluid accumulation also produces a gain in weight. One pint of accumulated fluid results in a weight gain of 1 pound. Thus, daily measurement of weight can be used as a means of assessing fluid accumulation in heart failure.

The peripheral edema is most pronounced in the lower extremities and in the area over the sacrum. As venous distention progresses, blood backs up in the hepatic veins that drain into the inferior vena cava, and the liver becomes engorged. In severe and prolonged

Table 20-1 Causes of Heart Failure

Impaired Cardiac Function	Excess Work Demands
Myocardial Disease	**Increased Pressure Work**
Cardiomyopathies	Systemic hypertension
Myocarditis	Pulmonary hypertension
Coronary insufficiency	Coarctation of the aorta
Myocardial infarction	
Valvular Heart Disease	**Increased Volume Work**
Stenotic valvular disease	Arteriovenous shunt
Regurgitant valvular disease	Excessive administration of
	intravenous fluids
Congenital Heart Defects	**Increased Perfusion Work**
	Thyrotoxicosis
	Anemia
Constrictive Pericarditis	

right-sided failure, liver function is frequently impaired, and liver cells may die. Congestion of the portal circulation may also lead to enlargement of the spleen with transudation of fluid into the peritoneal cavity (ascites). Congestion of the gut may cause gastrointestinal disturbances, including anorexia, abdominal pain, and loss of weight. In long-standing heart failure, severe weight loss may progress to cardiac cachexia.

Cyanosis may occur in either right- or left-sided heart failure. In right-sided failure, the blood flow is sluggish and extraction of oxygen from the blood as it passes through the capillaries is increased; the quantity of deoxygenated hemoglobin in the blood then increases.*

The jugular veins are above the level of the heart and are normally collapsed in the standing position. In severe right-sided failure, the external jugular veins become distended and can be visualized when the person is standing. The manifestations of right-sided heart failure are depicted in Figure 20-3.

Left-Sided Failure

The left side of the heart moves blood from the low-pressure pulmonary circulation into the high-pressure arterial side of the systemic circulation. With impairment of the left heart function, the blood tends to accumulate in the pulmonary circulation. An increase in pulmonary capillary pressure reflects the increased left atrial pressure and leads to pulmonary edema. In severe pulmonary

---

*The blue discoloration associated with cyanosis requires the presence of 5 g of deoxygenated hemoglobin. A severely anemic person may not have sufficient hemoglobin to permit 5 g to become deoxygenated. Some of the success credited to the bloodletting practices of the 18th and 19th centuries probably resulted from treating cyanosis by causing anemia.

edema, capillary fluid moves into the alveoli. The accumulated fluid in the alveoli and respiratory passages impairs the gas-exchange function of the lung. With the decreased ability of the lungs to oxygenate the blood, the hemoglobin leaves the pulmonary circulation without being fully oxygenated. Cyanosis and shortness of breath result.

Shortness of breath due to congestion and increased pressure in the capillaries of the lung is one of the major manifestations of left-sided heart failure. A perceived shortness of breath (breathlessness) is called *dyspnea*. Dyspnea related to an increase in activity is called *exertional dyspnea*. *Orthopnea* is shortness of breath that occurs when a person is supine, or lying down. The gravitational forces that cause fluid to become sequestered in the lower legs and feet when the person is sitting are not operational when the person is supine; the fluid is then mobilized and redistributed to an already distended pulmonary circulation. *Paroxysmal nocturnal dyspnea* is a sudden attack of dyspnea during sleep. It disrupts sleep, and the person awakens with a feeling of extreme suffocation. Bronchospasm due to congestion of the bronchial mucosa may be present, causing wheezing and difficulty in breathing. This condition is referred to as *cardiac asthma*.

Fatigue and limb weakness often accompany diminished output from the left ventricle. Cardiac fatigue is different from emotional fatigue in that it is not present in the morning but appears and progresses as activity increases during the day. In acute or severe left-sided failure, cardiac output may fall to levels that are insufficient for providing the brain with adequate oxygen, and there are indications of mental confusion and disturbed behavior. Confusion, impairment of memory, anxiety, restlessness, and insomnia are common in elderly persons with advanced heart failure, particularly in those with cerebral atherosclerosis.

Nocturia occurs relatively early in the course of congestive heart failure. During the day, when the person is in the upright position, the blood flow is redistributed away from the kidneys. At night, resting in the recumbent position produces an increase in cardiac output and blood flow to the kidneys; consequently, renal vasoconstriction diminishes and urine formation increases. When oliguria occurs, it is a late sign of suppression related to a severely reduced cardiac output.

Increased sympathetic activity, though a principal compensatory mechanism in heart failure, is also responsible for a number of physical signs. Peripheral vasoconstriction is manifested by pallor and coldness of the extremities and cyanosis of the digits. There may also be diaphoresis and tachycardia. Vasoconstriction may impede the loss of body heat and result in a low-grade fever.

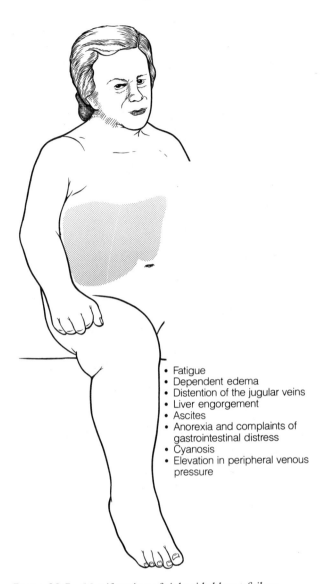

- Fatigue
- Dependent edema
- Distention of the jugular veins
- Liver engorgement
- Ascites
- Anorexia and complaints of gastrointestinal distress
- Cyanosis
- Elevation in peripheral venous pressure

Figure 20-3 *Manifestations of right-sided heart failure.*

■ Acute Pulmonary Edema

Acute pulmonary edema is a life-threatening condition. Although pulmonary edema is often associated with left heart failure, it can also result from increased permeability of the pulmonary capillary membrane, which in turn may be due to an infectious process, exposure to toxic gases, drug reactions, or other conditions. Hypervolemia due to rapid infusion of intravenous fluids or a blood transfusion in an elderly person or in a person with limited cardiac reserve may precipitate an episode of pulmonary edema. The following discussion centers on pulmonary edema due to heart failure.

With pulmonary edema due to left heart failure, the pulmonary capillary pressure rises severely. The rise can be measured using the Swan-Ganz catheter (see Chap.

18). This high level exceeds the osmotic pressure of the blood and results in transudation of fluid through the alveolar capillary walls into the alveoli and interstitial tissues. An episode of pulmonary edema usually happens at night when the person has been reclining for a period of time; gravitational forces are removed from the circulatory system, so that edema fluid that had been sequestered in the interstitial spaces in the lower extremities is returned to the vascular compartment and redistributed to the pulmonary circulation (as was discussed). Or an acute episode may be a complication of impaired cardiac pumping ability in myocardial infarction.

A person with pulmonary edema is usually seen sitting and gasping for air (Fig. 20-4). The apprehension is obvious. The pulse is rapid; the skin is moist and cool, and the lips and nail beds are cyanotic. As the lung edema worsens and oxygen supply to the brain falls off, confusion and stupor appear. Dyspnea and air hunger are accompanied by a cough productive of frothy and often

blood-tinged sputum—the effect of air mixing with the plasma and blood cells that have exuded into the alveoli. The movement of air through the alveolar fluid produces a fine crepitant sound, called *rales*, which can be heard through a stethoscope placed on the chest. As fluid moves into the larger airways, the breathing is louder. In the terminal stage it is called the *death rattle*. In severe pulmonary edema, persons literally drown in their own secretions.

In summary, congestive heart failure implies an accumulation of body fluids due to decreased cardiac function. In right-sided failure congestion of the systemic venous system occurs, and in left-sided failure pulmonary congestion occurs. Because the circulation forms a closed system, heart failure eventually affects both sides of the heart. Acute pulmonary edema represents a life-threatening accumulation of fluid in the lungs resulting from failure of the left ventricle.

■ Diagnosis and Treatment

As was stated earlier, heart failure is a manifestation of a number of heart diseases or other systemic pathologies. Diagnostic measures such as cardiac output, pulmonary capillary wedge pressure, and MUGA scans (described in Chap. 18) are used to identify the cause of heart failure and monitor the hemodynamic changes that occur during episodes of acute failure. The functional classification of the New York Heart Association is one guide to classifying the underlying problems (Table 20-2).

The treatment of heart failure is directed toward (1) correcting the cause, (2) improving cardiac function, (3) maintaining fluid volume within a compensatory range, and (4) arriving at an activity pattern consistent with individual limitations in cardiac reserve. It includes surgical treatment such as repair of a ventricular defect or replacement of a defective valve.

Medications Used in Treatment of Heart Failure

Medications such as digitalis preparations, diuretics, arterial and venous vasodilators, and angiotensin II enzyme inhibitors are prescribed. Digitalis is often prescribed to increase the heart's pumping efficiency. Restriction of salt intake and diuretic therapy facilitate the excretion of edema fluid. Counseling, health teaching, and other assistive measures help persons with heart failure to manage their activity patterns appropriately.

Digitalis

Digitalis has been a recognized treatment for congestive heart failure for the past 200 years. The various forms of digitalis are called *cardiac glycosides*. They improve cardiac

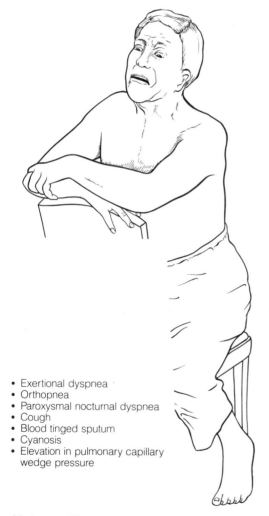

- Exertional dyspnea
- Orthopnea
- Paroxysmal nocturnal dyspnea
- Cough
- Blood tinged sputum
- Cyanosis
- Elevation in pulmonary capillary wedge pressure

Figure 20-4 *Manifestations of acute left-sided heart failure.*

Table 20-2   New York Heart Association Functional Classification of Patients with Heart Disease

Classification	Characteristics
Class I	Patients with cardiac disease but without the resulting limitations in physical activity. Ordinary activity does not cause undue fatigue, palpitation, dyspnea, or anginal pain.
Class II	Patients with heart disease resulting in slight limitations of physical activity. They are comfortable at rest. Ordinary physical activity results in fatigue, palpitation, dyspnea, or anginal pain.
Class III	Patients with cardiac disease resulting in marked limitation of physical activity. They are comfortable at rest. Less than ordinary physical activity causes fatigue, palpitation, dyspnea, or anginal pain.
Class IV	Patients with cardiac disease resulting in inability to carry on any physical activity without discomfort. The symptoms of cardiac insufficiency or of the anginal syndrome may be present even at rest. If any physical activity is undertaken, discomfort increases.

(From Criteria Committee of the New York Heart Association. Diseases of the Heart and Blood Vessels: Nomenclature and Criteria for Diagnosis. 6th ed, pp 112–113. Boston, Little, Brown, & Co. 1964)

function by increasing the force and strength of ventricular contraction. In addition, they slow the heart rate by decreasing SA node activity and decreasing conduction through the AV node, thus increasing diastolic filling time. These drugs cause a partial inhibition of the enzyme that activates the adenosine triphosphate (ATP) that supplies the energy for the operation of the sodium-potassium membrane pump. This causes decreased extrusion of calcium from cardiac cells following muscle contraction and results in increased availability of intracellular calcium for contractile processes and the development of muscle tension. Although not a diuretic, digitalis promotes urine output by improving renal blood flow. The margin between therapeutic and toxic doses of digitalis is very narrow. Low potassium levels predispose patients to digitalis toxicity, an important consideration in patients who are on digitalis since many of them are also taking diuretics, which promote potassium losses.

Digitalis toxicity can be described by its effect on three body systems—the heart, gastrointestinal tract, and central nervous system. The most serious effect is digitalis-induced arrhythmias. These arrhythmias can take many forms and can mimic most disturbances of cardiac rhythm. Anorexia, nausea, and vomiting are common gastrointestinal indications of toxicity. They may occur in patients receiving parenteral digitalis,

which suggests that they are a result of disturbances in the central nervous system rather than direct irritation of the gastrointestinal tract. Psychic and visual problems are signs of toxicity to the central nervous system. Some patients have described the visual disturbance as "looking through yellow-green glasses." A recent advance in laboratory methods allows the monitoring of serum digitalis levels.

Diuretics

Diuretics promote the excretion of edema fluid, and in emergencies they are often administered intravenously. The diuretic furosemide (Lasix) appears to have a biphasic effect on pulmonary congestion. When given intravenously, it appears to produce venous dilatation almost immediately with increased venous pooling of blood and a decrease in venous return to the right heart. The decrease in venous tone that occurs when furosemide is administered intravenously precedes its diuretic action by about 30 to 60 minutes.[7]

Vasodilator drugs

Vasodilator drugs cause relaxation of smooth muscle. These drugs induce venous pooling of blood, relax the pulmonary arterial and venous vessels, and reduce resistance in the systemic arterial vessels. With pooling of blood in the peripheral veins, there is less blood available to the right heart for delivery to the pulmonary circulation. Relaxation of the pulmonary vessels diminishes the pressure in the pulmonary capillaries and allows fluid to be reabsorbed from the interstitium of the lung and from the alveoli. (The reader is referred to Chap. 26 for a discussion of edema formation.) With a decrease in the resistance of the systemic arterial vessels, there is less pressure against which the left heart must pump, and thus the work of the left ventricle is decreased. Table 20-3 lists some vasodilator drugs used to treat acute pulmonary edema. Note that some of them exert their major action on the arterial system, some on the venous system, and some on both the arterial and venous systems.

Table 20-3   Vasodilator Drugs Used in Pulmonary Edema

Drugs	Site of Action	
	Arteries	Veins
Hydralazine	X	
Phentolamine	X	
Nitrates		X
Nitroprusside	X	X
Prazosin	X	X
Trimethaphan	X	X
Hexamethonium	X	X

(From Giles D: Principles of vasodilator therapy in left ventricular congestive heart failure. Heart Lung 9, No. 2:274, 1980)

Angiotensin-converting enzyme inhibitors

In heart failure, renin activity is frequently elevated because of decreased renal blood. The net result is an increase in angiotensin II, which causes vasoconstriction and increased aldosterone production (Chap. 16). Both of these mechanisms increase the work load of the heart. Converting enzyme inhibitors (captopril or Capoten), which prevent the conversion of angiotensin I to angiotensin II, may be used in the treatment of heart failure.

Treatment of Acute Pulmonary Edema

Treatment is directed toward reducing the fluid volume in the pulmonary circulation. This can be accomplished by reducing the amount of blood that the right heart delivers to the lungs or by improving the work performance of the left heart.

A number of measures are available that decrease the blood volume in the pulmonary circulation; the seriousness of the pulmonary edema will determine which are to be used. One of the simplest measures to relieve orthopnea is to assume the seated position. For many persons, sitting up or standing is almost a reflex and may be sufficient to relieve the symptoms associated with mild accumulation of fluid.

Measures to *improve left heart performance* focus on (1) decreasing the preload by reducing the filling pressure of the left ventricle and (2) reducing the afterload against which the left heart must pump. This can be accomplished through the use of *vasodilator drugs, treatment of arrhythmias* that impair cardiac function, and improving the contractile properties of the left ventricle with digitalis. *Rapid digitalization* may be accomplished with intravenous digitalis.

Oxygen therapy affords oxygenation of the blood and helps relieve anxiety. *Positive-pressure breathing* increases the intra-alveolar pressure that opposes the capillary filtration pressure in the pulmonary capillaries and is a temporary measure to decrease the amount of fluid moving into the alveoli.

Although its mechanisms of action are unclear, *morphine sulfate* is usually a drug of choice in acute pulmonary edema. Morphine relieves anxiety and depresses the pulmonary reflexes that cause spasm of the pulmonary vessels. It also increases venous pooling. Aminophylline is another drug, administered intravenously, that may be useful. It reduces bronchospasm, increases the glomerular filtration rate, and promotes urinary excretion of sodium and water. This drug relieves Cheyne-Stokes respirations, which sometimes occur in severe heart failure. Relief is due not to the theophylline itself, but to the ethylenediamine in which the theophylline is solubilized.

Another means of reducing pulmonary blood volume in severe life-threatening situations is venesection or alternating tourniquets. Fortunately, with modern pharmacologic treatments, there is less need for these treatment methods. Venesection consists of removing 300 ml to 500 ml of blood from the body. (It seems likely that the success of the barbershop surgeon with his bloodletting practices was due at least partly to the temporary relief of symptoms of pulmonary congestion.) Alternating tourniquets afford a means of trapping venous blood in the extremities. The tourniquets are inflated to levels between the arterial and venous pressures; this permits some inflow of arterial blood to the tissues while preventing outflow of venous blood to the heart. Four cuffs are used: one cuff is alternately deflated every 15 to 20 minutes so that venous flow from any one extremity is occluded only for a period of 45 to 60 minutes. Alternating tourniquets are an interim measure to be used while other forms of treatment are being initiated. Care must be taken when discontinuing the use of the tourniquets so that the heart is not suddenly confronted with an increase in venous return.

In summary, heart failure is the end result of a number of different types of heart disorders. Therefore, identification of the cause of heart failure is an important part of the treatment plan. Treatment is directed toward (1) correcting the cause whenever possible, (2) improving cardiac function, (3) maintaining the fluid volume within a compensatory level, and (4) developing an activity pattern that is consistent with individual limitations in cardiac reserve. Among the medications used in the treatment of heart failure are digitalis, diuretics, vasodilator drugs, and angiotensin II-converting enzyme inhibitors. Treatment of acute pulmonary edema is directed toward reducing the fluid volume in the pulmonary circulation. Emergency measures often focus on translocating the excess fluid from the pulmonary to the systemic circulations.

■ Study Guide

After you have studied this chapter, you should be able to meet the following objectives:

☐ Explain the effect of cardiac reserve on symptom development in heart failure.

☐ Explain how the compensatory mechanisms of increased sympathetic stimulation, fluid retention, and myocardial hypertrophy maintain cardiac reserve.

☐ Describe the effects of backward and forward failure on the circulation.

☐ Compare the hemodynamic and clinical manifestations of right-sided heart failure and left-sided heart failure.

☐ State why the presence of cyanosis is not a good indicator of hypoxia in persons with severe anemia.

☐ Use the Starling curve to explain the development of dyspnea in heart failure.

☐ Explain the mechanisms involved in paroxysmal nocturnal dyspnea.

☐ Describe the clinical picture of pulmonary edema.

☐ Describe the actions of digitalis and their effects on cardiac function.

☐ Explain the action of furosemide (Lasix) in relieving the signs and symptoms of acute pulmonary edema.

☐ Describe the action of vasodilating drugs in relieving the symptoms of heart failure and acute pulmonary edema.

☐ Relate the action of angiotensin II enzyme inhibitors to the improvement of cardiac function in persons with heart failure.

☐ Explain the rationale for placing a person with pulmonary edema in the seated position.

■ References

1. Gorlin R: Incidence, etiology, and prognosis of heart failure. Cardiovasc Rev Rep 6:765, 1983
2. Sidd JJ: Congestive heart failure. Orthop Clin North Am 9, No 3:744, 1978
3. Iseri LT, Benvenuti DJ: Pathogenesis and management of congestive heart failure—Revisited. Am Heart J 105:346, 1983
4. Chidsey CA, Harrison DC, Braunwald E: Augmentation of plasma norepinephrine response to exercise in patients with congestive heart failure. N Engl J Med 267:650, 1962
5. Chidsey CA, Braunwald E, Morrow AG: Catecholamine excretion and cardiac stores of norepinephrine in congestive heart failure. Am J Med 39:442, 1965
6. Braunwald E: The sympathetic nervous system in heart failure. Hosp Pract 5, No 12:31, 1970
7. Ditshit K et al: Renal and extrarenal effects of furosemide in congestive heart failure after acute myocardial infarction. N Engl J Med 288:1087, 1973

■ Additional References

Heart failure

Artman M, Graham TP: Congestive heart failure in infancy: Recognition and management. Am Heart J 103:1040, 1982

Atkins FL: New therapies in the management of congestive heart failure. J Kansas Med Soc 81(2):83-85, 1980

Bing RJ: The biochemical basis of myocardial failure. Hosp Pract 9:93, 1983

Blasco VV: Features of hepatic involvement in congestive heart failure. Cardiovasc Rev Rep 4:963, 1983

Brigham KL: Pulmonary edema: Cardiac and noncardiac. Am J Surg 138:361-367, 1979

Brigham KL: Lung vascular permeability and primary pulmonary edema. Western J Med 130(3):222-226, 1979

Bristow MR, Ginsburg R, Minobe W, Cubicciotti RS, Sageman WS, Lurie K, Billingham ME, Harrison DC, Stinson EB: Decreased catecholamine sensitivity and adrenergic-receptor density in failing human hearts. N Engl J Med 307:205, 1982

Cannon PJ: The kidney in heart failure. N Engl J Med 296:26, 1977

Carlet J, Francoual M, Lhoste F, Regnier B, Lemaire F: Pharmacological treatment of pulmonary edema. Intensive Care Med 6:113-122, 1980

Chatterjee K: Vasodilators and angiotensin-converting enzyme inhibitors in the treatment of heart failure. Cardiovasc Rev Rep 4:779, 1983

Dack S: Acute pulmonary edema. Hosp Med 14, No 3:112, 1978

DeSanctis RW, Atkinson AJ, Mullins CB: Congestive heart failure: Diagnosis and treatment today. Emerg Med 11:108-114+, 1979

Dickenson CJ, Marks J: Heart failure: Pathophysiological considerations. In Developments in Cardiovascular Medicine, pp 213-232 MTP Press, Lancaster, England, 1978

Hildner FJ: Pulmonary edema associated with low left ventricular filling pressures. Am J Cardiol 44:1410-1411, 1979

Jodice J: Management of acute pulmonary edema. J Emerg Nurs 4:19-22, 1978

Maskin CS, Le Jemtel TH, Kugler J, Sonnenblick EH: Inotropic therapy in the management of congestive heart failure. Cardiovasc Rev Rep 3:837, 1982

Recent developments in pulmonary edema. UCLA Conference reprinted in Ann Int Med 99:808, 1983

Ross J: The failing heart and the circulation. Hosp Pract 18:151, 1983

Segal BL: New approaches to therapy of acute heart failure. Am Fam Physician 21, No 2:131-135, 1980

Snashall PD: Pulmonary edema. Br J Dis Chest 74, No 2:2-22, 1980

Sochocky S: Pulmonary edema. Br J Clin Pract 33, No 5:127, 1979

Sonnenblick EH, Factor S, Le Jemtel TH: The rationale for inotrophic therapy in heart failure. Cardiovasc Rev Rep 4:910, 1983

Sparkes RS: The adrenergic nervous system in heart failure. N Engl J Med 311:850, 1984

Spooner B, Cross BW, Hasko BA: Diverse implications of laboratory values in congestive heart failure. Crit Care Quart 2:37-45, 1979

An update of congestive heart failure in infants. Issues Comp Pediatr Nurs 3:5-22, 1979

Weber KT, Janicki JS: The heart as a muscle-pump system and the concept of heart failure. Am Heart J 98, No 3:371-384, 1979

Willerson JT: What is wrong with the failing heart? N Engl J Med 307:243, 1982

Zak R: Cardiac hypertrophy: Biochemical and cellular relationships. Hosp Pract 18 No 3:85, 1983

Chapter 21

Circulatory Shock

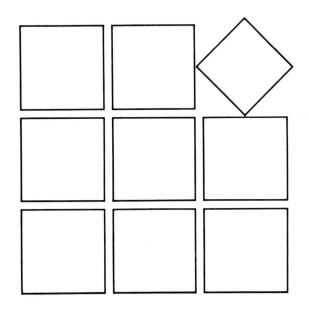

Circulatory shock is not a specific disease; it can occur in the course of many life-threatening traumatic or disease states. Shock can be due to trauma, blood loss, myocardial infarction, hypersensitivity reactions, or infections. Nor is shock a simple state of hypotension. Rather, circulatory shock implies a failure of the circulatory system. It has been defined as a clinical condition characterized by *"an inadequate blood flow to vital organs or the inability of the body cell mass to metabolize nutrients normally."*[1]

Although blood flow relies on blood pressure, the two are not synonymous. Blood flow relies not only on pressure, but on a vessel diameter that is large enough to facilitate flow and on sufficient blood to fill the vascular compartment. In shock, compensatory mechanisms that cause vasoconstriction often serve to maintain blood pressure while compromising blood flow.

In 1895 a Harvard surgeon published what has come to be recognized as the classic manifestations of irreversible shock.

> A patient is brought into the hospital with a compound comminuted fracture . . . , where the bleeding has been slight. As the litter is gently deposited on the floor he makes no effort to move or look about him. He lies staring at the surgeon with an expression of complete indifference as to his condition. There is no movement of the muscles of the face; the eyes, which are deeply sunken in their sockets, have a weird, uncanny look. The features are pinched and the face shrunken. A cold, clammy sweat exudes from the pores of the skin, which has an appearance of profound anaemia. The lips are bloodless and the fingers and nails are blue. The pulse is almost imperceptible;

a weak, threadlike stream may, however, be detected in the radial artery. The thermometer, placed in the rectum, registers 96° or 97°F. The muscles are not paralyzed anywhere, but the patient seems disinclined to make any muscular effort. Even respiratory movements seem for the time to be reduced to a minimum. Occasionally the patient may feebly throw about one of his limbs and give vent to a hoarse, weak groan. There is no insensibility . . . , but he is strangely apathetic, and seems to realize but imperfectly the full meaning of the questions put to him. There is no use to attempt an operation until appropriate remedies have brought about a reaction. The pulse, however, does not respond; it grows feebler and finally disappears, and "this momentary pause in the act of death" is soon followed by the grim reality. A post-mortem examination reveals no visible changes in the internal organs.[1]

■ Types of Shock

Adequate perfusion of body tissues depends on the pumping ability of the heart, a vascular circuit that transports blood to the cell and back to the heart, a sufficient amount of blood to fill the circulatory system, and tissues that are able to use and extract oxygen and nutrients from the blood delivered to the capillaries of the microcirculation. There are several ways to classify shock. For our purposes the following classification is useful: (1) hypovolemic, (2) cardiogenic, (3) peripheral pooling, and (4) septic shock. The four types of shock are summarized in Table 21-1.

Hypovolemic Shock

Hypovolemic shock occurs when there is an acute loss of 15% to 20% of the circulating blood volume. The decrease may be due to a loss of whole blood (hemorrhage), plasma (severe burns), or extracellular fluid (gastrointestinal fluids lost in vomiting or diarrhea). Hypovolemic shock can also occur with third-space losses, when extracellular fluid is trapped outside the vascular compartment. Often blood and fluid losses are concealed. One source cites the case of an elderly man who suffered severe crushing injuries of both legs. The patient had no external evidence of bleeding yet required 8 liters of blood over a period of 7 hours for stabilization of vital signs.[1]

Of the four types of shock, hypovolemic shock has been the most widely studied and usually serves as a prototype in discussions of the manifestations of shock. The severity and clinical findings associated with hypovolemic shock are summarized in Table 21-2.

The progression of hypovolemic shock can be divided into four stages. There is an *initial stage* during which the circulatory blood volume is decreased but not enough to cause serious effects. The second stage is the

---

Table 21-1   Classification of Shock

1. **Hypovolemic**
   Loss of whole blood
   Loss of plasma
   Loss of extracellular fluid
2. **Cardiogenic**
   Failure of the heart as a pump (myocardial damage)
   Severe alterations in rhythm (heart block or severe bradycardia)
   Inability to fill properly (cardiac tamponade)
   Obstruction to outflow (pulmonary embolus or thoracic aortic aneurysm)
3. **Peripheral Pooling**
   Loss of sympathetic vasomotor tone
   Presence of vasodilator substances in the blood (anaphylactic shock)
4. **Septic Shock**
   Vasodilatation
   Arteriovenous shunting
   Failure of body cells to utilize oxygen

(Based on data from MacLean LD: Shock: Causes and management of circulatory collapse. In Sabiston, DC (ed): Davis–Christopher Textbook of Surgery. 12th ed, p 67. Philadelphia, WB Saunders, 1981)

Table 21-2 Correlation of Clinical Findings and the Magnitude of Volume Deficit in Hemorrhagic Shock

Severity of Shock	Clinical Findings	Percent Reduction in Blood Volume* (ml in parentheses)
None	None; normal blood donation	Up to 10 (500 ml)†
Mild	Minimal tachycardia Slight decrease in blood pressure Mild evidence of peripheral vasoconstriction with cool hands and feet	15–25 (750–1250)
Moderate	Tachycardia, 100–120 bpm Decrease in pulse pressure Systolic pressure, 90–100 mm Hg Restlessness Increased sweating Pallor Oliguria	25–35 (1250–1750)
Severe	Tachycardia over 120 bpm Blood pressure below 60 mm Hg systolic and frequently unobtainable by cuff Mental stupor Extreme pallor, cold extremities Anuria	Up to 50 (2500)

*Blood volume changes based on the clinical observations of Beecher et al.
†Based on blood volume of 7% in a 70-kg male of medium build.
(From Weil M, Shubin H: Diagnosis and Treatment of Shock, p 118. Baltimore, Williams & Wilkins, 1967)

compensatory stage; although the circulating blood volume is reduced, compensatory mechanisms are able to maintain blood pressure and tissue perfusion at a level sufficient to prevent cell damage. The third stage is the *progressive stage* or *stage of decompensated shock.* At this point unfavorable signs begin to appear: the blood pressure begins to fall, blood flow to the heart and brain is impaired, capillary permeability is increased, fluid begins to leave the capillary, blood flow becomes sluggish, and the body cells and their enzyme systems are damaged. The fourth and final stage of shock is the *irreversible stage.* In irreversible shock, even though the blood volume may have been temporarily restored and vital signs stabilized, death ensues eventually. Although the factors that determine recovery from severe shock have not been clearly identified, it appears that they are related to blood flow at the level of the microcirculation.

Compensatory mechanisms

Three major compensatory mechanisms are activated in hypovolemic shock: (1) vasoconstrictor response, (2) shift of fluid from the interstitial to the intravascular compartment, and (3) increased pumping efficiency of the heart. The compensatory mechanisms in hypovolemic shock are summarized in Figure 21-1.

Within seconds after the onset of hemorrhage or the loss of blood volume signs of *sympathetic* and *adrenal medullary activity* appear. During the early stages, vasoconstriction causes a reduction in the size of the vascular compartment and an increase in peripheral vascular resistance. This response is usually all that is needed when the injury is slight, and blood loss is arrested at this point. Ten percent of a person's total volume of blood can be removed without significantly affecting blood pressure—the reader is reminded that the average blood donor loses a pint of blood without suffering adverse effects. Figure 21-2 shows how blood loss influences cardiac output and blood pressure. It can be seen that the changes in blood pressure lag behind the drop in cardiac output. This is due to the vasoconstriction and increase in heart rate that occur as blood leaves the circulatory system. It is also apparent that cardiac output and tissue blood flow will decrease before signs of hypotension occur.

As shock progresses, the heart rate and cardiac contractility increase and vasoconstriction becomes more

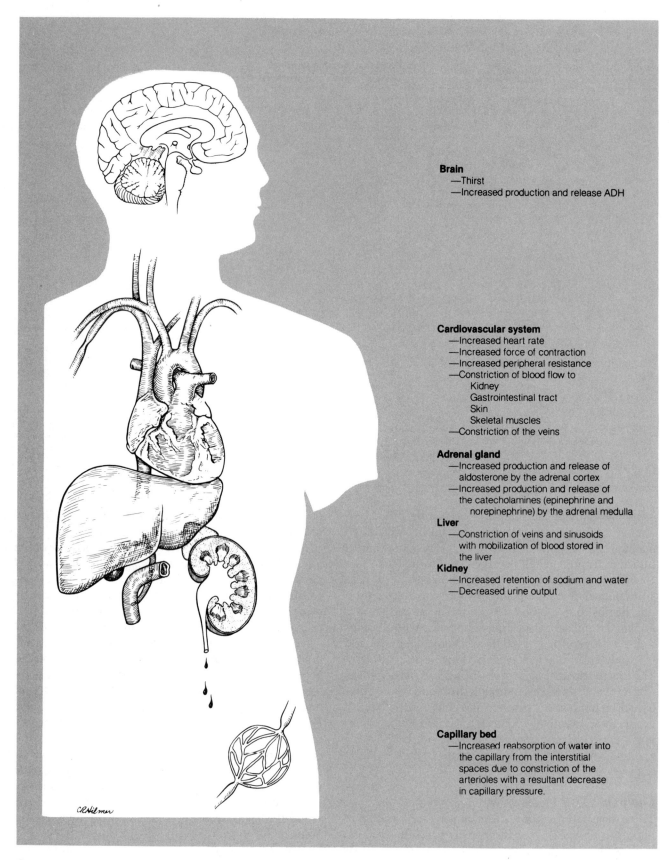

Brain
—Thirst
—Increased production and release ADH

Cardiovascular system
—Increased heart rate
—Increased force of contraction
—Increased peripheral resistance
—Constriction of blood flow to
    Kidney
    Gastrointestinal tract
    Skin
    Skeletal muscles
—Constriction of the veins

Adrenal gland
—Increased production and release of
    aldosterone by the adrenal cortex
—Increased production and release of
    the catecholamines (epinephrine and
        norepinephrine) by the adrenal medulla

Liver
—Constriction of veins and sinusoids
    with mobilization of blood stored in
    the liver

Kidney
—Increased retention of sodium and water
—Decreased urine output

Capillary bed
—Increased reabsorption of water into
    the capillary from the interstitial
    spaces due to constriction of the
    arterioles with a resultant decrease
    in capillary pressure.

Figure 21-1 *Conpensatory mechanisms in hypovolemic shock.*

intense. The blood flow to the skin, skeletal muscles, kidneys, and abdominal organs decreases. The sympathetic vasoconstrictor response affects both the arterioles and the veins. Arteriolar constriction helps to maintain blood pressure by increasing the total peripheral resistance, whereas venous constriction mobilizes blood that has been stored in the capacitance side of the circulation. There is considerable capacity for blood storage in the large veins of the abdomen and the liver. About 350 ml of blood that can be mobilized in shock is stored in the liver.

The compensatory changes in heart rate, cardiac contractility, and vascular tone developing in shock are mediated through the sympathetic nervous system. In the absence of sympathetic reflexes, only about 15% to 20% of the blood can be removed over a period of 30 minutes before death occurs, compared with the 30% to 40% that can be removed over a similar time period with intact sympathetic innervation.[2] Sympathetic stimulation does not cause constriction of the cerebral and coronary vessels, and blood flow through the heart and brain is maintained at essentially normal levels as long as the mean arterial pressure remains above 70 mm Hg.[2]

As has been stated, vasoconstriction causes a reduction in the size of the vascular compartment, so that it can be adequately filled by a smaller blood volume. Compensatory mechanisms designed to replace fluid lost from the vascular compartment also exist. During shock, a decline in capillary pressure causes water to be drawn into the vascular compartment from the interstitial spaces. The maintenance of vascular volume is further enhanced by renal mechanisms that conserve fluid. The previously described decrease in renal blood flow resulting from sympathetic vasoconstriction causes both a decrease in the glomerular filtration rate and an increase in the reabsorption of sodium and water, due to activation of the renin-angiotensin-aldosterone mechanism. The decrease in blood volume also stimulates the centers in the hypothalamus that regulate ADH and thirst; a decrease in blood volume of 10% is sufficient to activate both of these mechanisms.[3]

Cardiogenic Shock

Cardiogenic shock implies failure of the heart to adequately pump blood. It differs from hemorrhagic shock in that the cardiac output fails despite a normal or elevated blood volume and cardiac pressures. Cardiogenic shock can occur because of damage to the heart that occurs during myocardial infarction, ineffective pumping due to cardiac arrhythmias, obstruction of blood flow through the heart (cardiac tamponade), acute disruption of valvular function, or problems associated with open-heart surgery. In all of these cases there is a failure

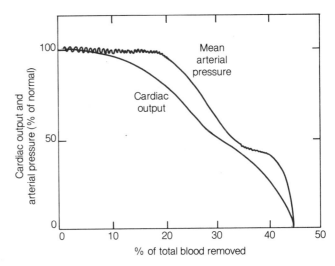

Figure 21-2 *Effect of hemorrhage on cardiac output and arterial pressure. (Guyton AC: Textbook of Medical Physiology, 6th ed. Philadelphia, WB Saunders, 1981)*

to eject blood from the heart, hypotension, and inadequate cardiac output. Often increased peripheral vascular resistance is present and contributes to the deterioration of cardiac function by increasing afterload.

The most common cause of cardiogenic shock is myocardial infarction. It develops in 15% to 20% of persons admitted to hospitals with a diagnosis of myocardial infarction, and its severity and progression appear to be related to the amount of myocardium that is involved.[3,4] Patients dying of cardiogenic shock generally have lost at least 40% of the contracting muscle of the left ventricle because of either a recent infarct or a combination of recent and old infarcts.

Cardiogenic shock can also follow other types of shock associated with inadequate coronary blood flow, or it can develop because substances released from ischemic tissues impair cardiac function. One such substance, myocardial toxic factor (MTF), is released into the circulation during severe shock. The MTF has a severe depressant effect on myocardial contractility, frequently reducing the cardiac contractile efficiency by as much as 50%. The MTF is thought to originate in the pancreas as the result of cellular ischemia in that organ.[2]

Treatment of cardiogenic shock requires a precarious balance between improving cardiac output, reducing the work load (and oxygen needs) of the myocardium, and preserving coronary perfusion. There is a need to regulate fluid volume within a level that maintains the filling pressure (venous return) of the heart and maximum utilization of the Frank–Starling mechanism without causing pulmonary congestion. Use of the Swan–Ganz balloon-tipped catheter has provided a means for monitoring the pulmonary capillary wedge or pulmonary artery end-diastolic pressure (Chap. 18). The catecholamines increase cardiac contractility but must be used with caution, because they also produce vaso-constriction and increase the afterload. The openings for the coronary arteries are located in the aorta just distal to the aortic valve. The major portion of coronary blood flow occurs during diastole and depends largely on aortic diastolic pressure. Unfortunately, an increase in aortic pressure needed to improve coronary perfusion pro-duces an increase in the afterload and myocardial oxygen consumption that may cause further myocardial ischemia and necrosis. The aortic balloon pump (to be discussed later) provides a means of increasing aortic diastolic pressure so as to maintain coronary and peripheral blood flow without increasing systolic pressure and the after-load, against which the left ventricle must pump.

Peripheral Pooling

With loss of blood vessel tone, the capacity of the vas-cular compartment expands to the extent that a normal volume of blood does not fill the circulatory system. Loss of vessel tone has two main causes: (1) a decrease in the sympathetic control of vasomotor tone and (2) the pres-ence of vasodilator substances in the blood. There is a decrease in venous return in peripheral pooling, which leads to a diminished cardiac output, but no decrease in the total blood volume; hence this type of shock is often referred to as *normovolemic shock.*

The term *neurogenic shock* describes shock due to decreased sympathetic control of blood vessel tone; there may be a defect in vasomotor center function in the brain stem or in the sympathetic outflow to the blood vessels. Output from the vasomotor center can be interrupted by brain injury, the depressant action of drugs, hypoxia, or lack of glucose (*e.g.,* insulin reaction). Fainting due to emotional causes is a transient form of neurogenic shock. General anesthetic agents can depress the vasomotor center, and spinal anesthesia or spinal cord injury can interrupt the transmission of outflow from the vaso-motor center. In contrast to hypovolemic shock, in neu-rogenic shock the heart rate is often slower than normal and the skin is dry and warm.

Vasodilator substances in the blood can produce massive vasodilatation with peripheral blood pooling. This in fact is what happens in *anaphylactic shock.* This type of shock is due to a hypersensitivity reaction in which histamine and histaminelike substances are released into the blood (Chap. 10). These substances cause dilatation of both arterioles and venules along with a marked increase in capillary permeability. The vascular response in anaphylactic shock is accompanied by the contraction of other nonvascular smooth muscle such as the bronchioles. Penicillin, shellfish, insect stings, animal sera, and plant pollens are antigens that are common causes of anaphylactic shock.

Anaphylactic shock is usually of sudden origin; death can occur within a matter of minutes unless appro-priate medical intervention is promptly instituted. Signs and symptoms associated with impending anaphylactic shock include abdominal cramps, apprehension, burn-ing and warm sensation of the skin, itching, urticaria (hives), coughing, choking, wheezing, tightness of the chest, and difficulty in breathing. Once blood begins to pool peripherally, there is a precipitous drop in blood pressure and the pulse becomes so weak that it is difficult to detect. Airway obstruction may ensue as a result of laryngeal edema.

Prevention of anaphylactic shock is always preferable to treatment. Once a patient has been sensitized to an anti-gen the risk of a fatal outcome always exists. All persons with known hypersensitivities should carry some form of warning to alert medical personnel should they become unconscious or unable to relate this information. Infor-mation about Medic Alert bracelets and tags is available through most pharmacies. Patients should be carefully questioned about any earlier drug reactions and should be told what medications they are to receive before the medications are administered. It is also recommended that persons being treated as outpatients remain in the facility for 30 minutes following any injection of medica-tion known to produce anaphylaxis, as most serious reactions occur within this period of time.

Unfortunately, it is not always possible to prevent anaphylactic shock. Therefore, all health care personnel should be aware of the characteristic signs and symptoms so that appropriate care can be instituted promptly. Epi-nephrine constricts the blood vessels and relaxes the smooth muscle in the bronchioles; it is usually the first drug to be given to a patient believed to be experiencing an anaphylactic reaction. Other treatment measures include the administration of oxygen, antihistamine drugs, and hydrocortisone. Resuscitation measures may be required. It is often helpful to institute measures to decrease absorption when the antigenic agent has been injected into the tissues. This can be accomplished by application of ice, which constricts the blood vessels. Measures to reduce absorption should not replace other treatment measures, but they may be particularly helpful in situations in which medical treatment is not immedi-ately available; for example, application of ice may delay the absorption of the antigen from a bee sting so that there is time to secure medical attention.

Septic Shock

Only in the past 30 years has septic shock come to be recognized as a clinical entity. Its incidence has increased in recent years. At present it has a mortality rate of about

50%. Septic shock is most frequently associated with gram-negative bacteremia, although it can be caused by gram-positive bacilli and other microorganisms.[5]

Unlike other types of shock, septic shock is often associated with pathologic complications such as pulmonary insufficiency (shock lung) and disseminated intravascular clotting (DIC). Septic shock often presents with fever, vasodilatation, and warm, flushed skin. Mild hyperventilation, respiratory alkalosis, and abrupt alterations in personality and inappropriate behavior (due to reduction in cerebral blood flow) may be the earliest signs of septic shock. These signs, which are thought to be a primary response to the bacteremia, often precede the usual signs and symptoms of sepsis by several hours or days.

Two major predisposing factors are involved in the development of septic shock: access to the vascular compartment by an infectious agent and a susceptible host. The elderly and those with extensive trauma and burns, neoplastic disease, and diabetes are particularly susceptible to infection and the development of septic shock. Another cause is the presence of an indwelling urinary or intravenous catheter. It has been proposed that the rising incidence of septic shock is related to (1) the widespread use of antibiotics, with development of a reservoir of virulent and resistant organisms; (2) concentration in hospitals of larger numbers of infections; (3) more extensive operations on elderly and high-risk patients; (4) an increase in the number of patients suffering from severe trauma; and (5) use of steroids and immunosuppressant and anticancer drugs.[6]

There appear to be two basic hemodynamic patterns associated with septic shock, dependent on the patient's vascular volume at the onset of shock.[1] The first pattern is a hyperdynamic circulatory response in patients with a normal blood volume at the onset of sepsis. These patients have a high cardiac output, normal or increased central venous pressure, increased pulse pressure, and warm and flushed skin. This response is seen most frequently in young healthy persons, for example, young women who have had a septic abortion. The second response pattern is seen in patients who have a decreased blood volume at the onset of sepsis. They present with a low cardiac output, low central venous pressure, and cold, cyanotic extremities.

The causes of septic shock are unclear. There is evidence suggesting that sepsis causes a cellular defect that inhibits oxygen utilization and occurs before hemodynamic changes such as hypotension occur.[1] In this situation, a hyperdynamic circulatory response is probably a compensatory mechanism to increase the blood flow and oxygen supply to the deficient cells. Another possibility is that toxins from the sepsis-producing organisms incite an immune reaction, which leads to

changes in the vascular tone and permeability. In experimental animals, shock may be induced by the injection of purified endotoxin, which has a protein lipopolysaccharide composition.[7] The polysaccharide component of the endotoxin produces a complement-consuming anaphylaxislike reaction during which vasoactive substances such as histamine and serotonin are liberated. Whether or not the reactions to endotoxins seen in animals hold true for humans is at present a subject of controversy.

It seems probable that various organisms may produce septic shock through different mechanisms; this would account for the different hemodynamic responses seen in hyperdynamic, or warm, septic shock and those seen in hypodynamic, or cold, septic shock.

Toxic shock syndrome

In recent years toxic shock syndrome has become recognized as a life-threatening event. It is characterized by extreme hypotension, high fever, headache, dizziness, myalgia, confusion, skin rash, conjunctivitis, sore throat, vomiting, and watery diarrhea. Desquamation (peeling) of the skin on the hands and feet frequently occurs during convalescence.

Although some cases of toxic shock syndrome have been reported in men and children, by far the greatest number of cases occur in menstruating women. In one study of 37 cases reported during a 5-year period in Wisconsin, 35 occurred in menstruating women, and at least 10 of these women had one recurrent episode during subsequent menstrual periods.[8] The majority of these women were tampon users. *Staphylococcus aureus* was the organism most frequently cultured from the cervix and vagina.[9] Onset of menstrual toxic shock syndrome occurs 1 to 11 days after vaginal bleeding begins, the median interval being 2 days.[10] Nonmenstrual toxic shock syndrome has been associated with surgical infections; nonsurgical infections of the skin, subcutaneous, or osseous tissues; and childbirth or abortion.

Although the pathogenesis of toxic shock syndrome is not fully understood, several contributing factors have been postulated.[9] The acute febrile illness, which is similar to endotoxic shock, suggests a toxin-mediated process. Toxins produced by *Staphylococcus aureus* are known to produce fever, hypotension, and death in laboratory animals. It seems possible that toxin-producing staphylococci previously colonized in nasal passages or on the skin could be introduced into the vagina by way of the fingers or tampon applicator. Since the menstrual flow is a good medium for bacterial growth, multiplication of the bacteria occurs, with production of large quantities of the toxin. The toxin then diffuses from the hyperemic vaginal mucosa into the circulation, triggering complement, coagulation, kallikrein, and prostaglandin mechanisms that act in concert to produce the hypotension and other manifestations of toxic shock syndrome. The skin rash characteristic of the disorder may represent a hypersensitivity reaction to the toxin.

In summary, shock is an acute emergency situation in which body tissues are either deprived of oxygen or cellular nutrients or are unable to use these materials in their metabolic processes. Shock may develop because there is not enough blood in the circulatory system (hypovolemic shock), because the heart fails as a pump (cardiogenic shock), because blood is pooled in the periphery (vasogenic or neurogenic shock), or because the tissues are unable to utilize oxygen and nutrients (septic shock).

■ Manifestations

Pathophysiologic Changes

The compensatory mechanisms that the body recruits in shock are not intended for long-term use. When injury is severe or its effects are prolonged, the compensatory mechanisms begin to have detrimental effects. The intense vasoconstriction causes a decrease in tissue perfusion, impaired cellular metabolism, liberation of lactic acid, and cell death. Once circulatory function has been reestablished at the onset of shock, whether the shock will be irreversible or the patient will survive is determined largely at the cellular level.

Flow in the microcirculation

Delivery of oxygen and nutrients to body cells and removal of metabolic waste products depend on adequate blood flow throughout the capillaries of the microcirculation. There are two types of capillary flow—*nutrient flow* and *nonnutrient flow* (see Chap. 14, Fig. 14-11). Nutrient flow describes flow in the true capillary pathways that supply cells with oxygen and nutrients. In nonnutrient flow, blood is shunted directly from the arterial to the venous side of the circulation without passing through the true capillary pathways. Nonnutrient flow provides warmth, but not oxygen and nutrients, to the tissues. In septic shock, nonnutrient flow is increased and the skin is warm and flushed. On the other hand, both nutrient and nonnutrient flow are decreased in hypovolemic shock and the skin is cool and clammy.

In severe and prolonged shock, the vascular system fails. When this occurs, there is relaxation of the arterioles and venules, a fall in arterial pressure, and

venous pooling of blood. At the capillary level, hypoxia and products of cell deterioration cause increased capillary permeability, stagnation of blood flow, and the formation of small blood clots.

Cellular changes

At the cellular level, oxygen and nutrients supply the energy needed to maintain cellular function. Within the cell, oxygen and fuel substrates are converted to adenosine triphosphate (ATP), the cell's energy source. The cell uses ATP for a number of purposes including protein synthesis and operation of the sodium and potassium membrane pump that extrudes sodium from the cell while returning potassium to its interior.

The cell uses two pathways to convert nutrients to energy (Chap. 1). The first is the *anaerobic* (nonoxygen) *glycolytic* pathway, which is located in the cytoplasm. Glycolysis converts glucose to pyruvate. The second pathway is the *aerobic citric acid cycle* (Krebs cycle), which is located in the mitochondria. When oxygen is available, pyruvate from the glycolytic pathway moves into the mitochondria and enters the citric acid cycle where it is transformed into ATP and metabolic byproducts (carbon dioxide and water). Breakdown products of fatty acids and proteins can also be metabolized in the mitochondrial pathway. When oxygen is lacking, pyruvate does not enter the citric acid cycle; instead, it is converted to ATP, and the byproduct is *lactic acid*. In severe shock, cellular metabolic processes are essentially anaerobic, which means that excess amounts of lactic acid accumulate in both the cellular and extracellular compartments.

The anaerobic pathway, while allowing energy production to continue in the absence of oxygen, is relatively inefficient—it produces only two ATP units, whereas the citric acid cycle produces 36 ATP units. Without sufficient energy production, normal cell function cannot be maintained (Fig. 21-3). The activity of the cell membrane pump is impaired—potassium leaves the cell and there is an influx of sodium and water. The cell swells and the membrane becomes more permeable. The mitochondria swell and the lysosomal membranes rupture. This is followed by cell death and the release of intracellular contents into the serum. Last, there is reason to believe that the release of lysosomal enzymes and their products (*e.g.*, MTF from pancreatic enzymes) and vasoactive peptides leads to changes in the microcirculation that adversely affect recovery from shock.

Signs and Symptoms

The signs and symptoms of shock are closely related to low peripheral blood flow and excessive sympathetic stimulation. For purposes of discussion, the manifestations of shock have been divided into the following

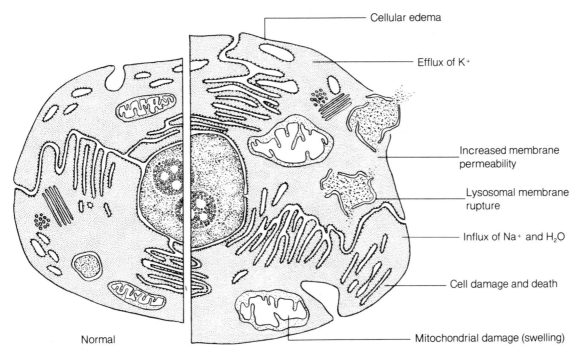

Figure 21-3 Cellular effects of shock.

categories: (1) thirst, (2) skin and body temperature changes, (3) arterial and venous pressure, (4) pulse, (5) urine output, and (6) changes in sensorium.

Thirst

Thirst is an early symptom in hypovolemic shock, easily overlooked in situations in which concealed bleeding occurs. Explanations regarding the causes of thirst are many, although the underlying cause is probably related to decreased blood volume and increased osmolarity (Chap. 25). Patients with trauma frequently have a decreased renal blood flow, due to an intense adrenal medullary response, along with an increase in ADH levels, which causes water retention. Water should, therefore, be given cautiously because water intoxication can occur in a patient who continues to drink water in the face of altered renal function.

Skin and body temperature

The skin reflects the existence of two different peripheral responses to shock. In one, sympathetic stimulation leads to intense vasoconstriction of the skin vessels with activation of the sweat glands—the skin is cool and moist. In the other, there is vasodilatation—the skin is warm and flushed. The former can be observed in hypovolemic and cardiogenic shock, the latter in hyperdynamic septic shock. In cardiogenic shock, the lips, nail beds, and skin are cyanotic because of stagnation of blood flow and increased extraction of oxygen from the hemoglobin as it passes through the capillary bed. In hemorrhagic shock the loss of red blood cells leaves the skin and mucous membranes pale.

The decrease in body temperature, often observed in shock, reflects a decrease in the body's metabolic rate. There is a reported correlation between the temperature in the great toe (great toe temperature minus environmental temperature) and the survival rate in shock, in that patients who had increases in toe temperature during dopamine treatment for shock had the highest survival rate. These differences were not accounted for by a simultaneous increase in rectal temperature and were therefore thought to reflect differences in peripheral blood flow to the distal extremities.[11] In septic shock, body temperature may be elevated because of infection and the skin may be warm because of nonnutrient shunting of blood flow in the capillary beds of the skin and peripheral tissues.

Pressures and pulses

There has been considerable controversy over the value of blood pressure measurements in the diagnosis and management of shock. This is because compensatory mechanisms tend to preserve blood pressure until shock is relatively far advanced. Furthermore, an adequate arterial pressure does not ensure the adequate perfusion of vital structures such as the liver and kidneys. This is not to imply that blood pressure should not be measured in patients at risk for developing shock, but it does indicate the need for other assessment measures by which shock may be detected at an earlier stage.

In shock, blood pressure is often measured intra-arterially, as the sphygmomanometer may not always provide an accurate means; systolic pressures measured by the cuff method are consistently lower than those measured intra-arterially. This is because, in shock, the increased vascular resistance in the upper extremities prevents the hemodynamic events that normally produce Korotkoff sounds. Thus, the first tapping sounds detectable with the stethoscope will be heard at a pressure considerably lower than that measured from the artery. The *Doppler method*, in which blood pressure is measured noninvasively by ultrasound, often provides a more accurate estimate of Korotkoff sounds when they are no longer audible through the stethoscope. In some instances, this method may be used as an alternative to continuous intra-arterial monitoring.

An increase in heart rate is often an early sign of shock. Like vasoconstriction, the tachycardia of early shock is a sign of sympathetic nervous system response to injury. Tachycardia may also reflect emotional aspects surrounding the injury or the pain associated with the trauma. Blood volume and vessel tone are reflected in the quality of the pulse. A weak and thready pulse indicates vasoconstriction and a reduction in filling of the vascular compartment.

Urine output

Urine output decreases in the initial stages of shock, as was discussed earlier. Compensatory mechanisms decrease renal blood flow as a means of diverting blood flow to the heart and brain. Oliguria of 20 ml/hour or less is indicative of severe shock and inadequate renal perfusion. Continuous measurement of urine output is essential for assessing the circulatory status of the patient in shock.

Sensorium

Restlessness and apprehension are common behaviors in early hypovolemic shock. As the shock progresses and blood flow to the brain decreases, the restlessness of an earlier stage is replaced by apathy and stupor. During this latter stage, there is no longer an expression of concern about the outcome of the injury, and complaints of pain and discomfort cease. If shock is unchecked, the apathy will progress to coma. Coma due to blood loss alone and not related to head injury or other factors is usually an unfavorable sign; it usually means that the patient has sustained a lethal blood loss.[5]

In summary, the manifestations of shock are related to a low peripheral blood flow and excessive sympathetic stimulation. The low peripheral blood flow produces (1) thirst, (2) changes in skin temperature, (3) a fall in blood pressure and an increase in heart rate, (4) changes in venous pressure, (5) decreased urine output, and (6) changes in the sensorium. Signs and symptoms such as changes in skin temperature (increased in septic shock and decreased in hypovolemic and other forms of shock)

may differ with the type of shock. The intense vasoconstriction that serves to maintain blood flow to the heart and brain causes a decrease in tissue perfusion, impaired cellular metabolism, liberation of lactic acid, and eventual cell death. Once circulatory function has been reestablished at the onset of shock, whether the shock will be irreversible or the patient will survive is determined largely by changes that occur at the cellular level.

■ Complications of Shock

Wiggers, a noted circulatory physiologist, has aptly stated, "Shock not only stops the machine, but it wrecks the machinery."[12] Indeed, many body systems are wrecked by severe shock. Four major complications of severe shock are (1) shock lung, (2) acute renal failure, (3) gastrointestinal ulceration, and (4) disseminated intravascular clotting. Thus, the complications of shock are serious, often fatal.

Shock Lung

Shock lung or *adult respiratory distress syndrome* (ARDS) is a potentially lethal form of respiratory failure that can follow severe shock (Chap. 24). The term *shock lung* was introduced during the Vietnam War to describe the progressive pulmonary failure seen in soldiers who suffered major trauma. The symptoms do not usually develop until 24 to 48 hours after the initial trauma, in some instances later. ARDS is thought to result from increased permeability of the pulmonary capillaries to water and plasma proteins. Protein-rich fluids leak into the alveolar and interstitial spaces, impairing gas exchange and making the lung stiffer and more difficult to inflate. Some patients develop a hyaline membrane similar to that seen in respiratory distress syndrome in the newborn. The respiratory rate and effort of breathing increase. Arterial blood gases establish the presence of profound hypoxemia with hypercarbia, resulting from impaired matching of ventilation and perfusion and from the greatly reduced diffusion of blood gases across the thickened alveolar membranes.

The exact cause of ARDS is unknown. It has been suggested that the problem results from (1) a decrease in lung perfusion and ischemia of the type II alveolar cells, which produce surfactant, (2) oxygen toxicity, (3) neurogenic factors that cause pulmonary venoconstriction and pulmonary edema due to sympathetic nervous factors, (4) fluid overload with stretching and disruption of the pulmonary capillaries, or (5) damage to the lung by endotoxins and substances released as the result of sepsis. One widely accepted cause of ARDS is disseminated intravascular clotting—the presence of thromboemboli in the pulmonary microcirculation. It is possible that multiple mechanisms operate to cause a similar pattern of injury or to trigger a common response (*e.g.,* intravascular clotting), which, in turn, produces the pulmonary damage.

Acute Renal Failure

The renal tubules are particularly vulnerable to ischemia, and *renal failure* is one important late cause of death in severe shock. In fact, sepsis and trauma account for the majority of cases of acute renal failure. The endotoxins that are implicated in septic shock are powerful vasoconstrictors, capable of activating the sympathetic nervous system and causing intravascular clotting. They have been shown to trigger all of the separate physiologic mechanisms that contribute to the onset of acute renal failure. The degree of renal damage is related to the severity and duration of shock; the normal kidney is able to tolerate severe ischemia for a period of 15 to 20 minutes. The renal lesion most frequently seen after severe shock is *acute tubular necrosis*. Acute tubular necrosis is usually reversible, although return to normal renal function may require weeks or months (see Chap. 27 for further discussion). *Continuous monitoring of urine output during shock provides a means of assessing renal blood flow.*

Gastrointestinal Ulceration

The gastrointestinal tract is particularly vulnerable to ischemia because of the circulatory pattern of its mucosal surface. In shock there is widespread constriction of blood vessels supplying the gastrointestinal tract; this causes a redistribution of blood flow such that mucosal perfusion is severely diminished. Superficial mucosal lesions of the stomach and duodenum can develop within hours of severe trauma, sepsis, or burn. (Stress ulcers associated with burns are called Curling's ulcers.) Bleeding is a common sign of gastrointestinal ulceration due to shock. Hemorrhage has its onset usually within 2 to 10 days following the original insult, and often it gives no warning.

Disseminated Intravascular Clotting (DIC)

Disseminated intravascular clotting, a complication of septic shock, is characterized by the formation of small clots in the microcirculation. Consumption and depletion of platelets, fibrinogen, and other clotting factors occur, leading to the disruption of the normal clotting process with abnormal bleeding or hemorrhage (see Chap. 12).

In summary, the complications of shock result from the deprivation of circulation to vital organs or systems such as the lungs, kidneys, gastrointestinal tract, and blood coagulation system. Shock lung or adult respiratory distress syndrome produces lung changes that occur with shock. It is characterized by changes in permeability of the alveolar-capillary membrane with the development of interstitial edema and severe hypoxia that does not respond to oxygen therapy. The renal tubules are particularly vulnerable to ischemia, and acute renal failure is an important complication of shock. Gastrointestinal bleeding occurs as a complication of gastrointestinal ischemia. Disseminated intravascular clotting is characterized by the formation of small clots in the circulation. It is thought to be caused by sluggish blood flow in the microcirculation or inappropriate activation of the coagulation cascade because of toxins or other products that are released as a result of the shock state.

■ Treatment Measures

The treatment of shock is directed toward *correcting* or *controlling the underlying cause* and *improving tissue perfusion.* This discussion presents an overview of commonly employed treatments.

In *hypovolemic shock,* the goal of treatment is to *restore vascular volume.* This can be accomplished through *intravenous administration of fluids and blood.* The plasma expanders (*dextrans* and *colloidal albumin solutions*) have a high molecular weight, do not necessitate blood typing, and remain in the circulation for longer periods of time than the crystalloids such as glucose and saline. The *dextrans must be used with caution, however, as they may induce serious or fatal reactions, including anaphylaxis.*

Circulatory Assistance

In *cardiogenic shock*, treatment measures are directed toward reducing the work of the heart while improving its pumping efficiency. An intra-aortic balloon pump may be used to supplement cardiac pumping in situations of severe cardiogenic shock. The balloon pump is inserted retrograde into the thoracic aorta through a peripheral artery. The balloon, filled with helium, is synchronized to inflate during diastole and deflate during systole. Diastolic inflation creates a diastolic pressure wave that results in increased perfusion to all the organs, including the myocardium. The sudden release of pressure at the onset of systole lowers resistance to ejection of blood from the left ventricle, thereby increasing the heart's pumping efficiency without increasing the afterload and myocardial oxygen consumption.

Vasoactive Drugs

Vasoactive drugs are agents capable of either constricting or dilating blood vessels. Currently, there is considerable controversy about the advantages or disadvantages related to use of these drugs. The major vasoactive drugs used to treat shock are summarized in Table 21-3.

There are two types of receptors for the sympathetic nervous system—alpha and beta. Beta receptors are further subdivided into beta-1 and beta-2. In the cardiorespiratory system, stimulation of the alpha receptors causes vasoconstriction; stimulation of beta-1 receptors causes an increase in heart rate and the force of myocardial contraction; and stimulation of beta-2 receptors produces vasodilatation of the skeletal muscle beds and relaxation of the bronchioles. Currently, dopamine is prescribed to treat shock because it induces a more favorable array of alpha and beta receptor actions than many of the adrenergic drugs. Dopamine is thought to increase blood flow to the kidneys, liver, and other abdominal organs while maintaining vasoconstriction of less vital structures such as the skin and skeletal muscles. *Nitroprusside* (Nipride), a vasodilator drug, is used to treat cardiogenic shock. It causes both arterial and venous dilatation, thus a decrease in venous return to the heart with a reduction in arterial resistance against which the left heart must pump. The arterial pressure is maintained by an increased ventricular stroke volume that is ejected against a lowered resistance; this allows blood to be redistributed from the pulmonary vascular bed to the systemic circulation.

In summary, the treatment of shock is dependent on the cause and type of shock that is present. It focuses on correcting or controlling the cause and improving tissue perfusion. In hypovolemic shock the goal of treatment is to restore vascular volume. In cardiogenic shock, treatment is directed toward reducing the work load of the heart while improving its pumping efficiency. Vasoactive drugs, capable of either constricting or dilating blood vessels, may be used.

■ Study Guide

After you have studied this chapter, you should be able to meet the following objectives:

☐ State a clinical definition of *shock*.

☐ List the chief characteristics of hypovolemic shock, cardiogenic shock, peripheral pooling, and septic shock.

☐ List and describe the four stages of hypovolemic shock.

☐ Trace the compensatory mechanisms that are activated in hypovolemic shock.

☐ State the basis of cardiogenic shock.

☐ State the rationale for the use of the vasodilator drugs and the intra-aortic balloon pump in cardiogenic shock.

Table 21-3 Vasoactive Drugs Used in Treatment of Shock

Drug	Mechanism	Action*
Epinephrine (Adrenalin)	Alpha	Vasoconstriciton (specific for anaphylactic shock)
	Beta 1 and 2	Increase in heart rate and cardiac contractility
		Causes a decrease in renal and splanchnic blood flow while increasing skeletal muscle flow
Norepinephrine (Levophed)	Alpha	Vasoconstriction
	Beta 1	Increase in heart rate and cardiac contractility
Isoproterenol (Isuprel)	Beta 1	Increase in heart rate and cardiac contractility
	Beta 2	Vasodilatation and perfusion of cerebral and renal tissue
Metaraminol (Aramine)	Alpha	Vasoconstriction
	Beta 1	Increase in heart rate and cardiac contractility
Dopamine (Intropin)	Alpha	Vasoconstriction with large doses
	Beta 1	Increased heart rate and cardiac contractility
	Dopaminergic	Vasodilatation of splanchnic and renal vessels
Dobutamine	Beta 1	Increases cardiac contractility with minimal increase in heart rate (specific in cardiogenic shock)
Nitroprusside (Nipride)	Dilator of venous and arterial smooth muscle	Decreases venous return to the heart causing a decrease in end-diastolic volume and pressure
		Decreases systemic vascular resistance with a resultant decrease in left ventricular stroke work (specific for cardiogenic shock)

*This list is not intended to be inclusive; it encompasses the drug actions related only to treatment of shock.

☐ State the common features of normovolemic shock, neurogenic shock, and anaphylactic shock.

☐ State a proposed mechanism for the development of toxic shock.

☐ List immediate treatment measures that health care professionals should take in anaphylactic shock.

☐ Differentiate nutrient flow from nonnutrient flow.

☐ Trace the conversion of oxygen and fuel substrates to ATP.

☐ State the physiologic basis of thirst in shock.

☐ State the manifestations of shock revealed in the skin and the body temperature.

☐ Describe the central problem involved in measuring blood pressure in shock.

☐ Describe changes in pulse rate, urinary output, and sensorium that are indicative of shock.

☐ Describe the pathology seen in shock lung.

☐ Describe the damage to the renal system and the gastrointestinal system associated with shock.

☐ State the rationale for treatment measures to correct and reverse shock.

■ References

1. MacLean FL: Shock: Causes and management of circulatory shock. In Sabiston DC (ed): Davis-Christopher's Textbook of Surgery, 12th ed, pp 58, 59, 62, 78. Philadelphia, WB Saunders, 1981

2. Guyton AC: Textbook of Medical Physiology, 6th ed, pp 333, 336, 441. Philadelphia, WB Saunders, 1981

3. Makabali C, Weil M, Henning RJ: An update on the therapy for shock: Current concepts in mechanisms and management of circulatory shock. Cardiovasc Rev Rep 3:899, 1982

4. Wilson RF: The pathophysiology of shock. Intensive Care Med 6:89, 1980

5. Shires TG, Canizaro PC, Carrico CJ et al: In Schwartz SI, Shires TG, Spencer FC et al (eds): Principles of Surgery, pp 176, 136. New York, McGraw-Hill, 1980

6. Altemeier WA, Todd JC, Inge WW: Gram-negative septicemia: A growing threat. Ann Surg 166:530, 1967

7. Weil M: Current understanding of mechanisms and treatment of circulatory shock caused by bacterial infection. Ann Clin Res 9:181, 1977

8. Davis JP, Chesney MD, Wand PJ et al: Toxic-shock syndrome. N Engl J Med 303:1429, 1980

9. Tofte RW, Williams DN: Toxic shock syndrome. Postgrad Med 73, No 1:175, 1983

10. Shands KN, Schmid GP, Bruce BD: Association of tampon use and staphylococcus aureus and clinical features in 52 cases. N Engl J Med 303:1436, 1980

11. Ruiz CE, Weil MH, Carlson RW: Treatment of circulatory shock with dopamine. JAMA 242, No 2:167, 1979

12. As cited in Smith JJ, Kampine JP: Circulatory Physiology, p 298. Baltimore, Williams & Wilkins, 1980

■ Additional References

Chaudry IH: Cellular mechanisms in shock and ischemia and their correction. Am J Physiol 245:R117, 1983

Foster SB, Canty KA: Pump failure following myocardial infarction: An overview. Heart Lung 9, No 2:293, 1979

Ganem D: Toxic shock syndrome. Medical Staff Conference, University of California, San Francisco. West J Med 135:383, 1981

Gysler M: Toxic shock syndrome—A synopsis. Pediatr Clin North Am 28:422, 1981

Loegering DJ: Intravascular hemolysis and RES phagocytic and host defense functions. Circ Shock 10:383, 1983

McCaffree RD: Shock: How to recognize its early stages and what to do about it. Med Times 107, No 9:25, 1979

Mohr JA, Coussons T: Septic shock. Med Times 107, No 9:39, 1979

Pepine CJ, Nichols WW, Alexander JA: Guidelines to evaluation and management of shock. Hosp Med 15, No 3:88, 1979

Pinsky MR: Cause-specific management of shock. Postgrad Med 73:127, 1983

Rackley CE et al: Cardiogenic shock. Med Times 107, No 9:33, 1979

Rice V: The clinical continuum of septic shock. Crit Care Nurse 4:86, 1984

Schlievert PM, Shands KN, Dan BB, Schmid GP, Nishimura RD: Identification and characterization of an exotoxin from *Staphylococcus aureus* associated with toxic-shock syndrome. J Infect Dis 143:509, 1981

Whitsett TL: Medical management of shock: Drugs of choice and their choice. Med Times 107, No 9:59, 1979

Wilson RF: The diagnosis and management of severe sepsis and septic shock. Heart Lung 5, No 3:422, 1976

Wilson RF: The pathophysiology of shock. Intensive Care Med 6:89, 1980

Zamora B: Management of hemorrhagic shock. Hosp Med 15, No 7:6, 1979

Chapter 22

Control of Respiratory Function

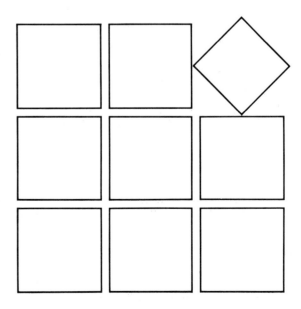

Respiration provides the body with a means for gas exchange. Respiration includes gas exchange at the cellular level (internal respiration), as well as the exchange of gases between the internal and external environments (external respiration). Respiration can be divided into three parts: (1) ventilation; (2) perfusion, or flow of blood in the pulmonary circulation; and (3) diffusion of gases between the alveoli and the blood in the pulmonary circulation. The discussion in this chapter focuses on the structure and function of the respiratory system as it relates to these three aspects of respiration. Included in the chapter is a discussion of breathing, breathing assessment, and coughing which is needed for an understanding of the content in subsequent chapters.

Structural Organization of the Respiratory System

The respiratory system consists of the airways (nasal passages, mouth, nasopharynx, larynx, and trachea), the lungs, and the chest cage. The chest cage is a closed compartment, bounded at the top by the neck muscles and at the bottom by the diaphragm. The outer walls of the chest cage are formed by the 12 pairs of ribs, the sternum, the thoracic vertebrae, and the intercostal muscles that lie between the ribs. The inside of the chest cage is called the *thoracic,* or *chest, cavity.* The lungs are cone-shaped organs located side by side in the thoracic cavity (Fig. 22-1). They are separated from each other by the

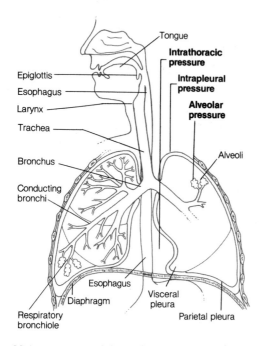

Figure 22-1 *Structures of the respiratory system and respiratory pressures.*

mediastinum (the space between the lungs) and its contents (the heart, great vessels, esophagus, thymus, lymph nodes, and the vagus, cardiac, and phrenic nerves). The lungs lie free, invested in a transparent serous membrane called the *pleura,* except for attachments to the heart and trachea. The upper part of the lung, which lies against the top of the thoracic cavity, is called the *apex,* and the lower part, which lies against the diaphragm, is called the *base.* The right lung is divided into three lobes and the left lung into two lobes.

The respiratory system can be divided into two parts: the conducting airways and the respiratory tissues, where gas exchange takes place. The conducting portion of the respiratory tract consists of the nose, nasopharynx, larynx, trachea, bronchi, and bronchioles (Fig. 22-1). The true respiratory portion of the lung consists of the alveolar structures and the pulmonary capillaries.

Conducting Airways

The conducting airways are lined with a pseudostratified columnar epithelium, which contains serous glands, mucus-secreting goblet cells, and hairlike projections called cilia (Fig. 22-2). The mucus produced by these cells forms a blanketlike layer, the *mucociliary blanket,* which protects the respiratory system and entraps dust and other foreign particles as they move through the conducting airways. The cilia, which are in constant motion, move the mucous blanket with its entrapped particles escalator fashion toward the pharynx from where it is either expectorated or swallowed.

The function of the mucous escalator in clearing the lower airways and alveoli is optimal at normal oxygen levels and is impaired by hypoxia and hyperoxia. Clearance is stimulated by coughing and adrenergic bronchodilators such as epinephrine. It is impaired by drying, for example, by heated but unhumidified indoor air during winter. Cigarette smoking also slows down or paralyzes the mucociliary escalator.[1] This slowing allows the residue from tobacco smoke, dust, and other particles to accumulate in the lungs, decreasing the efficiency of this pulmonary defense mechanism. There is also evidence that smoking causes hyperplasia of the goblet cells, which results in an increase in respiratory tract secretions, and increases the susceptibility and incidence of respiratory infections in smokers, as opposed to nonsmokers. As is discussed in Chapter 23, these changes are thought to contribute to the development of chronic bronchitis and emphysema.

Nasal passages

The nose is the preferred airway for the entrance of air into the respiratory tract during normal breathing. As air passes through the nasal passages, it is filtered, warmed,

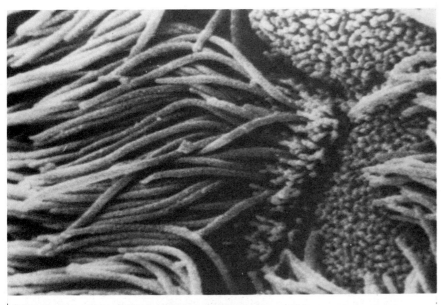

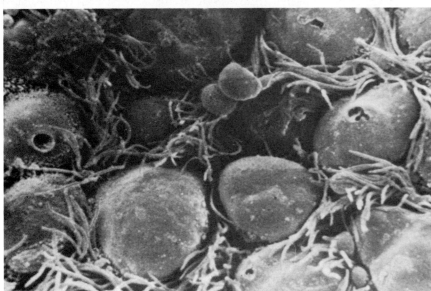

Figure 22-2 (Top) *Scanning electron micrograph showing cilia (longer projections) that are in constant motion, moving the mucociliary blanket upward in a conveyor-belt fashion toward the pharynx. The small, flat clusters are the microvilli, which transport fluid across the bronchial lining.* (Bottom) *Scanning electron micrograph of the small, round goblet cells that secrete mucus.* (Courtesy of Janice Nowell of the University of California, Santa Cruz, California)

and humidified. The outer part of the nasal passages is lined with coarse hair that aids in filtering dust and large particles from the air. The upper portion of the nasal cavity is lined with mucous membrane supplied with a rich network of small blood vessels, and it is this portion of the nasal cavity that supplies warmth and moisture to the air breathed.

The capacity of the air to contain water vapor without condensation occurring increases as the temperature rises. The *relative humidity* is the percentage of water vapor in the air at a specific temperature in relation to the maximum capacity of the air at that same temperature. The air in the alveoli, which is maintained at body temperature, is completely saturated with water vapor (rela-

tive humidity 100%) and usually contains considerably more water than is present in the air breathed. The difference between the water vapor contained in the air breathed and that found in the alveoli is drawn from the moist surface of the mucous membranes that line the respiratory passages and is a source of insensible water loss (Chap. 25). Under normal conditions, about a pint of water per day is lost in the process of humidifying the air breathed.[2] The amount of moisture required to humidify the air is increased when a person breathes dry air. It is also increased during fever due to the temperature-associated increase in water vapor pressure within the lungs. In addition, an increase in the respiratory rate usually accompanies fever, so that more air passes through the airways, withdrawing moisture from its mucosal surface. As water is removed from these secretions to humidify the air, the respiratory secretions often become thick preventing free movement of the cilia. Thus, the protective function of the mucociliary blanket may become impaired. This is particularly true of persons in whom the water intake is inadequate. With mouth breathing or breathing through a tracheotomy (opening in the throat), air entering the lungs is not warmed, filtered, or humidified as it would be when breathing through the nose. On the other hand, continuous airway ventilation (using humidified air) can lead to fluid overload by decreasing or eliminating the normal insensible water losses that occur with respiration.

Mouth and pharynx

The mouth serves as an alternative airway when the nasal passages are plugged or when there is need for the exchange of large amounts of air, such as occurs during exercise. The pharynx is the only opening between the nasal and mouth openings and the lungs. Consequently, obstruction of the pharynx leads to immediate cessation of ventilation. Neural control of the tongue and pharyngeal muscles is impaired in coma and in certain types of neurologic disease. In these conditions, the tongue tends to fall back into the pharynx and obstruct the airway, particularly if the person is lying on the back. Swelling of the pharyngeal structures due to injury or infection also predisposes a person to airway obstruction, as does the presence of a foreign body.

Larynx

The larynx connects the pharynx with the trachea. The epiglottis is a thin leaf-shaped structure that aids in covering the larynx during the act of swallowing to prevent food and fluids from entering the larynx and trachea. The walls of the larynx are supported by cartilaginous structures that prevent collapse during inspiration. The functions of the larynx can be divided into two categories: (1) those associated with speech and (2) those associated with protecting the lungs by preventing the entrance of substances other than air.

The larynx is located in a strategic position between the upper airways and the lungs, and is sometimes referred to as the watchdog of the lungs. When confronted with a substance other than air, the laryngeal muscles contract and close off the airway. At the same time, the cough reflex is initiated as a means of removing the foreign substance from the airway. Paralysis of the laryngeal muscles predisposes to aspiration of foreign materials into the lungs.

Tracheobronchial tree

The trachea, or windpipe, is a continuous tube that connects the larynx and the major bronchi of the lungs (Fig. 22-3). It is about 2.0 cm to 2.5 cm in diameter and about 10 cm to 12 cm in length. The walls of the trachea are supported by horseshoe-shaped cartilages that prevent it from collapsing during inspiration when the pressure in the thorax is negative.

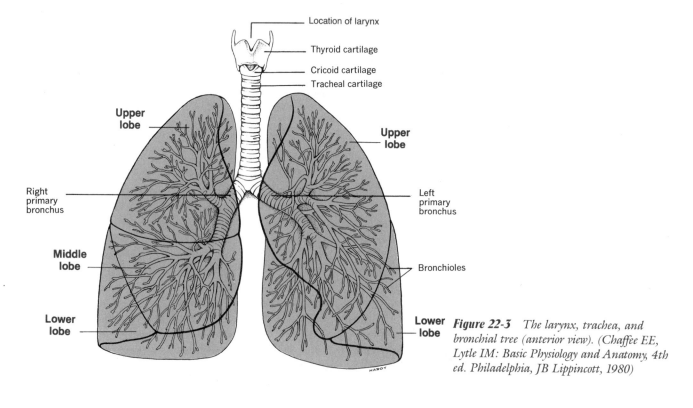

Figure 22-3 *The larynx, trachea, and bronchial tree (anterior view). (Chaffee EE, Lytle IM: Basic Physiology and Anatomy, 4th ed. Philadelphia, JB Lippincott, 1980)*

The trachea divides to form the right and left *primary* bronchi. Each bronchus enters the lung through a slit called the *hilus*. The point at which the trachea divides is called the *carina*. The carina is heavily innervated, and coughing and bronchospasm may result when this area is stimulated. The right primary bronchus is shorter and wider and continues at a more vertical angle with the trachea than the left primary bronchus, which is longer and narrower, and continues from the trachea at a more acute angle. This makes it easier for foreign bodies to enter the right main bronchus rather than the left. For this reason, when an endotracheal tube is inserted to maintain a patent airway and facilitate ventilation, it is essential to secure the tube properly. If the tube should slip into the right main bronchus, it would prevent air from entering the left lung, causing it to collapse (atelectasis).

Each primary bronchus divides into *secondary,* or *lobar, bronchi,* which supply each of the lobes of the lungs—*three in the right lung* and *two in the left.* The right middle lobe bronchus is of relatively small caliber and length and sometimes bends sharply near its bifurcation. It is surrounded by a collar of lymph nodes that drain both the middle and lower lobes and is particularly subject to obstruction, recurrent infection, and atelectasis. The secondary bronchi divide to form the segmental bronchi, which supply the bronchopulmonary segments of the lung. There are ten segments in the right lung and nine segments in the left lung. These segments are identified according to their location in the lung (*e.g.,* the apical segment of the right upper lobe) and are the smallest named units in the lung. Lung lesions such as atelectasis and pneumonia are often localized to a particular bronchopulmonary segment.

The bronchi continue to branch, forming *smaller bronchi,* until they become the *terminal bronchioles,* the smallest of the conducting airways. The structure of the primary bronchi is similar to that of the trachea in that both of these airways are supported by *cartilaginous rings.* As the bronchi become smaller, however, the cartilaginous support thins out until it disappears at the level of the bronchioles. Instead, the bronchioles are encircled with a *spiraling layer of smooth muscle fibers* (Fig. 22-4). Bronchospasm, or contraction, of these muscles causes narrowing of the bronchioles and impairs air flow.

Bronchial smooth muscle tone is controlled by the autonomic nervous system. Afferent fibers from receptors in the smooth muscle are carried in the vagus nerve to respiratory control centers in the brain stem. Activation of parasympathetic outflow to bronchial smooth muscle through vagal efferent fibers produces bronchoconstriction. Sympathetic stimulation produces relaxation of bronchial smooth muscle and is mediated by means of beta-adrenergic receptors (β_2). Studies have

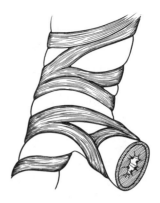

Figure 22-4 *Arrangement of smooth muscle fibers that surround the bronchioles.*

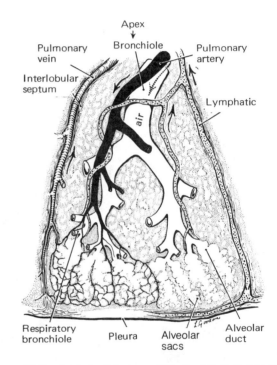

Figure 22-5 *A lobule of the lung. (Chaffee EE, Lytle IM: Basic Physiology and Anatomy, 4th ed. Philadelphia, JB Lippincott, 1980)*

shown that few, if any, sympathetic nerve fibers directly innervate the airways and release neuromediators.[3] The β receptors are stimulated by exogenous catecholamines or by epinephrine and norepinephrine that have been produced in the adrenal gland.

Respiratory Tissues

The lobules are the functional units of the lung where gas exchange takes place. Each lobule is supplied with structures that provide for both gas exchange and the circulation of blood (Fig. 22-5). The gas exchange structures consist of a bronchiole and the alveolar ducts and sacs. Blood enters the lobule through a pulmonary artery and then exits through a pulmonary vein. Lymphatic structures surround the lobule and aid in removal of plasma proteins and other particles from the interstitial spaces.

The alveolar sacs are cup-shaped, thin-walled structures separated from each other by thin alveolar septa. Most of the septa are occupied by a single network of capillaries, so that the blood is exposed to air on both sides. It has been estimated that there are about 300 million alveoli in an adult lung with a surface of about 50 m² to 100 m².[4] Unlike the bronchioles, which are tubes with their own separate walls, the alveoli are interconnecting spaces that have no separate walls (Fig. 22-6). As a result of this arrangement, the air between the alveolar structures mixes continually. Small discontinuities in the alveolar wall, the pores of Kohn, probably contribute to the mixing of air under certain conditions.

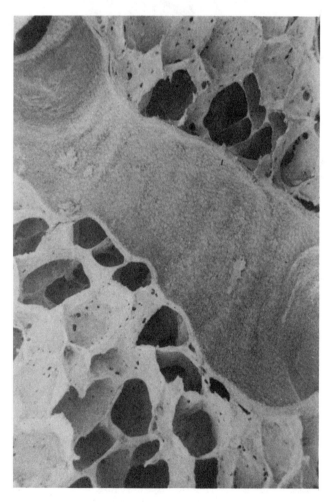

Figure 22-6 *A close-up of a cross section of a small bronchus and surrounding alveoli. (Courtesy of Janice A. Nowell of the University of California, Santa Cruz, California)*

The alveolar structures are composed of three types of cells—the alveolar macrophages, the type I alveolar cells, and the type II alveolar cells. The alveolar macrophages are responsible for the removal of offending matter from the alveolar epithelium. Available evidence suggests that smoking impairs the function of the macrophages. The type I alveolar cells are flat squamous epithelial cells, across which gas exchange takes place. The type II alveolar cells produce surfactant, a lipoprotein substance that decreases the surface tension within the alveoli. This action allows for greater ease of lung inflation and helps to prevent the collapse of the smaller airways (to be discussed later).

Pleura

A thin, transparent, double-layered serous membrane, called the pleura, lines the thoracic cavity and encases the lungs. The outer parietal layer lies adjacent to the chest wall, and the inner visceral layer adheres to the surface of the lung. A thin film of serous fluid separates the two pleural layers, and this allows the two layers to glide over each other and yet hold together, so that there is no separation between the lungs and the chest wall. This adherence is similar to what occurs when a glass of water is placed on a thin film of water that has been spilled on a table top. The pleural cavity is a potential space in which serous fluid or inflammatory exudate can accumulate. *Pleural effusion* is an abnormal collection of excess fluid or exudate in the pleural cavity.

The pressure within the pleural cavity is always negative in relation to alveolar pressure (about −4 mm Hg when the alveolar spaces are open to the atmosphere, *i.e.,* between breaths when the glottis is open). Both the lungs and the chest wall have elastic properties, each pulling in the opposite direction. If removed from the chest, the lungs would contract to a smaller size; and the chest wall, if freed from the lungs, would expand. The opposing forces of the chest wall and lungs create a pull against the visceral and parietal layers of the pleura, causing the pressure within the pleural cavity to become negative. During inspiration, the elastic recoil of the lung increases, causing intrapleural pressure to become more negative than during expiration. Without the negative intrapleural pressure holding the lungs against the chest wall, their elastic recoil properties would cause them to collapse. Collapse of the lungs due to air in the pleural cavity is called *pneumothorax*.

In summary, the function of the respiratory system is to oxygenate and remove carbon dioxide from the blood. The respiratory system can be divided into two parts: the conducting airways and the respiratory tissues where gas exchange takes place. The conducting airways include the nasal passages, mouth, nasopharynx, larynx, and tracheobronchial tree. The conducting airways are lined with pseudostratified columnar epithelium, which contains serous glands, goblet cells, and hairlike projections called cilia. The mucus produced by these cells forms the mucociliary blanket, which aids in removing dust and other foreign particles from the respiratory tract. The exchange of gases between the external environment and the blood takes place in the lobules of the lungs, which are supplied with gas exchange structures (bronchiole, alveolar duct, and alveolar sac) and capillary blood flow, which enters through a pulmonary artery and exits through a pulmonary vein. The pleura, which is a transparent double-layered membrane, invests the lungs. A thin layer of fluid separates the two layers of the pleura and allows them to adhere and slide effortlessly over each other. The opposing elastic forces of the lungs and chest wall pull on the pleura, creating a negative pressure within the pleural cavity. Without this negative pressure, which holds the lungs against the chest wall, the elastic properties of the lungs would cause them to collapse.

Exchange of Gases between the Atmosphere and the Alveoli

Respiratory Environment

There is nothing mystical about ventilation; it is a purely mechanical event that obeys the laws of physics as they relate to the behavior of gases. Some of these principles are summarized for the reader's review.

Atmospheric and respiratory pressures

At sea level, the atmospheric pressure is 760 mm Hg, or 14.7 pounds psi. In measuring respiratory pressure, atmospheric pressure is assigned a value of zero. A pressure of +15 mm Hg means that the pressure is 15 mm Hg above atmospheric pressure, and a pressure of −15 mm Hg is 15 mm Hg less than atmospheric.

Pressure–volume relationship

Boyle's law states that the pressure of a gas will vary inversely with the volume of the container, provided the temperature is kept constant. This means that if equal amounts of a gas are placed into two containers, one with a smaller volume than the other, the pressure of the gas in the container with the smaller volume will be greater than the pressure of the gas in that with the larger volume. The movement of gases is always from an area of greater pressure to one of lesser pressure. In the example just given, if a connection were placed between the two containers, air would move from the smaller volume to the larger volume.

Law of partial pressures

The pressure resulting from any particular gas is called the *partial pressure*, or *tension*. The capital letter P followed by the subscript for the chemical name of the gas (PO_2) is used to denote its partial pressure. The law of partial pressures states that the total pressure of a mixture of gases is equal to the sum of the partial pressures of the separate gases in the mixture. If the concentration of oxygen at 760 mm Hg is 20%, then its partial pressure is 152 mm Hg (760 × 0.20).

Water vapor pressure

The amount of water vapor contained in a gas mixture is determined by the temperature of the gas and is unrelated to atmospheric pressure. Air in the lungs is completely saturated (100% humidity) with water vapor. At a normal body temperature of 98.6°F, the pressure of water vapor in the lungs is 47 mm Hg. The water vapor pressure must be included in the sum of the total pressure of the gases in the alveoli (*i.e.*, the total pressure of other gases in the alveoli is 760 − 47 = 713 mm Hg).

Ventilation

Ventilation is concerned with the movement of gases into and out of the lung. It is dependent on a system of open airways and movement of the thoracic cage by the respiratory muscles—diaphragm, intercostals, and accessory muscles. The diaphragm is the principal muscle of inspiration. It is innervated by the phrenic nerve roots that arise from the cervical level of the spinal cord—mainly from C4, but also from C3 and C5. The intercostal muscles receive their innervation from the thoracic level of the spinal cord. When speaking of ventilation, the combined function of neuromuscular components and skeletal structures of the thoracic cage is often referred to as the *respiratory pump*.

Mechanics of breathing

During inspiration the volume of the thoracic cavity is increased and air moves into the chest. This increase in volume is brought about mainly by contraction of the diaphragm. When the diaphragm contracts, the abdominal contents are forced downward and the chest expands from top to bottom (Fig. 22-7). During normal levels of inspiration, the diaphragm moves about 1 cm, but this can be increased up to 10 cm on forced inspiration and expiration. Paralysis of the diaphragm causes it to move up rather than down during inspiration because of the negative pressure in the chest. This is called *paradoxical movement* and can be demonstrated on fluoroscopy when the patient sniffs.

The external intercostal muscles connect to the adjacent ribs and slope downward and forward. When they

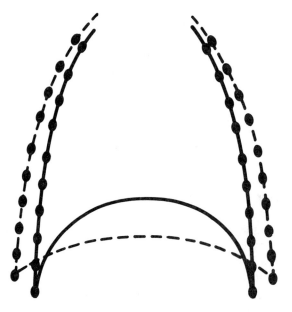

Figure 22-7 *Action of the diaphragm. The diaphragm is shown as a curved line across the bottom of the rib cage. At end-expiration, indicated by solid lines, the rib cage diameter is small and the dome of the diaphragm is sharply curved. As the diaphragm contracts, the dome descends and becomes flatter, while the lower border of the rib cage is simultaneously pushed upward and outward. (Guenter CA, Welch MH: Pulmonary Medicine, 2nd ed. Philadelphia, JB Lippincott, 1982)*

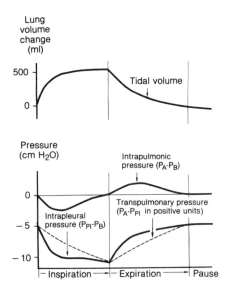

Figure 22-8 *Changes and interrelationships of lung volume, intrapulmonary pressure, intrapleural pressure, and transpulmonary pressure during a breathing cycle. (P_B = barometric pressure; P_A = alveolar pressure; P_{Pl} = pleural pressure.) (Slonin NB, Hamilton LH: Respiratory Physiology, 4th ed. St Louis, CV Mosby, 1981)*

contract, they raise the ribs and rotate them slightly so that the sternum is pushed forward; this enlarges the chest from side to side and from front to back. Paralysis of the intercostal nerves does not seriously affect respiration because of the effectiveness of the diaphragm.

The accessory muscles of inspiration include the scaline muscles, which elevate the first two ribs, and the sternocleidomastoid muscles, which raise the sternum. These muscles contribute little to quiet breathing but contract vigorously during exercise. Other muscles that play a minor role in inspiration are the alae nasi, which produce flaring of the nostrils during obstructed breathing.

During expiration, the elastic components of the chest wall and the lung structures that were stretched during inspiration recoil passively, causing lung volume to decrease so that the pressure within the lungs is greater than the atmospheric pressure; therefore, air moves out of the lungs. Normally, expiration is a passive event that contributes little to the work of breathing. Instead, energy is expended in the work of enlarging the chest during inspiration. When needed, the abdominal and internal intercostal muscles can be used to increase expiratory effort. The increase in intra-abdominal pressure that accompanies the forceful contraction of the abdominal muscles pushes the diaphragm upward and results in an increase in intrathoracic pressure. The internal intercostals move inward, pulling the chest downward, and are also used to increase expiratory effort.

Respiratory pressures. The pressure inside the airways and the alveoli of the lung is called the *intrapulmonary pressure*. The pressure within the alveoli can also be called the *alveolar pressure*. The gases within this area of the lung are in communication with atmospheric pressure. When the glottis is open and no air is moving into or out of the lungs (prior to inspiration or expiration) the intrapulmonary pressure is zero or equal to atmospheric pressure (atmospheric pressure − intrapulmonary pressure = 0). The pressure in the pleural cavity is called the *intrapleural pressure*. It is always less than, or negative in relation to, the intrapulmonary and atmospheric pressures. It is this negative pressure that overcomes the elastic recoil properties of the lungs and prevents the lungs from collapsing. The *intrathoracic* pressure is the pressure within the thoracic cavity. It is equal to intrapleural pressure and is the pressure to which the heart and great vessels are exposed. The locations of the different respiratory pressures are illustrated in Figure 22-1.

The intrapulmonary and intrapleural pressures change with ventilation (Fig. 22-8). They become negative as the chest enlarges during inspiration and positive as the chest becomes smaller during expiration. During inspiration there is a greater decrease in intrapleural pressure than in intrapulmonary pressure. The resultant increase in transpulmonary pressure (difference between airway and intrapleural pressure) pulls the airways open, facilitating the air flow. During expiration the reverse is true: there is a proportionately greater decrease in the airway pressure than in the intrapleural pressure; the transpulmonary pressure is less and the airways become smaller.

Lung volumes and capacities. The amount of air that is inhaled or exhaled from various lung volumes can be measured with a spirometer (Fig. 22-9). With the type of

spirometer depicted, the bell, which is inverted over a water bath, moves down during inspiration and up during expiration, causing the pen to move up and down and mark the chart paper.

Lung volumes can be subdivided into four components: tidal volume, inspiratory reserve volume, expiratory reserve volume, and residual volume. The *tidal volume* (TV), usually about 500 ml, is the amount of air that moves into and out of the lungs during normal breathing. The maximum amount of air that can be inspired in excess of the normal tidal volume is called the *inspiratory reserve volume* (IRV), and the maximum

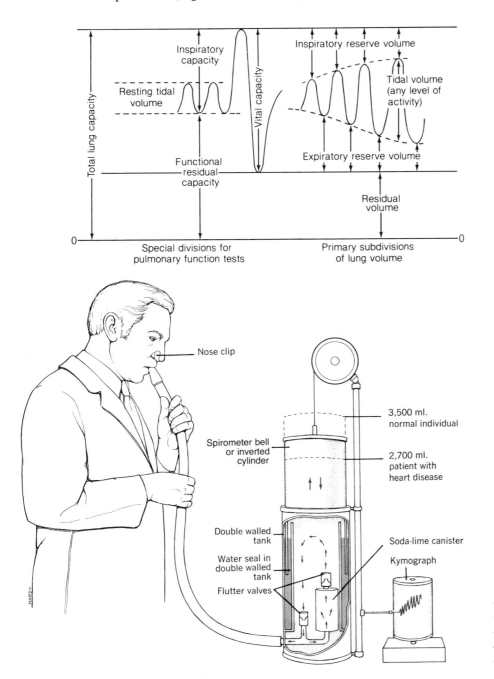

Figure 22-9 *Measurement of vital capacity using a spirometer. (Chaffee EE, Lytle IM: Basic Physiology and Anatomy, 4th ed. Philadelphia, JB Lippincott, 1980)*

amount that can be exhaled in excess of the normal tidal volume is the *expiratory reserve volume* (ERV). Some air always remains in the lungs following forced expiration—approximately 1200 ml; this air is the *residual volume* (RV). The residual volume tends to increase with age because more air is trapped in the lungs at the end of expiration.

Lung capacities include two or more components of the total lung volume. The *vital capacity* (VC) is a measure of respiratory reserve and is the amount of air that can be inhaled and forcibly exhaled in a single breath (usually about 4600 ml). The *inspiratory capacity* (IC) is the maximum volume of air that can be inspired after maximal expiration. The *functional residual capacity* (FRC) is the sum of the RV and ERV; it is the volume of air remaining in the lungs at the end-expiratory position.

The *total lung capacity* (TLC) is the sum of all the volumes in the lung. The residual volume cannot be measured with the spirometer because this air cannot be expressed from the lungs. The RV is measured by indirect methods such as the helium dilution method, the nitrogen washout method, or body plethysmography (see a respiratory physiology text for a description of these tests). Lung volumes and capacities are summarized in Table 22-1.

Pulmonary function studies. The previously mentioned lung volumes and capacities are anatomic or static lung volumes, measured without relation to time. The spirometer is also used to measure dynamic lung function (ventilation with respect to time); these tests are often used in assessing pulmonary function. Pulmonary function is measured for a variety of clinical purposes, including diagnosis of respiratory disease, preoperative surgical and anesthetic risk evaluation, and symptom and disability evaluation for legal or insurance purposes. The tests are often used in the evaluation of dyspnea, cough, wheezing, and abnormal x-ray or laboratory findings.

The *maximum voluntary ventilation (MVV)* measures the volume of air that a person can move into and out of the lungs during maximum effort lasting for 12 to 15 seconds. This measurement is usually converted to liters per minute. The *forced expiratory vital capacity (FVC)* involves full inspiration to total lung capacity followed by forceful maximal expiration. Obstruction of airways will produce an FVC that is lower than that observed with more slowly performed vital capacity measurements. The expired volume is plotted against time. The $FEV_{1.0}$ is the *forced expiratory volume* that can be exhaled in 1 second. Frequently, the $FEV_{1.0}$ is expressed as a percentage of the FVC. The $FEV_{1.0}$ and the FVC are used in the diagnosis of obstructive lung disorders. The *forced inspiratory vital flow (FIF)* measures the respiratory response during rapid maximal inspiration. Calculation of the airflow during the middle half of inspiration (FIF 25–75%) relative to the forced midexpiratory flow rate (FEF 25–75%) is used as a measure of respiratory muscle dysfunction, because the inspiratory flow is more dependent on effort than expiration. The pulmonary function tests are summarized in Table 22-2.

Table 22-1   Lung Volumes and Capacities

Volume	Symbol	Measurement
Tidal volume (about 500 ml at rest)	TV	Amount of air that moves into and out of the lungs with each breath
Inspiratory reserve volume (approximately 3000 ml)	IRV	Maximum amount of air that can be inhaled from the point of maximum expiration
Expiratory reserve volume (approximately 1100 ml)	ERV	Maximum volume of air that can be exhaled from the resting end-expiratory level
Residual volume (approximately 1200 ml)	RV	Volume of air remaining in the lungs after maximum expiration. This volume cannot be measured with the spirometer; it is measured indirectly using methods such as the helium dilution method, the nitrogen washout technique, or body plethysmography
Functional residual capacity (approximately 2300 ml)	FRC	Volume of air remaining in the lungs at end-expiration (sum of RV and ERV)
Inspiratory capacity (approximately 3500 ml)	IC	Sum of IRV and TV
Vital Capacity (approximately 4600 ml)	VC	Maximum amount of air that can be exhaled from the point of maximum inspiration
Total lung capacity (approximately 5800 ml)	TLC	Total amount of air that the lungs can hold; it is the sum of all the volume components after maximal inspiration. This value is about 20% to 25% less in females than in males.

Lung compliance

Lung compliance describes the ease with which the lungs can be inflated and is related to their elasticity. It is similar to blowing up a new and noncompliant balloon and one that is compliant from having been blown up before. Specifically, it refers to a change in lung volume that occurs with a given change in respiratory pressures.

$$\text{compliance} = \frac{\text{change in volume}}{\text{change in pressure}}$$

For example, it takes less negative pressure, and thus less inspiratory effort, to inflate a compliant lung than it does to inflate a stiff and noncompliant lung. Lung compliance is decreased in lung diseases such as interstitial lung disease and pulmonary fibrosis, which cause the lungs to become stiff and lose their elasticity. Pulmonary congestion and edema produce a reversible decrease in pulmonary compliance. Pulmonary compliance is increased in the elderly and in persons with emphysema, probably because of changes in elastic tissues. Although increased compliance would seem to be advantageous because the lung can be inflated more easily, this is not the case. Instead, increased compliance reduces the transpulmonary pressure that holds the airways open. Less change in intrapleural pressure is needed to inflate the lung, and as a result the difference between intrapleural and airway pressure is decreased. This tends to cause airway closure and the trapping of gases in the alveoli. Lung compliance can be evaluated by using lung volumes and esophageal pressures, which are used as a measurement for intrapleural pressure. Lung volumes are measured using the spirometer, and esophageal pressures are measured by passing a tube with a small balloon attached into the esophagus.

Surface tension

An important factor in lung inflation is the surface tension of the liquid film that lines the alveoli. It arises because the forces that hold the molecules of the liquid film together are much stronger than those between the liquid–gas interface; the result is that the liquid surface area tends to become as small as possible. The same behavior is seen in soap bubbles. The surface of the bubble contracts to form a sphere as the bubble is being blown. The pressure in the alveoli (which are modeled as spheres with open airways leading from them) can be predicted using Laplace's law (pressure = 2 × surface tension/radius). Thus, if the surface tension were equal throughout the lung, the alveoli with the smallest radii would have the greatest pressure, and this would cause them to empty into the larger alveoli. This does not occur, however, because of the surface-tension reducing properties of the surfactant molecules that line the inner surface of the alveoli.

The pulmonary surfactants are a group of phospholipids that are synthesized within the type II alveolar cells and secreted into the alveoli where they become part of the lining layer. The surfactant molecule has two ends:

Table 22-2 Pulmonary Function Tests[a]

Test	Symbol	Measurement
Maximal voluntary ventilation	MVV	Maximum amount of air that can be breathed in a given time
Forced vital capacity	FVC	Maximum amount of air that can be rapidly and forcefully exhaled from the lungs following full inspiration. The expired volume is plotted against time.
Forced expiratory volume achieved in 1 sec	$FEV_{1.0}$	Volume of air expired in the first second of FVC.
Percentage of forced vital capacity	$FEV_{1.0}/FVC\%$	Volume of air expired in the first second, expressed as a percentage of FVC.
Forced midexpiratory flow rate	FEF25–75%	The forced midexpiratory flow rate determined by locating the points on the volume–time curve recording obtained during FVC corresponding to 25% and 75% of FVC and drawing a straight line through these points. The slope of this line represents the average midexpiratory flow rate.
Forced inspiratory flow rate	FIF25–75%	FIF is volume inspired from RV at the point of measurement. FIF25–75% is the slope of a line between the points on the volume pressure tracing corresponding to 25% and 75% of the inspired volume.

*By convention, all the lung volumes and rates of flow are expressed in terms of body temperature and pressure and saturated with water vapor (BTPS), which allows for a comparison of the pulmonary function data from laboratories with different ambient temperatures and altitudes.

a hydrophobic (water-insoluble) and a hydrophilic (water-soluble) end. The hydrophilic end attaches to fluid molecules and the hydrophobic end to the gas molecules, interrupting the forces between the fluid molecules that are responsible for creating the surface tension. Surfactant exerts three important effects on lung inflation: (1) it increases lung compliance, or ease of inflation; (2) it provides stability and more even inflation of the alveoli; and (3) it assists in keeping the alveoli dry. Without surfactant, lung inflation would be extremely difficult, requiring intrapleural pressures of -20 mm Hg to -30 mm Hg, compared with the -3 mm Hg to -5 mm Hg normally needed to maintain inflation of the alveoli.[5] Surfactant not only reduces the surface tension in the alveoli, but it does so more effectively in the small alveoli, which have the greatest tendency to empty into the larger alveoli and collapse. It is thought that the surface-active molecules of surfactant are more densely packed at the surface of the small alveoli, and hence the surface-tension reducing ability is greater than in larger alveoli where the density of the molecules is less. Surfactant also helps to keep the alveoli dry. The surface tension forces tend to suck fluid into the alveoli from the capillaries; by reducing these forces, surfactant prevents the transudation of this fluid across the alveolar–capillary membrane.

The type II alveolar cells that produce surfactant do not begin to mature until weeks 26 to 28 of gestation, and consequently, many premature babies are born with poorly functioning type II alveolar cells and have difficulty producing sufficient amounts of surfactant. In these babies, the collapse of the lungs because of a lack of surfactant is called respiratory distress syndrome (RDS), or hyaline membrane disease. The production of surfactant also requires adequate amounts of oxygen and blood flow for delivery of substrates such as fatty acids. Among infants predisposed to develop RDS are premature infants, infants of diabetic mothers, infants born by cesarean section (when performed prior to the 38th week of gestation), and those suffering from hypoxia, acidosis, and hypothermia.

When it is necessary to consider the early delivery of an infant, an estimate of the maturity of the type II alveolar cells can be obtained by measuring the *lecithin* to *sphingomyelin* (L/S) ratio in the amniotic fluid through amniocentesis. In this way, it is often possible to delay the delivery of an infant until the type II alveolar cells are sufficiently mature to permit its survival. The incidence of RDS among premature babies born through vaginal delivery appears to be less than among those born by cesarean section, and it has been hypothesized that the stress of vaginal delivery may increase the babies' cortisol levels. A number of studies have shown that cortisol can accelerate the maturation of type II cells.[6] These observa-

tions have led to the clinical use of corticosteroid drugs before delivery in mothers with babies at high risk for developing RDS.

Surfactant production is also impaired in adult respiratory distress syndrome (ARDS), or shock lung, discussed in Chapter 21.

Airway resistance

Airway resistance refers to the impediment that air encounters as it moves through the airways. The volume of air that moves into and out of the alveoli is directly related to the pressure gradient between the alveoli and the atmosphere and inversely related to the resistance of the airways. The resistance of the airways, in turn, is inversely proportional to the fourth power of the airway radius. Normally, resistance to airflow is so small that only minute changes in pressure are needed to move large volumes of air into the lungs. For example, the average pressure gradient during a normal breath of 500 ml of air is less than 1 mm Hg. Because a change in the size of the airway radius produces a 16-fold change in airflow, small changes in airway caliber, such as those caused by pulmonary secretions or bronchospasm, can produce a marked increase in airway resistance. For persons with these conditions to maintain the same rate of airflow as before the onset of increased airway resistance, an increase in driving pressure (respiratory effort) is needed.

The airway resistance is greatly affected by lung volumes, being less during inspiration than during expiration. This is because the airways are pulled open by traction from the surrounding lung tissue; as the lungs expand the airways are pulled open, and as the lungs deflate the elastic fibers of the airways recoil and their diameters decrease in size. This is one of the reasons persons with conditions such as bronchial asthma, which cause abnormal airway resistance, often have less difficulty in inhaling than exhaling.

Laminar and turbulent airflow. There are two types of airflow: laminar and turbulent. Laminar, or streamlined, airflow occurs in straight circular tubes with the gas in the center of the tube moving twice as fast as the average velocity because the gas at the periphery must overcome the resistance to flow. In contrast to laminar flow, turbulent flow is disorganized flow in which the molecules of the gas move laterally, collide with each other, and change their velocities. Whether or not turbulence develops depends on the radius of the airways, the interaction of the gas molecules, and the velocity of airflow. It is most apt to occur when the radius of the airways is large and the velocity of flow is high. Turbulent flow occurs regularly in the trachea. Turbulence of airflow accounts for the respiratory sounds that are heard during chest auscultation (listening to the chest with a stethoscope).

In the bronchial tree with its many branches, laminar airflow probably occurs only in the very small airways where velocity of flow is low. Because the small airways contribute so little resistance, they constitute a silent zone. In small airway disease, it is probable that considerable abnormalities are present before the condition can be detected using the usual measurements of airway resistance.

Dynamic airway compression. Whether one starts to exhale forcefully or begins to exhale slowly and then accelerates, the volume of air that is exhaled over a given period of time remains the same (Fig. 22-10). This occurs because the forced expiratory effort reduces the transpulmonary pressure needed to hold the airways open. Before inspiration has begun, the transpulmonary pressure (intrapleural pressure − airway pressure) is about − 4 mm H$_2$O. The traction forces associated with increased lung expansion produce further increases in transpulmonary pressure during inspiration. During forced expiration, transpulmonary pressure is decreased because of a disproportionate increase in intrapleural pressure compared with airway pressure. As air moves out of the lung the drop in airway pressure causes a further decrease in the transpulmonary pressure (Fig. 22-11). If this drop in airway pressure is sufficiently great, the surrounding intrapleural pressure will compress the airway, interrupting the airflow and trapping air in the alveoli. Although this type of expiratory flow limitation is seen only during forced expiration in normal persons, it may occur during normal breathing in persons with lung diseases such as emphysema, which magnify the pressure drop along the smaller airways and increase the intrabronchial pressure needed to maintain airway patency. Measures such as pursed lip breathing increase the airway pressure and improve the expiratory flow rates. Another factor that increases airway closure is low lung volumes, which reduce the transpulmonary driving pressure.

Efficiency and work of breathing

The *minute volume* is the amount of air that is exchanged in 1 minute; it is determined by the metabolic needs of the body. The minute volume is equal to the tidal volume multiplied by the respiratory rate, which is about 6000 ml (500 ml tidal volume × respiratory rate of 12 breaths per minute) during normal activity. The pattern of breathing—the tidal volume and the rate of breathing—is usually determined by the ease of lung expansion (compliance) and the effort needed to move air through the conducting airways. For example, in persons with stiff and noncompliant lungs, expansion of the lungs is

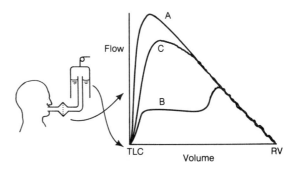

Figure 22-10 *Flow-volume curves. In A, a maximal inspiration was followed by a forced expiration. In B, expiration was initially slow and then forced. In C, expiratory effort was submaximal. The descending portions of all three curves are almost superimposed. (West JB: Respiratory Physiology, 2nd ed. Baltimore, Williams & Wilkins, 1979)*

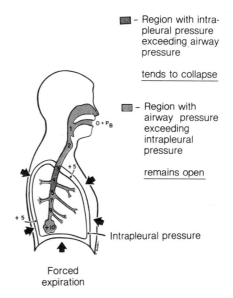

- Region with intrapleural pressure exceeding airway pressure

  tends to collapse

- Region with airway pressure exceeding intrapleural pressure

  remains open

Intrapleural pressure

Forced expiration

Figure 22-11 *Mechanism that limits maximal expiratory flow rate. Forced expiration increases intrapleural pressure, reversing the transpulmonary pressure relationship. This reversal collapses nonrigid airways to produce an expiratory "check-valve." (Slonin NB, Hamilton LH: Respiratory Physiology, 4th ed. St Louis, CV Mosby, 1981)*

difficult, and these persons usually find it easier to breathe if they keep their tidal volume low and breathe at a more rapid rate (*i.e.,* 300 × 20 = 6000 ml) to achieve their minute volume and meet their oxygen needs.

minute volume = tidal volume × respiratory rate

On the other hand, persons with airway disease usually find it less difficult to inflate the lungs but expend more energy in moving air through the airways. As a result, these persons tend to take deeper breaths and to breathe at a slower rate (*i.e.,* 600 × 10 = 6000 ml) to achieve their oxygen needs.

Dead air space

Dead air space refers to the air that must be moved with each breath but *does not participate in gas exchange*. Movement of air through dead air space contributes to the work of breathing but not to gas exchange. There are two types of dead air space: that contained in the *conducting airways (anatomic),* and that contained in the *respiratory portion of the lung (physiologic dead space)*. The volume of airway dead space is fixed and is approximately 150 ml to 200 ml, depending on body size. It constitutes air contained in the nose, pharynx, trachea, bronchi, and so on. If the alveloi are ventilated but deprived of blood flow, they do not contribute to gas exchange and thus constitute alveolar, or physiologic, dead space. The total dead space is equal to the airway and alveolar dead air space. The effective minute volume is equal to the minute ventilation minus the physiologic dead air space. Creation of a tracheotomy decreases the dead space of the airways and can have the effect of decreasing the work of breathing.

In summary, ventilation provides the means for the exchange of gases (renewal of oxygen and removal of carbon dioxide) between the lungs and the atmosphere. It is dependent on a system of open airways and movement of the thoracic cage by the respiratory muscles—the diaphragm and intercostals. The energy that is used for respiration is expended in enlarging the chest during inspiration. Expiration involves the recoil of the elastic components of the chest wall that were stretched during inspiration and is largely passive, thus contributing very little to the work of breathing. Lung compliance describes the ease with which the lungs can be inflated. A spirometer is used to measure lung volumes and capacities. Pulmonary function tests measure ventilation with respect to time.

■ Exchange and Transport of Gases in the Body

Pulmonary Blood Flow

The lungs have a dual blood supply, the bronchial and the pulmonary circulations. The *pulmonary circulation* provides for the gas exchange function of the lungs, whereas the *bronchial circulation* provides cells of the lungs with blood to meet their nutritional needs.

The *bronchial arteries* arise from the thoracic aorta and enter the lungs with the major bronchi, dividing and subdividing along with the bronchial tubes supplying them and the other lung structures with oxygen. The capillaries of the bronchial circulation drain into the *bronchial veins,* the larger of which empties into the vena cava and returns blood to the right heart. The smaller of the bronchial veins empties into the pulmonary veins. This blood is unoxygenated, because the bronchial circulation does not participate in gas exchange. As a result, this blood dilutes the oxygenated blood returning to the left heart from the lungs and reduces the saturation of hemoglobin, so that it is less than 100% saturated as it leaves the left heart and moves into the systemic circulation.

The primary function of the pulmonary circulation is to facilitate gas exchange. The pulmonary circulation serves several important functions in addition to gas exchange; it filters all the blood that moves from the right to the left side of the circulation, it removes most of the thromboemboli, and it serves as a reservoir of blood for the left side of the heart. In order to accomplish this, there must be a continuous flow of blood through the respiratory portion of the lungs. Unoxygenated blood enters the lung through the pulmonary artery, which has its origin in the right heart and enters the lung at the hilus, along with the primary bronchus. The pulmonary arteries branch in a manner similar to that of the airways. The small pulmonary arteries accompany the bronchi as they move down the lobules and branch to supply the capillary network that surrounds the alveoli (see Fig. 22-5).

The meshwork of capillaries in the respiratory portion of the lung is so dense that the flow in these vessels is often described as being similar to a sheet of flowing blood. The oxygenated capillary blood is collected in the small pulmonary veins of the lobules, and from there it moves to the larger veins to be collected finally in the four large pulmonary veins that empty into the left atrium. The term *perfusion* is used to describe the flow of blood through the pulmonary capillary bed.

The pulmonary vessels are thinner and more compliant than those in the systemic circulation, and the pressures in the pulmonary system are much lower (22/8 mm Hg versus 120/70 mm Hg). The low-pressure, low-resistance characteristics of this system serve to accommodate the delivery of varying amounts of blood from the systemic circulation without producing signs and symptoms of congestion. The volume in the pulmonary circulation is about 500 ml, with about 100 ml of this volume being located in the pulmonary capillary bed. When the output of the right ventricle and the input of the left ventricle are equal, the pulmonary blood flow remains constant. However, small differences between the input and output can result in large changes in the pulmonary volume if the differences continue for many heartbeats. The movement of blood through the pulmonary capillary bed requires that the mean pulmonary arterial pressure be greater than the mean pulmonary venous pressure. Pulmonary venous pressure increases in left-sided heart failure, and this causes the blood to accumulate in the pulmonary capillary bed, resulting in transudation of capillary fluid into the alveoli. Acute pulmonary edema is discussed in Chapter 30.

Ventilation–Perfusion Relationships

The distribution of pulmonary blood flow and ventilation differs along the distance of the lung from top to bottom. This distribution is normally altered by changes in position and exercise. It is also altered by bed rest and diseases of the heart and lungs.

Distribution of blood flow

The distribution of pulmonary blood flow is greatly affected by body position. In the upright position, the distance of the upper apices of the lung above the level of the heart often exceeds the perfusion capabilities of the mean pulmonary arterial pressure (about 12 mm Hg), and therefore blood flow in the upper part of the lung is less than in the base or bottom part of the lung. In the supine position, the lungs and heart are at the same level and blood flow to the apices and base of the lung become more uniform. In this position, however, blood flow to the posterior or dependent portions (*e.g.*, bottom of the lung when lying on the side) exceeds the flow in the anterior or nondependent portions of the lung. In persons with pulmonary vascular congestion, rales develop in the dependent portions of the lungs exposed to increased blood flow.

Pulmonary blood flow can be markedly altered by disease conditions of the lung. Persons with chronic lung disease often have marked alterations in the pulmonary blood flow that contributes to problems with oxygenating blood (Chap. 23). Alveolar hypoxia is a potent constrictor of pulmonary vasculature. Bronchial asthma often causes marked reduction in the blood flow to regions of the lung because of the hypoxic vasoconstriction of the poorly ventilated areas. Clinically, the effect of hypoxia on pulmonary blood vessels may result in the marked elevation of pulmonary arterial blood pressure.

Distribution of ventilation

Changes in posture affect ventilation as well as blood flow. At normal lung volumes, ventilation decreases per unit volume with increased distance up the lung at normal lung volumes. During inspiration, the movement of the ribs increases the lung volume proportionately more at the base of the lung than at the apex and the downward movement of the diaphragm expands the lower lobes of the lung more than the upper lobes. As a result, more air moves into the lower portions of the lung. As with blood flow, the difference in ventilation is abolished in the supine position, and the posterior (bottom) portion of the lung is better ventilated than the anterior (upper) portion. The same holds true for the lateral position.

At low lung volumes, however, the pattern of ventilation that occurs at normal and high lung volumes is reversed. With a small inspiration air goes to the apex rather than the base of the lung. As with blood flow, this uneven distribution of ventilation is thought to result from gravity and from distortion of the lungs and chest wall by their weight, which causes changes in lung expansion and the intrapleural pressure. At the end of maximal expiration at low lung volumes, the intrapleural pressure at the base of the lung exceeds the airway pressure, causing airway collapse, so that air moves into the top part of the lungs. At larger lung volumes, there is greater chest expansion with greater decreases in the intrapleural pressure at the base of the lung, so that the airways remain open and air moves preferentially into that portion of the lung.

It is important to recognize that even at low lung volumes some air remains in the alveoli of the lower portion of the lungs, preventing their collapse. According to the law of Laplace (discussed previously) the pressure needed to overcome the tension in the wall of a sphere or an elastic tube is inversely related to its radius (pressure = 2 × tension/radius); therefore, the small airways close first, trapping some gas in the alveoli. Trapping of air in the alveoli of the lower part of the lungs may be increased in older individuals and in persons with lung disease (*e.g.*, emphysema). This is thought to be due to a loss in the elastic recoil properties of the lungs, so that the intrapleural pressure (created by the elastic recoil of the lung and chest wall) becomes less negative. In these persons, airway closure occurs at the end of normal lung volumes, trapping larger amounts of air. Eventually the air trapping causes an increase in the anterior-posterior chest dimensions.

Ventilation–perfusion ratio

The gas exchange properties of the lung are dependent on the matching of ventilation and perfusion, so that there are equal amounts of air and blood entering the respiratory portion of the lungs. Two factors may interfere with the matching of ventilation and perfusion—hypoventilation and shunt. Shunt refers to blood that moves from the venous to the arterial system without being oxygenated. There are two types of shunts: physiologic and anatomic. In a physiologic shunt, the blood moves through the lung without going through the

Normal

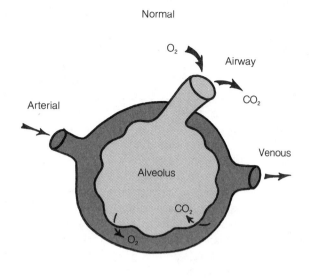

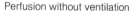

Perfusion without ventilation

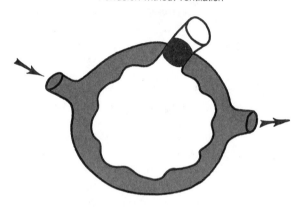

Ventilation without perfusion

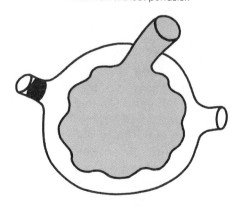

Figure 22-12 *Matching of ventilation and perfusion.*

ventilated portion of the lung. In an anatomic shunt, the blood moves from the venous to the arterial side of the circulation without moving through the lung. Anatomic intracardiac shunting of blood because of congenital heart defects is discussed in Chapter 19. Physiologic shunting of blood usually results from destructive lung disease, which impairs ventilation, or from heart failure in which there is interference with the movement of blood through sections of the lungs.

There are many causes of mismatched ventilation and perfusion, of which the most obvious are illustrated in Figure 22-12. Diagram A illustrates the desired ventilation and perfusion pattern in which normal ventilation of the alveoli and normal blood flow through the pulmonary capillary that surrounds it occur. Diagram B illustrates a situation of hypoventilation in which perfusion is normal while ventilation is lacking because of airway obstruction. This is the type of situation that occurs in atelectasis (Chap. 23). In diagram C ventilation is normal, but the pulmonary artery supplying the lobule is obstructed. An example of this situation is pulmonary embolism. Most of the situations in which ventilation and perfusion are mismatched are less obvious. In lung disease, for example, there may be altered ventilation in one area of the lung and altered perfusion in another area.

Alveolar Gas Exchange

Gas exchange takes place in the alveoli. Here gases diffuse across the alveolar–capillary membrane moving from an area of higher concentration to one of lower concentration. Oxygen moves from the alveoli into the capillary, and carbon dioxide moves from the capillary network into the alveoli. There is rapid equilibration between the gases in the alveoli and those in the blood, so that the partial pressure of the blood gas at the venous end of the pulmonary capillary is approximately the same as that in the alveoli.

The diffusion of gases in the lung is influenced by four factors: (1) the surface area available for diffusion, (2) the thickness of the alveolar–capillary membrane through which the gases diffuse, (3) the differences in the partial pressure of the gas on either side of the membrane, and (4) the characteristics of the gas. Diseases that destroy lung tissue or increase the thickness of the alveolar–capillary membrane influence the diffusing capacity of the lung. Removal of one lung, for example, reduces the diffusing surface by one-half. The thickness of the alveolar capillary membrane and the distance for diffusion are increased in pulmonary edema and pneumonia. Administration of high concentrations of oxygen increases the difference in pressure on the two sides of the alveolar–capillary membrane and increases the diffusion of the gas. The characteristics of the gas and its molecular weight and solubility determine how rapidly it diffuses through the respiratory membranes. Carbon dioxide diffuses 20 times more rapidly than oxygen, because of its greater solubility in the respiratory membranes. The factors that affect alveolar–capillary gas exchange are summarized in Table 22-3.

The *diffusing capacity of the lung* (D_L) is a measure of the rate of transfer of gases through the alveolar–capillary membrane (measured in milliliters per minute). It is measured using a gas that readily diffuses across the membrane, is easily analyzed, and is affected by the same factors that influence oxygen diffusion. Carbon monoxide, which meets these criteria, is usually used for this purpose. The test is done by having a person breathe a known concentration of carbon monoxide (usually for a 10-second breathhold or short measured interval of time). The volume of carbon monoxide that diffuses across the alveolar–capillary membrane is calculated from measurements of lung volume and changes in carbon monoxide level of inspired and expired air. Because blood levels of carbon monoxide are usually zero, there is no back diffusion of the gas and the difference between the inspired and expired carbon monoxide reflects the diffusion of the gas. The diffusing capacity for oxygen can be calculated using the diffusing capacity for carbon monoxide and known information about the solubility of the two gases. Persons who smoke or are exposed to carbon monoxide may have appreciable amounts of the gas in their lungs, invalidating the test results. The diffusing capacity of the lung is affected by conditions that alter the permeability of the alveolar–capillary membrane and the ability of the red blood cells to bind and transport the gas.

Gas Transport

The lungs enable inhaled air to come in close proximity to blood flowing through the pulmonary capillaries so that exchange of gases between the internal environment of the body and the external environment can take place. They thus restore the oxygen content of the arterial blood and remove the carbon dioxide from the venous blood. The red blood cells, in turn, facilitate transport of gases as they move between the lungs and the tissues.

Oxygen transport

Oxygen is transported in two forms—in chemical combination with hemoglobin and physically dissolved in blood plasma. The *partial pressure* (PO_2), or *oxygen tension,* is the level of the *dissolved gas,* much like the dissolved carbon dioxide in a capped bottle of a carbonated soft drink. It is the dissolved form of oxygen that crosses the cell membrane and participates in cell metabolism.

Table 22-3 Factors Affecting Alveolar–Capillary Gas Exchange

Factors Affecting Gas Exchange	Examples
Surface area available for diffusion	Removal of a lung or diseases such as emphysema and chronic bronchitis, which destroy lung tissue or cause mismatching of ventilation and perfusion
Thickness of the alveolar–capillary membrane	Conditions such as pneumonia, interstitial lung disease, and pulmonary edema, which increase membrane thickness
Partial pressure of alveolar gases	Ascent to high altitudes where the partial pressure of oxygen is reduced. In the opposite direction, increasing the partial pressure of a gas in the inspired air (*e.g.,* oxygen therapy) will increase the gradient for diffusion
Solubility and molecular weight of the gas	Carbon dioxide, which is more soluble in the cell membranes, diffuses across the alveolar capillary membrane more rapidly than oxygen

Hemoglobin in the red blood cell is the transport vehicle, binding oxygen in the pulmonary capillaries and releasing it into the tissue capillaries. The released oxygen becomes dissolved in the plasma as it moves between the red blood cell and the tissue cells.

Dissolved oxygen. Only about 1% of the oxygen carried in the blood is in the dissolved state; the remainder is carried with the hemoglobin. The amount of oxygen that will dissolve in plasma is determined by two factors: (1) the solubility of oxygen in plasma and (2) the partial pressure of the gas in the alveoli. The solubility of oxygen in plasma is fixed and is very small. For every *1 mm Hg* PO_2 present in the alveoli, *0.003 ml of oxygen becomes dissolved in 100 ml of plasma.* This means that at a normal alveolar PO_2 of 100 mm Hg the blood carries only 0.3 ml of dissolved oxygen in every 100 ml of plasma. As will be discussed, this amount is very small compared with the amount that can be carried in an equal amount of blood when oxygen is attached to hemoglobin.

Athough the oxygen carried in plasma is insignificant, as just described, it may be a lifesaving mode of transport in carbon monoxide poisoning when most of the hemoglobin sites are occupied by carbon monoxide and are unavailable for transport of oxygen. The hyperbaric chamber, in which 100% oxygen at high atmospheric pressures is administered to treat certain disorders, increases the amount of oxygen that can be carried in the dissolved state, so that sufficient oxygen may be made available to prevent the death of vital structures such as brain cells. The reader may want to calculate the amount of oxygen that can be carried in the plasma when a person breathes 100% oxygen at 3 atmospheres, the pressure frequently employed in hyperbaric chambers.*

Hemoglobin transport. In the lung, oxygen moves across the alveolar capillary membrane, through the plasma, and into the red blood cell where it forms a loose and reversible bond with the hemoglobin molecule (Fig. 22-13). In the normal lung, this process is rapid, so that even with a fast heart rate, the hemoglobin is almost completely saturated with oxygen during the short time that it spends in the pulmonary capillary bed. A small amount of unoxygenated blood from the bronchial circulation is mixed with the oxygenated blood in the pulmonary veins and as a result, the hemoglobin is only about 95% to 97% saturated as it moves into the arterial circulation.

Hemoglobin is a highly efficient carrier of oxygen, and approximately 98% to 99% of the oxygen used by body tissues is carried in this manner. *Each gram of hemoglobin is capable of carrying about 1.34 ml of oxygen when completely saturated.* This means that a person with a hemoglobin of 14 gm/100 ml of blood carries 18.8 ml of oxygen in each 100 ml of blood in the form of oxyhemoglobin.

The oxygenated hemoglobin is transported in the arterial blood to the peripheral capillaries where the oxygen is released and made available to the tissues for use in cell metabolism. As the oxygen moves out of the capillaries in response to the needs of the tissues, the hemoglobin saturation, which was about 95% to 97% as the blood left the left heart, drops to about 75% as the mixed venous blood returns to the right heart.

Oxygen–hemoglobin dissociation. Oxygen that remains bound to hemoglobin cannot participate in tissue metabolism. The efficiency of the oxygen transport system is dependent on the ability of the hemoglobin molecule to bind oxygen in the lung and release it on demand. The affinity of hemoglobin refers to its capacity to bind oxygen, thus, the hemoglobin binds oxygen readily when affinity is increased and releases oxygen when affinity is decreased.

Hemoglobin's affinity for oxygen is influenced by pH, in that it binds oxygen under alkaline conditions and releases it under acid conditions. Carbon dioxide moves out of the blood in the lungs, raising the pH and thereby

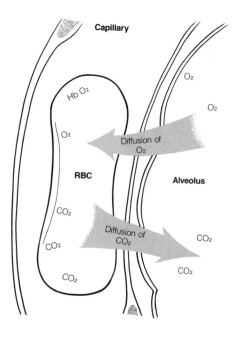

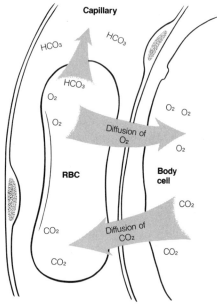

Figure 22-13 *Transport of oxygen by the red blood cell. (A) Oxygen moves from the alveoli to the hemoglobin, and carbon dioxide moves from the red cell to the alveoli. (B) Oxygen moves from the red blood cell to the capillary fluid and then into the interstitial fluid, where it becomes available to the cell, while carbon dioxide moves in the opposite direction.*

*2280 (760 mm Hg × 3 atmospheres) × 0.003 (solubility of O_2 in plasma) = 6.8 ml/100 ml of plasma. The actual value would be slightly less than this, because the calculation does not take into account the partial pressure of carbon dioxide or water vapor pressure in the alveoli.

increasing the oxygen affinity. In the tissues, a decrease in pH because of cellular release of carbon dioxide and metabolic acids lowers hemoglobin affinity for oxygen and thereby enhances its release.

The relationship between the oxygen carried in combination with hemoglobin and the PO_2 of the blood is described by the *oxygen–hemoglobin dissociation curve*, which is pictured in Figure 22-14. The curve is S-shaped, with the top *flat portion* representing the binding of oxygen to the *hemoglobin in the lung* and the *steep portion* representing its *release into the tissue capillaries*. At about 100 mm Hg PO_2, a plateau occurs at which point the hemoglobin is 100% saturated. Increasing the alveolar PO_2 above this level will have no further effect in increasing hemoglobin saturation. Even at high altitudes, when the partial pressure of oxygen is considerably decreased, the hemoglobin remains relatively well saturated. At 60 mm Hg PO_2 the hemoglobin is still 89% saturated.

The steep portion of the dissociation curve—between 60 mm Hg and 40 mm Hg—represents the removal of oxygen from the hemoglobin as it moves through the tissue capillaries. This portion of the curve is of great importance for it permits considerable transfer of oxygen from hemoglobin to the tissues with only a small drop in oxygen tension. Normally the tissues remove about 5 ml of oxygen per 100 ml of blood, and the hemoglobin of mixed venous blood as it returns to the right heart is about 75% saturated (PO_2 40 mm Hg). In this portion of the dissociation curve, the rate at which oxygen is released from the hemoglobin is determined largely by tissue utilization. During strenuous exercise, for example, the muscle cells may remove as much as 15 ml of oxygen per 100 ml of blood from the hemoglobin.

Hemoglobin can be regarded as an oxygen buffer system that regulates oxygen pressure in the tissues. Thus, hemoglobin affinity for oxygen must change with the metabolic needs of the tissues. This change is represented by a shift in the dissociation curve to the right or the left as pictured in Figure 22-13.

As the curve shifts to the right, the tissue PO_2 is greater for any given level of hemoglobin saturation. A shift to the right is usually caused by conditions such as fever, acidosis, or an increase in PCO_2, which reflects increased tissue metabolism. Hypoxia also causes the dissociation curve to shift to the right. The red blood cells, unlike other tissues, contain high levels of the glycolytic intermediate 2,3-diphosphoglycerate (2,3-DPG), the levels of which increase during hypoxia; this reduces hemoglobin affinity for oxygen and favors its release to the tissues. A shift to the right because of an increase in 2,3-DPG occurs in various conditions of hypoxia, including those resulting from high altitude, pulmonary insufficiency, heart failure, and severe anemia.

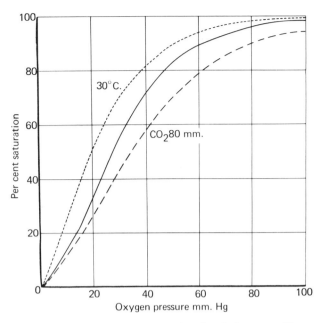

Figure 22-14   *The oxygen–hemoglobin dissociation curve. Note that when the carbon dioxide is increased or when the blood pH is decreased, the curve is shifted to the right, and therefore the hemoglobin binds less oxygen for any partial pressure of oxygen. When the curve is shifted to the left, as occurs when the carbon dioxide is decreased or the pH is increased, the opposite occurs. (Chaffee EE, Lytle IM: Basic Physiology and Anatomy, 4th ed. Philadelphia, JB Lippincott, 1980)*

A shift to the left of the dissociation curve represents an enhanced affinity of hemoglobin for oxygen and occurs in situations associated with a decrease in tissue metabolism, such as alkalosis, decreased body temperature, and decreased carbon dioxide levels. The degree of change in affinity is indicated by the P_{50}, or the partial pressure of oxygen that is needed to achieve a 50% saturation of hemoglobin. Returning to Figure 22-13, the reader will note that the dissociation curve on the left has a P_{50} of about 20 mm Hg; the normal curve, a P_{50} of 26; and the curve on the right, a P_{50} of 35 mm Hg.

Cyanosis.   Reduced hemoglobin—hemoglobin from which the oxygen has been removed—is purple. Cyanosis is the purplish discoloration of the skin, nail beds, and mucous membranes because of the presence of excessive reduced hemoglobin in the superficial capillaries. Cyanosis does not occur until there is at least 5 gm of reduced hemoglobin per 100 ml of blood in these capillaries. The appearance of cyanosis depends on the thickness and pigment of the skin, the peripheral blood flow, and the amount of hemoglobin present. Consequently, cyanosis is not always a sensitive index of hypoxia. It is difficult to detect in persons with dark skin. Cyanosis is deceiving; it can occur when there is a local decrease in blood flow and does not necessarily reflect the oxygen content of blood flow in other parts of the body. For example, it is common for the fingers to turn blue during exposure to cold. This is because of the sluggish blood flow with increased extraction of oxygen from the blood as it flows through the superficial vessels. Because cyanosis appears when there is 5 gm of reduced hemoglobin in 100 ml of blood, a person with polycythemia (an excess of red blood cells) may easily carry 5 gm of reduced hemoglobin per 100 ml of blood without evidence of hypoxia. A person with anemia, on the other hand, may not have sufficient hemoglobin that 5 gm/100 ml can be present in the reduced state; in this case the person will be hypoxic but not cyanotic. The undersurface of the tongue is a reliable area to check for central cyanosis because of heart or lung disease[7] (cyanosis resulting from abnormal peripheral circulation does not occur here).

Carbon dioxide transport

Carbon dioxide is a by-product of tissue metabolism. It is transported in the blood in three forms—*attached to hemoglobin, as dissolved carbon dioxide,* and *as bicarbonate.* About 4 ml of CO_2 is transported from the tissues to the lungs in each 100 ml of blood. Carbon dioxide is much more soluble in plasma than oxygen, and, as a result, larger quantities are carried in the extracellular fluid as bicarbonate (60%–70%) and in the dissolved form (about 10%). The remainder of the carbon dioxide is transported as carbaminohemoglobin. How dissolved carbon dioxide and bicarbonate influences acid–base balance is discussed in Chapter 27.

Blood gases

To accurately measure blood gases, arterial blood is required. Venous blood is not used because venous levels of oxygen and carbon dioxide reflect the metabolic requirements of the tissues rather than the gas exchange properties of the lungs. The PO_2 of arterial blood is normally above 80 mm Hg, and the PCO_2 is in the range of 35 mm Hg to 45 mm Hg.

Hypoxia

Hypoxia refers to a reduction in tissue oxygenation. It can result from an inadequate amount of oxygen in the air, disease of the respiratory system, alterations in circulatory function, anemia, or the inability of the cells to utilize oxygen. The causes of hypoxia can be divided into four categories: (1) hypoxemic hypoxia in which the oxygen content of the blood is reduced; (2) stagnant, or ischemic hypoxia, in which circulation of oxygen in the blood is impaired; (3) anemic hypoxia, in which the ability to transport oxygen in the blood decreases; and (4) histotoxic hypoxia, in which the cells are unable to utilize oxygen (*e.g.,* cyanide poisoning). The categories, mechanisms of production, and causes of hypoxia are summarized in Table 22-4.

Acute hypoxia

The partial pressure of oxygen decreases as one ascends above sea level and much of what is known about acute hypoxia has been learned from high altitude and aviation studies. The partial pressure of oxygen, which constitutes 21% of the total gases in the air, falls from 159 mm Hg at sea level (760 mm Hg barometric pressure) to 110 mm Hg at 10,000 feet to 73 mm Hg at 20,000 feet.[6] Denver, Colorado, with an altitude of 5250 feet, has an oxygen content of 121 mm Hg. Atmospheric oxygen is diluted with water vapor and carbon dioxide in the lung. As a result, alveolar oxygen pressure is less than that in the environment; it falls from about 104 mm Hg at sea level to 67 mm Hg at 10,000 feet to 40 mm Hg at 20,000 feet. The ceiling for breathing air is approximately 23,000 feet; this can be doubled to about 47,000 feet when breathing pure oxygen. The use of pressurized cabins in aircraft allows for safe travel at high altitudes. In the clinical setting, acute hypoxia can occur at sea level in persons with sudden blood loss, carbon monoxide poisoning, acute circulatory disorders, respiratory disease, or other disorders that interfere with the exchange or transport of oxygen.

Table 22-4   Types, Mechanisms of Production, and Causes of Hypoxia

Type	Mechanisms of Production	Causes
Hypoxemic hypoxia	Insufficient oxygen reaching the blood	Decreased oxygen in the atmosphere Pulmonary disease Airway obstruction Neuromuscular disease
Stagnant hypoxia	Failure to transport oxygen because of impaired blood flow	Heart Failure Circulatory shock Local disruption of blood flow
Anemic hypoxia	Reduction in the oxygen-carrying capacity of the blood	Decrease in red blood cells Abnormal hemoglobin Carbon monoxide poisoning
Histotoxic hypoxia	Impaired utilization of oxygen by the cell	Cellular poisons such as cyanide Tissue edema Abnormal tissue needs

Severe hypoxia causes cyanosis, cardiovascular signs such as tachycardia, and central nervous system signs such as mental clouding. The signs of hypoxia are usually mild until the PO_2 falls below 60 mm Hg, and the symptoms do not become severe until the PO_2 falls to 40 mm Hg to 50 mm Hg. One of the earliest signs of acute hypoxia is a chemoreceptor-mediated increase in ventilation. The chemoreceptors (to be discussed later in this chapter) are particularly sensitive to changes in PO_2 (blood oxygen levels) in the range of 60 mm Hg to 30 mm Hg. Important early effects of acute hypoxia are decreases in judgment and motor proficiency. These manifestations become more acute with prolonged exposure to hypoxic conditions. For example, mental proficiency is decreased to half of normal after 1 hour of sudden exposure to the barometric pressures at 15,000 feet and decreased to one-fifth after 18 hours.[6] Other signs of acute hypoxia include dyspnea, fatigue, headache, nausea and vomiting, and decreased visual acuity. Cyanosis of the lips and nail beds is usually present in persons with adequate hemoglobin levels. Cheyne–Stokes breathing and insomnia are common problems in unacclimated persons during the first several days of exposure to high altitudes. Disorientation, hallucinations, convulsions, and coma occur with extreme levels of hypoxia. It has been speculated that some of the symptoms, such as insomnia and Cheyne–Stokes breathing, associated with ascent to high altitudes are related to the decreased carbon dioxide levels resulting from hyperventilation.

Chronic hypoxia

Chronic hypoxia induces changes similar, albeit of a lesser degree, to those observed in acute hypoxia. Dyspnea, fatigue, and cyanosis are common problems associated with a long-term impairment in the oxygenation of tissues. In addition, there is evidence of adaptive mechanisms, such as pulmonary hypertension and polycythemia.

The body adapts to hypoxia by increased ventilation, pulmonary vasoconstriction, and increased production of red blood cells. Hyperventilation results from the hypoxic stimulation of the chemoreceptors. The stimulus for the increased production of red blood cells results from the release of erythropoietin from the kidneys in response to hypoxia (Chap. 13). Polycythemia increases the red blood cell concentration and the oxygen carrying capacity of the blood. Pulmonary vasoconstriction occurs as a local response to alveolar hypoxia; it increases pulmonary arterial pressure and serves to improve the matching of ventilation and blood flow. Other adaptive mechanisms include a shift in the oxygen dissociation curve to the right as a means of increasing oxygen release to the tissues. An increase in oxidative enzymes in the cell serves as a means of increasing the efficiency of oxygen utilization.

In summary, the lungs enable inhaled air to come in close proximity with the blood flowing through the pulmonary capillaries, so that the exchange of gases between the internal environment of the body and the external environment can take place. The blood provides the means for the transport of gases in the body. Oxygen is transported in two forms: (1) in chemical combination with hemoglobin and (2) physically dissolved in plasma (PO_2). Hemoglobin is an efficient carrier of oxygen, and about 98% to 99% of oxygen is transported in this manner. Carbon dioxide is carried in three forms—as carbaminohemoglobin, dissolved carbon dioxide, and bicarbonate. Seventy percent to 80% of carbon dioxide in the plasma is in the bicarbonate or dissolved form. Hypoxia refers to an acute or chronic reduction in tissue oxygenation. It can result from decreased oxygen content of the blood (hypoxemic hypoxia), impaired blood flow (stagnant hypoxia), reduced oxygen-carrying capacity of the blood (anemic hypoxia), or impaired cellular utilization of oxygen (histotoxic hypoxia).

■ Control of Respiration

Neural Control Mechanisms

Unlike the heart, which has inherent rhythmic properties and can beat independently of the nervous system, muscles controlling respiration require continuous input from the nervous system. The movement of the diaphragm, intercostal muscles, sternocleidomastoid, and other accessory muscles controlling ventilation is integrated by neurons located in the pons and medulla. These neurons are collectively referred to as the *respiratory center.* Previous beliefs regarding separate inspiratory and expiratory centers are probably no longer applicable. Instead, it is now believed that the respiratory center consists of two dense bilateral aggregates of respiratory neurons involved in both initiating inspiration and expiration and incorporating afferent impulses into motor responses of the respiratory muscles. The first, or dorsal, group of neurons in the respiratory center is concerned primarily with inspiration. These neurons control the activity of the phrenic nerves and drive the second, or ventral, group of respiratory neurons. In addition, they probably integrate impulses from the lungs and airways into the ventilatory response. The second group of neurons, which contains both inspiratory and expiratory neurons, controls the spinal motor neurons of the intercostal and abdominal muscles. The pacemaker properties of the respiratory center result from the cycling of the two groups of respiratory neurons. The nature and mechanism of this cycling is still under investigation.

Axons from the neurons in the respiratory center cross in the midline and descend in the ventrolateral columns of the spinal cord. The tracts that control expiration and inspiration are spatially separated in the cord, as are the tracts that transmit specialized reflexes (*e.g.*, coughing and hiccuping) and voluntary control of ventilation. Only at the level of the spinal cord are the respiratory impulses integrated to produce a reflex response. The neural control of ventilation is depicted in Figure 22-15.

The control of breathing has both automatic and voluntary components. The automatic regulation of ventilation is controlled by input from two types of sensors or receptors: chemoreceptors, which monitor the blood levels of oxygen, carbon dioxide, and *p*H and adjust ventilation to meet the changing metabolic needs of the body; and lung receptors, which monitor breathing patterns and lung function. Voluntary regulation of ventilation integrates breathing with voluntary acts such as speaking, blowing, and singing. These acts, initiated by

the motor and premotor cortex, cause the temporary suspension of automatic breathing. It has been suggested that alterations in the control of automatic and voluntary regulation of breathing may contribute to various forms of sleep apnea. This is discussed in Chapter 24.

The automatic and voluntary components of respiration are regulated by afferent impulses coming to the respiratory center from a number of sources. Afferent input from higher brain centers is evidenced by the ability to consciously alter the depth and rate of respiration. Fever, pain, and emotion exert their influence through lower brain centers. Vagal afferents from sensory receptors in the lungs and airways are integrated in the dorsal area of the respiratory center.

Chemoreceptors

Tissue needs for oxygen and the removal of carbon dioxide are regulated by chemoreceptors that monitor blood levels of these gases. Input from these sensors is transmitted to the respiratory center, and ventilation is adjusted to maintain the arterial blood gases within a normal range.

There are two types of chemoreceptors: central and peripheral chemoreceptors. The most important chemoreceptors for sensing changes in blood carbon dioxide content are the central chemoreceptors. These receptors are actually chemosensitive regions located in the medulla near the respiratory center and are bathed in cerebrospinal fluid. Although the central chemoreceptors monitor carbon dioxide levels, the actual stimulus for these receptors is provided by hydrogen ions that are present in the cerebrospinal fluid. This fluid is separated from the blood by the blood–brain barrier, which permits the free diffusion of carbon dioxide but not of bicarbonate or hydrogen ions. The carbon dioxide, in turn, combines rapidly with water to form carbonic acid, which dissociates into hydrogen ions. Thus, the carbon dioxide content in the blood regulates ventilation through its effect on the *p*H of the extracellular fluid of the brain. These chemoreceptors are extremely sensitive to short-term changes in carbon dioxide. The effect of an increase in plasma carbon dioxide levels on ventilation reaches its peak within a minute or so and then declines if the CO_2 level remains elevated. With long-term elevation in carbon dioxide, a compensatory increase in bicarbonate secretion into the cerebral spinal fluid occurs, which acts as a buffer for the hydrogen ions. Thus, persons with chronically elevated levels of carbon dioxide no longer respond to this stimulus for increased ventilation but rely on the stimulus provided by a decrease in the blood oxygen levels.

The arterial oxygen levels are monitored by peripheral chemoreceptors located in the carotid and aortic bodies. Although these chemoreceptors also monitor carbon dioxide, they play a much more impor-

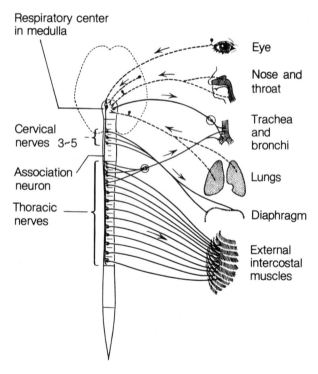

Figure 22-15 *Activity in the respiratory center. Impulses traveling over afferent neurons activate central neurons, which in turn activate the efferent neurons that supply the muscles of respiration. Thus, respiratory movements may be altered by a variety of stimuli. (Chaffee EE, Greisheimer EM: Basic Physiology and Anatomy, 3rd ed. Philadelphia, JB Lippincott, 1974)*

Respiratory center in medulla

Eye

Nose and throat

Cervical nerves 3–5

Trachea and bronchi

Association neuron

Lungs

Thoracic nerves

Diaphragm

External intercostal muscles

tant role in monitoring arterial blood oxygen levels. These receptors exert little control over ventilation until the PO_2 has dropped to below 60 mm Hg. Hypoxia is the main stimulus for ventilation in persons with chronic hypercarbia. If these persons are given oxygen therapy at a level sufficient to increase the PO_2 above that needed to stimulate the peripheral chemoreceptors, their ventilation may be seriously depressed.

Lung receptors

There are three types of lung receptors: stretch, irritant, and juxtacapillary (J) receptors. Stretch receptors are located in the smooth muscle layers of the conducting airways. They respond to changes in pressure within the walls of the airways. When the lung is inflated, these receptors inhibit inspiration and promote expiration (Hering–Breuer reflex). They are important in establishing breathing patterns and in minimizing the work of breathing by adjusting the respiratory rate and tidal volume to accommodate changes in lung compliance and airway resistance. Irritant receptors have a distribution similar to that of the stretch receptors. They can be mechanically stimulated by increases in airway pressure, changes in lung inflation, and changes in bronchial smooth muscle tone. Stimulation of the irritant receptors leads to airway constriction and a pattern of rapid, shallow breathing. This pattern of breathing probably protects respiratory tissues from the damaging effects of toxic inhalants. It is also thought that the mechanical stimulation of receptors may serve to ensure more uniform lung expansion by initiating periodic sighing and yawning. The function of the J receptors is uncertain; at present, it is thought that they sense lung congestion. These receptors may be responsible for the rapid, shallow breathing that occurs with pulmonary edema, pulmonary embolism, and pneumonia.

Alterations in Breathing Patterns

The act of breathing is normally effortless and does not require conscious thought. In an adult, the normal rate of respiration is about 16 to 18 per minute, with about one breath for every four heartbeats. This rate increases with exercise and other activities that increase body metabolism. In normal breathing, expiration is largely passive and is accomplished within 4 to 6 seconds.

Respiratory movements are normally smooth, with equal expansion of both sides of the chest. In men, respiratory movements tend to be primarily diaphragmatic, whereas in women, there tends to be greater movement of the intercostal muscles. When breathing becomes labored, the accessory muscles of the neck come into play, and there may be flaring of the nares.

The suffix *pnea* denotes a relationship to breathing. *Tachypnea* is rapid breathing, and *hyperpnea* is an increase in both the rate and depth of respiration. Hyperpnea is normal during exercise. *Bradypnea* is an abnormally slow respiratory rate. *Hyperventilation* is ventilation in excess of that needed to maintain a normal level of arterial PCO_2. Hyperventilation causes a decrease in PCO_2 and tends to lead to respiratory alkalosis (Chap. 27).

Periodic breathing

Periodic breathing describes a breathing pattern in which there are episodes of apnea, or absence of breathing. *Cheyne–Stokes breathing* is a type of periodic breathing characterized by periods of slowly waxing and waning respirations, separated by a period of apnea that lasts up to 30 seconds. Cheyne–Stokes breathing is thought to be caused by impaired function of the central feedback mechanisms that buffer the respiratory center's response to carbon dioxide. In order for Cheyne–Stokes respirations to occur, the hyperpneic and apneic phases of the breathing pattern must be long enough for sufficient changes in the carbon dioxide content of the blood to occur. During the hyperpneic phase of Cheyne–Stokes breathing, carbon dioxide levels fall, leading to a decreased stimulus for ventilation and finally to apnea. The period of apnea, in turn, causes the carbon dioxide content of the blood to accumulate, and this leads to the hyperpneic phase of the respiratory pattern. Two types of disease conditions cause predisposition to Cheyne–Stokes breathing. One is congestive heart failure, in which there is a great delay in moving blood with its altered carbon dioxide content from the lungs to the chemoreceptors in the brain that control ventilation. The other is impaired function of the brain centers regulating the feedback mechanisms that control respiration. An area of the brain stem controls the feedback gain of the respiratory center in response to changes in carbon dioxide level. Cheyne–Stokes respirations may be seen in persons who have brain lesions that affect this area. Cheyne–Stokes breathing is also seen in healthy individuals as an adaptive response to high altitudes, especially during sleep.

Dyspnea

Dyspnea is a subjective sensation of difficulty in breathing that includes both the perception of labored breathing and the reaction to that sensation.[8] The terms *dyspnea, breathlessness,* and *shortness* of breath are often used interchangeably. Dyspnea is observed in at least three different major cardiopulmonary disease states: primary lung diseases such as pneumonia, asthma, and emphysema; heart disease that is characterized by pulmonary congestion; and neuromuscular disorders such as myasthenia gravis and muscular dystrophy that affect the respiratory muscles. Although dyspnea is often associated with respiratory disease, its presence does not necessarily imply pathology; dyspnea occurs during exercise, particularly in untrained individuals.

The cause of dyspnea is unknown. Four types of mechanisms have been proposed to explain the sensation: (1) stimulation of lung receptors, (2) increased sensitivity to changes in ventilation perceived through central nervous system mechanisms, (3) reduced ventilatory capacity or breathing reserve, and (4) stimulation of neural receptors in the muscle fibers of the intercostals and diaphragm and of receptors in the skeletal joints.[9] The first of the suggested mechanisms is stimulation of the previously described lung receptors. These receptors are stimulated by the contraction of bronchial smooth muscle, the stretch of the bronchial wall, pulmonary congestion, and conditions that decrease lung compliance. The second category of proposed mechanisms focuses on central nervous system mechanisms that transmit information to the cortex regarding respiratory muscle weakness or a discrepancy between the increased effort of breathing and inadequate respiratory muscle contraction. The third type of mechanism focuses on a reduction in ventilatory capacity or breathing reserve. As a general rule, a reduction in breathing reserve (maximum voluntary ventilation not being used during a given activity) to less than 65% to 75% correlates well with dyspnea. The fourth possible mechanism is stimulation of muscle and joint receptors in the respiratory musculature because of a discrepancy in the tension generated by these muscles and the tidal volume that results.

Table 22-5 Instrument to Measure Dyspnea*

A. Degree of Shortness of Breath Graded from 0 to 3

Grade	Description
0	No unusual shortness of breath compared to other persons of same age, height, and sex
1	More shortness of breath than a person of same age when walking up hills or hurrying on level ground
2	Shortness of breath when walking on level ground
3	Shortness of breath at rest or while dressing

B. Visual Analog Scale

```
   0 _____ 10
                  10 cm
No difficulty                        Unable to
  breathing                          breathe
```

*For use in illness trajectory.
(From Carrieri VK, Jansen-Bjerklie S, Jacobs S: Thje sensation of dyspnea: A review. Heart Lung 13, No 4:441, 1984)

These receptors, once stimulated, transmit signals that bring about an awareness of the breathing discrepancy.

Like other subjective symptoms, such as fatigue and pain, dyspnea is difficult to quantify because it relies on a person's perception of the problem. The most common method for measuring dyspnea is a retrospective determination of the level of daily activity at which a person experiences dyspnea. A number of scales are available for this use. One of these uses four grades of dyspnea to evaluate disability (Table 22-5).[9] The visual analog scale is used to assess breathing difficulty that occurs with a given activity such as walking a certain distance. It can also be used to assess dyspnea over time. The treatment of dyspnea depends on the cause. The techniques used clinically to reduce dyspnea include those to reduce anxiety, breathing retraining, and energy conservation measures.

Cough Reflex

The cough reflex protects the lung from accumulation of secretions and from entry of irritating and destructive substances; it is one of the primary defense mechanisms of the respiratory tract.

The cough reflex is initiated by receptors located in the tracheobronchial wall; they are extremely sensitive to irritating substances and to the presence of excess secretions. Afferent impulses from these receptors are transmitted through the vagus to the medullary center, which integrates the cough response.

Coughing itself requires the rapid inspiration of a large volume of air (usually about 2.5 liters), followed by rapid closure of the glottis. This is followed by forceful contraction of the abdominal and expiratory muscles. As these muscles contract, there is a marked elevation of intrathoracic pressures to levels of 100 mm Hg or more. The rapid opening of the glottis, at this point, leads to an explosive expulsion of air.

There are many conditions that may interfere with the cough reflex and its protective function. The reflex is impaired in persons with *weakness of the abdominal or respiratory muscles*. This can be caused by disease conditions that lead to muscle weakness or paralysis or by prolonged inactivity or it may be an outcome of surgery involving these muscles. Bed rest interferes with expansion of the chest and limits the amount of air that can be taken into the lungs in preparation for coughing, so the cough is weak and ineffective. Disease conditions that *prevent effective closure of the glottis and laryngeal muscles* interfere with accomplishment of the marked increase in intrathoracic pressure that is needed for effective coughing. The presence of a nasogastric tube, for example, may prevent closure of the upper airway structures. The presence of such a tube may also fatigue the receptors for the cough reflex that are located in the area. Last, the cough reflex is impaired when there is *depressed function of the medullary centers* in the brain that integrate the cough reflex. Interruption of the central integration aspect of the cough reflex can arise as the result of diseases of this part of the brain or the action of drugs that depress the cough center.

Although the cough reflex is basically a protective mechanism, frequent and prolonged coughing can be exhausting and painful and can exert undesirable effects on the cardiovascular and respiratory systems and on the elastic tissues of the lungs. This is particularly true in young children and the elderly.

Sputum

Sputum consists of respiratory secretions that are ejected from the mouth during coughing and expectoration. A cough is said to be productive or nonproductive depending on the amount of sputum produced.

Sputum contains mucus produced by the epithelial cells that line the respiratory tract as well as any debris that has been inhaled. The normal adult produces about 100 ml of sputum per day, most of which is swallowed as it is propelled into the pharynx by the action of the mucociliary blanket. With infection of the respiratory tract, the sputum often contains infecting organisms and inflammatory debris and becomes purulent. The color of the sputum is an important sign. Yellow sputum, for example, may indicate infection. The presence of verdoperoxidase, liberated from the polymorphonuclear cells in the sputum, causes stagnant pus to turn green. Patients with lower respiratory tract infections may report having a green sputum upon arising in the morning that turns yellow as the day progresses. Pulmonary edema often causes exudation of red blood cells into the alveoli, thus producing frothy blood-tinged sputum. The coughing up of blood-tinged sputum is called hemoptysis.

Methods of cough relief fall into three categories. The *first is correction of the underlying cause*. When this fails or cannot be accomplished immediately, a *second method, administration of a drug with a cough suppressant action*, may be initiated, as long as the agent does not disrupt elimination of tracheobronchial secretions. The *third method relies on the use of expectorant drugs (or procedures)*, to increase the quantity of bronchial secretions or to liquefy them; this facilitates removal of secretions from the respiratory system and hence diminishes the need to cough. Table 22-6 lists various cough preparations and summarizes their mechanism of action.

Cough suppressants (antitussive drugs)

Narcotics such as *morphine, hydromorphone*, and *levorphanol* cause potent suppression of the cough reflex at the level of the medullary cough center. These drugs also inhibit the ciliary action of the respiratory mucous

Table 22-6 Medications Used in the Treatment of Cough

Classification of Preparations	Mechanism of Action
Antitussive Drugs	
Narcotics	Act centrally on the medullary cough center to suppress the cough
Codeine	
Hydrocodone	
Non-narcotic	Acts centrally on the medullary cough center to suppress the cough
Dextromethorphan	
Antihistamine	Acts centrally on the cough center
Diphenhydramine	
Peripherally and centrally acting antitussive	Local anesthetic that acts peripherally on the stretch receptors in the lung and centrally to suppress the cough reflex
Benzonatate	
Peripherally acting demulcents	Coat the irritated mucosal surface of the pharynx
Honey	
Glycerin	
Expectorants	
Gastric reflex stimulants	Increase the production of respiratory tract secretions by causing gastric irritation, which stimulates the gastric reflex and production of respiratory secretions
Potassium iodide	
Syrup of ipecac	
Guaifenesin	
Ammonium chloride	
Bronchial secretory cell stimulant	Acts on bronchial secretory glands to stimulate increased production of respiratory tract secretions
Elixir of terpin hydrate	
Mucolytic agent	Reduces the viscosity of mucus by depolymerizing (breaking down) mucopolysaccharides in mucus
Acetylcysteine (Mucomyst)	

membrane and depress respiration. Therefore, persons receiving these drugs for control of pain need to be observed for development of respiratory complications, which can arise from depression of respiration and impairment of the cough reflex and other respiratory defense mechanisms.

The narcotics *codeine* and *hydrocodone* also act as cough suppressants but have fewer side-effects and are therefore sometimes used as *antitussive drugs*. Some of the *non-narcotic agents such as dextromethorphan* are effective in suppressing the cough without creating drug dependence or other undesirable effects. It is these centrally acting non-narcotic antitussive drugs that are usually contained in over-the-counter preparations.

Another group of drugs *act peripherally* to reduce stimulation of the afferent receptors of the cough reflex. One of these, *benzonatate (Tessalon)*, is believed to have a local anesthetic effect. Another group of locally acting agents are the demulcents, such as glycerin and honey, which act by coating the irritated pharyngeal structures. Many cough syrups and lozenges contain a demulcent.

Expectorants

Expectorants are drugs or substances that increase the secretion of mucus in the bronchi and reduce its viscosity, making it easier to move the secretions toward the mouth so that they can be disposed of.

Water is probably one of the most effective and is certainly one of the best expectorants. In addition to its use to increase hydration, water is also effective in the form of inhaled steam or moisture.

A number of expectorants are believed to act reflexly by causing gastric irritation, which in turn stimulates respiratory tract secretion. The reader is undoubtedly familiar with the increase in salivation and respiratory tract secretions that accompanies nausea and vomiting. Among the expectorants that act by causing gastric irritation are *potassium iodide, ammonium chloride, syrup of ipecac,* and *guaifenesin* (Table 22-6). Potassium iodide preparations leave a brassy taste in the mouth and lead to unpleasant hypersecretion from the eyes, nose, and mouth. It can also cause painful swelling of the parotid gland and an acneiform skin rash. Iodine preparations influence thyroid function and persons who use these medications over long periods may have changes in thyroid function. *Syrup of ipecac* is nauseating and is a useful emetic in small children. It is included, in dilute forms, in some cough preparations. Guaifenesin is incorporated into many over-the-counter cough medications, although its effectiveness as an expectorant is controversial. *Elixir of terpin hydrate* is thought to have a direct stimulatory effect on the bronchial secreting cells and is often combined with codeine in cough syrups. The mucolytic agent acetylcysteine is administered to liquefy the viscid mucus seen in cystic fibrosis.

In summary, the respiratory system requires continuous input from the nervous system. The movement of the diaphragm, intercostal muscles, and other respiratory muscles is controlled by neurons of the respiratory center located in the pons and medulla. The control of breathing has both automatic and voluntary components. The automatic regulation of ventilation is controlled by two types of receptors: lung receptors, which protect respiratory structures, and the chemoreceptors, which monitor the gas exchange function of the lung by sensing changes in blood levels of carbon dioxide, oxygen, and *pH*. There are three types of lung receptors: stretch receptors, which monitor lung inflation; irritant receptors, which protect against the damaging effects of toxic inhalants; and J receptors, which are thought to sense lung congestion. There are two groups of chemoreceptors: central chemoreceptors and peripheral chemoreceptors. The central chemoreceptors are the most important in sensing changes in carbon dioxide levels; and the peripheral chemoreceptors, in sensing arterial blood oxygen levels. Voluntary respiratory control is needed for integrating breathing and actions such as speaking, blowing, and singing. These acts, which are initiated by the motor and premotor cortex, cause temporary suspension of automatic breathing.

Alterations in breathing patterns include tachypnea (rapid breathing), hyperpnea (increase in both the rate and depth of respiration), bradypnea (abnormally slow respiratory rate), and hyperventilation (respiration in excess of that needed to maintain a normal level of PCO_2). Periodic breathing is manifested by periods of apnea. Dyspnea is a subjective sensation of difficulty in breathing. The cough reflex protects the lungs from accumulation of secretions and injury from irritating substances. It is initiated by airway receptors and transmitted to the medullary cough center, which integrates the cough response. The protective functions of the cough reflex are impaired by weakness of the expiratory muscles, by conditions that prevent closure of the glottis, and by depressed function of the medullary cough center. The cough reflex can be suppressed by medications that (1) depress the medullary cough center, (2) soothe the irritated mucosal surface of the pharynx, or (3) act peripherally on the stretch receptors in the lung. Expectorants are drugs that decrease the viscosity of the respiratory tract secretions and thereby facilitate their expulsion from the respiratory tract.

■ Study Guide

After you have studied this chapter, you should be able to meet the following objectives:

☐ State the three major components of respiration.

☐ List the structures of the conducting airways and respiratory tissues.

☐ Describe the function of the mucociliary blanket.

☐ Define the term water vapor pressure.

☐ Cite the source of water for humidification of air as it moves through the airways.

☐ Explain the mechanisms whereby fever causes an increase in the viscosity of respiratory secretions.

☐ Relate the differences in anatomic structure of the right and left primary bronchi to the effect of foreign body aspiration and displacement of an endotracheal tube.

☐ Compare the supporting structures of the large and small airways in terms of cartilaginous and smooth muscle support.

☐ Describe the autonomic nervous system innervation of the airways.

☐ Relate the elastic properties of the lungs and chest wall to the creation of a negative intrapleural pressure.

☐ State the function of the three types of alveolar cells.

☐ Relate Boyle's law to inspiration and expiration.

☐ Explain how the law of partial pressure can be used to determine the pressure of a gas when its percentage of the total is known.

☐ Explain the effect that water vapor pressure has on the partial pressure of other alveolar gases.

☐ Compare atmospheric, airway, alveolar, and intrapleural pressures during the inspiratory and expiratory phases of ventilation.

☐ Define the terms inspiratory reserve, expiratory reserve, vital capacity, and residual volume.

☐ Describe the method for measuring FEV_1.

☐ State the formula for determining lung compliance.

☐ Use the law of Laplace to explain the need for surfactant in maintaining the inflation of small alveoli.

☐ State the major determinant of airway resistance.

☐ Explain why increasing lung volume (taking deep breaths) reduces airway resistance.

☐ Explain the effect of forced and normal expiratory effort on the volume of air that can be exhaled in a given period of time.

☐ Cite the difference between physiologic and anatomic dead air space.

☐ Trace the exchange of gases in the alveoli.

☐ Compare the distribution of blood flow and ventilation in the top and the bottom of the lungs in the standing and lying positions.

☐ Explain why ventilation and perfusion must be matched.

☐ List four factors that affect alveolar–capillary gas exchange.

☐ Explain the difference between PO_2 and hemoglobin-bound oxygen.

☐ Describe the transport of oxygen by hemoglobin.

☐ Explain the significance of *shift to the right* versus *shift to the left* in the oxygen-dissociation curve.

☐ State the significance of blood hemoglobin levels and the development of cyanosis.

☐ Explain why venous blood samples are not usually used for the measurement of blood gases.

☐ Define hypoxia.

☐ List the four types of hypoxia.

☐ State the manifestations of acute hypoxia.

☐ Explain how the body adapts to chronic hypoxia.

☐ Describe the difference between automatic and voluntary control of ventilation.

☐ Compare the role of the central and peripheral chemoreceptors in monitoring the PO_2 and PCO_2 levels of the blood.

☐ Cite the function of the lung receptors.

☐ Define four terms that are used to denote alterations in normal breathing.

☐ Describe the type of periodic breathing known as Cheyne–Stokes breathing.

☐ Define dyspnea.

☐ List three types of conditions in which dyspnea occurs.

☐ State the purpose of the cough reflex.

☐ Trace the physiologic mechanisms involved in coughing from the inhalation of an irritating substance to the actual expulsion effort of the cough.

☐ List four conditions that interfere with coughing.

☐ Compare the physiologic basis for the use of cough suppressants with that for the use of expectorants.

■ References

1. Ayres SM: Cigarette smoking and lung diseases. Basics of RD 5, No 5, 1975
2. Ham AW: Histology, 7th ed, p 719. Philadelphia, JB Lippincott, 1979
3. Berne RM, Levy MN: Physiology, p 655. St. Louis, CV Mosby, 1983

4. West JB: Respiratory Physiology, p 10. Baltimore, Williams & Wilkins, 1974

5. Robbins SL, Cotran RS, Kumar V: Pathologic Basis of Disease, 5th ed, p 484. Philadelphia, WB Saunders, 1984

6. Guyton A: Textbook of Medical Physiology, 6th ed, p 477, 542, 544. Philadelphia, WB Saunders, 1981

7. Branin PK: Physical assessment in acute respiratory failure. Crit Care Quart 1:27, 1979

8. Howell JBL, ed: Breathlessness. Philadelphia, FA Davis, 1966

9. Carrieri VK, Jansen-Berjklie S: The sensation of dyspnea: A critical review. Heart Lung 13:437, 1984

Chapter 23

Alterations in Respiratory Function

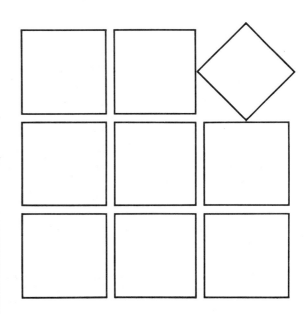

Respiratory illnesses represent one of the more common reasons for visits to the physician, admission to the hospital, and forced inactivity among all age groups. Forty-seven million Americans—children and adults—suffer from one or more chronic respiratory diseases. Each year more than 30,000 children under 5 years of age die of respiratory disease, more than 15,000 in the first year of life.[1] For purposes of discussion, the respiratory disorders included in this chapter have been divided into six groups: (1) infections, (2) disorders of the pleura, (3) obstructive lung disorders, (4) interstitial lung disease, (5) pulmonary vascular disease, and (6) lung cancer. Alterations in ventilation and respiratory failure are discussed in Chapter 24.

■ Respiratory Infections

The respiratory tract is susceptible to infectious processes caused by many types of microorganisms. For the most part, the signs and symptoms of respiratory tract infections depend on the function of the structure involved, the severity of the infectious process, and the person's age and general health. The discussion in this section of the chapter focuses on the common cold, acute respiratory tract infections in children, pneumonia, tuberculosis, and fungal infections of the lung.

The Common Cold

The common cold occurs more frequently than any other respiratory tract infection. Most adults have 2 to 4 colds per year; children may have up to 12 per year.[2] The condition usually begins with a feeling of dryness and stuffiness affecting mainly the nasopharynx; it is accompanied by excessive production of nasal secretions and lacrimation, or tearing of the eyes. Usually the secretions remain clear and watery. The mucous membranes of the upper respiratory tract become reddened, swollen, and bathed in mucous secretions. Involvement of the pharynx and larynx causes sore throat and hoarseness. Headache and generalized malaise may be present. In severe cases there may be chills, fever, and marked prostration. The disease process is usually self-limiting, lasting about 7 days.[2]

Although the condition can be caused by a number of viruses, the rhinovirus has been shown to cause the greatest percentage of diagnosed colds.[3] The first step in the spreading of a cold is the shedding of viruses, the area of greatest potential being the nasal mucosa. In infected individuals, the number of rhinoviruses was found to be 10 to 100 times greater in the nasal mucus than in pharyngeal secretions.[4] Studies have shown that colds are spread most frequently in the home or school.[5,6] The fingers are the most incriminated source of spread and

the nasal mucosa and conjunctival surface of the eyes the most important portals of entry of the virus. Cold viruses have been found to survive for 3.5 hours on the skin and hard surfaces, such as wood and plastic; survival is poor on facial tissue and porous cloth. The most highly contagious period of time is during the first 3 days following the onset of symptoms with an incubation period of about 5 days. Studies suggest that the aerosol spread of colds through coughing and sneezing is much less important than the spread by fingers picking up the virus from contaminated surfaces and carrying it to the nasal membranes and eyes.[6,7] This suggests that careful attention to hand washing is one of the most important preventive measures for avoiding the common cold.

A large number of over-the-counter remedies are available for treating the common cold. Because the common cold is an acute and self-limiting illness in persons who are otherwise healthy, treatment with antibiotics and other medications that are potentially harmful is contraindicated. Symptomatic treatment with rest and antipyretic drugs is all that is usually needed. Controversy exists regarding the use of vitamin C to reduce the incidence and severity of colds and influenza. Several studies have shown a reduced incidence,[8,9] whereas others have found that vitamin C had no effect on the number or severity of colds.[10] Antihistamines are popular over-the-counter drugs because of their action in drying nasal secretions. As with vitamin C, there is no evidence that antihistamines shorten the duration of the cold, and they may cause dizziness, drowsiness, and impaired judgment. They may also dry up bronchial secretions and worsen the cough. Decongestant drugs (sympathomimetic agents) are available in over-the-counter nasal sprays, drops, and oral cold medications. These drugs constrict the blood vessels in the swollen nasal mucosa and reduce nasal swelling. Rebound nasal swelling can occur with indiscriminate use of nasal drops and sprays. Oral preparations containing decongestants may cause systemic vasoconstriction and elevation of blood pressure when given in doses large enough to relieve nasal congestion; therefore, they should be avoided by persons with hypertension, heart disease, hyperthyroidism, diabetes mellitus, and other health problems.

Acute Respiratory Infections in Children

In children, respiratory tract infections are common; although they are troublesome, they are usually not serious. Frequent infections occur because the immune system of infants and small children has not been exposed to many common pathogens; consequently, they tend to develop infections with each new exposure. Although most such infections are not serious, the small size of an infant or child's airways tends to promote impaired airflow and obstruction. For example, an infection that causes only sore throat and hoarseness in an adult may result in serious airway obsruction in a small child.

Upper airway infections

Obstruction of the upper airways secondary to infection tends to exert its greatest effect during the inspiratory phase of respiration. Movement of air through an obstructed upper airway, particularly the vocal cords in the larynx, tends to produce a crowing sound called *stridor*. Impairment of the expiratory phase of respiration can also occur; this causes a *wheezing* (whistling) sound as air moves through the obstructed area. With mild to moderate obstruction, inspiratory stridor is more prominent than expiratory wheezing because the airways tend to dilate with expiration. When the swelling and obstruction become severe, the airways can no longer dilate during expiration and both stridor and wheezing occur.

Cartilaginous support of the trachea and the larynx is poorly developed in infants and small children. As a result, these structures are soft and tend to collapse when there is airway obstruction and a child cries, causing the inspiratory pressures to become more negative. When this happens both the stridor and inspiratory effect are increased. The phenomenon of airway collapse in the small child is analogous to what happens when a thick beverage, such as a milkshake, is drunk through a soft paper straw. The straw will collapse when the negative pressure produced by the sucking effort exceeds the flow of liquid through the straw.

The marked decrease in intrathoracic pressure resulting from increased inspiratory effort in the presence of airway obstruction also tends to cause retraction (sucking in) of the softer chest structures, such as the supraclavicular spaces, the sternum, the epigastrium, and the intercostal spaces. The increased inspiratory effort also causes flaring of the nares.

There are two upper respiratory tract infections of early childhood that are serious—croup and epiglottitis. Croup is the more common one, and it is usually benign and self-limiting. Epiglottitis, on the other hand, is rapidly progressive and life-threatening. The characteristics of both infections are described in Table 23-1.

Croup. Croup is a viral infection that affects the larynx, trachea, and bronchi. It is generally seen in children aged 3 months to 3 years. Because the subglottic area is normally the narrowest part of the respiratory tree in this age group, the obstruction is usually greatest in this area.[11]

Croup is characterized by inspiratory stridor, hoarseness, and a barking cough. The British use the term *croup* to describe the cry of the crow or raven, and this is undoubtedly how the term originated. One form of croup, spasmodic croup, characteristically occurs at night. The episode usually lasts several hours and may recur several nights in a row. Spasmodic croup tends to recur with subsequent respiratory infections.

Although the respiratory manifestations of croup often appear suddenly, they are usually preceded by upper respiratory infections that cause rhinorrhea (runny nose), coryza (common cold), hoarseness, and a low-grade fever. The symptoms usually subside when the child is exposed to moist air. For example, letting the bathroom shower run and then taking the child into the bathroom often brings prompt and dramatic relief of

Table 23-1 Characteristics of Epiglottitis, Croup, and Bronchiolitis in Small Children

Characteristics	Epiglottitis	Croup	Bronchiolitis
Common causative agent	*Hemophilus influenzae*, type B bacterium	Parainfluenza virus	Respiratory syncytial virus most common
Most commonly affected age group	1–5 years	3 months to 3 years	Less than 18 months (most severe in infants under 6 months)
Onset and preceding history	Sudden onset	Usually follows symptoms of a cold	Preceded by stuffy nose and other signs
Prominent features	Child appears very sick and toxic Sits with mouth open and chin thrust forward Low-pitched stridor, difficulty swallowing, fever, drooling, anxiety *Danger of airway obstruction and asphyxia*	Stridor and a wet, barking cough Usually occurs at night Relieved by exposure to cold or moist air	Breathlessness, rapid shallow breathing, wheezing, cough, and retractions of lower ribs and sternum during inspiration
Usual treatment	Intubation or tracheotomy Treatment with appropriate antibiotic	Mist tent or vaporizor Administration of oxygen	Supportive treatment, administration of oxygen and hydration

symptoms. A mist tent or vaporizer is used for more continuous treatment. Exposure to cold air also seems to relieve the airway spasm; often, the severe symptoms will be relieved simply because the child is exposed to cold air on the way to the hospital emergency room.

Other treatments may be required when a mist tent is ineffective. One method is to administer a racemic mixture of epinephrine (L-epinephrine and D-epinephrine) by positive pressure breathing through a face mask. A second method involves administration of the anti-inflammatory adrenal corticosteroid hormones. Establishment of an artificial airway may become necessary in severe airway obstruction.

Epiglottitis. Acute epiglottitis is caused by *Hemophilus influenzae*, type B bacterium. It is characterized by inflammatory edema of the supraglottic area, which includes the epiglottis and pharyngeal structures. It comes on suddenly bringing danger of airway obstruction and asphyxia; the child with epiglottitis requires immediate hospitalization.

The child appears pale, toxic, and lethargic and assumes a distinctive position—sitting up with the mouth open and the chin thrust forward. Difficulty in swallowing, a muffled voice, drooling, fever, and extreme anxiety are present.

Immediate establishment of an airway by either endotracheal tube or tracheotomy is usually needed. If epiglottitis is suspected, the child should never be forced to lie down because this causes the epiglottis to fall backward and may lead to complete airway obstruction. Examination of the throat with a tongue blade or other instrument may cause fatal airway obstruction and should be done only by medical personnel experienced in intubation of small children. It is also unwise to attempt any procedure, such as drawing blood, that would heighten the child's anxiety because this, too, could precipitate airway spasm and cause death.

Recovery from epiglottitis is usually rapid and uneventful once an adequate airway has been established and appropriate antibiotic therapy has been initiated.

Lower airway infections

Lower airway infections produce air trapping with prolonged expiration. Wheezing results from bronchospasm, mucosal inflammation, and edema. The child presents with increased expiratory effort, increased respiratory rate, and wheezing. If the infection is severe, there will also be marked intercostal retractions and signs of impending respiratory failure.

Bronchiolitis. Bronchiolitis is a viral infection of the lower airways, most commonly caused by the respiratory syncytial virus. Other viruses, such as adenovirus, para-

influenza, and rhinovirus, have also been implicated as causative agents. The infection produces inflammatory obstruction of the small airways and necrosis of the cells lining the airways. The child is usually able to take in sufficient air but has trouble exhaling it. Air becomes trapped in the lung distal to the site of obstruction and interferes with gas exchange. Hypoxemia and, in severe cases, hypercapnia may develop. Airway obstruction may produce air trapping and hyperinflation of the lungs or collapse of the alveoli. Bronchiolitis is usually seen in children under 18 months of age, the most serious cases occurring in babies under 6 months of age.

Babies with acute bronchiolitis have a typical appearance, marked by breathlessness with rapid respirations, a distressing cough, and retraction (drawing in) of the lower ribs and sternum. Crying, feeding, and activity exaggerate these signs. Wheezing and rales may or may not be present depending on the degree of airway obstruction. In infants with severe airway obstruction, wheezing decreases as the airflow diminishes. Generally the most critical phase of the disease is the first 24 to 72 hours.[12] Cyanosis, pallor, listlessness, and sudden diminution or absence of breath sounds indicate impending respiratory failure.

Treatment is supportive and includes administration of humidified oxygen to relieve hypoxia. A position that facilitates respiratory movements (elevation of the head) and avoids airway compression is used. Unnecessary handling is kept at a minimum to avoid tiring. Because the infection is viral, antibiotics are not effective and are given only for a secondary bacterial infection. Dehydration may occur as the result of increased insensible water losses because of the rapid respiratory rate and feeding difficulties, and measures to ensure adequate hydration are needed. Recovery begins after the first 48 to 72 hours and is usually rapid and complete.[13]

Signs of impending respiratory failure

Respiratory problems of infants and small children are often of sudden origin, and recovery is usually rapid and complete. However, children are at risk for development of airway obstruction and respiratory failure resulting from obstructive disorders or lung infection. The child with epiglottitis is at risk for development of airway obstruction; the child with bronchiolitis, for development of respiratory failure resulting from impaired gas exchange. The signs and symptoms of impending respiratory failure are listed in Chart 23-1.

Pneumonias

The term *pneumonia* describes inflammation of parenchymal structures of the lung, such as the alveoli and the bronchioles. Etiologic agents include both infectious

Chart 23-1 *Signs of Respiratory Distress and Impending Respiratory Failure in the Infant and Small Child*

- Cyanosis that is not relieved by administration of oxygen (40%)
- Heart rate of 150 per minute or greater and increasing
- Bradycardia
- Very rapid breathing (rate 60 per minute in the newborn to 6 months or above 30 in children 6 months to 2 years)
- Very depressed breathing (rate 20 per minute or below)
- Retractions of the supraclavicular area, sternum, epigastrium, and intercostal spaces
- Extreme anxiety and agitation
- Fatigue
- Decreased level of consciousness

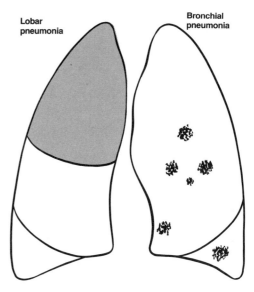

Figure 23-1 *Distribution of lung involvement in lobar and bronchial pneumonia.*

and noninfectious agents. For example, inhalation of irritating fumes or aspiration of gastric contents can result in severe pneumonia. Recently subtle changes have occurred in the spectrum of microorganisms causing infectious pneumonias, namely, a decrease in pneumonias caused by *Streptococcus pneumoniae* and an increase in pneumonias caused by other microorganisms such as *Pseudomonas, Candida* and other fungi, and nonspecific viruses. Many of these pneumonias occur in persons with impaired immune defenses. *Pneumocystis carinii,* a virulent type of pneumonia, has recently surfaced as a disease associated with an acquired immunodeficiency state.[16]

Pneumonias are usually classified according to their etiologic agent and their anatomic distibution. The anatomic distribution can be considered under three general headings: (1) lobar, (2) bronchial, and (3) interstitial. In lobar pneumonia, there is involvement of a large portion or an entire lobe of a lung (Fig. 23-1). With bronchopneumonia, there is a patchy consolidation with involvement of multiple lobules. These lesions vary in size from 3 cm to 4 cm and, because of gravity, are more common in the lower and posterior portions of the lung. In interstitial pneumonia, the inflammatory process is more or less confined to the area within the wall that surrounds the alveoli and bronchioles. This type of pneumonia is generally caused by viral or mycoplasma infections.

Although antibiotics have significantly reduced mortality due to pneumonias, these diseases remain an important immediate cause of death in the elderly and in persons with debilitating diseases. In 1981 pneumonia was the sixth leading cause of death in the United States.[14]

The normal lung is sterile. Most of the agents that cause pneumonia are inhaled into the lung in the air breathed. Depending on the population being examined, pneumococci have been shown to be present in the nasopharynx in 5% to 59% of healthy persons;[15] normally, respiratory tract defense mechanisms would prevent these organisms from entering the lung. Loss of the cough reflex, damage to the ciliated endothelium that lines the respiratory tract, and lowered resistance to infection all increase susceptibility to pneumonia. Persons with immunologic deficiencies, congestive heart failure, or hypostatic pulmonary edema are particularly prone to develop pneumonia. Table 23-2 summarizes respiratory tract defense mechanisms and factors that impair their effectiveness and thereby are predisposing factors to pneumonia.

Lobar pneumonia

Approximately 90% to 95% of cases of lobar pneumonia are caused by the pneumococcus *Streptococcus pneumoniae.*[17] Classically, lobar pneumonia occurs in otherwise healthy adults and is relatively uncommon in infants and the elderly.

The tissue changes in lobar pneumonia are consistent with signs of acute inflammation. This acute inflammatory response can be divided into four stages:(1) congestion, (2) red hepatization, (3) gray hepatization, and (4) resolution. Often its progress is modified by antibiotic therapy. The *congestive stage* represents the initial inflammatory response and is characterized by vascular engorgement of the alveolar vessels and transudation of serous fluid into the alveoli. The period of congestion lasts for about 24 hours and is followed by the stage of *red hepatization.* During this stage, there is extravasation of red blood cells and fibrin into the alveoli, and the lungs become firm and red with a liverlike

Table 23-2 Respiratory Defense Mechanisms and Conditions that Impair Their Effectiveness

Defense Mechanism	Function	Factors that Impair Effectiveness
Nasopharyngeal defenses	Remove particles from the air; contact with surface lysosomes and immunoglobulins (IgA) protect against infection	IgA deficiency state, hay fever, common cold, trauma to the nose, others
Glottic and cough reflexes	Protect against aspiration into tracheobronchial tree	Loss of cough reflex due to stroke or neural lesion, neuromuscular disease, abdominal or chest surgery, depression of the cough reflex due to sedation or anesthesia, presence of a nasogastric tube (tends to cause adaptation of afferent receptors)
Mucociliary blanket	Removes particles from the respiratory tract	Smoking, viral diseases, chilling, inhalation of irritating gases
Pulmonary macrophages	Remove microorganisms and foreign particles from the lung	Chilling, alcohol intoxication, smoking, anoxia

appearance—hence the term red hepatization. The stage of *gray hepatization* is characterized by an accumulation of fibrin and the beginning disintegration of the inflammatory white and red cells. Sometimes the infection extends into the pleural cavity causing *empyema*—pus in the pleural cavity. In untreated pneumonia, the stage of *resolution* occurs in about 8 to 10 days and represents the enzymatic digestion and removal of the inflammatory exudate from the infected lung area. The exudate is either coughed up or removed by macrophages.

The signs and symptoms of lobar pneumonia coincide with the stage of the disease. The onset is usually sudden and is characterized by malaise, a severe shaking chill, and fever. The temperature may go as high as 106°F. During the congestive stage, coughing brings up a watery sputum; and breath sounds are limited, with fine crepitant rales. As the disease progresses, the character of the sputum changes; it may be blood tinged (or rust colored) to purulent. Pleuritic pain, a sharp pain that is more severe with respiratory movements, is common. With antibiotic therapy, fever usually subsides in about 48 to 72 hours and recovery is uneventful.

Bronchopneumonia

Bronchopneumonia is considered to be a disease of the very young, the very old, and the debilitated—the very young because their immunologic reserve and respiratory defense mechanisms have not as yet developed and the very old because of a decline in immunity and because many have other diseases that predispose them to pneumonia.

Virtually any pathogenic organism can cause bronchopneumonia. Hospitalized patients are susceptible to bacteria present in the environment. These infections have been reported to occur in 0.5% to 5.0% of all hospitalized patients and in 12% of those sick enough to be admitted to intensive care units.[18] These nosocomial (hospital-acquired) infections are usually due to gram-negative microorganisms and are resistant to microbial therapy. Proper hand washing and decontamination of inhalation equipment is important in preventing these infections.

In contrast to lobar pneumonia, which has a rapid onset, the early manifestations of bronchopneumonia are often insidious and in most cases include a low-grade fever along with a cough and inspiratory rales. Complications include formation of a lung abscess, empyema, and bacteremia.

Viral or mycoplasmal pneumonias

Viral pneumonias can occur as a primary infection or as a complication of other diseases, such as chickenpox and measles. The influenza virus is the most common cause of viral pneumonia. In the adult, chickenpox is associated with pneumonia in 10% to 15% of cases, with a mortality rate of about 20%.[19] The mycoplasmas are the smallest free-living agents of disease, having characteristics of both viruses and bacteria. Pneumonias due to the mycoplasmas are sometimes called *primary atypical pneumonias*.

Viral or atypical pneumonias involve the interstitium of the lung and may masquerade as chest colds, with manifestations often confined to fever, headache, and muscle aches and pains. Viruses impair the respiratory tract defenses and are predisposing factors to secondary bacterial infections.

Immunization

Vaccines are available to protect against the influenzal infections and pneumococcal pneumonia. These vaccines are recommended for high-risk groups who, because of their age or underlying health problems, are unable to cope well with these infections and often require medical attention, including hospitalization. For example, influenza outbreaks in nursing homes resulted in infection rates as high as 60%, with mortality rates of 30% or more.[20]

Influenza immunization.   Several strains of the influenza virus are responsible for epidemics of the disease. These strains undergo small changes over time that affect their antigenicity and the host protection afforded by previous immunization. The greatest impact of influenza is normally seen when new strains appear against which the population lacks immunity. Therefore, the formulation of the influenza vaccine must be changed yearly in anticipation of changes in the influenza virus. Each year the Public Health Advisory Committee on Immunization Practices updates its recommendations for the composition of the vaccine.

Currently, the Immunization Practices Advisory Committee recommends annual vaccination using inactivated influenza vaccine to prevent or minimize the effect of influenza infections in high-risk groups.[20,21] The high-risk group has been classified into three categories according to priority of need. The highest-priority groups are adults and children with chronic cardiovascular or pulmonary system disorders severe enough to have required regular medical follow-ups or hospitalization during the preceding year and residents of nursing homes and other chronic-care facilities. Of second priority are medical personnel working with high-risk patients. Although not proven, it is believed that these personnel may transfer influenza infections to their patients. The third-priority group includes otherwise healthy individuals who are over 65 years of age and adults and children with chronic metabolic diseases such as diabetes mellitus, kidney dysfunction, anemia, or asthma severe enough to have required regular medical checkups or hospitalization during the previous year.

Pneumococcal immunization.   Like influenza, pneumococcal pneumonia causes significant morbidity and mortality in high-risk groups. A 23-valent pneumococcal vaccine, composed of antigens from 23 types of *Streptococcus Pneumoniae* (pneumococcus) was licensed in the United States in 1983, replacing the 14-valent type licensed in 1977. At present, pneumococcal vaccine is given only once; revaccination is not recommended. This is because local and systemic reactions are common among persons who receive second doses. At present, it is also recommended that persons who have received the 14-valent type of vaccine should not be revaccinated with the 23-valent vaccine.[22]

Vaccination with the pneumococcal vaccine is recommended for adults with chronic illnesses, particularly cardiovascular and pulmonary diseases, who sustain increased morbidity with respiratory infections. Vac-

cination is also recommended for adults with other chronic illnesses associated with increased risk of pneumococcal infections and for otherwise healthy older adults, especially those aged 65 and over. Children aged 2 years and older with chronic illnesses such as sickle cell disease, splenectomy, nephrotic syndrome, cerebrospinal fluid leaks, or conditions associated with immunosuppression should also be immunized.[22]

Tuberculosis

Tuberculosis is an infectious disease caused by *Mycobacterium tuberculosis*. The mycobacteria are slender rod-shaped, acid-fast, aerobic organisms. There are two forms of tuberculosis that pose a particular threat in humans—*Mycobacterium tuberculosis* and *Mycobacterium bovis*. Bovine tuberculosis is acquired by drinking milk from infected cows and has its initial effects on the gastrointestinal tract. This form of tuberculosis has been virtually eradicated in North America and other developed countries as a result of rigorous controls of dairy herds and pasteurization of milk. There has been a recent increase in the United States of atypical mycobacterial infections, including those caused by Group I, *Mycobacterium kansasii*, and Group III, *Mycobacterium intracellularis*.

The incidence of tuberculosis in the United States has decreased markedly during the past several decades, with active cases falling from 76.7 per 100,000 in 1932 to 11.0 per 100,000 in 1982.[23] At present most infected persons are over age 30, and it has been suggested that most new cases will arise in persons already exposed to the disease. It has been estimated that 95% of children living in the United States will reach full maturity without ever having been exposed to the disease.[24]

Transmission

Tuberculosis is an airborne infection spread by *droplet nuclei*—minute, invisible particles harbored in the respiratory secretions of persons with active tuberculosis. Although the secretions often contain many larger particles, these larger particles tend to be filtered out of the air by gravity. If the larger particles are inhaled, they are usually trapped in the nasopharyngeal area and are removed by the action of the mucociliary blanket. Consequently, it is only the droplet nuclei that contribute to the transmission of the disease. These nuclei remain suspended in air and are circulated by air currents. They are so small that when inhaled they travel directly to the alveoli.

Pathogenesis

The destructiveness of tuberculosis is due not to the inherently destructive tubercle bacillus, but to the hypersensitivity response it evokes. For purposes of discussion, tuberculosis can be divided into primary and secondary infections; the initial infection is classified as primary tuberculosis and subsequent infections as secondary tuberculosis.

Primary tuberculosis is usually initiated in the alveolar wall as a result of inhaling tubercle bacilli. Primary tuberculosis has sometimes been called childhood tuberculosis, probably because contact with the disease occurred during childhood. The process begins as an acute inflammatory response and progresses to a chronic granulomatous inflammation (Chap. 8). Cell-mediated immunity and hypersensitivity reactions contribute to the evolution of the disease.

The initial response of the involved alveolar tissue is a local nonspecific pneumonitis. With initiation of the inflammatory response, polymorphonuclear leukocytes enter the area and phagocytize the bacilli but do not kill them. Within about 24 to 48 hours the polymorphonuclear cells are replaced by macrophages (histiocytes). Many of the bacilli engulfed by the macrophages remain viable and proliferate. At some time, approximately days 10 to 20, the infiltrating macrophages begin to elongate and fuse together to form an epithelioid cell tubercle, which becomes surrounded by lymphocytes. One or more tubercles may form. Following this period of time, the central portion of the lesion undergoes necrosis and forms a yellow cheesy mass called *caseous necrosis*. The tuberculin skin test becomes positive at about the time that the caseous necrosis occurs, suggesting that the necrosis results from the hypersensitivity response. Healing of the tubercular lesion occurs as collagenous scar tissue forms and encapsulates the lesion. In time most of these lesions become calcified and are visible on a chest x-ray film. The primary lesion is known as a *Ghon focus*, and the combination of the tubercle lesion and the involved lymph nodes is the *Ghon complex*. The Ghon complex may contain viable organisms.

Occasionally, primary tuberculosis may progress, eroding into a bronchus and there discharging the contents of its necrotic center. An air-filled cavity forms, permitting bronchogenic spread of the disease. In rare instances, tuberculosis may erode into a blood vessel, giving rise to hematogenic dissemination. *Miliary tuberculosis* decribes minute lesions resulting from this type of dissemination and may involve almost any organ, particularly the brain, meninges, liver, kidney, and bone marrow.

Secondary tuberculosis usually results from reactivation of a previously healed primary lesion. It often occurs in situations of impaired body defense mechanisms. The partial immunity that follows initial exposure affords protection against reinfection and to some extent aids in localizing the disease should secondary infection occur. The hypersensitivity reaction, on the other hand, is an aggravating factor in secondary tuberculosis, as evidenced by the frequency of cavitation and bronchial dissemination. The cavities may coalesce to a size of up to 10 cm to 15 cm in diameter. Pleural effusion and tuberculous empyema are common as the disease progresses.

Clinical manifestions

Primary tuberculosis is usually asymptomatic, the only evidence of the disease being a positive tuberculin skin test and the presence of calcified lesions on the chest x-ray film. Secondary tuberculosis may also be asymptomatic, particularly when the lesion is confined to the apices or upper portions of the lung. Often, however, there is an insidious onset of afternoon elevation of temperature, night sweats, slight cough with mucoid sputum, weakness, fatigability, and loss of appetite and weight. As the disease advances, there may be dyspnea and orthopnea.

Diagnostic measures

The most frequently used screening methods for tuberculosis are the tuberculin skin tests and chest x-ray studies. Cultures (bacteriologic studies) of the sputum or gastric contents determine the presence of the organism. Gastric contents are aspirated after a fast of 8 to 10 hours, usually as the patient arises in the morning. These secretions contain tubercle bacilli swallowed during the night.

The tuberculin skin test was introduced by Robert Koch in the late 19th century. The test measures delayed hypersensitivity (cell-mediated, type IV) that follows exposure to the tubercle bacillus. It is important to recognize that a positive reaction to the skin test does not mean that a person has tuberculosis, only that there has been exposure to the bacillus and that cell-mediated immunity to the organism has developed.

There are two skin tests, the multiple puncture technique and the intercutaneous technique. In the multiple puncture technique, use of purified protein derivative (PPD)—for example, in the Aplitest, SlavoTest PPD, Heaf test, or old tuberculin (Tine, MonoVacc) test—is the preferred method. A positive response is manifested by vesicle formation at the test site. The quantity of tuberculin introduced under the skin using the multiple puncture technique cannot be precisely controlled. For this reason the multiple puncture methods are not intended as diagnostic tests but are used as initial screening procedures in asymptomatic persons who have not been exposed to someone with tuberculosis. Verification of the reaction to a multiple puncture test is recommended by the standard Mantoux test unless vesicle formation is present.[25] The intercutaneous or Mantoux test (Aplisol or Tubersol) is the standard test for suspected tuberculosis. A positive reaction is evidenced by a discrete area of skin elevation of 10 mm or more. In tuberculosis, the areas of induration usually are between 15 mm and 20 mm or more.

Classification

The general classification of tuberculosis, published in 1980 by the American Thoracic Society, is as follows:[26]

0.   No tuberculosis exposure, not infected. No history of exposure, reaction to tuberculin skin test not significant.
1.   Tuberculosis exposure, no evidence of infection. History of exposure, reaction to tuberculin skin test not significant.
2.   Tuberculosis infection, no disease. Significant reaction to tuberculin skin test, negative bacteriologic studies (if done), no clinical or x-ray evidence of tuberculosis.
3.   Tuberculosis, current disease. Tuberculosis cultured (if done), otherwise both a significant reaction to the tuberculin test and clinical or x-ray evidence of current tuberculosis infection. The status of patient's tuberculosis is described by: location of disease, bacteriologic status, chemotherapy status, x-ray findings, and tuberculin skin test reaction. A person remains in Class 3 until treatment for the current episode of the disease has been completed.
4.   Tuberculosis, no current disease. History of previous episode of tuberculosis or x-ray findings in a person with significant reaction to tuberculin skin test, negative bacteriologic studies, no clinical or x-ray evidence of current disease.
5.   Tuberculosis suspect, diagnosis pending.

In some cases, additional features—x-ray findings and the tuberculin skin test reaction—are included.

Treatment

Tuberculosis is an unusual disease in that chemotherapy is required for a long time. The tubercle bacillus is an aerobic organism that multiplies slowly and remains relatively dormant in oxygen-poor caseous material. It undergoes a high rate of mutation and tends to develop a resistance to any one drug. For this reason, multiple drug regimens are used, except for prophylaxis. The primary drugs used in the treatment of tuberculosis are isoniazid (INH), rifampin, ethambutol, and streptomycin. Secondary drugs include aminosalicylic acid (PAS), ethionamide, capreomycin, kanamycin, pyrazinamide, and viomycin. The secondary drugs are usually considered only when resistance to the primary choice drugs develops. All of these drugs act by inhibiting the growth of the tubercle bacillus.

Isoniazid is remarkably potent against the tubercle bacillus and is probably the most widely used drug in tuberculosis. Although its exact mechanism of action is unknown, it apparently combines with an enzyme that is needed by the INH-susceptible strains of the tuberculous bacillus. Resistance to the drug develops rapidly, and combination with other effective drugs delays the development of resistance. Rifampin inhibits RNA synthesis in bacteria. Although ethambutol is known to inhibit the growth of the tubercle bacillus, its mechanism of action is unknown. Streptomycin, the first drug found to be effective against tuberculosis, must be given parenterally, which limits its usefulness particularly in long-term therapy. It remains an important drug in tuberculosis therapy and is used primarily in individuals with severe, possibly life-threatening forms of tuberculosis.

Two groups of persons meet the criteria established for the use of antimycobacterial therapy for tuberculosis: the first consists of those who have contact with cases of active tuberculosis and who are at risk for developing an active form of the disease (classification 1 or 2); the second group includes persons with active tuberculosis (classification 3).

INH is commonly used prophylactically in the first group. This group includes persons with a positive skin test who (1) have had close contact with active cases of tuberculosis, (2) have converted from a negative to positive skin test within two years, (3) have a history of untreated tuberculosis or x-ray evidence of asymptomatic tuberculosis, (4) have special risk factors such as immunosuppression or silicosis, and (5) are 35 years of age or under with a positive reaction of unknown duration. Because INH can cause hepatitis, persons being treated with the drug should be followed closely and warned of symptoms of the disease.[27,28]

Based on several recent trials, a marked change in chemotherapy for uncomplicated tuberculosis has developed. Short-course programs of therapy (usually 9 months) have replaced the traditional 18-to-24-month traditional multidrug regimens. The goals of short-course treatment are to achieve rapid elimination of the organism (as indicated by sputum culture) and to prevent relapse. Therapy is usually initiated with INH and rifampin. If drug resistance is possible, ethambutol is added to the regimen until sensitivity studies are obtained. If the organism is found to be sensitive to INH and rifampin, ethambutol is discontinued. The drug therapy should be continued for 6 months after the sputum culture is negative. Because 90% of patients have a negative culture by 3 months, the total duration of the treatment is usually 9 months. After the therapy is completed, the patients are followed for a minimum of 12 months.[26,29]

Fungal Infections of the Lung

Although the spores of fungi are constantly present in the air we breathe, only a few reach the lung and cause disease. The most common of these are histoplasmosis coccidioidomycosis, and blastomycosis. These infections are usually mild and self-limiting and are seldom noticed unless they produce local complications or progressive dissemination occurs. The signs and symptoms of these infections commonly resemble tuberculosis.

Histoplasmosis

Histoplasmosis, caused by the dimorphic fungus (Chap. 7) *Histoplasma capsulatum,* is the most common fungal infection in the United States. On the basis of skin testing surveys, 18% to 20% of persons in the United States have been infected with the disease.[30] Most cases occur along the major river valleys of the Midwest—the Ohio, the Mississippi, and the Missouri. The organism grows in soil and other areas that have been enriched with bird excreta: old chicken houses, pigeon lofts, barns, and trees where birds roost. The infection is acquired by inhaling the fungal spores that are released when the dirt or dust from the infected areas is disturbed. The spores convert to the parasitic yeast phase when exposed to body temperature in the alveoli. The organisms are then carried to the regional lymphatics and from there they are disseminated throughout the body in the bloodstream. They are removed from the circulation by fixed macrophages of the reticuloendothelial system. When delayed hypersensitivity develops (Chap. 10), the macrophages are usually able to destroy the fungi.

The manifestations of histoplasmosis are strikingly similar to those of tuberculosis. Depending on the host resistance and immunocompetence, the disease usually takes one of four forms: (1) latent asymptomatic disease, (2) self-limiting primary disease, (3) chronic pulmonary disease, or (4) disseminated infection. The average incubation period for the infection is about 14 days. Only 40% of infected persons have symptoms and only about 10% of these are ill enough to see a physician.[31] *Asymptomatic latent histoplasmosis* is characterized by evidence of healed lesions in the lungs or hilar lymph nodes accompanied by a positive histoplasmin skin test (analogous to the tuberculin test). *Primary pulmonary histoplasmosis* occurs in otherwise healthy people as a mild, self-limiting, febrile, respiratory infection. Its symptoms include muscle and joint pains and a nonproductive cough. Erythema nodosum (subcutaneous nodules) or erythema multiforme (hivelike lesions) sometimes appear. During this stage of the disease, chest x-rays usually show single or multiple infiltrates.

Chronic histoplasmosis is similar to secondary tuberculosis. Infiltration of the upper lobes of one or both lungs with cavitation occurs. This form of the disease is more common in middle-aged men who smoke and in persons with chronic lung disease. The most common manifestations are productive cough, fever, night sweats, and weight loss. In many persons, the disease may be self-limiting. In others there is progressive destruction of lung tissue and dissemination of the disease.

Disseminated histoplasmosis can follow either primary or chronic histoplasmosis but most often develops as an acute and fulminating infection in the very old or the very young, or in persons with compromised immune function. Although the macrophages of the reticuloendothelial system can remove the fungi from the bloodstream, they are unable to destroy them.[31] Characteristically this form of the disease produces a high fever, generalized lymph node enlargement, hepatosplenomegaly, muscle wasting, anemia, leukopenia, and thrombocytopenia. There may be hoarseness, ulcerations of the mouth and tongue, nausea, vomiting, diarrhea, and abdominal pain. Often, meningitis becomes a dominant feature of the disease.

Absolute diagnosis of histoplasmosis requires cultural identification of the organism. The infection incites a delayed hypersensitivity immune response and the histoplasmin skin test is used to test for exposure to the disease. This test remains positive after the initial infection has occurred and does not indicate whether the disease is of recent or past origin. In addition to the delayed response, the humoral immune system responds to the acute infection by producing antibodies. Though these antibodies are not protective, they serve as markers of infection. These antibodies can be measured by means of the complement fixation (CF) test. An immunodiffusion (ID) test can also be used as a test for the antibodies. Both the CF and ID become positive 2 weeks after the onset of symptoms. The antifungal drugs amphotericin B and ketoconazole are used for persons with disease severe enough to require treatment or those with compromised immune function who are at risk for developing disseminated disease. Amphotericin B is given intravenously and is usually the drug of choice in severe disease. The drug can impair kidney and liver function and produce anemia. Ketoconazole is given orally and takes up to 3 weeks to produce its effect.

Coccidioidomycosis

Coccidioidomycosis is a common fungal infection caused by inhaling the spores of *Coccidioides immitis.* An estimated 100,000 new cases occur annually.[31] It is most prevalent in the southwestern United States. About 80% of persons in the San Joaquin Valley are coccidioidin positive.[17] Because of its prevalence in this area, the disease is sometimes referred to as San Joaquin fever or valley fever. The disease resembles tuberculosis, and its mechanisms of infection are similar to those of histoplasmosis.

The disease most commonly occurs as an acute, primary self-limiting pulmonary infection with or without systemic involvement, but in some cases it progresses to a disseminated disease. About 60% of exposed persons only manifest a positive skin test (either coccidioidin skin test or spherulin skin test) and are unaware of the infection.[31] In the other 40% the illness usually resembles influenza. There may be fever, a cough, and pleuritic pain, accompanied by erythema multiforme or erythema nodosum. The skin lesions are usually accompanied by arthralgias or arthritis without effusion, particularly of the ankles and knees. The terms desert bumps and desert arthritis are used to describe these manifestations. The presence of skin and joint manifestations indicates strong host defenses, because persons who have had them seldom develop disseminated disease. Disseminated disease occurs in 1 out of 6000 infected persons or in fewer than 0.5% of persons with symptomatic disease. The commonly affected structures in disseminated disease are the lymph nodes, meninges, spleen, liver, kidney, skin, and adrenals. Meningitis is the most common cause of death.

Positive diagnosis of coccidioidomycosis can be made by direct visualization of spherules (multinucleated parasitic *Coccidioides immitis* cells) in the expectorated sputum after application of 10% potassium hydroxide. Although cultures can be used to identify the fungus, it is positive in only about half of the cases. Furthermore, extreme caution is needed when handling this fungus because laboratory personnel can be easily infected. Two serologic tests, the tube-precipitin (TP) test and the complement-fixation (CF) test, are considered to be extremely useful in establishing a diagnosis of coccidioidomycosis. The CF test may be used in following the progress of the disease; an elevated CF titer is considered to indicate risk of disease dissemination. The skin tests with coccidioidin and spherulin do not indicate whether the disease is recent or has occurred in the past. Their main value is in epidemiologic studies and for confirmation of the diagnosis in persons who convert from a negative to a positive test during an illness. As with histoplasmosis, the antifungal drugs amphotericin B and ketoconazole are used in the treatment of progressive or disseminated diseases.

Blastomycosis

Blastomycosis is caused by the organism *Blastomyces dermatitidis*. It is characterized by local suppurative and granulomatous lesions of the lungs and skin. The disease is most commonly found in North America and is particularly prevalent in the southeastern and south central states.

The symptoms of acute infection are similar to those of acute histoplasmosis, including fever, cough, aching of the joints and muscles, and, uncommonly, pleuritic pain.

In contrast to histoplasmosis, the cough in blastomycosis is often productive and the sputum is purulent. Acute pulmonary infections are usually self-limiting or progressive. Extrapulmonary spread most commonly involves the skin, bones, or prostate gland. These lesions may provide the first evidence of the disease.

The diagnosis of blastomycosis is more difficult than that of histoplasmosis. Visualization of the yeast in the sputum after application of 10% potassium hydroxide provides a presumptive diagnosis. When this fails, cultural isolation of the fungus is often attempted. The blastomycin skin test lacks specificity and is no longer available. The treatment of the progressive or disseminated form of the disease includes the use of amphotericin B or ketoconazole.

In summary, respiratory infections are the most common cause of respiratory illness. They include the common cold, respiratory infections common to children, pneumonias, and tuberculosis. The common cold occurs more frequently than any other respiratory infection. The fingers are the most incriminated source of transmission, and the most common portals of entry are the nasal mucosa and the conjunctiva of the eye. Because of the smallness of the airway of infants and children, respiratory tract infections in them are often more serious. Infections that may cause only a sore throat and hoarseness in the adult may produce serious obstruction in the child. Among the respiratory tract infections that affect small children are croup, epiglottitis, and bronchiolitis. Epiglottitis is a life-threatening supraglottic infection carrying the danger of airway obstruction and asphyxia. Pneumonia describes an infection of the parenchymal tissues of the lung. Lobar pneumonia involves a large portion or lobe of the lung and is usually caused by the *Pneumococcus*. Bronchopneumonia is caused by a number of agents. It is characterized by patchy consolidation of multiple lobes of the lung and frequently affects persons with other debilitating diseases. It can be caused by numerous agents. Viral or atypical pneumonia can occur as a primary infection, such as that caused by influenza virus, or as a complication of other viral infections, such as measles. Viral and atypical pneumonias involve the interstitium of the lung and often masquerade as chest colds. Vaccines are available for the immunization of persons in high-risk groups for the development of influenzal or pneumococcal pneumonias. Tuberculosis is a chronic respiratory infection caused by the *Mycobacterium tuberculosis*. The incidence of tuberculosis, which is now being treated effectively with chemotherapeutic drugs, has decreased sharply in the past four to five decades. Infections caused by the fungi *Histoplasma capsulatum* (histoplasmosis), *Coc-*

cidioides immitis (coccidioidomycosis), and *Blastomyces dermatitidis* (blastomycosis) resemble tuberculosis. These infections are common but seldom serious unless they produce progressive destruction of lung tissue or the infection disseminates outside the lungs.

Disorders of the Pleura

The pleura is a thin double-layered membrane that encases the lungs. The inner visceral pleura lies adjacent to the lung; the outer parietal layer covers the inner aspect of the chest wall, the superior aspect of the diaphragm, and the mediastinum. The visceral and parietal pleurae are separated by a thin layer of serous fluid, and the potential space between the two layers is called the *pleural cavity*. The space between the right and left pleural cavities is completely separated by the mediastinum, which contains the heart and other thoracic structures. Because of the inward elastic recoil forces of the lung and the outward elastic recoil of the chest wall, the pressure within the pleural space is negative. It becomes more negative as the chest expands during inspiration and less negative as the chest contracts during expiration. It is the negative pressure within the pleural cavity that keeps the lungs from collapsing. Disorders of the pleura include pain, pneumothorax, and pleural effusion.

Pleural Pain

Pain is one of the most common symptoms of conditions that cause inflammation of the pleura. Most commonly the pain is abrupt in onset, that is, the person experiencing it can cite almost to the minute when the pain started. It is usually unilateral, and tends to be localized to the lower and lateral part of the chest. Although the pain may radiate to the shoulder or abdomen, it does not usually originate from the substernal, paravertebral, or any other central part of the chest. The pain is usually made worse by chest movements, such as coughing and deep breathing, that exaggerate pressure changes within the pleural cavity and increase movement of the inflamed or injured pleural surfaces. Because deep breathing is painful, tidal volumes are usually kept small and breathing becomes rapid. Reflex muscle splinting usually occurs on the affected side, causing a lesser excursion of the affected side during respiration and development of atelectasis.

It is usually important to differentiate pleural pain from pain produced by other conditions, such as musculoskeletal strain of chest muscles, bronchial irritation, and myocardial disease. Musculoskeletal pain may occur as the result of frequent forceful coughing. This type of pain is usually bilateral and located in the inferior portions of the rib cage where the abdominal muscles insert into the anterior rib cage. It is usually made worse by those movements associated with contraction of the abdominal muscles. The pain associated with irritation of the bronchi is usually substernal and dull in character, rather than sharp; it is usually worse with coughing but is not affected by deep breathing. Myocardial pain, which was discussed in Chapter 19, is usually located in the substernal area and is not associated with respiratory movements.

Although analgesic and narcotic drugs reduce awareness of pleural pain, they usually do not entirely relieve the discomfort associated with coughing and deep breathing. The nonsteroidal antiinflammatory drug indomethacin has been used successfully for relieving pain and facilitating effective coughing.[30]

Pneumothorax

Pneumothorax refers to an accumulation of air within the pleural cavity with a resultant partial or complete collapse of the affected lung. *Spontaneous pneumothorax* occurs when an air-filled bleb, or blister, on the lung surface ruptures and air leaks into the pleural cavity. In *secondary pneumothorax*, air enters the pleural space as the result of injury to the chest wall, respiratory structures, or esophagus. *Tension pneumothorax* describes the condition in which the pressure within the pleural space is greater than the atmospheric pressure during the entire respiratory cycle.

What causes the air-filled blebs responsible for spontaneous pneumothorax and why they rupture are unknown. The incidence of spontaneous pneumothorax is greatest in young men. It may also occur in lung diseases, such as chronic obstructive lung disease, which cause trapping of gases and destruction of lung tissue. Because the pressure in the pleural space is normally negative in relation to the pressure within the alveoli, rupture of the lung surface allows air to enter the pleural space; the lung collapses as a result of its own recoil. The air leak will usually continue until the decline in lung size causes it to seal.

Secondary pneumothorax may be caused by penetrating or nonpenetrating injuries. Fractured or dislocated ribs with penetration of the pleura is the most common cause of pneumothorax due to nonpenetrating chest injuries. An accompanying hemothorax is common with these types of injuries. Pneumothorax may also occur because of fracture of the trachea or major bronchus or rupture of the esophagus. Persons with pneumothorax due to chest trauma frequently have other complications and may require chest surgery.

A tension pneumothorax is a life-threatening situation. It occurs when injury to the chest or respiratory structures permits air to enter but not leave the pleural space, with the lesion acting as a one-way valve (Fig. 23-2). This results in a rapid increase in pressure within the chest, a compression atelectasis of the unaffected lung, a shift in the mediastinum to the opposite side of the chest, and compression of the vena cava with impairment of venous return to the heart. Emergency treatment of tension pneumothorax involves the prompt insertion of a large-bore needle or chest tube into the affected side of the chest along with water-seal drainage or continuous chest suction to aid in lung reexpansion. The sucking of air into the thoracic cavity through an open chest wound can often be prevented by promptly covering the area with an airtight covering (*e.g.,* Vaseline gauze or a firm piece of plastic). It is essential, however, that the covering be secured in a manner that seals the wound during inspiration and allows air to exit during expiration.

Manifestations

The manifestations of pneumothorax depend on its size and the integrity of underlying lung. In spontaneous pneumothorax, manifestations of the disorder include development of pleuritic pain in an otherwise healthy individual. There is an almost immediate increase in respiratory rate as a result of the activation of receptors that monitor lung volume; this may be accompanied by dyspnea. An asymmetry of the chest may be present because of the presence of increased air trapped in the pleural cavity of the affected side. The asymmetry of the affected side may be evidenced during inspiration as a lag in the movement of the affected side (the affected side of the chest does not begin to move until after the unaffected side has reached the same degree of inflation as the lung with the air trapped in the pleural space). Percussion of the chest produces a more hyperresonant sound because of an increased air-to-fluid ratio, and breath sounds are decreased over the area of the pneumothorax. If the pneumothorax is large, the structures in the mediastinal space will shift toward the unaffected side of the chest (Fig. 23-2). When this occurs, the position of the trachea, normally located in the midline of the neck, deviates with the mediastinum. The position of the trachea can be used as a means of assessing this portion of the chest. There may be distention of the neck veins and subcutaneous emphysema (movement of air into the subcutaneous tissues of the chest and neck) and clinical signs of shock.

Hypoxemia usually develops immediately after a large pneumothorax followed by vasoconstriction of the blood vessels in the affected lung, causing the blood flow to shift to the unaffected lung. In persons with spontaneous pneumothorax, this mechanism usually returns oxygen saturation to normal within about 24 hours.

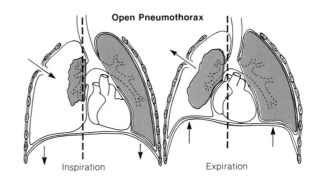
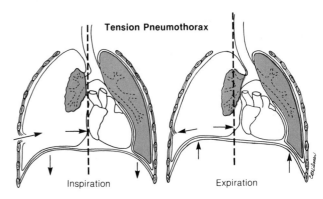

Figure 23-2 *Open or communicating pneumothorax (top) and tension pneumothorax (bottom). In an open pneumothorax, air enters the chest during inspiration and exits during expiration. There may be slight inflation of the affected lung due to a decrease in pressure as air moves out of the chest. In tension pneumothorax, air can enter but not leave the chest. As the pressure in the chest increases the heart and great vessels are compressed and a shift occurs in the mediastinal structures toward the unaffected side of the chest. The trachea is pushed from its normal midline position toward the unaffected side of the chest and the unaffected lung is compressed.*

Diagnosis and treatment

Diagnosis of pneumothorax can be confirmed by chest x-ray. The treatment of pneumothorax varies with the extent of the disorder. Even without treatment, air within the pleural space usually reabsorbs once the pleural leak seals. In small spontaneous pneumothoraces, the air usually reabsorbs spontaneously and only observation and follow-up chest x-rays are required. In larger pneumothoraces, the air is removed by needle aspiration or underwater seal drainage with or without an aspiration pump. This type of drainage system allows the air to exit the pleural space through a tube that is immersed in water, with the water acting as a one-way valve to prevent the air from reentering the chest. In secondary pneumothorax, surgical closure of the chest wall defect, ruptured airway, or perforated esophagus may be required.

Pleural Effusion

Normally only a thin layer (usually less than 10 ml-20 ml) of serous fluid separates the visceral and parietal layers of the pleural cavity. Pleural effusion refers to a collection of fluid in the pleural cavity. The fluid may be a transudate, exudate, chyle, or blood.

Like edema developing elsewhere in the body, pleural effusion occurs when the rate of fluid formation exceeds the rate of its removal (see Chap. 26). Five mechanisms have been linked to the abnormal collection of fluid in the pleural cavity: (1) increased capillary pressure, as in congestive heart failure; (2) increased capillary permeability, which occurs with inflammatory conditions; (3) decreased colloidal osmotic pressure, such as the hypoalbuminemia occurring with liver disease and nephrosis; (4) increased intrapleural negative pressure, which develops with atelectasis; and (5) impaired lymphatic drainage of the pleural space, which is usually due to obstructive processes such as mediastinal carcinoma.[32]

Pleural effusion may involve the presence of a transudate or exudate, depending on the protein content of the fluid. A transudate has a protein content of less than 3.0 gm/ml and an exudate a protein content greater than 3.0 gm/ml. Additional criteria that may be used to define a pleural exudate are (1) a pleural fluid-to-serum-protein ratio greater than 0.5, (2) a pleural lactic dehydrogenase (LDH) exceeding 200 IU, or (3) a pleural fluid-to-serum-LDH ratio exceeding 0.6.[33] The LDH is a protein marker and is easily measured. Conditions that produce exudative pleural effusions are infections, pulmonary infarction, malignancies, rheumatoid arthritis, and lupus erythematosus. *Empyema* refers to pus in the pleural cavity; it can be caused by direct spread from adjacent bacterial pneumonia, rupture of a lung abscess into the pleural space, invasion from a subphrenic infection, or infection associated with trauma.

Noninflammatory collections of serous fluid are called *hydrothorax*. The condition may be either unilateral or bilateral. The most common cause of hydrothorax is congestive heart failure. Other causes of hydrothorax include renal failure, nephrosis, liver failure, malignancy, and myxedema.

Chylothorax refers to the presence of chyle in the thoracic cavity. Chyle, a milky fluid containing chylomicrons is found in the lymph fluid originating in the gastrointestinal tract. The thoracic duct transports chyle to the central circulation. Chylothorax results from trauma, inflammation, or malignant infiltration obstructing chyle transport from the thoracic duct into the central circulation.

Hemothorax is the presence of blood in the thoracic cavity. Bleeding may arise from chest injury, a complication of chest surgery, malignancies, or rupture of a great vessel such as an aortic aneurysm. Hemothorax may be classified as minimal, moderate, or large.[30] A minimal hemothorax involves the presence of 300 ml to 500 ml of blood in the pleural space. Small amounts of blood are generally absorbed from the pleural space and a minimal hemothorax generally clears in 10 to 14 days without complication. A moderate hemothorax (500 ml-1000 ml of blood) fills about one-third of the pleural space and may produce signs of lung compression and loss of intravascular volume. It requires immediate drainage and replacement of intravascular fluids. A large hemothorax fills half or more of the hemithorax; it indicates the presence of 1000 ml or more of blood in the thorax and is usually caused by bleeding from a high-pressure vessel such as an intercostal or mammary artery. It requires immediate drainage and, if the bleeding continues, surgery to control the bleeding. One of the complications of untreated moderate or large hemothorax is fibrothorax— or the fusion of the pleural surfaces by fibrin, hyalin, and connective tissue—and in some cases calcification of the fibrous tissue, which causes restriction in lung expansion.

Manifestations

The manifestations of pleural effusion vary with the cause. Hemothorax may be accompanied by signs of blood loss, and empyema by fever and other signs of inflammation. Fluid in the pleural cavity acts as a space-occupying mass; it causes a decrease in lung volume on the affected side that is proportional to the size of fluid collection. The effusion causes a mediastinal shift toward the contralateral side with a decrease in lung volume on that side as well. Characteristic signs of pleural effusion are dullness or flatness to percussion and diminished breath sounds. Pleuritic pain usually occurs only when inflammation is present, although a constant type of discomfort may be felt with large effusions. Usually 2000 ml or more of fluid must be present before dyspnea occurs. A minimum of 250 ml of unilateral fluid accumulation must be present before the condition can be detected on chest x-ray.

Treatment

Thoracentesis, the aspiration of fluid from the pleural space, is used for both diagnostic and therapeutic purposes. It is often used to obtain a sample of pleural fluid for diagnostic studies. The treatment of pleural effusion is directed at the cause of the disorder. With large effusions, thoracentesis may be used to allow for the reexpansion of the lung. A palliative method of treatment used when pleural effusion is due to a malignancy is the injection of a sclerosing agent into the pleural cavity; this causes obliteration of the pleural space and prevents the reaccumulation of fluid.

In summary, disorders of the pleura include pain, pneumothorax, and pleural effusion. Pain is a common symptom associated with conditions that produce inflammation of the pleura. Characteristically, it is unilateral, abrupt in onset, and exaggerated by respiratory movements. Pneumothorax refers to an accumulation of air in the pleural cavity with the partial or complete collapse of the lung. It can result from rupture of an air-filled bleb on the lung surface or from penetrating or nonpenetrating injuries. A tension pneumothorax is a life-threatening event in which air progressively accumulates within the thorax, causing not only the collapse of the lung on the injured side but also a progressive shift of the mediastinum to the opposite side of the thorax, producing severe cardiorespiratory impairment. Pleural effusion refers to the collection of fluid in the pleural cavity. The fluid may be a transudate (hydrothorax), exudate (empyema), blood (hemothorax), or chyle (chylothorax).

■ Obstructive Lung Disorders

The function of the airways is to facilitate the movement of gases into and out of the lungs. As the airways branch out from the major bronchi they decrease in size and lose their cartilaginous support. At the point where the cartilaginous support disappears and the diameter is reduced to about 1 mm, the bronchi become bronchioles. Rings of smooth muscle joined by diagonal muscle fibers surround the epithelial lining of the bronchioles. Contraction and relaxation of the smooth muscle layer, which extends into the wall of the alveolar ducts, control the resistance to airflow through the bronchioles. The bronchioles are lined with simple columnar and cuboidal epithelium, which contains ciliated and secretory cells. The smooth muscle layer of the bronchioles is richly innervated and sensitive to catecholamines and other chemical mediators. Airway obstruction can result in thickened secretions (mucous plugs), spasm of the bronchial smooth muscle (bronchospasm), or disease conditions that disrupt the structure of the bronchioles and alveoli. This section of the chapter includes a discussion of atelectasis, bronchial asthma, and chronic lung disease.

Atelectasis

Atelectasis refers to the incomplete expansion of a lung or portion of a lung. It can be caused by airway obstruction, lung compression such as occurs in pneumothorax or pleural effusion, or the increased recoil of the lung because of loss of pulmonary surfactant (discussed in Chap. 22). The disorder may be present at birth (primary atelectasis), or it may develop in the neonatal period or in later life (secondary atelectasis). Primary atelectasis of the newborn implies that the lung has never been inflated. It is seen most frequently in premature and high-risk infants. A secondary form of atelectasis can occur in infants who established respiration and subsequently developed impairment of lung expansion. Among the causes of secondary atelectasis in the newborn are the respiratory distress syndrome associated with lack of surfactant and airway obstruction due to aspiration of amniotic fluid or blood.

In the older child or adult atelectasis is commonly caused by airway obstruction. With the complete obstruction of the airway absorption of oxygen from the dependent alveoli occurs, followed by collapse of that portion of the lung. A bronchus can be obstructed by a *mucous plug* that forms within the airway or by *external compression* due to fluid, tumor mass, exudate, or other matter in the area surrounding the airway. A small segment of lung or an entire lung lobe may be involved in atelectasis, and both chest expansion and breath sounds are decreased on the affected side. If the collapsed area is large, the trachea will deviate to the affected side. Signs of respiratory distress will be proportional to the extent of lung collapse.

The danger of atelectasis increases following surgery. Anesthesia, pain, administration of narcotics, and immobility tend to promote retention of viscid bronchial secretions and hence airway obstruction. Encouraging a patient to cough and to take deep breaths along with frequent change of position, adequate hydration, and early ambulation decrease the likelihood of atelectasis developing.

Bronchial Asthma

Conservative estimates indicate that between 8 million and 10 million Americans suffer from bronchial asthma. The disease affects individuals of all ages and is the most common cause of chronic illness in children under age 17.[34]

The disease is characterized by bronchial hyperreactivity to various stimuli, causing reversible bronchospasm, edema of the mucosal surface of the bronchioles, and increased production of mucus. Wheezing and dyspnea occur because of airway obstruction. In severe cases there is hyperinflation of the lungs and an imbalance between ventilation and perfusion, with impairment of gas exchange. The attacks differ from person to person, and between attacks many persons are symptom free. Both immune mechanisms (extrinsic asthma) and autonomic nervous system imbalances (intrinsic asthma) play a role in the associated bronchospasm; these are described in the section entitled Types of Asthma.

Etiologic mechanisms

Immune response. Allergic asthma results primarily from a type I, IgE immune response (Chap. 10). The mast cells of the bronchial tissues contain granules of chemical mediators—histamine, slow-reacting substance of anaphylaxis (SRS-A), eosinophil chemotactic factor, platelet-activating factor, and prostaglandins—that can provoke bronchospasm, vascular permeability, and increased mucus secretion and in other ways may trigger an asthmatic attack. The granules from the sensitized mast cells are released on exposure to the offending allergen. Common allergens include house dust, pollen from trees, grass, and weeds, animal danders, and mold spores.

Autonomic nervous system (ANS) imbalance. The autonomic nervous system influences both bronchial smooth muscle and mediator release from the mast cells. The ANS parasympathetic component produces bronchoconstriction and promotes mediator release, whereas the sympathetic component produces bronchial relaxation and inhibits mediator release. Normally no chronically active bronchial relaxant (sympathetic) forces are in operation; rather, a slight, vagally mediated bronchoconstrictor tone predominates. Hence a modest increase in sympathetic activity during periods of stress and increased oxygen need can bring about a marked decrease in airway resistance; this makes breathing easier and allows for increased ventilation.

The effect of the sympathetic nervous system on bronchial smooth muscle tone and mast cell function is mediated by beta$_2$ sympathetic nervous system receptors. The smooth muscle tone and inflammatory mediator release from the mast cells are modulated by intracellular levels of the cyclic nucleotides, particularly adenosine monophosphate (cAMP). When the level of this second messenger (cAMP) falls, bronchial smooth muscle contracts. Beta-adrenergic agonists such as epinephrine augment the cAMP levels in the mast cells so there is less mediator release from the mast cell granules. The interaction between autonomic nervous system influences, cAMP levels, and drugs used for asthma is depicted in Figure 23-3.

Types of asthma

There are two types of asthma, extrinsic and intrinsic. *Extrinsic* or allergic *asthma* is caused by release of inflammatory mediators from sensitized mast cells. Generally, this form of asthma is seen in persons with a family history of allergy and its onset occurs during childhood or adolescence. Persons with allergic asthma may also have other allergies such as hay fever. Attacks are related to exposure to specific allergens. Skin tests for the offending allergens are positive. *Intrinsic asthma* is characterized by an absence of clearly defined precipitating factors. Onset is usually after age 35. The attacks are frequently precipitated by factors such as infection, weather changes, exercise, emotion, exposure to bronchial irritants, and various drugs, including aspirin.

There is a small group of asthmatics in whom aspirin sensitivity is associated with severe asthmatic attacks, presence of nasal polyps, and recurrent episodes of rhinitis.[35] In addition, the yellow food dye tartrazine and nonsteroidal anti-inflammatory drugs, such as aminopyrine, phenylbutazone, ibuprofen, and indomethacin, may provoke attacks.

Exercise-induced asthma is seen in both intrinsic and extrinsic asthma, although the relationship between exercise and bronchial spasm is not understood. The response is often exaggerated when the person exercises in a cold environment; wearing a mask over the nose and mouth often minimizes the attack or prevents it. It appears that the proper selection of a mask could be important for persons subject to exercise-induced asthma, because it has been shown that increasing the humidity of the inhaled air is more important than simply heating the air.[36]

Manifestations

Persons with asthma exhibit a wide range of signs and symptoms, from chest tightness to an acute immobilizing attack. Many sufferers are asymptomatic between attacks.

With progressive airway obstruction occurring during an attack, expiration becomes prolonged. The $FEV_{1.0}$ is decreased. Air becomes trapped in the lungs, increasing the residual volume (Chap. 22). The asthmatic must now breathe at a higher lung volume, and more energy is needed to overcome the tension already present in the lungs. Fatigue follows. Both inspiratory reserve capacity and vital capacity diminish. Because air is trapped in the alveoli and inspiration is occurring at higher lung volumes, the cough becomes less effective. As the condition progresses, the effectiveness of alveolar ventilation declines with mismatching between ventilation and perfusion. Exchange of gases is impaired and cyanosis develops.

During an *acute attack*, the asthmatic generally prefers to sit up. There is visible use of the accessory muscles. The skin is often moist, and anxiety and apprehension are obvious. The person wheezes during both inspiration and expiration, often audibly. The breath sounds may be coarse and loud. Vesicular breath sounds become quite distant because of trapping of air. Dyspnea may be severe, and often the person is able to speak only one or two words before taking a breath. A cough may accompany the wheezing. At the point where airflow is markedly decreased, the cough becomes ineffective despite being repetitive and hacking; this point often marks the onset of respiratory failure.

Treatment

Two modalities are used in the management of bronchial asthma. One method focuses on prevention, the other on treatment during an attack. Figure 23-3 diagrams the action of various therapeutic drugs in relieving asthmatic bronchospasm.

Preventive measures include *avoidance of bronchial irritants* such as allergens or breathing of cold air that are known to precipitate an attack. A careful history is often needed to identify all the contributory factors. When the offending agent cannot be avoided (*e.g.,* house dust), a *program of desensitization* may be undertaken (Chap. 10). The drug *cromolyn sodium* is sometimes effective in preventing allergic reactions. The drug is administered by inhalation. It *stabilizes the mast cells,* thereby preventing release of the inflammatory mediators that cause the

attack. This drug must be given prophylactically and is of no benefit when taken during an attack.

During the attack itself, bronchodilators are used. These include the *beta-adrenergic agonists (e.g.,* epinephrine) and theophylline preparations. The adrenergic agents relax bronchial smooth muscle and relieve congestion of the broncial mucosa. Certain forms of these drugs may be given by inhalation for rapid onset of action. *Ipatropium* is a synthetic atropine analog that is administered by inhalation. It produces bronchodilatation by direct action on the large airways and does not change the composition or viscosity of the bronchial mucus. At the time of this writing, ipatropium has not been approved for use in the United States. *Theophylline* also acts by relaxing smooth muscle. Theophylline preparations can be administered by oral, rectal, or intravenous route. The adrenergic drugs and theophylline preparations have different mechanisms of action and are therefore complementary. The adrenergic drugs directly increase the levels of cAMP in the bronchial smooth

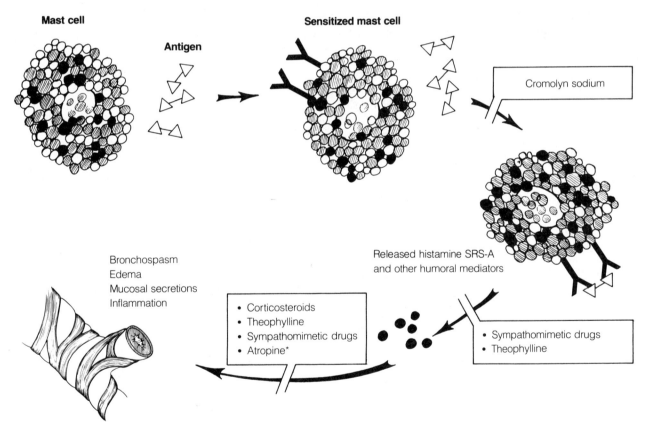

Figure 23-3 *The site of action of drugs used in treatment of bronchial asthma. Cromolyn sodium prevents mast cell degranulation and mediator release. The sympathomimetic drugs (beta-adrenergic agonists) and theophylline inhibit mediator production by the mast cells. The adrenal corticosteroid hormones, theophylline, sympathomimetic drugs, and atropine reduce or prevent bronchospasm, edema, excess mucosal secretions, and inflammation.*

muscle, whereas theophylline decreases the metabolism of cAMP and increases diaphragmatic contractility.[37] The *adrenocorticosteroid* drugs are also used to treat acute asthmatic attacks. It is thought that these drugs stabilize the lysosomes of the inflammatory cells, prevent the accumulation of histamine in mast cells, sensitize the beta-adrenergic receptors, and exert other anti-inflammatory actions. The effects of these drugs are described in greater detail in Table 23-3.

Relaxation techniques and *controlled breathing* help to allay the panic and anxiety that aggravate breathing difficulties. In a child, measures to encourage independence as it relates to symptom control, along with those directed at helping to develop a positive self-concept, are essential.

Chronic Obstructive Pulmonary Disease

In the United States, chronic lung disease ranks second to coronary heart disease as a cause of disability subject to Social Security payment. In 1981, chronic lung disease was the fifth leading cause of death in the United States.[38]

The terms chronic obstructive lung disease (COLD), chronic obstructive pulmonary disease (COPD), and chronic obstructive airway disease (COAD) denote a group of respiratory disorders characterized by obstruction to airflow in the lung. The abbreviation COPD will be used in this chapter. The most prevalent of these disorders are chronic bronchitis and emphysema. In chronic bronchitis there is excessive mucus production by the mucosal cells of the bronchi and chronic productive cough (2 tablespoonsful of sputum a day or more) that has persisted for at least 3 months per year for 2 successive years or more. Pulmonary emphysema is an abnormal dilatation of the air spaces distal to the terminal bronchioles with destruction of the alveolar walls. In addition to these two types of COPD, this section presents a brief description of two other causes of chronic obstructive lung disease—bronchiectasis and cystic fibrosis.

Both the episodic (asthma) and persistent (chronic

Table 23-3   Bronchodilator Drugs Used in the Treatment of Asthma and Chronic Obstructive Pulmonary Diseases

Drug	Action	Route of Administration
Adrenergic Drugs	Drugs with a beta$_2$ action produce relaxation of the bronchial smooth muscle by acting at the level of adenyl cyclase to increase cAMP; beta$_1$ agonists stimulate the heart, causing tachycardia and danger of arrhythmias; drugs with an alpha action cause vasoconstriction and raise blood pressure	
Epinephrine	Stimulates both alpha and beta receptors, producing tachycardia and blood pressure changes as well as bronchial dilatation	Usually given by inhalation or subcutaneous injection Intramuscular suspension preparations are available
Ephedrine (and related preparations such as pseudoephedrine)	Not a catecholamine; acts by inducing catecholamine release; has disadvantage of causing central nervous system stimulation and cardiovascular side-effects	Usually given orally, often in combinations of theophylline and a sedative
Isoproterenol	Both beta$_1$ and beta$_2$ actions	Usually given by inhalation Can be given sublingually
Metaproterenol	Mainly beta$_2$; can cause troublesome muscle tremors; may produce tachycardia and blood pressure changes	Oral and inhalation
Terbutaline	Beta$_2$ actions; may produce troublesome muscle tremors. May also produce tachycardia and blood pressure changes	Oral; subcutaneous, inhalation
Isoetharine	Mainly beta$_2$	Inhalation
Albuterol	Mainly beta$_2$	Inhalation
Theophylline Preparations		
Theophylline Aminophylline (86% theophylline) Oxtriphylline (65% theophylline)	Produce bronchodilatation by inhibiting metabolism of cAMP; can cause nausea and vomiting, which is mediated through the central nervous system; may produce seizures at high levels, particularly in children	Usually given orally as a single agent, or occasionally as a combination preparation with an adrenergic drug and a sedative May be given intravenously or rectally

bronchitis and emphysema) disorders of the lung give rise to *hyperinflation of the lung, prolongation of the expiratory phase of respiration,* and *impaired gas exchange* due to disproportion between ventilation and perfusion. The forced vital capacity (FVC) is the amount of air that can be forcibly exhaled following maximal inspiration. In a normal young adult, this should be achieved in 4 to 6 seconds.[39] The forced expiratory volume that can be achieved in 1 second is termed the $FEV_{1.0}$. In chronic lung disease the time required for FVC is increased, the $FEV_{1.0}$ is decreased, and the ratio of the $FEV_{1.0}$ to the FVC is decreased. These and other measurements of expiratory flow are determined by spirometry and are used in diagnosis of COPD (Chap. 22).

Chronic bronchitis and pulmonary emphysema are closely related. Among persons with COPD, many will be found to have both chronic bronchitis and emphysema; some will have only chronic bronchitis; others will have emphysema.

For descriptive purposes, the euphemisms *blue bloaters* and *pink puffers* have been used to differentiate the clinical manifestations of chronic bronchitis and pulmonary emphysema. The reader will find that in actual practice, the distinction between them is not as vivid as is presented here. This is because many individuals with COPD have combinations of both conditions. Characteristically, the secretions of chronic bronchitis obstruct airflow, causing an imbalance in ventilation and perfusion. For some unknown reason, persons with this form of COPD do not increase their total minute ventilation

to compensate for the imbalance in ventilation and perfusion; consequently, they develop hypoxemia, cyanosis, and eventually cor pulmonale with systemic edema. These are the "blue bloaters." They are also known as "nonfighters." With pulmonary emphysema there is a proportional loss of both ventilation and perfusion area in the lung. For whatever reason, these persons are "fighters"—able to struggle and overventilate, and thus to maintain relatively normal blood gas levels until late in the disease. They are the "pink puffers." The important features of these two forms of COPD are described in Table 23-4.

Chronic bronchitis

A chronic productive cough is the prominent feature of chronic bronchitis, and it is often present for many years before the onset of other symptoms. It is seen most commonly in middle-aged men and is associated with chronic irritation from inhaled substances and recurrent infections. In the United States, smoking is the most important cause of chronic bronchitis.

The disease involves both the major and the small airways, and is characterized by inflammation, edema, hyperplasia of the bronchial glands, and overproduction of mucus. Viral and bacterial infections are common and are thought to be a result of rather than a cause of the problem.

Shortness of breath on exertion and finally at rest is due to airway obstruction. Airway obstruction leads to an imbalance between ventilation and perfusion, with

Table 23-4   Characteristics of Chronic Bronchitis and Emphysematous Types of Chronic Lung Disease

Characteristic	Chronic Bronchitis ("Blue Bloaters")	Pulmonary Emphysema ("Pink Puffers")
Smoking history	Usual	Usual
Age of onset	Relatively young	Relatively old
Clinical features		
Barrel chest (hyperinflation of the lungs)	May be present	Often dramatic
Weight loss	Infrequent	May be severe in advanced disease
Shortness of breath	Predominant early symptom, insidious in onset, exertional	May be absent early in disease
Decreased breath sounds	Variable	Characteristic
Wheezing	Variable	Usually absent
Rhonchi	Often prominent	Usually absent or minimal
Sputum	Frequent early manifestation, frequent infections, abundant purulent sputum	May be absent or may develop late in the course
Cyanosis	Often dramatic	Often absent, even late in the disease when there is low PO_2
Blood gases	Hypercapnia may be present Hypoxemia may be present	Relatively normal until late in the disease process
Cor pulmonale	Frequent Peripheral edema	Only in advanced cases
Polycythemia	Frequent	Only in advanced cases
Prognosis	Numerous life-threatening episodes due to acute exacerbations	Slowly debilitating disease

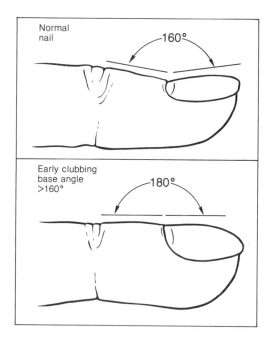

Figure 23-4   *Clubbing of the finger.*

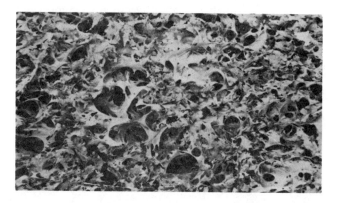

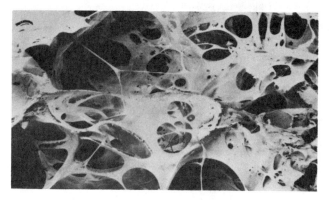

Figure 23-5   *Transmission electron micrograph of lung tissue.* (Top) *Normal tissue;* (bottom) *emphysematous tissue (both at same magnification). Note the enlargement of air spaces in the emphysematous lung. (Courtesy of Kenneth Siegesmund, PhD. Anatomy Department, The Medical College of Wisconsin)*

hypoxemia and *cyanosis*. Then *pulmonary hypertension* ensues, associated with right heart failure, or *cor pulmonale*, and peripheral edema. The hypoxemia acts as a stimulus for red blood cell production with a resultant *polycythemia*. As the disease progresses, breathing is labored, even when the person is at rest. The expiratory phase of respiration is prolonged, and expiratory rhonchi and rales can be heard on auscultation. Another common finding in chronic bronchitis is *clubbing of the fingers*, a condition in which the tips of the fingers become bulbous, resembling drumsticks (Fig. 23-4). Normally there is an obtuse angle of about 160° between the base of the nail and the adjacent dorsal surface of the finger; with clubbing, this angle exceeds 180°. In contrast with persons with emphysema, those with chronic bronchitis tend to maintain normal or elevated body weight.

Emphysema

In emphysema enlargement and destruction of the air spaces distal to the terminal bronchioles occur. Note the loss of alveolar tissue demonstrated in Figure 23-5. The two principal types of emphysema are centrilobular and panlobular. The centrilobular type affects the respiratory bronchioles, with initial preservation of the alveolar ducts and sacs. In the panlobular form the peripheral alveoli are involved. Figure 23-6 depicts the alveolar involvement associated with centrilobular and panlobular emphysema.

There are several known or suspected causes of emphysema, the most important of which is cigarette smoking. The risk of emphysema increases with the number of cigarettes smoked.[40] A second cause of emphysema is a deficiency of alpha$_1$-antitrypsin. Alpha$_1$-antitrypsin is a proteinase inhibitor; it blocks the action of the proteolytic enzymes that are destructive to elastin and other substances in the alveolar wall. The deficiency is an inherited autosomal recessive disorder. Approximately 70% to 80% of persons with a homozygous pattern of inheritance for alpha$_1$-antitrypsin deficiency have COPD.[41] The severity of the condition and age at onset may vary from individual to individual. There is now evidence that cigarette smoking reduces the body stores of alpha$_1$-antitrypsin over time. Therefore, smoking and repeated respiratory tract infections (which also impede normal secretion) tend to contribute to the development of emphysema in persons with an alpha$_1$-antitrypsin deficiency.

Emphysema causes trapping of air in the alveoli. Afflicted persons have marked *dyspnea and struggle to maintain normal blood gas levels with increased ventilatory effort*. The work of breathing is greatly increased and eating is often difficult. As a result, there is often considerable *weight loss*. With hyperinflation of the lungs, there is an increase in the anterior–posterior dimensions of the chest—which yields the appearance of the so-called barrel chest typical of the person with emphysema. Usually the seated position is preferred because it serves to stabilize the chest structures. The expiratory phase of respiration may be accomplished through *pursed lips*. With hyperinflation of the lungs, there is a tendency toward airway collapse during expiration. The pursed-lip breathing serves to increase the airway pressure and thereby prevents such collapse. One popular test to assess the severity of obstructive airway disease that is employed in emphysema is the *match test*. In this test, a lit match is held 6 inches from the mouth, and the patient is asked to extinguish it. Ability to extinguish the match indicates a maximum voluntary ventilation of 60 liters/minute and a forced expiratory volume at 1 second of 1.6 liters.[30]

Treatment

The treatment of COPD can be described under seven headings: (1) avoidance of smoking and environmental irritants, (2) prevention and control of respiratory infections, (3) maintenance of optimal nutritional status and fluid balance, (4) medications, (5) physical therapy and psychosocial rehabilitation, (6) control of shortness of breath, and (7) administration of oxygen or other methods of respiratory therapy. Obviously, not all persons with COPD have the same treatment needs.

Because COPD is a chronic disease, the outcomes of treatment are largely dependent on self-care measures that involve both the afflicted person and the family members. These persons need to have a complete understanding of the disease process and the manner in which it affects respiratory function, as well as the purpose of the prescribed treatment measures.

Control of the environment. Avoidance of cigarette smoke and other environmental airway irritants is a must. Vocational counseling may be needed if there is occupational exposure. Monitoring of air pollution levels and adjusting activities accordingly will aid in controlling shortness of breath. Wearing a cold weather mask often prevents dyspnea and bronchospasm due to cold air and wind exposure.

Control of infection. Respiratory tract infections can prove fatal to persons with severe COPD. A person with COPD should avoid exposure to others with known respiratory tract infections and should avoid attending large gatherings during periods of the year when influenza or respiratory tract infections are prevalent. Immunization for influenza and pneumococcal infections will decrease the likelihood of their occurrence. Persons with COPD should be taught to monitor their sputum for signs of infection, so that treatment can be instituted at the earliest sign of infection.

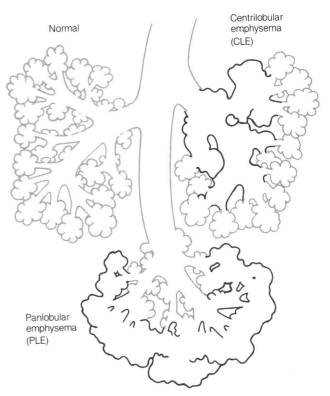

Figure 23-6 *The changes in alveolar structure associated with centrilobular and panlobular emphysema.*

Maintenance of nutrition and fluid balance. Because so much effort goes into breathing, many persons with COPD find it difficult to chew their food and to manage the effort of a large meal. This situation, combined with impaired diaphragm descent, air-swallowing, and medications that cause anorexia and nausea, impairs nutrition and promotes weight loss. Small, frequent, nutritious, and easily swallowed feedings aid in maintaining good nutrition and preventing weight loss. Vitamin supplements may be called for. Water is the most readily available expectorant for liquefying secretions, so fluid intake should be encouraged, particularly in persons who have thick, tenacious sputum. Fluid that is either too hot or too cold may aggravate breathing problems.

Medications. Several groups of medications are used in long-term management of COPD, including adrenergic (adrenalin-related) drugs, theophylline preparations, and expectorants. Adrenal corticosteroid hormones may be used in some cases. Expectorants are discussed in Chapter 22. Both *adrenergic* and *theophylline* preparations act by relaxing bronchiolar smooth muscle. Combination drugs, most often consisting of an adrenergic drug, a theophylline preparation, and a sedative to counteract CNS stimulation by the adrenergic drug, may be helpful. However, because sedative drugs depress the respiratory center, the combination drugs are used less frequently than in the past. In addition, the combination of theophylline and adrenergic drugs may lead to a higher incidence of adverse effects. Also, with the development of *adrenergic drugs* that act specifically on the *beta₂ receptors* of the lung and cause less central nervous system stimulation than the older adrenergics such as ephedrine and pseudoephedrine, there is less need for the combination drugs. The beta₂ agonists also have less effect on the cardiovascular system.

Theophylline preparations can be administered orally, rectally, or intravenously. There is wide variability from case to case in the absorption and metabolism of these preparations; therefore, theophylline blood level serves as a guide in arriving at an effective dosage schedule. Although the adrenal corticosteroids are not routinely prescribed for long-term treatment of COPD, some persons do require them. The adrenal corticosteroids are available for local use in aerosol form minimizing the undesirable effects that often accompany systemic use. Table 23-3 lists some of the common adrenergic drugs, their mechanisms of action, and their side-effects.

Many adrenergics are available in aerosol form for inhalation, and in this form they are particularly useful in controlling bronchospasm. Because they are convenient and effective, they can be abused by improper administration and overuse. Of special concern is the potential for development of cardiac arrhythmias.

Rehabilitation and breathing training. The maintenance or improvement of physical and psychosocial functioning is an essential component in the treatment plan for persons with COPD. A long-term pulmonary rehabilitation program can significantly reduce episodes of hospitalization and add measurably to a person's ability to manage and cope with his or her impairment in a positive way. Breathing exercises and retraining focus on restoring the function of the diaphragm, reducing the work of breathing, and improving gas exchange. Physical conditioning, with a gradual increase in activity, improves exercise tolerance. Psychosocial rehabilitation must be individualized to meet the specific needs of persons with COPD and their families. These needs will vary with age, occupation, financial resources, social and recreational interest, and interpersonal and family relationships. Work simplification strategies may be needed when impairment is severe.

Breathing exercises and retraining are designed to increase respiratory muscle strength and endurance, thereby improving exercise performance. The diaphragm and other inspiratory muscles form a muscle pump that is as vital to the respiratory functions of the body as the heart is to the circulatory functions. During inspiration the diaphragm contracts and descends; during expiration it passively ascends, causing air to leave the lungs. In normal respiration, the diaphragm contributes 65% to the work of breathing, while the accessory muscles contribute about 35%.[42] In emphysema, the contribution of the diaphragm to the work of breathing is largely diminished because of loss of lung elasticity, with air trapping and lung distention. In order to compensate for this deficiency, persons with emphysema use their accessory muscles for breathing. Breathing is laborious, and the work of breathing increases. This labored breathing pattern may progress to the point that the diaphragm contributes only about 30% to the effort of breathing, and the accessory muscles carry 70% of the load.[42] Recent studies have shown that although respiratory muscles may be weakened in COPD, it is possible to strengthen them through inspiratory muscle training using either resistive loading during inspiration or normocapnic hypernia.[43,44] Resistive loading is accomplished by having the person breathe through an inspiratory breathing device that increases the resistance to airflow during inspiration. Hand-held devices that can be used at home are available for this purpose. Isocapnic hyperneic exercise uses exercises that increase ventilation, trains expiratory as well as inspiratory muscles, and is best suited for the development of respiratory muscle endurance. Isocapnic hyperneic exercise requires the use of a special rebreathing circuit to maintain normal carbon dioxide levels. At present, the rebreathing equipment needed for this type of exercise is not available for home use, which limits the usefulness of this type of exercise.

Postural drainage provides a means for removing excess secretions from the lungs. It is done by positioning the patient's body according to the distribution and configuration of the tracheobronchial tree so that gravity causes secretions to drain into the larger airways from which they can be effectively removed. The effectiveness of postural drainage may be enhanced by percussion or vibration of the chest wall, done with vibrating or tapping motions of the hands or electronic vibrators or ultrasound generators. The reader is referred to other reference sources, some of which are listed at the end of the chapter, for a more complete description of these exercises and treatments.

Oxygen therapy. In advanced cases of COPD, the imbalance between ventilation and perfusion causes hypoxemia. Hypoxemia, with arterial PO_2 levels below 55 mm Hg, causes polycythemia and reflex vasoconstriction of the pulmonary vessels, with resultant pulmonary hypertension and further impairment of gas exchange in the lung. These patients are at risk for developing cor pulmonale.

In such severe cases, administration of continuous low-flow (1-2 liters/minute) oxygen often increases the arterial oxygen levels, decreases dyspnea and pulmonary hypertension, and improves neuropsychological function and exercise tolerance. Portable oxygen administration units, which allow for mobility and the performance of activities of daily living, are usually used. The Nocturnal Oxygen Therapy Trial Group study of persons with advanced disease—particularly those with heart failure associated with COPD—performed at six centers in the United States and Canada has clearly shown that oxygen is more effective when given almost continuously than when it is given roughly 50% of the time. The survival rate of persons receiving continuous oxygen therapy was almost two times that of those receiving 12-hour nocturnal therapy.[45]

It has been found that persons with COPD may have episodes of hypoxemia both at night and during daytime naps. These persons do not, however, experience the daytime hypersomnolence and loud snoring that is usually associated with sleep apnea (Chap. 24). The hypoxemia that occurs during sleep in persons with COPD is usually associated with slow and shallow breathing rather than with periods of apnea. Cardiac arrhythmias and other electrocardiographic evidence of myocardial ischemia may accompany the episodes of hypoxemia.[46] Sleep studies, in which arterial oxygen saturation is measured using an ear oximeter, may be done when nocturnal hypoxemia is suspected in a person with COPD. Although these persons do not usually experience severe hypoxemia during waking hours and do not meet the criteria for continuous low-flow oxygen therapy, they may benefit from nocturnal oxygen therapy.[47]

Oxygen administration in persons with COPD must be undertaken with a certain amount of caution. The saying, "A little bit is good, a whole lot is better," does not hold true for oxygen administration in COPD. The flow rate (in liters per minute) is usually titrated to provide an arterial PO_2 of about 60 mm Hg. Because the ventilatory drive associated with hypoxic stimulation of the peripheral chemoreceptors does not occur until the arterial PO_2 has been reduced to about 60 mm Hg or less, increasing the arterial oxygen above that level tends to depress stimulation for ventilation and often leads to hypoventilation and carbon dioxide retention.

Intermittent positive pressure breathing. For those who need additional assistance in clearing secretions from the respiratory tract, mechanical devices that deliver medications in the form of a mist may be used. Hand-held nebulizers and, rarely, intermittent positive pressure breathing (IPPB) are employed. IPPB is accomplished by machines that deliver nebulized air to the lungs under increased pressure during inspiration. Bronchodilator drugs are usually added to the nebulizer.

Cystic fibrosis

Cystic fibrosis is a hereditary disease transmitted as an *autosomal recessive trait*. It affects approximately 1 in 2000 children. Homozygotes (persons with two defective genes) have all, or substantially all, of the clinical symptoms of the disease; whereas, heterozygotes are carriers of the disease but have no recognizable symptoms. It is an exocrine gland disorder involving both the mucus-secreting and the eccrine glands. Because cystic fibrosis involves production of a thick tenacious mucus, it is sometimes referred to as mucoviscidosis.

Clinically, cystic fibrosis is characterized by elevation of sodium chloride in the sweat, pancreatic insufficiency, and chronic lung disease. Abnormalities in pancreatic function are present in about 80% of affected children. The pancreatic insufficiency gives rise to malabsorption and steatorrhea. In the newborn, meconium ileus may cause intestinal obstruction. Respiratory manifestations are due to an accumulation of viscid mucus in the bronchi, which produces bronchial obstruction and dilatation. Mucus plugs can result in the total obstruction of an airway, causing atelectasis.

Diagnosis and treatment. Early diagnosis and treatment are important in that they may delay the onset of chronic illness. The diagnosis is generally based on an abnormal pilocarpine iontophoresis sweat chloride test. The test is usually done on sweat obtained from a child's forearm or from an infant's thigh. A small electric current is used to carry the drug pilocarpine, which increases sweat production, into the skin. Sweat is collected using an absorbent paper or gauze sponge and then analyzed in the laboratory. The test is often inaccurate in the newborn because the quantity of sweat that they produce is insufficient for testing. Babies with the disorder often taste salty when they are kissed. A new device that simplifies the sweat test and reduces its cost has recently been introduced on the market. The device, which looks like an oversized wristwatch, uses pilocarpine iontophoresis to induce sweating. It is a battery-operated unit that uses disposable patches that change color when sweat chloride levels are elevated.

The treatment of cystic fibrosis usually consists of replacement of pancreatic enzymes, physical measures to improve the clearance of tracheobronchial secretions (postural drainage and chest percussion), and prompt treatment of respiratory tract infections. Progress of the disease is variable. With improved medical management the survival rate, which at present is about 20 years of age, has increased.

Bronchiectasis

Bronchiectasis is an abnormal dilatation of the bronchioles associated with chronic necrotizing infection of the bronchi. To be diagnosed as bronchiectasis the dilatation must be permanent, because reversible bronchial dilatation may accompany viral and bronchial pneumonias. There are a number of causes of bronchiectasis, including bronchial obstruction due to conditions such as tumors and foreign bodies; congenital abnormalities in which abnormal development of the bronchi occurs; cystic fibrosis, in which airway obstruction is caused by impairment of normal mucociliary function; immunologic deficiencies, which predispose to respiratory tract infections; and exposure to toxic gases, which cause airway obstruction. Two conditions, obstruction and infection, are present in all of these disorders and both contribute to the development and progression of the disease. Bronchial obstruction causes atelectasis, which results in smooth muscle relaxation and dilatation of the walls of the airways that remain patent. Infection produces inflammation, weakening, and further dilatation of the walls of the bronchioles.

Diagnosis and treatment.   Bronchiectasis is associated with an assortment of abnormalities that profoundly affect respiratory function, including atelectasis, obstruction of the smaller airways, and diffuse bronchitis. There is coughing, fever, recurrent bronchopulmonary infection, and expectoration of foul-smelling, purulent sputum. The quantity of sputum can often amount to cupsful. The physiologic abnormalities that occur in bronchiectasis are similar to those seen in chronic bronchitis and emphysema. As in both of these conditions, chronic bronchial obstruction leads to marked dyspnea and cyanosis. Clubbing of the fingers sometimes develops.

The basic therapy consists of early recognition and treatment of infection along with regular postural drainage and chest physical therapy. Persons with this disorder benefit from many of the same rehabilitation and treatment measures used in the treatment of chronic bronchitis and emphysema.

In summary, airway obstruction occurs in a number of reversible and chronic conditions. Atelectasis refers to an incomplete expansion of the lung. Although it is often caused by airway obstruction, it can also result from the compression of lung structures, such as occurs in pneumothorax or from recoil of the lung due to loss of surfactant. Bronchial asthma is characterized by hyper-

sensitivity of the bronchial smooth muscle to various stimuli. It causes reversible bronchospasm, edema of the mucosal surface of the bronchioles, and increased production of mucus. Chronic obstructive pulmonary disease describes a group of conditions characterized by obstruction to airflow in the lungs. Among the conditions associated with COPD are chronic bronchitis, emphysema, cystic fibrosis, and bronchiectasis. The condition is manifested by hyperinflation of the lungs, increased time required for the expiratory phase of respiration, and mismatching of ventilation and perfusion. As the condition advances, signs of respiratory distress and impaired gas exchange are evident, with development of hypercapnia and hypoxemia.

■ Interstitial Lung Disorders

The interstitial lung diseases are a diverse group of lung disorders with similar clinical and pathophysiologic features. They include the occupational lung diseases, lung diseases caused by toxic drugs and radiation, and lung diseases of unknown etiology. These lung diseases are currently thought to affect more than 10 million people in the United States.[48]

The interstitial lung diseases produce varying degrees of inflammation, fibrosis, and disability. The disorders may be acute or insidious in onset; they may be rapidly progressive, slowly progressive, or static in their course. Because they result in a stiff and noncompliant lung, they are commonly classified as fibrotic or restrictive lung disorders. The most common of the interstitial lung diseases are those caused by exposure to occupational and environmental inhalants and sarcoidosis, the cause of which is unknown. Examples of interstitial lung diseases and their etiologies are listed in Table 23-5.

In contrast to the obstructive lung diseases, which primarily involve the airways of the lung, the restrictive lung disorders exert their effect on the collagen and elastic connective tissue found between the airways and the blood vessels of the lung. In addition, many of these diseases also involve the airways, arteries, and veins. In general, these lung diseases share a pattern of lung dysfunction that includes diminished lung volumes, reduced diffusing capacity of the lung, and varying degrees of hypoxemia.

Regardless of the cause, current theory suggests that the majority of interstitial lung diseases have a common pathogenesis. It is thought that these disorders are initiated by some type of injury to the alveolar epithelium, followed by an inflammatory process that involves the alveoli and interstitium of the lung. An accumulation of inflammatory and immune cells causes continued damage of lung tisue and the replacement of normal, functioning lung tissue with fibrous scar tissue.[49]

Manifestations

Interstitial lung disease is characterized by an insidious onset of breathlessness; initially it occurs during exercise and may progress to the point that the person is totally incapacitated. Typically, a person with a restrictive lung disease breathes with a pattern of rapid shallow respirations. This tachypneic pattern of breathing, in which the respiratory rate is increased and the tidal volume is decreased, leads to a reduction in the work of breathing, because it takes less work to move air through the airways at an increased rate than it does to stretch a stiff lung to accommodate a larger tidal volume. A nonproductive cough is also present in many individuals, particularly if there is continued exposure to the inhaled irritant. Basilar rales may be present in the lungs, and clubbing of the fingers and toes may occur.

Lung volumes, including vital capacity and total lung capacity, are reduced. In contrast to chronic obstructive lung disease, in which expiratory flow rates are reduced, the FEV_1 is usually preserved in interstitial lung disease, although the ratio between the FEV_1 and the vital capacity may increase. Although resting arterial blood gases are usually normal early in the course of the disease, arterial oxygen levels may fall during exercise, and in cases of advanced disease, hypoxemia is often present even at rest. In the late stages of the disease, hypercapnia and respiratory acidosis develop. The impaired diffusion of gases that occurs in persons with interstitial lung disease is thought to be due primarily to an increase in physiologic dead space resulting from unventilated regions of the lung.

Diagnosis and Treatment

The diagnosis of interstitial lung disease requires a careful personal and family history, with particular emphasis on exposure to environmental, occupational, and other injurious agents. Chest x-rays may be used as an initial diagnostic method, and serial chest films are often used in following the progress of the disease. A biopsy specimen for histologic study and culture may be obtained by means of surgical incision or by bronchoscopy using a fiberoptic bronchoscope. Bronchoalveolar lavage involves the instillation of fluid into the alveoli through a bronchoscope and its subsequent suction removal as a means of obtaining inflammatory and immune cells for laboratory study. Gallium lung scans are often used to detect and quantify the chronic alveolitis that occurs in interstitial lung disease. Gallium does not localize in

Table 23-5   Causes of Interstitial Lung Diseases

Etiology	Examples
Known	
Occupational and environmental inhalants	
Inorganic dusts	Silicosis
	Asbestosis
	Talcosis
	Coal miner's pneumoconiosis
	Berylliosis
Organic dusts	Farmer's lung (moldy hay)
	Pigeon breeder's lung (bird serum, excreta, and feathers)
	Air-conditioner lung (bacteria found in humidifiers and air conditioners)
	Baggassosis (contaminated sugarcane)
Gases, fumes, aerosols	Silo filler's lung (nitrogen dioxide, chlorine, ammonia, phosgene, sulfur dioxide
Drugs	Cancer chemotherapeutic drugs, (*e.g.*, bleomycin), nitrofurantoin
Radiation	External radiation, inhaled radioactive materials
Infections	Widespread tuberculosis
Poisons	Paraquat
Diseases of other organ systems	Chronic pulmonary edema
	Chronic uremia
Unknown	
	Sarcoidosis
	Idiopathic pulmonary fibrosis
	Connective tissue diseases, such as lupus erythematosus, scleroderma, and rheumatoid arthritis

normal lung tissue, and increased uptake of the radionuclide occurs in interstitial lung disease and other diffuse lung diseases.

The treatment goals for interstitial lung diseases focus on identifying and removing the injurious agent, suppressing the inflammatory response, preventing progression of the disease, and providing supportive therapy for persons with advanced disease. Generally, the treatment measures vary with the type of lung disease that is present. Corticosteroid drugs are frequently used to suppress the inflammatory response. Many of the supportive treatment measures used in the late stages of the disease, such as oxygen therapy and measures to prevent infection, are similar to those discussed for persons with chronic obstructive lung disease.

Occupational Lung Diseases

The occupational lung diseases can be divided into two major groups: the pneumoconioses and the hypersensitivity diseases. The pneumoconioses are caused by the inhalation of inorganic dusts and particulate matter. The hypersensitivity diseases result from the inhalation of organic dusts and related occupational antigens. A third type of occupational lung disease, byssinosis, a disease that affects cotton workers, has characteristics of both the pneumoconioses and hypersensitivity lung disease.

Among the pneumoconioses are silicosis (found in hard-rock miners, foundry workers, sandblasters, pottery makers, and workers in the slate industry), coal miner's pneumoconiosis (found in coal miners), asbestosis (in asbestos miners, manufacturers of asbestos products, and installers and removers of asbestos insulation), talcosis (in talc miners or millers and in infants and small children who accidentally inhale powder containing talc), and berylliosis (in ore extraction workers and alloy production workers). The danger of exposure to asbestos dust is not confined to the workplace. The dust pervades the general environment because it was used in the construction of buildings and in other applications before its health hazards were realized. It has been mixed into paints and plaster, wrapped around water and heating pipes, used to insulate hair dryers, and woven into theater curtains, hot pads, and ironing board covers.

Important etiologic determinants in the development of the pneumoconioses are (1) the size of the dust particle, its chemical nature, and its ability to incite lung destruction and (2) the concentration of and length of exposure to the dust. The most dangerous particles are those in the range of 1–5 μm. These small particles are carried through the inspired air into the alveolar structures, whereas larger particles are trapped in the nose or mucous linings of the airways and removed by the mucociliary blanket. Exceptions are asbestos and talc particles, which range in size from 30 to 60 μm but find their way into the alveoli because of their density. All particles within the alveoli must be cleared by the lung macrophages. Macrophages are thought to transport engulfed particles from the small bronchioles and the alveoli, which have neither cilia nor mucus-secreting cells, to the mucociliary escalator or to the lymphatic channels for removal from the lung. This clearing function is hampered when the function of the macrophage is impaired by factors such as cigarette smoking, consumption of alcohol, and hypersensitivity reactions. This helps to explain the increased incidence of lung disease among smokers exposed to asbestos. In silicosis the ingestion of silica particles leads to the destruction of the lung macrophages and the release of substances that produce fibrosis. Tuberculosis and other diseases caused by the mycobacteria are common in persons with silicosis. Because the macrophages are responsible for protecting the lungs from tuberculosis, the destruction of macrophages accounts for the increased susceptibility to tuberculosis in persons with silicosis.

With some dusts there is a fine line between the concentration of dust in the environment and the effect that it will have on the lung. For example, acute silicosis is seen only in persons whose occupations entail intense exposure to silica dust over a short period of time. It is seen in sandblasters, who use a high-speed jet of sand to clean and polish bricks and the insides of corroded tanks, in tunnelers, and in rock drillers, particularly if they drill through sandstone.[50] Acute silicosis is a rapidly progressive disease, usually leading to severe disability and death within 5 years of diagnosis. In contrast to acute silicosis, which is caused by exposure to extremely high concentrations of silica dust, the symptoms related to chronic low-level exposure to silica dust often do not begin to develop until after many years of exposure, and then the symptoms are often insidious in onset and slow to progress.

The hypersensitivity occupational lung disorders (hypersensitivity pneumonitis) are caused by intense and often prolonged exposure to inhaled organic dusts and related occupational antigens. Affected persons have a heightened sensitivity to the antigen. Unlike bronchial asthma, this type of hypersensitivity reaction involves primarily the alveoli. These disorders cause progressive fibrotic lung disease, which can be prevented by the removal of the environmental agent. The most common causes of hypersensitivity pneumonitis are farmers' lung, which results from exposure to moldy hay; pigeon breeders' lung, provoked by exposure to the serum, excreta, or feathers of birds; baggassosis, from contaminated sugarcane; and humidifier or air-conditioner lung, caused by bacteria in the water reservoirs of these appliances.

Sarcoidosis

Sarcoidosis, sometimes called Boeck's sarcoid, is a multisystem granulomatous disorder of unknown etiology. An alteration in T-lymphocyte function is thought to contribute to the disorder.[51]

The disease predominantly affects young adults, aged 20 to 40 years, although it may occur in older groups. The annual incidence of sarcoidosis in the United States is about 22,500 cases; it is 10 to 20 times more common in blacks and is more prevalent in both blacks and whites living in the southeastern part of the country.[52]

Sarcoidosis is a disease of variable manifestations and an unpredictable course of progression that can affect any organ system. The three systems that most commonly present symptoms are the lungs, the skin, and the eyes. Table 23-6 lists the systems of extrathoracic involvement in sarcoidosis. More than 40% of persons with sarcoidosis report nonspecific symptoms such as fever, sweating, anorexia, weight loss, fatigue, and myalgia. Although only about 60% of persons with sarcoidosis have respiratory symptoms, almost all have abnormal chest x-rays. In about 25% of cases, the disease is first detected on a routine chest x-ray. The roentgenographic manifestations of the disorder can be classified into four stages.[53]

Stage 0 no roentgenographic abnormalities.
Stage 1 bilateral hilar adenopathy.
Stage 2 bilateral hilar adenopathy with parenchymal infiltrates.
Stage 3 parenchymal infiltrates without hilar adenopathy.

In persons with stage 0 disease, that is, with other symptomatology but no x-ray findings, the rate of spontaneous recovery approaches 100%. The x-ray abnormalities will clear in about 65% of persons with stage 1, 50% of persons with stage 2, and 20% of persons with stage 3 disease.

   The diagnosis of sarcoidosis is usually made using the transbronchial lung biopsy, bronchial lavage, the Kveim skin test, and serum angiotensin-converting enzyme (SACE) test. The Kveim test is a skin test that uses antigen from human sarcoid tissue injected intradermally into the flexor surface of the forearm. The injection site is observed for the development of a nodule during the 6 weeks following injection of the antigen. If a nodule develops, it is examined through biopsy for sarcoid tissue. In active sarcoidosis the SACE level is elevated. The SACE test is used to evaluate the progress of the disease and the effectiveness of treatment. When treatment is indicated, the corticosteroid drugs are used. These agents produce clearing of the chest x-ray and improve pulmonary function, but it is not known whether they affect the long-term outcome of the disease.

In summary, the interstitial lung diseases are characterized by fibrosis and decreased compliance of the lung. They include the occupational lung diseases, lung diseases caused by toxic drugs and radiation, and lung diseases of unknown etiology, such as sarcoidosis. These disorders are thought to result from an inflammatory process that begins in the alveoli and extends to involve the interstitial tissues of the lung. In contrast with chronic obstructive pulmonary diseases, which affect the airways, interstitial lung diseases affect the supporting collagen and elastic tissues that lie between the airways and blood vessels. These lung diseases produce a decrease in lung volumes, reduced diffusing capacity of the lung, and varying degrees of hypoxia. Because of a

Table 23-6 Sites of Extrathoracic Involvement in Sarcoidosis

Site	Approximate Incidence (%)	Manifestations
Liver	90 (biopsy)	Hepatomegaly, abnormal liver function tests
Eye	15–20	Lacrimal gland involvement, iridocyclitis, keratoconjunctivitis, cataract formation, glaucoma
Skin	20	Erythema nodosum, cosmetically unattractive and disfiguring skin lesions
Spleen	10	Splenomegaly, abdominal pain, anemia, leukopenia, thrombocytopenia
Central nervous system	5	Chronic meningitis, involvement of cranial nerves, *e.g.,* Bell's palsy; endocrine disorders due to involvement of hypothalamus or pituitary gland, *e.g.,* diabetes insipidus
Bone	4	Arthritis of large weight-bearing joints, bone cysts
Abnormal calcium metabolism	15	Hypercalcemia, hypercalciuria

reduction in lung compliance, persons with this form of lung disease breathe with a pattern of rapid and shallow respirations.

■ Pulmonary Vascular Disorders

The renewal of blood oxygen levels and the removal of carbon dioxide occur as blood moves through the lung. They are dependent on the matching of ventilation and perfusion. This section discusses two major problems of the pulmonary circulation, pulmonary embolism and pulmonary hypertension. Pulmonary edema, another major problem of the pulmonary circulation, is discussed in Chapter 20.

Pulmonary Embolism

Pulmonary embolism develops when a blood-borne substance lodges in a branch of the pulmonary artery and obstructs the flow. The embolism may consist of a thrombus, air that has accidentally been injected during intravenous infusion, fat that has been mobilized from the bone marrow following a fracture or from a traumatized fat depot,[54] or amniotic fluid that has entered the maternal circulation following rupture of the membranes at the time of delivery. This discussion is limited to the most common form of pulmonary embolism, thromboembolism.

In the United States approximately 630,000 cases of thromboembolism occur annually.[54] About 67,000 of these persons die within the first hour, before a diagnosis can be made and treatment instituted. Another 120,000 deaths occur in persons in whom the condition went unrecognized. Pulmonary embolism is uncommon before adulthood and increases in incidence with age, so that at age 80, about 70% of autopsied patients have emboli.[30]

Almost all pulmonary emboli are due to deep vein thrombosis. Therefore, persons at risk for developing venous thrombosis are the same persons who are at risk for developing thromboemboli.

The outcome of embolism in relation to cardiopulmonary function depends on the size and location of the obstruction. Small emboli that become lodged in the peripheral branches of the pulmonary artery may exert little effect, whereas sudden death occurs when a large embolus causes total occlusion of the pulmonary artery. Depending on size, pulmonary embolism causes (1) obstruction of pulmonary blood flow, with pulmonary arterial hypertension and right heart failure, (2) breathlessness, (3) hypoxemia, and (4) lung infarction.

Manifestations

Dyspnea, abrupt in onset, is the most common symptom of pulmonary embolism, and the breathing pattern is often rapid and shallow. With obstruction of pulmonary blood flow, there is severe apprehension and crushing substernal chest pain similar to that of myocardial infarction; the neck veins are distended, and cyanosis, diaphoresis, syncope, mental confusion, and other signs of shock follow. Pulmonary infarction often causes pleuritic pain that changes with respiration, being more severe on inspiration and less severe on expiration. With lung infarction there may be hemoptysis.

Diagnosis and treatment

Diagnosis of pulmonary embolism is based on blood gases, lung scan, laboratory studies, chest x-ray films, electrocardiogram (ECG), and, in selected cases, angiography. The arterial oxygen tension (PO_2) is almost always decreased when significant-sized emboli are present in the lung. This is because of the mismatching of ventilation and perfusion. The lung scan is a widely used diagnostic test. In this test, radioactive iodinated serum albumin is injected intravenously and collects in the pulmonary circulation. A scintillation counter is passed over the chest to provide a picture of blood flow in the various lung segments. The laboratory studies and chest x-ray films are useful in ruling out other conditions that might give rise to similar symptoms. The ECG may show signs of right heart strain due to pumping against an increase in pulmonary vascular resistance caused by the presence of emboli. Angiography involves the passage of a venous catheter through the heart and into the pulmonary artery under fluoroscopy. An embolectomy is sometimes performed during this procedure.

The treatment goals for pulmonary emboli focus on (1) the prevention of deep vein thrombosis and the development of thromboemboli, (2) the protection of the lungs from exposure to thromboemboli when they occur, and (3) in the case of large and life-threatening pulmonary emboli, sustaining of life and restoration of pulmonary blood flow.

Prevention focuses on (1) identification of persons at risk, (2) avoidance of venous stasis and hypercoagulability states, and (3) early detection of venous thrombosis. In patients at risk, low-dose subcutaneous heparin may be administered to decrease the likelihood of deep vein thrombosis, thromboembolism, and fatal pulmonary embolism following major surgical procedures.

There are two surgical procedures for protecting the lung from thromboemboli: venous ligation to prevent the embolus from traveling to the lung and vena caval plication. The plication, done with a suture, or by insertion of a clip, filter, or sieve, permits blood to flow while trapping the embolus.

Restoration of blood flow in persons with life-threatening pulmonary emboli can be accomplished through the surgical removal of the embolus or emboli. In the case of multiple pulmonary emboli, the thrombolytic drug streptokinase may be used. The drug is administered intravenously or directly into the pulmonary artery. Fibrolytic therapy is followed by administration of heparin and then warfarin.

Pulmonary Hypertension

Pulmonary hypertension describes the elevation of pressure in the pulmonary arterial system. The pulmonary circulation is a low pressure system designed to accommodate varying amounts of blood delivered from the right heart and to facilitate gas exchange. The normal mean pulmonary artery pressure is about 15 (28 systolic/8 diastolic) mm Hg. Pulmonary artery hypertension can be caused by an elevation in left atrial pressure, increased pulmonary blood flow, or increased pulmonary vascular resistance. Although pulmonary hypertension can develop as a primary disorder, most cases develop secondary to some other condition.

Etiologic mechanisms

Increased left atrial pressure. In conditions such as mitral valve stenosis and left ventricular heart failure, the elevation in left atrial pressure is transmitted to the pulmonary circulation and results in a passive elevation of pulmonary arterial pressures. Continued increases in left atrial pressure can lead to medial hypertrophy and intimal thickening of the small pulmonary arteries, causing sustained hypertension.

Increased pulmonary blood flow. Increased pulmonary blood flow results from increased flow through left-to-right shunts in congenital heart diseases such as atrial or ventricular septal defects and patent ductus arteriosus. If the high flow state is allowed to continue, morphologic changes will occur in the pulmonary vessels, leading to sustained pulmonary hypertension. The pulmonary vascular changes that occur with congenital heart disorders are discussed in Chapter 19.

Increased pulmonary vascular resistance. Unlike the vessels in the systemic circulation, which generally dilate in response to hypoxemia and hypercapnia, the pulmonary vessels constrict. The stimulus for constriction seems to originate in the air spaces in the vicinity of the small branches of the pulmonary arteries. In situations in which hypoventilation of certain regions of the lung occurs, the response is adaptive in that it diverts blood flow away from the poorly ventilated areas to more adequately ventilated portions of the lung. This effect, however, becomes less beneficial as more and more areas of the lung become poorly ventilated.

Pulmonary hypertension may develop at high altitudes in persons with normal lungs. It is also a common problem in persons with advanced chronic bronchitis and emphysema. In interstitial lung diseases, the fibrotic process may actually cause obliteration of pulmonary vessels, leading to pulmonary hypertension. Persons who experience marked hypoxemia during sleep, that is, those with sleep apnea, may experience marked elevations in pulmonary arterial pressure.

Primary pulmonary hypertension. Primary pulmonary hypertension is a rare, often lethal, form of pulmonary hypertension, the etiology of which is unknown. It is characterized by marked intimal fibrosis of the pulmonary arteries and arterioles. The disease can occur at any age, and familial occurrences have been reported. Persons with the disorder usually have a steadily progressive downhill course, with death occurring in 3 to 4 years. The recent use of the vasodilators hydralazine and diazoxide for the treatment of this form of pulmonary hypertension has met with some degree of success.

Cor Pulmonale

The term cor pulmonale refers to heart failure resulting from primary lung disease and and long-standing pulmonary hypertension. It involves hypertrophy and the eventual failure of the right ventricle. The manifestations of cor pulmonale include the signs and symptoms of the primary lung disease and the signs of right-sided heart failure. There is shortness of breath and a productive cough, which becomes worse during periods of heart failure. Failure of the right ventricle and elevation of intrathoracic pressure resulting from airway obstruction cause venous distention and peripheral edema. Plethora (redness) and cyanosis and warm moist skin may be present because of the compensatory polycythemia and desaturation of arterial blood that occur with chronic lung disease. Drowsiness and altered consciousness may occur as the result of carbon dioxide retention. Management of cor pulmonale focuses on the treatment of both the lung disease and the heart failure (Chap. 20). Low-flow oxygen therapy may be used to reduce the pulmonary hypertension and polycythemia associated with severe hypoxemia due to chronic lung disease.

In summary, pulmonary vascular disorders include pulmonary embolism and pulmonary hypertension. Pulmonary embolism develops when a blood-borne substance lodges in a branch of the pulmonary artery and obstructs blood flow. The embolus can consist of a thrombus, air, fat, or amniotic fluid. The most frequent form is a thromboembolus arising from the deep venous channels of the lower extremities. Pulmonary hypertension is the elevation of pulmonary arterial pressure. It can be caused by an elevated left atrial pressure, increased pulmonary blood flow, or increased pulmonary vascular resistance secondary to lung disease. The term cor pulmonale describes right heart failure caused by primary pulmonary disease and long-standing pulmonary hypertension.

■ Cancer of the Lung

In the United States, lung cancer strikes an estimated 130,000 persons every year,[55] most commonly those between 40 and 70 years of age. Lung cancer is a leading cause of death among men and a steadily increasing cause among women. These consistent increases over the past 50 years have coincided closely with the increase in cigarette smoking over the same span. It has been estimated that 85% of lung cancer cases are due to cigarette smoking.[56] Many studies have shown that the risk of developing lung cancer increases with the number of cigarettes smoked and that the average male smoker is ten times more likely to develop lung cancer than the non-smoker.[57] Industrial hazards also contribute to the incidence of lung cancer. A commonly recognized hazard is exposure to asbestos, with the mean risk of lung cancer among asbestos workers significantly greater than in the general population. Tobacco smoke contributes heavily to the development of lung cancer in persons exposed to asbestos; the risk in this population group is estimated to be 92 times greater than that for nonsmokers.[58]

Bronchogenic carcinoma is the cancer type seen in 90% to 95% of cases. These tumors can be further subdivided into epidermoid or squamous cell carcinoma (35%-50%); adenocarcinoma (15%-35%); small cell anaplastic (oat cell) carcinoma (20%-25%); and large cell carcinoma (10%-15%).[57]

The tracheobronchial tree is lined with at least five types of epithelial cells that form the pseudostratified cell layer of these airways (Chap. 1). There are three types of columnar cells—the mucus-secreting goblet cells, the ciliated cells, and the brush cells. The basal cells are small, multiple, potential stem cells parallel to the basement membrane on which the pseudostratified cell layer rests. One group of basal cells probably acts as reserve cells for the columnar cells; the other group, termed Kulchitsky (or K-type) cells, appears to be neuroendocrine in origin and is believed to have the capacity to secrete hormones. These cell characteristics would account for the paraneoplastic syndromes that occur in some forms of bronchogenic carcinoma. Squamous cell carcinoma probably arises from the basal reserve cells, adenocarcinoma from the mucin-secreting cells, and small cell and bronchial carcinoid cancers from the K-type cells.[58]

Manifestations

Cancer of the lung develops insidiously, often giving little if any warning of its presence. Because its symptoms are similar to those associated with smoking and chronic bronchitis, they are often disregarded.

The manifestations of lung cancer can be divided into four categories: (1) local respiratory disturbances, (2) the effects of local spread and metastasis, (3) nonspecific effects such as weight loss, and (4) the nonmetastatic endocrine, neurologic, and connective tissue disorders.[30]

Lung cancers produce their local effects through the irritation and obstruction of airways and invasion of the mediastinum and pleural space. The earliest symptoms are chronic cough, shortness of breath, and wheezing due to airway irritation and obstruction. Hemoptysis (blood in the sputum) occurs when the lesion erodes blood vessels. Pain receptors in the chest are limited to the parietal pleura, mediastinum, larger blood vessels, and peribronchial afferent vagal fibers.[30] Dull, intermittent, poorly localized retrosternal pain is common in

tumors that involve the mediastinum. Pain becomes persistent, localized, and more severe when the disease invades the pleura.

Tumors that invade the mediastinum may cause hoarseness (because of the involvement of the recurrens laryngeal nerve) and difficulty in swallowing (due to compression of the esophagus). An uncommon complication called the *superior vena cava syndrome* can occur in some persons with mediastinal involvement. Interruption of flow in this vessel usually results from compression by the tumor or involved lymph nodes. The disorder can interfere with venous drainage from the head, neck, and chest wall. The outcome is determined by the speed with which the disorder develops and the adequacy of the collateral circulation.

Tumors adjacent to the visceral pleura often insidiously produce pleural effusion. This effusion can compress the lung and cause atelectasis and dyspnea. It is less apt to cause fever, pleural friction rub, or pain than pleural effusion resulting from other causes.

Metastases are present in 50% of patients with lung cancer when they first present with evidence of lung cancer and develop inevitably in the majority (90%) of patients.[59] The most common sites of these metastases are the brain, bone, and liver.

Paraneoplastic disorders are those that are unrelated to metastasis. No other type of cancer produces such disorders as frequently as lung cancer. Neurologic or muscular symptoms often develop 6 months to 4 years before the lung tumor is detected. One of the more common of these problems is weakness and wasting of the proximal muscles of the pelvic and shoulder girdles with decreased deep tendon reflexes, but without sensory changes.[30]

Certain bronchogenic carcinomas produce hormones. It has been estimated that approximately 10% of persons with bronchogenic cancer have evidence of ectopic hormone production.[30] The most frequently produced hormones are parathormone (causing hypercalcemia, Chap. 25), antidiuretic hormone (syndrome of inappropriate secretion of ADH, Chap. 25), and ACTH (clinical Cushing's syndrome, Chap. 39).

Because cancer of the lung is usually far advanced before it is discovered, the prognosis is generally poor, with a 5-year survival rate of only 5% to 10%. The hope for the future rests with methods of earlier detection and with prevention.

Diagnosis and Treatment

The diagnosis of lung cancer is based on a careful history and physical examination and other tests such as chest x-ray, bronchoscopy, cytologic studies (Papanicolaou test) of the sputum or bronchial washings, percutaneous needle biopsy of lung tissue, scalene lymph node biopsy, radioisotope studies, and carcinoembryonic antigen enzyme titers. Radioisotope studies include technetium-99, which is used to detect superior vena caval obstruction and study pulmonary blood flow. Gallium and bleomycin scans become fixed to the tumor and can be used to detect its presence. The carcinoembryonic antigen (CEA) is produced by undifferentiated lung tumor cells; high CEA titers usually correlate with extensive disease. This test is often used to follow the progress of the disease and its response to treatment.

Like other types of cancer, lung cancers are classified according to cell type (squamous cell carcinoma, adenocarcinoma, small cell anaplastic carcinoma, and large cell carcinoma) and staged according to the TNM system (see Chap. 5). These classifications are used for treatment planning.

Treatment methods for lung cancer include surgery, radiotherapy, and chemotherapy.[59] These treatments may be used singly or in combination. Surgery is usually used for the removal of small localized tumors. It can involve a lobectomy, pneumonectomy, or segemental resection of the lung. Radiation can be used as a definitive or main treatment modality, as part of a combined treatment plan, or for palliation of symptoms. Because of the frequency of metastases, chemotherapy is frequently used in the treatment of lung cancer. Combination chemotherapy, which uses a regimen of several drugs, is usually used. Immunotherapy, using the bacille Calmette-Guérin (BCG) of the *Mycobacterium tuberculosis bovis*, has been used as an adjuvant treatment. Several other immunotherapy regimens are under investigation. The mechanisms of these treatment methods are discussed in Chapter 5.

In summary, cancer of the lung is a leading cause of death among men ages 40 to 70, and the death rate is increasing among women. In the United Staes this increase in death rate has coincided with the increase in cigarette smoking. Industrial hazards, such as exposure to asbestos, increase the risk of developing lung cancer. Of all forms of lung cancer, bronchogenic carcinoma is the most common, accounting for 90% to 95% of cases. Because lung cancer develops insidiously, it is often far advanced before it is diagnosed, a fact that is used to explain the poor 5-year survival rate for the cancer—only 5% to 10% of affected persons are alive and well 5 years after treatment.

■ Study Guide

After you have studied this chapter, you should be able to meet the following objectives:

☐ Describe the transmission of the common cold from one person to another.

☐ Explain why respiratory infections are common in young children.

☐ Compare croup, epiglottitis, and bronchiolitis in terms of incidence by age, site of infection, and signs and symptoms.

☐ Define the terms *wheezing* and *stridor*.

☐ Explain the mechanisms of sternal and chest wall retraction in small children with upper airway obstruction due to infection.

☐ Give the reason that children with epiglottitis require immediate medical care.

☐ List the signs of impending respiratory failure in small children.

☐ Differentiate between areas of the lung that are involved in lobar, bronchial, and viral pneumonias.

☐ Explain why bronchopneumonia is often seen at the extremes of age.

☐ Describe the four stages of lung involvement in lobar pneumonia.

☐ Explain why the formulation of the influenza vaccine must be changed from year to year.

☐ Cite the characteristics of three groups of persons for whom influenza vaccine is recommended.

☐ State why revaccination with pneumococcal vaccine is not recommended.

☐ Describe the transmission of tuberculosis.

☐ Differentiate between primary tuberculosis and secondary tuberculosis on the basis of their pathophysiology.

☐ State the significance of a positive reaction to the skin test for tuberculosis.

☐ State the American Thoracic Society classification of tuberculosis.

☐ Explain why multiple drug regimens are used in treatment of tuberculosis.

☐ State the mechanism for the transmission of fungal infections of the lung.

☐ State the characteristics of pleural pain.

☐ Explain why tension pneumothorax is a life-threatening situation.

☐ Describe five mechanisms that cause pleural effusion.

☐ Relate the pathologic changes that occur with pleural effusion to the production of signs and symptoms.

☐ Define the terms *hydrothorax*, *chylothorax*, and *hemothorax*.

☐ Explain why surgery increases the risk of atelectasis.

☐ State the feature common to chronic obstructive pulmonary diseases.

☐ State the effect that stimulation of the sympathetic and parasympathetic nervous systems have on bronchial smooth muscle.

☐ State the difference between extrinsic and intrinsic asthma.

☐ Relate the pathology that occurs in bronchial asthma to the production of signs and symptoms.

☐ Explain the distinction between chronic bronchitis and emphysema.

☐ State the function of alpha$_1$ antitrypsin in the prevention of chronic obstructive lung disease.

☐ Explain why cigarette smoking may cause emphysema.

☐ Explain the increase in chest dimensions that occurs in obstructive lung diseases.

☐ State the difference between chronic obstructive pulmonary diseases and interstitial lung diseases.

☐ Compare the breathing patterns of persons with chronic obstructive pulmonary disease and those of persons with interstitial lung disease.

☐ Explain the rationale for inspiratory muscle training in persons with chronic obstructive pulmonary disease.

☐ Describe the rationale for the use of low-flow oxygen in patients with severe hypoxemia due to chronic obstructive pulmonary disease.

☐ State the changes in ventilation that cause nocturnal hypoxemia in some persons with chronic obstructive pulmonary disease.

☐ Describe the abnormalities characteristic of cystic fibrosis.

☐ State the chief manifestations of bronchiectasis.

☐ Cite the characteristics of occupational dusts that determine their pathogenicity in terms of the production of pneumoconioses.

☐ Compare the hypersensitivity reactions that occur with bronchial asthma with those that occur in the hypersensitivity form of occupational lung diseases.

☐ State the immediate effects of pulmonary embolism.

☐ State three causes of pulmonary hypertension.

☐ Describe the alterations in cardiovascular function that are descriptive of cor pulmonale

☐ State two environmental factors that may cause bronchogenic cancer.

☐ List two symptoms of lung cancer that are related to the invasion of the mediastinum.

☐ Cite three paraneoplastic manifestations of lung cancer.

■ References

1. Facts About Lung Disease. New York, American Lung Association, 1980
2. Gwaltney JM Jr.: Epidemiology of the common cold. Ann NY Acad Sci 54, 1980
3. Hendley JA, Gwaltney JM Jr, Jordon WS: Rhinovirus infections in an industrial population. IV. Infections within the families of employees during two fall peaks of respiratory illness. Am J Epidemiol 89:184, 1969
4. Beem, MO: Acute respiratory illness in nursery school children. A longitudinal study of occurrence of illness and respiratory viruses. Am J Epidemiol 90:30, 1969
5. Klumpp TG: The common cold. Med Times 98:1s, 1980
6. Hendley JO, Wenzel RP, Gwaltney JM Jr: Transmission of rhinovirus colds by self-inoculation. N Engl J Med 288:1361, 1973
7. Gwaltney JM Jr, Moskalski PB, Hendley JO: Hand-to-hand transmission of rhinovirus colds. Ann Intern Med 88:464, 1978
8. Anderson TW, Reid BW, Beaton GH: Vitamin C and the common cold: A double blind study. Can Med Assoc J 107:503, 1974
9. Miller JZ, Nance WE, Norton JA et al: Therapeutic effect of vitamin C: A co-twin study. JAMA 237:248, 1977
10. Carr B, Einstein R, Lai LY, Martin NG, Starmer GA: Vitamin C and the common cold. Med J Aust 2:411, 1981
11. Simkins R: Croup and epiglottitis: Am J Nurs 81:519, 1981
12. Sims DG: Acute bronchiolitis in infancy. Nurs Times 75:1842, 1979
13. Simkins R: The crisis of bronchiolitis: Am J Nurs 81:514, 1981
14. Vital Statistics Report: Annual Summary of the United States, 1979, Vol 28, No 13. Washington DC, US Department of Health and Human Services, 1980
15. Dowling JN, Sheehe PR, Feldman H: Pharyngeal pneumococcal acquisitions in "normal" families: A longitudinal study. J Infect Dis 124, No 1:9, 1971
16. Fick RB, Reynolds HY: Changing spectrum of pneumonia—New media creation or clinical reality. Am J Med 74:1, 1983
17. Robbins SL, Cotran R, Kumar V: Pathologic Basis of Disease, 3rd ed, p 734. Philadelphia, WB Saunders, 1984
18. National Nosocomial Infection Study, Fourth Quarter, 1972. Atlanta, US Center for Disease Control, 1974
19. Jones DA: Viral infection of the respiratory system. Chest Heart Stroke J 3, No 5:48, 1979
20. Center for Disease Control: Prevention and control of influenza. MMWR 33 No 19, 1984

21. Prevention and control of influenza. Ann Intern Med 101:218, 1984
22. Center for Disease Control: Update: Pneumococcus polysaccharide vaccine usage—United States. MMWR 33 No 20, 1984
23. Tuberculosis Statistics, DHHS Publication No (CDC)81-8241. Bethesda, MD, US Department of Health and Human Services, 1980.
24. Youmans GP: Tuberculosis, p 356. Philadelphia, WB Saunders, 1979
25. American Thoracic Society, Ad Hoc Committee of the Scientific Assembly on Tuberculosis, Comstock GW Chr: The tuberculin skin test. Am Rev Respir Dis 124:356, 1982
26. American Thoracic Society, Scientific Assembly on Tuberculosis, Weg JG, Chr: Diagnostic standards and classification of tuberculosis and other mycobacterial diseases, 14th edition. Am Rev Respir Dis 124:343, 1981
27. Ad hoc Committee of the American Thoracic Society: Statement on preventive therapy of tuberculosis infection. Am Rev Respir Dis 110:371, 1974
28. Johnson JR: Chemoprophylaxis of pulmonary tuberculosis. Postgrad Med 74 No 3:64, 1983
29. Dall L: Chemotherapy for pulmonary tuberculosis. Postgrad Med 74 No 3:73, 1983
30. Guenther CA, Welch MH: Pulmonary Medicine, 2nd ed, pp 109, 433, 476, 526, 556, 810, 812, 821. Philadelphia, JB Lippincott, 1982
31. Davies SF, Sarosi GA: Fungal infections of the lung. Postgrad Med 73, No 6:242, 1983
32. Sahn SA: Pleural manifestations of pulmonary disease. Hosp Pract 16, No 3:73, 1981
33. Smith LH, Thier SO: Pathophysiology: The Biological Principles of Disease, p 1050. Philadelphia, WB Saunders, 1981
34. National Institute on Allergy and Infectious Diseases Task Force Report No 79-387, Bethesda, MD, p 7, 1979
35. Samter M, Beers RR: Intolerance to aspirin: Clinical studies and considerations of pathogenesis. Ann Intern Med 68:975, 1968
36. McFadden ER, Ingram RH Jr: Exercise-induced asthma. N Engl J Med 301:763, 1979
37. Auber M, DeTroyer A, Sampson M: Aminophylline improves diaphragmatic contractility. N Engl J Med 305:249, 1981
38. Vital Statistics Report: Annual Summary of the United States, 1981, Vol 33, No 3 Washington, DC, US Department of Health and Human Services, 1981
39. Chronic Obstructive Pulmonary Disease, 5th ed, inside front cover. American Lung Association and Medical Section, American Thoracic Society, 1977
40. The Health Consequences of Smoking. Washington DC, US Department of Health, Education and Welfare, 1971
41. Kueppers F, Black LP: Alpha-antitrypsin and its deficiency. Am Rev Respir Dis 110:176, 1974
42. Hodgkin JE et al: Chronic obstructive airway diseases: Current concepts in diagnosis and comprehensive care. JAMA 232, No 12:1253, 1975
43. Kim MJ: Respiratory muscle training: Implications for patient care. Heart Lung 13:333, 1984
44. Pardy RL, Rivington R, Daspas PJ et al: Inspiratory muscle training compared with physiotherapy in patients with chronic airflow limitations. Am Rev Respir Dis 123:421, 1981
45. Nocturnal Oxygen Therapy Group Trial: Continuous or nocturnal oxygen therapy in hypoxemic chronic obstructive lung disease. Ann Intern Med 93:391, 1980
46. Tirlapur DTM, Mir MA: Nocturnal hyoxemia associated with electrocardiographic changes in patients with chronic obstructive airways disease. N Engl J Med 306:125, 1982
47. Fletcher EC, Levin DC: Cardiopulmonary hemodynamics during sleep in subjects with chronic obstructive pulmonary disease. Chest 85 No 1:6, 1984
48. Luce JM: Interstitial lung disease. Hosp Pract 18, No 7:173, 1983
49. Crystal RG, Gadek JE, Ferrans VJ et al: Interstitial lung disease. Am J Med 70:542, 1981
50. Occupational Lung Disease: An Introduction. New York, American Lung Association, 1983
51. Crystal RG, Roberts WC, Hunninghake GW et al (moderators): Pulmonary sarcoidosis: A disease characterized and perpetuated by activated lung T-lymphocytes (report of the NIH conference). Ann Intern Med 94:73, 1981
52. Daniele RP: Sarcoidosis: Diagnosis and management. Hosp Pract 18, No 6:113, 1983
53. Whitcomb ME: The Lung: Normal and Diseased, p 150. St. Louis, CV Mosby, 1982
54. Dalen JE, Alpert JS: Natural history of pulmonary embolism. Prog Cardiovasc Dis 17:259, 1975
55. Cancer Facts 1984. New York, American Cancer Society, 1984
56. Progress against Cancer of the Lung, Publication No (NIH) 76-526, Washington, DC, US Department of Health, Education and Welfare, 1974
57. Smoking and cancer. MMWR 31, No 11:77 1982
58. Carr DT: Bronchiogenic carcinoma. Basics RD 5, No 5:55, 1977
59. Van Houte P, Salazar OM, Phillips CE et al: Lung Cancer. In Rubin P (ed): Clinical Oncology, 6th ed, p 142. New York, American Cancer Society, 1983

■ Additional References

Bilman MJ et al: The ventilatory muscles. Fatigue, endurance, and training. Chest 82:761, 1982

Brandstetter RD, Kazemi H: Aging and the respiratory system. Med Clin North Am 67 No 2:419, 1983

Clee MD, Clark RA: Medical problems associated with tobacco smoking. Pharmacol Ther 16:283, 1982

Gross D: New concepts in respiratory muscle function. Isr J Med Sci 19:383, 1983

King M: Mucus and mucociliary clearance. Basics RD 11 No 1, 1982

Macklem PT: The diaphragm in health and disease. Lab Clin Med 99:5, 1982

Mennies JH: Smoking: The physiologic effects. Am J Nurs 83:1143, 1983

Nadel JA: Bronchial reactivity. Adv Intern Med 28:207, 1983

Risser NL: Preoperative and postoperative care to prevent pulmonary complications. Heart Lung 9:57, 1980

Roussos C, Macklem PT: The respiratory muscles. N Engl J Med 307:786, 1982

Chronic pulmonary disease

Buckley JM: The problem patient: Exercise-induced asthma. Hosp Pract 14, No 5:119-120, 1979

Chakrin LW, Krell RD: Pathophysiology and pharmacotherapy of asthma: An overview. J Pharm Sci 69 No 2:236-238 1980

Cherniack NS: The control of breathing in COPD. Chest 77:291, 1980

Crystal RG, Bitterman PB, Rennard SI: Interstitial lung diseases of unknown cause (part 1 and part 2). N Engl J Med 310:154, 435, 1984

Elpern EH: Asthma update: Pathophysiology and treatment. Heart Lung 9 No 4:665-670, 1980

Flenley DD, Calverly PMA, Douglas NJ et al: Nocturnal hypoxemia and long-term domiciliary oxygen therapy in "blue and bloated" bronchitis. Chest 77 No 2:305-307, 1980

Ghory AC, Patterson R: Treating asthma in the elderly. Geriatrics 35:32-38, 1980

Gross NJ, Skorodin MS: Role of parasympathetic system in airway obstruction due to emphysema. N Engl J Med 311:421, 1984

Hale KA: Chronic airflow obstruction. Postgrad Med 73:259, 1983

Hiller, FC, Wilson FJ: Evaluation and management of acute asthma. Med Clin North Am 63 No 3:669, 1983

Horton FO, Mackenthun AV, Anderson PS et al: Alpha, antitrypsin heterozygotes (Pi type mz): A longitudinal study of the risk of development of chronic air flow limitation. Chest 77 No 2:261-264, 1980

Hudgel DW, Madsen LA: Acute and chronic asthma: A guide to intervention. Am J Nurs 80:1791-1795, 1980

Hunter AM, Carey MA, Larsh HW: The nutritional status of patients with chronic obstructive pulmonary disease. Am Rev Respir Dis 124:376, 1981

Jacobs MM, Bowers B: Protocol: Chronic obstructive lung disease. Nurs Pract 4 No 6:11, 24-28, 1979

Lee M, Gentry AF, Schwartz R, et al: Tartrazine-containing drugs. Drug Intell Clin Pharm 15:782, 1981

Massaro D: Clinical implications of the effect of breathing pattern on the lung. Respiratory Care 25 No 3:377-380, 1980

Matthews JJ: Chronic obstructive pulmonary disease. Topics Emerg Med 2:13-24, 1980

Peter RH, Rubin L: The pharamacologic control of the pulmonary circulation in pulmonary hypertension. Adv Intern Med 29:495, 1984

Petty TL: Long-term outpatient oxygen therapy in advanced chronic obstructive pulmonary disease. Chest 77 No 2:304, 1980

Reed CE: Physiology and pharmacology of beta$_2$ adrenergic agents. Chest 73 No 6:914-926, 1978

Schwartz SH: Asthma therapy. Postgrad Med 73:269, 1983

Snider GL: Control of bronchospasm in patients with chronic obstructive pulmonary diseases. Chest 73 No 6:927-934, 1978

Tattersfield AE: Bronchodilator drugs. Pharmacol Ther 17:299, 1982

Ted Tse CS: Food products containing tartrazine. N Engl J Med 306:681, 1982

Tomashefski JF: Symposium: Definition, differentiation and classification of COPD. Postgrad Med J 62 No 1:88-97, 1977

Unger KM, Moser KM, Hansen P: Selection of an exercise program for patients with chronic obstructive pulmonary disease. Heart Lung 9 No 1:68-76, 1980

Wood BA, Mazow JB, Jackson D: The terrible triad—Asthma, nasal polyps, and sensitivity to aspirin. Heart Lung 12:554, 1983

Respiratory disorders in children

Barker GA: Current management of croup and epiglottitis. Pediatr Clin North Am 26 No 3:565,1979

Cramblett HG: American Academy of Pediatrics Proceedings: Croup—Present-day concept. Pediatrics 25:1071, 1980

Evans HE: Lung Diseases in Children. New York, American Lung Association, 1979

Jones R, Santos JI, Overall JC Jr: Bacterial tracheitis. JAMA 242:721, 1979

Larter N: Cystic fibrosis. Am J Nurs 81:527, 1981

Mathews LW, Drotar D: Cystic Fibrosis—A long-term chronic disease. Med Clin North Am 31 No 1:133, 1984

Mendelsohn J: Pediatric respiratory emergencies. Top Emerg Med 2:25, 1980

Milner AD: Acute airway obstruction in children under 5. Thorax 37:641, 1982

Page HS: Croup and epiglottitis: Sudden trouble for young children. Am Lung Assoc Bull 67 No 2:9, 1981

Pinney M: pneumonia. Am J Nurs 81:517, 1981

Simkins R: Asthma: Reactive airway disease. Am J Nurs 81:523, 1981

Simkins R: Croup and epiglottitis. Am J Nurs 81:519, 1981

Simkins R: The crisis of bronchiolitis. Am J Nurs 81:514, 1981

Respiratory tract infections

Austrian R: A reassessment of pneumococcal vaccine. N Engl J Med 310:651, 1984

Drutz DJ, Catanzar A: Coccidioidomycosis. Am Rev Respir Dis 117:559, 1978

Fick RB, Reynolds HY: Changing spectrum of pneumonia—New media creation or clinical reality. Am J Med 74:1, 1983

Finland M: Pneumonia and pneumococcal infections, with special reference to pneumococcal pneumonia. Am Rev Respir Dis 120:481-502, 1979

Frame PT: Acute infectious pneumonia in the adult. Basics RD 10 No 3, 1982

Goodwin RA Jr, Loyd JE, Des Pres RM: Histoplasmosis in normal hosts. Medicine (Baltimore) 60:231, 1981

Hendley JO, Sande MA, Stewart PM, Gwaltney JM Jr: Spread of streptococcus pneumoniae in families: I. Carriage rates and distribution of types. J Infect Dis 132 No 1:55-61, 1975

Kesarwala HH: Pneumonia: A clinical review. J Med Soc NJ 77 No 1:43-46, 1980

Kilbourn JP: Bacterial flora of the respiratory tract. J Am Med Tech 42:218-226, 1980

Murray BE, Moellering RC: Antimicrobial agents in pulmonary infections. Med Clin North Am 64 No 3:319-320, 1980

Murray HW, Tuazon C: Atypical pneumonias. Med Clin North Am 64 No 3:507-527, 1980

Reichman RC, Dolin R: Viral pneumonias. Med Clin North Am 64 No 3:491-505, 1980

Sarosi GA, Dacies SF: Blastomycoses. Am Rev Respir Dis 120:911, 1979

Tuazon C: Gram-positive pneumonias. Med Clin North Am 64 No 3:343-361, 1980

Lung cancer

Anderson RW, Artenzen CE: Carcinoma of the lung. Surg Clin North Am 60 No 4, 1980

MacMahon H et al: Diagnostic methods in lung cancer. Semin Oncol 10:20, 1983

Whimster WF: Lung tumors: Differentiation and classification. Pathol Annu 18 Pt 1:121, 1983

Chapter 24

Alterations in Control of Ventilation and Respiratory Failure

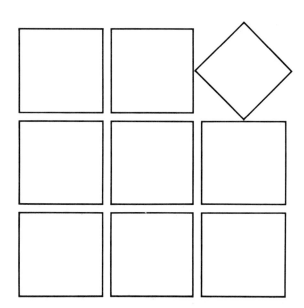

The major function of the lungs is to oxygenate and remove carbon dioxide from the blood as a means of supporting the metabolic functions of body cells. Hypoventilation and respiratory failure result in hypoxia and hypercapnia, whereas hyperventilation causes hypocapnia. The discussion in this chapter focuses on alterations in ventilatory control and respiratory failure.

■ Alterations in Control of Ventilation

Normally breathing involves a smooth and regular sequence of inspiration and expiration at a rate and depth regulated to maintain the arterial partial pressures of O_2 and CO_2 at relatively constant levels. Unlike the action of the heart, which beats independently of the nervous system, the inflation and deflation of the lungs require continuous input from the nervous system (see Chap. 22). A number of different types of disorders may alter neural control of ventilation. The ventilatory drive can be depressed by drugs, rendered ineffective in neu-

romuscular disorders affecting the respiratory muscles, and increased in hyperventilation syndrome. In sleep apnea abnormalities in the coordination of ventilation occur during sleep. Sudden infant death syndrome (SIDS) has been attributed to abnormalities in ventilatory drive.

Drug-Induced Respiratory Depression

Impaired function of the respiratory muscles can be caused by drugs that depress the central nervous system and the respiratory center; neuromuscular blocking drugs such as *d*-tubocurarine and succinylcholine (used to effect muscle relaxation during surgery) that block the transmission of impulses at the level of the myoneural junction; or drugs that act peripherally at a site beyond the myoneural junction, possibly by interfering with calcium release from the sarcoplasmic reticulum (Table 24-1).

Almost all the drugs known to cause depression of the central nervous system have been associated with decreased alveolar ventilation. Stupor and coma caused by depressant drug poisoning present as a picture of metabolic coma, progressing from class O to IV (Chap. 47). Overdoses of barbiturates, hypnotics, narcotics, and antidepressant drugs are common causes of admission to respiratory intensive care units. Airway obstruction due to involvement of the muscles of the oropharynx and loss of the cough reflex precedes or accompanies loss of ventilatory drive and complicates the condition. Insertion of an endotracheal tube with mechanical ventilatory support may be needed when hypoventilation causes hypercapnia. It is important to recognize that small doses of drugs that depress the respiratory center may cause further impairment of ventilation and lead to hypercapnia in persons with preexisting respiratory disease. Therefore, these drugs should be used with great caution in persons with chronic lung disease and respiratory muscle weakness.

Weakness of the Respiratory Muscles

Weakness of the respiratory muscles can result from conditions that denervate the muscles (*e.g.*, spinal cord injury or poliomyelitis), affect the myoneural junction (*e.g.*, myasthenia gravis), or cause direct involvement of the muscles themselves (*e.g.*, muscular dystrophy). Disorders of the respiratory muscles are characterized by decreased vital capacity and maximum voluntary ventilation, while measures of expiratory flow are well maintained. Many persons with these disorders may be able to maintain adequate ventilation for brief periods of time, but sustaining normal minute ventilation may impose an

---

Table 24-1 Drugs with Respiratory Depressant Actions*

Functional Drug Groups†	Mechanisms of Action
Anesthetic Agents	
General anesthesia	Depression of CNS function including medullary respiratory center
Spinal anesthesia	Production of ascending muscle paralysis to level of respiratory muscles
Drugs Affecting Brain Stem Respiratory Mechanisms	
Opiates and narcotic analgesics	Depression of brain stem respiratory mechanisms, causing a decrease in ventilatory drive
Barbiturates and sedatives	
Tricyclic antidepressants	
Alcohol	
Drugs Affecting Myoneural Junction	
Muscle relaxants	Production of impulse blockade at level of myoneural junction in skeletal muscle, including respiratory muscles
Aminoglycoside antibiotics‡	
Polymixin antibiotics‡	
Quinine‡	
Quinidine‡	
Drugs Affecting Muscle Contraction	
Dantrolene	Reduction of excitation –contraction coupling within skeletal muscle fiber, causing muscle weakness

*The respiratory effects of these drugs are usually dose dependent.
†This list of drugs is not inclusive.
‡The respiratory effects of these drugs usually occur at toxic doses.

excessive load on the weakened and fatigued muscles, and hypoventilation may result. Persons with impaired respiratory muscle function show extreme sensitivity to respiratory depressant drugs.

Sleep Apnea

Apnea is defined as the cessation of airflow through the nose and mouth for a period of 10 seconds or longer. The diagnosis of sleep apnea depends on the occurrence of 30 or more apneic periods during 7 hours of sleep.[1] Typically, the apneic periods last for 15 to 120 seconds and some persons may have as many as 500 apneic periods per night.

Sleep stages and respiration

Sleep is not a constant, uniform state, but rather a pattern of sequential stages with a periodicity of about 90 minutes. These stages are associated with electroencephalographic (EEG), behavioral, and physiologic changes that affect the control of breathing. Two sleep states have been defined: rapid eye movement (REM), also referred to as active sleep, and non-REM sleep, or quiet sleep.

Non-REM sleep is encountered when one first becomes drowsy; it has four stages reflecting an increasing depth of sleep. Stage 1 consists primarily of low-voltage, mixed-frequency EEG activity; it reflects the drowsy state. Stage 2 is a deeper sleep during which EEG activity is characterized by bursts of high-frequency (12–14 cycles/second) and high-amplitude waves called K complexes. Stages 3 and 4 are often referred to as slow-wave sleep because the EEG is dominated by high-voltage, low-frequency (1–2 cycles/second) waves. Stages 1 and 2 of non-REM sleep are often characterized by a pattern of breathing in which there is cyclic waning and waxing of tidal volume and respiratory rate, which may include brief periods (5–15 seconds) of apnea. Although the amount of periodic breathing that occurs during the first two stages of non-REM sleep differs among healthy persons, it is more common in persons over age 40.[2] Periodic breathing during sleep is very common at high altitudes because of a change in set point of the PO_2 chemoreceptors. Once sleep becomes stabilized during stages 3 and 4 of non-REM sleep, breathing becomes more regular. During slow-wave sleep, ventilation is usually 1 liter to 2 liters/minute less than during quiet wakefulness; the PCO_2 levels are 4 mm Hg to 8 mm Hg greater; the PO_2 levels are 3 mm Hg to 10 mm Hg less; and the pH is 0.03 to 0.05 units less.[2] Control of breathing during non-REM sleep is dominated by automatic control mechanisms—responses to hypercapnia, hypoxia, and lung inflation are intact and critically important to maintaining ventilation.

REM sleep resembles wakefulness in many ways: the EEG is unsynchronized with low-voltage and mixed-frequency waves, and there are frequent muscular and rapid eye movements. Autonomic nervous system activity changes during REM sleep: the heart rate and blood pressure may fluctuate rapidly and the cerebral blood flow and metabolic rate decrease. Respiration becomes irregular (but not periodic) and may include periods of apnea lasting as long as 15 to 20 seconds in healthy adults and 10 seconds in infants. Breathing during REM sleep has many of the features of the voluntary type of control associated with talking, walking, and swallowing. Automatic control of breathing remains during REM sleep, but its influence is diminished.

During all the stages of sleep the tone of most skeletal muscles decreases, with the exception of the diaphragm.[3] This loss of muscle tone is most pronounced during REM sleep. In the awake state, intercostal muscle activity tends to stiffen the rib cage. With the absence of this tone during sleep, the negative intrapleural pressure caused by contracton of the diaphragm can cause paradoxical motion of the rib cage (the rib cage moves inward during inspiration rather than outward) and a decrease in functional residual capacity. The loss of tone in the upper airways can cause airway obstruction. Negative airway pressure produced by contraction of the diaphragm tends to bring the vocal cords together, collapse the pharyngeal wall, and suck the tongue back into the throat. Airway collapse is increased in persons with conditions that cause narrowing of the upper airway or weakness of the throat muscles.

Types of sleep apnea

Sleep apnea can be classified as obstructive, central, or mixed. Obstructive apnea is caused by the obstruction of the upper airway. With central apnea the respiratory drive ceases and there is no movement of the chest or abdominal muscle. Mixed apnea constitutes a mixture of central and obstructive apnea. Because breathing seems to be controlled by different mechanisms during REM and non-REM sleep, different causes are associated with the different types of sleep apnea.

Obstructive sleep apnea. Obstructive sleep apnea is commonly associated with obesity and disorders that compromise the patency of the airway. It occurs most commonly in middle-aged men. Although androgens are suspected of contributing to the disorder, their mechanism of action is at present unknown. The Pickwickian syndrome, named after the fat boy in Charles Dickens' *The Posthumous Papers of the Pickwick Club,* published in 1837, is characterized by obesity, hypersomnolence, periodic breathing, hypoxemia, and right heart failure. Alcohol and other drugs that depress the central nervous system seem to increase the severity of obstructive apneic episodes.

Obstructive sleep apnea is characterized by loud snoring interrupted by periods of silence. Abnormal gross motor movements during sleep are common. In many cases, the snoring precedes by many years the onset of other signs of sleep apnea. There are often complaints of morning headache and nausea and persistent daytime sleepiness. The hypersomnolence can lead to occupational and driving accidents. Psychological problems associated with impotence, intellectual deterioration, and depression are also part of the symptom complex. The signs and symptoms of sleep apnea are summarized in Chart 24-1. In children, a decline in school performance may be the only indication of the problem.

In addition to the sleep disturbances, a number of cardiovascular problems are associated with sleep apnea syndromes. A number of cardiac arrhythmias have been observed in individuals with sleep apnea. Frequent apneic periods may result in increased pulmonary and systemic blood pressures. More than two-thirds of the sleep apneic patients in one study had daytime hypertension.[4] In severe cases, pulmonary hypertension, polycythemia, and cor pulmonale may develop.

Central sleep apnea. Central sleep apnea is associated with disorders that affect the central nervous system and respiratory neurons, such as encephalitis, brain stem infarction, and bulbar poliomyelitis. With central sleep apnea sleep is difficult to maintain and several awakenings occur during the night. There may be some daytime fatigue, depression, and impaired sexual functioning. In contrast to persons with obstructive sleep apnea, persons with central sleep apnea tend to be of normal weight.

Diagnosis and treatment

Sleep apnea is usually suspected from a history of snoring, disturbed sleep, and daytime sleepiness. A definitive diagnosis is accomplished with sleep studies done using polysomnography.[5] This procedure consists of (1) an EEG and electro-oculogram to determine the sleep

---

Chart 24-1 Signs and Symptoms of Sleep Apnea

Noisy snoring
Insomnia
Abnormal movements during sleep
Morning headaches
Excessive daytime sleepiness
Intellectual and personality changes
Sexual impotence
Systemic hypertension
Pulmonary hypertension, cor pulmonale
Polycythemia

---

stages, (2) monitoring of the airflow, (3) an ECG to detect arrhythmias, (4) impedance pneumography, intercostal electromyography, or esophageal manometry to monitor respiratory effort, and (5) ear oximetry or transcutaneous oxygen monitoring to detect changes in oxygen saturation.

The treatment of sleep apnea is determined by the type of apnea that is present. Weight loss is often beneficial in persons with obstructive apnea. Severe cases may require a tracheostomy. The successful use of nocturnal nasal-airway pressure has been reported recently as a means of treating obstructive sleep apnea.[6] The drug protriptyline, a nonsedative tricyclic antidepressant that reduces REM sleep, has also been used successfully to reduce apneic episodes in some persons.[7] In cases of central apnea, a variety of medications have been used to increase the central respiratory drive, including theophylline, acetazolamide, clomipramine, and medroxyprogesterone. In severe cases, the most effective treatment is electrical stimulation of the phrenic nerves with implanted electrodes.

Sudden Infant Death Syndrome

Sudden infant death syndrome (SIDS), or crib death, is the most common cause of death in infants 1 to 12 months of age and is most common between the ages of 3 and 18 weeks.[8] The incidence is about 2 per 1000 infants; it is less common in whites, greater in blacks, and greatest in Native Americans.[9] Male infants are at greater risk than female infants, and infants born prematurely are at greater risk than full-term infants. There is an increased incidence of SIDS among infants born to young unmarried mothers who had little prenatal care, as well as among infants of mothers who were narcotic addicts. Although there is no evidence of genetic transmission, SIDS has occurred three and even four times in the same family, and twins and triplets have a greater incidence of SIDS.[9]

The usual history of an infant with SIDS is one of a previously healthy infant who is found dead after going to sleep for a nap or for the night. In the past, these deaths have often been attributed to infanticide, allergic responses, infections, or suffocation. Current theory, however, suggests that an abnormal control of ventilation places the infant at particular risk for this disorder. The ventilatory response of an infant varies from that of the adult in several ways.[10] Unlike the adult, the newborn infant responds to hypoxemia with a temporary increase in ventilation, followed by a sustained decrease in ventilation. The hypoxemia may induce periodic breathing with periods of apnea lasting from 10 to 20 seconds. Even prior to birth, hypoxemia such as that produced by cigarette smoking in the mother has been observed to cause a decrease in the breathing movements of the fetus.

Episodes of periodic breathing are most severe in premature and high-risk infants. Periodic breathing in infants occurs primarily during sleep and may be partly related to the compliant chest wall of the infant. During REM sleep, which constitutes about 50% to 80% of sleep in infants, there is loss of the intercostal muscle tone; this leads to an exaggeration of the paradoxical chest motion and airway collapse as the diaphragm contracts and pulls the chest cage inward. It has been suggested that partial obstruction of the airways or inadequacy of the ventilatory pump of infants at risk for SIDS causes alveolar hypoxia, which leads to hyperplasia of pulmonary vascular smooth mucle and hypoxemia, which leads to changes in brain stem cells.[9] Both pulmonary vascular hyperplasia and changes in the brain stem cells have been observed on autopsy in infants who died of SIDS. As the pulmonary vascular muscularity increases, pulmonary vasoconstriction becomes more intense, increasing the afterload burden of the right heart enough to promote cardiac failure and even more severe hypoxia. The brain stem changes promote hypoventilation and hypoxemia, causing further brain stem injury.

Diagnosis and treatment

Measures for the management and treatment of SIDS have focused on methods of identifying those infants at risk. High-risk infants (*e.g.*, those with near-miss SIDS and infants who have been successfully resuscitated) are placed on home monitoring programs, and the parents are trained in both monitoring and cardiorespiratory resuscitation methods.

Hyperventilation Syndrome

The hyperventilation syndrome involves overbreathing, reduction in PCO_2, and respiratory alkalosis. In 1871 De Costa provided the first account of the syndrome in the medical literature when he reported on the cases of 300 Civil War soldiers affected with the disorder. The disorder has subsequently been labeled soldier's heart, irritable heart, De Costa's syndrome, and neurocirculatory asthenia. De Costa noted that the affected soldier "got out of breath, could not keep up with his comrades, was annoyed with dizziness and palpitation, and with pain in the chest; his accouterments oppressed him, and all through this he appeared well and healthy." The nervous manifestations of the syndrome were "headache, dizziness, and disturbed sleep."[11] Removal from the stress of active duty along with enforced rest reduced the symptoms, but even with removal from active duty, the "irritability of the heart remained."[11]

Causes

The causes of the disorder have been categorized into four groups: (1) organic, (2) physiologic, (3) emotional, and (4) habitual.[12] Organic causes include such things as

drug effects and central nervous system lesions, such as meningitis. Altitude acclimation, heat, and exercise constitute physiologic causes of hyperventilation.[13] Emotional states that predispose to hyperventilation are hysteria, anxiety, depression, and anger. Whereas stress may trigger the initial event, anxiety and fear over the symptoms may perpetuate the syndrome.[16] Because the symptoms of hyperventilation syndrome commonly involve the heart and head, the person experiences intense anxiety, often accompanied by a fear of death or of losing control. The condition occurs in children as well as adults.[14]

Manifestations

The hyperventilation syndrome commonly causes symptoms such as headache, dyspnea, numbness and tingling sensations, lightheadedness, chest pain, palpitations, and sometimes syncope. There are often complaints of dyspnea and being unable to take a full deep breath. Persons with a full constellation of the syndrome breathe with rapid, shallow breaths marked by irregularity in the depth and rate of respiration. Sighing is common. Hyperventilators are primarily thoracic rather than abdominal breathers. There is a tendency to breathe using the upper chest wall intercostal muscles, which may cause dull aching soreness in the left precordial area, mimicking angina. It has been suggested that the alkalosis associated with hyperventilation syndrome can induce coronary artery spasm in persons with Prinzmetal's angina [15, 16] and in some individuals with atherosclerotic coronary artery disease.[16, 17] It has also been observed that S–T wave changes can occur with hyperventilation.[14]

For many persons afflicted with the hyperventilation syndrome there may not be a continuously symptomatic state but recurrences of symptoms with or without recognizable provocative stresses. In others, a more chronic form of the disorder may occur in which the respiratory center is reset to allow for lower levels of PCO_2 to persist in spite of a normal pH.[18] This may explain the chronicity of the disorder and the easy provocation of symptoms associated with hyperventilation in individuals who are chronically hypocapnic. Sympathetic nervous system stimulation provokes a hyperventilatory response and may increase the occurrence of symptoms in persons with chronic hyperventilation problems.

Diagnosis and treatment

A provocative test, in which a person purposefully hyperventilates, can be done to demonstrate occurrence of the symptoms.[11] Arterial blood gases may be obtained to study the pH and carbon dioxide levels. Electrocardiograph monitoring is done during the test on persons who have complained of chest pain, and caution should be used when performing the test on persons with known or suspected coronary heart disease. The treatment focuses on educating the person and his family about the disorder, relaxation therapy, and training to overcome faulty breathing patterns. Rebreathing into a paper bag can be used to control the symptoms. For many individuals, the realization that they can control their symptoms and nothing is seriously wrong reduces their anxiety and helps them to control the disorder.

In summary, alterations in the control of ventilation include drug-induced disorders, respiratory muscle weakness, sleep apnea, SIDS, and the hyperventilation syndrome. Almost all the drugs known to cause depression of the respiratory system have been associated with impairment of ventilation. Drugs can act centrally to depress the respiratory center, or they may act peripherally at the level of the myoneural junction. Weakness of the respiratory muscles can result from conditions that denervate the muscles, affect the myoneural junction, or cause direct involvement of muscle tissue. Sleep apnea involves 30 or more apneic spells characterized by the cessation of airflow through the nose and mouth for a period of 10 seconds or longer. It can result from disorders that compromise the patency of the airways during sleep (obstructive sleep apnea) or disorders that affect the central nervous system and respiratory neurons (central sleep apnea). SIDS is the most common cause of death in infants 1 to 12 months of age. Although its cause is unknown, current theory suggests that these infants have immature or impaired ventilatory control mechanisms. The hyperventilation syndrome consists of overbreathing, reduction in PCO_2, and respiratory alkalosis. It can result from organic causes such as drug effects and central nervous system lesions, physiologic changes such as heat exposure and exercise, emotional states, or habit. It can cause a number of signs and symptoms such as headache, dyspnea, numbness and tingling sensations, lightheadedness, palpitations, and sometimes syncope.

■ Acute Respiratory Failure

Respiratory failure occurs when the lungs are unable to adequately oxygenate the blood or prevent undue retention of carbon dioxide even at rest. Respiratory failure can develop acutely in persons whose lungs previously had been normal or may be superimposed on chronic disease of the lung or chest wall. It has been reported that obstructive lung disease accounts for about one-third of the cases of acute respiratory failure in intensive care units.[19]

There is no absolute definition of the levels of arterial PO_2 and PCO_2 that indicate respiratory failure.

As a general rule, respiratory failure refers to a PO_2 level of 50 mm Hg or less and hypercapnia (hypercarbia) to a PCO_2 level greater than 50 mm Hg. These values are not altogether reliable when dealing with persons who have chronic lung disease, because many of these persons are alert and functioning with blood gas levels outside this range. Table 24-2 compares the normal values for blood gases with those of respiratory failure.

Causes

Respiratory failure is not a specific disease. It is associated with a number of disorders in which the lungs fail to deliver sufficient oxygen to the arterial blood or to remove sufficient carbon dioxide. Three types of conditions contribute to the hypoxemia in respiratory failure: hypoventilation, impaired diffusion across the alveolar capillary membrane, and mismatching of ventilation and perfusion. These conditions include impaired ventilation due to upper airway obstruction, weakness or paralysis of the respiratory muscles, chest wall injury, and disease of the pulmonary airways and lungs. Respiratory failure can also arise when diffusion of gases across the alveolar capillary membrane is impeded. The causes of respiratory failure are summarized in Table 24-3; many are discussed in other parts of the text.

Manifestations

Respiratory failure may be seen in previously healthy persons as the result of acute disease or trauma involving the respiratory system, or it may develop in the course of a chronic respiratory disease. The presenting signs and symptoms are different in each of these situations. The common manifestations of respiratory failure are *hypoxemia* and *hypercapnia*. Various types of respiratory failure are associated with different degrees of hypoxemia and carbon dioxide retention. In the respiratory syndrome that causes impaired diffusion across the alveolar capillary membrane, hypoxemia becomes severe, whereas arterial PCO_2 decreases or remains normal because carbon dioxide is more soluble in the alveolar capillary membrane than oxygen. In conditions such as chronic obstructive pulmonary disease in which respiratory failure is superimposed on lung disease, severe mismatching of ventilation and perfusion often results in both hypoxemia and hypercapnia.

Hypoxemia

In hypoxemia, the blood oxygen levels are insufficient to meet the oxidative requirements of body tissues. These tissues vary considerably in their vulnerability to hypoxia; those with the greatest need are the nervous system and heart.

Table 24-2   Blood Gases in Respiratory Failure Compared with Normal Values

Arterial Blood Gas Value	Normal Value	Respiratory Failure
PO_2	Above 80 mm Hg	50 mm Hg or less
PCO_2	35–45 mm Hg	50 mm Hg or above

Table 24-3   Causes of Respiratory Failure

Category of Impairment	Examples
Impaired Ventilation	
Upper airway obstruction	Laryngospasm
	Foreign body aspiration
	Tumor of the upper airways
	Infection of the upper airways (*e.g.,* epiglottitis)
Weakness or paralysis of the respiratory muscles	Drug overdose
	Injury to the spinal cord
	Poliomyelitis
	Guillain-Barré syndrome
	Muscular dystrophy
	Disease of the brain stem
Chest wall injury	Rib fracture
	Burn eschar
Impaired Matching of Ventilation and Perfusion	
	Chronic obstructive lung disease
	Restrictive lung disease
	Severe pneumonia
	Atelectasis
Impaired Diffusion	
Pulmonary edema	Left heart failure
	Inhalation of toxic materials
Respiratory distress syndrome	Respiratory distress syndrome in the newborn
	Adult respiratory distress syndrome (shock lung)

The signs and symptoms of hypoxemia can be grouped into two categories: those resulting from impaired function of vital centers and those resulting from the activation of compensatory mechanisms. Central nervous system hypoxia produces symptoms similar to acute intoxication. There may be personality changes, restlessness, agitation to combative behavior, muscle incoordination, euphoria, impaired judgment, delirium, and eventual coma. The neurologic manifestations are frequently the presenting clinical features in acute respiratory failure. Tachycardia, cool skin (peripheral vasoconstriction), diaphoresis, and a mild increase in blood pressure result from the recruitment of sympathetic compensatory mechanisms. Although cyanosis may be evident, its presence cannot be relied on. Its detection requires a concentration of approximately 5 gm/100 ml in the circulating blood (Chap. 22). When the hemoglobin concentration is normal, this means that the arterial saturation must be reduced to below 70% and the arterial PO_2 to less than 35 mm Hg, hence it is a late sign of hypoxemia.[20] This is especially critical in someone with anemia. Hypotension and bradycardia are often preterminal events in hypoxemia, indicating the failure of compensatory mechanisms. The signs and symptoms of hypoxemia are listed in Chart 24-2.

Hypoxemia may be insidious in onset, and its symptoms may be attributed to other causes, particularly in chronic lung disease. Decreased sensory function, such as impaired vision or fewer complaints of pain may be an early sign of hypoxia. This is probably because the involved sensory neurons have the same need for high levels of oxygen as do other parts of the nervous system.

Hypercapnia

Carbon dioxide has a direct vasodilatory effect on many blood vessels and a sedative effect on the nervous system. When the cerebral vessels are dilated, headache will develop. The conjunctiva are hyperemic and the skin flushed. Hypercapnia has nervous system effects similar to those of an anesthetic—hence the term *carbon dioxide narcosis*. There is progressive somnolence, disorientation, and, if untreated, coma. Mild to moderate increases in blood pressure are common. The signs and symptoms

---

Chart 24-2   *Signs and Symptoms of Hypoxemia*

Arterial blood gas levels below 50 mm Hg
Tachycardia
Mild increase in blood pressure
Cool and moist skin
Confusion
Delirium
Difficulty in problem solving
Loss of judgment
Euphoria
Unruly or combative behavior
Sensory impairment
Mental fatigue
Drowsiness
Stupor and coma (late)
Hypotension (late)
Bradycardia (late)

---

of hypercapnia are summarized in Chart 24-3. The body adapts to chronic increases in blood levels of carbon dioxide, hence persons with chronic hypercapnia may not develop symptoms until the PCO_2 is markedly elevated. Elevated levels of PCO_2 are characterized by respiratory acidosis, discussed in Chapter 27.

Chart 24-3   Signs and Symptoms of Hypercapnia

Headache
Conjunctival hyperemia
Flushed skin
Increased sedation
   Drowsiness
   Disorientation
   Coma
Tachycardia
Diaphoresis
Mild to moderate increase in blood pressure

Treatment

Treatment of respiratory failure is directed toward correcting the cause and relieving the hypoxemia and hypercapnia; and for this purpose a number of treatment modalities are available, including establishment of an airway, use of bronchodilators, antibiotics for respiratory infections, and others. Controlled oxygen therapy and mechanical ventilation are measures that are used in treating blood gas abnormalities associated with respiratory failure.

Oxygen therapy

Oxygen may be given by nasal cannula, catheter, Venturi mask, or mask–bag combination. Oxygen may also be administered directly into an endotracheal or tracheostomy tube. A high-flow administration system is one in which the flow rate and reserve capacity are sufficient to provide all of the inspired air. A low-flow oxygen system delivers less than the total inspired air. The oxygen must be humidified as it is being administered. The flow rate (liters per minute) is based on the arterial PO_2. The rate must be carefully monitored in persons with chronic lung disease because marked increases in PO_2 (above 60 mm Hg) are apt to depress the ventilatory drive. There is also the danger of oxygen toxicity with high concentrations of oxygen. Continuous breathing of high concentrations can lead to diffuse parenchymal lung injury. Persons with normal lungs begin to experience respiratory symptoms ranging from substernal distress to paresthesias, nausea and vomiting, general malaise, and fatigue after breathing 100% oxygen (at 1 atmosphere) for 6 to 30 hours.[20]

Mechanical ventilation

Should oxygen therapy and other conservative methods prove ineffective in situations in which the PO_2 cannot be maintained at 50 mm Hg and respiratory acidosis is out of control, use of a mechanical ventilator may be a life-saving measure. Mechanical ventilators are of two types—pressure-controlled units and volume-controlled units. The pressure-controlled ventilator delivers a tidal volume determined by the airway pressure while the flow rate is being controlled. The volume-controlled ventilator delivers a preselected tidal volume while the pressure is monitored. The tidal volume and respiratory rate are adjusted to maintain ventilation at a given minute volume. A nasotracheal, orotracheal, or tracheotomy tube is inserted into the trachea to provide the patient with the airway needed for mechanical ventilation.

Adult Respiratory Distress Syndrome

The adult respiratory distress syndrome (ARDS) is an extreme form of noncardiac pulmonary edema and is the final common pathway through which many serious localized and systemic disorders exert their effect on the respiratory system. Approximately 140,000 cases of ARDS occur each year in the United States, and at least 50% of these persons die despite the most sophisticated intensive medical care.[21]

The exact cause of ARDS is unknown. It is thought to result from injury to the microcirculation (small blood vessels and capillaries) of the lung. Numerous insults are associated with its development. The term *shock lung* (Chap. 21) has been used to describe the respiratory distress syndrome associated with trauma and hypovolemic or septic shock. It may also result from aspiration, infectious processes, hematologic disorders, metabolic events, and reactions to drugs and toxins (Chart 24-4). It is not known whether multiple pathogenic mechanisms operate to cause a similar pattern of injury or common mechanisms triggered by diverse mechanisms are responsible.[22]

Although a number of conditions may lead to ARDS, they all produce similar pathologic lung changes. The permeability of the alveolar capillary membrane increases which permits large protein molecules to move out of the vascular compartment into the interstitium and alveoli of the lung. The increased protein concentration in the interstitial spaces contributes to the entry of water. The surface tension in the alveoli may increase markedly because of the inactivation of surfactant by the plasma proteins and injury to the surfactant-producing cells. This and the increased pressure caused by excess fluid in the interstitial spaces cause alveolar collapse and make the lung stiff and difficult to inflate. The compliance of the lung decreases, and the work of breathing increases. Hyaline membranes develop and line the alveolar ducts and alveoli, compromising the diffusion of respiratory gases.

Clinically, the syndrome consists of progressive respiratory distress, an increase in respiratory rate, and signs of respiratory failure. X-ray findings usually show exten-

Chart 24-4   *Conditions in Which the Respiratory Distress Syndrome Can Develop**

Aspiration
  Gastric acid
  Near-drowning
Reaction to drugs and toxins
  Chlordiazepoxide
  Heroin
  Methadone
  Propoxyphene
  Chloroform
  Colchicine
  Barbiturates
  Inhaled gases
    Ammonia
    Phosgene
    Ozone
    Oxygen (high concentrations)
    Smoke
Hematologic disorders
  Multiple blood transfusions
  Disseminated intravascular clotting (DIC)
  Exposure to cardiopulmonary bypass
Infectious causes
  Bacterial pneumonia
  Fungal and *Pneumocystis carinii* pneumonias
  Gram-negative sepsis
  Tuberculosis
  Viral pneumonia
Immune reactions
  Anaphylactic shock
  Allergic reactions to inhaled substances
Metabolic disorders
  Diabetic ketoacidosis
  Uremia
Trauma
  Burns
  Fat embolus
  Head trauma
  Chest trauma and lung injury
  Shock

*This list not intended to be inclusive.

sive bilateral consolidation of the lung tissue. Severe hypoxemia persists in spite of increased inspired oxygen levels.

The treatment goals in ARDS are to supply oxygen to vital organs and provide supportive care until the condition causing the pathologic process has been reversed and the lungs have had a chance to heal. Assisted ventilation using high concentrations of oxygen may be required to overcome the hypoxemia. Positive end-expiratory pressure (PEEP) breathing, which increases the pressure in the airways during expiration, may be used to assist in reinflating the collapsed areas of the lung and improve the matching of ventilation and perfusion.

In summary, respiratory failure is a condition in which the lungs fail to adequately oxygenate the blood or prevent undue retention of carbon dioxide. The causes of respiratory failure are many: it may arise acutely in persons with previously healthy lungs or may be superimposed in chronic lung disease. It is generally defined as a PO_2 of 50 mm Hg or less and a PCO_2 of 50 mm Hg or more. Hypoxemia incites sympathetic nervous system responses such as tachycardia and produces symptoms similar to those of alcohol intoxication. Hypercapnia causes vasodilatation of blood vessels, including those in the brain, and has an anesthetic effect (carbon dioxide narcosis). Adult respiratory distress syndrome (ARDS) is an extreme form of noncardiogenic pulmonary edema that results in respiratory failure. The condition can be caused by a number of serious localized and systemic disorders that cause damage to the alveolar capillary membrane of the lung. It results in interstitial edema of lung tissue, an increase in surface tension due to inactivation of surfactant, collapse of the alveolar structures, a stiff and noncompliant lung that is difficult to inflate, and impaired diffusion of the respiratory gases with severe hypoxemia that is resistant to oxygen therapy.

■ Study Guide

After you have studied this chapter, you should be able to meet the following objectives:

☐ List at least three categories of drugs that can depress respiratory function.

☐ Cite a common characteristic related to ventilatory impairment that occurs in disorders of the respiratory muscles.

☐ Define sleep apnea.

☐ Compare the respiratory activities that occur during each of the four stages of sleep.

☐ List the behaviors that are characteristic of REM sleep.

☐ Differentiate between the alterations in respiratory function that account for the cessation of breathing in central and obstructive sleep apnea.

☐ State the signs and symptoms of sleep apnea.

☐ Compare the characteristics of persons at risk for developing obstructive sleep apnea with those of persons at risk for developing central sleep apnea.

☐ Describe methods that might be used in the diagnosis of sleep apnea.

☐ Compare the control of breathing and response to hypoxia in infants and adults.

☐ Cite four general causes of hyperventilation syndrome.

☐ State the signs and symptoms of hyperventilation syndrome.

☐ Relate the alterations in arterial carbon dioxide levels to the production of altered body function in hyperventilation syndrome.

☐ Describe the measures used in the treatment of the hyperventilation syndrome.

☐ State a general definition for acute respiratory failure.

☐ Explain the pathology of respiratory failure by citing clinical examples.

☐ Describe the clinical manifestations of hypoxemia and hypercapnia.

☐ Explain why cyanosis cannot be used as a diagnostic criteria for hypoxemia.

☐ Describe the pathologic lung changes that occur in ARDS.

☐ List the conditions that are associated with ARDS.

☐ Relate the clinical manifestations of ARDS with the pathologic changes that occur.

■ References

1. Morgan EJ, Hobbs WR: Sleep apnea syndromes. W Va Med J 75, No 1:14, 1979
2. Phillipson EA: Breathing disorders during sleep. Basics RD 7, No 3:102, 1979
3. Cherniack NA: Respiratory dysrythmias during sleep. N Engl J Med 305 No 6:325, 1981
4. Guilleminault C, Cummeninsky J, Dement WC: Sleep apnea: Recent advances. Adv Intern Med 25:347, 1980
5. Burroughs BJ, Knudson RJ, Quan SF: Respiratory Disorders, 2nd ed, p 132. St Louis, CV Mosby, 1983
6. Rapoport DM, Sorkin B, Garay SM et al: Reversal of the "Pickwickian Syndrome" by long-term use of nocturnal nasal-airway pressure. N Engl J Med 307, No 15:931, 1982
7. Brownell LG, West P, Sweatman P et al: Protriptyline in obstructive sleep apnea. N Engl J Med 307, No 17:1038, 1982
8. Valdes-Dapena MA: Sudden infant death syndrome: A review of the medical literature 1974–1979. Pediatrics 66, No 4:597, 1980
9. Shannon DC, Kelly DH: SIDS and near-SIDS. N Engl J Med 306, No 17:1022, 1982
10. Kryger MH (ed): Pathophysiology of Respiration, p 265. New York, Wiley, 1981
11. Magarian GJ: Hyperventilation syndromes: Infrequently recognized common expression of anxiety and stress. Medicine 61, No 4:219, 1982
12. Pfeffer JM: The aetiology of the hyperventilation syndrome. Psychosomatics 30:47, 1978
13. Lum LC: Hyperventilation: The tip of the iceberg. J Psychosom Res 19:375, 1975
14. Herman SP, Stickler GB, Lucas AR: Hyperventilation syndromes in children and adolescents: Long-term follow-up. Pediatrics 67:183, 1981
15. Mortenson SA, Vihelmson R, Sande E: Prinzmetal's variant angina (PVA), circadian variation in response to hyperventilation. Acta Med Scand (Suppl) 644:38, 1981
16. Yasue H, Nagao M, Omote S et al: Coronary artery spasm and Prinzmetal's variant of angina induced by hyperventilation and tris-buffer infusion. Circulation 58:56, 1978
17. Yasue H, Omote S, Takizawa A et al: Alkalosis-induced coronary vasoconstriction: Effects of calcium, diliazem, nitroglycerin and propranolol. Am Heart J 102:206, 1981
18. Gennari FJ, Goldstein MB, Schwartz WB: The nature of renal adaptation to chronic hypocapnia. J Clin Invest 51:1722, 1972
19. Rogers RM, Weiler C, Ruppenthal B: The impact of intensive care unit on survival of patients with acute respiratory failure. Heart Lung 1:475, 1973
20. Pierce AK: Oxygen toxicity. Basics RD 1, No 2, 1972
21. Rogers RM: Acute respiratory failure. Med Times 106, No 7:26, 1979
22. Spragg RG: Adult respiratory distress syndrome. Hosp Med 14 No 3:31, 1979

■ Additional References

Alexander JA, Rodgers BM: Diagnosis and management of pulmonary insufficiency. Surg Clin North Am 60, No 4:983, 1980

Balk R, Bone RC: The adult respiratory distress syndrome. Med Clin North Am 67 No 3:685, 1983

Balk R, Bone RC: Classification of acute respiratory failure. Med Clin North Am 67 No 3:551, 1983

Berger AJ, Mitchell RA, Severinghaus JW: Medical progress: Regulation of respiration (first of three parts). N Engl J Med 297, No 2:92–97, 1977

Berger AJ, Mitchell RA, Severinghaus JW: Medical progress: Regulation of respiration (second of three parts). N Engl J Med 297, No 3:138–142, 1977

Berger AJ, Mitchell RA, Severinghaus JW: Medical progress: Regulation of respiration (third of three parts). N Engl J Med 297, No 4:194–201, 1977

Block AJ: Dangerous sleep: Oxygen therapy for nocturnal hypoxemia. N Engl J Med 306:166, 1982

Block AJ: Respiratory disorder during sleep. Heart Lung 9:1011, 1980

Bone RC, Stober G: Mechanical ventilation in respiratory failure. Med Clin North Am 67 No 3:598, 1983

Compernolle T, Hooglduin K, Loele L: Diagnosis and treatment of the hyperventilation syndrome. Psychosomatics 20:612, 1979

Cherniack NS: The control of breathing in COPD. Chest 77, No 2:291–293, 1980

Demling DH, Nerlich M: Acute respiratory failure. Surg Clin North Am 63, No 2:337, 1983

Fletcher EC, Levin DC: Cardiopulmonary hemodynamics during sleep in subjects with chronic obstructive pulmonary disease. Chest 85:6, 1984

Fromm G: Using basic laboratory data to evaluate patients with acute respiratory failure. Crit Care Q 1:43–51, 1979

Harman E, Wynne JW, Block AJ et al: Sleep-disordered breathing and oxygen desaturation in obese patients. Chest 79:256, 1981

Koss JA, Christoph C: Oxygen therapy and other respiratory therapy in acute respiratory failure. Crit Care Q 1:53–63, 1979

Luce JM: Respiratory complications of obesity. Chest 78:626, 1980

Martin RJ: The treatment of acute respiratory failure without mechanical ventilation. Med Times 106, No 7:31–37, 1978

Mechanical ventilation (series of 4 articles). Am J Nurs 84:1372, 1984

McMichan JC, Piepgras DG, Gracey DR et al: Electrophrenic respiration. Mayo Clin Proc 54:662, 1979

Radwan L, Defmats H: Variations of arterial oxygen and carbon dioxide tensions during 24 hours in chronic respiratory insufficiency. Scand J Respir Dis 55:99–104, 1974

Remolina C, Khan AU, Santiago TV et al: Positional hypoxemia in unilateral lung disease. N Engl J Med 304:523, 1981

Rhodes ML: Acute respiratory failure in chronic obstructive lung disease. Crit Care Q 1:1–14, 1979

Rochester DF, Arora NS: Respiratory muscle failure. Med Clin N Am 67, No 3:573, 1983

Sprung CL, Pons G, Elser B et al: The adult respiratory distress syndrome. Postgrad Med 74, No 1:253, 1983

Tisi GM: Strategies of care in acute respiratory failure. Med Times 107, No 5:43–51, 1979

Unit IV

Alterations in Body Fluids

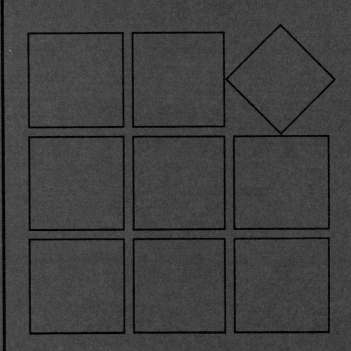

Chapter 25

Alterations in Body Fluids and Electrolytes

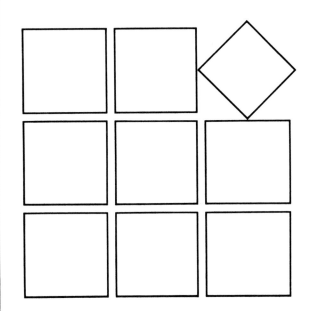

Body fluids consist of water and electrolytes. The precise regulation of these fluids within a very narrow physiologic range is essential to life. Normally, the volume and composition of these fluids remain relatively constant in the presence of a wide range of changes in intake and output. Environmental stresses and disease states often increase losses, impair intake, and otherwise interfere with mechanisms that regulate body fluid volume and composition. This chapter is divided into three parts: (1) regulation of body fluids, (2) alterations in body water, and (3) alterations in the electrolyte composition of body fluids.

■ Regulation of Body Fluids

Distribution

Body fluids are distributed between two body compartments. The *intracellular compartment* contains the fluid within all of the body's billions of cells (Fig. 25-1). The *extracellular compartment* contains all of the fluid located

outside of the cells. Included in the extracellular compartment are the *interstitial fluids* (fluids that surround the cells), *intravascular fluids,* cerebral spinal fluid, and fluid contained within the various body spaces such as the pleural cavity and the joint spaces. Even the water contained in the anterior chamber of the eye is considered to be extracellular fluid.

Electrical Properties

Body fluids contain both water and chemical compounds. In solution, these chemical compounds can remain either intact or separate in a process known as *dissociation. Electrolytes* are compounds that dissociate in solution to form *charged particles,* or *ions.* For example, a sodium chloride molecule dissociates to form a positively charged sodium (Na^+) and a negatively charged chloride (Cl^-) ion. Substances such as glucose and urea remain intact and are called *nonelectrolytes.*

Positively charged ions are called *cations* because they are attracted to the *cathode* of a wet electric cell. Similarly, *negatively charged ions* are called *anions* because they are attracted to the *anode.* The ions found in body fluids carry either one charge *(a monovalent ion)* or two charges *(a divalent ion).*

The location of electrolytes is influenced by their electrical charges. You will recall that *ions* with *like* charges *repel* and *ions* with *opposite* charges *attract.* This attraction or repulsion can cause electrolytes to move from one body compartment to another. In other words, an excess of positively charged ions in a body compartment attracts negatively charged ions in an attempt to balance the electrical charge.

In general, the positive charge from one cation is no different from the positive charge of another; for example, the positive charge from a sodium ion is equivalent to the positive charge from a potassium ion. As a general rule, however, the total number of cations in the body equals the total number of anions.

The unit that expresses the charge equivalency of a given weight of an electrolyte is milliequivalents per liter (mEq/liter). One milliequivalent of sodium will have the same number of charges as 1 mEq of chloride regardless of molecular weight (only sodium will be positive and chloride will be negative). The number of milliequivalents in a substance can be derived from the following formula:

$$mEq/liter = \frac{mg/100\ ml \times 10 \times valence}{atomic\ weight}$$

The International System of Units expresses electrolytes as millimoles per liter (mmol/liter).

$$mmol/liter = \frac{mEq/liter}{valence}$$

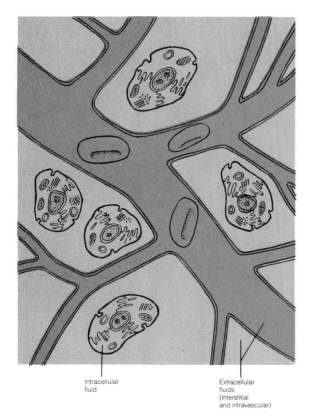

Intracellular
fluid

Extracellular
fluids
(Interstitial
and intravascular)

Figure 25-1   *Distribution of body water—the extracellular space includes the vascular compartment and the interstitial spaces.*

This means that 1 mEq will equal 1 mmol of a monovalent electrolyte. Laboratory reports of serum electrolytes and electrolyte composition of intravenous solutions and other medications are expressed as either mEq/liter or mmol/liter.

Chemical Properties

In a biologic system, the concentration of dissolved particles in a solution influences water movement and controls cell size. *Diffusion* is the movement of charged or uncharged particles along a *concentration gradient*. The addition of sugar to a container of water is an example of diffusion. Initially, the concentration of sugar will be greatest at the point where it comes in contact with the water. Moments later, however, the sugar will have diffused so that its concentration has been equalized throughout the container. Many small molecules move from one body compartment to another along a concentration gradient.

Most of the membranes in the body are semipermeable. This means that they allow water and small uncharged particles to diffuse freely through their pores while partially or completely preventing the passage of charged ions and large molecules. In diffusing through a semipermeable membrane, water moves from the side with the lesser number of nondiffusible particles to the side that has the greater number (Fig. 25-2). The pressure due to water movement is called the *osmotic pressure*. The osmotic activity, or work potential, that dissolved particles exert in drawing water from one side of the membrane to another is measured through use of a unit called a *milliosmol per liter* (mOsm/liter).

> One gram mol of a nondiffusible
> and nonionizable substance
> is equal to 1 osmol.

A milliosmol is equal to one-thousandth of an osmol. If a substance dissociates to form two ions, then 0.5 gm mol of the substance will equal 1 osmol. Each nondiffusible particle, large or small, is equally effective in its ability to pull water through a semipermeable membrane. Thus, the osmotic activity of a solution is determined by the number, rather than the size, of the dissolved particles.

The osmotic activity of a solution may be expressed as either osmolarity or osmolality. Osmolarity refers to the osmolar concentration in 1 liter of solution (mOsm/liter), whereas osmolality refers to the osmols dissolved in 1 kg of water (mOsm/kg H_2O). Although the terms *osmolarity* and *osmolality* are often used interchangeably, most clinical laboratories report osmotic activity as osmolality. The normal serum osmolality of body serum is approximately 280 mOsm/kg H_2O.

The movement of water across a cell membrane by means of osmosis can cause the cell to either swell or

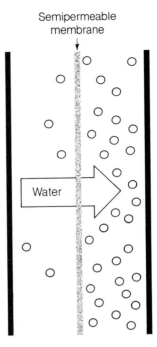

Figure 25-2 *Movement of water across a semipermeable membrane. Water movement is from the side that has the lesser number of nondiffusible particles to the side that has the greater number.*

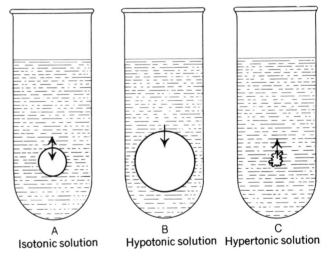

Figure 25-3 *Osmosis: (A) red cells undergo no change in size in isotonic solutions, (B) they increase in size in hypotonic solutions, and (C) they decrease in size in hypertonic solutions. (Chaffee EE, Greisheimer EM: Basic Physiology and Anatomy, 3rd ed. Philadelphia, JB Lippincott, 1974)*

shrink (Fig. 25-3). By definition, a *hypertonic* solution is one that causes a cell to shrink or become crenated. A *hypotonic* solution causes a cell to swell. An *isotonic* solution is one that does not cause cells to either shrink or swell.

In summary, body fluids are distributed between the intracellular and extracellular compartments of the body. The extracellular fluid compartment contains the intravascular fluid, interstitial fluid, and the fluid contained in the extracellular spaces such as the pleural cavity. Body fluids contain water, charged particles called *electrolytes,* and noncharged particles called *nonelectrolytes.* Electrolytes are measured in *mEq,* a measurement unit that expresses the charge equivalency of a given weight of an electrolyte. *Diffusion* is the movement of charged and noncharged particles along a concentration gradient. Both electrolytes and nonelectrolytes move between body compartments by diffusion. The movement of water across the semipermeable membranes of the body is controlled by the nondiffusible particles on either side of the membrane in a process called *osmosis.* Osmosis is regulated by the number rather than the size of the nondiffusible particles.

■ Alterations in Body Water

There is a continuous movement of water and electrolytes both into and out of the body and among the various body structures and compartments. As a general rule, the level of body water and electrolytes present at any given time is directly related to the amount taken into the body minus the amount lost from the body.

$$\frac{\text{level of water}}{\text{and electrolytes}} = \frac{\text{amount}}{\text{taken in}} - \frac{\text{amount lost}}{\text{from the body}}$$

For example, the total amount of sodium chloride present in the body at any given time will reflect the oral or parenteral intake, or both, minus what has been lost from the body through the skin, kidneys, and bowel.

As a method for approaching the study of fluids and electrolytes, it is recommended that the reader consider

---

Chart 25-1   Functions of Water

Provides form for body structures
Acts as a transport vehicle for
   nutrients
   electrolytes
   blood gases
   metabolic wastes
   heat
   electrical currents
Provides insulation
Aids in the hydrolysis of food
Acts as a medium and reactant for chemical reactions
Acts as a lubricant
Cushions and acts as a shock absorber

---

(1) the purpose or function that water or a given electrolyte serves in the overall body function, (2) the basal or minimum body requirements, (3) the sources of gain and loss, (4) the effect of age on volume and regulation, and (5) the mechanisms responsible for regulating body levels of water or specific electrolytes. The causes and manifestations of fluid and electrolyte imbalances can be related to these mechanisms for easier understanding of the subject.

Functions

Because of its ubiquitous nature, the functions of water in the human body are many (see Chart 25-1). Water adds to the structure of the body, acts as a transport vehicle, lubricates and cushions, acts to hydrolyze food in the digestive system, and is necessary for chemical reactions that occur within the cell.

It is water that gives the body its *structure.* One has only to compare the dry and wrinkled skin of an elderly person with that of a child to become aware of the extent to which water contributes to the overall form and appearance of the body. Water adds a resiliency to the skin and underlying tissues that is often referred to as *skin* or *tissue turgor.* Tissue turgor is assessed by pinching a fold of skin between the thumb and forefinger. Normally, the skin immediately returns to its normal configuration when the fingers are released. A loss of 3% to 5% of body water causes the resiliency of the skin to be lost, and the tissue will remain raised for several seconds.

The transport of body nutrients, wastes, electrical currents, and heat depends on fluid movement both in the interstitial spaces and in the vascular compartment. In relation to *body temperature,* water not only transports heat from the inner core of the body to the periphery where it can be released into the external environment, but it also *insulates* the body against changes in the external temperature. Were it not for the insulation afforded the body by its water content, the body would be much like a rock, gaining heat during the day and losing it at night.

Water *hydrolyzes* the food eaten, breaking it down into particles that can be digested and then absorbed across the gastrointestinal tract wall. In addition, many of the *chemical reactions* that occur within the body require water as a medium or reactant.

Water also lubricates and cushions. Synovial fluid lubricates the joints, and pericardial fluid prevents the heart from rubbing against the pericardial sac. The act of swallowing would be difficult, if not impossible, were it not for the lubricating properties of the mucus that lines the gastrointestinal tract. The cerebral spinal fluid acts to cushion the brain. During pregnancy, amniotic fluid acts as a shock absorber and protects the delicate fetus.

Requirements

Regardless of age, all normal individuals require approximately 100 ml of water per 100 calories metabolized. This means that a person expending 1800 calories requires approximately 1800 ml of water for metabolic purposes. The metabolic rate increases with fever and there is a 13% increase in metabolic rate for every 1°C (7%/1°F) increase in body temperature.

Effect of Age

The body is largely water, and therefore body water is usually expressed as a percentage of body weight. Total body water varies with age, decreasing from infancy to old age. In the full-term infant, body water constitutes as much as 75% to 80% of body weight, whereas body water accounts for only 60% to 70% of body weight in the adult. The premature infant has greater amounts of body water, the elderly person much less in relation to body weight. Because fat is essentially water free, obesity tends to decrease the percentage of water that the body contains, sometimes reducing these levels to values as low as 45% of body weight.

Body water is distributed between the intracellular and extracellular compartments. The intracellular compartment contains about two-thirds of the body's water and the extracellular compartment about one-third. In the adult, intracellular water constitutes about 45% of body weight and extracellular fluid about 15% (Fig. 25-4).

Despite its greater body water content, the infant is more likely to develop fluid imbalances than the adult. This is because the infant has both a higher metabolic rate and a larger surface area in relation to its body mass than an older child or adult. Also, the infant has more difficulty in concentrating its urine because its kidney structures are immature. This means that the infant has greater skin and urine losses and that more water is needed to transport metabolic wastes. The infant, therefore, both ingests and excretes greater volumes of water in relation to its size than the adult. For example, an infant may exchange one-half of its extracellular fluid volume in a single day, whereas an adult exchanges only about one-sixth of this volume during the same period of time. By the third year of life, the percentages and distribution of body water in the young child approach those of the adult.

Gains and Losses

The main source of water gain is that which is absorbed from the gastrointestinal tract; this includes water obtained from fluids, ingested foods, tube feedings, and

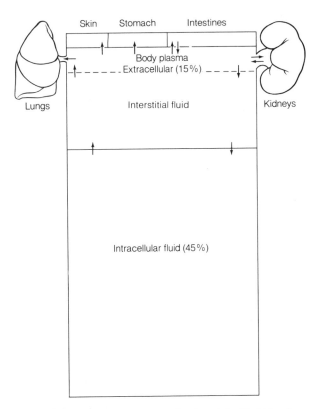

Figure 25-4 *Fluid compartments in the adult. Fluid in the intracellular compartment constitutes about 45% of body weight, whereas fluid in the extracellular compartment constitutes about 15% of body weight. Fluid from the extracellular compartment moves into the gastrointestinal tract, skin, lungs, and kidneys.*

sometimes water used in rectal irrigation. Water gain also includes water derived from cellular oxidation of foodstuffs. This quantity varies from 150 ml to 250 ml depending on the rate of metabolism.

Water losses occur through the kidneys, skin, lungs, and gastrointestinal tract. Even when oral and parenteral intake has been withheld, the kidneys continue to produce urine as a means of ridding the body of metabolic wastes. The urine output that is required to eliminate these wastes is called the *obligatory urine output*. The obligatory urine loss is about 300 ml to 500 ml/day.

Water losses that occur from the skin and respiratory tract are termed *insensible water losses* because the individual is not aware that they are occurring. Under normal conditions, water vapor lost from the skin and lungs approximates 500 ml/m^2 of surface area per day. Skin losses include the water that continually diffuses through the pores in the skin as well as the water lost in the process of sweating. Respiratory losses consist of water vapor that is withdrawn from the mucous membranes to humidify the inspired air and then is lost to the environment during expiration. For readers who have lived in a cold climate, the frosty breath that they see on a cold day is evidence of water losses that occur with respiration. Sources of water gain and loss are summarized in Table 25-1.

Regulation

Two physiologic mechanisms assist in regulating body water levels; one of these is *thirst* and the other is the *kidneys' ability to concentrate urine.* Thirst is primarily a regulator of intake, renal concentrating mechanisms is a regulator of output. Both mechanisms respond to changes in extracellular volume and osmolality.

Thirst

The thirst center is located in the lateral preoptic area of the hypothalamus (Fig. 25-5). Nerve cells, called osmoreceptors, which are located in or near the thirst center, respond to changes in extracellular osmolality by either swelling or shrinking. Thirst occurs when an increase in extracellular osmolality causes these cells to shrink. Thirst is one of the earliest symptoms of water loss, occurring when water loss is equal to 2% of body weight.

The most common cause of thirst is an increase in the osmotic concentration of the extracellular fluids. A second cause of thirst is severe hypokalemia, which causes significant defects in the kidneys' ability to concentrate urine. This results in polyuria followed by polydipsia. Hypokalemia is known to stimulate prostaglandin E synthesis. Inasmuch as prostaglandin E is known to stimulate thirst, it is also possible that polydipsia secondary to hypokalemia is mediated by prostaglandins. A third cause of thirst is a decrease in blood volume, which may or may not be associated with a decrease in serum osmolality. Thirst is one of the earliest symptoms of hemorrhage, often being present long before other signs of blood loss begin to appear. Last, dryness of the mouth produces a sensation of thirst that is not necessarily associated with the body's state of hydration, for example, the thirst that a lecturer experiences as the mouth dries during speaking. It is interesting to note

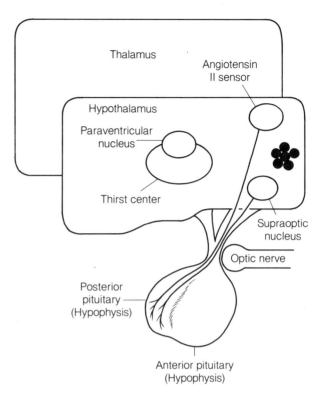

Figure 25-5 *The center of the hypothalamus and pituitary gland, which are involved in water balance.*

that in animal experiments in which salivary secretion was blocked, excessive drinking did not occur unless the animals were eating food.[1] This same effect has been reported in humans with salivary glands that did not secrete saliva, suggesting that the lubricating properties of water are needed for swallowing food.

Alterations in thirst mechanisms. Excessive thirst is called *polydipsia.* Polydipsia is normal when it accompanies conditions of water deficit. Although infrequent, a water excess can occur as the result of excess intake that is unrelated to need. An example of excessive water intake occurs in psychogenic polydipsia. Persons afflicted with this disorder drink water in excess of what the kidneys can excrete. A 1977 news story related the fatal outcome of a 29-year-old woman with a diagnosis of chronic schizophrenia who was drinking 4 gallons of water a day to "cleanse her body of cancer."[2] The thirst mechanism may also be depressed. This sometimes occurs in elderly individuals.

Renal concentrating mechanisms

The kidneys control the concentration of most of the constituents in body fluids, including water and electrolytes. Each kidney has about 1 million functional units called nephrons (see Chap. 29). Water and electrolytes

Table 25-1   Sources of Body Water Gains and Losses in the Adult

Gains		Losses	
		Urine	1500 ml
Oral intake		Insensible losses	
As water	1000 ml	Lungs	300 ml
In food	1300 ml	Skin	500 ml
Water of oxidation	200 ml	Feces	200 ml
Total	2500 ml	Total	2500 ml

are filtered from the blood in the *glomerulus* and are then selectively reabsorbed in the *tubules*. The rate at which water and electrolytes can be removed from the body is determined by renal blood flow and the glomerular filtration rate; urine output declines during shock as renal blood flow falls. As the urine filtrate moves through the tubule, water and electrolytes that are needed for maintaining the volume and composition of body fluids are reabsorbed into the extracellular fluid and those that are not needed are excreted in the urine.

Antidiuretic hormone

The reabsorption of water by the kidneys is regulated by the antidiuretic hormone (ADH), also known as *vasopressin*. The antidiuretic hormone is synthesized by cells in the supraoptic and paraventricular nuclei of the hypothalamus (Fig. 25-5). The hormone is transported along a neural pathway (the hypophyseal tract) to the neurohypophysis (posterior pituitary) and is then stored for future release. A rise in ADH levels causes increased reabsorption of water from the distal tubules and collecting ducts of the kidneys. As with thirst, ADH levels are controlled by volume and osmolar changes in the extracellular fluids. Osmoreceptors in the hypothalamus sense changes in extracellular osmolality and stimulate the production and release of ADH. A small increase in serum osmolality of 1% to 2% is sufficient to cause ADH release. Likewise, stretch receptors in the great veins, atria, and carotid sinus area sense changes in blood volume or blood pressure and input from these receptors aids in regulation of ADH release.

Stress situations tend to cause an increase in ADH release. Severe pain, trauma, surgery, certain anesthetic agents, and some analgesic drugs increase ADH levels. Nicotine stimulates ADH release. Alcohol, on the other hand, inhibits ADH release. Table 25-2 lists drugs that are known to affect ADH release.

Two important conditions serve to alter ADH levels: diabetes insipidus and inappropriate secretion of ADH. Because of their effect on water balance, both of these conditions are discussed in this chapter.

Diabetes insipidus. Diabetes insipidus means "tasteless diabetes" as opposed to diabetes mellitus, or "sweet diabetes." Diabetes insipidus occurs because of a defect in the synthesis or release of ADH *(central diabetes insipidus)* or because the kidneys do not respond to ADH *(nephrogenic diabetes insipidus)*. About 60% of diabetes insipidus seen clinically results from tumors or lesions in the hypophyseal tract.[3] Temporary diabetes insipidus can result following surgery in the area of the hypophyseal tract or head injury. A person with diabetes insipidus excretes large quantities of urine, usually 3 liters to 15 liters per day. This large urine output is

Table 25-2 Drugs that Affect ADH Levels

Drugs that Decrease ADH Levels/Action	Drugs that Increase ADH Levels/Action
Demeclocycline	Acetaminophen
Ethanol	Analgesics (morphine and meperidine)
Glucocorticoids	Anesthetics (most)
Lithium carbonate	Antipsychotic tranquilizers
Morphine antagonists	Cancer drugs (vincristine and cyclophosphamide)
Norepinephrine	Carbamazepine
Phenytoin	Chlorpropamide
Reserpine, chlorpromazine	Clofibrate
	Isoproterenol
	Nicotine
	Phenobarbital
	Thiazide diuretics (chorothiazide)
	Tricyclic antidepressants

accompanied by excessive thirst; as long as the thirst mechanism is normal and fluid is readily available, there is little or no alteration in the fluid levels in persons with diabetes insipidus. The danger arises when the condition develops in an unconscious person, because an inadequate fluid intake rapidly leads to hypertonic dehydration and increased serum osmolality.

Diagnosis of diabetes insipidus is based on measurements of urine and serum osmolality. These tests may be used to evaluate the response to an infusion of a hypertonic saline solution or to pharmacologic preparations of ADH. Persons with nephrogenic diabetes insipidus do not respond to pharmacologic preparations of the hormone; this method is used to differentiate between the two forms of the disease. Diagnostic measures for diabetes insipidus include those that rule out psychogenic polydipsia as a reason for the excessive thirst and increased urine output. A recently developed radioimmunoassay test for ADH can be used for this purpose. When central diabetes insipidus is suspected, diagnostic methods such as skull x-rays and computed tomographic (CT) scans of the pituitary hypothalamic area are done to determine the cause of the disorder.

The treatment of central diabetes insipidus consists of treating any underlying disorder and supplying the body with pharmacologic preparations that contain the missing hormone. These preparations must be administered parenterally or nasally; they are not given by mouth because they are destroyed in the gastrointestinal tract. New nonhormonal forms of therapy have recently been introduced for cases in which ADH release is still present. The oral hypoglycemic agent chlorpropamide (Diabinese) may be used to stimulate ADH release in central diabetes insipidus. Other drugs that are under investigation for use with this form of diabetes insipidus are carbamazepine (Tegretol) and clofibrate. In nephrogenic diabetes insipidus, the thiazide diuretics are now the specific form of therapy. These drugs probably act predominantly by causing an increase in sodium excretion by the kidneys, which lowers the glomerular filtration rate and increases reabsorption of fluid in the proximal tubule.[4]

Syndrome of inappropriate ADH. The syndrome of inappropriate ADH (SIADH) results from a failure of the negative feedback system that regulates ADH release and inhibition. The secretion of ADH continues in the presence of decreased serum osmolality; this leads to a marked retention of water in excess of sodium, causing a dilutional hyponatremia. An increase in the glomerular filtration rate resulting from an increased plasma volume causes further increases in sodium loss. Urine osmolality is high and serum osmolality low. Urine output decreases despite adequate or increased fluid intake and the resultant water retention produces an acute gain in body weight. Serum sodium, hematocrit, and blood urea nitrogen are all decreased because of the expansion of the extracellular fluid volume.

The SIADH can be caused by a number of conditions including lung tumors and chest lesions, central nervous system (CNS) disorders, and various pharmacologic agents. The first report of SIADH was made in the late 1950s in association with lung cancer. Tumors, particularly bronchogenic carcinoma, are known to produce and release ADH independent of hypothalamic control mechanisms. Other intrathoracic conditions, such as tuberculosis, pneumonia, and positive pressure breathing, are also known to cause SIADH. The suggested mechanism for SIADH in these cases is decreased atrial filling with activation of the atrial volume receptors. Disease and injury to the CNS can cause direct pressure on or direct involvement of the hypothalamic-posterior pituitary structures. Examples include brain tumors, hydrocephalus, head injury, meningitis, and encephalitis. Other stimuli such as pain, stress, and temperature changes are capable of stimulating ADH release through the limbic system. Drugs induce SIADH in different ways; some drugs are thought to increase hypothalamic production and release, whereas others are believed to act directly on the renal tubules to potentiate the action of ADH.

SIADH may occur as a transient condition, as in a stress situation, or as a chronic condition resulting from a lung tumor. The severity of symptoms is usually proportional to the extent of sodium depletion and water intoxication. Symptoms of mild SIADH (serum sodium levels around 130 mEq/liter) include thirst, headache, anorexia, muscle cramps, general fatigue, and dulling of the sensorium. In severe SIADH (serum sodium levels below 126 mEq/liter) neurologic symptoms of acute water intoxication begin to appear; they include nausea, vomiting, muscular twitching, seizure, and coma.

The treatment of SIADH depends on its severity. In mild cases the treatment consists of fluid restriction. If fluid restriction is not sufficient, diuretics such as mannitol or furosemide (Lasix) may be given to promote diuresis and free water clearance. Lithium and the antibiotic demeclocycline inhibit the action of ADH on the renal collecting ducts and are sometimes used in treating the disorder. In cases of severe sodium depletion, a hypertonic (3% or 5%) sodium chloride solution may be administered intravenously.

Extracellular Fluid Deficit

Body-fluid levels are dependent on both sodium and water balance. Water provides about 90% to 93% of the volume of body fluids, and sodium salts comprise 90% to 95% of the solute in the extracellular fluids. This means that the total volume of fluid in the extracellular compartment is controlled by the osmotic effect of sodium. The concentration of sodium, on the other hand, is determined by the water volume. There are two major types of alterations in extracellular fluid: one involves proportionate changes in both sodium and water (isotonic contraction or expansion of the extracellular fluid volume), and the other is a change in water as it relates to sodium concentration (dilutional hyponatremia, in which sodium is excessively diluted, and dilutional hypernatremia, in which sodium is insufficiently diluted).

An extracellular fluid volume deficit occurs when the body water is reduced. It can consist of an isotonic depletion of body fluids in which the losses of water and electrolytes are proportional or in which the water losses are in excess of the sodium losses (dilutional hypernatremia). Extracellular fluid deficit ultimately causes a loss of cellular fluids. Fluid deficit is a serious threat to all individuals, especially those with limited ability to conserve water. For example, dehydration caused by diarrhea continues to be one of the leading causes of death among children.

Causes

There are two main causes of an extracellular fluid deficit: (1) a decrease in the intake of fluids and electrolytes and (2) an increased loss. The extracellular fluid compartment is the source of all body secretions, including sweat, urine, and gastrointestinal secretions. This means that excessive losses of any of these fluids afford the potential for extracellular fluid deficit (Table 25-3).

Table 25-3 Extracellular Fluid Deficit

Causes	Signs and Symptoms
Decreased Fluid Intake	**Acute Weight Loss (% of total weight)**
Unconsciousness or inability to express thirst	Mild extracellular deficit: 2% loss
Oral trauma or inability to swallow	Moderate extracellular deficit: 2%–5% loss
Impaired thirst mechanism	Severe extracellular deficit: 6% or more loss
Withholding fluids for therapeutic purposes	**Thirst**
Increased Fluid Losses	**Decreased Urine Output**
Gastrointestinal losses	In water deficit
Vomiting	Increased urine osmolality
Diarrhea	Increased specific gravity
Gastrointestinal suction	In sodium and water deficit
Fistula drainage	Normal specific gravity and osmolality
Urine losses	Low sodium chloride content
Diuretic therapy	**Decreased Serum Volume**
Osmotic diuresis (hyperglycemia)	Increased serum osmolality
Adrenal insufficiency	Increased hematocrit
Salt-wasting renal disease	Increased BUN
Skin losses (salt and water)	**Decreased Vascular Volume**
Fever	Tachycardia
Exposure to hot environment	Weak and thready pulse
Burns and wounds that remove skin	Postural hypotension
Third space losses (sodium and water)	Decreased vein filling and vein refill time
Intestinal obstruction	Hypotension and shock
Edema	**Decreased Volume in Extracellular Spaces**
Ascites	Depressed fontanel in an infant
Burns (first several days)	Sunken eyes and soft eyeballs
	Loss of Intracellular Fluid
	Dry skin and mucous membrane
	Cracked and fissured tongue
	Decreased salivation and lacrimation
	Neuromuscular
	Weakness
	Fatigue

Gains and losses

Increased surface losses. The skin acts as an exchange surface for body heat and as a vapor barrier to prevent water from leaving the body. Body surface losses of sodium and water increase when there is excessive sweating or when large areas of the skin have been damaged. Fever and hot weather increase sweating. During heavy exercise in a hot environment, sweat losses may exceed 3.5 liters/hour.[1] Both respiratory rate and sweating are usually increased as body temperature rises. As much as 3 liters of water may be lost in a single day as a result of fever. Burns are another cause of excess fluid loss. Evaporative losses range from 0.8 ml to 2.6 ml/kg percent burn area. This loss can approach a level of 6 liters to 8 liters per day.[5]

Gastrointestinal losses. There is a continuous exchange of fluid between the extracellular compartment and the lumen of the gastrointestinal tract. In a single day, 8 liters to 10 liters of extracellular fluid is secreted into the gastrointestinal tract; most of this fluid is reabsorbed as the bowel contents move toward the anus. Vomiting and diarrhea interrupt the reabsorption process and in some situations lead to increased secretion of fluid (in excess of 8–10 liters) into the gastrointestinal tract; the presence of irritating or hypertonic contents increases the movement of fluid into the bowel, exaggerating fluid losses. In many forms of diarrhea, the rate of fluid secretion into the gastrointestinal tract is increased because of the osmotic or irritating effects of the causative agent. In Asiatic cholera, death can occur within a matter of hours as irritating substances formed by the cholera organism cause excessive amounts of fluid to be secreted into the bowel; these fluids are then lost as vomitus or diarrheal fluid.

Third space losses. Third space losses refer to the sequestering of extracellular fluids in an area that is physiologically unavailable to the body—in the serous cavities or the lumen of the gut. For example, fluid deficits can develop in intestinal obstruction as water and electrolytes pool in the distended bowel. The capillaries that supply the third space often have an increased permeability and there is a concomitant movement of plasma proteins into the sequestered area. The osmotic gradient associated with the presence of these colloids causes additional water to move into the third space area.

Renal losses. The kidneys normally regulate the volume and solute concentration of the extracellular fluid—promoting diuresis in situations of fluid excess and conserving fluids when extracellular fluid volume is decreased. Extracellular fluid deficit can result from osmotic diuresis or the injudicious use of diuretic therapy. In hyperglycemia, serum sodium is diluted as the osmotic effects of the elevated glucose cause water to be pulled out of body cells. The presence of glucose in the urine filtrate prevents reabsorption of water by the renal tubules; this causes increased losses of both sodium and water. The degree of hyponatremia, or serum sodium decrease, resulting from hyperglycemia can be estimated by assuming a 1.6 mEq/liter decrease in serum sodium for every 100 mg/ml rise in blood sugar above normal values.[6]

Manifestations

The signs and symptoms of fluid deficit are closely associated with the functions of water that were discussed earlier in the chapter. A discussion of the signs and symptoms associated with extracellular fluid deficit is complicated by the fact that fluid deficit may present as an isotonic depletion of fluid volume or as a situation in which water losses exceed sodium loss. The signs and symptoms presented in this section of the chapter consider both situations.

Body weight. A decrease in body weight is one of the best indicators of fluid loss. One liter of water weighs 1 kg (2.2 lb). A mild extracellular fluid deficit exists when weight loss equals 2% of body weight; in a person weighing 68 kg (150 lb) this percentage of weight loss equals 1.4 liters of water. Severe fluid deficit exists when weight loss is in excess of 6% of body weight. To be accurate, weight must be measured at the same time each day, with an equal amount of clothing being worn. Because extracellular fluid is trapped within the body in persons with third space losses, body weight may not decrease when extracellular fluid loss occurs for this reason.

Intake and output. Intake and output affords a second method for assessing fluid balance. Although these measurements provide insight into the causes of fluid imbalance, they are often inadequate in measuring actual losses and gains. This is because accurate measurements of intake and output are often difficult to obtain and insensible losses are difficult to estimate. Pflaum reported a mean error in intake and output calculations of 800 ml per day compared with daily weight measurements.[7]

Thirst. Thirst is an early symptom of water deficit, occurring when water losses are equal to 1% to 2% of body weight. Unfortunately, infants and persons who are unconscious or who cannot communicate are unable to express this need. Also, thirst is not always present in isotonic fluid deficit that is caused by sodium depletion.

Urine output. Urine output usually decreases and urine osmolality and specific gravity increase during periods of water deficit. An exception to this rule occurs in situations in which the fluid deficit occurs as a result of renal mechanisms in situations in which the kidneys' ability to concentrate urine has been impaired or when diuresis occurs for other reasons. Normally, the ratio of urine osmolality to serum osmolality in a 24-hour urine sample exceeds 1 and after an overnight fast should be greater than 3 to 1. A dehydrated patient (one who has a loss of water) may have a urine osmolality that exceeds 1000 mOsm/kg H_2O. In persons who have difficulty concentrating their urine, for example, those with diabetes insipidus or chronic renal failure, the urine to serum ratio is often less or equal to 1. Urine specific gravity compares the weight of urine with that of water, providing an index for solute concentration. A change in specific gravity of 1.010 to 1.020 (water is considered to be 1.000) is an increase of 400 mOsm/kg H_2O. In the sodium-depleted state, the kidney will usually try to conserve sodium; urine specific gravity will be normal and urine sodium and chloride concentrations will be low.

Serum osmolality. The normal serum osmolality is 275 to 295 mOsm/kg H_2O. Because the serum in the extracellular compartment is roughly 90% to 93% water, the concentration of blood cells and other solutes will increase as extracellular water decreases. This is true of hematocrit and blood urea nitrogen (BUN). Serum sodium will also increase when fluid deficit is due primarily to a water loss.

Extracellular fluids. Arterial and venous volumes decline during periods of fluid deficit. There is a change in both the pulse and blood pressure that occurs as the volume in the arterial system declines. The heart rate increases and the pulse becomes weak and thready. Postural hypotension is an early sign of fluid deficit, characterized by a blood pressure that is at least 10 mm Hg lower when one is sitting and standing than lying down. When volume depletion becomes severe, signs of shock and vascular collapse appear. On the venous side of the circulation, the veins become less prominent and venous refill time increases. A simple test to determine venous refill time consists of compressing the distal end of a vein on the dorsal aspect of the hand (when the hand is not in the dependent position). The vein is then emptied by "milking" the blood toward the heart. Normally, the vein will refill almost immediately when the occluding finger is removed. When venous volume is decreased, as occurs in fluid deficit, the venous refill time will increase.

The fluid in all of the body spaces decreases in fluid deficit. Although most body spaces are not visible, a decrease in cerebral spinal fluid in the infant causes depression of the anterior fontanel. Likewise, the eyes assume a sunken appearance and feel softer than normal when the fluid content in the anterior chamber of the eye is decreased.

Intracellular fluids. As fluid is lost from the extracellular compartment in excess of solute, the osmolality of the extracellular fluid becomes hypertonic in relation to the fluid in the intracellular compartment. When this happens, the water is pulled out of body cells. The skin and mucous membranes become dry, and there is a decrease in the activity of the cells in the salivary and lacrimal glands. The tongue becomes dry and fissured. Swallowing is difficult. A reliable method for testing for dryness of the mouth is to place your finger on the mucous membranes where the gums and the cheek meet. When a fluid deficit is present, you will find that your finger does not glide easily because of the dryness. This method works well in infants and in persons who are unresponsive.

One of the most serious aspects of a fluid deficit is the dehydration of brain and nerve cells. Generalized muscle weakness, muscle rigidity, and muscle tremors often occur in severe fluid deficit as water is removed from the cells in the nervous system. Delirium, hallucinations, and maniacal behavior may also develop in situations of severe fluid deficit.

Body temperature. Dehydration is known to produce a rise in body temperature. Part of this elevation in temperature probably results from a lack of available fluid for sweating. It also appears that dehydration has a direct effect on the hypothalamus, because dehydration can cause fever even in a cold environment. Body temperature may reach 105°F when dehydration is severe.[8]

Treatment

The treatment of fluid deficit consists of replacement therapy, which includes replacing both the water and the electrolytes that have been lost. Replacement fluids can be given orally or intravenously. The oral route is usually preferable.

Oral glucose–electrolyte replacement solutions are available for the treatment of infants with diarrhea.[9] Until recently, these solutions were prescribed either early in the diarrhea illness to prevent dehydration or as a first step in reestablishing oral intake after parenteral replacement therapy. These solutions are now being widely used as replacements for intravenous fluids in the treatment of dehydration due to diarrhea in small children, especially in developing countries where the availability of intravenous fluids is limited and diarrhea is the leading cause of death.[10] However, intravenous replacement fluids continue to be the treatment of choice for severe fluid deficit.

Extracellular Fluid Excess (Isotonic)

In extracellular fluid excess, there is usually retention of both sodium and water with an isotonic expansion of fluid in the extracellular compartment.

Causes

Extracellular fluid excess is generally caused by conditions that favor the retention of sodium and water, such as heart failure, cirrhosis of the liver, and kidney disease (Table 25-4). Circulatory overload can occur during administration of intravenous fluids or blood; this is particularly true when blood is given to a patient with a normal blood volume. The elderly and patients with heart disease require careful observation because even small amounts of blood may overload the circulatory system. Although extracellular fluid excess often accompanies disease, this is not always the case. For example, a compensatory increase in extracellular fluid occurs during hot weather, and premenstrual fluid retention is caused by hormonal changes.

Manifestations

Development of edema is characteristic of extracellular fluid excess.* Just as weight loss is a good indicator of extracellular fluid deficit, so also is weight gain a good indicator of fluid excess. In situations in which fluid excess occurs gradually, edema fluid may mask weight loss that is due to actual loss of tissue mass; this often happens in debilitating disease states and in starvation. The edema associated with excess extracellular fluid may be generalized or it may be confined to dependent areas of the body such as the legs and feet. Often the eyelids are puffy when the person awakens. When excess fluid accumulates in the lungs, there is shortness of breath, complaints of dyspnea, rales, and a productive cough. An increase in vascular volume causes the pulse to have a full and bounding quality.

*The causes and mechanisms associated with edema are discussed in Chapter 26.

Table 25-4 Extracellular Fluid Excess

Causes	Signs and Symptoms
Excess Sodium and Water Intake	**Acute Weight Gain (in excess of 5%)**
Excess dietary intake	**Increased Extracellular Fluid**
Medications or home remedies containing sodium	Pitting edema of the extremities
Administration of parenteral solutions that	Puffy eyelids
contain sodium	Pulmonary edema
Decreased Renal Losses	Shortness of breath
Renal disease	Rales
Increased corticosteroid levels	Dyspnea
Aldosterone	Cough
Glucocorticoids	Full and bounding pulse
Congestive heart failure	Venous distention
Cirrhosis	

In summary, an isotonic fluid deficit is characterized by a reduction in the extracellular fluid volume that is caused by a loss of both sodium and water. Extracellular fluid volume deficit causes thirst, decreased vascular volume and urine output, increased specific gravity, and signs related to loss of fluid from the cellular compartment. The causes and manifestations of extracellular fluid volume deficit are summarized in Table 25-3. An extracellular fluid volume excess describes an isotonic expansion of the extracellular compartment. It is seen in conditions that favor reabsorption of sodium and water by the kidneys. Although extracellular fluid excess is frequently seen in disease states, it can occur as a compensatory mechanism during hot weather or as an indication of cyclic changes in hormonal balance, such as premenstrual fluid retention. The causes and manifestations of extracellular fluid excess are summarized in Table 25-4.

■ Electrolyte Disorders

Although water provides volume for the body fluids, it is the electrolytes that contribute to the function of these fluids. Electrolytes serve many functions. They (1) assist in regulating water balance, (2) participate in acid–base regulation, (3) contribute to enzyme reactions, and (4) play an essential role in neuromuscular activity. This section focuses on the alterations in body function that are associated with disturbances in sodium, potassium, calcium, phosphate, and magnesium balance. Alterations in bicarbonate and chloride concentrations are discussed in Chapter 27.

There are marked differences in the composition of intracellular and extracellular electrolytes (Table 25-5). The reader will note that the sodium concentration is greatest in the extracellular compartment, whereas potassium is concentrated within the cells. Blood tests measure the concentration of electrolytes in the extracellular compartment rather than the intracellular compartment. The suffix *-emia* refers to blood. Hyponatremia, for example, denotes a decreased sodium concentration in the blood. Although blood levels are usually representative of the total body levels of an electrolyte, this is not always the case, particularly with potassium, which is approximately 28 times more concentrated inside the cell than outside.

Alterations in Sodium Balance

Sodium affects many body functions. Regulation of serum sodium is essential for maintaining (1) the osmolality of the extracellular fluids, (2) normal neuromuscular function, (3) acid–base balance, and (4) numerous vital chemical reactions. As the major cation in the extracellular compartment, sodium and its attendant anions (chloride and bicarbonate) account for about 93% of the osmotic activity that is present in the extracellular fluids. Sodium is a component of sodium bicarbonate and, as such, is very important in regulating acid–base balance.

Gains and losses

Sodium intake is normally derived from dietary sources. Body needs can usually be met by as little as 500 mg/day.* In the United States, the average salt intake is about 6 gm to 15 gm/day or 12 to 30 times the daily requirement. Other sources of sodium are intravenous saline infusions and medications that contain sodium. An often-forgotten source of sodium is the sodium bicarbonate or other sodium-containing home remedies that are used to treat upset stomach or other ailments. Sodium ingestion in excess of what the kidneys can

*In the absence of sweating.

excrete is an unlikely occurrence in healthy individuals, probably because taste prohibits this from occurring and because of the kidneys' remarkable ability to regulate sodium. Sodium excess has occurred, however, in persons receiving intravenous saline infusions and in persons unable to monitor their oral intake. The accidental substitution of salt for sugar in infant formulas has been known to produce severe hypernatremia, causing brain damage and death.

The body loses sodium through the kidneys, skin, and gastrointestinal tract. The kidneys are extremely efficient in regulating sodium output, and when sodium intake is limited or conservation of sodium is needed, the kidneys are able to reabsorb almost all of the sodium that has been filtered by the glomerulus. This results in an essentially sodium-free urine. Conversely, urinary losses of sodium will increase as intake is increased. For practical purposes, the 24-hour urinary excretion of sodium is assumed to be equal to sodium intake.

Renal losses.   Alterations in kidney function can cause either an increase or a decrease in sodium losses. Sodium deficit with an accompanying loss of extracellular fluid occurs in salt-wasting kidney disease. On the other hand, many forms of kidney disease cause sodium retention. A decrease in renal blood flow causes increased sodium retention by means of the renin–angiotensin–aldosterone mechanism. Sodium retention is therefore increased in nonrenal diseases that lead to a decrease in renal blood flow. In congestive heart failure, renal blood flow is decreased because the heart does not pump properly.

Skin losses.   Although skin losses of sodium are usually negligible, sweat losses can be extensive during exercise and periods of exposure to a hot environment. A person who sweats profusely can lose as much as 15 gm to 30 gm of sodium per day; this amount decreases to as little as 3 gm to 5 gm with acclimatization.[1] Loss of skin surface, such as occurs in extensive burns, also leads to excessive skin losses of sodium.

Gastrointestinal losses.   Sodium moves freely between the extracellular fluid and the contents of the gastrointestinal tract. In the upper part of the gastrointestinal tract, the concentration of sodium is very similar to that of serum. Sodium is reabsorbed as the contents of the gut move through the lower part of the bowel, so that the concentration of sodium in the stool is normally only about 32 mEq/liter. Sodium losses increase with vomiting, diarrhea, fistula drainage, and gastrointestinal suction. Irrigation of gastrointestinal tubes with distilled water removes sodium from the gastrointestinal tract as do repeated tap water enemas.

Table 25-5   Concentration of Intracellular and Extracellular Electrolytes

Electrolytes	Intracellular Concentration (mEq/liter)	Extracellular Concentration (mEq/liter)
Sodium	10	137–147
Potassium	141	3.5–5.0
Chloride	4	100–106
Bicarbonate	10	24–31
Phosphate	75	1.7–3.6
Calcium	1	4.5–5.3
Magnesium	58	1.5–2.5

Regulation

The normal serum concentration of sodium ranges from 135 to 147 mEq/liter. It is important for the reader to recognize that serum sodium values reflect the concentration of sodium in the extracellular fluids, expressed as milliequivalents per liter, rather than an absolute amount. This means that dehydration will cause the concentration of sodium to increase even though the total body sodium remains unchanged. Likewise, fluid excess will cause sodium levels to decrease even though sodium has not been lost from the body.

Aldosterone.   Renal absorption of sodium by the kidney is largely regulated by aldosterone levels. Aldosterone is a mineralocorticoid hormone (remember that sodium and potassium are minerals) that is produced by the adrenal cortex. The hormone promotes the reabsorption of sodium into the blood and the secretion of potassium into the distal tubule of the kidney, allowing potassium to be lost in the urine. Several mechanisms are known to control aldosterone levels: (1) extracellular sodium concentrations, (2) extracellular potassium levels, (3) angiotensin II, and (4) the adrenocorticotropic hormone (ACTH). A reduction in renal blood flow increases aldosterone by means of the renin–angiotensin mechanism. Although aldosterone increases sodium reabsorption by the kidney and thereby contributes to what might be called the short-term regulation of sodium balance, it seems to play only a minor role in the long-term regulation of sodium levels. This is because an increase in sodium reabsorption through the aldosterone mechanism ultimately leads to an increase in vascular volume, which causes an increase in the renal blood flow and glomerular filtration rate, with a subsequent decrease in renin release.

Addison's disease is a condition of chronic adrenal insufficiency in which there is unregulated loss of sodium in the urine with increased retention of potassium. The *glucocorticoids* from the adrenal cortex also have mineralocorticoid activity. *Cushing's syndrome* characterizes a condition in which there are increased levels of glucocorticoids. The fact that these hormones increase salt and water retention helps to explain why persons who are being treated with drugs that contain exogenous forms of these hormones often develop hypertension and edema. Alterations in the adrenocortical hormones are discussed in Chapter 39.

Sodium deficit

Sodium deficit in the extracellular fluids (hyponatremia) occurs when the sodium concentration in the blood falls below 137 mEq/liter. Sodium deficit may constitute an actual loss of sodium from the body, or it may occur because of the dilution of sodium resulting from a gain of extracellular water. Usually, sodium is lost from the body.

Causes. Normally, homeostatic mechanisms make it almost impossible to produce an increase in body water when renal function is adequate and ADH and aldosterone levels are normal. Excess water is retained, however, when a person has an elevation in ADH levels. Although uncommon, water excess can occur as the result of excessive water intake. As was mentioned earlier in the chapter, drinking water in excess of what the kidneys can excrete occurs in patients with psychogenic polydipsia. Water intoxication in the psychiatric patient may be aggravated by treatment with antipsychotic drugs that increase ADH levels.

Excessive sodium losses occur with excessive sweating, gastrointestinal losses, and diuresis. Excessive sweating in hot weather leads to loss of sodium and water. Hyponatremia develops when fluids lost in sweating are replaced by the drinking of tap water.* Repeated administration of tap water enemas or frequent irrigation of gastrointestinal tubes with distilled water leads to removal of sodium chloride from the gastrointestinal tract. Salt depletion also occurs with adrenal insufficiency and diuresis due to vigorous use of diuretics (see Table 25-6).

Manifestations. In hyponatremia, the osmotic pressure of the extracellular fluids becomes less than that in the cells and water moves out of the extracellular compartment into the cells. The signs and symptoms of hyponatremia depend on the rapidity of onset and the severity of the sodium dilution. If the condition develops slowly, the signs and symptoms are usually not apparent until serum sodium levels approach 125 mEq/liter. The brain and nervous system are the most seriously affected by increases in intracellular water, and neurologic signs and symptoms progress rapidly once the serum sodium levels fall below 120 mEq/liter. Swelling of the brain can

* Salt tablets (0.5 gm/500 ml water) may be used to replace excessive sweat losses. Oral electrolyte solutions, such as Gatorade (Stokely Van Camp), Sportade punch concentrate (Becton, Dickinson) and Bike Half-time Punch Mix (Kendall) can also be used to replace water and electrolytes lost through excessive perspiration.

Table 25-6 Sodium Deficit

Causes	Signs and Symptoms
Excess Water Intake or Gain	**Laboratory Values**
Administration of excess sodium-free parenteral solutions	Serum sodium below 137 mEq/liter
Psychogenic polydipsia	Decreased serum osmolality
Ingestion of tap water during periods of sodium deficit	Dilution of other blood components, including chloride, hematocrit, and BUN
Repeated administration of tap water enemas	**Increased Water Content of Brain and Nerve Cells**
Decreased Water Losses	Headache
	Depression
Kidney disease that impairs water elimination	Personality changes
Increased ADH levels	Confusion
Trauma, stress, pain	Apprehension and feeling of impending doom
SIADH	Lethargy
Use of medications that increase ADH release	Stupor
	Coma
	Convulsions
	Gastrointestinal Disturbances
	Anorexia
	Abdominal cramps
	Diarrhea
	Increased Intracellular Fluid
	Fingerprinting over sternum

cause headache, mental depression, apprehension, personality changes, gross motor weakness, and even hemiplegia. Convulsions and coma occur when serum sodium levels reach extremely low levels. An acute increase in intracellular water is often of sudden onset and should be suspected in any postoperative or posttrauma patient who suddenly behaves in a bizarre fashion.

An increase in intracellular water produces another interesting finding. The increased intracellular water content causes tissues to have a plastic consistency that is similar to that of modeling clay. This permits fingerprinting of the skin. If you roll your finger over the sternum, your fingerprint will become visible on the patient's skin. This is different from the tissue indentation that occurs with pitting edema.

Sodium excess

Sodium excess in the extracellular fluids (hypernatremia) occurs when sodium levels rise above 47 mEq/liter.

Causes.   Serum sodium excess almost always follows a loss in body fluids that contains more water than sodium.* This can occur (1) in diabetes insipidus, in which urinary losses of water are increased, (2) when respiratory losses are increased as during tracheo-

---

*The reader will note that the causes and manifestations of hypernatremia are similar to those of water deficit.

bronchitis, (3) in situations of watery diarrhea, and (4) when osmotically active tube feedings are given with inadequate amounts of water. The therapeutic administration of sodium-containing solutions may also cause hypernatremia. Cardiopulmonary resuscitation often requires the administration of large doses of sodium bicarbonate (50 mEq/50 ml). Hypernatremia will develop unless an additional 850 ml of water accompanies each three ampules that are administered.[6] Intraamniotic instillation of hypertonic saline for therapeutic abortion may inadvertently be injected intravenously, causing hypernatremia.

Generally hypernatremia, with an accompanying water deficit, will stimulate thirst and increase water intake. Hypernatremia is therefore more apt to occur in infants and persons who are unable to express their thirst or obtain water to drink. The unconscious person is particularly at risk for developing hypernatremia (see Table 25-7).

Manifestations.   The *clinical manifestations* of hypernatremia are largely related to an increase in serum osmolality; this causes water to be pulled out of body cells. With hypernatremia, urine output is decreased because of renal conserving mechanisms. Thirst is excessive. Body temperature is frequently elevated and the skin becomes warm and flushed. The mucous membranes are dry and sticky and the tongue is rough and dry. The subcutaneous tissues assume a firm and rubbery texture.

Table 25-7 Hypernatremia

Causes	Signs and Symptoms
Excess Sodium Intake	**Laboratory Findings**
Rapid or excess administration of parenteral sodium chloride or sodium bicarbonate solutions	Serum sodium above 147 mEq/liter
	Increased serum osmolality
Excess oral intake	**Thirst**
Decreased Extracellular Water	**Urine Output**
Increased water losses	Oliguria or anuria
Diuretic therapy	High specific gravity
Adrenal cortical hormone excess	**Intracellular Dehydration**
Diabetes insipidus	Skin and mucous membranes
Tracheobronchitis	Skin dry and flushed
Watery diarrhea	Mucous membranes dry and sticky
Hypertonic tube feedings	Tongue rough and dry
Decreased water intake	Subcutaneous tissue
Unconsciousness or inability to relate thirst	Firm and rubbery
Oral trauma or inability to swallow	Central nervous system
Impaired thirst mechanism	Agitation and restlessness
Withholding of water for therapeutic reasons	Decreased reflexes
	Maniacal behavior
	Convulsions and coma
	Increased body temperature
	Decreased vascular volume
	Tachycardia
	Decreased blood pressure
	Weak and thready pulse

The vascular volume decreases; the pulse becomes rapid; and the blood pressure drops. Most significantly, water is pulled out of the cells in the central nervous system; this causes decreased reflexes, agitation, and restlessness. Coma and convulsions may develop as hypernatremia progresses. Permanent brain damage has occurred in infants recovering from severe hypernatremia.

Alterations in Potassium Balance

Potassium is the major cation in the intracellular compartment. Potassium affects many body functions and (1) contributes to maintenance of intracellular osmolality, (2) is necessary for neuromuscular control and the precise regulation of skeletal, cardiac, and smooth muscle activity, (3) influences acid–base balance, and (4) participates in many intracellular enzyme reactions. For example, potassium contributes to the intricate chemical reactions that transform carbohydrates into energy, change glucose into glycogen, and convert amino acids to proteins.

Gains and losses

Potassium intake is normally derived from dietary sources. In healthy individuals, potassium balance can usually be maintained by a daily dietary intake of 50 mEq to 100 mEq. Additional amounts of potassium are needed during periods of trauma and stress. The kidneys are the main source of potassium loss. Normally about 80% to 90% of potassium losses occur in the urine and the remaining losses occur in the stool and sweat.

Regulation

Potassium is essentially an intracellular cation. This means that serum levels of potassium, which normally range from 3.5 to 5.0 mEq/liter will not always reflect the intracellular potassium content; however, they do accurately reflect the concentration in the extracellular fluid. Potassium moves freely between the interstitial and vascular compartments. When body cells are injured or when cellular activity becomes catabolic, potassium is released into the extracellular compartment and is then lost in the urine. Subsequently, with chronic potassium deficiency, the kidneys' ability to conserve potassium improves and the loss is reduced to as little as 5 mEq/liter. When this happens, serum levels of potassium are likely to remain within normal levels even though total body potassium has decreased. However, serum potassium levels tend to fall when tissue breakdown ceases and cellular activity becomes anabolic, causing potassium to move back into the cellular compartment. This is because potassium is needed for glycogen storage and protein synthesis.

Aldosterone regulation.   Aldosterone plays an important role in regulating extracellular potassium concentrations. Urinary losses of potassium increase under the influence of aldosterone, whereas sodium retention is increased. The feedback regulation of aldosterone levels, in turn, is strongly regulated by serum potassium levels; for example, an increase in potassium ion concentration of less than 1 mEq/liter will cause aldosterone levels to triple. Furthermore, this increased secretion will continue for as long as the elevated potassium levels are present.

Potassium balance can be seriously affected by disorders of aldosterone secretion. Primary aldosteronism is caused by a tumor in the cells of the adrenal cortex (in the zona glomerulosa) that secrete aldosterone. Excess secretion of aldosterone by the tumor cells causes severe potassium losses and a decrease in serum potassium levels. Patients with this disorder may develop muscle paralysis as a result of the low serum levels of potassium. Adrenal insufficiency (Addison's disease) causes the opposite effect; these patients have elevated serum potassium levels due to an aldosterone deficiency.

Potassium–hydrogen ion exchange.   The hydrogen ion concentration (pH) of the extracellular fluid contributes to compartmental shifts of potassium. In acidosis, the movement of hydrogen ions into body cells is used as a means of buffering pH changes in the extracellular fluids. Generally, the serum potassium concentration rises 0.6 mEq/liter for each 0.1 unit fall in blood pH. When a hydrogen ion moves into the cell, another positively charged ion (potassium) must leave, to maintain the cell's neutrality. This means that potassium tends to move out of the intracellular compartment in acidosis and into the intracellular compartment in alkalosis.

A potassium and hydrogen exchange also occurs in the distal tubule of the kidney. When the extracellular concentration of potassium is high, tubular secretion of potassium into the urine is increased and hydrogen excretion is decreased, causing an increase in serum pH (metabolic acidosis). Conversely, when extracellular concentrations of potassium are low, tubular secretion of potassium into the urine is decreased and hydrogen ion secretion is increased; this tends to lead to metabolic alkalosis.

Potassium deficit

Hypokalemia refers to a decrease in serum potassium levels below 3.5 mEq/liter. Because potassium moves freely between the intracellular and extracellular compartments, hypokalemia can occur as the result of a loss of total body potassium or because extracellular potassium has moved into the intracellular compartment. Usually both intracellular and extracellular potassium concentrations are decreased simultaneously.

Causes. Potassium deficit can occur for three reasons: (1) intakes inadequate, (2) losses are excessive, or (3) extracellular potassium has moved into body cells (Table 25-8).

With an acute loss of potassium, the kidneys are unable to conserve potassium, and even in time of great need the kidneys continue to excrete potassium. This means that a potassium deficit can develop rather quickly if intake is inadequate. Unfortunately, intake is frequently impaired at the time that potassium losses are increased, as following surgery or during prolonged diarrhea. The elderly are particularly likely to develop a potassium deficit. This is because they often have poor eating habits as a consequence of living alone; they have

limited income, which makes buying foods high in potassium difficult; they have difficulty in chewing many of the foods that have a high potassium content because of poorly fitting dentures; or they may have problems with swallowing. Furthermore, medical problems in the elderly often require treatment with drugs, such as diuretics, that tend to increase potassium losses.

The kidneys are the main source of potassium loss. Normally about 80% to 90% of potassium losses occur in the urine and the remaining losses in the stool and sweat. Unfortunately, the kidneys do not have the homeostatic mechanisms needed to conserve potassium during acute decreased intake. An adult on a potassium-free diet will continue to lose approximately 5 mEq to 15 mEq of potassium daily. Following trauma, and in stress situations, urinary losses of potassium are greatly increased, sometimes approaching levels of 150 to 200 mEq/day. Diuretic therapy (with the exception of

---

Table 25-8 Potassium Deficit

Causes	Signs and Symptoms
Inadequate Intake	**Laboratory Values**
Inability to eat	Serum potassium below 3.5
Diet deficient in potassium	mEq/liter
Administration of potassium-free parenteral solutions	**Skeletal Muscles**
Excessive Gastrointestinal Losses	Fatigue
Vomiting	Muscle tenderness or
Diarrhea	paresthesias
Suction	Weakness
Fistula drainage	Muscle flabbiness
Excessive Renal Losses	Paralysis
Diuretic phase of renal failure	**Cardiovascular System**
Diuretic therapy (except triamterene and spironolactone)	Postural hypotension
Increased mineralocorticoid levels	Increased sensitivity to digitalis
Cushing's syndrome	Arrhythmias
Primary aldosteronism	**Gastrointestinal Tract**
Treatment with glucocorticoid hormones	Anorexia
Intracellular Shift	Vomiting
Treatment for diabetic acidosis	Abdominal distension
Alkalosis, either metabolic or respiratory	Paralytic ileus
	Respiratory Muscles
	Shortness of breath
	Shallow breathing
	Kidneys
	Polyuria
	Low osmolality and specific
	gravity of urine
	Nocturia
	Thirst
	Central Nervous System
	Function
	Confusion
	Depression
	Acid–Base Balance
	Metabolic alkalosis

spironolactone and triamterene) results in additional urinary losses of potassium.

Although potassium losses through the skin and gastrointestinal tract are usually minimal, these losses can become excessive under certain conditions. For example, burns increase surface losses of potassium and sweat losses can become markedly increased in persons who are acclimated to a hot climate. In other situations, gastrointestinal losses become excessive; this occurs with vomiting and diarrhea and in situations in which gastrointestinal suction is being used.

Manifestations.   Potassium deficit results in impaired function of skeletal, cardiac, and smooth muscle. Often the signs and symptoms of potassium deficit are gradual in onset and for that reason go undetected for a considerable period of time.

Renal function.   Important abnormalities of renal function occur in hypokalemia. The kidneys become unable to concentrate urine normally. Urine output is increased, urine specific gravity is decreased, and serum osmolality is increased. The patient complains of polyuria, nocturia, and thirst.

Gastrointestinal function.   Hypokalemia causes numerous signs and symptoms associated with gastrointestinal function. These include anorexia, nausea, vomiting, abdominal distention, absence of bowel sounds, and paralytic ileus. When gastrointestinal symptoms occur gradually and are not severe, they often serve to impair potassium intake.

Neuromuscular function.   At least three defects in skeletal muscle function occur with potassium deficiency: (1) alterations in the resting membrane potential (see Chap. 1), (2) alterations in glycogen synthesis and storage, and (3) impaired ability to increase blood flow during strenuous exercise.[11] With hypokalemia there is hyperpolarization of neuromuscular tissue with decreased responsiveness to stimulation. Neuromuscular signs and symptoms appear when serum potassium levels fall to approximately 2.5 mEq/liter. Muscle weakness appears first, followed by paralysis. Leg muscles, particularly the quadriceps, are most prominently affected. Some patients complain of muscle tenderness and paresthesias rather than weakness. In chronic potassium deficiency, actual muscle atrophy may occur and contribute to muscle weakness. Familial periodic paralysis is a disorder in

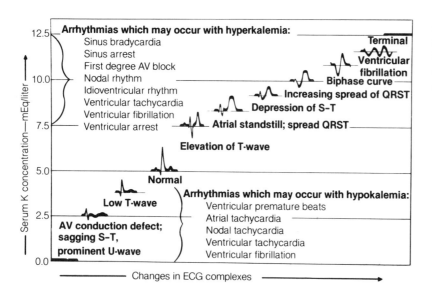

Figure 25-6   *ECG changes at various levels of serum potassium concentration. (Krupp MA, Chatton MJ (eds): Current Medical Diagnosis and Treatment. Copyright 1974, Lange Medical Publications, Los Altos, CA)*

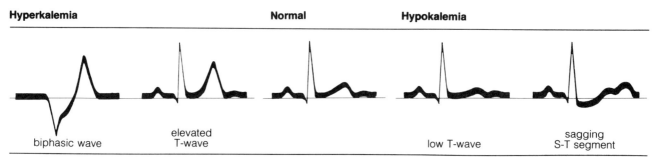

which episodes of hypokalemia cause attacks of flaccid paralysis that last from a few minutes to several hours. The paralysis may be precipitated by situations that reduce serum potassium levels, such as a high carbohydrate meal or administration of insulin, epinephrine, or glucocorticoid drugs. The paralysis is often reversed by potassium therapy. Severe hypokalemia may affect the respiratory muscles. When this happens, the diaphragm is usually affected earlier than the intercostal muscles.

Normal concentrations of intracellular potassium are necessary for glycogen synthesis in muscle cells. This means that potassium deficiency has the potential for interfering not only with the electrical activity of skeletal muscle but also with muscle metabolism, especially under exercise conditions that rely heavily on anaerobic pathways. Release of potassium from muscle is thought to contribute to the autoregulation of blood flow during exercise. Thus, potassium deficiency can interfere with the release of potassium ions from exercising muscle, impair blood flow, and consequently impose a risk of ischemic injury to muscle cells during intense physical exercise.[11]

Cardiovascular function.   Potassium deficiency also affects cardiovascular function. Postural hypotension is common. *Of particular importance is the fact that hypokalemia increases the risk of digitalis toxicity.* The dangers associated with digitalis toxicity are compounded in patients who are receiving both digitalis and diuretics. Serious cardiac arrhythmias that result from hypokalemia are described in Figure 25-6.

Treatment.   Potassium deficits are treated by increasing the intake of foods high in potassium content—meats, dried fruits, fruit juices (particularly orange juice), and bananas. The reader is referred to a nutrition text for a description of foods that are high in potassium.

Potassium supplements are prescribed for persons whose intake of potassium is insufficient in relation to losses. This is particularly true of persons who are on diuretic therapy and who are taking digitalis.

Potassium is given intravenously when the oral route is not tolerated or when rapid replacement is needed. The rapid infusion of a concentrated potassium solution has been known to cause death due to cardiac arrest. It is suggested that all health personnel who assume responsibility for administering intravenous solutions containing potassium be fully aware of all the precautions pertaining to its dilution and flow rate. Pharmacology texts, drug company package inserts, fluid and electrolyte texts, and pharmacists serve as useful resources for this information.

Potassium excess

Hyperkalemia refers to an increase in blood levels of potassium in excess of 5.5 mEq/liter. In general it can be said that serum potassium excess occurs whenever potassium gains exceed losses.

Causes.   The major causes of potassium excess are (1) renal failure, (2) adrenal insufficiency, and (3) excess potassium gains due to tissue trauma or intravenous administration of potassium at a rate that exceeds the kidneys' ability to control serum potassium levels (Table 25-9). It is difficult to increase potassium intake to the point of causing hyperkalemia when sufficient aldosterone is present and renal function is adequate. An exception to this rule is when potassium solutions are being infused intravenously—*severe and fatal incidents of hyperkalemia have resulted from the intravenous infusion of potassium. Intravenous solutions containing potassium should never be started until urine output has been assessed and renal function deemed to be adequate;* this is because the kidneys control potassium losses. Movement of

---

Table 25-9   Potassium Excess

Causes	Signs and Symptoms
Excessive Intake or Gain	**Laboratory Values**
Excessive oral intake	Serum potassium above 5.5 mEq/liter
Excessive or rapid parenteral infusion	**Neural and Skeletal Muscle Activity**
Tissue trauma, burns, and massive crushing injuries	Paresthesias
Decreased Renal Losses	Weakness and dizziness
Renal failure	Muscle cramps
Adrenal insufficiency	**Smooth Muscle Activity of the Gastrointestinal Tract**
Addison's disease	Nausea, diarrhea
Potassium-sparing diuretics (spironolactone and triamterene)	Intestinal colic and gastrointestinal distress
	Cardiac Electrophysiology
	Peaked T waves, depressed S–T segment
	Depressed P wave and widening of QRS segment
	Cardiac arrest

potassium out of body cells into the extracellular fluids also affords the potential for the elevation of blood potassium. For example, burns and crushing injuries cause potassium to be liberated into the extracellular fluid. Often these same injuries cause a decrease in renal function, which contributes to the development of hyperkalemia.

Manifestations.   The signs and symptoms of potassium excess are closely related to the alterations in neuromuscular function that accompany potassium deficit. Although the mechanisms responsible for the altered neuromuscular function observed in hypo- and hyperkalemia are different, the end results are similar. The first symptom associated with hyperkalemia is often a paresthesia; this may appear when potassium levels reach 6 mEq/liter. The most serious effect of hyperkalemia is cardiac arrest. The electrocardiographic changes that occur with alterations in serum potassium levels are described in Figure 25-6.

Treatment.   The treatment of potassium excess focuses on (1) decreasing or curtailing intake, (2) increasing renal excretion, and (3) increasing cellular uptake. Decreased intake can be accomplished by restricting dietary sources of potassium. It should be mentioned here that the major ingredient in most of the salt substitutes is potassium chloride, and they should not be given to patients with renal problems. Increasing potassium output is often more difficult. Persons with renal failure may require hemodialysis or peritoneal dialysis to reduce the serum potassium levels. A sodium polystyrene sulfonate resin may also be used to remove potassium ions from the colon. The sodium ions in the resin are replaced by potassium ions and then the potassium-containing resin is excreted in the stool.

Emergency methods usually focus on measures that cause serum potassium to move into the cell. The intravenous infusion of insulin and glucose is sometimes used for this purpose.

Alterations in Calcium and Phosphate Balance

There is a close link between the regulation of calcium and of phosphate ions in the body. A change in the concentration of one ion leads to a change in the concentration of the other. Therefore, calcium and phosphate are discussed together in this chapter.

Calcium and phosphate salts are deposited in the organic matrix of bone—bone is essentially 30% matrix and 70% salts. In the extracellular fluid the concentration of calcium and phosphate is reciprocally regulated—when calcium levels are high, phosphate levels are low

and *vice versa*. Normal serum levels of calcium (9.0–10.6 mg/dl) and phosphate (3.0–4.5 mg/dl) are regulated so that their product (calcium × phosphate) is maintained at a value of approximately 35. This reciprocal relationship is important because the concentrations of calcium and phosphate are considerably greater than those required to cause precipitation. Precipitation of calcium and phosphate salts is normally prevented by inhibitors that are present in most tissues.

Gains and losses
Calcium and phosphate enter the body through the gastrointestinal tract, are stored in bone, and are excreted through the kidney. The major source of calcium is milk and milk products. Phosphate is derived from many sources, including milk and meats. Only about 30% to 50% of dietary calcium is absorbed in the duodenum and upper jejunum; the remainder is excreted in the stool. Phosphate, on the other hand, is absorbed exceedingly well.

Normally, the kidney controls calcium and phosphate losses. The two ions are filtered in the glomerulus and are selectively reabsorbed in the renal tubules. The amount of phosphate that is lost in the urine is directly related to phosphate concentrations in the blood. When serum phosphate levels rise above a critical level, the rate of phosphate loss in the urine reflects the excess blood phosphate levels. Calcium excretion is reciprocally related to phosphate excretion. In renal failure, phosphate excretion is impaired and as a result serum calcium levels decline as blood phosphate levels rise.

Regulation
Serum calcium and phosphate are regulated by vitamin D, parathyroid hormone, and calcitonin. The body contains a supply of exchangeable calcium that is in equilibrium with calcium in the extracellular fluids. Most of this exchangeable calcium is found in bone. It is this exchangeable pool that serves as a storage site for calcium. Movement of calcium between the blood and the exchangeable pool is rapid—it usually occurs within minutes to 1 hour. The regulation of phosphate levels is closely linked to calcium metabolism. The phosphate ion is freely absorbed from the intestine, and changing the serum phosphate levels to as high as three to four times the normal value does not seem to have an immediate effect on body function. Bone metabolism and the actions of vitamin D, parathyroid hormone, and calcitonin are discussed in Chapter 52.

Extracellular calcium
Calcium can be found in several forms in the body. Ninety-nine percent of body calcium is found in bone, where it provides the strength and stability for the collagen and ground substance that form the structural

matrix of the skeletal system. The other 1% is located in the tissues and extracellular fluids. The calcium salts in bone serve as a reservoir of tissue and serum calcium.

Extracellular calcium exists in three forms. About 50% of serum calcium is bound to plasma proteins and cannot pass through the capillary wall to leave the vascular compartment. Five percent of serum calcium is combined with substances such as citrate, phosphate, and sulfate. This form is not ionized. The remaining 45% of serum calcium is ionized. It is the ionized calcium that is able to leave the capillary and enter the intercellular spaces, and it is this form of calcium that is physiologically important.

Serum calcium serves a number of functions. First, ionized calcium helps to maintain the permeability of cell membranes. Nerve cell membranes are less permeable and less excitable when sufficient ionized calcium is present. Second, calcium participates in a number of enzyme reactions. Third, calcium aids in blood clotting. The calcium ion is required for all but the first two steps of the intrinsic pathway for blood coagulation. Removal of ionized calcium is often used as a method to prevent clotting in blood that has been removed from the body. For example, citrate is often used to prevent clotting in blood that is to be used in transfusion. Fortunately, calcium ion concentrations in the body never fall to levels that affect blood clotting.

Most of the nondiffusible calcium is bound to albumin with only about 10% to 15% of the protein-bound fraction associated with globulin. Thus, the total serum calcium will change with changes in serum albumin. As a general rule, the total serum calcium is decreased 0.8 mg/dl for every gram per deciliter from normal that occurs in the serum albumin level. Hypocalcemia associated with decreased serum albumin levels results in a decrease in protein-bound rather than ionized calcium and is usually asymptomatic. An alkaline *p*H will increase binding of calcium to protein, lowering the ionized calcium while the total serum calcium remains unchanged. Hyperventilation can produce an effective hypocalcemia with tetany by increasing the protein-binding of calcium without altering the total calcium concentrations.[12]

Calcium deficit

Serum calcium levels are protected by bone stores and do not usually require a continual daily intake.

Causes. The causes of hypocalcemia, or deficit in ionized calcium, are (1) impaired ability to mobilize calcium from bone stores, (2) abnormal binding of calcium so that greater proportions of calcium are in the un-ionized form, (3) abnormal losses of calcium by the kidney, and (4) decreased absorption of calcium from the intestine (Table 25-10).

The ability to mobilize calcium from bone stores is impaired in hypoparathyroidism. A parathyroid hormone (PTH) deficiency occurs in primary hypoparathyroidism and in accidental surgical removal of the parathyroid glands during thyroid surgery. All patients who have had a thyroidectomy should be observed for signs of calcium deficit during the early postoperative period. A pseudohypoparathyroidism occurs when there is end-organ refractoriness to PTH.

The electrolyte or ionized form of calcium is decreased as serum calcium binds to plasma proteins or other substances. For example, serum *p*H affects the ionization of calcium; ionization is increased in acidosis and decreased in alkalosis. As mentioned previously, citrate combines with calcium and is often used as an anticoagulant for blood transfusions. Theoretically, excess citrate in donor blood could combine with the

Table 25-10   Calcium Deficit

Causes	Signs and Symptoms
Decreased Serum Levels	**Laboratory Values**
Intestinal malabsorption	Serum calcium below 4.5
Rapid dilution of serum by parenteral administration of calcium-free solutions	mEq/liter
	Increased Nerve Excitability
Hypoparathyroidism	Paresthesias, especially numbness
Vitamin D deficiency (or impaired activation of vitamin D)	or tingling
Increased Serum Losses	Skeletal muscle cramps
Sequestering of calcium in tissue *e.g.,* massive infections of subcutaneous tissue	Abdominal spasms and cramps
	Hyperactive reflexes
Decreased ionization (alkalosis or rapid correction of acidosis)	Carpopedal spasm
	Tetany
Citrate binding due to excessive administration of citrated blood	Laryngeal spasm
	Positive Chvostek's test
Acute pancreatitis	Positive Trousseau's test
Hyperphosphatemia (in renal insufficiency)	
Decrease in Serum Albumin Levels	

calcium in the recipient's blood, causing hypocalcemia and tetany. Normally, however, this does not occur because the liver removes the citrate from the blood within a matter of minutes. Therefore, when blood transfusions are given at a slow rate (less than 1 liter/hour in the adult) there is little danger of hypocalcemia due to citrate binding.[1] Hypocalcemia is a common finding in acute pancreatitis. It is not known whether the calcium is precipitated in the pancreas as a result of fat necrosis or calcium is sequestered elsewhere.

There is an inverse relationship between calcium and phosphate excretion by the kidneys. Phosphate is retained in renal failure, causing serum calcium levels to decrease and PTH levels to increase. Hypocalcemia and hyperphosphatemia occur when the glomerular filtration rate falls below 25 ml to 30 ml/minute, the normal being 100 ml to 120 ml/minute.

Intestinal absorption of calcium decreases with a deficiency of vitamin D. Vitamin D deficiency because of lack of intake is seldom seen today because many foods are fortified with vitamin D. Vitamin D deficiency is more apt to occur in malabsorption states, such as biliary obstruction, pancreatic insufficiency, and celiac disease in which the ability to absorb fat and fat-soluble vitamins is impaired. Vitamin D (inactivated form) is stored in the liver. In subsequent steps the liver and the kidneys convert inactive vitamin D to the activated form (1,25-dihydroxycholecalciferol). Vitamin D remains in the body only a short time once it has been activated. This means that patients with renal failure will have problems with the absorption of calcium because of impaired activation of vitamin D. Fortunately, the activated form of the hormone has been synthesized and is now available (calcitriol) for use in the treatment of calcium deficit in patients with renal failure.

Manifestations. Acute hypocalcemia ordinarily causes no significant signs and symptoms aside from those associated with neural excitability. This is because tetany will lead to death before other effects can develop. Ionized calcium stabilizes neuromuscular excitability. In severe hypocalcemia, increased neuromuscular excitability can cause tetany, laryngeal spasm, convulsions, and death. Both the Chvostek's and the Trousseau's signs are utilized to observe for an increase in neuromuscular excitability and tetany. The Chvostek's sign is elicited by tapping the face just below the temple at the point where the facial nerve emerges. Tapping the face over the facial nerve causes spasm of the lip, nose, or face when the test is positive. An inflated blood pressure cuff is used to test for Trousseau's sign. The cuff is inflated to a point which temporarily occludes the circulation of the hand, usually for a period of 1 to 5 minutes. Contraction of the fingers and hands (carpopedal spasm) indicates the presence of tetany.

Treatment. The treatment of calcium deficit is directed toward increasing the intake or absorption from the intestine. One glass of milk contains about 300 mg of calcium. An intravenous infusion containing calcium gluconate is used when tetany is present or anticipated because of a decrease in serum calcium. The active form of vitamin D is administered when the liver or kidney mechanisms needed for hormone activation are impaired.

Calcium excess

A serum calcium excess (hypercalcemia) results from excessive bone resorption and from intestinal absorption that exceed the ability of the kidney to excrete the excess calcium ions (Table 25-11).

Causes. The most common causes of increased bone resorption (or destruction) are neoplasms, hyperparathyroidism, and prolonged immobility. There are a number of malignant tumors, including carcinoma of the lungs, kidneys, bone, and ovaries that have been associated with hypercalcemia. Some tumors actually destroy the bone, while others produce a parathyroidlike hormone. Intestinal absorption of calcium increases with excessive doses of vitamin D. Fortunately, the liver can store vitamin D; and it is reported that 1000 times the normal quantities can be ingested with only a threefold increase in serum levels of the active vitamin.[1] Another cause of excessive calcium absorption is the milk–alkali syndrome. The milk–alkali syndrome occurs in patients with peptic ulcers who are being treated with excessive amounts of milk and alkaline antacids, particularly calcium carbonate preparations. Excess calcium carbonate taken without milk has also been known to produce an increase in calcium levels. The thiazide diuretics produce an increase in total serum calcium of 0.5 to 1.0 mg/dl in otherwise healthy persons.[12] This reflects the indirect effects of hemoconcentration and the direct effects of bone resorption. In most persons, the calcium levels return to normal after several weeks of therapy. However, the thiazide diuretics may cause hypercalcemia in persons with underlying bone disorders and increased bone resorption.

Manifestations. The signs and symptoms associated with calcium excess originate from three sources: (1) a decrease in neuromuscular activity, (2) reabsorption of calcium from bone, and (3) exposure of the kidney to high concentrations of calcium. Neural excitability is decreased in hypercalcemia. There may be a dulling of consciousness, stupor, weakness, and muscle flaccidity. Acute psychoses are common when calcium levels rise above 16 mg/100 ml. The heart responds to elevated levels of calcium with increased contractility and ventricular arrhythmias. Digitalis causes these responses to

Table 25-11   Calcium Excess

Causes	Signs and Symptoms
Increased Serum Gains	**Serum Calcium above 5.5 mEq/liter**
Increased intestinal absorption	**Altered Neural and Muscular Activity**
Excessive vitamin D	Muscle weakness and atrophy
Excessive calcium in diet	Ataxia, loss of muscle tone
Milk–alkali syndrome	Lethargy
Increased bone resorption	Stupor and coma
Immobility	Personality or behavioral changes
Increased levels of parathyroid hormone	**Associated with Increased Bone Resorption**
Malignant neoplasms including leukemia and lymphomas	Deep bone pain
Thiazide diuretics	Pathologic fractures
Decreased Losses	**Renal**
Hyperparathyroidism	Signs of renal insufficiency (acute reversible)
	Polyuria
	Flank pain
	Signs of kidney stones
	Increased losses of sodium and potassium
	Cardiovascular
	Hypertension
	Shortening of the QT interval, AV block on electrocardiogram
	Gastrointestinal
	Anorexia
	Nausea
	Vomiting
	Constipation

be accentuated. High calcium concentrations in the urine impair the ability of the kidney to concentrate urine by interfering with the action of ADH. This causes salt and water diuresis and an increased sensation of thirst. Hypercalciuria also predisposes to the development of renal calculi.

Hypercalcemic crisis describes an acute increase in serum calcium levels above 8 to 9 mEq/liter or (4–4.5 mmol/liter). Malignant disease and hyperparathyroidism are major causes of hypercalcemic crisis. In hypercalcemic crisis, polyuria, excessive thirst, volume depletion, fever, altered levels of consciousness, azotemia (nitrogenous wastes in the blood), and a disturbed mental state accompany other signs of calcium excess. Symptomatic hypercalcemia is associated with a high mortality rate; death is often due to cardiac arrest.

Treatment.   The treatment of calcium excess is usually directed toward correcting or controlling the condition that is causing the disorder. Diuretics and sodium chloride can be administered in emergency treatment of hypercalcemia. Corticosteroids and mithramycin are used to treat hypercalcemia due to malignancy.

Phosphate

Phosphate is an integral part of all body tissues. About 85% of phosphorus is located in bone; most of the remaining 15% is located intracellularly. In the adult, the normal serum phosphate level is 3.0 to 4.5 mg/100 ml of serum. These values are slightly higher in children (4.0–7.0 mg/100 ml).

The functions of phosphate can be grouped into four categories: (1) phosphate plays a major role in bone formation; (2) it is essential to metabolic processes, that is, it is incorporated into adenosine triphosphate (ATP) as well as into enzymes needed for glucose, fat, and protein metabolism; (3) it is an essential component of several vital parts of the cell, being incorporated into the nucleic acids and into the cell membrane; and (4) it acts as an acid–base buffer in the extracellular fluid and in renal excretion of hydrogen ions. Delivery of oxygen by the red cell depends on organic phosphates in ATP and 2,3-diphosphoglycerate (2,3-DPG). Phosphate is also needed for normal function of other blood cells, including the white cells and platelets.

Phosphate deficit

Only recently has the importance of phosphate depletion been recognized.

Causes.   Phosphate depletion is associated with antacid use, malnutrition, alcoholism, ketoacidosis, and hyperthyroidism. Antacids that contain aluminum hydroxide, aluminum carbonate, and calcium carbonate bind with phosphate, causing increased phosphate losses in the stool. Aluminum hydroxide is sometimes used therapeutically to decrease phosphate levels in chronic renal failure. Alcoholism is commonly recognized as a cause of hypophosphatemia. One study reports that 42% of alcoholic patients who were admitted to the hospital had low serum phosphate levels.[13] The mechanisms underlying hypophosphatemia in the alcoholic are not clearly undertood; it may be related to malnutrition or to hypomagnesemia. Malnutrition and diabetic ketoacidosis increase phosphate excretion and phosphate loss from the body. Refeeding of malnourished patients increases phosphate incorporation into nucleic acids and phosphorylated compounds in the cell. The same thing happens when diabetic ketoacidosis is reversed with insulin therapy. The intracellular shift of phosphate causes the serum phosphate levels to drop. Parathyroid hormone decreases the serum phosphate levels through a different mechanism: it increases the renal excretion of phosphate. Alkalosis has an indirect effect on serum phosphate levels. The increase in pH causes increased binding of calcium, which in turn leads to a decrease in ionized calcium and an increase in the release of PTH.

Manifestations. Hypophosphatemia causes signs and symptoms related to altered neural function, disturbed musculoskeletal function, and hematologic disorders. Neural manifestations include intentional tremors, paresthesias, hyporeflexia, stupor, coma, and seizures (Table 25-12). Anorexia and dysphagia can occur. There may be muscle weakness, stiffness of the joints, bone pain, and osteomalacia. Red cell metabolism is impaired in phosphate deficiency; the cells become rigid and have increased hemolysis and diminished ATP and 2,3-DPG levels. Chemotaxis and phagocytosis by white blood cells is impaired. Platelet function is also disturbed.

Treatment. The treatment of hypophosphatemia includes replacement therapy. This may be accomplished with dietary sources high in phosphate (one glassful of milk contains about 250 mg phosphate) or with oral or intravenous replacement solutions. Phosphate supplements are usually contraindicated in hypercalcemia and renal failure. Treatment with phosphate supplements can lead to disseminated calcification.

Phosphate excess

Hyperphosphatemia usually results from renal failure or a decrease in PTH. Hyperphosphatemia has been reported in children following use of a single sodium phosphate/biphosphate enema.[14]

Hyperphosphatemia is associated with a decrease in serum calcium; thus, many of the signs and symptoms of a phosphate excess may be related to a calcium deficit (see Table 25-10).

Alterations in Magnesium

Magnesium is the second most abundant intracellular cation. Fifty percent of the total magnesium content of the body is stored in bone, 49% is contained in the body

---

Table 25-12 Phosphate Deficit

Causes	Signs and Symptoms
Increased Loss from the Gastrointestinal Tract	**Serum Levels Below 3.0 mg/100 ml in Adults and 4.0 mg/100 ml in Children**
Antacids (aluminum and calcium)	**Altered Neural Function**
Severe diarrhea	Intention tremor
Lack of vitamin D	Ataxia
Increased Renal Excretion	Paresthesias
Alkalosis	Hyporeflexia
Hyperparathyroidism	Confusion
Diabetic ketoacidosis	Stupor
Renal tubular defects	Coma
Decreased Intake	Seizures
Malnutrition	**Altered Musculoskeletal Function**
Alcoholism	Muscle weakness
Increased Movement into the Cell	Joint stiffness
Intravenous hyperalimentation	Bone pain
Recovery from malnutrition	Osteomalacia
Administration of insulin for ketoacidosis	**Gastrointestinal Symptoms**
	Anorexia
	Dysphagia
	Hematologic Disorders
	Hemolytic anemia
	Platelet dysfunction with bleeding disorders
	Impaired function of white blood cells

cells, and the remaining 1% is dispersed in the extracellular fluids. The normal serum concentration of magnesium is 1.5 to 2.5 mEq/liter.

Regulation

Only recently has the importance of magnesium to the overall function of the body been fully recognized. The functions of magnesium can be grouped into three categories. First, magnesium acts as a cofactor in many enzyme reactions, particularly those that involve transfer of a phosphate group. Second, magnesium exerts an effect similar to that of calcium on neuromuscular function, in that neuromuscular activity is increased when magnesium levels are decreased. Third, magnesium deficiency is associated with both a potassium and a calcium deficiency state. Renal excretion of potassium is increased in magnesium deficiency. The actions of PTH in maintaining normal serum calcium levels appear to be impaired in hypomagnesemia.

Gains and losses

The average American diet contains about 180 mg to 300 mg of magnesium. All green vegetables contain abundant amounts of magnesium. Although controversial, it is generally agreed that the minimum daily requirement for magnesium in the adult is 250 mg (150 mg in the infant and 400 mg in pregnant or lactating women).[15] Magnesium is absorbed from the intestine and excreted by the kidney. Calcium and magnesium compete for absorption in both the intestine and renal tubules; that is, factors that increase calcium absorption will cause a decrease in magnesium absorption. Although the mechanisms are unclear, the actions of PTH and magnesium levels appear to be related. Hyperparathyroidism increases the renal excretion of magnesium. It has also been suggested that the action of PTH

in regulating calcium metabolism is impaired in hypomagnesemia; that is, hypomagnesemia is associated with hypocalcemia.[16]

Magnesium deficit

Magnesium deficiency usually results from impaired magnesium absorption in the intestine or from increased urinary losses. One of the most common causes of hypomagnesemia is alcoholism. Multiple factors lead to hypomagnesemia in alcoholism, including low intake and gastrointestinal losses from diarrhea. The effects of hypomagnesemia are exaggerated by other electrolyte disorders, such as hypokalemia, hypocalcemia, and metabolic acidosis, often seen in chronic alcoholism. Magnesium levels are also decreased in conditions that cause malabsorption, in malnutrition, and in patients receiving parenteral hyperalimentation in which magnesium is inadequate. Prolonged diarrhea may also lead to severe magnesium deficiency. Excessive intake of calcium will impair magnesium absorption by competing for the same transport site. Magnesium losses are increased in diabetic ketoacidosis, diuretic therapy, and hyperaldosteronism (Table 25-13).

The signs and symptoms of magnesium deficit are characterized by personality change and an increase in neuromuscular irritability. Tremors; athetoid or choreiform movements; positive Babinski's, Chvostek's, or Trousseau's signs; tachycardia; hypertension; and ventricular arrhythmias are signs and symptoms associated with the increase in neuromuscular irritability.

Magnesium excess

Magnesium excess is rare. The signs and symptoms occur only when serum magnesium levels exceed 4 mEq/liter.[11] When it does occur it is usually related to renal insufficiency or to injudicious use of magnesium sulfate as a

---

Table 25-13 Magnesium Deficit

Causes	Signs and Symptoms
Impaired Intake or Absorption	**Laboratory Findings**
Alcoholism	Serum magnesium less than 1.4 mEq/liter
Malabsorption	
Small-bowel bypass surgery	**Neuromuscular Hyperirritability**
Malnutrition or starvation	Personality change
Parenteral hyperalimentation of inadequate mg^{++}	Athetoid or choreiform movements
High dietary intake of calcium without	Positive Babinski's sign
concomitant increase in mg^{++}	Nystagmus
	Tetany
Increased Losses	Positive Chvostek's or Trousseau's signs
Diabetic ketoacidosis	
Diuretic therapy	**Cardiovascular Manifestations**
Hyperparathyroidism	Tachycardia
Hyperaldosteronism	Hypertension
Magnesium-wasting renal disease	Ventricular arrhythmias

laxative. Hypermagnesemia causes sedation of the nervous system with muscle weakness, confusion, and respiratory paralysis. There is a decrease in blood pressure and the electrocardiogram shows an increase in the PR interval, a broadening of the QRS complex, and elevation of the T wave. The treatment of hypermagnesemia includes cessation of magnesium administration. Calcium is a direct antagonist of magnesium, and intravenous administration of calcium may be used. Peritoneal dialysis or hemodialysis may be required.

In summary, electrolytes serve many functions. They (1) assist in regulating body water balance, (2) participate in acid–base balance, (3) contribute to enzyme reactions, and (4) play an essential role in neuromuscular activity. Serum levels of an electrolyte represent its concentration (mEq/liter) in the extracellular compartment.

Sodium is the major cation in the extracellular fluid. Serum sodium levels are strongly affected by extracellular water levels: sodium concentration is increased in water deficit and decreased in water excess. Normal levels of sodium are essential to maintenance of the osmolality of the extracellular fluids; many of the manifestations of altered sodium balance are caused by swelling (hyponatremia) or shrinking (hypernatremia) of body cells, including those of the central nervous system. Sodium also contributes to neuromuscular excitability, acid–base balance, and numerous chemical reactions that occur in the body. Potassium is the major intracellular cation. It contributes to the maintenance of intracellular osmolality, is necessary for normal neuromuscular function, and influences acid–base balance. Because potassium is poorly conserved by the body, adequate daily intake is needed. Most of the body's potassium loss occurs through the kidneys; hence, potassium imbalances can occur rapidly in situations of diuresis (hypokalemia) or renal failure (hyperkalemia). Alterations in potassium balance affect skeletal, cardiac, and smooth muscle function. There is a close link between the regulation of calcium and the regulation of phosphate in the body (*e.g.*, an elevation of serum phosphate produces a decrease in serum calcium). Of the three forms of extracellular calcium (protein bound, citrate bound, and ionized), only the ionized form can cross the cell membrane and contribute to cellular function. Ionized calcium has a number of functions: it contributes to neuromuscular function, serves a vital function in the blood clotting process, and participates in a number of enzyme reactions. Alterations in ionized calcium levels produce changes in neural excitability: it is increased in hypocalcemia and decreased in hypercalcemia. Phosphate is largely an intracellular anion. It is incorporated into the nucleic acids and into ATP. A phosphate deficit causes signs and symptoms of altered neural function,

disturbed musculoskeletal function, and hematologic disorders. Phosphate excess occurs with renal failure and PTH deficit; it is associated with decrease in serum calcium. Magnesium is the second most abundant intracellular cation. It acts as a cofactor in many enzyme reactions and exerts an effect similar to that of the calcium ion on neuromuscular function.

■ Study Guide

After you have studied this chapter, you should be able to meet the following objectives:

☐ Differentiate between the intracellular compartment and the extracellular compartment.

☐ Define *electrolyte*.

☐ State the formula for deriving the number of milliequivalents in a substance.

☐ Explain the term *concentration gradient*.

☐ State the parameters that determine the level of body water and electrolytes.

☐ Explain why water is essential to life by summarizing its functions in the body.

☐ State the source(s) of water gain and of water loss.

☐ Describe the means by which thirst is manifested.

☐ Explain how ADH regulates renal reabsorption of water.

☐ Compare the pathophysiologic defect in diabetes insipidus with that in SIADH.

☐ Describe the pathology of extracellular fluid volume deficit with reference to its manifestations in the skin, gastrointestinal tract, the third space, and the urinary tract.

☐ Relate the signs and symptoms of fluid volume deficit to the functions of water.

☐ Describe the effect of fluid deficit on arterial and venous volumes and on the brain and nerve cells.

☐ Relate the causes of extracellular fluid excess to its clinical manifestations.

☐ Relate the effect of body water on sodium concentration in the extracellular fluids.

☐ Describe the role of the kidneys in regulating serum sodium.

☐ State the effect of renal disease on serum sodium.

☐ Compare Cushing's syndrome with Addison's disease with reference to serum aldosterone level.

☐ State the criterion for hyponatremia.

☐ Relate the causes of hyponatremia to its clinical manifestations.

☐ Describe the clinical manifestations of hypernatremia.

☐ State the functions of potassium.

☐ Describe the relationship of pH to potassium balance.

☐ Describe the feedback regulation of serum aldosterone.

☐ List the causes of potassium deficit.

☐ State the sources of potassium loss.

☐ Relate hypokalemia to its clinical manifestations in four major body systems.

☐ State the role of the kidneys in regulating serum potassium.

☐ Compare hypokalemia and hyperkalemia.

☐ Explain the interaction between serum calcium and serum phosphate.

☐ Describe the role of vitamin D in regulating serum calcium and phosphate.

☐ Compare the physiologic actions of PTH and calcitonin.

☐ List the functions of serum calcium.

☐ Describe the clinical manifestations of decreased serum calcium gains compared with those of increased serum calcium losses.

☐ Describe the clinical manifestations of hypercalcemic crisis.

☐ List the functions of phosphate.

☐ Relate the causes of hypophosphatemia to its clinical manifestations.

☐ State the relationship between hyperphosphatemia and serum calcium.

☐ Describe the neuromuscular manifestations of hypomagnesemia.

References

1. Guyton A: Textbook of Medical Physiology, pp 441, 392, 890, 89, 974. Philadelphia, WB Saunders, 1981
2. Lawrence SV: Woman's death by water intoxication ruled suicide. Clin Psych News 5:3, 1977
3. Baker AB, Baker LH: Clinical neurology, Vol. 2. In Haymaker W, Anderson E (eds): Disorders of the Hypothalamus and Pituitary Gland, pp 18, 24, 25. New York, Harper & Row, 1976
4. Moses M, Miller M, Streeten DHP: Pathology and pharmacologic alterations in release and actions of ADH. Metabolism 25:705, 1976
5. Pruit BA: Other complications of burn injury. In Artz CP et al: Burns, p 518. Philadelphia, WB Saunders, 1979
6. Narins RG, Jones ER, Stom MC: Diagnostic strategies in disorders of fluid, electrolyte and acid–base balance. Am J Med 72:496, 1982
7. Pflaum SS: Investigation of intake–output as a means of assessing body fluid balance. Heart Lung 8:498, 1979
8. Goldberger E: A Primer on Water, Electrolytes, and Acid–Base Syndromes, 6th ed, p 34. Philadelphia, Lea & Febiger, 1980
9. Snyder JD: From pedalyte to popsicles: A look at oral rehydration therapy in the United States. Am J Clin Nutr 35:157, 1982
10. The Medical Letter Vol 25, No 629:19, 1983
11. Knockel JP: Neuromuscular manifestations of electrolyte disorders. Am J Med 72:521, 1982
12. Agus LS, Wasserstein A, Goldfarb S: Disorders of calcium and magnesium homeostasis. Am J Med 72:473, 1982
13. Stein JH, Smith WO, Ginn HE: Hypophosphatemia in acute alcoholism. Am J Med Sci 252:78, 1966
14. Davis RF, Eichner J, Archie W et al: Hypocalcemia, hyperphosphatemia and dehydration following a single hypertonic phosphate enema. J Pediatr 90, No 3:484, 1977
15. Metheny NM, Snively WD: Nurses' Handbook of Fluid Balance, 4th ed, p 59. Philadelphia, JB Lippincott, 1983
16. Sodeman WA, Sodeman TM: Pathologic Physiology, p 993. Philadelphia, WB Saunders, 1980

■ Additional References

Fluid balance

Anderson BJ: Antidiuretic hormone: Balance and imbalance. J Neurosurg Nurs 11, No 2:71, 1979

Coleman P: Antidiuretic hormone: Physiology and pathophysiology—A review. J Neurosurg Nurs 11, No 4:199, 1979

Grant M, Kubo R: Assessing a patient's hydration status. Am J Nurs 75, No 8:199, 1975

Gennari FJ: Serum osmolality: Uses and limitations. N Engl J Med 310:102, 1984

Hays RM: Principles of ion and water transport in the kidney. Hosp Pract 13, No 9:79, 1978

Humes DH, Narins RG, Brenner BM: Disorders of water balance. Hosp Pract 14, No 3:133, 1979

Kee JL: Clinical implications of laboratory studies in critical care. Crit Care Quart 2:1, 1979

Knochel JP: Neuromuscular manifestations of electrolyte disorders. Am J Med 72:521, 1982

Kubo WR, Grant MM: The syndrome of inappropriate secretion of antidiuretic hormone. Heart Lung 7, No. 3:469, 1978

Kubo WR: Fluid and electrolyte problems. Crit Care Update 19, 1979

Miller PR, Krebs RA, Neal BJ et al: Hypodipsia in geriatric patients. Am J Med 73:354, 1982

Newsome HH Jr: Vasopressin: Deficiency, excess and the syndrome of inappropriate antidiuretic hormone secretion. Nephron 23:125, 1979

Ricci MM: Water and electrolyte metabolism in patients with intracranial lesions. J Neurosurg Nurs 9, No 4:165, 1979

Robertson GL: Thirst and vasopressin function in normal and disordered states of water balance. J Lab Clin Med 101:351, 1983

Robertson GL, Aycinena P, Zerbe RL: Neurogenic disorders of osmoregulation. Am J Med 73:339, 1982

Rosenbaum JF, Rothman JS, Murray GB: Psychosis and water intoxication. Clin J Psych 40:287, 1979

Skorecki KL, Brenner BM: Body fluid homeostasis in man: A contemporary overview. Am J Med 70:77, 1981

Twombly M: The shift into third space. Nursing 78:38, 1978

Wilson RF: Tips on managing fluid and electrolyte problems. Consultant 31, 1977

Calcium, magnesium, and phosphate balance

Chan JCM: Clinical disorders of calcium, phosphate, magnesium and hydrogen ion metabolism. Urology 13, No 2:122, 1979

Fitzgerald F: Clinical hypophosphatemia. Annu Rev Med 29:177, 1978

Juan D: Differential diagnosis of hypercalcemia. Postgrad Med 66, No 4:72, 1979

Juan D: Hypocalcemia. Arch Intern Med 139:1166, 1979

Kreisber RA: Phosphorus deficiency and hypophosphatemia. Hosp Pract 12, No 3:121, 1977

Recker RR, Saville PD: Hypercalcemia and hypocalcemia in clinical practice. Hosp Med 15, No 9:74, 1979

Roberts A: Systems of life. Calcium homeostasis: Regulation. Nurs Times 75:center pages, 1977

Roberts A: Systems of life. Calcium homeostasis: Clinical disorders. Nurs Times 75:center pages, 1979

Swales JD: Magnesium deficiency and diuretics. Br Med J 2:1377, 1982

Zeluff GW, Suki WN, Jackson D: Hypercalcemia—Etiology, manifestations and management. Heart Lung 9, No 1:146, 1980

Zeluff GW, Suki WN, Jackson D: Depletion of body phosphate—Ubiquitous, subtle, dangerous. Heart Lung 6, No 3:519, 1977

Potassium balance

Adrogue HJ, Madias NE: Changes in potassium concentrations during acute acidosis. Am J Med 71:456, 1981

Harrington JT, Isner JM, Kassirer JP: Our national obsession with potassium. Am J Med 73:155, 1982

Cohen J: Disorders of potassium balance. Hosp Pract 15, No 1:119, 1979

Layzer RB: Periodic paralysis and the sodium–potassium pump. Ann Neurol 11:547, 1982

Morgan DB, Davidson C: Hypokalemia and diuretics: An analysis of publications. Br Med J 1:905, 1980

Nardone DA, McDonald WJ, Girard DE: Mechanisms of hypokalemia: Clinical correlation. Medicine 57, No 5:435, 1978

Rao TL, Mathru KM, Salem MR et al: Serum potassium levels following transfusion of frozen erythrocytes. Anesthesiology 52:170, 1982

Sopko JA, Freeman RM: Salt substitutes as a source of potassium. JAMA 238:608, 1977

Sterns RH, Cox M, Feig PU et al: Internal potassium balance and the control of the plasma potassium concentration. Medicine 60:339, 1981

Tannen RL: Effects of potassium on blood pressure control. Ann Intern Med 98 p 2:773, 1983

Vee R: The role of potassium in health and disease. Crit Care Nurs 2 No 3:54, 1982

Zeluff GW, Suki WN, Jackson D: Hypokalemia—Cause and treatment. Heart Lung 7, No 5:854, 1978

Sodium balance

Adlard JM, George JM: Hyponatremia. Heart Lung 7, No 4:587, 1978

Arieff AI, Francisco L, Massry S: Neurological manifestations and morbidity of hyponatremia: Correlation with brain and electrolytes. Medicine 55, No 2:121, 1976

Arieff AI, Guisado R: Effects on the central nervous system of hypernatremic and hyponatremic states. Kidney Int 10:104, 1976

Burke MD: Electrolyte studies. 1. Sodium and water. Postgrad Med 64, No 4:147, 1978

Levy M: The pathophysiology of sodium balance. Hosp Pract 13, No 11:95, 1978

Moses AM, Miller M: Drug-induced hyponatremia. N Engl J Med 291, No 23:1234, 1974

Chapter 26

Alterations in Distribution of Body Fluids: Edema

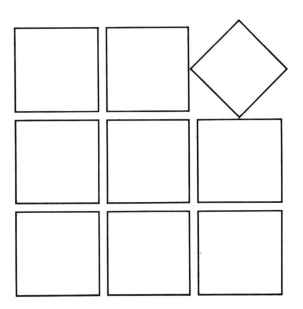

Normally, about 5% of the total body water is contained in the interstitial, or tissue, spaces. This water acts as a transport vehicle for gases, nutrients, wastes, and other materials that need to be transported between body cells and the vascular compartment. Interstitial fluid also provides a reservoir from which vascular volume can be maintained during periods of hemorrhage or loss of vascular volume. A tissue gel, or spongelike material composed of large quantities of mucopolysaccharides, fills the tissue spaces and aids in the even distribution of interstitial fluid. This tissue gel decreases with age and is thought to account in part for the wrinkled appearance that occurs with aging.

Several factors contribute to alterations in the distribution of extracellular water. Because of the nonspecific nature of these alterations and the frequency with which they occur, this chapter focuses on *increases* in interstitial fluid, or *edema*.

■ Regulation of Interstitial Fluid Volume

The interchange of cellular and vascular fluid occurs at the capillary level, with fluid leaving the capillary bed, traversing the interstitial spaces, and entering the cell and vice versa. Normally, the movement of fluid between the capillary bed and the interstitial spaces is continuous. A state of equilibrium exists as long as equal amounts of fluid both enter and leave the interstitial spaces. White blood cells, plasma proteins, and other molecules which are too large to reenter the capillary rely on the loosely structured wall of the lymphatic vessels for return to the vascular compartment. About 10% of the filtered fluid is returned to the circulation through the lymphatics.

$$\frac{\text{fluid leaving}}{\text{the capillary}} = \frac{\text{fluid reentering}}{\text{the capillary}} + \text{lymphatic flow}$$

Capillaries are microscopic vessels one layer thick that connect the arterioles of the arterial system with venules of the venous system. Small cuffs of smooth muscle, the precapillary sphincters, are positioned at the arterial end of the capillary. The smooth muscle tone of the arterioles, venules, and precapillary sphincters serves to control blood flow through the capillary bed (see Fig. 26-1).

Two types of mechanisms control the movement of capillary fluid—outward and inward forces (Fig. 26-1). The outward forces, those that cause fluid to move out of the capillary into the tissue spaces, include (1) the capillary filtration (or capillary) pressure, (2) the negative tissue fluid pressure, and (3) the colloid osmotic pressure exerted by plasma proteins that are in the tissue spaces. The inward movement of fluid is controlled largely by the colloid osmotic pressure within the capillary.

Capillary Filtration Pressure

The capillary filtration pressure is the force that pushes water through the capillary pores into the interstitial spaces. Capillary filtration pressure reflects the arterial

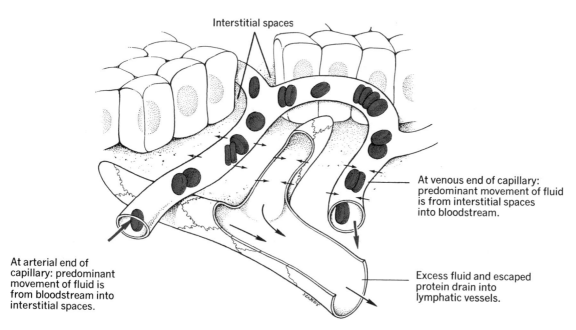

At arterial end of capillary: predominant movement of fluid is from bloodstream into interstitial spaces.

Interstitial spaces

At venous end of capillary: predominant movement of fluid is from interstitial spaces into bloodstream.

Excess fluid and escaped protein drain into lymphatic vessels.

Figure 26-1 *Exchanges through capillary membranes in the formation and removal of interstitial fluid. (From Chaffee EE. Lytle IM: Basic Physiology and anatomy, 4th ed. Philadelphia, JB Lippincott, 1980)*

pressure, the venous pressure, and the hydrostatic effects of gravity (Fig. 26-2).

The *arterial pressure* decreases as blood moves away from the heart. Nevertheless, the pressure at the arterial end of the capillary is normally higher than the pressure at its venous end. This pressure difference, or gradient, contributes to the exchange of fluid at the capillary level. *Venous pressure* is freely transmitted back to the capillary because there are no sphincters at this end of the capillary. This means that increases in venous pressure, such as those that occur with heart failure, will eventually lead to an increase in intracapillary pressure. Capillary pressure also reflects changes in *capillary volume*. Capillary volume is controlled by the precapillary flow (tone of the pre-capillary sphincters and the arterioles that supply the capillary) and the postcapillary (venule and small vein) resistances. Selective constriction of the venules will cause capillary pressures to rise, whereas constriction of the arterioles and precapillary sphincters leads to a decrease in pressure. The pressure due to gravity is called the *hydrostatic pressure*. In a person in the standing position, the weight of the blood in the vascular column causes an increase of 1 mm Hg in pressure for every 13.6 mm of distance from the heart.* Gravity has no effect on blood pressure in a person in the recumbent position because the blood vessels are then at the level of the heart. Often the terms capillary pressure and hydrostatic pressure are used interchangeably; this is because of the passive nature of pressure in the capillary bed. In this chapter, for purposes of discussion, hydrostatic pressure is considered to be the result of gravity and is presented separately from other factors that affect capillary pressure.

Colloid Osmotic Pressure

Colloids are particles that become evenly dispersed when placed in solution, much as cream particles become dispersed when milk is homogenized. The term *colloid osmotic pressure* is used to distinguish the osmotic effects of the colloids from those of the dissolved crystalloids such as sodium. The plasma proteins are large colloid molecules that disperse in the blood and occasionally escape into the tissue spaces. Because the capillary membrane is almost impermeable to the plasma proteins, these particles exert a force that draws fluid into the capillary and offsets the pushing force of the capillary filtration pressure. The plasma contains a mixture of plasma proteins, including albumin, the globulins, and fibrinogen. Albumin, which is the smallest and most

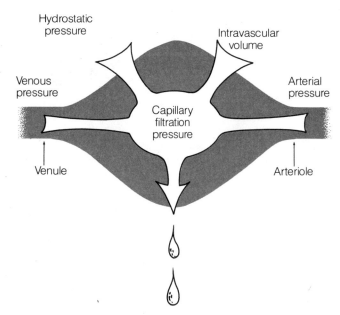

Figure 26-2 *The forces that influence capillary filtration pressure.*

abundant of the plasma proteins, accounts for about 70% of the total osmotic pressure. The reader is reminded that it is the number, and not the size of the particles in solution, that controls the osmotic pressure. One gram of albumin (molecular weight 69,000) contains almost six times as many molecules as 1 gm of fibrinogen (molecular weight 400,000).†

Lymph Flow

Normally, slightly more fluid leaves the capillary than can be reabsorbed at the venous end. This excess fluid is returned to the circulation by way of the lymph channels; almost all body tissues have lymph channels. The structure of the lymph capillary is unique in that the junctions between the endothelial cells of the vessels are loosely connected to form valves and are attached by anchoring filaments to the surrounding tissue (Fig. 26-3). These valves allow fluid to enter the lymph channel. Once the fluid has entered the lymph channel, however, it cannot leave because the valve prevents backward flow. The anchoring filaments serve to pull the valve open when tissue fluid increases. Contraction of smooth muscles in the lymph channels (lymph pump) causes the lymph fluid to empty into the veins in the chest. Compression of tissues and muscle movements contributes to the movement of fluid in the lymph channels.

---

*The hydrostatic pressure in the veins of an adult male can reach a level of 90 mm Hg. This pressure is then transmitted to the capillary bed.

†The normal values for the plasma proteins are (1) albumin 4.5 gm per 100 ml, (2) globulins 2.5 gm per 100 ml, and (3) fibrinogen 0.3 gm per 100 ml.

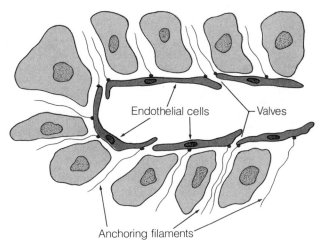

Figure 26-3 *Special structure of the lymphatic capillaries that permits passage of substances of high molecular weight back into the circulation. (From Guyton AC: Textbook of Medical Physiology, 6th ed. Philadelphia, WB Saunders, 1981)*

In summary, exchange of fluids between the vascular compartment and the interstitial spaces occurs at the capillary level. The capillary filtration pressure pushes fluids out of the capillaries, and the colloidal osmotic pressure exerted by the plasma proteins pulls fluids back into the capillaries. Albumin, which is the smallest and most abundant of the plasma proteins, provides the major osmotic force for return of fluid to the vascular compartment. Normally, slightly more fluid leaves the capillary bed than can be reabsorbed. This excess fluid is returned to the circulation by way of the lymphatic channels.

■ Edema

Edema refers to excess interstitial fluid in the tissues. Edema is not a disease but rather the manifestation of altered physiologic function.

Causes

The alterations in physiologic function that lead to edema are (1) increases in capillary filtration pressure, (2) decreases in capillary colloid osmotic pressure, (3) increases in capillary permeability, and (4) obstruction to lymph flow. Edema can occur in healthy as well as sick individuals, for example, the swelling of the hands and feet that occurs in hot weather. The causes of edema are summarized in Table 26-1.

Table 26-1 Causes of Edema

Increased Capillary Pressure
  Arteriolar dilatation
    Allergic responses (hives and angioneurotic edema)
    Inflammation
  Venous obstruction
    Hepatic obstruction
    Heart failure
    Thrombophlebitis
  Increased vascular volume
    Heart failure
    Increased levels of adrenal cortical hormones
    Increased premenstrual sodium retention
    Pregnancy
    Environmental heat stress
  Effects of gravity
    Prolonged standing

Decreased Colloid Osmotic Pressure
  Decreased production of plasma proteins
    Liver disease
    Starvation or severe protein deficiency
  Increased loss of plasma proteins
    Protein-losing kidney diseases
    Extensive burns

Increased Capillary Permeability
  Inflammation
  Immune responses
  Neoplastic disease
  Tissue injury and burns

Obstruction of Lymphatic Flow
  Infection or disease of the lymphatic structures
  Surgical removal of lymph nodes

Increased capillary presssure

Edema develops when an increase in capillary pressure causes excess movement of fluid from the capillary bed into the interstitial spaces. Among the factors that cause an increase in capillary pressures are (1) <u>decreased resistance to flow through the arterioles and capillary sphincters that supply the capillary bed,</u> (2) <u>increased resistance to outflow at the venous end of the capillary</u> bed, (3) increased extracellular fluid volume associated <u>with an increase in intravascular volume,</u> and (4) <u>increased gravitational forces.</u> In hives and other allergic or inflammatory conditions, localized edema develops because of a histamine-induced dilatation of the precapillary sphincters and arterioles that supply the swollen area. Impaired venous outflow from the capillary causes a retrograde increase in capillary pressure. Thrombophlebitis, or the presence of venous blood clots, leads to edema of the affected part. In right-sided heart failure, blood dams up throughout the entire systemic venous system, causing organ congestion and edema of the dependent extremities. Increased reabsorption of sodium and water by the kidney leads to an increase in extracellular volume with an increase in capillary pressure and subsequent movement of fluid into the tissue spaces. In hot weather dilatation of the superficial blood vessels occurs and sodium and water retention increases, which causes swelling of the hands and feet. Edema of the ankles and feet becomes more pronounced during prolonged periods of standing when the forces of gravity are superimposed on the heat-induced vasodilatation and the increase in extracellular fluid volume.

Decreased colloid osmotic pressure

The plasma proteins exert the osmotic force that is needed to move fluid back into the capillary from the tissue spaces. Edema develops when plasma protein levels become inadequate because of abnormal losses or inadequate production. The glomerulus of the kidney nephron is a network of capillaries. In certain conditions, these capillaries may become permeable to the plasma proteins. When this happens, large amounts of plasma proteins are filtered out of the blood and then lost in the urine. An excess loss of plasma proteins also occurs when large areas of skin are injured or destroyed. Edema is a common problem during the early stages of a burn, resulting from both capillary injury and loss of plasma proteins.

Plasma proteins are synthesized from amino acids. In starvation and malnutrition, edema develops because of a lack of amino acids for use in plasma proteins production. In starvation, edema may actually mask the loss of tissue mass. Finally, because plasma proteins are synthesized in the liver, severe liver dysfunction causes decreased plasma protein synthesis with the development of edema and ascites. Liver disease also contributes to edema formation by causing obstruction to venous flow through the portal circulation and through impaired metabolism of hormones, such as aldosterone, which increase sodium retention.

It is now possible to measure the colloid osmotic pressure of the plasma (25.4 is normal).[1] Infusion of albumin can be used to raise colloidal osmotic pressure as a means of restoring intravascular volume or reversing interstitial fluid losses.

Increased capillary permeability

In situations of increased capillary permeability, the capillary pores become enlarged or the integrity of the capillary wall is destroyed. Injury due to burns, mechanical distention, inflammation, and immune responses are known to increase capillary permeability. Once an increase in capillary permeability has been established, plasma proteins and other osmotically active particles leak out into the interstitial spaces and perpetuate the accumulation of tissue fluid.

Obstruction of lymphatic flow

The osmotically active plasma proteins and other large particles rely on the lymphatics for movement back into the circulatory system from the interstitial spaces. Lymphedema occurs when there is obstructed lymph flow. Malignant involvement of lymph structures or removal of lymph nodes at the time of cancer surgery are common causes of lymphedema. Another cause of lymphedema is infection. Elephantiasis (filariasis) is a tropical infection in which nematodes of the superfamily Filarioidea invade the lymph nodes, causing massive swelling of a body part. This infection has been reported to cause a single leg to swell to such proportions that it weighs almost as much as the rest of the body.

Effects

The effects of edema are determined largely by its location. Edema of the brain, larynx, and lung is an acute, life-threatening situation. On the other hand, swelling of the ankles and feet is often insidious in onset and may or may not be associated with disease. Edema may interfere with movement, limiting motion, or making opening of the eyes difficult. Edema can also be disfiguring. In terms of psychologic effects and self-concept, edema often causes a distortion of body features, creating problems ir obtaining proper-fitting clothing and shoes.

At the tissue level, edema increases the distance for diffusion of oxygen, nutrients, and wastes. Edematous tissues are usually more susceptible to injury and to development of ischemic tissue damage, including pressure sores. The skin of a severely swollen finger can act as a tourniquet, shutting off the blood flow to the finger.

In chronic edema, the tissue spaces become stretched like an old balloon so that less filtration pressure is needed to push fluids into the interstitial spaces. The stretching of the tissue spaces makes correction or permanent reversal of edema difficult.

Pitting edema

Pitting edema occurs when the accumulation of interstitial fluid exceeds the absorptive capacity of the tissue gel. In pitting edema, the tissue water is mobile and can be translocated with pressure exerted by a finger. Imagine, if you will, a sponge that is supersaturated with water. To test for pitting edema, the observer applies firm finger pressure to the edematous areas. Pitting edema is present if an indentation remains after the finger has been removed.

Nonpitting edema

Nonpitting edema usually represents a situation in which serum proteins that have accumulated in the tissue spaces coagulate. Often the area is firm and discolored.

Brawny edema describes a type of nonpitting edema in which the skin thickens and hardens. Nonpitting edema is seen most frequently following local infection or trauma.

Assessment

Methods for assessing edema include visual inspection, including the use of digital pressure to determine the degree of pitting that is present. Pitting edema is evaluated on a scale of $+1$ to $+4$. Daily weight is also a useful index of interstitial fluid gain. A third assessment measure involves measuring the circumference of an extremity (or the abdomen).

Treatment

The treatment of edema is usually directed toward (1) maintaining life in situations in which the swelling involves vital structures, (2) correcting or controlling the cause, and (3) preventing tissue injury. Diuretic therapy is often used to treat edema. The reader is again reminded that edema is not always associated with disease and that normal compensatory increases in tissue fluid may respond to such simple measures as elevating the feet.

Elastic support stockings and sleeves are applied to increase the resistance to the outward flow of fluid from the capillary. These support devices are often prescribed in situations such as lymphatic or venous obstruction and are most efficient if applied before the tissue spaces have filled with fluid, as in the morning before the effects of gravity have caused fluid to move into the ankles.

Accumulation of Fluid in the Serous Cavities

The serous cavities are potential spaces located in strategic body areas where there is continual movement of body structures—the joints, the pericardial sac, and the pleural cavity. The exchange of extracellular fluid between the capillaries, the interstitial spaces, and the potential space of the serous cavity is similar to capillary exchange mechanisms that exist elsewhere in the body. The potential spaces are closely linked with lymphatic drainage systems. The milking action of the moving structures continually forces fluid and plasma proteins back into the circulation, keeping these cavities empty. One of the factors that contributes to fluid accumulation in a potential space is obstruction to lymph flow.

The prefix *hydro-* may be used to indicate the presence of excessive fluid, as in hydrothorax, which means excessive fluid in the pleural cavity. Or the term *effusion*

may be used, as in pleural effusion, referring to an accumulation of fluid in the pleural cavity.

The fluid accumulated in a serous cavity may be either serous or exudative. A common cause of fluid accumulation in serous cavities is infection. In infection, white cells and cellular debris collect and obstruct lymph flow, causing osmotically active proteins to accumulate. A second cause of fluid accumulation is a malignant tumor; malignant tumors may invade the lymph channels that drain the serous cavity, and thus contribute to fluid accumulation.

Ascites is an accumulation of fluid in the peritoneal cavity. Because of its location in relation to the portal circulation, the peritoneal cavity is more susceptible to excess fluid accumulation than are other body cavities. This is because anytime there is a significant increase in pressure in the liver sinusoids, serum exudes through the capillaries on the surface of the liver and passes into the peritoneal cavity. Congestive heart failure, cirrhosis, and carcinoma of the liver are examples of conditions that obstruct hepatic blood flow and cause fluid to move into the peritoneal cavity. Because the portal vein receives blood from the peritoneal surface, portal hypertension creates an increase in the filtration pressure of the capillaries that line the peritoneal cavity.

Excess fluid may be aspirated or removed from a serous cavity. The term paracentesis refers to removal of fluid through a puncture site. Usually a needle or similar instrument is inserted into the cavity and the fluid is withdrawn. Analysis of the fluid for the presence of infectious organisms and malignant cells often aids in diagnosis of the disease responsible for the fluid accumulation.

In summary, edema occurs in healthy as well as sick individuals. The physiologic mechanisms that predispose to edema formation are (1) increased capillary pressure, (2) decreased capillary colloidal osmotic pressure, (3) increased capillary permeability, and (4) obstruction of lymphatic flow. The effect that edema exerts on body function is determined by its location—cerebral edema can be a life-threatening situation, whereas swollen feet can be a normal discomfort that accompanies hot weather.

■ Study Guide

After you have studied this chapter, you should be able to meet the following objectives:

☐ Describe the role of the capillaries in regulating interstitial fluid volume.

☐ Explain the use of the term *colloid osmotic pressure.*

☐ Describe lymph flow.

☐ Describe the pathologic basis of increased capillary pressure.

☐ Explain the relationship between plasma protein levels and edema formation.

☐ List the causes of increased capillary permeability.

☐ State the clinical manifestations of lymphedema.

☐ Compare pitting edema and nonpitting edema.

☐ State the goal in treatment of edema.

☐ Explain why the serous cavities are referred to as *potential spaces*.

■ Reference

1. Morissette MP: Colloid osmotic pressure: Its measurement and clinical value. Can Med Assoc J 116:897, 1977

■ Additional References

Burch E: Cardiac edema. Consultant, April 227, 1980
Guyton AC: Textbook of Medical Physiology, ed 6, pp 358, 370. Philadelphia, WB Saunders, 1981

Chapter 27

Alterations in Acid–Base Balance

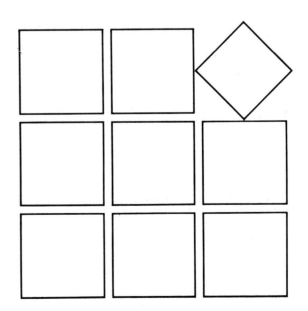

Normal body function is dependent on the precise regulation of acid–base balance. The metabolic activities that take place in the body require the regulation of pH so that enzyme systems and chemical reactions can proceed at an optimal rate. Two types of acids are produced during the metabolic processes that transform carbohydrates, fats, and proteins into cellular energy: volatile and nonvolatile. Carbonic acid, which is volatile, results from dissolved carbon dioxide; it is called a respiratory acid because it is eliminated through the lungs. All of the other acids formed in the body or that enter the body through the gastrointestinal tract or parenteral route are referred to as metabolic acids. These nonvolatile metabolic acids are derived mainly from protein breakdown. The hydrogen ions from the metabolic acids are excreted through the kidneys.

Many conditions, pathologic and otherwise, afford the potential for altering body pH. This chapter focuses on metabolic and respiratory-induced changes in acid–base balance.

■ Regulation of Acid–Base Balance

The symbol pH refers to the concentration of hydrogen ions, or more specifically to the negative logarithm (p) of the hydrogen (H^+) in milliequivalents per liter. The hydrogen ion and carbon dioxide content of the body are normally regulated so that the pH of the extracellular fluids is maintained within the narrow range of 7.35 to 7.45.

Carbon Dioxide

The carbon dioxide content of the blood is transported in three forms: (1) attached to hemoglobin, (2) dissolved carbon dioxide (PCO_2), and (3) bicarbonate (HCO_3^-) (see Fig. 27-1). Normally, about 23% of the carbon dioxide is transported in the red blood cell where it is attached to the hemoglobin molecule. A small percentage of carbon dioxide dissolves in the plasma to form the volatile acid carbonic acid (H_2CO_3), and the rest of the carbon dioxide is carried as the bicarbonate ion. Collectively, dissolved carbon dioxide and bicarbonate constitute about 77% of the carbon dioxide that is transported in the extracellular fluid.

Carbon dioxide content in blood can be calculated using the *solubility coefficient* for carbon dioxide. Under normal physiologic conditions, this coefficient has been shown to have a value of 0.03. This means that the H_2CO_3 content of the venous blood, which has a PCO_2 value of 45 mm Hg, will be 1.35 mEq/liter (45 times 0.03 = 1.35).

Carbon dioxide also combines with water to form *bicarbonate* ($CO_2 + H_2O = H^+ + HCO_3^-$). This reaction is catalyzed by the enzyme carbonic anhydrase, which is present in large quantities in the red blood cell and in other tissues of the body. The rate of the reaction between carbon dioxide and water is increased about 5000 times by the presence of carbonic anhydrase. Were it not for this enzyme, the reaction would occur too slowly to be of any significance. Base bicarbonate is formed when the cations sodium, potassium, calcium, and magnesium combine with the bicarbonate ion.

Metabolic Acids

Metabolic acids are the main source of hydrogen ions in the body. The two major metabolic acids are phosphoric acid and sulfuric acid, which are formed in the process of protein breakdown. They are strong acids and are dissociated in H^+, SO_4^{--}, HPO_4^{--} and $H_2PO_4^-$. Other acids that are produced through metabolic processes are lactic acid and the ketoacids.

Lactic acid is formed when insufficient oxygen is available to convert metabolic end products to water and carbon dioxide. The ketoacids are metabolic acids that are produced when carbohydrates are not available for use in cell metabolism or when cells are unable to use carbohydrates, for example, in diabetes mellitus. Intracellular hydrogen ions are buffered by cell proteins and extracellular ions by the bicarbonate-carbonic acid buffer system.

Control Mechanisms

The body has two major mechanisms for controlling pH. One is the regulation of pH by renal and respiratory mechanisms that act to selectively release hydrogen and carbon dioxide into the external environment. The other is a system for buffering excess acid and alkali to protect the body against extreme changes in pH.

Blood buffer systems

The ability of the body to maintain the pH of the extracellular fluids within the physiologic range is dependent on the blood buffer systems. These buffers are immediately available for combination with excess acids and alkalis and thus prevent large changes in pH from occurring. The body has several blood buffer systems—the phosphate, hemoglobin, and bicarbonate systems. Of these systems, the bicarbonate buffer system assumes the major role in the regulation of extracellular pH.

A buffering system consists of a weak acid and the alkali salt of that acid or a weak base and its acid salt. In the bicarbonate buffer system, carbon dioxide combines with water in a reversible reaction to form the weak acid, carbonic acid ($CO_2 + H_2O \rightleftharpoons H_2CO_3 \rightleftharpoons H^+ + HCO_3^-$). The carbonic acid dissociates into a bicarbonate (HCO_3^-) ion and a hydrogen (H^+) ion. The alkali salt of carbonic acid is sodium bicarbonate ($Na\,HCO_3$). The bicarbonate buffer system is unique in that its acid is volatile and can be released into the air through the respiratory system.

Respiratory mechanisms

The respiratory system plays a major role in the regulation of dissolved carbon dioxide. This is accomplished through changes in ventilation. Increased carbon dioxide produces an increase in respiration, causing CO_2 to be expired into the air from the lung. Respiratory compensation is rapid and effective but seldom returns pH completely to normal.

Renal Mechanisms

Renal mechanisms regulate acid–base balance by causing the excretion of hydrogen. These mechanisms take longer to develop than respiratory mechanisms, but they are able to return the pH to normal. The kidneys can produce an acid or an alkaline urine as a means for controlling pH. This is accomplished through the secretion of hydrogen ions into the tubular fluid and the reabsorption of bicarbonate ions into the extracellular fluid (Fig. 27-2). The process of hydrogen ion secretion begins when carbon dioxide moves into the tubular cell. The carbon dioxide combines with water in a carbonic anhydrase-catalyzed reaction that yields a bicarbonate ion and a hydrogen ion. The bicarbonate ion is then absorbed into the extracellular fluid and the hydrogen ion is secreted into the tubular fluid in a coupled reaction that involves the reabsorption of a sodium ion. The hydrogen ion, once it enters the tubular fluid, combines with a bicarbonate ion to form carbon dioxide and water. The water then passes into the urine and the carbon dioxide diffuses back into the tubular cell.

Normally, only a few hydrogen ions remain in the tubular fluid for passage into the urine. This is because

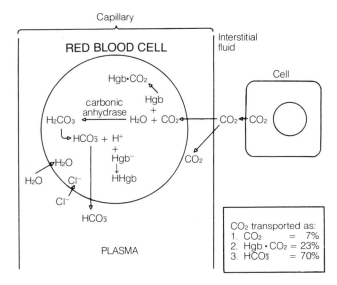

Figure 27-1 *Mechanisms of carbon dioxide transport. (From Guyton AC: Textbook of Medical Physiology, 6th ed. Philadelphia, WB Saunders, 1981)*

the tubular secretion of hydrogen ions is roughly equal to the number of bicarbonate ions that are filtered in the glomerulus. When excess carbon dioxide is present, such as occurs during periods of decreased ventilation, hydrogen ion secretion will exceed bicarbonate filtration, and the urine will become acidic. On the other hand, filtration of bicarbonate in excess of hydrogen ion secretion produces an alkaline urine.

An extremely acid urine is damaging to the structures in the urinary tract. Therefore, the maximum decrease in pH that the kidneys can excrete is 4.5; this limits the number of hydrogen ions that the kidneys can excrete. The kidneys use two other buffer systems for excreting hydrogen ions when the need to eliminate acids exceeds the pH limits of the urine. One of these is the phosphate buffer system and the other is the ammonia buffer system.

The *phosphate buffer system* consists of monohydrogen phosphate (HPO_4^{--}) and dihydrogen phos-

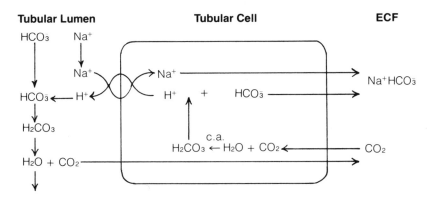

Figure 27-2 *Hydrogen ion (H^+) secretion and bicarbonate ion (HCO_3^-) retrieval in a renal tubular cell. Carbon dioxide (CO_2) diffuses into the tubular cell from the blood where it combines with water in a carbonic anhydrase (c.a.) catalyzed reaction that yields carbonic acid (H_2CO_3). The H_2CO_3 dissociates to form H^+ and HCO_3^-. The H^+ is secreted into the tubular fluid in exchange for Na^+. The Na^+ and HCO_3^- enter the extracellular fluid. (From Chaffee EE, Lytle IM: Basic Physiology and Anatomy, 4th ed. Philadelphia, JB Lippincott, 1980)*

phate ($H_2PO_4^-$). The combination of H^+ with HPO_4^{--} to form $H_2PO_4^-$ allows the kidney to increase its excretion of hydrogen ions (Fig. 27-3).

The *ammonia buffer system* allows the hydrogen ion to combine with ammonia (NH_3) to form an ammonium ion (NH_4^+). The ammonium ion is excreted in the urine as ammonium chloride (Fig. 27-4). Ammonia is synthesized by the renal tubules from amino acids. In contrast to the rapidly occurring changes in respiration that compensate for pH changes, the renal ammonia buffer system requires two to three days to become optimally effective.

The phosphate and ammonia systems have a two-fold effect in returning pH toward a more normal value in acidosis. You will note in Figures 27-3 and 27-4 that these two buffer systems not only remove a hydrogen ion from the extracellular fluid but also add a bicarbonate ion to the blood buffer pool by converting carbon dioxide to bicarbonate.

Determination of pH

The pH of the extracellular fluid is determined by the bicarbonate to carbonic acid ratio and the degree to which carbonic acid dissociates to form a hydrogen and a bicarbonate ion. The dissociation constant (K) is used to describe the degree to which an acid dissociates. The

symbol pK refers to the negative logarithm of the dissociation constant. At normal body temperature the pK for the bicarbonate buffer system is 6.1. The use of a negative logarithm for the dissociation constant allows pH to be expressed as a positive value.

The Henderson-Hasselbalch equation computes the serum pH by using the logarithm of the dissociation constant and the logarithm of the bicarbonate and dissolved carbon dioxide ratio. In its simplest form this equation states that

$$pH = pK + \log \frac{HCO_3}{H_2CO_3}$$

As a point of emphasis, it is the ratio rather than the absolute values for bicarbonate and carbonic acid that determines pH. Let us consider two examples to emphasize this point. The first situation uses normal serum values and the second uses increased concentrations of both bicarbonate and carbonic acid.

Situation 1

$$pH\ 7.4 = 6.1 + \log$$
$$\frac{27\ mEq/liter\ HCO_3}{1.35\ mEq/liter\ H_2CO_3}$$
$$ratio\ 27{:}1.35 = \underline{20{:}1}*$$

*The log of 20 is 1.3.

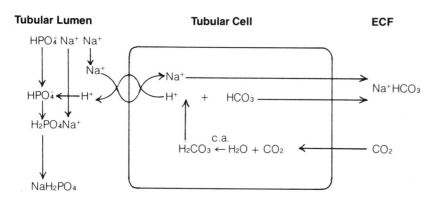

Figure 27-3 *The renal phosphate buffer system. The monohydrogen phosphate ion (HPO_4^{--}) enters the renal tubular fluid in the glomerulus. A H^+ combines with the HPO_4^{--} to form $H_2PO_4^-$ and is then excreted into the urine in combination with Na^+. The HCO_3^- moves into the extracellular fluid along with the Na^+ that was exchanged during secretion of the H^+ (From Chaffee EE, Lytle IM: Basic Physiology and Anatomy, 4th ed. Philadelphia, JB Lippincott, 1980)*

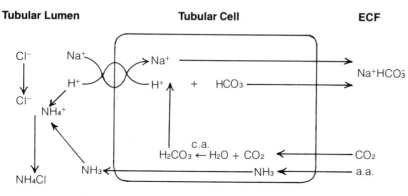

Figure 27-4 *The ammonia buffer system in a renal tubular cell. The tubular cell synthesizes ammonia (NH_3) from amino acides (a.a.). The NH_3 is secreted into the tubular fluid, where it combines with a H^+ to form an ammonium ion (NH_4^+). The ammonium ion combines with chloride for excretion in the urine. The HCO_3^- moves into the extracellular fluid along with the Na^+ that was exchanged during secretion of the H^+. (From Chaffee EE, Lytle IM: Basic Physiology and Anatomy, 4th ed. Philadelphia, JB Lippincott, 1980)*

Situation 2

$$pH\ 7.4 = 6.1 + \log$$
$$\frac{48 \text{ mEq/liter HCO}_3}{2.40 \text{ mEq/liter H}_2\text{CO}_3}$$
$$\text{ratio } 48{:}2.4 = 20{:}1^*$$

These examples demonstrate that *p*H will remain relatively stable over a wide range of changes in bicarbonate and carbonic acid concentrations as long as the ratio values for the two concentrations approach a ratio value of 20 to 1. Plasma *p*H will decrease when the ratio is less than 20 to 1 (for example, the log of 10 is 1; when the ratio of HCO$_3$ to H$_2$CO$_3$ is equal to 10, the *p*H of the blood will be 7.1) and it will increase when the ratio is greater than 20 to 1.

Correction Versus Compensation

There are two mechanisms for regulating *p*H changes. One mechanism corrects the underlying cause and the other compensates for the disorder.

Correction of acid–base disorders requires that the primary causative factor be controlled or corrected. Improved ventilation is a corrective measure in respiratory acidosis. In diabetic ketoacidosis, administration of insulin is corrective in that it prevents further breakdown of fats with formation of organic acids.

Compensation for acid–base disorders can be either respiratory or renal. The respiratory system can compensate for changes in *p*H by either increasing or decreasing ventilation. Respiratory compensation is rapid but it is seldom complete. The kidney, as mentioned earlier, compensates for *p*H changes by producing either an acid or an alkaline urine. It normally takes longer to recruit renal compensatory mechanisms than respiratory mechanisms. Renal mechanisms are more efficient, however, because they continue to operate until the *p*H has returned to normal or near normal levels.

Compensatory mechanisms usually provide a means to control *p*H in situations in which correction is impossible or cannot be immediately achieved. Often, compensatory mechanisms are interim measures that permit survival while the body attempts to correct the primary disorder. It is important for the reader to recognize that compensation requires the use of mechanisms that are different from those that caused the primary disorder. In other words, the lungs cannot compensate for respiratory acidosis that is caused by lung disease, nor can the kidneys compensate for metabolic acidosis that occurs because of kidney failure. The body can, however, use renal mechanisms to compensate for respiratory-induced changes in *p*H and it can use respiratory mechanisms to compensate for metabolically induced changes in acid–base balance.

Effects of Potassium on pH

Potassium and hydrogen are interchangeable cations that move freely between the intracellular and extracellular compartments. This means that excess hydrogen ions can move into the intracellular compartment for buffering. When this happens potassium moves out of the cell into the extracellular fluids. Conversely, in hypokalemia potassium moves out of the cell into the extracellular fluid and hydrogen moves into the cell; this causes alkalosis.

Hydrogen and potassium also compete for excretion into the urine. In the distal tubules of the kidney, potassium or hydrogen is secreted into the tubular fluid as sodium is reabsorbed into the extracellular fluid. For example, in hypokalemia, there are fewer potassium ions available for secretion into the urine, which means that there will be a predominance of hydrogen-ion secretion into the urine. This tends to cause alkalosis because the secreted hydrogen ions are removed from the extracellular fluid. On the other hand, hyperkalemia tends to cause *p*H to decrease as the kidney secretes potassium ions in excess of hydrogen ions.

Effects of Chloride on pH

Chloride and bicarbonate can substitute for each other when anion exchange is needed. For example, serum bicarbonate levels normally increase as chloride is secreted into the stomach following a heavy meal, causing what is termed the postprandial alkaline tide. Later, as the chloride is reabsorbed from the intestine, the *p*H returns to normal. Hypochloremic alkalosis refers to an increase in *p*H that is induced by a decrease in serum chloride levels. Hyperchloremic acidosis occurs when excess levels of chloride are present.

Assessment

The terms acidemia and alkalemia refer only to the *p*H of the blood as measured on a *p*H meter and give little information about the cause of the acid–base disorder. It was pointed out earlier that *p*H can be relatively normal within a wide range of changes in dissolved carbon dioxide and base bicarbonate levels. A number of laboratory tests can be used to provide a better description of acid–base disorders.

*The log of 20 is 1.3.

Carbonic acid

As mentioned previously, carbonic acid levels can be determined from blood gas measurements using the PCO_2 and the solubility coefficient for carbon dioxide (normal arterial PCO_2 is 38 mm Hg to 42 mm Hg).

Bicarbonate

More than 70% of the carbon dioxide content is in the form of bicarbonate. The serum bicarbonate level can be determined from the carbon dioxide content in the blood. The normal range of values for venous bicarbonate is 24 to 33 mEq/liter.

Base excess or deficit

Base excess or deficit measures the level of all the buffer systems in the blood—hemoglobin, protein, phosphate, and bicarbonate. The normal base excess is assigned a value of 0. Base excess or deficit describes the amount of a fixed acid or base that must be added to a blood sample to achieve a pH of 7.4 (normal -2.5 to $+2.5$ mEq/liter). For practical purposes, base excess is a measurement of bicarbonate excess or deficit. A positive result (bicarbonate excess) indicates metabolic alkalosis and a negative result (bicarbonate deficit) indicates metabolic acidosis.

Anion gap

The anion gap describes the difference between the sodium ion concentration and the sum of the measured anions (Cl^- and HCO_3^-). This difference represents the concentration of unmeasured anions such as phosphates, sulfates, organic acids, and proteins that are present in the extracellular fluid (Fig. 27-5). Normally, the anion gap is about 12 mEq/liter. (A value of 16 mEq is normal if the potassium concentration is used to calculate the anion gap.)

In summary, normal body function is dependent on the precise regulation of acid–base balance. In regulating acid–base balance, the pH (negative logarithm of the hydrogen ion concentration) of the extracellular fluid is normally regulated within a narrow range of 7.35 to 7.45. Metabolic processes produce volatile and nonvolatile acids that must be buffered and eliminated from the body. Dissolved carbon dioxide forms a volatile acid (carbonic acid), which is eliminated through the lungs. The nonvolatile acids, most of which are excreted by the kidneys, are derived mainly from protein and noncarbohydrate metabolism. The ability of the body to maintain the pH within the normal physiologic range is dependent on blood buffer systems, the most important of which is the bicarbonate buffer system. It is the ratio of the bicarbonate ion concentration to dissolved carbon dioxide (carbonic acid concentration) that determines body pH. When this ratio is 20:1, the pH is 7.4. In situations of altered acid–base balance, the regulation of pH depends on both corrective and compensatory mech-

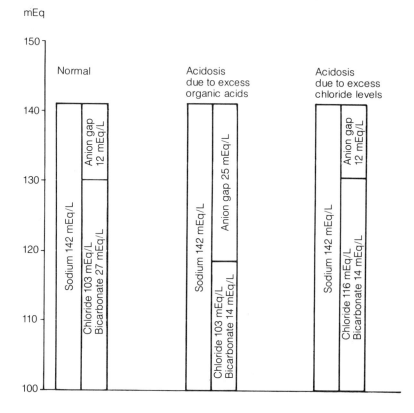

Figure 27-5 *The anion gap in acidosis due to excess metabolic acids and excess serum chloride levels. Unmeasured anions such as phosphates, sulfates, and organic acids increase the anion gap because they replace bicarbonate (this assumes there is no change in sodium content).*

anisms. When possible, mechanisms that correct the disorder causing the imbalance are used; when correction is not immediately possible, regulation of pH is accomplished through compensatory mechanisms.

Alterations in Acid–Base Balance

The terms acidosis and alkalosis describe the clinical conditions that arise as the result of changes in pH, dissolved carbon dioxide, and bicarbonate concentrations. Acidosis and alkalosis involve the *primary defect*, or the initiating event, that causes the acid–base disorder and the *compensatory state* that results from homeostatic mechanisms that attempt to prevent large changes in pH.

A primary defect in acid–base balance can be either *respiratory* or *metabolic* in origin. Cell metabolism regulates carbon dioxide and bicarbonate. Therefore, primary alterations in the bicarbonate portion of the bicarbonate-carbonic acid ratio are referred to as metabolic acid–base disorders (Chart 27-1). Carbonic acid is a volatile acid that is eliminated from the body through the respiratory tract. It follows that primary disorders of the carbonic acid portion of the bicarbonate-carbonic acid ratio are classified as respiratory pH disorders.

Both primary and compensatory mechanisms often are operational in acid–base disorders. For example, a patient may have a primary metabolic acidosis as a result of an accumulation of ketoacids and a compensatory respiratory alkalosis as a result of increased ventilation. Figure 27-6 illustrates the PCO_2, bicarbonate, and pH changes that occur in acute and chronic disorders of acid–base balance.

Most of the manifestations of acid–base disorders fall into three main categories: (1) those associated with the primary disorder that caused the pH disturbance, (2) those related to the altered pH, and (3) those that occur because of the body's attempt to compensate for the altered pH. Many of the alterations in body function associated with acid–base disturbances are directly related to the pH change and its effect on the excitability

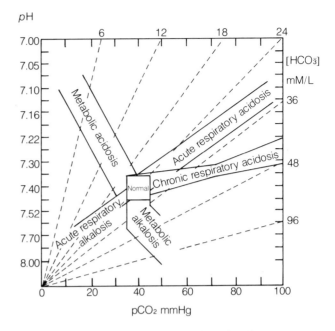

Figure 27-6 *Acute and chronic acid–base disorders as determined by PCO_2, bicarbonate, and pH values. (Adapted from Masoro EJ, Siegel PD: Acid–Base Regulation: Its Physiology, Pathophysiology and Interpretation of Blood Gas Analysis. Philadelphia, WB Saunders, 1977)*

of the nervous system. The hydrogen ion tends to stabilize the nerve membrane rendering it less excitable. The ionization of serum calcium is also affected by changes in pH, and this too contributes to the excitability of the nervous system. For example, ionization of serum calcium is increased in acidosis, and this tends to decrease nerve excitability. Conversely, alkalosis causes a decrease in ionized calcium levels with a resultant increase in neural excitability.

Metabolic Acidosis

Metabolic acidosis refers to a primary deficit in base bicarbonate. In metabolic acidosis, the pH falls below 7.35, and the plasma bicarbonate decreases to less than 24 mEq/liter.

Chart 27-1 *Primary Defects in Acid–Base Balance*

↓ HCO_3^-	Metabolic acidosis represents a decrease in bicarbonate (HCO_3 deficit)
↑ H_2CO_3	Respiratory acidosis represents an increase in carbonic acid (H_2CO_3 excess)
↑ HCO_3^-	Metabolic alkalosis represents an increase in bicarbonate (HCO_3 excess)
↓ H_2CO_3	Respiratory alkalosis represents a decrease in carbonic acid (H_2CO_3 deficit)

Causes

The causes of metabolic acidosis can be divided into two groups: increased production of metabolic acids and decreased bicarbonate. The first group is characterized by disorders that cause an increase in metabolic acids (lactic acid and ketoacids). Patients in this group have an increased anion gap because of an accumulation of unmeasured metabolic acids. The second group has a decreased serum bicarbonate; persons in this group have an increased chloride level and a normal anion gap. The causes of metabolic acidosis are described in Table 27-1.

Increased production of metabolic acids.   Metabolic acids tend to accumulate and increase when (1) metabolic demands are in excess of carbohydrate stores or when body cells are not able to use carbohydrates normally, (2) body cells are forced to metabolize carbohydrates without a sufficient supply of oxygen, or (3) the kidneys are unable to excrete metabolic acids.

Formation of ketoacids.   The production of the metabolic ketoacids is increased when carbohydrate stores are low or when the body cannot use available carbohydrates as a fuel. When this happens, the body is forced to mobilize fatty acids as a means of producing ketones, which are then used in the metabolic process. Ketone production is high during periods of *fasting, starvation,* and *uncontrolled diabetes mellitus.** Ketoacidosis also develops in persons who are following a ketogenic diet for weight control or for other purposes. The ketogenic diet is high in fat content and low in carbohydrates.

Salicylate toxicity.   Salicylate overdose causes two types of acid–base disorders. Initially, the salicylates stimulate the respiratory center causing marked hyperventilation and development of respiratory alkalosis. Renal mechanisms compensate for the increased pH by causing increased excretion of the bicarbonate ion and other basic salts. Salicylates also interfere with carbohydrate metabolism, which leads to an increased production of metabolic acids; this usually occurs several hours after acute intoxication.

*The reader is referred to Chapter 39 (Alterations in Endocrine Control of Growth and Metabolism) and Chapter 40 (Diabetes Mellitus) for additional information on the metabolic events that surround ketone production.

Table 27-1   Metabolic Acidosis

Laboratory Findings

Primary Defect (Uncompensated)		Compensation
pH Decreased	Bicarbonate Decreased	PCO$_2$ Decreased

Causes	Manifestations
Increase in Metabolic Acids (Increased Anion Gap)	**Altered Gastrointestinal Function**
Excess production of metabolic acids	Anorexia
Fasting and starvation	Nausea
Ketogenic diet	Vomiting
Diabetic ketoacidosis	Abdominal pain
Lactic acidosis	**Depression of Neural Function**
Alcoholic ketoacidosis	Weakness
Salicylate poisoning	Lethargy
Decreased loss of metabolic acids	General malaise
Renal failure	Confusion
Increase in Bicarbonate Loss (Normal Anion Gap)	Stupor
	Coma
Loss of intestinal secretions	Depression of vital functions
Diarrhea	**Skin**
Intestinal suction	Warm and flushed
Intestinal or biliary fistula	**Signs of Compensation**
Decreased renal losses	Kussmaul breathing
Renal tubular acidosis	Acid urine
Treatment with acetazolamide	Increased ammonia in urine
Increased chloride levels	Increased serum potassium
Abnormal chloride reabsorption by the kidney	
Sodium chloride infusions	
Treatment with ammonium chloride	
Parenteral hyperalimentation	

Formation of lactic acid. The accumulation of lactic acid in the body occurs for two reasons: (1) because of excess lactic acid production and (2) because of decreased removal of lactic acid from the blood by the liver. Lactic acid is produced during periods of anaerobic metabolism when cells do not receive sufficient oxygen for converting body fuel sources to carbon dioxide and water. Blood flow to skeletal muscles, liver, and other tissues is decreased during shock and heart failure. Lactic acid also accumulates during periods of excessive oxygen need, such as during strenuous exercise when blood flow and oxygen delivery cannot keep pace with the increased needs of the exercising muscle. Because the liver removes lactic acid from the blood and converts it to glucose, lactic acidosis can occur in liver disease or in situations that impair the liver's ability to convert lactic acid to glucose.

Impaired renal excretion of hydrogen. The excretion of metabolic acids occurs through the kidney. In renal failure there is loss of both glomerular and tubular function with retention of nitrogenous wastes and metabolic acids. Bicarbonate losses are increased when renal tubular cells are unable to secrete hydrogen ions or when bicarbonate reabsorption is decreased. In a condition called renal tubular acidosis, there is normal glomerular function, but the tubular secretion of hydrogen or reabsorption of bicarbonate is abnormal. Treatment with the drug acetazolamide (Diamox) also leads to increased renal losses of bicarbonate. This drug, which is an inhibitor of carbonic anhydrase, interferes with the formation of carbonic acid in the renal tubular cells; this leads to increased losses of bicarbonate, sodium, and chloride.

Increased bicarbonate losses. Intestinal secretions have a high bicarbonate concentration. Consequently, excessive losses of bicarbonate occur with increased losses of intestinal secretions, as in severe diarrhea, small bowel or biliary fistula drainage, ileostomy drainage, and intestinal suction. In diarrhea of microbial origin, bicarbonate is secreted into the bowel to neutralize the metabolic acids that are produced by the organisms causing the diarrhea.

Chloride ion excess. When the anion gap is within normal limits, there is a reciprocal relationship between serum chloride concentrations and serum bicarbonate levels; when chloride levels are elevated, the bicarbonate concentration will decrease. Hyperchloremic acidosis can occur as the result of abnormal reabsorption of chloride by the kidney or as the result of treatment with chloride-containing medications (sodium chloride, amino acid–chloride hyperalimentation solutions, and ammonium chloride). Ammonium chloride is broken down into an ammonium (NH_4) and a chloride ion. The ammonium ion is converted to urea in the liver. This leaves the chloride ion free to react with hydrogen to form hydrochloric acid. The administration of intravenous sodium chloride or parenteral hyperalimentation solutions that contain an amino acid–chloride combination can cause acidosis in a similar manner.

Manifestations

The signs and symptoms of metabolic acidosis usually begin to appear when plasma bicarbonate is 20 mEq/liter (mmol/liter) or less. The manifestations of metabolic acidosis fall into three categories:

1. Signs and symptoms of the disorder causing the acidosis.
2. Alterations in function resulting from the decreased *p*H.
3. Changes in function due to recruitment of compensatory mechanisms.

The first category of signs and symptoms is related to the primary disorder. With diabetic ketoacidosis there is an increase in blood and urine sugars and the breath has the characteristic smell of acetone. In patients in renal failure, blood urea nitrogen and tests of renal function are abnormal.

The second category of symptoms relates to alterations in body function that result from a decrease in *p*H. These signs and symptoms occur regardless of the cause of the *p*H disorder. A patient with metabolic acidosis will often complain of weakness, fatigue, general malaise, and a dull headache. There may also be anorexia, nausea, vomiting, and abdominal pain. The anorexia associated with mild metabolic acidosis may be viewed as advantageous for persons who are trying to lose weight through use of a ketogenic diet. On the other hand, the gastrointestinal symptoms may be misleading in a patient with undiagnosed diabetes mellitus. For example, such a patient may be thought to have gastrointestinal flu or some other form of abdominal pathology, such as appendicitis.

Neural activity becomes depressed as the *p*H declines. As acidosis progresses the level of consciousness decreases and stupor and coma develop. The skin is often warm and flushed because the skin vessels become less responsive to the vasoconstrictor input from the sympathetic nervous system. Tissue turgor is impaired and the skin is dry in situations in which fluid deficit accompanies acidosis. When the *p*H falls to 7.0 the heart also becomes unresponsive to the catecholamines (norepinephrine and epinephrine). At this point both heart rate and cardiac output decrease. Acidosis develops rapidly following cardiac arrest—both lactic acid and carbonic acid accumulate. Therefore, it is necessary to infuse sodium bicarbonate during cardiopulmonary resuscitation procedures.

A third group of signs and symptoms seen in metabolic acidosis are those related to the recruitment of renal and respiratory compensatory mechanisms. When renal mechanisms are operative, the urine pH will decrease and urine ammonia levels will rise. The respiratory system compensates by increasing ventilation; this is accomplished through deep and often rapid respirations called *Kussmaul breathing*. Kussmaul breathing removes carbon dioxide from the blood as evidenced by a low PCO_2. For descriptive purposes, it can be said that Kussmaul breathing resembles the hyperpnea of exercise—the person appears to have been running.

Treatment

The treatment of metabolic acidosis focuses on correcting the condition that caused the disorder and on restoring the fluid and electrolytes that have been lost from the body.

Lactic acidosis

Lactic acidosis is a rare but serious form of metabolic acidosis. Because of its clinical importance and because it is not discussed elsewhere in the book, lactic acidosis is discussed separately in this chapter. Lactic acid is the end product of the anaerobic metabolism of glucose. Although the normal person produces lactate ions, they are removed by the liver and converted to pyruvate so that they can be converted to glucose or oxidized in the citric-acid cycle. This means that they do not accumulate in the extracellular fluid. The potential for development of lactic acidosis exists during periods of excess production or when lactate is not removed from the blood.

Lactic acidosis is seen most frequently in situations in which acute cellular hypoxia is present, such as shock or severe heart failure. The condition is also seen in severe liver failure, pulmonary insufficiency, and pulmonary edema. Although lactate levels rise during severe exercise, the blood is usually promptly cleared of the excess lactic acid when the activity is stopped. The oral hypoglycemic drug, phenformin (DBI), is known to cause lactic acidosis by interfering with the liver's ability to convert lactate to glucose. Phenformin has been withdrawn from general use, although it is still available for investigational purposes. Lactic acidosis can also occur following the ingestion of a number of toxic agents, including the salicylates, ethylene glycol, paraldehyde, and methanol. Ethanol also interferes with the liver's ability to remove lactate from the blood; and when consumed in large amounts, it affords the potential for causing lactic acidosis.

Arterial lactate concentrations are elevated (about 2 mEq/liter) in lactic acidosis, the serum pH is decreased, and the anion gap is increased. Furthermore, urine tests of acetone are usually negative or only slightly positive.

The intravenous infusion of methylene blue, which facilitates the conversion of lactic acid to pyruvic acid, is sometimes used in the treatment of lactic acidosis. Sodium bicarbonate may also be given to correct the acidosis; this drug is the treatment of choice in cardiac arrest.

Metabolic Alkalosis

Metabolic alkalosis refers to a primary increase in base bicarbonate. In metabolic alkalosis, serum pH is above 7.45, plasma bicarbonate is above 29 mEq/liter, and base excess is above +2.5 mEq/liter. The causes of metabolic alkalosis are described in Table 27-2.

Causes

Bicarbonate increase. An increase in bicarbonate ion concentration can occur as the result of (1) excessive ingestion of alkaline drugs, (2) rapid decrease in extracellular fluid volume, or (3) rapid correction of compensated respiratory acidosis. The medicinal use of sodium bicarbonate or other alkaline salts increases bicarbonate intake. The milk-alkali syndrome occurs in patients with peptic ulcer who are being treated with excessive amounts of milk and alkaline antacids. Renal reabsorption of sodium and bicarbonate is increased when the extracellular fluid volume decreases suddenly; this is called *contraction alkalosis* and can occur in the course of diuretic therapy. Respiratory acidosis causes a compensatory loss of hydrogen and chloride ions in the urine along with retention of base bicarbonate. If the cause of the respiratory acidosis is corrected abruptly, metabolic alkalosis may develop.

Hydrogen and chloride loss. Hydrogen and chloride losses are increased (1) during vomiting or gastric suctioning, (2) in hypokalemia, and (3) with excessive levels of aldosterone. Vomiting and gastric suctioning remove both hydrogen and chloride from the body, causing increased retention of sodium bicarbonate. In hypokalemia, renal excretion of hydrogen is increased as the kidney focuses on conserving potassium. Chloride and potassium losses are also increased with the excessive use of organic mercurial, thiazide, and loop diuretics (furosemide and ethacrynic acid). Increased aldosterone levels cause increased reabsorption of sodium and bicarbonate and increased urinary losses of potassium and chloride.

Manifestations

The signs and symptoms of metabolic alkalosis are related to the primary cause of the disorder, to the associated changes in pH, and to accompanying decreases in

Table 27-2 Metabolic Alkalosis

Laboratory Findings

Primary Defect (Uncompensated)		Compensation
pH Increased	Bicarbonate Increased	PCO$_2$ Increased

Causes	Manifestations
Increase in Gain of Bicarbonate	**Altered Gastrointestinal Function**
Ingestion of sodium bicarbonate or alkaline salts	Anorexia
Milk–alkali syndrome	Nausea
Contraction alkalosis (loss of body fluids)	Painless vomiting
Increase in Hydrogen Ion Loss	**Increased Excitability of the Nervous System**
Loss of chloride (hydrogen) with bicarbonate retention	Confusion
Vomiting	Hyperactive reflexes
Gastric suctioning	Muscle hypertonicity
Potassium deficit with hydrogen ion excretion	Tetany
Diuretic therapy	Convulsions
Excessive levels of adrenal cortical hormones	**Signs of Compensation**
Decreased potassium intake	Decreasd rate and depth of respiration
Increased potassium losses	Increased urine pH

potassium. Anorexia, nausea, and vomiting often occur as the result of metabolic alkalosis. Alkalosis causes increased excitability of the nervous system. Consequently, the patient may be confused and mentally unreliable. Hypertonic reflexes, tetany, and carpopedal spasm may occur. Metabolic alkalosis may also lead to a compensatory hypoventilation with development of respiratory acidosis. The pH of the urine is usually increased as the kidney attempts to decrease the pH levels.

Treatment

The treatment of metabolic alkalosis is usually directed toward correcting the condition that has caused the disorder. Potassium chloride is often administered when there is a potassium deficit. The chloride anion replaces the bicarbonate anion, and administration of potassium allows the kidneys to conserve hydrogen in exchange for the excretion of potassium ions.

Respiratory Acidosis

Respiratory acidosis is due to an accumulation of carbonic acid or dissolved carbon dioxide. In respiratory acidosis plasma pH is below 7.35 and PCO$_2$ is above 50 mm Hg.

Causes

Respiratory acidosis can occur as an acute or a chronic disorder in acid–base balance. The causes of respiratory acidosis include any respiratory problem that impairs ventilation (See Chap. 24). Acute respiratory infections, narcotic or bicarbonate overdose, chest injuries, and pulmonary edema are examples of conditions that lead to acute respiratory acidosis. Acute respiratory acidosis can also result from breathing air that has a high carbon dioxide content. Chronic obstructive lung disease causes chronic respiratory acidosis (Table 27-3).

Manifestations

An *acute episode* of severe respiratory acidosis in a person suffering from chronic lung disease often results in what is called *carbon dioxide narcosis*. Carbon dioxide narcosis occurs in patients in whom the respiratory center in the brain has become adapted to increased levels of carbon dioxide. In these patients, the decreased oxygen content of the blood serves as the major stimulus for respiration. If oxygen is administered at a flow rate that is sufficient to suppress the stimulus, the rate and depth of respiration will decrease and the carbon dioxide content of the blood will increase. The signs and symptoms of carbon dioxide narcosis are varied. There may be psychologic disturbances, including irritability, depression, euphoria, paranoia, and hallucinations. Muscle twitching may occur, and reflexes may be decreased or absent. As the PCO$_2$ rises, impairment of consciousness can range from lethargy to coma. Paralysis of the extremities may occur and there may be respiratory depression. Less severe forms of acidosis are often accompanied by such signs as a warm and flushed skin, headache, weakness, and tachycardia.

Chronic respiratory acidosis is often seen in patients with chronic respiratory problems; it is often accompanied by varying degrees of hypoxia. Weakness and a dull headache are common manifestations of chronic respiratory acidosis.

The treatment of acute and chronic respiratory acidosis is directed toward improving ventilation.

Table 27-3   Respiratory Acidosis

Laboratory Findings

Primary Defect (Uncompensated)		Compensation
pH Decreased	PCO$_2$ Increased	Bicarbonate Increased

Causes	Manifestations

Increased Carbon Dioxide Inhalation
  Breathing air that is high in carbon dioxide content
Decreased Ventilation
  Depression of the central nervous system
    Drug overdose
    Head injury
  Diseases of the airways or lungs
    Bronchial asthma
    Emphysema
    Chronic bronchitis
    Respiratory distress in the newborn
    Pneumonia
    Pulmonary edema
Disorders of Chest Wall or Respiratory Muscles
  Paralysis of respiratory muscles
  Chest injuries
  Treatment with curare
	Depression of Neural Function
	  Headache
	  Weakness
	  Confusion and disorientation
	  Behavioral changes
	    Depression
	    Paranoia
	    Hallucinations
	  Tremors
	  Paralysis
	  Stupor and coma
	Skin
	  Warm and flushed
	Compensatory Mechanisms
	  Increased loss of hydrogen in the urine
	    (metabolic alkalosis)

Respiratory Alkalosis

Respiratory alkalosis is caused by a decrease in dissolved carbon dioxide or a carbonic acid deficit. In respiratory alkalosis, the *p*H is above 7.45, arterial PCO$_2$ is below 35 mm Hg, and serum bicarbonate levels are usually below 24 mEq/liter. Because respiratory alkalosis can occur suddenly, bicarbonate level may not change before correction has been accomplished.

Causes

The causes of respiratory alkalosis focus on situations that produce hyperventilation. Hyperventilation means that the respiratory rate is in excess of that needed to maintain normal PCO$_2$ levels and should not be confused with the hyperpnea that occurs with exercise. The most common cause of hyperventilation is anxiety. The hyperventilation syndrome, which is characterized by recurring episodes of hyperventilation, is described in Chapter 24. Other causes of hyperventilation are fever, oxygen deficiency, early salicylate toxicity, and encephalitis. Salicylate toxicity and encephalitis produce hyperventilation by directly stimulating the respiratory center. Hyperventilation can also occur during anesthesia or with use of mechanical ventilatory devices (Table 27-4).

Manifestations

The signs and symptoms of respiratory alkalosis are associated with hyperexcitability of the nervous system. There is often a feeling of lightheadedness, dizziness, tingling, and numbness of the fingers and toes. There may also be sweating, palpitations, panic, air hunger, and dyspnea. Chvostek's and Trousseau's signs may be positive, and tetany and convulsions may occur. Because carbon dioxide provides the stimulus for short-term regulation of respiration, short periods of apnea may occur in persons with acute episodes of hyperventilation.

The treatment of respiratory alkalosis focuses on measures to increase the PCO$_2$. Attention is directed toward correcting the disorder that caused the overbreathing. Rebreathing of small amounts of expired air (breathing into a paper bag) may prove useful in restoring PCO$_2$ levels in persons with anxiety-produced respiratory alkalosis.

In summary, acidosis describes a decrease in *p*H, and alkalosis describes an increase in *p*H. Acid–base disorders may be caused by alterations in the body's volatile acids (respiratory acidosis or respiratory alkalosis) or nonvolatile acids (metabolic acidosis or metabolic alkalosis). Metabolic acidosis is defined as a decrease in bicarbonate, and metabolic alkalosis as an increase in bicarbonate. Metabolic acidosis is caused by either an excessive production and accumulation of metabolic acids or an excessive loss of bicarbonate. Metabolic alkalosis is caused by an increase in bicarbonate gain or a decrease in hydrogen ion or chloride ion levels. Respiratory acidosis reflects an increase in carbon dioxide levels and is caused by conditions that produce hypoventilation. Respiratory alkalosis is caused by conditions that

Table 27-4　Respiratory Alkalosis

Laboratory Findings

Primary Defect (Uncompensated)		Compensation
pH Increased	PCO$_2$ Decreased	Bicarbonate Decreased

Causes	Manifestations
Increased Ventilation **(Hyperventilation)** 　Stimulation of respiratory center 　　Elevated blood ammonia 　　Salicylate toxicity 　　Encephalitis 　　Anxiety 　Reflex stimulation 　　Hypoxemia 　Lung disease that reflexly stimulates ventilation 　　Local lung lesions 　Mechanical ventilation	**Increased Excitability of the Nervous System** 　Numbness and tingling of fingers and toes 　Dizziness, panic, and lightheadedness 　Tetany 　Positive Chvostek's and Trousseau's signs 　Convulsions

cause hyperventilation and a reduction in carbon dioxide levels. The signs and symptoms of acidosis and alkalosis reflect (1) alterations in body function associated with the disorder causing the acid–base disturbance, (2) the effect of the pH change on body function, and (3) the body's attempt to correct and maintain the pH within a normal physiologic range. In general, neuromuscular excitability is decreased in acidosis and increased in alkalosis.

■ Study Guide

After you have studied this chapter, you should be able to meet the following objectives:

☐ Describe carbon dioxide transport.

☐ Describe the role of the respiratory system in control of pH.

☐ Describe hydrogen ion secretion by renal mechanisms.

☐ Describe the renal phosphate buffer system and the ammonia buffer system.

☐ Describe the blood buffer systems.

☐ State the Henderson-Hasselbalch equation and explain its use.

☐ Compare corrective versus compensatory mechanisms for regulation of changes in pH.

☐ Describe the role of potassium in pH regulation.

☐ Explain the postprandial alkaline tide.

☐ Define the *anion gap*.

☐ Describe a clinical situation involving an acid-base disorder in which both primary and compensatory mechanisms might be active.

☐ Describe the effect of metabolic acidosis on the renal and gastrointestinal systems.

☐ Categorize the following signs and symptoms of metabolic acidosis: Kussmaul breathing, odor of acetone on the breath, decrease in heart rate and output.

☐ State the cause of lactic acidosis.

☐ List the causes of metabolic alkalosis.

☐ Describe the clinical manifestations of metabolic alkalosis.

☐ Explain the relationship between respiratory disorders and respiratory acidosis.

☐ Explain the relationship between hyperventilation and respiratory alkalosis.

■ Additional References

Ackerman GL, Arruda JA: Acid–base and electrolyte imbalance in respiratory failure. Med Clin North Am 67 No 3:645, 1983

Adrogue HJ, Madias NE: Changes in plasma potassium concentration during acute acid–base disturbances. Am J Med 71:456, 1981

Adrogue HJ, Wilson H, Boyd AE et al: Plasma acid–base patterns in diabetic ketosis. N Engl J Med 307:1603, 1982

Broughton JD: Understanding blood gases. In Hudak C et al: Critical Care Nursing, 2nd ed. Philadelphia, JP Lippincott, 1977

Cahill GF, Jr: Ketosis. Kidney Int 20:416, 1981

Chan JCM: Acid–base, calcium, potassium and aldosterone metabolism in renal tubular acidosis. Nephron, 23:152, 1979

Cogan MC, Fu-Ying Liu, Berger BE et al: Metabolic alkalosis. Med Clin North Am 67 No 4:903, 1983

Cohen S, Miller M, Sherman RL: Metabolic acid–base disorders: Part 1—Chemistry and physiology. Am J Nurs 77, No 10:1619, 1977

Cohen S, Miller M, Sherman RL: Metabolic acid–base disorders. Am J Nurs 78, No 1:87, 1978

Dubose TD: Clinical approach to patients with acid–base disorders. Med Clin North Am 67 No 4:799, 1983

Emmett M, Narins RG: Clinical use of the anion gap. Medicine 56:38, 1977

Hassan H: Hypercapnia and hyperkalemia. Anaesthesia 34:897, 1979

Hill J: Salicylate intoxication. N Engl J Med 288:1110, 1973

Kaehny WD: Respiratory acid–base disorders. Med Clin North Am 67 No 4:915, 1983

Kreisberg RA: Lactate homeostasis and lactic acidosis. Ann Intern Med 92:227, 1980

Laski ME: Normal regulation of acid–base balance: Renal and pulmonary response and other extrarenal buffering mechanisms. Med Clin North Am 67 No 4:771, 1983

Lum LC: Respiratory alkalosis and hypocarbia. Chest Heart Stroke J, 3:31, 1978-1979

Martinez-Maldonado M, Sanchez-Montserrat R: Respiratory acidosis and alkalosis. Clin Nephrol 7, No 5:191, 1977

Narins RG, Jones ER, Stom MC et al: Diagnostic strategies in disorders of fluid, electrolytes and acid–base homeostasis. Am J Med 72:496, 1982

Oh MS, Carroll JH: The anion gap. N Engl J Med 297:814, 1977

Sabatini S, Arruda JA, Kurtzman NA: Disorders of acid–base balance. Med Clin North Am 62, No 6:1223, 1978

Tannen RL: Ammonia and acid-base homeostasis. Med Clin North Am 67 No 4:781, 1983

Chapter 28

Control of Renal Function

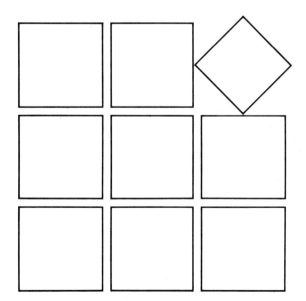

It is no exaggeration to say that the composition of the blood is determined not so much by what the mouth takes in as by what the kidneys keep (Homer W. Smith, *From Fish to Philosopher*).[1] The kidneys are two remarkable organs. Each is smaller than a man's fist, yet in one day they filter about 1700 liters of blood and combine its waste products into about 1 liter of urine. As a part of their function, the kidneys filter physiologically essential substances, such as sodium and potassium ions, from the blood and selectively reabsorb those that are needed to maintain the normal composition of the internal body fluids. Substances not needed for this purpose pass into the urine. In regulating the volume and composition of body fluids, the kidneys perform both excretory and endocrine functions. The renin–angiotensin mechanism participates in the regulation of blood pressure and the maintenance of circulatory blood volume, and erythropoietin indirectly stimulates the formation of red blood cells. The discussion in this chapter focuses on the structure and function of the kidneys, tests of renal function, and actions of diuretics.

■ Kidney Structure and Function

Gross Structure

The kidneys are paired, bean-shaped organs that lie outside the peritoneal cavity in the back of the upper abdomen, one on each side of the vertebral column at the level of the twelfth thoracic to third lumbar vertebrae (Fig. 28-1). The right kidney is normally lower than the left, presumably because of the position of the liver. In the adult each kidney measures about 10 cm to 12 cm in length, 5 cm to 6 cm in width, and 2.5 cm in depth and weighs about 4 ounces to 6 ounces. Usually only the lower edge of the right kidney is palpable on abdominal examination. Alterations in kidney size and shape are frequently associated with disease states.

The medial border of the kidney is indented by a deep fissure called the *hilus*. It is here that blood vessels and nerves enter and leave the kidney. The ureters, which connect the kidney with the bladder, also enter the kidney at the hilus.

On longitudinal section, the outer third of the kidney can be seen to have a brownish red hue. This is the cortex (Fig. 28-2). The medulla, or inner portion, of the kidney consists of light-colored cone-shaped masses, the renal pyramids, that are divided by the columns of the cortex (columns of Bertin). Each pyramid, topped by a region of the cortex, forms a lobe of the kidney. The apexes of the pyramids form the papillae (8–18 per kidney) which are perforated by the openings of the collecting ducts of Bellini. The renal pelvis is a wide funnel-shaped structure at the upper end of the ureter. It is made up of calyces or cuplike structures that drain the upper and lower halves of the kidney.

Each kidney is ensheathed in a fibrous external capsule and is surrounded by a mass of fatty connective tissue, especially at its ends and borders. The adipose

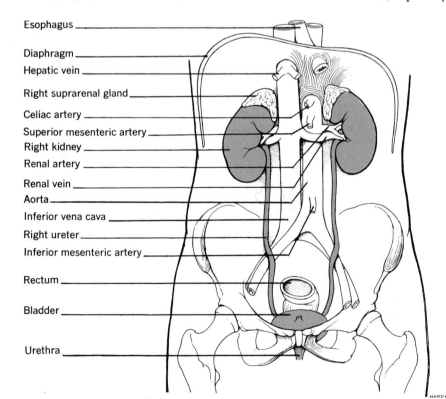

Esophagus

Diaphragm

Hepatic vein

Right suprarenal gland

Celiac artery

Superior mesenteric artery

Right kidney

Renal artery

Renal vein

Aorta

Inferior vena cava

Right ureter

Inferior mesenteric artery

Rectum

Bladder

Urethra

Figure 28-1 *The kidneys, ureter, and bladder. (From Chaffee EE, Creisheimer EM: Basic Physiology and Anatomy, 3rd ed. Philadelphia, JB Lippincott, 1974)*

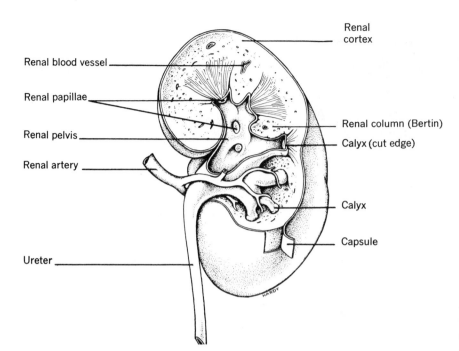

Renal cortex

Renal blood vessel

Renal papillae

Renal pelvis

Renal artery

Ureter

Renal column (Bertin)

Calyx (cut edge)

Calyx

Capsule

Figure 28-2 *The internal structure of the kidney. (From Chaffee EE, Lytle IM: Basic Physiology and Anatomy, 4th ed. Philadelphia, JB Lippincott, 1980)*

tissue protects the kidney from mechanical blows, and assists, together with the attached blood vessels and fascia, in holding the kidney in place. If this fat is absorbed, as can occur during severe weight loss, the kidney may slip out of position, compressing the ureter and obstructing urine flow. Although the kidneys are relatively well protected, they may occasionally be bruised by blows to the loin or by compression between the lower ribs and the ilium. Because the kidneys are outside the peritoneal cavity, injury and rupture do not produce the same threat of peritoneal involvement as does rupture of organs such as the liver or spleen.

Nephron

Each kidney is composed of more than a million tiny, closely packed functional units called *nephrons*. Each nephron consists of a vascular component (a glomerulus) and a tubular component (Fig. 28-3). The nephron is supplied by two capillary beds, the glomerulus and the peritubular network. The glomerulus is a unique high-pressure filtration system that is located between two arterioles, the afferent and efferent arterioles. The peritubular capillary network is a low-pressure reabsorptive system originating from the efferent arteriole. These capillaries are distributed around all portions of the tubules, an arrangement that permits rapid movement of solutes and water between the tubule lumen and the capillaries. The peritubular capillaries rejoin to form the venous channels by which blood ultimately leaves the kidneys.

Glomerular structure and function

The glomerulus consists of a network of capillaries encased in a thin-walled sac, *Bowman's capsule*. Fluid and particles from the blood are filtered through the membrane of the glomerulus into Bowman's capsule, which extends to form the tubules of the nephron. The mass of capillaries and its surrounding epithelial capsule are collectively referred to as the *renal corpuscle* (Fig. 28-4).

The glomerular capillary membrane is composed of three layers: (1) the capillary endothelial layer, (2) the basement membrane, and (3) the single-celled capsular epithelial layer. The endothelial layer lines the glomerulus and interfaces with blood as it moves through the capillary. It is perforated by many small holes called *fenestrations*. The basement membrane consists of a homogeneous acellular meshwork of collagen fibers, glycoproteins, and mucopolysaccharides. The epithelial layer that covers the glomerulus is continuous with the epithelium that lines Bowman's capsule. The epithelial layer that covers the glomerulus is called the *visceral epithelium* to differentiate it from the *parietal layer* that lines Bowman's capsule. The visceral epithelial cells have unusual octopuslike structures in that they possess a large number of extensions, or foot processes (podocytes), that are embedded in the basement membrane (Fig. 28-5). These foot processes form slit pores through which the glomerular filtrate passes.

Because both the endothelial and epithelial layers of the glomerular capillary have porous structures, it is the basement membrane that determines the permeability of the glomerular capillary membrane. The spaces between

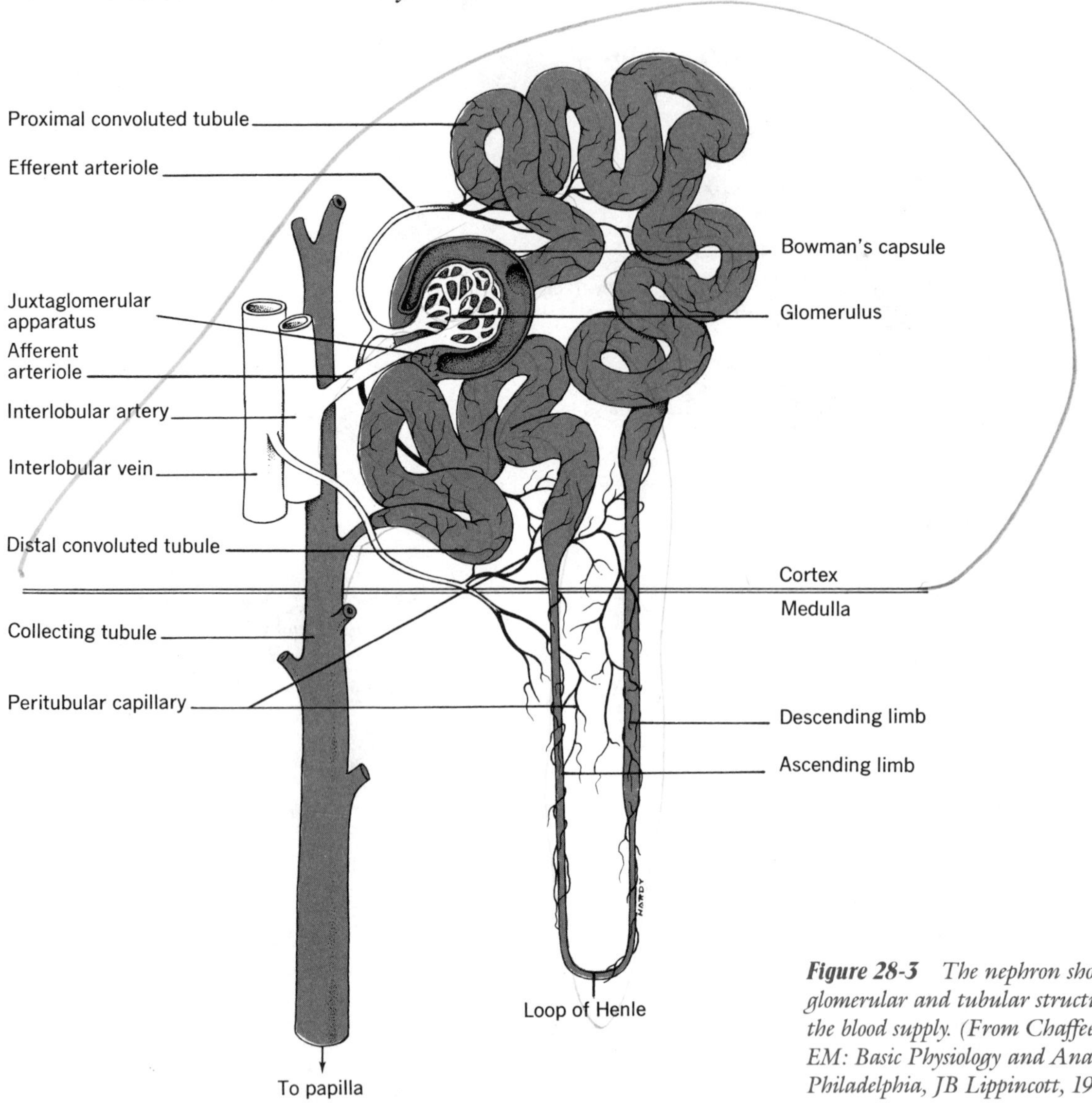

Figure 28-3 *The nephron showing the glomerular and tubular structures along with the blood supply. (From Chaffee EE, Greisheimer EM: Basic Physiology and Anatomy, 3rd ed. Philadelphia, JB Lippincott, 1974)*

the fibers that make up the basement membrane represent the pores of a filter and determine the size-dependent permeability barrier of the glomerulus. The size of the pores in the basement membrane normally prevents red blood cells and plasma proteins from passing through the glomerular membrane into the urine filtrate. There is evidence that the epithelium plays a major role in forming the basement membrane components, and it is probable that the epithelial cells are active in forming new basement membrane material throughout life. Because material is being added to the exterior of the basement membrane, it seems reasonable to assume that equal amounts are being removed from the inner surface to keep it from becoming unduly thick.[2] Alterations in the structure and composition of the glomerular basement membrane are responsible for the leakage of proteins and blood cells that occurs with many forms of glomerular disease.

Another important component of the glomerulus is the mesangium. There are areas where the capillary endothelium and basement membrane do not completely surround each capillary. Mesangial cells, which lie between the capillary tufts, provide support for the glomerulus in these areas (see Fig. 28-4, *B*). The mesangial cells produce an intercellular substance that is similar to that of the basement membrane, and it is this substance that covers the endothelial cells where they are not covered by epithelially derived basement membrane. The mesangial cells possess (or can develop) phagocytic properties and remove macromolecular materials that enter the intercapillary spaces. Mesangial cells also exhibit contractile properties in response to neurohumoral substances and are thought to contribute to the regulation of blood flow through the glomerulus. In normal glomeruli, the mesangial area is narrow and contains only a small number of cells. Mesangial hyperplasia and increased mesangial matrix occur in a number of glomerular diseases.

Tubular structure and function

Although the plasma is filtered in the glomerulus, it is the tubular structures that transform the filtered fluid into urine. The nephron tubule is divided into four segments: a highly coiled segment called the *proximal convoluted tubule,* which originates in Bowman's capsule; a thin, looped structure called the *loop of Henle;* a distal coiled portion called the *distal convoluted tubule;* and the final segment called the *collecting tubule,* which joins with several tubules to collect the urine filtrate. The filtrate passes through each of these segments before reaching the pelvis of the kidney.

Nephrons can be roughly grouped into two categories. About 85% of the nephrons originate in the superficial part of the cortex and are called *cortical nephrons.* They have short and thick loops of Henle that penetrate only a short distance into the medulla. The remaining 15% are called *juxtamedullary nephrons.* They originate deeper in the cortex and have longer and thinner loops of Henle that penetrate the entire length of the medulla. The juxtamedullary nephrons are largely concerned with urine concentration.

Throughout its course, the tubule is composed of a single layer of epithelial cells resting on a basement membrane. The structure of the epithelial cells varies with tubular function. The cells of the proximal tubule have a fine villous structure that increases the surface area for reabsorption; they are also rich in mitochondria, which support active transport processes. The epithelial layer of the thin segment of the loop of Henle is thin, with very few mitochondria, indicating minimal metabolic activity and active reabsorptive function.

About 65% of all reabsorptive and secretory processes that occur in the tubular system take place in the proximal tubule.[3] There is almost complete reabsorption of nutritionally important substances such as glucose, amino acids, and vitamins; electrolytes such as sodium, potassium, chloride, and bicarbonate are about 80% reabsorbed in this tubular segment. As solutes are transported out of the tubular cells, their concentration within the lumen decreases, and their concentration outside the tubule increases, providing a concentration gradient for the osmotic reabsorption of water. The proximal tubule is highly permeable to water, and the osmotic movement of water occurs so rapidly that the concentration difference of solutes on either side of the membrane is seldom more than a few milliosmols.

The thin segment of the loop of Henle is important in maintaining the concentrating capabilities of the nephron. As its name implies, the epithelial cells of this tubular segment are very thin, contributing to their

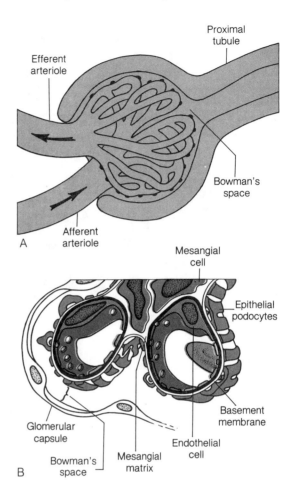

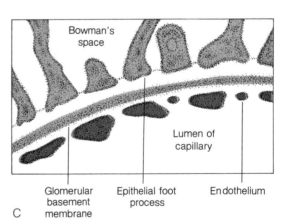

Figure 28-4 *Renal corpuscle. (A) Structures of the glomerulus. (B) Position of the mesangial cells in relation to the capillary loops and Bowman's capsule. (C) Cross section of the glomerular membrane illustrating the position of the endothelium, basement membrane, and epithelial foot processes.*

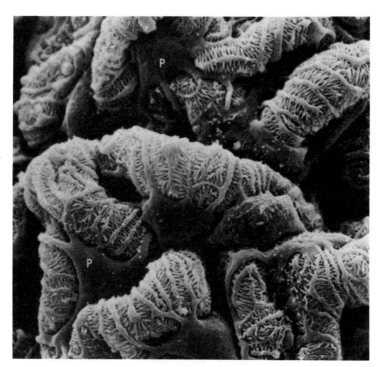

Figure 28-5 *Scanning electron micrograph of a glomerulus from the kidney of a normal rat. The visceral epithelial cells, or podocytes (P), extend multiple processes outward from the main cell body to wrap around individual capillary loops. Immediately adjacent pedicels, or foot processes, arise from different podocytes (magnification × 4800). (From Brenner BM, Rector FC: The Kidney, Philadelphia, WB Saunders, 1981. Reprinted by permission.)*

permeability characteristics. The descending limb is highly permeable to water and moderately permeable to urea, sodium, and other ions. The ascending limb, in contrast to the descending limb, is far less permeable to urea and water but capable of active sodium transport. As will be explained later, these differences in permeability and sodium transport are responsible for the production of a countercurrent mechanism that concentrates solutes in the interstitial fluids surrounding the collecting ducts, a condition necessary for the antidiuretic hormone (ADH)-mediated reabsorption of water.

The distal tubule begins in the ascending limb of Henle where the epithelial cells become thickened. This portion of the ascending limb is often called the *thick segment of the ascending limb of Henle.* The distal tubule is divided into two segments: the *diluting segment* and the *late distal tubule.* The diluting segment includes the entire thick portion of the loop of Henle and about half of the convoluted portion of the distal tubule. The cells of the thick segment are specifically adapted for reabsorption of chloride from the tubular lumen into the extracellular fluid for return to the bloodstream. The reabsorption of the negative chloride ions creates an

electrical gradient, which results in the passive reabsorption of sodium. Certain diuretic drugs act by inhibiting this transport system. The diluting segment is almost entirely impermeable to water and urea, and consequently the outward transport of sodium and chloride dilutes the tubular fluid, a condition that is necessary for production of a dilute urine. The later distal tubule is adapted for the active transport of sodium and other positive ions. It is here and in the collecting tubule that potassium ions are secreted into the tubular fluid and aldosterone exerts its effects on sodium and potassium reabsorption.

Like the distal tubule, the collecting duct is divided into two segments: *the cortical collecting tubule* and *the inner medullary collecting duct.* The cortical segment begins in the renal cortex at the termination of the convoluted distal tubule. It fuses with cortical tubules from several other nephrons before it turns downward from the cortex toward the renal papillae. As the cortical collecting duct passes through the medullary portion of the kidney, it becomes the inner medullary collecting duct. The epithelium of the collecting duct is well designed to resist extreme changes in the osmotic or *p*H characteristics of tubular fluid, and it is here that the urine becomes highly concentrated, highly diluted, highly alkaline, or highly acidic. The permeability of the epithelium to water in both portions of the collecting duct is determined mainly by the concentration of ADH. When large quantities of the hormone are present, the tubular epithelium becomes very permeable to water, and most of the water that is in the tubular fluid is reabsorbed from the tubule and returned to the blood. Very little water is reabsorbed in the absence of the hormone. Alterations in body fluids due to disorders of ADH levels are discussed in Chapter 25.

Urine formation

Urine formation begins with the filtration of essentially protein-free plasma through the glomerular capillaries into Bowman's capsule. The movement of fluid through the glomerular capillary bed is determined by the factors (capillary pressure and colloidal osmotic pressure) that affect fluid movement through other capillaries in the body (see Chap. 26). About 125 ml of fluid, the glomerular filtration rate (GFR), is filtered each minute. This amount can vary from a few milliliters to as high as 200 ml/minute.

The location of the glomerulus, between two arterioles, allows for the maintenance of a high-pressure filtration system. The capillary filtration pressure (60 mm Hg) in the glomerulus is about two to three times higher than that of other capillary beds in the body. The filtration pressure and the glomerular filtration rate are regulated by the constriction and relaxation of the afferent and efferent arterioles. Constriction of the efferent arteriole increases resistance to outflow from the glomeruli and increases the glomerular pressure and the glomerular filtration rate. On the other hand, constriction of the afferent arteriole causes a reduction in the renal blood flow, glomerular filtration pressure, and glomerular filtration rate. Both the afferent and efferent arterioles are innervated by the sympathetic nervous system. During periods of strong sympathetic stimulation, such as occurs during shock, the filtration pressure can be reduced to a point at which the glomerular filtration rate falls to almost zero.[3]

From Bowman's capsule the glomerular filtrate moves into the tubular segments of the nephron. In its movement through the lumen of the tubular segments, the glomerular filtrate is changed considerably by the transtubular transport of water and solutes. Tubular transport occurs in both inward and outward directions as tubular reabsorption and tubular secretion (Fig. 28-6). The basic mechanisms of transport through the tubular membrane are similar to those of other membranes in the body and include both passive and active transport. Water and urea are passively absorbed along

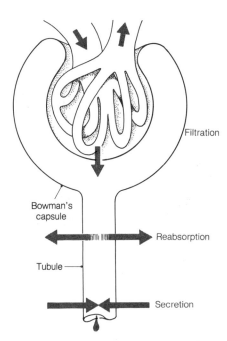

Figure 28-6 *Mechanisms of urine formation. The plasma is filtered in the glomerulus, and urine is formed as substances are reabsorbed or secreted into the filtrate.*

concentration gradients. Sodium, potassium, chloride, calcium, phosphate, and urate ions, glucose molecules, and amino acids are actively absorbed through the tubular membrane. Some substances such as hydrogen, potassium, and urate ions are actively secreted into the tubular fluids. Under normal conditions only about 1 ml of the 125 ml/minute that is filtered by the glomerulus is excreted as urine. The other 124 ml is reabsorbed in the tubules. This means that the average output of urine is about 60 ml/hour.

Renal clearance

Renal clearance describes the ability of the kidneys to remove or clear the blood of a particular substance. It is determined by the particle size, the particle's ability to be filtered through the glomeruli, and the capacity of the renal tubules to reabsorb or secrete the substance. Inulin, which is a large polysaccharide, is freely filtered in the glomeruli and is neither reabsorbed nor secreted by the tubular cells. Because of these properties, inulin can be used as a measure of the glomerular filtration rate. Other substances such as glucose, which are freely filtered in the glomeruli but completely reabsorbed by the tubular cells, have a low renal clearance.

Renal threshold (transport maximum)

Many substances such as glucose are freely filtered in the glomerulus and reabsorbed by special tubular transport systems. The maximum amount that these transport systems can reabsorb, called the *transport maximum,* is usually sufficient for all of the filtered substance to be reabsorbed and none to appear in the urine. The point at which the substance appears in the urine is also called the *renal threshold*. There are, however, situations in which the amount of substance filtered in the glomerulus exceeds the transport maximum for the substance. For example, when blood sugar is elevated in uncontrolled diabetes mellitus, the amount that is filtered in the glomerulus often exceeds the transport maximum (320 mg/minute) for glucose, and sugar spills into the urine.

Control of urine concentration

The kidneys are able to produce either a concentrated or a dilute urine depending on the composition and volume of the extracellular fluids. The concentration or dilution of the urine occurs in the collecting tubules and is depen-

dent on (1) the increased solute concentration in the medullary area surrounding the collecting ducts and (2) the selective permeability of the collecting tubules, which is controlled by ADH.

In about one-fifth of the nephrons (juxtamedullary nephrons), the loops of Henle and peritubular capillaries (the vasa recta) descend into the renal medulla. Here a countercurrent mechanism controls water and solute flow. As a result, water is kept out of the peritubular area surrounding the tubules, and sodium and urea are retained. A consequence of these processes is that a high concentration of the osmotically active particles collect in the interstitium of this portion of the kidney (Fig. 28-7). It is here, where the kidney surrounds the collecting tubules, that the presence of these osmotically active particles facilitates the ADH-mediated reabsorption of water.

During periods of dehydration, the kidney plays a major role in maintaining water balance. Osmoreceptors in the hypothalamus sense the increase in osmolality of extracellular fluids and stimulate the release of ADH. The collecting tubules, under the influence of ADH, become permeable to water. Once the permeability of the collecting tubules has been established, water moves out of the tubular lumen and into the interstitium of the medullary area, where it enters the peritubular capillaries for return to the vascular system. This serves to maintain extracellular volume by returning water to the vascular compartment and leads to the production of a concentrated urine by removing water from the tubular filtrate. In the absence of ADH, the renal tubules remain impermeable to water, and a dilute urine is formed.

Sodium elimination

The excretion of sodium by the kidney is highly variable. Sodium is freely filtered in the glomerulus and then reabsorbed as fluid moves through the tubules. Its level in urine reflects both the GFR and tubular reabsorption. Excretion is increased when the GFR is high and tubular reabsorption is low. Sodium reabsorption in the distal tubule is highly variable and is dependent on the presence of aldosterone. In the presence of aldosterone, almost all the sodium from the distal tubular fluid is reabsorbed, and the urine becomes essentially sodium-free. Virtually no sodium is reabsorbed from the distal tubule in the absence of aldosterone. The remarkable ability of the distal tubular cells to alter sodium reabsorption in relation to changes in aldosterone allows the kidney to excrete urine with sodium levels that range from a few tenths of a gram to 40 gm.

Potassium elimination

Like sodium, potassium is freely filtered in the glomerulus; but unlike sodium, potassium is both reabsorbed from and secreted into the tubular fluid. The

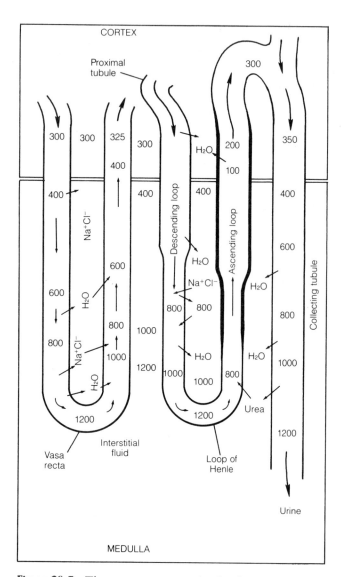

Figure 28-7 *The countercurrent mechanism for concentrating urine. Antidiuretic hormone controls the permeability of the collecting tubule.*

secretion of potassium into the tubular fluid occurs in the distal tubule and is regulated by aldosterone. Only about 70 mEq of potassium are delivered to the distal tubule each day, yet the average person consumes this much and more potassium in the diet. Excess potassium that is not filtered in the glomerulus and delivered to the distal tubule must therefore be secreted into the tubular fluid for elimination from the body. In the absence of aldosterone (as in Addison's disease), potassium secretion becomes minimal, and in this situation, potassium reabsorption exceeds secretion, causing blood levels of potassium to increase.

Regulation of pH

Neither the blood buffer systems nor the respiratory control mechanisms for carbon dioxide elimination can eliminate hydrogen ions (H^+) from the body. This is accomplished by the kidneys. The average American diet results in the liberation of 40 mmol to 80 mmol of hydrogen ions each day. Virtually all of the hydrogen ions that are excreted in the urine are secreted into the tubular fluid by means of tubular secretory mechanisms. As described in Chapter 27, the ability of the kidney to excrete hydrogen depends on buffers in the urine that combine with the ion. The three major buffers are bicarbonate (HCO_3^-), phosphate (HPO_4^{--}), and ammonia (NH_3). Bicarbonate is both filtered into the tubular fluid and reformed in the renal tubular cells in a process that uses carbonic anhydrase as a catalyst. The HPO_4^{--} is filtered in the tubular fluid and is not reabsorbed. Ammonia is synthesized in tubular cells by the deamination of certain amino acids. It diffuses into the tubular fluid and combines with the hydrogen ion. An important aspect of this buffer system is that the deamination process increases whenever the hydrogen concentration of the body remains elevated for 1 to 2 days.

Uric acid elimination

Uric acid is a product of purine metabolism (Chap. 53). Excess blood levels (hyperuricemia) can cause gout, and excess urine levels can cause kidney stones. Uric acid is freely filtered in the glomerulus, completely reabsorbed in the proximal convoluted tubule, secreted into the tubular fluid in the middle section of the proximal tubule, and finally reabsorbed in the loop of Henle. Uric acid uses the same transport systems as other anions such as aspirin, sulfinpyrazone, and probenecid. Small doses of aspirin compete with uric acid for secretion into the tubular fluid and reduce uric acid secretion, whereas large doses compete with uric acid for reabsorption and increase uric acid excretion in the urine. Because of its effect on uric acid secretion, aspirin is not recommended for treatment of gouty arthritis. Thiazide and loop diuretics (furosemide and ethacrynic acid) can also cause

hyperuricemia (and gouty arthritis), presumably through a decrease in extracellular fluid volume and enhanced uric acid reabsorption.

Urea elimination

Urea is an end product of protein metabolism. The normal adult produces 25 gm to 30 gm per day;[1] but the quantity rises when a high-protein diet is consumed, when there is excessive tissue breakdown, or in the presence of gastrointestinal bleeding. In the presence of gastrointestinal bleeding, the blood protein is broken down in the intestine and the urea is absorbed into the blood. The kidneys, in their role of regulators of blood urea nitrogen (BUN) levels, filter the urea in the glomeruli and then reabsorb it in the tubules. This allows for maintenance of a normal BUN, which is in the range of 8 mg to 25 mg per 100 ml of blood. Blood urea nitrogen becomes concentrated during periods of dehydration, and its excretion is markedly decreased when the glomerular filtration rate drops. The renal tubules are permeable to urea, which means that the longer the tubular fluid remains in the kidney, the greater the reabsorption of urea into the blood. Hence, only small amounts of urea are reabsorbed into the blood when the glomerular filtration rate is high; whereas, relatively large amounts of urea are returned to the blood when the glomerular filtration rate is reduced.

Renal Blood Flow

Each kidney is supplied by a renal artery that arises on either side of the aorta. Upon entering the kidney, each renal artery divides into the segmental and then the lobar arteries that supply the upper, middle, and lower parts of the kidney. The lobar arteries further subdivide to form the interlobar arteries at the level of the cortical medullary junction (Fig. 28-8). These arteries arch across the pyramids to form the arcuate arteries, which give rise to the intralobular arteries. The afferent arterioles that supply the glomeruli arise from the interlobular arteries.

In the adult the kidneys are perfused with about 1300 ml of blood per minute, or about 25% of the cardiac output. This large blood flow is not needed for renal metabolism but to ensure sufficient glomerular filtration for the removal of waste products from the blood. Blood flow to the kidneys remains relatively constant with the mean arterial blood pressure range of 80 mm Hg to 180 mm Hg. The constancy of flow is maintained by a process called autoregulation (discussed in Chap. 14). For autoregulation to occur, the resistance of blood flow through the kidney must be varied in direct proportion to the arterial pressure. The exact mechanisms responsible for the intrarenal regulation of blood flow are still unclear. It seems likely that the intrarenal release of substances capable of regulating local vascular

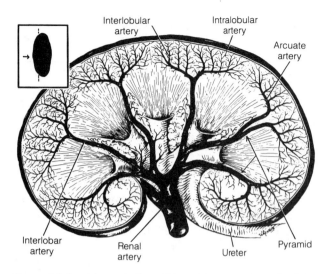

Interlobular artery

Intralobular artery

Arcuate artery

Interlobar artery

Renal artery

Ureter

Pyramid

Figure 28-8 *Schematic illustration of the arterial supply of the kidney, simplified for clarity. (From Ham AW, Cormack DH: Histology, 8th ed, p 775. Philadelphia, JB Lippincott, 1979)*

resistance may play a role.[4] Although nearly all the blood flow to the kidney passes through the cortex, less than 10% is directed to the medulla, and only about 1% goes to the papillae. Under conditions of decreased renal blood flow or increased sympathetic nervous system stimulation, blood flow is redistributed away from the cortex toward the medulla. This redistribution of blood flow decreases glomerular filtration while maintaining the urine concentrating ability of the kidneys, a factor that is important during conditions such as shock.

Endocrine Function

At present it is known that the kidney is concerned with either producing or activating renin, erythropoietin, and vitamin D.

Renin–angiotensin mechanism

Renin is released by special cells located near the glomerulus (juxtaglomerular cells) in response to a reduction in the glomerular filtration rate or as a result of sympathetic stimulation (Fig. 28-9). Renin combines with *angiotensinogen,* a plasma protein that circulates in the blood, to form *angiotensin I,* which is subsequently converted to *angiotensin II. Angiotensin II* is a potent *vasoconstrictor* and *stimulator* of *aldosterone release.* The role of the renin–angiotensin–aldosterone mechanism in control of blood pressure is discussed in Chapter 16.

Regulation of red blood cell formation

Erythropoietin is released in response to hypoxia. It acts on bone marrow to stimulate production and release of red blood cells (Chap. 13). Although the role of the

kidney in erythropoietin production is not fully understood, it is believed that the kidney responds to hypoxia by producing a substance or enzyme that converts a circulating plasma protein to an active form of erythropoietin. As a result, persons with chronic hypoxia often have increased red blood cell levels (polycythemia) because of increased erythropoietin levels. This occurs in persons with congestive heart failure, chronic lung disease, or in those living at a high altitude.

Activation of vitamin D

Vitamin D is activated in the kidney. Cholecalciferol (vitamin D_3) is transformed to 25-hydroxycholecalciferol in the liver and then converted to active 1,25-dihydroxycholecalciferol in the kidney. The role of vitamin D in calcium metabolism is discussed in Chapter 25.

In summary, the kidneys perform both excretory and endocrine functions. In the process of excreting wastes, the kidneys filter the blood and then selectively reabsorb those materials that are needed to maintain a stable internal environment. The kidneys (1) rid the body of metabolic wastes, (2) regulate fluid volume, (3) regulate the composition of electrolytes, (4) assist in maintaining acid–base balance, (5) aid in regulation of blood pressure through the renin–angiotensin–aldosterone mechanism and control of extracellular fluid volume, (6) regulate red blood cell production through erythropoietin, and (7) aid in calcium metabolism by activating vitamin D.

■ Tests of Renal Function

The function of the kidneys is to filter the blood, selectively reabsorb those substances that are needed to maintain the constancy of body fluid, and excrete metabolic wastes. Therefore, the composition of the urine and blood provides valuable information about the adequacy of renal function. Radiologic tests, endoscopy, and renal biopsy are procedures that afford a means of viewing the gross and microscopic structures of the kidneys and urinary system.

Urinalysis

Urine is a clear, amber-colored fluid that is about 95% water and 5% dissolved solids. The kidneys normally produce about 1.5 liters of urine a day. Normal urine contains metabolic wastes and few, if any, plasma proteins, blood cells, and glucose molecules. Urine tests can be performed on a single urine specimen or on a 24-hour urine sample. Table 28-1 describes urinalysis values for normal urine.

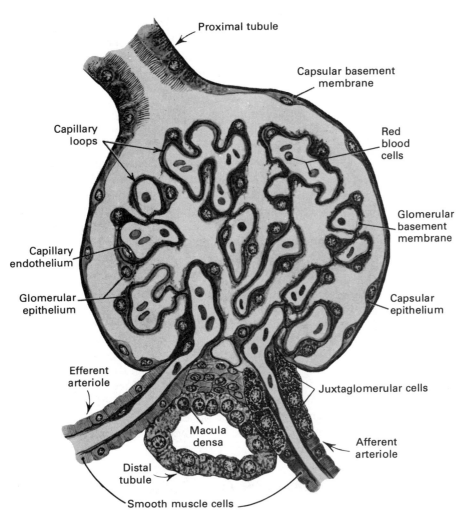

Figure 28-9   *The renal capsule showing the close contact of the distal tubule with the afferent arteriole and the macula densa and juxtaglomerular apparatus. (From Ham AW, Cormack DH: Histology, 8th ed. Philadelphia, JB Lippincott, 1979)*

Table 28-1   Normal Values for Routine Urinalysis

General Characteristics and Measurements	Chemical Determinations	Microscopic Examination of Sediment
Color: yellow–amber; indicates a high specific gravity and small output of urine	Glucose—negative Ketones—negative Blood—negative Protein—negative Bile-bilirubin— negative	Casts negative— occasional hyaline casts Red blood cells negative Crystals negative White blood cells negative
Turbidity: clear		
Specific gravity: 1.015–1.025 with a normal fluid intake		
*p*H: 4.6–8; average person has a *p*H of about 6 (acid)		

(From Fishbach F: A Manual of Laboratory Diagnostic Tests, p 112, Philadelphia, JB Lippincott, 1980)

Casts are molds of the distal nephron lumen. A gellike substance called Tamm and Horsfall mucoprotein, which is formed in the tubular epithelium, forms the matrix of casts. Casts composed of this gel but devoid of cells are called *hyaline casts*. These casts tend to develop when the protein concentration of the urine is high (as in nephrotic syndrome) and urine osmolality is high and urine *p*H is low. The inclusion of granules or cells in the matrix of the protein gel leads to formation of various other types of casts.

Specific gravity

The *specific gravity* (or osmolality) of urine varies with its concentration of solutes. Urine specific gravity provides a valuable index of the hydration status and functional ability of the kidneys. Although there are more sophisticated methods for measuring specific gravity, it can be easily measured using an inexpensive piece of equipment called a urinometer (Fig. 28-10). Healthy kidneys can produce a concentrated urine with a specific gravity of 1.030 to 1.040. During periods of marked hydration, the specific gravity can approach 1.000. With diminished renal function, there is a loss of renal concentrating ability, and the urine specific gravity may fall to levels of 1.006 to 1.010. These low levels are particularly significant if they occur during periods that follow a decrease in water intake (*e.g.*, during the first urine specimen on arising in the morning).

Blood Tests

Blood tests can provide valuable information about the kidney's ability to remove metabolic wastes from the blood and to maintain normal electrolyte and *p*H composition of the blood. Normal blood values are listed in Table 28-2. Serum potassium, phosphate, blood urea nitrogen (BUN), and creatinine tend to increase in renal failure. Serum calcium, *p*H, and bicarbonate tend to decrease in renal failure. The effect of renal failure on the concentration of serum electrolyte and metabolic end products is discussed further in Chapter 30.

Creatinine

Creatinine is a product of *creatine* metabolism in muscles; therefore, its formation and release is relatively constant and proportional to the amount of muscle mass present. Because creatinine is filtered in the glomeruli but not reabsorbed in the tubules, its blood values depend closely on the glomerular filtration rate. In addition to its use in calculating the glomerular filtration rate, the creatinine level is useful in estimating the functional capacity of the kidney (Fig. 28-11). The creatinine value for a woman with a small frame is approximately 0.5 mg per 100 ml of blood, for a normal adult man about 1.0 mg per 100 ml of blood, and for a muscular man about 1.4 mg per 100 ml of blood. A normal serum creatinine usually is indicative of normal renal function. If the value doubles, the glomerular filtration rate—and renal function—probably have fallen to half their normal state. A rise in blood creatinine level to three times the normal value suggests that there is a 75% loss of renal function, and with creatinine values of 10 mg per 100 ml or more, it can be assumed that about 90% of renal function has been lost.

Glomerular Filtration Rate

The glomerular filtration rate provides a measure to assess renal function and can be measured clinically by collecting timed samples of blood and urine. Creatinine, a product of creatine metabolism by the muscle, is filtered by the kidneys but not reabsorbed in the renal tubule. Therefore, one of the substances that are measured in calculating the GFR is creatinine. The clearance rate for such a substance is the amount that is completely cleared by the kidneys in 1 minute. The formula is expressed as follows:

$$C = \frac{UV}{P}$$

where C = clearance rate
U = urine concentration
V = urine volume
P = plasma concentration

The normal creatinine clearance is 115 to 125 ml/minute and is corrected for body surface area, which reflects the muscle mass where creatinine metabolism takes place. The test may be done on a 24-hour basis with blood

Table 28-2   Normal Blood Chemistry Levels

Substance	Normal Value
BUN	8.0 mg/100 ml to 25.0 mg/100 ml
Creatinine	0.5 mg/dl to 1.5 mg/dl
Sodium	137 mEq/liter to 147 mEq/liter
Chloride	100 mEq/liter to 106 mEq/liter
Potassium	3.5 mEq/liter to 5 mEq/liter
Carbon dioxide (CO$_2$ content)	24 mEq/liter to 30 mEq/liter
Calcium	4.5 mEq/liter to 5.3 mEq/liter
Phosphate	1.7 mEq/liter to 3.6 mEq/liter
Uric acid	3.0 mg/100 ml to 8.5 mg/100 ml
*p*H	7.35 to 7.45

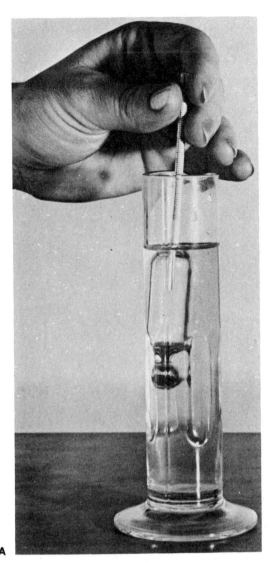
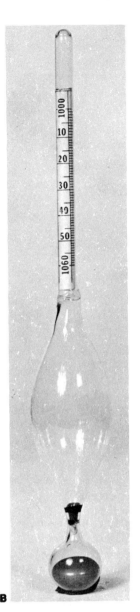

Figure 28-10 (A) *Urinometer, used for measuring the specific gravity of urine;* (B) *urinometer scale. (From Metheny NM, Snively WD Jr: Nurses' Handbook of Fluid Balance, 3rd ed. Philadelphia, JB Lippincott, 1979)*

drawn at the time the urine collection is completed. In another method two 1-hour urine samples can be collected with a blood sample drawn between.

Cystoscopy

Cystoscopy provides a means for direct visualization of the urethra, bladder, and ureteral orifices. It relies on the use of a cystoscope, an instrument with a lighted lens. The cystoscope is inserted through the urethra into the bladder. Biopsy specimens, lesions and small stones, and foreign bodies can be removed from the urethra, bladder, and ureters by this means.

Ultrasound Studies

Ultrasound studies use the reflection of ultrasonic or high-frequency waves to visualize the deep structures of the body. The procedure is painless and noninvasive and it requires no patient preparation. Ultrasound is used to

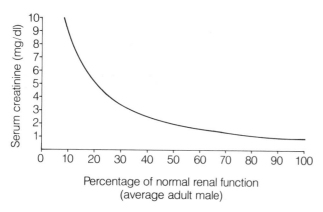

Figure 28-11 *Relationship between percentage of renal function and serum creatinine levels. (Drawn from data in Mitch WE, Walser M: A simple method of estimating progression of chronic renal failure. Lancet 1326, December 18, 1976)*

visualize the structures of the kidneys and has been proved useful in the diagnosis of many urinary tract disorders, including congenital anomalies, renal abscesses, hydronephrosis, and kidney stones. It can differentiate between a renal cyst and a renal tumor.[4] The use of ultrasound also permits accurate needle placement for renal biopsy and catheter placement through the skin (percutaneous nephrostomy).

Radiologic Studies

Radiologic studies include a simple flat plate (x-ray) of the kidneys, ureters, and bladder (KUB) that can be used to determine the size, shape, and position of the kidneys and to note any radiopaque stones that may be in the kidney pelvis or ureters. An excretory urogram, or intravenous pyelogram (IVP), is done by injecting a radiopaque dye into a peripheral vein; this dye is then filtered by the glomerulus and excreted into the urine, and x-ray films are taken as it moves through the kidneys and ureters. The IVP is used to detect space-occupying lesions of the kidneys, pyelonephritis, hydronephrosis, vesicoureteral reflux, and kidney stones. Some individuals are highly allergic to the radiographic dye used for the IVP and may develop an anaphylactic reaction following administration of the dye. Therefore, all individuals undergoing IVP studies should be questioned about previous reactions to the dye or to similar dyes. If the test is considered essential, premedication with antihistamines and corticosteroids may be used. The dye also reduces renal blood flow; acute renal failure can occur, particularly in persons with vascular disease or preexisting renal insufficiency.[4]

Other radiologic tests include computerized axial tomography, radionuclide imaging, and renal arterio-

grams. Computerized axial tomography (CT scans) refers to x-ray films taken by rotating tubes that sharply delineate tissue at any level they radiate. CT scans may be used to outline the kidney and detect renal masses and tumors. Radionuclide imaging involves the injection of a radioactive material that is subsequently detected externally by a scintillation camera, which detects the radioactive emissions. Radionuclide imaging is used to evaluate renal function and structures as well as the ureters and bladder. It is particularly useful in evaluating the function of renal transplant kidneys. Renal arteriography provides x-ray pictures of the blood vessels supplying the kidney. It involves the injection of a radiopaque dye directly into the renal artery. Usually a catheter is introduced through the femoral artery and advanced under fluoroscopic view into the abdominal aorta; the catheter tip is then maneuvered into the renal artery and the dye is injected. This test is used in evaluating persons suspected of having renal artery stenosis, abnormalities of renal blood vessels, or vascular damage to the renal arteries following trauma.

In summary, urinalysis and blood tests that measure levels of by-products of metabolism and electrolytes provide informaton about renal function. Cystoscopic examinations can be used for direct visualization of the urethra, bladder, and ureters. Ultrasound can be used to determine kidney size and renal radionuclide imaging to evaluate the kidney structures. Radiologic methods such as the excretory urogram or intravenous pyelogram provide a means by which kidney structures such as the renal calyces, pelvis, ureters, and bladder can be outlined.

■ Action of Diuretics

In some disease states, it is desirable to increase the urine output through the use of diuretics. Diuresis is the rapid passage of urine through the kidneys. Water reabsorption in the kidneys is largely passive and is dependent on sodium reabsorption. Therefore, most diuretics exert their action by interfering with sodium reabsorption. Only those substances that have a direct impact on the kidneys are regarded as diuretics. For example, digitalis preparations increase urine output in persons with heart failure by increasing cardiac output, renal blood flow, and the glomerular filtration rate but are not diuretics. Because of diuretics' mechanism of action, it is logical to include a discussion of them in this chapter. There are four types of diuretics: (1) osmotic, (2) inhibitors of urine acidification, (3) inhibitors of sodium transport, and (4) aldosterone antagonists. Table 28-3 describes the sites and mechanisms of action and untoward effects of these classes of diuretics. (See Fig. 28-12.)

Table 28-3   Diuretic Actions*

Diuretic	Site of Action	Untoward Actions
Osmotic diuretics	Cause water diuresis by creating an osmotic gradient, which serves to hold water in the tubular fluid; osmotic diuretics are filtered in the glomerulus but not reabsorbed in the tubule	Cause dehydration and electrolyte imbalance
Inhibitors of urine acidification (carbonic anhydrase inhibitors)	Impair hydrogen ion secretion in the tubular exchange system where sodium reabsorption is linked to hydrogen secretion	Increase potassium and bicarbonate losses; cause systemic acidosis
Mercurial diuretics	Prevent sodium reabsorption in the proximal tubule	Cause sodium depletion because of site of action; excess chloride loss can lead to hypochloremic alkalosis
Aldosterone antagonists	Block sodium reabsorption in the potassium–sodium exchange site of the distal tubule	Can increase potassium levels
Thiazide diuretics	Prevent sodium chloride reabsorption at the site between ascending loop of Henle and aldosterone-governed site	Cause increased potassium loss; may increase uric acid levels and impair glucose metabolism
Loop diuretics	Prevent sodium reabsorption in the active transport site of the ascending loop of Henle	Increase potassium losses and uric acid retention; ethacrynic acid has been associated with eighth nerve damage and deafness

*The reader is referred to a pharmacology text for specific examples of each of these diuretics.

Osmotic Diuretics

Osmotic diuretics such as mannitol are substances that are filtered in the glomerulus but not reabsorbed in the tubules. Because they are not reabsorbed, they serve to increase the osmolality of the tubular filtrate and cause a decrease in water reabsorption. The osmotic diuretics maintain a high urine volume following a hemolytic reaction or the ingestion of toxic substances, such as salicylates or barbiturates, that are excreted in the urine. Osmotic diuretics have a dehydrating effect on body tissues and may be useful in reducing intracranial or intraocular pressure. In diabetes mellitus, the renal tubular cells are unable to reabsorb all of the glucose that is filtered in the glomerulus, and this glucose acts as an osmotic diuretic.

Inhibitors of Urine Acidification

Acetazolamide (Diamox), a *carbonic anhydrase inhibitor,* impairs the reaction that converts carbon dioxide and water to bicarbonate and hydrogen ions. Bicarbonate is poorly absorbed in the renal tubules; rather, it combines with hydrogen that is secreted into the tubule to form carbon dioxide and water. The carbon dioxide is then reabsorbed into the tubular cells where it combines with water, in a carbonic anhydrase-catalyzed reaction, to form bicarbonate and hydrogen ions. When hydrogen ion secretion is blocked by the action of acetazolamide, both the bicarbonate ion and the sodium ion that accom-

pany it are lost in the urine. The loss of bicarbonate results in a mild systemic acidosis, and as this occurs the kidneys resume secreting hydrogen ions, overcoming the effect of the carbonic anhydrase inhibition. Therefore, the action of acetazolamide is of short duration, and this drug has been replaced by more effective diuretics, such

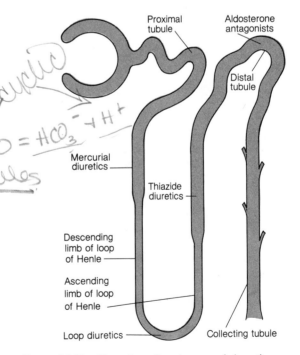

Figure 28-12 *Sites where diuretics exert their action.*

as the thiazides. Acetazolamide also decreases the formation of aqueous humor and cerebral spinal fluid, and it continues to be used for that purpose.

Inhibitors of Sodium Transport

Sodium reabsorption occurs in the proximal tubule, the ascending loop of Henle, the tubular area between the ascending loop of Henle, and the distal tubule where aldosterone regulates sodium and potassium exchange. Diuretics that alter sodium transport can act at any of these levels.

Mercurial diuretics (*e.g.,* mercaptomerin and meralluride) act to inhibit enzymes needed for sodium transport that are located in the *proximal convoluted tubules,* where 70% to 80% of the filtered sodium is reabsorbed. With use of the mercurial diuretics, there is also decreased reabsorption of the chloride ion, causing excess chloride losses in the urine with a resultant development of hypochloremic alkalosis. The mercurial diuretics are poorly absorbed from the gastrointestinal tract and they almost always cause gastrointestinal irritation. Therefore, they are given by injection.

Thiazide diuretics (*e.g.,* chlorothiazide [Diuril] chlorthalidone (Hygroton), and hydrochlorothiazide [Hydro-Diuril]) exert their action by preventing the reabsorption of sodium chloride in the area of the tubular structures located *between the ascending loop of Henle and the distal tubular site,* where aldosterone exerts its action. The thiazides cause increased loss of potassium in the urine, uric acid retention, and some impairment of glucose tolerance. They are given orally and are very suitable for long-term therapy.

Furosemide (Lasix), ethacrynic acid (Edecrin), and bumetanide (Bumex) are sometimes called *loop diuretics* because they exert their major effect on sodium reabsorption occurring in the *ascending loop of Henle.* About three-fourths of the sodium remaining after passage through the proximal tubule is absorbed in the ascending loop of Henle. This means that diuretics that act at these sites can cause potent diuresis. Impairment of sodium reabsorption in the loop of Henle causes a decrease in the osmolarity of the interstitial fluid surrounding the collecting ducts and further impedes the kidney's ability to concentrate urine. Both of these drugs cause potassium loss, increase uric acid retention, and tend to impair glucose tolerance. Both drugs also afford the potential for the development of hypovolemia. Ethacrynic acid is associated with eighth nerve damage and deafness. Because of its ability to produce arteriolar vasodilatation and diuresis when given intravenously, furosemide is often administered in emergency treatment of pulmonary edema.

Aldosterone Antagonists

Spironolactone (Aldactone), triamterene (Dyrenium), and amiloride (Moduretic) are *aldosterone antagonists,* which block the action of aldosterone on the distal tubular exchange site. In this way they increase the loss of sodium in the urine while enhancing potassium retention. Because of this action, these diuretics are sometimes called *potassium-sparing diuretics.* Spironolactone, in particular, has the potential for causing hyperkalemia.

In summary, diuretics are drugs that increase urine output. Diuretics, with the exception of osmotic diuretics, exert their action by altering sodium transport. Osmotic diuretics are filtered in the glomerulus and reabsorbed in the tubules. They act by increasing the osmolarity of tubular fluid. Inhibitors of urine acidification, such as acetazolamide, prevent bicarbonate reabsorption and with it accompanying sodium reabsorption. The mercurial and thiazide diuretics, as well as furosemide, ethacrynic acid, and bumetanide, inhibit sodium transport at different tubular sites. The aldosterone antagonists, spironolactone, triamterene, and amiloride, block the action of aldosterone in the distal tubule. These diuretics decrease sodium reabsorption while causing potassium retention. They are sometimes called potassium-sparing diuretics.

■ Study Guide

After you have studied this chapter, you should be able to meet the following objectives:

☐ Describe the anatomy of the normal kidney.

☐ State the reason that injury to the kidney does not usually produce peritonitis.

☐ Describe the structure and function of the glomerular capillary membrane including the endothelial layer, basement membrane, and epithelial layer.

☐ List the parts of the tubule.

☐ Differentiate between glomerular filtration, tubular reabsorption, and tubular secretion.

☐ Trace the elimination of uric acid by the kidney and explain the effect of small doses of aspirin on uric acid elimination.

☐ Describe the determinants of blood flow in the kidney.

☐ Define renal clearance.

☐ Explain how the kidney produces a concentrated urine.

☐ Describe the role of aldosterone in regulating sodium and potassium.

☐ Explain the endocrine function of the kidneys.

☐ Describe the characteristics of normal urine.

☐ Explain the significance of casts in the urine.

☐ Explain the value of the urine specific gravity in evaluating renal function.

☐ Explain the value of serum creatinine levels in evaluating renal function.

☐ Explain the concept of the glomerular filtration rate.

☐ Describe the methods used in cystoscopic examination of the urinary tract, ultrasound studies of the urinary tract, CT scans, IVP studies, and renal artery arteriogram.

☐ State the basis for the action of osmotic diuretics.

☐ Describe the actions of acetazolamide.

☐ Explain why mercaptomerin and meralluride alter sodium transport.

☐ Describe the actions of furosemide and ethacrynic acid.

☐ Give another term for aldosterone antagonists and one example of an aldosterone antagonist.

☐ Name and describe three tests of renal function.

■ References

1. Robbins SL, Cotran RS, Kumar V: Pathologic Basis of Disease, 2nd ed, p 993. Philadelphia, WB Saunders, 1984
2. Ham AW, Cormack DH: Histology, 8th ed, p 767. Philadelphia, JB Lippincott, 1979
3. Guyton A: Textbook of Medical Physiology, 6th ed, p 411. Philadelphia, WB Saunders, 1981
4. McConnell EA, Zimmerman MF: Care of the Patient with Urologic Problems, p 19. Philadelphia, JB Lippincott, 1983

Chapter 29

Alterations in Renal Function

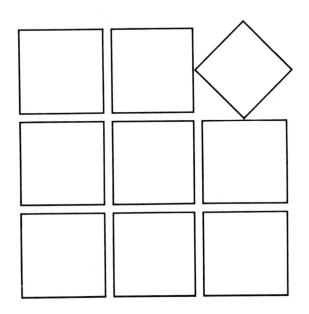

In 1975, an estimated 80,000 to 110,000 deaths were due to renal diseases. During that same period another 1.2 million Americans were afflicted with nonfatal but disabling urological disorders such as urinary tract infections, kidney stones, and obstructive disorders.[1] The number of persons with chronic and disabling renal disease has increased, in part because of recent advances in dialysis and renal transplant methods that are now keeping alive persons who would formerly have died of renal failure.

The urinary tract is subject to much the same types of disorders as other parts of the body, including developmental defects, infections, altered immune responses, and neoplasms. The kidney filters blood from all parts of the body, and although many forms of renal disorders originate within the kidney, there are some that arise as a consequence of disease or functional states of other systems of the body such as hypertension and diabetes. The discussion in this chapter focuses on each of these categories of urinary tract disease, and Chapter 30 discusses acute and chronic renal failure. The effects of other disease conditions, such as hypertension, shock, and diabetes mellitus, are discussed in other sections of the text.

■ Congenital Disorders of the Kidney

About 10% of persons are born with potentially significant malformations of the urinary system.[2] Unlike other organs, which develop in a direct and continuous process, the kidneys evolve through the differentiation of three sets of excretory organs, with the third set remaining as the permanent kidneys. In the process of development, the secretory or nephronic components of the kidney develop independently of the collecting system, and the two then are joined. It is during these complex stages of development that structural abnormalities may occur. The permanent kidneys develop early in the fifth week of gestation and begin to function about 3 weeks later. The urine produced by the fetal kidneys mixes with the amniotic fluid, and the fetus drinks it and reabsorbs it through the gastrointestinal tract. In conditions in which the kidneys fail to develop, the amount of amniotic fluid is very small. In other defects, which impair swallowing by the fetus, there are excessive amounts of amniotic fluid.

Congenital defects of the kidney can take several forms. They can result in a decrease in the amount of kidney tissue that is present (agenesis or hypoplasia), alterations in the form and position of the kidneys (kidney displacement or horseshoe kidney), or alterations in the differentiation of kidney structures (renal cysts and polycystic kidney disease).

Agenesis and Hypoplasia

The term agenesis refers to the absence of an organ due to failure to develop. *Unilateral agenesis* of the kidneys is relatively common, and persons with this defect are often unaware of its presence as long as the single kidney functions normally. *Agenesis of both kidneys* is rare. It is incompatible with life, and infants with this defect are either stillborn or die shortly after birth. In renal *hypoplasia,* the kidneys do not develop to normal size. Like agenesis, hypoplasia more commonly affects only one kidney. When both kidneys are affected, there is progressive development of renal failure, and children with this condition often die of renal failure unless sustained on dialysis.

Alterations in Kidney Position and Form

The developmental process can result in kidneys that lie outside their normal position, usually just above the pelvic brim or within the pelvis. Because of the abnormal position, kinking of the ureters and obstruction of urine flow may occur. One of the most common alterations in kidney form is the horseshoe kidney. This abnormality occurs in about 1 out of 600 persons and is characterized by fusion of the kidneys at the midline. It usually does not cause problems unless there is an associated defect in the renal pelvis or kidneys that favors obstruction to renal flow.

Alterations in Differentiation

One of the common characteristics of alterations in the differentiation of kidney structures is the formation of cysts.[3] These cysts are thought to result from developmental defects that cause partial intratubular obstruction with dilatation of nephron structures that are proximal to the obstruction or from a basement membrane defect that prevents its stretching to accommodate varying amounts of tubular fluids.[4] Cystic diseases of the kidney are reasonably common, and some forms, such as polycystic kidney disease, are major causes of renal failure.

Polycystic disease of the kidneys is characterized by the presence of *bilaterally* enlarged and cyst-filled kidneys. Polycystic kidney disease is categorized into infantile and adult types. *Infantile polycystic kidney disease* is inherited as an autosomal recessive trait. The kidneys are nonfunctional at birth, and fetuses with this defect are stillborn or, if born alive, usually die shortly thereafter. The *adult form of polycystic kidney disease* is fairly common, affecting about 1 in 500 persons. It is manifested as an autosomal dominant trait. The disease is characterized by enlarged palpable cyst-filled kidneys that can reach the size of a football. The disease usually gives rise to signs of renal failure during the third or fourth decade of life, although some persons may begin to have symptoms in their teens and others not until they reach 70 or 80 years of age. In the members of an affected family, polycystic kidney disease tends to cause kidney failure at the same age; families in whom it becomes manifest early in life are thus more aware of the family history than those in whom the disease becomes manifest later in life. A very common early symptom is a dull, aching pain of the abdomen or back, which is thought to be caused by pressure from the large cysts. Persons with polycystic kidney disease often have cysts in the liver and intracranial aneurysms. Although the liver cysts seldom cause problems, the intracranial aneurysms may have serious consequences, especially if coupled with hypertension. Fifteen percent of deaths in persons with polycystic kidney disease are caused by these aneurysms.[4]

In summary, approximately 10% of persons are born with potentially significant malformations of the urinary system. These abnormalities can range from bilateral renal agenesis, which is incompatible with life, to hypogenesis of one kidney, which usually causes no problems unless the function of the single kidney is impaired. Polycystic kidney occurs as the result of an inherited trait. Infantile polycystic kidney is inherited as a recessive trait and results in nonfunctional kidneys, which are present at birth. The adult form of polycystic kidney disease is inherited as an autosmal dominant trait and is not manifested until later in life.

■ Urinary Tract Infections and Pyelonephritis

Urinary tract infections are the second most common type of bacterial infections seen by the physician (respiratory tract infections are first). More women than men have urinary tract infections; about 20% of all women will develop at least one urinary tract infection during their lifetime.[1] These infections range from simple bacteriuria (bacteria in the urine) to severe kidney involvement with irreversible loss of kidney function. *Cystitis,* an acute infection of the bladder, is considered a lower urinary tract infection. *Pyelonephritis,* an infection of the kidney pelvis and interstitium, is an upper urinary tract infection. For all patients who must go on dialysis to sustain life, infections are the cause of the situation in 13% to 22%.

Bacteriuria

Normal urine is clear amber in color and has a distinctive aroma. Bacteria convert urea to ammonia, increasing the *p*H of the urine and causing it to have a strong and pungent smell. Although normally these changes occur in urine that has been allowed to stand for a period of time, they are also present in the freshly voided urine of persons with a urinary tract infection. Depending on the type and extent of infection, the urine may contain mucus shreds and may be discolored, thick, and cloudy.

The presence of 100,000 or more organisms per milliliter of urine is consistent with bacteriuria. Three types of methods are commonly used to detect the presence of bacteria in the urine: microscopic examination of the sediment from a centrifuged sample of urine, urine culture, and chemical tests.

Four chemical tests are available to detect the presence of bacteria in the urine: (1) the nitrate (Griess) test, based on the reduction of nitrate to nitrite by the bacteria; (2) the glucose oxidase test, which relies on the removal of residual glucose in the urine by bacterial action; (3) the catalase test, which detects the presence of enzymes produced by the bacteria; and (4) the reduction of tetrazolium salts by the bacteria after standardized incubation of voided urine. Of these, the nitrate test (or nitrate test combined with tetrazolium salts) is done most widely in this country. Individual test strips (Microstix–Nitrite or Bac–U–Dip) are available for home use or in screening programs. The test is most reliable if done on the first morning specimen, because incubation time in the bladder is needed for bacterial reduction of nitrate to nitrite, and should be carried out on three consecutive mornings.[5] Positive findings are usually confirmed by microscopic or culture methods.

Care is needed in collecting urine specimens that are representative of bladder urine, that is, the sample must be examined and cultured promptly. Specimens kept for longer than 1 hour must be refrigerated to prevent the contaminating organisms from multiplying. Catheterized specimens, once common, have been largely replaced by clean voided specimens. To obtain a clean voided specimen, the area around the urethral meatus is carefully cleansed and a midstream specimen is obtained by having the person void directly into a sterile container. This method is usually adequate and eliminates the risk of introducing organisms into the bladder during insertion of a catheter. In infants, a suprapubic needle aspiration may be done when there is indication of bacteriuria.

Pyuria, the presence of pus cells (polymorphonuclear leukocytes) in the urine, has long been believed to represent infection of the urinary tract; however, about 50% of persons with bacteriuria do not have significant pyuria.

Host Resistance

Most urinary tract infections ascend the urinary tract through the urethra; occasionally, entry may be through the bloodstream or lymphatics. Obstruction and reflux of urinary flow are important contributing factors in the development of urinary tract infections.

The urine formed in the kidneys and found in the bladder is normally sterile, whereas the distal portion of the urethra often contains pathogens. The bacteria responsible for most urinary tract infections are *Escherichia coli (E. coli), Enterobacter, Klebsiella, Pseudomonas,* and *Proteus.* It has been estimated that 80% to 90% of all initial urinary tract infections are caused by *E. coli,* whereas in persons who have been treated with antimicrobial drugs or have been subjected to catheterization or other urological procedures other organisms, such as *Proteus* or enterocoli, are more apt to be the causative pathogens.

In women, the urethra is short and in close proximity to the vagina and rectum, offering little protection against entry of microorganisms into the bladder. There is a peak incidence of these infections in the 15-to-24-year age group, suggesting that hormonal and anatomic changes associated with puberty as well as sexual activity contribute to urinary tract infections. The role of sexual activity in the development of urethritis and cystitis is controversial. The well-documented "honeymoon cystitis" suggests that sexual activty may contribute to such infections in susceptible women. Various preventive measures have been recommended for sexually active women who are bothered with frequent urinary tract infections. These measures include drinking a glassful or two of water and emptying the bladder soon after intercourse on the assumption that this will wash the bacteria out of the urethra and bladder. Women are also more likely to develop urinary tract infections during pregnancy, possibly because of related anatomic and physiologic changes. For example, the ureters and renal pelvis dilate during most normal pregnancies.

In men, the length of the urethra and the antibacterial properties of the prostatic fluid provide some protection from ascending urinary tract infections until age 50. After this age, prostatic hypertrophy becomes more common, and with it may come obstruction and urinary tract infection.

One common cause of urinary tract infections is reflux or obstruction of urine flow. Under normal conditions, bacteria are removed from the bladder with each voiding. The bladder mucosa has antibacterial properties that further protect against urinary tract infections, and host factors including phagocytosis aid in the removal of bacteria from the urinary tract. Thus, inability to empty the bladder completely with each voiding impedes removal of bacteria from the bladder.

In women, a *urethrovesical reflux* can occur during coughing and sneezing, when an increase in intrathoracic pressure causes the urine to be squeezed into the urethra and then to flow back into the bladder as the pressure decreases. This also happens when the act of voiding is abruptly interrupted for any reason. Because the urethral orifice is frequently contaminated with bacteria, the reflux mechanism may cause bacteria to be drawn back into the bladder.

A second type of reflux mechanism can occur at the level of the bladder and the ureter. This reflux mechanism is called the *vesicoureteral reflux.* It is commonly seen in children with urinary tract infections and is believed to occur because of congenital defects in length, diameter, muscle structure, or innervation of the submucosal segment of the ureter.[6] It is also seen in adults with obstruction to bladder outflow. There is a question whether the renal scarring often observed in association with vesicoureteral reflux is due primarily to infection or to the pressure and presence of urine constituents that reflux into the kidney.

Urinary catheters are tubes made of rubber or plastic. They are inserted through the urethra into the bladder for the purpose of urinary drainage. They are a source of urethral irritation and provide a means for entry of microorganisms into the urinary tract. Indwelling catheters are used in about 10% of patients admitted to general hospitals.[5] A *closed drainage system* (closed to the entrance of air and other sources of contamination) and careful attention to perineal care (cleansing of the area around the urethral meatus) will help to prevent infection in persons who require an indwelling urinary catheter. Careful handwashing and early detection and treatment of urinary tract infections are also essential. When an indwelling catheter is employed, the risk of infection is increased with use of broad-spectrum antibiotics and catheter irrigations—in fact, hospital patients themselves are cited as the most common reservoir of infection.[7] The Center for Disease Control[7] recommends that patients with urinary catheters not share a room unless special requirements for intensive care make this necessary. This recommendation follows the observation that an increased incidence of urinary tract infections has been reported in catheterized patients sharing a room.

Cystitis

An acute episode of cystitis is characterized by frequency of urination (sometimes as often as every 20 minutes), lower abdominal discomfort, and burning and pain on urination (dysuria). There may also be systemic signs of infection, with fever and generalized malaise. If there are no complications, the symptoms disappear within 48 hours. This type of cystitis is mainly a disorder of young women.

Pyelonephritis

Pyelonephritis refers to an infection of the kidneys and renal pelvis. In its earliest stages it is characterized by inflammatory foci that are interspersed throughout the renal interstitium. Small abscesses may form on the surface of the kidney. In time the lesions are replaced by scar tissue. There are two forms of pyelonephritis, acute and chronic. Because pyelonephritis affects the tubules and interstitium of the kidney, it is classified as a tubulointerstitial kidney disease.

Acute pyelonephritis represents an acute suppurative inflammation of renal tubulointerstitial tissues caused by bacterial infection. Infection may occur through the bloodstream or ascent from the bladder. Among the factors contributing to the development of acute pyelonephritis are catheterization and urinary tract instrumentation, vesicoureteral reflux, pregnancy, preexisting renal disease, and diabetes mellitus. The higher incidence of pyelonephritis in diabetics has been attributed to more frequent urinary tract instrumenation, increased susceptibility to infection, and more frequent occurrence of neurogenic bladder.

The onset of acute pyelonephritis is usually abrupt, with chills and fever, headache, back pain, tenderness over the costovertebral angle, and general malaise. The accompanying signs of bladder irritation, such as dysuria, frequency, and urgency, are usually present. Pyuria is present, but is not diagnostic, because it also occurs in lower urinary tract infections. It is now possible to localize the site of both upper and lower urinary tract infections by detecting the presence of *antibody coating* on the bacteria.[8] Antibody coating is an imune response of the kidney and is easily detected by the immunofluorescence test. The finding of leukocyte casts in the urine indicates that the infection is in the kidney rather than the lower urinary tract. Acute pyelonephritis is treated with appropriate antimicrobial drugs. Unless obstruction or other complications are present, the symptoms usually disappear within several days. Hospitalization during initial treatment may be necessary. Depending on the cause, recurrent infections are possible.

Chronic pyelonephritis is both chronic and progressive. There is scarring and deformation of the renal calyces and pelvis. The disorder appears to involve a bacterial infection superimposed on obstructive abnormalities or the vesicoureteral reflux. Recent evidence suggests that autoimmune mechanisms may contribute to the pathogenesis of chronic pyelonephritis.[9] The condition may cause many of the same symptoms as acute pyelonephritis, or its onset may be insidious. Loss of tubular function and the ability to concentrate urine gives rise to polyuria and nocturia, and mild proteinuria is common. Severe hypertension is often a contributing factor in the progress of the disease. Chronic pyelonephritis is a significant cause of renal failure. It is thought to be responsible for 25% of all cases of renal insufficiency and end-stage renal disease.[9]

Diagnosis and Treatment

Early diagnosis and treatment are essential to preventing permanent kidney damage. Screening of high-risk groups and attention to care of patients with indwelling catheters are important measures. Pregnant women and persons with diabetes or renal problems who are at risk for developing urinary tract infections can be followed in the physician's office. The availability of reliable diagnostic tests makes screening of large populations possible. Although not a common practice, it would be feasible to screen school-age girls because it has been estimated that 5% to 6% of girls will have at least one episode of bacteriuria between the time of entering first grade and graduation from high school.[5]

Lower urinary tract infections are usually treated successfully with single-dose antimicrobial therapy and increased fluid intake.[10] A follow-up urine culture is essential when single-dose therapy is used. Failure of single-dose therapy is suggestive of the presence of renal infection, and this method of treatment can be used as a means of localizing urinary tract infections to the kidneys. Because there is risk of permanent kidney damage with pyelonephritis, these infections are treated much more aggressively. Treatment with an appropriate antimicrobial is usually continued for 10 to 14 days. Hospitalization is often recommended during the early stages of the infection until a response to treatment is observed.

Chronic infections are more difficult to treat. Because they are often associated with obstructive uropathy or reflux flow of urine, diagnostic tests are usually performed to detect such abnormalities. When possible, the condition causing the reflux flow or obstruction is corrected.

In summary, urinary tract infections are the second most common cause of bacterial infection seen by the practicing physician. These infections range from bacteriuria to severe kidney infections that ultimately cause irreversible kidney damage. Most upper urinary tract infections ascend from the urethra and bladder, and urinary obstruction and reflux are factors predisposing to their development.

■ Obstructive Disorders

Urinary obstruction can occur in persons of any age and can involve any of the urinary tract structures, from the renal tubules to the urinary meatus. Ninety percent of obstructions are located below the level of the glomeruli, and most cause impairment of urine flow. Obstruction to urine flow can result from developmental defects, calculi, normal pregnancy, benign prostatic hypertrophy, infection and inflammation with development of scar tissue, and neurologic disorders such as spinal cord injury and diabetic neuropathy.

The effects of urinary obstruction are threefold: (1) heightened susceptibility to infection, (2) greater likelihood that calculi will develop, and (3) permanent kidney damage. The extent of these effects is determined by the severity and duration of the obstruction. When urine flow is obstructed, the filtration of urine continues, the calyces of the kidney become distended, and the kidney pelvis becomes dilated and its pressure is elevated. The elevated pressure is transmitted back through the collecting ducts to the cortex where it causes compression of blood vessels. If the obstruction is complete, serious and irreversible kidney damage occurs after about 3 weeks and, if incomplete, after about 3 months.[4]

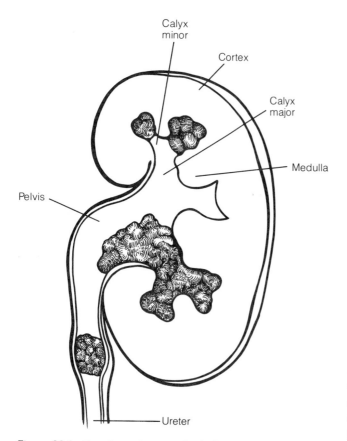

Figure 29-1 *Locations where renal calculi may form.*

Hydronephrosis is a dilatation of the renal pelvis with progressive renal atrophy caused by obstruction to urine flow through the ureter or lower parts of the urinary tract. At autopsy, hydronephrosis is found in 3% to 4% of adults and 2% of children.[3]

Diagnosis is made on the basis of intravenous pyelography, cystography, or cystoscopy. Ultrasound has proved to be a useful noninvasive diagnostic method for use in the detection of urinary tract obstructions.

Urolithiasis

Urolithiasis refers to calculi, or stones, that occur in the urinary tract. Nephrolithiasis (kidney stones) is the third most common urinary disorder in hospitalized patients. Kidney stones are three times more common in males than females. Although stones can form in any part of the urinary tract, most develop in the kidney (Fig. 29-1). A small stone may become trapped in a minor calyx and cause no symptoms. However, occasionally a stone will fill the entire renal pelvis; its shape gives it its name—*staghorn* stone. Stones passing into the ureter obstruct urine flow, causing colicky pain. Bladder stones are seen more frequently in elderly men and often are associated with prostatic hypertrophy.

The development of nephrolithiasis requires the presence of a nidus, or nucleus, for stone formation and a urinary environment that supports the continued precipitation of stone components. It is thought that the kidneys normally produce substances that inhibit stone formation. Currently three major theories are used to explain stone formation: the saturation theory, the deficiency of stone formation inhibitors theory, and the matrix theory.[11] The saturation theory states that the risk of stone formation is increased when the urine is saturated with stone components (calcium salts, uric acid, magnesium ammonium phosphate, or cystine). The stone inhibitor theory states that persons who have a deficiency of these inhibitors are at increased risk for stone formation. The matrix theory states that organic materials such as mucopolysaccharides that are derived from tubular cells act as a nidus for stone formation. This theory is based on the observation that organic matrix materials can be found in all layers of kidney stones. At present it is not known whether the matrix material contributes to the initiation of stone formation or the material is merely entrapped in the stone as it forms.

Calcium (oxalate or phosphate) stones, magnesium ammonium phosphate stones, uric acid stones, and cystine stones are the four types of renal stones. The causes and treatment measures for each of these types of stones are described in Table 29-1. By far the largest number of kidney stones (80%–90%) are calcium—calcium oxalate, calcium phosphate, or a combination of

Table 29-1 Composition, Contributing Factors, and Treatment of Kidney Stones

Type of Stone	Contributing Factors	Treatment
Calcium (oxalate and phosphate)	Hypercalcemia and hypercalciuria Immobilization Hyperparathyroidism Vitamin D intoxication Diffuse bone disease Milk–alkaline syndrome Renal tubular acidosis Hyperoxaluria Intestinal bypass surgery	Treatment of underlying conditions Thiazide diuretics Increased fluid intake
Magnesium ammonium phosphate (struvite)	Urea-splitting urinary tract infections	Treatment of urinary tract infection Acidification of the urine Increased fluid intake
Uric acid (urate)	Formed in acid urine with *p*H of approximately 5.5 Gout High-purine diet	Increased fluid intake Allopurinal for hyperuricuria Alkalinization of urine
Cystine	Cystinuria (inherited disorder of amino acid metabolism)	Increased fluid intake Alkalinization of urine

the two. Calcium stones are usually associated with increased blood and urinary concentrations of calcium. Excessive bone reabsorption caused by immobility, bone disease, hyperparathyroidism, and renal tubular acidosis are all predisposing contributory conditions. Very high oxalate concentrations in the blood and urine may promote the formation of oxalate stones. Magnesium ammonium phosphate (struvite) stones are caused by the urea-splitting action of bacteria. Staghorn stones are almost always associated with urinary tract infections and a persistently alkaline urine. The presence of gout, along with a high concentration of uric acid, increases development of uric acid stones. Unlike radiopaque calcium stones, uric acid stones are not visible on x-ray films. Cystine stones are rare. They are seen in cystinuria in which a genetic defect of renal transport of cystine occurs.

Manifestations

The presence of renal stones may give rise to a condition called *renal colic*. The symptoms of renal colic are due to stones that are 1 cm to 5 cm in diameter that are able to move into the ureter and obstruct urine flow. Classic ureteral colic is manifested by acute, excruciating pain in the flank and upper outer quadrant of the abdomen on the affected side. The pain may radiate to the lower abdominal quadrant, the bladder area, the perineum, and the scrotum in the male. The skin may be cool and clammy, and nausea and vomiting are often present. The colicky nature of the pain, which comes and then subsides, is due to the ball-valve action of the stone.

Diagnosis and Treatment

An intravenous pyelogram is usually used as a means of confirming the diagnosis and determining the location of the stone.

Treatment of acute renal colic is supportive for the most part. It includes measures to relieve the pain, promote passage of the stone, and prevent urinary tract infection and renal damage. An occasional stone will necessitate surgery for removal. All urine should be strained during an attack of renal colic in the hope of retrieving the stone for chemical analysis. Recently, the percutaneous dissolution method for removing struvite and cystine stones has been accomplished. With this method of treatment, a large catheter is inserted into the lower part of the kidney through the skin, and the kidney is irrigated with a stone-dissolving solution. The time from onset of irrigation to the end of solvent infusion has ranged from 6 days to 45 days.[12] This method of treatment does not work for calcium stones. Treatment measures are also directed at preventing further stone formation; the type of stone and the factors that contributed to its formation need to be identified. This information, along with a careful history and laboratory tests, affords the basis for long-term preventive measures.

In summary, obstruction of urine flow can occur at any level of the urinary tract. Obstructive disorders tend to increase urinary tract infection and calculi and can cause permanent damage to renal structures. Among the causes of urinary obstruction are developmental defects, normal pregnancy, infection and inflammation, neurologic defects, and nephrolithiasis, or kidney stones. There are four types of stones: calcium (oxalate and phosphate) stones, which are associated with increased blood or urine levels of calcium; magnesium ammonium phosphate (struvite) stones, which are associated with urinary tract infections; uric acid stones, which are related to elevated uric acid levels; and cystine stones, which are seen in cystinuria.

■ Disorders of the Nephron

Diseases of the Glomerulus

Within the glomeruli, the capillary network of the kidneys, blood is filtered and the urine filtrate formed. The glomerular membrane is composed of three layers: (1) the endothelial layer lining the capillary, (2) the basement membrane, and (3) a layer of epithelial cells forming the outer surface of the capillary and lying adjacent to Bowman's capsule. The membrane is selectively permeable, allowing water, electrolytes, and dissolved particles, such as glucose and amino acids, to enter, and preventing larger particles, such as the plasma proteins and blood cells, from entering the urine filtrate.

Diseases of the glomeruli disrupt glomerular filtration and alter the capillary membrane, so that it is permeable to plasma proteins and blood cells. Because the glomerulus lies in a strategic position between the afferent and efferent arterioles that connect with the peritubular capillaries, glomerular disease affords the potential for structural damage to the tubules, blood vessels, and interstitial tissues. The glomeruli may be injured by immune mechanisms associated with primary or secondary glomerulonephritis, by metabolic diseases such as diabetes mellitus, and by vascular disorders such as hypertension. Only during the past several decades has an understanding of the various forms of glomerular pathology emerged. Much of this understanding can be attributed to advances in immunobiology and electron-microscopy, development of animal models, and increased use of renal biopsy during the early stages of glomerular disease.

The cellular changes that occur with glomerular disease include proliferative and sclerotic changes. The term *proliferation* refers to an increase in cells in the glomerulus, regardless of origin; *sclerosis* refers to an increase in the noncellular components of the glomerulus. Glomerular changes can be diffuse, involving all glomeruli and all parts of the glomeruli, focal, involving only a certain proportion of glomeruli, segmental, involving only a certain segment of each glomerulus, or mesangial, affecting only the mesangial layer.[4]

Glomerulonephritis

The term *glomerulonephritis*, which means inflammation of the glomerulus, is used to describe a group of diseases in which glomerular pathology is dominant but interstitial disease is also present. It is now accepted that immune mechanisms are probably responsible for most, if not all, forms of glomerulonephritis. Two basic types of antibody-associated injury are thought to be associated with the immune response: (1) injury caused by soluble circulating antigen–antibody complexes that become deposited in the glomerulus and (2) injury caused by antibodies reacting with fixed antigens that are either produced by glomerular tissues or planted there from the circulation.

Manifestations. Glomerulonephritis causes injury to the glomeruli; it disrupts glomerular filtration and alters the capillary membrane, so that it is permeable to plasma proteins and blood cells. This leads to proteinuria, hematuria, pyuria, oliguria, edema, hypertension, and azotemia. Proteinuria, predominantly albuminuria, provides the most important evidence of glomerular injury. With progression from mild to severe glomerular injury, progressively greater amounts of larger plasma proteins, such as gamma globulins, are found in the urine. Hematuria can result from bleeding that occurs anywhere in the urinary tract. With glomerular disease, the red blood cells are either entrapped in casts or the action of tubular enzymes causes degradation of the red cells so that the urine is smoke or cola colored. Passage of polymorphonuclear white blood cells through the glomerular membrane causes pyuria. Oliguria (decrease in urine output) occurs when glomerular injury is severe enough to produce a marked decrease in the glomerular filtration rate. With glomerular disease, the causes of edema are twofold: there is a hypoalbuminemia that results from loss of albumin in the urine and a retention of sodium and water (see Chap. 26). Hypertension results from an increased vascular volume that occurs secondary to increased sodium and water retention and from increased renin levels. Azotemia, or increased levels of nitrogenous wastes in the blood, results from both a reduced filtration of urea and other nitrogenous wastes in the glomeruli and increased tubular reabsorption of these substances because of renal hypoperfusion.

Types. There are four basic types of glomerulonephritis: (1) acute glomerulonephritis, (2) rapidly progressive glomerulonephritis, (3) glomerulonephritis characterized by nephrosis, and (4) chronic glomerulonephritis.

Acute glomerulonephritis. Acute glomerulonephritis involves an acute inflammatory response and is characterized by hematuria, red cell casts in the urine, oliguria, and azotemia. Proteinuria and hypertension may also be present, although not usually as severe as in the nephrotic syndrome, discussed later in this chapter. Acute glomerulonephritis can occur as a primary renal disease or as an integral component of a systemic disease, such as systemic lupus erythematosus. The most common type is acute proliferative, or poststreptococcal, glomerulonephritis.

The most commonly recognized form of acute proliferative glomerulonephritis is that which follows infections by strains of group A, beta-hemolytic streptococci. In this type of glomerulonephritis, there is an abnormal immune reaction, causing circulating immune complexes to become entrapped in the glomerular membrane, which incites an inflammatory response. Proliferation of the endothelial cells lining the glomerulus and the mesangial cells lying between the endothelium and epithelium of the capillary membrane follows (Fig. 29-2). The capillary membrane swells and is then permeable to plasma proteins and blood cells. Although the disease is seen primarily in children, adults of any age can also be affected.

This type of glomerulonephritis follows a streptococcal infection by about 10 days to 2 weeks—the time needed for formation of antibodies. As the glomerular membrane swells, oliguria is one of the early symptoms. Salt and water retention gives rise to edema, particularly of the face and hands, and frequently to hypertension. Proteinuria and hematuria follow from the increased capillary permeability. In a child, the cola-colored urine may be the first sign of the disorder. Important laboratory findings include an elevated streptococcal exoenzyme (antistreptolysin-O) titer, a decline in C3 complement (see Chap. 9), and the presence of cryoglobulins (antigen-complexed globulins) in the serum.

Treatment of acute poststreptococcal glomerulonephritis is largely symptomatic. The acute symptoms usually begin to subside in about 10 days to 2 weeks, although in some children the proteinuria may persist for several months. The immediate prognosis is favorable, and approximately 95% recover spontaneously. The outlook is less favorable for adults. About 60% recover completely. In the remainder of cases, the lesions resolve eventually but there may be permanent kidney damage.

Rapidly progressive glomerulonephritis.

As the name implies, this type of glomerulonephritis is rapidly progressive, with renal failure occurring within a matter of weeks or months. It is characterized by focal and segmental proliferation of epithelial cells with formation of crescent-shaped structures that accumulate in Bowman's space. Persons with this disorder often have evidence of

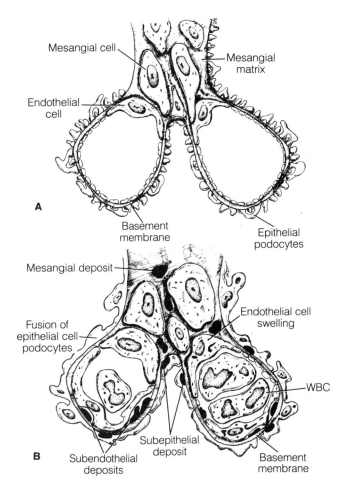

Figure 29-2 *Schematic representation of glomerulus:* (A) *normal;* (B) *localization of immune deposits (mesangial, subendothelial, subepithelial) and changes in glomerular architecture associated with injury. (From Whitley K, Keane WF, Vernier RL: Acute glomerulonephritis: A clinical overview. Med Clin North Am 68, No 2:263, 1984)*

antibodies directed against the basement membrane. This form of glomerulonephritis is associated with glomerular diseases that include systemic lupus erythematosus, acute poststreptococcal glomerulonephritis (usually in adults), and Goodpasture's syndrome among others. There is extensive inflammation of the proliferated epithelial layer of the glomerular membrane that lines Bowman's capsule. Clinically, there is an insidious onset of signs related to fluid retention and uremia. Ultimately, dialysis or renal transplant is required because the outlook for recovery is poor.

Goodpasture's syndrome is a form of rapidly progressive glomerulonephritis in which antiglomerular membrane antibodies bind to both lung and kidney tissue, giving rise to pulmonary hemorrhage and glomerulonephritis.

Nephrotic syndrome. Certain types of glomerulonephritis are characterized by a condition called the *nephrotic syndrome,* which is manifested by excessive permeability of the glomerular membrane. It is characterized by massive proteinuria with a daily loss of 3.5 gm or more of protein. There is an associated *hypoalbuminemia* (less than 3 gm per 100 ml), *generalized edema,* and *hyperlipidemia.* The edema is due to a decrease in capillary colloidal osmotic pressure that accompanies the loss of plasma proteins. Both cholesterol and triglyceride levels are usually increased, as part of the hyperlipidemia. It is believed that the hyperlipidemia results from compensatory increases in the production of albumin by the liver, which serves as a stimulus for increased synthesis of low-density lipoproteins. Because of the elevated levels of cholesterol and triglycerides, persons with the nephrotic syndrome run an increased risk of developing atherosclerosis. The loss of immunoglobulins in the urine is believed to increase susceptibility to infection, especially infection due to the staphylococcus and the pneumococcus.

Nephrosis can occur as a result of primary glomerular disease or secondary to glomerular changes that result from systemic diseases such as diabetes mellitus or lupus erythematosus. Among the primary glomerular diseases that give rise to the nephrotic syndrome are minimal change disease, focal sclerosis, membranous glomerulonephritis, and proliferative membranous glomerulonephritis.

Minimal change disease, or *lipid nephrosis,* is characterized by diffuse loss of the foot processes in the epithelial layer of the glomerular membrane. Although an immune mechanism has not been identified in this type of glomerulonephritis, there is increasing evidence that one does exist. It is the main form of nephrotic syndrome in children, with a peak incidence in those 2 to 3 years of age. Approximately 75% of children with the nephrotic syndrome have this form. It is highly responsive to glucocorticosteroids, and in 90% of cases is completely reversed by a fairly short course of oral glucocorticosteroid therapy. Nevertheless, some children have further relapses and some will become steroid-dependent. The long-term prognosis is generally good, however, with complete remission in many cases.

Focal sclerosis takes its name from the fact that it affects only one segment of the glomerulus. It accounts for about 10% to 15% of cases of nephrosis. There is persistent proteinuria, and response to glucocorticoids is poor. Renal failure ensues within 10 years of diagnosis in more than 50% of the cases.

Membranous glomerulonephritis is characterized by a progressive thickening of the glomerular wall on the epithelial side of the basement membrane. Although it can develop at any age, it is more common after age 40.

This form of the disease is thought to result from an immune complex phenomenon. Approximately 10% of persons with lupus erythematosus also have membranous glomerulonephritis. Various infections such as syphilis, malaria, or hepatitis-B virus, exposure to heavy metals, and certain tumors are associated with the condition. However, in most cases the underlying cause is unknown.

The first indications of the presence of disease are hypoalbuminemia and hyperlipidemia, and the course of the disease varies from case to case. In 70% to 90% of cases the changes are irreversible, progressing finally to renal failure within 2 to 20 years.

Proliferative membranous glomerulonephritis involves membranous changes of the epithelial layer of the glomerulus and proliferative changes in the mesangium. It accounts for 5% to 10% of cases of idiopathic nephrotic syndrome. The course is relentlessly progressive, with chronic renal failure developing within 10 years in some 50% of cases.[4]

Chronic glomerulonephritis. Chronic glomerulonephritis is the end-stage of the many different types of glomerulonephritis. It rarely develops in children with acute poststreptococcal glomerulonephritis and is frequently seen in persons who survive the acute phase of rapidly progressive glomerulonephritis. However, in about one-fourth of the persons who present with chronic glomerulonephritis, there is no history of glomerular disease.[4] In most cases, chronic glomerulonephritis develops insidiously and is characterized by signs of chronic renal failure (see Chap. 30). The disease is progressive, but at widely varying rates.

Diabetic glomerulosclerosis

Diabetic nephropathy, or kidney disease, is a major complication of diabetes mellitus. It has been estimated that 30% of persons with type I insulin-dependent diabetes develop end-stage renal disease.[4] The glomerulus is the most commonly affected structure in diabetic nephropathy; thickening of the glomerular basement membrane and development of diffuse or nodular glomerulosclerosis are the most prominent types of pathology. Widespread thickening of the glomerular capillary basement membrane occurs in almost all diabetics and can occur without evidence of proteinuria.[4] Diffuse glomerulosclerosis involves an increase in the mesangial matrix and thickening of the glomerular basement membrane. In nodular glomerulosclerosis, also known as *Kimmelstiel–Wilson disease,* there is nodular deposition of hyaline in the mesangial portion of the glomerulus. As the sclerotic process progresses in both the diffuse and nodular forms of glomerulosclerosis, complete obliteration of the glomerulus occurs, with impairment of renal function. Although the mechanisms of glomerular changes in diabetes are uncertain, they are thought to represent defective synthesis of the basement membrane and mesangial matrix with an inappropriate incorporation of glucose into the noncellular components of these glomerular structures.

The manifestations of diabetic glomerulosclerosis include recurrent proteinuria with slow but steady progression to renal failure. The condition occurs more frequently in poorly controlled diabetics, which emphasizes the need for adherence to treatment methods that improve metabolic control.

Hypertensive glomerular disease

Hypertension is associated with a number of changes in glomerular structures, including sclerotic changes. As the glomerular vascular structures thicken and perfusion diminishes, the blood supply to the nephron decreases, causing the kidneys to lose some of their ability to concentrate the urine. This may be evidenced by nocturia. Blood urea nitrogen (BUN) levels may also become elevated, particularly during periods of water deprivation. Proteinuria may occur as a result of changes in glomerular structure. Renal failure and azotemia occur in 1% to 5% of persons with long-standing hypertension. They are more common in malignant or accelerated forms of hypertension.[4]

Disorders of the Renal Tubules

A number of disorders affect tubular structures, including the proximal and distal tubules. Most of these diseases also affect the interstitial tissue that surrounds the tubules, and thus the disorders are often called *tubulointerstitial diseases.* These disorders include acute tubular necrosis (Chap. 30), the previously discussed chronic pyelonephritis and urinary obstruction, and the effects of drugs and toxins.

Drug-related nephritis

Drug-related nephropathies involve functional or structural changes in the kidney that occur following exposure to a drug. The kidney is exposed to a high rate of delivery of any substance that is in the blood, because of its large blood flow and high filtration pressure. The kidney is also very active in the metabolic transformation of drugs and is therefore exposed to a number of toxic metabolites. Some drugs and toxic substances damage the kidneys by causing a decrease in blood flow, others directly damage tubulointerstitial structures, and still others cause damage by producing hypersensitivity reactions. The tolerance to drugs varies with age and is dependent on renal function, state of hydration, blood pressure, and the *p*H of the urine. Because of a decrease in physiologic

function, the elderly are particularly susceptible to renal damage due to drugs and toxins. The dangers of nephrotoxicity are increased when two or more drugs capable of producing renal damage are given at the same time.

Acute drug-related hypersensitivity reactions produce tubulointerstitial nephritis, with damage to the tubules and to the interstitium. It was initially observed in patients who were sensitive to the sulfonamide drugs; currently it is more frequently observed to result from use of methicillin and other synthetic antibiotics, as well as furosemide and the thiazides, in persons who are sensitive to these drugs. The condition begins about 15 days after exposure to the drug (the period may vary from 2 to 40 days).[4] At the onset there is fever, eosinophilia, hematuria, mild proteinuria, and in about one-fourth of cases a rash. In about 50% of the cases oliguria and signs of acute renal failure develop. Withdrawal of the drug is usually followed by complete recovery, but there may be permanent damage in some cases, usually in older persons. Drug nephritis may not be recognized in its very early stage because it is rare.

Chronic analgesic nephritis, which is seen in relation to analgesic abuse, causes interstitial nephritis with renal papillary necrosis.[4] When first observed, it was attributed to phenacetin, a then-common ingredient of over-the-counter pain medications containing aspirin, phenacetin, and caffeine. Although phenacetin is no longer contained in these preparations, it has been suggested that other ingredients such as aspirin and acetaminophen may also contribute to the disorder. How much analgesic it takes to produce papillary necrosis is not known; ingestion of 2 kg to 30 kg of these analgesic compounds over a period of years has been known to result in papillary necrosis.[4] Headache, anemia, gastrointestinal symptoms, and hypertension are associated with the condition.

In summary, diseases of the nephron include disorders of the glomerulus and the renal tubules. Diseases of the glomerulus disrupt glomerular filtration and alter the permeability of glomerular capillary membrane to plasma proteins and blood cells. Glomerulonephritis is a term used to describe a group of diseases that cause inflammation and injury of the glomerulus. These diseases disrupt the capillary membrane and cause proteinuria, hematuria, pyuria, oliguria, edema, hypertension, and azotemia. Almost all, if not all, types of glomerulonephritis are due to immune mechanisms. Chronic glomerulonephritis represents the end-stage of the many types of glomerulonephritis and is characterized by an insidious onset of renal failure. Glomerulosclerosis, a form of diabetic nephropathy, is a major complication of diabetes mellitus. The disorder is characterized by progressive thickening of the glomerular basement membrane with obliteration of the glomerulus and impairment of renal function. Tubulointerstitial diseases affect both the tubules and the surrounding interstitium. These disorders include acute tubular necrosis, chronic pyelonephritis, urinary obstruction, and the effects of drugs and toxins.

■ Neoplasms

There are two major groups of renal neoplasms: adult kidney cancers and embryonic kidney tumors (Wilms' tumor), which occur during childhood.

Adult Kidney Cancers

Adult kidney cancer accounts for 2% of all cancers. An estimated 18,100 new cases of kidney cancer are diagnosed each year, and approximately 8300 persons die annually from this type of cancer.[13] The availability of computed tomography (CT) scanning has contributed significantly to earlier diagnosis and more accurate staging of renal cancers.

Renal cell carcinoma (hypernephroma) accounts for approximately 85% of kidney tumors, with transitional or squamous cell cancers of the renal pelvis accounting for most of the remaining cancers. The etiology of hyperneophroma remains unclear. It occurs most often in older individuals in the sixth or seventh decade. Males are affected twice as frequently as females. Some of these tumors are thought to occur as a result of chronic irritation associated with kidney stones. Epidemiologic evidence suggests a correlation between smoking and renal cancer.[13]

The manifestations of kidney cancer include hematuria, costovertebral pain, presence of a palpable mass, polycythemia, and fever. Hematuria, which occurs in 70% to 90% of cases, is the most reliable of these signs. It is, however, intermittent and may be microscopic; as a result, the tumor may reach a considerable size before it is detected. In about one-third of the cases, metastases are present at the time of diagnosis.

Renal cancer is suspected when hematuria and a renal mass are found. Renal ultrasonograhy, CT scanning, intravenous pyelograms, and renal arteriography are used to confirm the diagnosis. Surgery (radical nephrectomy with lymph node dissection) is the treatment of choice for all resectable tumors. Preoperative irradiation may be used. Single-agent and combination chemotherapy have been used with limited success. The 5-year survival rate for hypernephroma ranges from 30% to 50%.

Wilms' Tumor (Nephroblastoma)

Wilms' tumor is one of the most common malignant tumors of children; 75% of cases occur in children under 5 years of age.[13] Epithelial, muscle, and bone tissue are components of the tumor. The common presenting signs are a large abdominal mass and hypertension. Treatment involves surgery, chemotherapy, and radiotherapy (the tumor is radiosensitive). Two-year survival rates for children under 2 years of age have increased to about 73% with this aggressive plan of treatment. The survival rate for older children is less.

In summary, there are two major groups of renal neoplasms: adult kidney cancers and embryonic kidney tumors (Wilms' tumor) that occur during childhood. Adult kidney cancers account for 2% of all cancers. The most common manifestation of kidney cancer is hematuria. Renal ultrasonography has contributed significantly to earlier diagnosis and more accurate staging of renal cancers. Wilms' tumor is the most common malignant tumor of children. The most common presenting signs are a large abdominal mass and hypertension. The 2-year survival rate for children with Wilms' tumor is about 73% with an aggressive plan of treatment.

■ Study Guide

After you have studied this chapter, you should be able to meet the following objectives:

- ☐ Explain the basis of congenital malformations of the urinary system.
- ☐ State the pathologic changes that occur with polycystic kidney disease.
- ☐ Cite the organism that is most often responsible for urinary tract infections.
- ☐ Explain what is meant by the term *clean voided specimen*.
- ☐ Explain why urinary tract infections are more common in women than in men.
- ☐ Describe three measures aimed at reducing urinary infections due to the use of urinary catheters.
- ☐ State the symptoms of cystitis.
- ☐ Compare acute pyelonephritis and chronic pyelonephritis.
- ☐ Describe the effects of urinary tract obstruction on renal structure and function.
- ☐ Describe the three major theories used to explain the formation of kidney stones.

☐ Define *hydronephrosis*.

☐ List appropriate treatment measures for acute renal colic.

☐ Relate the proteinuria, hematuria, pyuria, oliguria, edema, hypertension, and azotemia that occur with glomerulonephritis to changes in glomerular structure.

☐ Compare acute proliferative glomerulonephritis and rapidly progressive glomerulonephritis.

☐ Describe the general clinical manifestations of the nephrotic syndrome and name three primary glomerular disorders that are representative of the syndrome.

☐ Describe the form of diabetic nephropathy known as diabetic glomerulosclerosis.

☐ Explain the vulnerability of the kidney to injury due to drugs and toxins.

☐ List the major manifestations of renal cancer.

☐ Describe a renal cancer found most frequently in young children.

■ References

1. Report of the Coordinating Committee: Research Needs in Nephrology and Urology, Vol. 1. National Institute of Health, National Institute of Arthritis, Metabolism, and Digestive Disorders, Public Health Service, 1978. DHEW Publication No (NH) 78–1481

2. Holiday MA: Developmental abnormalities of the kidney in children. Hosp Pract 13, No 6:101, 1978

3. Report of the Coordinating Committee: Research Needs in Nephrology and Urology, Vol 5, p 3. National Institute of Health, National Institute of Arthritis, Metabolism, and Digestive Disorders, Public Health Service. DHEW Publication No (NIH) 78–1485

4. Robbins SL, Cotran RS, Kumar V: Pathologic Basis of Disease, 2nd ed, pp 999, 1000, 1051, 1003, 1018, 1020, 1022, 1023, 1046, 1036. Philadelphia, WB Saunders, 1984

5. Kunin C: Detection, Prevention and Management of Urinary Tract Infections, 3rd ed, pp 41, 99, 157. Philadelphia, Lea & Febiger, 1979

6. Hodson J, Kincaid–Smith P: Reflux Nephrology, p 3. New York, Masson Publishing, 1979

7. Center for Disease Control: Epidemics of nosocomial urinary tract infections caused by multiple resistant gram-negative bacilli: Epidemiology and control. J Infect Dis 133, No 3:363–366, 1976

8. Jones SR, Smith JW, Sanford JP: Localization of urinary tract infections by detection of antibody-coated bacteria in urine sediment. N Engl J Med 290, No 11:591, 1974

9. Mayrer AR, Winter P, Andriole VT: Immunopathologenesis of chronic pyelonephritis. Am J Med 73, No 7:59, 1983

10. Stamm WE, Turck M: Urinary tract infection. Adv Intern Med 24:141, 1983

11. Abraham PA, Smith CL: Medical evaluation and management of calcium nephrolithiasis. Med Clin North Am 68, No 2:281, 1984

12. Dretler SP, Pfister RC: Percutaneous dissolution of renal calculi. Annu Rev Med 34:359, 1983

13. Frank I, Keys M, McCure CS: Urological and male genital cancers. In Rubin P(ed): Clinical Oncology, 6th ed, p 198. American Cancer Society, 1983

■ Additional References

Brenner B, Hostetter TH, Hume DH: Molecular basis of proteinuria of glomerular origin. N Engl J Med 298:826, 1978

Brenner B, Meyer TW, Hostetter TH: Dietary protein intake and the progressive nature of kidney disease. N Engl J Med 307:652, 1982

Clayman RV, Surya V, Miller RP et al: Pursuit of the renal mass: Is ultrasound enough? Am J Med 77:218, 1984

Coe F: Nephrolithiasis: Causes, classification and management. Hosp Pract 16, No 4:33–45, 1981

Coe FL: Treatment and prevention of renal stones. Consultant 18, No 10:47–50, 1978

Coltman K: Urinary tract infections: New thoughts on an old subject. Practitioner 223:351, 1979

Cornfeld D: Nephrosis in childhood. Hosp Med 14, No 3:98–111, 1978

Cotran RS: Tubulointerstitial nephropathies. Hosp Pract 17, No 1:79, 1982

Culpepper RM, Andreoli TE: The pathophysiology of glomerulonephropathies. Adv Intern Med 28:161, 1983

Derrick FC, Carter WC: Kidney stone disease. Postgrad Med 66, No 4:115–125, 1979

Donadio JV: Glomerulonephritis: Approach to diagnosis and treatment. Hosp Med 14, No 4:36–33, 1978

Dubach CD, Rosner B, Pfister E: Epidemiologic study of abuse of analgesics containing phenacetin: Renal morbidity and mortality (1968–1979). N Engl J Med 308:357, 1983

Fairly KF, Whitworth JA: Problems in the treatment of urinary tract infections. Drugs 19:190–194, 1980

Fer MF, McKinney TD, Richardson RL et al: Cancer and the kidney: Renal complications of neoplasms. Am J Med 71:704, 1981

Gabow PA, Ikle DW, Holmes JH: Polycystic kidney disease: Prospective analysis of nonazotemic patients and family members. Ann Intern Med 101:238, 1984

Galloway E, Glassman AB, Haley WE: Acute glomerulonephritis. Am J Med Technol 45, No 8:694–700, 1979

Glassock RJ: The nephrotic syndrome. Hosp Pract 14, No 11:105–129, 1979

Gleckman RA: Recurrent urinary tract infections. Postgrad Med 65, No 2:156–159, 1979

Grob PR: Urinary tract infections in general practice. Practitioner 221, No 8:237–244, 1978

Hodson CJ, Cotran RS: Reflux nephropathy. Hosp Pract 17, No 4:133, 1982

Kaplan RA: Renal calculi. Hosp Med 14, No 8:52–67, 1978

Kirschbaum BB: Glomerular basement membrane and anti-GBM antibody disease. Nephron 29:205, 1981

Kleeman CR et al: Kidney stones. West J Med 132, No 4:313–332, 1980

Kunin C, Polyak F, Postel E: Periurethral bacterial flora in women. JAMA 243, No 2:134–139, 1980

Kurtz S: UTI in the elderly: Seeking solutions for special problems. Geriatrics 10:97–102, 1980

Lach PA, Elster AB, Roghmann KJ: Sexual behavior and urinary tract infection. Nurse Pract 5:27–32, 1980

Loening SA, Smiley JW, Smith CL: Kidney stones—Suspicion to therapy. Patient Care 14:26 + , 1980

Madaio MP: The diagnosis of acute glomerulonephritis. N Engl J Med 309:1299, 1983

Mauer SM, Steffes MW, Brown DM: The kidney in diabetes. Am J Med 70:603, 1981

Mowad JL: Pyuria: Guide to management. Hosp Med 15, No 12:34–37, 1979

Nagar D, Wathen RL: Nephrotic syndrome. Primary Care 6, No 3:541–560, 1979

Nemoy NJ: Axioms on renal calculi. Hosp Med 15, No 2:8–19, 1979

Pagana KD: The intrigue and challenge of Goodpasture's syndrome. Heart Lung 9, No 4:699–706, 1980

Peters DK: The major glomerulopathies. Hosp Pract 16, No 117, 1981

Platt R: Quantitative definition of bacteriuria. Am J Med 73:44, 1983

Robinson RL: Laboratory findings in the differential diagnosis of acute renal failure. Crit Care Q32, No 4:87–98, 1979

Sabbath LD: Urinary tract infections in the female. Obstet Gynecol 55, No 5:162s–165s, 1980

Sheldon CA, Gonzales R: Differentiation of upper and lower urinary tract infections: How and when. Med Clin North Am 68, No 2:321, 1984

Stamm WE: Measurement of pyuria and its relation to bacteriuria. Am J Med 75 (Suppl):53, 1983

Steinmetz PR, Koeppen BM: Cellular mechanisms of diuretic action along the nephron. Hosp Pract 19, No 9:125, 1984

Stillman MT, Napier J, Blackshear JL: Adverse effects of nonsteroidal anti-inflammatory drugs on the kidney. Med Clin North Am 68, No 2:371, 1984

Turek M: Urinary tract infections. Hosp Pract 15, No 1:49–58, 1980

Vogel CH: Postobstructive diuresis. Nursing '79 9, No 3:50–56, 1979

Walther PC, Lamm D, Kaplan GW: Pediatric urolithiases: A ten-year review. Pediatrics 65, No 6:1068–1072, 1980

Whitley K, Keane WF, Vernier RL: Acute glomerulonephritis. Med Clin North Am 68, No 2:259, 1984

Chapter 30

Renal Failure

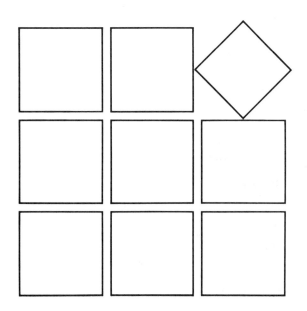

Renal failure is the situation in which the kidneys fail to remove the metabolic end products from the blood and to regulate the electrolyte and *p*H balance of the extracellular fluids. The underlying cause may be renal pathology, systemic disease, or urologic defects of nonrenal origin. Chronic renal failure is the end result of irreparable damage to the kidney. It develops slowly, usually over a number of years. By contrast, acute renal failure is abrupt in onset and is often reversible if recognized early and treated appropriately.

■ Acute Renal Failure

Azotemia

The term azotemia means an abnormally high level of nitrogenous wastes (blood urea nitrogen, uric acid, and serum creatinine) in the blood. Its presence reflects renal inability to filter these waste products from the blood. Azotemia is found in both acute and chronic renal failure. The normal concentration of urea in the plasma is

approximately 26 mg/100 ml. In renal failure this level may rise as high as 800 mg/100 ml.[1]

Acute renal failure refers to an acute suppression of renal function. The true incidence of acute renal failure is unknown, but it is thought to affect at least 10,000 persons annually in the United States.[2] The mortality is, unfortunately, about 60%. This is probably because older persons and those with severe illness and trauma are being kept alive by respirators and other extraordinary means until renal failure supervenes.

Causes of Acute Renal Failure

The conditions responsible for acute renal failure are usually described as prerenal, intrarenal, and postrenal (Table 30-1). This classification aids in identifying and treating the cause of the disorder.

Prerenal conditions

Prerenal causes of acute renal failure consist of those conditions that impair renal blood flow. This is the most common form of acute renal failure and is considered to be reversible if the basis of renal hypofunction can be identified and corrected within 24 hours.

The kidneys normally filter about 20% to 25% of the cardiac output. With a loss of blood volume or cardiac failure, this large blood flow to the kidneys may be sharply reduced. When the afferent arterial pressure falls much below 60 mm Hg to 70 mm Hg, glomerular filtration ceases, and little or no urine is formed. Thus, one of the early manifestations of prerenal failure is a sharp decrease in urine output. Normally, the ratio of serum BUN to creatinine is about 20 to 1, but in acute renal failure, there is a disproportionate elevation in BUN compared with serum creatinine. This is because the low glomerular filtration rate allows more time for smaller particles, such as urea, to filter back into the blood. Creatinine, being larger and nondiffusible, remains in the tubular fluid, and the total amount of creatinine that is filtered, although small, is excreted in the urine.

Intrarenal conditions

Intrarenal causes of acute renal failure can be grouped into five categories: ischemia, injury to the glomerular membrane (acute glomerulonephritis), acute tubular necrosis, intratubular obstruction, and acute pyelonephritis and necrotizing papillitis. Acute glomerulonephritis is discussed in Chapter 29, as is pyelonephritis.

Intratubular obstructions are due to the accumulation of casts and cellular debris, secondary to severe hemolytic reactions or myoglobinuria. Skeletal and cardiac muscle contains myoglobin, which accounts for their rubiginous color. Myoglobin corresponds to hemoglobin in function, serving as an oxygen reservoir within the muscle fibers. Myoglobin is not normally

---

Table 30-1 Causes of Acute Renal Failure

Prerenal
  Hypovolemia
    Dehydration
    Loss of gastrointestinal tract fluid
    Hemorrhage
    Fluid sequestration (*e.g.,* burns)
  Septicemia
    Septic shock
  Heart failure
  Interruption of renal blood flow due to surgery
    and other causes
Intrarenal
  Prolonged renal ischemia
  Exposure to nephrotoxic agents
    Aminoglycosides (*e.g.,* gentamicin, kanamycin, colistin)
    Heavy metals (*e.g.,* lead, mercury)
    Organic solvents (*e.g.,* carbon tetrachloride,
      ethylene glycol)
    Radiopaque contrast media
    Sulfonamides
  Acute glomerulonephritis
  Intratubular obstruction
    Uric acid crystals
    Hemolytic reactions (*e.g.,* blood transfusion reactions)
    Precipitated proteins resulting from multiple myelomas
    Rhabdomyolysis
  Acute inflammatory conditions
    Acute pyelonephritis
    Necrotizing papillitis
Postrenal
  Ureteral obstruction (*e.g.,* calculi, tumors)
  Bladder outlet obstruction (*e.g.,* prostatic hypertrophy,
    urethral strictures)

found in the serum or urine. It has a low molecular weight of 17,000; should it escape into the circulation, it is rapidly filtered in the glomerulus. Myoglobinuria is most commonly due to muscle trauma but may result from extreme exertion, hyperthermia, sepsis, prolonged seizures, potassium or phosphate depletion, and alcoholism or drug abuse. Hemoglobin may also escape into the glomerular filtrate when serum levels are markedly increased as a result of a severe hemolytic reaction. Both myoglobin and hemoglobin cause discoloration of the urine, ranging from the color of tea to red, brown, or black.

Acute tubular necrosis is characterized by destructive changes in the tubular epithelium due to ischemia or exposure to nephrotoxic agents. Shock and heart failure, to name two such events, cause prerenal failure, tend to cause renal ischemia, and if allowed to progress, can produce tubular necrosis. As a rule, the blood supply to a normal kidney can be interrupted for about 30 minutes without inflicting damage on the kidney,[3] but in acute trauma, sepsis, and heart failure, for example, the interruption in blood flow is often both more severe and longer in duration.

Several drugs and other chemicals, including organic solvents and heavy metals, such as lead and mercury, can injure the renal tubular structures. The aminoglycosides, a group of antibiotics of which gentamicin, kanamycin, and colistin are examples, are all capable of impairing renal function. Several factors contribute to aminoglycoside toxicity, including a decrease in the glomerular filtration rate, which often occurs in the elderly, a preexisting renal disease, hypovolemia, and concurrent administration of other drugs that have a nephrotoxic effect. Contrast media used during cardiac catheterization and intravenous cholangiography, for example, may also be nephrotoxic. The risk of renal damage due to radiopaque contrast media is greatest in elderly persons, in persons with diabetes mellitus, and in persons who for one reason or another are susceptible to kidney disease.

Postrenal conditions

Obstruction of the urinary system at any point from the renal calyces to the urinary meatus is the cause of postrenal failure. Prostatic hypertrophy is the most common underlying problem. Postrenal failure can also be caused by ureteral obstruction in persons who have only one functioning kidney. Obstructive uropathy is responsible for about 10% of cases of acute renal failure.[4]

Clinical Manifestations

The manifestations of acute renal failure are frequently superimposed on the signs and symptoms exhibited by the condition that caused the kidney failure—heart failure, shock, prostatic hypertrophy, and others. Because acute renal failure is potentially reversible, it is important that early signs be recognized so that appropriate treatment measures can be instituted promptly.

Acute renal failure causes marked impairment in the elimination of nitrogenous wastes, water, and electrolytes. Its course is frequently divided into two phases: the oliguric and the diuretic phase.

Oliguric phase

During the oliguric phase, urine output is greatly reduced. The magnitude of the azotemia that develops depends largely on urine output and on the degree of protein breakdown that is taking place. Although oliguria is usually associated with acute renal failure, there are situations in which urine output will be nearly normal, such as when intrarenal dysfunction impairs the ability of the renal tubular structures to concentrate the urine. In severe oliguria, which is accompanied by tissue breakdown, the BUN, creatinine, potassium, and phosphate serum levels increase rapidly, and metabolic acidosis develops. Fluid retention gives rise to edema, water intoxication, and pulmonary congestion. If the period of oliguria is prolonged, hypertension frequently develops and, with it, signs of uremia. When untreated, uremia's neurologic manifestations progress from neuromuscular irritability to convulsions, somnolence, and finally, coma and death. Hyperkalemia is usually asymptomatic until serum levels of potassium rise above 6.0 to 6.5 mEq/liter, at which point characteristic electrocardiographic changes and signs of muscle weakness are seen. Gastrointestinal bleeding and infection are serious complications of acute renal failure.

Diuretic phase

The diuretic phase of acute renal failure usually begins within a few days to 6 weeks of the oliguria, indicating that the nephrons have recovered to the point at which urine excretion is possible. Diuresis usually occurs before renal function has returned to normal. Consequently, BUN, serum creatinine, potassium, and phosphate may remain elevated or continue to rise even though urine output is increased. In some cases, the diuresis may be due to impaired nephron function and may cause excessive loss of water and electrolytes.

Treatment

A major concern in the treatment of acute renal failure is identifying and correcting the cause by improving renal perfusion or discontinuing nephrotoxic drugs. Fluids are carefully regulated in an effort to maintain normal fluid volume and electrolyte concentrations. Adequate caloric intake is needed to prevent the breakdown of body proteins that increases nitrogenous wastes. Parenteral hyperalimentation may be used for this purpose. Because secondary infections are a major cause of death in persons with acute renal failure, constant vigilance is needed to detect and prevent such infection. Dialysis may be indicated when nitrogenous wastes and water and electrolyte balance cannot be kept under control by other means.

In summary, acute renal failure is an acute reversible suppression of kidney function. It is generally classified as prerenal, intrarenal, or postrenal in origin. Typically, it progresses through an oliguric phase during which urine output is markedly diminished and fluid and end products of metabolism accumulate. During the second phase, that of diuresis, urine output increases as renal function begins to return. Usually, correction of the azotemia follows diuresis.

■ Chronic Renal Failure

Chronic renal failure differs from acute renal failure in that it represents progressive and irreversible destruction of kidney structures. In end-stage renal disease, the kidneys are often shrunken, and evidence of the underlying disease process has been obscured by the scar tissue and destructive changes that have occurred. Chronic renal failure can result from various conditions, including all of the renal diseases discussed in Chapter 29. Regardless of the cause, the consequences of nephron destruction culminate in progressive deterioration of the filtration, reabsorption, and endocrine functions of the kidneys. The rate of destruction differs from case to case and may range from several months to many years. In its final stages, chronic renal failure involves virtually every body organ and structure.

Uremia, which literally means urine in the blood, is the term used to describe the clinical manifestations of end-stage renal failure. It is different from azotemia, which refers to the accumulation of nitrogenous wastes in the blood and can occur without symptoms.

The person with uremia looks sick. The body is emaciated and there is extreme muscle wasting. A smell of urine clings to the body. The skin is a sallow brown. It is dry and, because of the uncontrolled itching, there are bruises and scratch marks everywhere. In the end, crystals of urea and other metabolic wastes, which are present even in the perspiration—the uremic frost—begin to precipitate on the skin. The respirations are deep and sighing and there is evidence of mild dyspnea. Anorexia, nausea, and vomiting are present. The tongue and mucous membranes are dry and cracked. Belching and hiccoughs are common. Often the fetid smell of digested blood is on the breath—the result of gastrointestinal tract ulceration and bleeding. Although initially there is a burning sensation in the feet, this is replaced by numbness, paresthesias, muscle cramps, and twitching. Muscle weakness is often overwhelming, and lethargy and difficulty in concentrating occur. Soon coma will ensue and then death.

As recently as 20 years ago, most patients in chronic renal failure progressed to the uremic stage and then died. But today, through dialysis and renal transplantation, patients in end-stage renal failure not only survive but may lead productive lives. In many such cases, the patients die not of uremia, but of complications such as cardiovascular disease.

Signs of renal failure do not begin to appear until extensive loss of function in both kidneys has occurred. This must be true, because many persons survive an entire lifetime with only one kidney, many of them unaware of this fact. Or a person in end-stage renal disease may receive a healthy kidney from a close relative, such as a parent or sibling, leaving the donor with only one kidney.

The kidney has tremendous adaptive capabilities. As nephrons are destroyed, the remaining nephrons undergo adaptive changes by which they compensate for the lost nephrons. In the process, each of the remaining nephrons filters more solute from the blood. Because these solute particles are osmotically active, they cause additional water to be lost in the urine. Along with this, the kidneys lose their ability to concentrate the urine. One of the earliest signs of renal failure is *isosthenuria*—polyuria with excretion of urine that is almost isotonic with plasma. Because the few remaining nephrons constitute the functional reserve of the kidneys, when the function of these remaining nephrons is disrupted, renal failure progresses rapidly.

All forms of renal failure are characterized by a marked reduction in the glomerular filtration rate. There are four stages in the progression of renal failure: renal impairment, renal insufficiency, renal failure, and uremia.[5] *Renal impairment* occurs when the glomerular filtration rate falls to 40% to 50% of normal. *Renal insufficiency* represents a reduction in the glomerular filtrate to a level of 20% to 40% of normal. During this stage, azotemia and mild anemia are present. *Renal failure* develops when the glomerular filtration rate drops to about 10% of normal. *Uremia* is the final stage and is characterized by the symptomatology of renal failure.

Clinical Manifestations

The signs and symptoms of renal failure can be divided as follows: (1) derangements in the chemical, electrolyte, and fluid balance that result directly from impaired

Table 30-2   Alterations in Body Function that Occur with Chronic Renal Failure

Body System	Altered Function	Manifestation
Body Fluids	Compensatory changes in tubular functions	Fixed specific gravity of urine; polyuria and nocturia
	Decreased ability to synthesize ammonia and conserve bicarbonate	Metabolic acidosis
	Inability to excrete potassium	Hyperkalemia
	Inability to regulate sodium excretion	Salt wasting or sodium retention
	Impaired ability of the kidney to excrete phosphate	Hyperphosphatemia
	Hyperphosphatemia and inability of the kidney to activate vitamin D	Hypocalcemia and increased levels of parathyroid hormone
Hematopoietic	Impaired synthesis of erythropoietin and effects of uremia	Anemia
	Impaired platelet function	Bleeding tendencies
Cardiovascular	Activation of renin–angiotensin mechanism, increased vascular volume, and failure to produce vasodepressor substances	Hypertension
	Fluid retention and hypoalbuminemia	Edema
	Excess extracellular fluid volume, anemia	Congestive heart failure; pulmonary edema
	Elevated BUN	Uremic pericarditis
Gastrointestinal	Liberation of ammonia	Anorexia, nausea, vomiting
	Decreased platelet function and increased gastric acid secretion due to hyperparathyroidism	Gastrointestinal bleeding
Neurologic	Fluid and electrolyte imbalance	Headache
	Increase in metabolic acids and other small, diffusible particles, such as urea	Signs of uremic encephalopathy: lethargy, decreased alertness, loss of recent memory, delirium, coma, seizures, asterixis, muscle twitching, and tremulousness
		Signs of neuropathy: restless leg syndrome, paresthesias, muscle weakness, and paralysis
Osteodystrophy	Hyperphosphatemia	Osteomalacia
	Hypocalcemia	Osteoporosis
	Hyperparathyroidism	Bone pain and tenderness
		Spontaneous fractures
	Calcium × phosphate product greater than 60	Metastatic calcifications
Skin	Salt wasting	Dry skin and mucous membranes
	Anemia	Pale, sallow complexion
	Hyperparathyroidism	Pruritus
	Decreased platelet function and bleeding tendencies	Ecchymosis and subcutaneous bruises
	High concentration of metabolic end products in body fluids	Uremic frost and odor of urine on skin and breath
Genitourinary	Impaired general health	
	Decreased testosterone	Impotence and loss of libido
	Decreased estrogen	Amenorrhea and loss of libido

nephron function and (2) the associated alterations in function in other parts of the body. These changes are summarized in Table 30-2.

Alterations in body fluids

One of the earliest signs of impaired renal function is the inability of the kidneys to regulate the concentration of the urine. In renal failure, the specific gravity of the urine becomes fixed (1.008-1.012) and varies little from spec-imen to specimen. Polyuria and nocturia are common. The first morning specimen is usually best for assessing the kidneys' ability to concentrate the urine, because this usually represents a period of time when fluid intake is minimal.

Renal ability to regulate sodium excretion is lost as renal function declines. Normally, the kidneys tolerate large variations in sodium intake (from 1 mEq to 900 mEq) while maintaining normal serum levels of sodium.[6] As renal function begins to fail, the kidneys lose the ability to excrete large amounts of sodium and to conserve small amounts. Consequently, the ingestion of excess sodium tends to cause hypertension and edema. Likewise, volume depletion and further decreases in the glomerular filtration rate occur when sodium intake is restricted or excess sodium is lost from the body due to diarrhea or vomiting.

Regulation of serum phosphate levels requires a daily urinary excretion of an amount equal to that ingested in the diet. With deteriorating renal function, phosphate excretion falls, and the phosphate level rises. Because of this, the serum calcium level must fall in order for the body to maintain the normal calcium times phosphate product (discussed in Chap. 25). This fall in serum calcium due to the hyperphosphatemia in turn acts as a stimulus for parathyroid release; calcium is then reabsorbed from the bones. The unrelieved hypocalcemia results in hyperplasia of the parathyroids.

The kidneys control vitamin D activity by converting the inactive form of vitamin D (25-hydroxycholecalciferol) to its active form (1,25-dihydroxycholecalciferol). In renal failure, however, the hypocalcemia is aggravated by the lack of vitamin D.

Phosphate-binding antacids are frequently administered to treat the hypocalcemia and hyperphosphatemia. They act by increasing fecal losses of phosphate, thereby reducing its absorption from the gastrointestinal tract. At the same time, milk and foods high in phosphate content are eliminated from the diet. In renal failure there is a rise in the plasma magnesium level. Because many antacids contain magnesium, these should not be given to treat the hyperphosphatemia. Once the phosphate level has been reduced, the active form of vitamin D (calcitriol) may be given for the hypocalcemia—there is a danger that tissue precipitation will occur if vitamin D is given before the phosphate level has been brought down.

About 90% of potassium excretion is through the kidneys. In renal failure, potassium excretion by each nephron increases as the kidney adapts to a decrease in the glomerular filtration rate. As a result, hyperkalemia usually does not develop until kidney function is severely compromised. Because of this adaptive mechanism, it is not usually necessary to restrict potassium intake in chronic renal failure until urinary output is less than 1000 ml per day and the glomerular filtration rate has dropped below 10 ml per minute.[6]

The kidneys are largely responsible for eliminating metabolic acids, which they do by secreting hydrogen ions, conserving bicarbonate, and producing ammonia, which acts as a buffer for hydrogen ions that are excreted in the urine. With a decline in renal function, these mechanisms become impaired, and *metabolic acidosis* is an almost inevitable complication. In long-term renal failure, the acidosis seems to stabilize as the disease progresses, probably as the result of the tremendous buffering capacity of bone. This buffering action is thought to increase bone reabsorption and to contribute to the skeletal defects that are present in chronic renal failure. If hypertension and edema are not a problem, the accompanying metabolic acidosis may be treated by administering appropriate doses of sodium bicarbonate.

Azotemia is an early sign of renal failure, usually seen before other symptoms become evident. Although urea is one of the first of the nitrogenous wastes to become elevated, it is unclear how urea alone causes symptoms. Gout is uncommon in renal failure, even though uric acid levels are increased. Much of the excess urate is excreted in the stool. Creatinine is not known to be toxic; its presence in the blood serves mainly as a useful indirect method for assessing the glomerular filtration rate and the extent of renal damage that has occurred.

Anemia

The kidney is the primary site of erythropoietin production. In renal failure, erythropoietin production is often insufficient to stimulate adequate red cell production by the bone marrow. Moreover, the accumulation of toxins further suppresses bone marrow red cell production, and the cells that are produced have a shortened life span. Both of these situations contribute to the anemia of chronic renal failure. This anemia, being based on lack of erythropoietin, is not relieved by dialysis. Androgenic steroids and iron supplements may be prescribed to treat this type of anemia.

Bleeding tendencies

It has been estimated that 17% to 20% of persons in chronic renal failure have a bleeding tendency.[3] Although platelet production is normal in number, platelet function is impaired, and this is the basis of the bleeding problem. Epistaxis, gastrointestinal bleeding, and bruising of the skin and subcutaneous tissues are seen.

Cardiovascular problems

As was stated earlier, renal failure gives rise to cardiovascular disorders, including hypertension, edema, congestive heart failure, and pericarditis.

Hypertension is a very common early manifestation of renal failure. This type of hypertension is believed to result from increased renin production (the renin-angiotensin mechanism) by the kidneys coupled with excess extracellular fluid volume. It is generally believed that the kidneys produce vasodepressor substances and that these may be reduced in renal disease. Even in advanced renal failure, enough functioning renal tissue remains to produce renin in quantity.[7] This hypertension is treated like other types of hypertension; generally, a diuretic along with one or more other medications is administered. In the later stages of renal failure, dialysis may be needed to maintain the extracellular fluid volume.

In chronic renal failure, the increased extracellular fluid volume consequent to sodium and water retention gives rise to edema; the associated proteinuria and hypoalbuminemia also contribute to the development of edema. The increase in extracellular fluid also contributes to the congestive heart failure and pulmonary edema that occur in the late stages of uremia.

Pericarditis is seen in as many as 50% of persons with chronic renal failure,[8] because of exposure of the pericardium to metabolic end products. A different form of pericarditis occurs in patients on dialysis, and this form, though not yet clearly defined, is believed to be due to the effects of stress, heparinization, or infection.

Gastrointestinal disturbances

Anorexia, nausea, and vomiting are common in uremia, and there is often a salty or metallic taste in the mouth that further depresses the patient's appetite. Ulceration and bleeding of the gastrointestinal mucosa may develop, and hiccoughs are common. The cause of the nausea and vomiting is unclear. It has been suggested that decomposition of urea by the intestinal flora may liberate ammonia, which irritates the lining of the gastrointestinal tract. Parathyroid hormone increases gastric acid secretion, and it has been proposed that this increase along with the bleeding tendency due to platelet dysfunction is a contributory factor.

Neurologic disorders

Neurologic disorders, which are common in uremia, may be categorized as uremic encephalopathy and peripheral neuropathies.

The central nervous system disturbances in uremia are similar to those caused by other metabolic and toxic disorders, such as portal-systemic encephalopathy, hypoxia, and water intoxication. These manifestations are more closely related to the progress of the uremic disorder than to the level of the metabolic end products.[9] For example, profound encephalopathy is common in *acute* renal failure and less common in *chronic* renal failure despite the more marked blood chemistry abnormalities seen in the latter. A reduction in alertness and awareness is probably the earliest and most significant indication of uremic encephalopathy. This is often followed by an inability to fix the attention, loss of recent memory, and perceptual errors in identifying persons and objects. Delirium and coma come late in the course, and finally convulsions are the preterminal event.

Disorders of motor function frequently accompany the neurologic manifestations of uremic encephalopathy. During the early stages, there is often difficulty in performing fine movements of the extremities; the gait becomes unsteady and clumsy. *Asterixis*—flapping movements of the hands and feet—often occurs as the disease progresses. It can be elicited by having the patient hold his or her arms hyperextended at the elbow and wrist, with the fingers spread apart. If asterixis is present, this position causes side-to-side flapping movements of the fingers. *Tremulousness* on movement of the extremities precedes asterixis.

Uremic encephalopathy is believed to result, at least in part, from an excess of toxic organic acids that overwhelm the normal mechanisms that prevent their entrance into the brain. The rapid reversal of the effects of uremic encephalopathy with dialysis suggests that this is the case.[9]

Neuropathy, or involvement of the peripheral nerves, is common. It affects the lower limbs more frequently than the upper, is usually symmetrical, and affects both sensory and motor function. The *restless legs syndrome* is one of the manifestations of peripheral nerve involvement; it consists of deep creeping, crawling, prickling, and itching sensations. These sensations are usually more intense at night, and moving the legs brings relief. A burning sensation of the feet, which may be followed by muscle weakness and atrophy, is a manifestation of uremia. The uremic neuropathies usually improve with dialysis or renal transplantation.

Osteodystrophy

Renal osteodystrophy is a condition resulting from chronic renal failure. It is characterized by derangements of serum calcium and serum phosphorus. The condition has sometimes been called *renal rickets*, because in children its manifestations resemble those of a vitamin D deficiency. The primary changes in renal osteodystrophy are osteomalacia and osteoporosis, in which the calcium and phosphate content of the bone decrease and loss of the supporting structural matrix occurs. Increased parathyroid function causes excessive reabsorption of bone along the long bones, distal ends of the clavicle, and small bones, which can be seen on x-ray films. In advanced osteodystrophy, cysts may develop in the bone, a condition called *osteitis fibrosa cystica*. The symptoms of renal osteodystrophy include pain, tenderness, and sometimes spontaneous fractures.

Soft-tissue calcification, or *metastatic calcification*, of the cornea, arteries, subcutaneous tissues, and muscle can occur when the phosphate times calcium product rises higher than 60. This is seen after dialysis has been instituted and is usually associated with a rapid rise in the serum calcium level, which precedes a fall in the phosphate level. Calcium deposits in the eye may cause conjunctivitis and are often evidenced by what is called "band" keratopathy. Calcium deposits in the skin cause intense itching.

Skin disorders

The skin is pale because of the anemia, and may have a sallow, yellow-brown hue. Subcutaneous bruising is common. The skin and mucous membranes are dry because of the salt wasting. An odor of urine exudes from the body. Pruritus is common, apparently due to the hyperparathyroidism, because it is usually relieved following parathyroidectomy. In the advanced stages of uremia, urea crystals may precipitate on the skin—the result of the high urea concentration that is present in the body fluids. There are changes in the fingernails, evidenced by a dark band just behind the leading edge of the nail, followed by a white band. This is known as Terry's nails.

Genitourinary changes

There is a reduction in testosterone and estrogen. A decrease in testicular size, male impotence, and amenorrhea are common findings. Related to these changes, loss of libido may be a very early indication of renal failure.

Effect of Renal Failure on Elimination of Drugs

The incidence of adverse drug reactions is known to increase in persons with renal failure. Decreased elimination by the kidneys allows drugs or their metabolites to accumulate in the body and requires that drug dosages be adjusted accordingly. This also means that patients with renal failure should be cautioned against the use of over-the-counter remedies.

In considering the effect of various drugs and medications on persons with renal disease, several factors about the drugs need to be taken into account: their absorption, distribution, metabolism, and excretion. The administration of large quantities of phosphate-binding antacids to control hyperphosphatemia and hypocalcemia in persons with advanced renal failure tends to interfere with the absorption of some drugs. Many drugs are bound to plasma proteins, such as albumin, for transport in the body, and the unbound portion of the drug is available to act at the various receptor sites and is free to be metabolized. Many persons have a decrease in plasma proteins, which are used for the binding and transport of drugs. In the process of metabolism, some drugs form intermediate metabolites that are toxic if not eliminated. This is true of meperidine, which is metabolized to the toxic intermediate normeperidine, which causes excessive sedation, nausea, and vomiting. Some drugs contain unwanted nitrogen, sodium, potassium, and magnesium and must be avoided in persons with renal failure. Penicillin, for example, contains potassium. Nitrofurantoin and ammonium chloride add to the body's nitrogen pool. Many antacids contain magnesium.

Treatment

The treatment of chronic renal failure can be divided into two stages: conservative management of renal insufficiency and dialysis or renal transplantation. The conservative treatment consists of measures to prevent or retard deterioration in renal function and to assist the body in compensating for the existing impairment. When conservative measures are no longer effective, dialysis or renal transplantation becomes necessary. The discussion in this chapter is limited to an overview of dietary management of renal failure and dialysis treatment methods. The reader is referred to specialized texts for a more complete discussion of renal failure and its management.

Dietary management

Regulating the intake of protein, calories, sodium, potassium, and fluids is of primary importance in controlling the adverse effects of renal insufficiency. In fact, it is often possible to delay the need for dialysis or transplantation through wise manipulation of food and fluid intake. The goal of dietary treatment is to provide optimum nutrition while maintaining tolerable levels of metabolic wastes. The specific diet prescribed depends on the type and severity of kidney disease that is present. Because of the severe restrictions placed on food and fluid intake, these diets may be complicated to prepare and unappetizing.

Proteins. Because proteins are broken down to form nitrogenous wastes, dietary restriction of protein is common. At present considerable controversy exists over the degree of restriction needed and the type of protein to be allowed. Usually, protein need not be restricted until renal insufficiency is relatively far advanced (glomerular filtration rate of 20 ml per minute or less). At this point, some clinicians recommend a protein intake of about 0.5 gm/kg of body weight or about 40 gm per day.[6] Other pioneers in the field of therapeutic diets for renal failure recommend a more stringent protein restriction. Giordano suggests that protein intake should be restricted to 25 gm per day or less.[10] With this more stringent limitation in protein intake, only those proteins that have a high biologic value are included. Proteins with a high biologic value are believed to promote the reutilization of endogenous nitrogen, decreasing the amount of nitrogenous wastes that are produced and thus ameliorating the symptoms of uremia. In reutilizing nitrogen, the proteins ingested in the diet are broken down into their constituent amino acids to be utilized in the synthesis of protein required by the body. A man weighing about 150 lb or 70 kg synthesizes at least 150 gm of protein daily, while ingesting only about 60 gm.[10] For this to be accomplished, amino acids must be recycled, and the ingestion of proteins that have a high biologic value makes it possible. Almost all of the amino acids in a whole egg are utilized in the synthesis of essential body proteins, hence, eggs are said to have a high biologic value. In contrast, fewer than half of the amino acids in cereal proteins are reutilized. Amino acids not reutilized to build body proteins are broken down and form the end products of protein metabolism, such as urea.

Calories. A second consideration in the dietary management of renal failure is the provision of adequate calories in the form of carbohydrates and fats to meet energy needs. This is particularly important when the protein content of the diet is severely restricted. If sufficient calories are not available, either the limited protein in the diet goes into energy production, or body tissue itself will be used for energy purposes.

Potassium. When the glomerular filtration rate falls to extremely low levels, the regulation of potassium is seriously compromised and dietary restriction of potassium becomes mandatory. Many patients in renal failure retain the ability to excrete potassium adequately, provided their intake is not excessive. Using salt substitutes that contain potassium or ingesting fruits, fruit juice, chocolate, potatoes, or other high-potassium foods carries the risk of hyperkalemia.

Sodium. The amount of sodium that is indicated in the diet depends on the kidneys' ability to excrete sodium and water and must be individually determined. For this assessment, the 24-hour urinary excretion of sodium is measured. Some patients will require 1 gm to 2 gm of sodium to prevent sodium depletion; some will require restriction to 250 mg to prevent edema and extracellular fluid excess. Generally, renal disease of glomerular origin is more likely to contribute to sodium retention, whereas tubular dysfunction causes salt wasting.

Fluids. As with sodium, fluid restriction varies with renal ability to excrete water. Fluid intake in excess of what the kidneys can excrete causes circulatory overload, edema, and water intoxication. Inadequate intake, on the other hand, causes volume depletion and hypotension as well as further decreases in the already compromised glomerular filtration rate. When fluid restriction is a requirement, a daily weight check and daily intake and output record will be made to determine the allowable quantity of water. It is common practice to allow a daily intake of 500 ml to 800 ml, which is equal to insensible (unperceived) water loss, plus a quantity equal to the previous 24-hour urine output.

Dialysis and renal transplantation

Dialysis and renal transplantation have become accepted methods for treatment of end-stage renal disease, and because they are closely linked, advances in these techniques are closely parallel. Theoretically, universal access to both types of treatment has become possible through public funding. In 1984, an estimated 55,000 people in the United States were receiving dialysis treatment at a cost of more than $3 million.[11]

The choice between dialysis and transplantation is dictated by age, related health problems, donor availability, and personal preference. Regardless of advances in transplantation technology, dialysis will probably continue to play a major role as a treatment method for end-stage renal disease. It is life-sustaining to the patient who is awaiting a suitable kidney transplant; it is needed during the postoperative transplant period and as a backup form of treatment if the transplantation is unsuccessful.

Hemodialysis. The basic principles of hemodialysis have remained unchanged over the years. A hemodialysis system, or artificial kidney, consists of three parts—a blood compartment, a dialysis fluid compartment, and a cellophane membrane that separates the two compartments. There are several types of dialyzers, all of which incorporate these parts, and all of which function in similar fashion. The cellophane membrane is semipermeable, permitting all molecules, except blood cells and plasma proteins, to move freely in both directions—from the blood into the dialyzing solution and from the dialyzing solution into the blood. The direction of flow is determined by the concentration of the substances contained in the two solutions. Normally, the waste products and the excess electrolytes in the blood diffuse into the dialyzing solution. If there is a need to replace or add substances, such as bicarbonate, to the blood, these can be added to the dialyzing solution (see Fig. 30-1).

During dialysis, the blood moves from an artery, through the tubing and blood chamber in the dialysis unit, and then back into the body through a vein. Access to the vascular compartment is made through tubing implanted into an artery and a vein (an external AV shunt) or through an internal AV fistula, which is created by anastamosing an artery and a vein. A connecting tube is placed between the implanted arterial and venous tubes of the AV shunt between dialysis treatments, so that blood flows directly from the artery into the vein. An

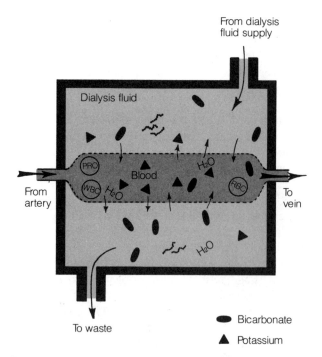

Figure 30-1 Schematic diagram of a hemodialysis system. The blood compartment and dialysis solution compartment are separated by a cellophane membrane. This membrane is porous enough to allow all of the constituents, except the plasma proteins and blood cells, to diffuse between the two compartments.

internal AV fistula requires puncture with a special wide-bore needle for the performance of each dialysis treatment. Heparin is used to prevent clotting within the dialysis system; it can be administered continuously, intermittently, or regionally. Most patients are dialyzed two to three times a week for 4 to 5 hours. Many persons can be managed on hemodialysis in their homes.

Peritoneal dialysis.   Peritoneal dialysis operates on the same principle as hemodialysis, but in this type of dialysis, the thin serous membrane of the peritoneal cavity serves as the dialyzing membrane. A sterile dialyzing solution (usually about 2 liters) is instilled into the peritoneal cavity through a special cannula or catheter over a period of 10 to 20 minutes. The solution is then allowed to remain, or dwell, in the peritoneal cavity for variable lengths of time, at least 30 to 45 minutes, during which the metabolic end products and extracellular fluid diffuse into the dialysate. At the end of the dwell time, the dialysate is drained by gravity out of the peritoneal cavity into a sterile bag. The procedure is repeated as necessary.

Peritoneal dialysis is effective in both acute and chronic renal failure. Less equipment is needed (unless the equipment is automated) and blood transfusion or anticoagulants are not routinely required. Persons living alone can monitor their dialysis, whereas hemodialysis usually requires that a second person assist. However, peritoneal dialysis does require more time than hemodialysis. It takes about six times as long to exchange the toxins and there is greater danger of infection (peritonitis).

Continuous ambulatory peritoneal dialysis (CAPD) is a self-care procedure. It is accomplished by means of a catheter implanted surgically into the peritoneal cavity. A prepackaged dialysis solution is connected to the catheter and allowed to drain into the peritoneal cavity by gravity. Once emptied, the bag is rolled up and secured under the clothing. When the exchange process has been completed, the bag is unrolled and lowered below the level of the catheter, allowing the waste-containing dialyzing solution to drain from the peritoneal cavity back into the bag. A solution exchange is usually performed every 4 to 6 hours during the daytime and every 8 hours at night. Each exchange, which involves draining the solution and infusing the new solution, requires about 30 to 45 minutes. The continuous rather than intermittent nature of ambulatory peritoneal dialysis avoids the rapid fluctuations in extracellular fluid volume associated with hemodialysis, and there is less need for dietary restrictions.

Renal transplantation.   Improvements in tissue typing and cross-match studies and in the preservation and transport of cadaver kidneys have contributed significantly to the success rate of renal transplants during the past two decades. Live donor transplants from family members with matching tissue types account for about 40% of all transplants in the United States; the remainder are cadaver transplants. The ethical aspect of accepting kidneys from family members is controversial, although no significant damaging effects have been detected 10 to 15 years after kidney donation. Recipients require immunosuppression to prevent rejection of the transplanted kidney. Among the drugs most commonly used for this purpose are cyclosporin and prednisone.

In summary, chronic renal failure represents the end-stage destructive effects of many different forms of kidney disease. Regardless of the cause, the consequences of nephron destruction present in end-stage renal disease result in progressive deterioration in the filtration, reabsorption, and endocrine functions of the kidney. In its advanced stages, renal failure affects almost every system in the body. It causes azotemia and alterations in sodium and water excretion and in body levels of potassium, phosphate, calcium, and magnesium. It also causes anemia, alterations in cardiovascular function, neurologic disturbances, gastrointestinal dysfunction, and discomforting skin changes. Within the past 20 years, dialysis and renal transplantation have allowed persons with what was once a fatal disorder to survive and lead a relatively normal and productive life.

Study Guide

After you have studied this chapter, you should be able to meet the following objectives:

☐ Describe the clinical manifestations of azotemia with reference to urea and creatinine.

☐ Classify the following conditions as prerenal, intrarenal, or postrenal: acute glomerulonephritis, prostatic hypertrophy, hemorrhage, septicemia, hemolytic reaction.

☐ Describe the two phases that are characteristic of the course of acute renal failure.

☐ Describe the alterations in serum sodium, serum phosphate, and potassium regulation that occur as renal function declines.

☐ Explain the relationship between hypertension and renal function.

☐ Describe the manifestations of renal failure as they apply to four or more major body systems.

☐ State the basis of drug sensitivity in persons with renal failure.

☐ State the goal in dietary management of chronic renal failure.

☐ Compare hemodialysis with peritoneal dialysis.

References

1. Guyton A: Textbook of Medical Physiology, 6th ed, p 424. Philadelphia, WB Saunders, 1981
2. Report of the Coordinating Council: Research Needs in Nephrology and Urology, Vol I, p 16. National Institute of Health, National Institute of Arthritis, Metabolism, and Digestive Diseases, Public Health Service, 1978. DHEW Publication No (NIH) 78-1481
3. Leaf A, Cotran R: Renal Pathophysiology, pp 167, 204. New York, Oxford University Press, 1980
4. Schrier RW: Acute renal failure: Pathogenesis, diagnosis and management. Hosp Pract 16, No 3:101, 1981
5. Mitchell JC: Axioms on uremia. Hosp Med 14, No 7:6, 1978
6. Orme BM: Chronic renal failure: Guide to management. Hosp Med 14, No 1:99, 105, 1978
7. Merrill JP, Hampters CL: Uremia. N Engl J Med 282, No 18:1014, 1970
8. Zeluff GW, Eknoyan G, Jackson D: Pericarditis in renal failure. Heart Lung 8, No 6:1139, 1979
9. Raskin NH, Fishman RA: Neurological disorders in renal failure. N Engl J Med 294, No 3:143, 147, 1976
10. Giordano C: The role of diet in renal disease. Hosp Pract 12, No 11:115-119, 1977
11. Rao KV: Status of renal transplantation. Med Clin North Am 68, No 2:427, 1984

Additional References

Bergstein JM: Acute renal failure in children. Crit Care Q 1:41-51, 1978

Chambers JK: Assessing the dialysis patient at home. Am J Nurs 81, No 4:750-754, 1981

Comty CM, Collins AJ: Dialytic therapy in management of chronic renal failure. Med Clin North Am 68, No 2:399, 1984

Diamond JR, Yoburn DC: Nonoliguric acute renal failure. Arch Intern Med 142:1882, 1982

Eknoyan G: Axioms on acute oliguria. Hosp Med 13 No. 12:32, 1977

Eknoyan G: Side effects of hemodialysis. N Engl J Med 311:915, 1984

Fisher JW: Mechanism of anemia of chronic renal failure. Nephron 25:106-111, 1980

Kafetz K: Renal impairment in the elderly: A review. J R Soc Med 76:398, 1983

Kanis JA: Osteomalacia and chronic renal failure. J Clin Pathol 34:1295, 1981

Kurtzman NA: Chronic renal failure: Metabolic and clinical consequences. Hosp Pract 17, No 8:107, 1982

Lazarus JM: Uremia: A clinical guide. Hosp Med 15, No 1:52-73, 1979

Leste GW: Nondialytic treatment of established acute renal failure. Crit Care Q 1:11-24, 1978

Lourie EG, Hampers CL: The success of Medicare's End-Stage Renal-Disease Program. N Engl J Med 305:434, 1981

Mitch WE, Wilcox CS: Disorders of body fluids, sodium and potassium in chronic renal failure. Am J Med 72:536, 1982

Mitchell JC: Axioms on uremia. Hosp Med 14, No 7:6-23, 1978

Orr ML: Drugs and renal disease. Am J Nurs 81, No 5:969-970, 1981

Platzer H: A patient suffering from chronic renal failure. Nursing Times 76:191-195, 1980

Rao KV: Status of renal transplantation. Med Clin North Am 68, No 2, 1984

Roberts SL: Renal assessment: A nursing point of view. Heart Lung 8, No 1:105-113, 1979

Robinson RL: Laboratory findings in the differential diagnosis of renal failure. Crit Care Q 1:87-99, 1979

Schrier R: Acute renal failure. Kidney Int 15:205-216, 1979

Sexauer CL, Matson JR: Anemia in chronic renal failure. Ann Clin Lab Sci 11:484, 1981

Sorkin MI: Acute renal failure. Med Times 107, No 10:33-39, 1979

Stark JL: BUN/creatinine: Your keys to kidney function. Nursing '80 10, No 5:33-38, 1980

Szwed JJ: Pathophysiology of acute renal failure: Rationale for signs and symptoms. Crit Care Q 1:1-9, 1978

Tilney NL, Lazarus JM: Acute renal failure in surgical patients. Surg Clin North Am 63, No 2:357, 1983

Weiss RA, Edelmann CM Jr: Children on dialysis. N Engl J Med 307:1574, 1982

Unit V

Alterations in Genitourinary Function

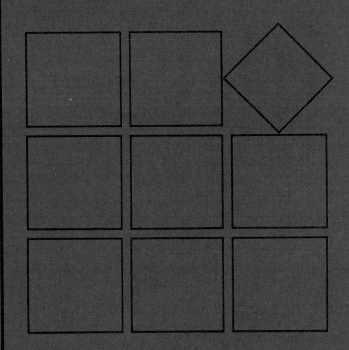

Chapter 31

Alterations in Urine Elimination

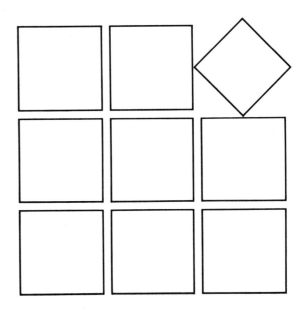

Although the kidneys control the formation of urine and regulate the composition of body fluids, it is the bladder that stores urine and controls its elimination from the body.[1] Alterations in the storage and expulsion functions of the bladder can cause incontinence accompanied by social and hygienic problems or obstruction of urinary flow with deleterious effects on ureteral and, ultimately, renal function. The discussion in this chapter focuses on normal control of urine elimination, urinary retention, incontinence, and bladder cancer. A discussion of urinary tract infections can be found in Chapter 29.

■ Control of Urine Elimination

The bladder (also known as the urinary vesicle) is a freely movable organ located behind the pelvic bone in the male and in front of the vagina in the female. The bladder consists of two parts: the fundus, or body, and the neck, or posterior urethra. In the male, the urethra continues anteriorly through the penis. Urine passes from the kidneys to the bladder through the ureters, which are 4 mm to 5 mm in diameter and about 30 cm in length. The ureters enter the bladder bilaterally at a location toward its base and in close proximity to the urethra (Fig. 31-1). The triangular area that is bounded by the ureters and the urethra is called the *trigone*. There are no valves at the ureteral openings, but as the pressure of the urine within the bladder rises, the ends of the ureters are compressed against the bladder wall to prevent the backflow of urine.

Bladder Structure

The bladder is composed of four layers: (1) an outer serosal layer, which covers the upper surface and is continuous with the peritoneum, (2) a network of smooth

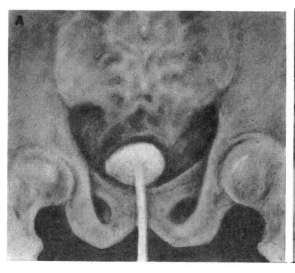
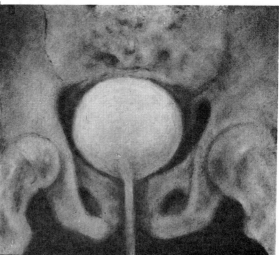
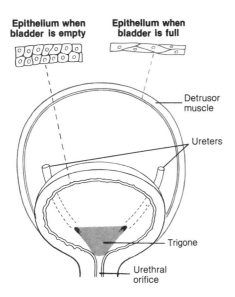

Figure 31-1 (Top) *Cystogram of male bladder, showing position and filling.* (Bottom) *Diagram of the bladder, showing the detrusor muscle, ureters, trigone area, and urethral orifice. Note the flattening of epithelial cells when the bladder is full and the wall is stretched. (From Chaffee EE, Lytle IM: Basic Physiology and Anatomy, 4th ed. Philadelphia, JB Lippincott, 1980)*

muscle fibers called the detrusor muscle, (3) a submucosal layer of loose connective tissue, and (4) an inner mucosal lining of transitional epithelium. The tonicity of the urine is often quite different from that of the blood and the transitional epithelial lining of the bladder acts as an effective barrier to prevent the passage of water between the blood and the bladder contents. The inner elements of the bladder form folds, or rugae. As the bladder expands during filling, these rugae spread out to form a single layer without disrupting the integrity of the epithelial lining.

Muscles in the bladder neck, sometimes referred to as the internal sphincter, are a continuation of the detrusor muscle. They run down obliquely behind the proximal urethra, forming the posterior urethra in males and the entire urethra in females. When the bladder is relaxed, these circular muscle fibers are closed and act as a sphincter. When the detrusor muscle contracts, the sphincter is pulled open simply by the changes that occur in bladder shape. In the female, the urethra (2.5–3.5 cm) is shorter than in the male (16.5–18.5 cm), and the urethral resistance also tends to be less in the female.

Another muscle important to bladder function is the circular skeletal muscle, the external sphincter, that surrounds the urethra distal to the base of the bladder. In general, the external sphincter operates as a reserve mechanism to stop micturition when it is occurring and to maintain continence in the face of unusually high bladder pressure. The skeletal muscle of the pelvic floor also contributes to the support of the bladder and the maintenance of continence. The diaphragm and abdominal muscles play a secondary role in micturition. Their contraction may further increase intravesicular pressure.

Neural Control of Bladder Function

The innervation of the bladder consists of a peripheral autonomic reflex that is subject to facilitation or inhibition by higher neurologic centers. There are three main levels of neurologic control for bladder function: (1) the spinal cord reflex centers, (2) the micturition center in the brain stem, and (3) the cortical and subcortical centers.

Spinal cord centers

The centers for reflex control of micturition are located in the sacral (S2–S4) and thoracolumbar (T11–L1) segments of the spinal cord (Fig. 31-2). Motor neurons for the detrusor muscle are located in the sacral cord; their axons travel to the bladder through the pelvic nerve. Lower motor neurons for the external sphincter are also located in the sacral segments of the spinal cord. These motor neurons communicate with the cerebral cortex via the pyramidal tracts and send impulses to the external sphincter via the pudendal nerve. The sympathetic motor

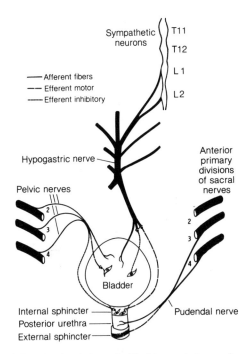

Figure 31-2 *Nerve supply to the bladder and the urethra. (From Chaffee EE, Lytle IM: Basic Physiology and anatomy, 4th ed. Philadelphia, JB Lippincott, 1980)*

fibers for the trigonal area of the bladder are located in the thoracolumbar segments of the spinal cord. Sensation from the urethra and bladder are returned to the CNS by means of fibers that travel with the parasympathetic (pelvic nerve), somatic (pudendal), and sympathetic (hypogastric) nerves. The pelvic nerve carries sensory fibers from the stretch receptors of the bladder; the pudendal nerve, sensory fibers from the external sphincter and pelvic muscles; and the hypogastric nerve, sensory fibers from the trigonal area.

Brain stem micturition center

The acute coordination of the normal micturition reflex occurs in the micturition center of the brain stem, facilitated by ascending and descending pathways from the reflex centers in the spinal cord (Fig. 31-3). This center is thought to coordinate the activity of the detrusor muscle and the external sphincter. The detrusor motor neurons of the sacral cord do not respond directly to afferent information generated by bladder filling. Instead, bladder emptying occurs only after afferent generation of a brain-stem-integrated micturition response. Direct reflex detrusor response to afferent pelvic nerve activity develops after spinal cord injury but does not occur normally.

Cortical and subcortical centers

Cortical brain centers allow for inhibition of the micturition center in the brain stem and conscious control of urination. Neural influences from the subcortical centers

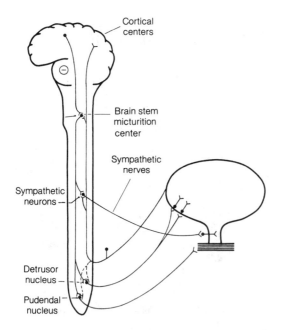

Figure 31-3 *Neuronal interactions between lower urinary tract and nervous system. Prior to micturition, the bladder afferents ascend to the micturition center, which is normally inhibited by higher centers. Efferents from the micturition center descend to the thoracolumbar sympathetic center and the detrusor and pudental nuclei to coordinate vesical contraction with relaxation of the smooth muscle and striated muscle sphincters. (From Krane RJ, Sirosky MB, (eds): Clinical Neuro-Urology, p 145. Boston, Little, Brown, & Co. © 1979. Used with permission.)*

in the basal ganglia, which are conveyed by extrapyramidal pathways, modulate the contractile response. They modulate and delay the detrusor contractile response during filling and then modulate the expulsive activity of the bladder to facilitate complete emptying.[2]

Micturition

In infants and small children micturition is an involuntary act that is triggered by a spinal cord reflex; when the bladder fills to a given capacity, the detrusor muscle contracts, and relaxation of the external sphincter occurs. As the bladder grows and increases in capacity, the tonicity of the external sphincter increases. At age 2 to 3 the child becomes conscious of the need to urinate and can learn to briefly contract the pelvic muscles in order to inhibit contraction of the detrusor muscle and thus delay urination. As the central nervous system continues to mature, inhibition of involuntary detrusor muscle activity takes place. Once continence has been achieved in the child, micturition becomes voluntary.

In order to maintain continence, or retention of urine, the bladder must function as a low-pressure storage system; that is, the pressure within the bladder must

remain lower than urethral pressure. For this to occur, bladder filling is accompanied by an almost imperceptible increase in intravesicular pressure. The volume in the bladder can vary from 10 ml to 400 ml with only a 5-cm to 10-cm H_2O increase in pressure.[3] Sustained elevations in intravesicular pressures (greater than 40 cm to 50 cm H_2O) are associated with ureteral dilatation and development of vesicoureteral reflux. While the pressure within the bladder is maintained at low levels, sphincter pressure remains high (45 cm to 65 cm H_2O) as a means of preventing loss of urine as the bladder fills. When the bladder is distended to 150 ml to 300 ml, the sensation of fullness is transmitted to the spinal cord and then to the cerebral cortex, allowing for conscious inhibition of the micturition reflex. During the act of micturition, the detrusor muscle of the bladder fundus and bladder neck contract down on the urine in the fundus; the ureteral orifices are forced shut; the bladder neck is widened and shortened as it is pulled up by the globular muscles in the bladder fundus; and the resistance of the internal sphincter in the bladder neck is decreased as urine moves out of the bladder.

Pharmacology of micturition

Both sympathetic and parasympathetic neuromediators contribute to the micturition reflex. The parasympathetic innervation of the bladder is mediated by the neuromediator acetylcholine. Two types of acetylcholine receptors effect various aspects of micturition—nicotinic and muscarinic. Nicotinic receptors are found in the autonomic ganglia, the neuromuscular end plates of the external sphincter and pelvic muscles, and the spinal cord. Muscarinic receptors are found in the postganglionic parasympathetic endings of the detrusor muscle.

Although sympathetic innervation is not essential to the act of micturition, it allows the bladder to store a large volume without the involuntary escape of urine—a mechanism that is consistent with the fight-or-flight function subserved by the sympathetic nervous system. The bladder is supplied with both alpha and beta (beta$_2$) sympathetic receptors. The beta receptors are found in the detrusor muscle; they produce relaxation of the detrusor muscle, increasing the bladder volume at which the micturition reflex is triggered.[4] Alpha receptors are found in the trigone area, including the intramural ureteral musculature, bladder neck, and internal sphincter. Activation of alpha receptors produces contraction of these muscles. A cessation of sympathetic activity occurs with activation of the micturition reflex. During ejaculation, which is mediated by the sympathetic nervous system, the musculature of the trigone area as well as that of the bladder neck and prostatic urethra contract and prevent the backflow of seminal fluid into the bladder.

Because of their effect on bladder function, drugs that selectively activate or block autonomic nervous system outflow or receptor activity have the potential for impairing urine elimination. Table 31-1 describes the action of drugs that can impair bladder function or can be used in the treatment of micturition disorders.

Diagnostic Methods of Evaluating Bladder Function

Bladder structures can be assessed by a number of methods. They can be visualized indirectly using x-rays of the abdomen, excretory urograms, or cystograms (see Fig. 31-1), which involve the use of a radiopaque dye, computerized tomography (CT scan), or ultrasound. Cystoscopy provides the means for direct visualization of the urethra, bladder, and ureteral orifices.

Urodynamic studies
Urodynamic studies are used to study bladder function and voiding problems. Three aspects of bladder function can be studied using urodynamic studies: (1) bladder, urethral, and intra-abdominal pressure changes, (2) characteristics of urine flow, and (3) the activity of the external sphincter and pelvic floor striated muscle. Specific urodynamic tests include uroflometry, cystometrography, urethral pressure profile, sphincter electromyography, and uroflow studies.

Uroflometry. Uroflometry measures the flow rate (milliliters/minute) during urination. It is commonly done using a weight-recording device located at the bottom of a commode receptable unit. As the person being tested voids, the weight of the commode receptable unit increases. This weight change is electronically recorded and then analyzed using both weight (converted to milliliters) and time.

Cystometrography. The cystometrogram (CMG) is used to measure bladder pressure during both filling and voiding. It provides valuable information about uninhibited bladder contractions, the sensation of bladder fullness and desire to urinate, and the ability to inhibit urination. The test uses either carbon dioxide or sterile

Table 31-1   Bladder Function and Drug Actions

Function	Drug Groups	Examples
Detrusor Muscle		
Increased tone and contraction	Cholinergic drugs (stimulate parasympathetic receptors that cause detrusor muscle contraction)	Bethanechol (Urecholine) Carbachol (Doryl) Methacholine (Mechoyl) Furethonium (Furethide)
	Anticholinesterase drugs (inhibit acetylcholine destruction)	Neostigmine (Prostigmin) Distigmine (Ubretid)
Inhibition of detrusor muscle relaxation during filling	Beta-adrenergic blocking drugs (block beta receptors that cause detrusor muscle relaxation)	Propranolol (Inderal)
Decreased tone	Anticholinergic drugs (block parasympathetic receptors that cause detrusor muscle contraction)	Atropine Methantheline (Banthine) Propantheline (Pro-Banthine) Oxybutynin (Ditropan)
	Adrenergic agonists (activate beta sympathetic receptors that cause detrusor muscle relaxation)	Isoproterenol Baclofen (Lioresal) Hydramitrazine (Lisidonil)
Internal Sphincter		
Increased tone	Alpha-adrenergic agonists (activate alpha receptors that cause contraction of muscles of the internal sphincter)	Phenylephrine (Neo-Synephrine) Ephedrine Phenylpropanolamine (Propadrine) Imipramine (Tofranil, Presamine)
Decreased tone	Alpha-adrenergic blocking drugs	Phenoxybenzamine
External Sphincter		
Decreased tone	Skeletal muscle relaxants	Baclofen (Lioresal) Dantrolene (Dantrium) Diazepam (Valium)

(Developed from information in: Bissada NK, Finkbeiner AE: Pharmacology of continence and micturition. Am Family Physician 20, No. 5:128, 1979)

water to fill the bladder and some means for continuous recording of pressure during bladder filling and voiding. In a normally functioning bladder, the pressure usually remains constant at 8 cm H_2O to 15 cm H_2O until 350 ml to 450 ml of fluid has been instilled in the bladder. At this point a definite sensation of fullness occurs and the pressure rises sharply to 40 cm H_2O to 100 cm H_2O, and voiding around the catheter occurs. Urinary continence requires that urethral pressure exceed bladder pressure. Usually bladder pressure rises 30 cm H_2O to 40 cm H_2O during voiding. If the urethral resistance is high because of obstruction, greater pressures will be required, a condition that can be detected through use of the CMG.

Urethral pressure profile. The urethral pressure profile (UPP) is used to evaluate the intraluminal pressure changes along the length of the urethra with the bladder at rest; it provides information about smooth muscle activity along the length of the urethra. This test can be done using the infusion method (the most commonly used), the membrane catheter method, or the microtip transducer. The infusion method involves inserting a small double-lumen urethral catheter, infusing fluid or carbon dioxide into the bladder, and measuring the changes in urethral pressure as the catheter is slowly withdrawn.

Sphincter electromyography. Sphincter electromyography (EMG) allows the activity of the striated (voluntary) muscles of the perineal area to be studied. Activity is recorded using anal (catheter or plug), urethral (catheter), or perineal (cup or paste) electrodes. Electrode placement is based on the muscle groups that need to be tested. The test is usually done along with urodynamic tests such as the CMG and uroflow studies.

It is often advantageous to evaluate several components of bladder function simultaneously. The most common combinations of studies are CMG, urethral sphincter EMG, and abdominal pressure; UPP and urethral sphincter EMG; and uroflometry, urethral sphincter EMG, and abdominal and bladder pressure (often referred to as a micturition study).[5] Rectal pressure is usually used as a measure of abdominal pressure.

In summary, although the kidneys function in the formation of urine and the regulation of body fluids, it is the bladder that stores and controls the elimination of urine. Micturition is basically a function of the peripheral autonomic nervous system, subject to facilitation or inhibition from higher neurologic centers. The parasympathetic nervous system controls the motor function of the bladder detrusor muscle and the tone of the internal sphincter; its cell bodies are located in the sacral spinal cord and communicate with the bladder through the pelvic nerve. Efferent sympathetic control originates at the level of segments T11 through L2 of the spinal cord and produces relaxation of the detrusor muscle and contraction of the internal sphincter. Skeletal muscle found in the external sphincter and the pelvic muscles that support the bladder are supplied by the pudendal nerve, which exits the spinal cord at the level of segments S2 through S4. The micturition center in the brain stem coordinates the action of the detrusor muscle and the external sphincter, whereas cortical centers permit conscious control of micturition. Bladder function can be evaluated using urodynamic studies that measure bladder, urethral, and abdominal pressures, urine flow characteristics, and skeletal muscle activity of the external sphincter.

■ Alterations in Bladder Function

Alterations in bladder function include both urinary obstruction with retention of urine and urinary incontinence with involuntary loss of urine. Although the two conditions have almost the opposite effects on urination, they can have similar causes. Both can result from either structural changes in the bladder, urethra, or surrounding organs or from impairment of neurologic control of bladder function.

Urinary Retention

Urinary retention occurs when urine is produced normally by the kidneys but is retained in the bladder.[5] Urinary retention can result from a number of conditions, including urethral obstruction, impaired innervation of the bladder (neurogenic bladder), and the effects of drug actions on the control of bladder function. Urinary retention is a serious disorder because it has the potential to produce kidney damage.

Urethral obstruction

Major structural urinary obstruction occurs through processes that cause intrinsic narrowing of or external compression of the urinary meatus or bladder outlet structures. In males, the most important cause of urinary obstruction is external compression of the urethra due to enlargement of the prostate gland (see Chap. 33). External obstructive processes are less common in females, and when they do occur, they are most often caused by a cystocele of the bladder (Chap. 35). Bladder tumors and secondary invasion of the bladder by tumors arising in structures that surround the bladder and urethra can compress the bladder neck or urethra and cause obstruction. Narrowing of the urethra due to congenital deformities or scar tissue from injury or infection can also obstruct urine flow. Congenital narrowings of the urinary meatus (meatal stenosis) are more common in boys, and obstructive disorders of the posterior urethra are more common in girls. Gonorrhea and other sexually transmitted diseases contribute to the incidence of infection-produced urethral strictures.

Compensatory changes. The body normally compensates for the obstruction of urine outflow with mechanisms designed to prevent urine retention. These mechanisms can be divided into three stages: irritability, a compensatory stage, and a decompensatory stage.[6] The degree to which these compensatory changes occur and their effect on bladder structure and urinary function depend on the extent of the obstruction, the rapidity with which it occurs, and the presence of other contributing factors, such as neurologic impairment and infection.

During the early stage of obstruction, the bladder begins to hypertrophy and becomes hypersensitive to afferent stimuli arising from bladder filling. The ability to suppress urination is diminished, and bladder contraction can become so strong it virtually produces bladder spasm. There is urgency, sometimes to the point of incontinence, and frequency both during the day and at night.

With continuation and progression of the obstruction, compensatory changes begin to occur. There is further hypertrophy of the bladder muscle, the thickness of the bladder wall may double, and the pressure generated by detrusor contraction can increase from a normal 20 cm to 40 cm H_2O to 50 cm to 100 cm H_2O in order to overcome the resistance from the obstruction. As the force needed to expel urine from the bladder increases, compensatory mechanisms may become ineffective, causing muscle fatigue before complete emptying can be accomplished. After a few minutes, voiding can again be initiated and completed, accounting for the frequency of urination.[5]

Normally the inner bladder surface is smooth. With continued outflow obstruction, this smooth surface is replaced with coarsely woven structures (hypertrophied smooth muscle fibers) called trabeculae. Small pockets of mucosal tissue, called cellules, commonly develop between the trabecular ridges.[6] These pockets form diverticula when they extend between the actual fibers of the bladder muscle (Fig. 31-4). Because the diverticula have no muscle, they are unable to contract and expel their urine into the bladder, and secondary infections due to stasis frequently occur.

Along with hypertrophy of the bladder wall, there is hypertrophy of the trigone area and the interureteric ridge, which is located between the two ureters. This

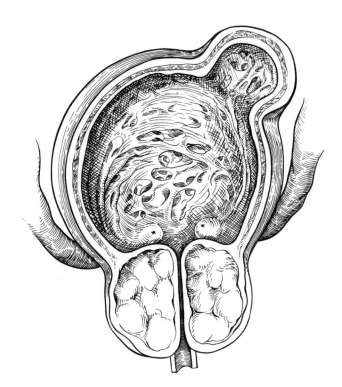

Figure 31-4 *Destructive changes of the bladder wall with development of diverticulum due to benign prostatic hypertrophy.*

causes back pressure on the kidneys, the development of hydroureters (Fig. 31-5), and eventual kidney damage.

When compensatory mechanisms are no longer effective, signs of decompensation begin to occur. The contraction of the detrusor muscle becomes too short to completely expel the urine, and residual urine results. At this point the symptoms of obstruction become pronounced. Frequency of urination, hesitancy, a need to strain to initiate urination, a very weak and small stream, and termination of the stream before the bladder is completely emptied occur. The amount of residual urine may increase up to 1000 ml to 3000 ml, and overflow incontinence occurs. There may also be acute, or sudden, complete retention of urine. The signs of urinary retention are summarized in Chart 31-1.

Chart 31-1 Signs of Urethral Obstruction and Urine Retention

Bladder distention
Hesitancy
Straining when initiating urination
Small and weak stream
Frequency
Feeling of incomplete bladder emptying
Overflow incontinence

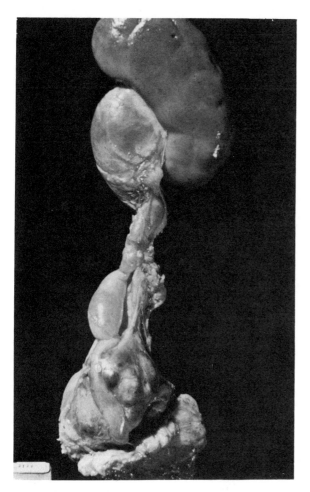

Figure 31-5 *Hydroureter caused by ureteral obstruction in a woman with cancer of the uterus.*

Treatment. The immediate treatment of outflow obstruction is relief of bladder distention. This is usually accomplished through urinary catheterization (discussed later in this chapter). Long-term treatment is directed toward correcting the problem causing the obstruction.

Neurogenic Bladder

The innervation of the bladder can be interrupted at any level and can selectively involve either sensory or motor innervation or both. Neurogenic disorders of the bladder are usually manifested in one of two ways: by detrusor muscle hyperreflexia or by detrusor muscle areflexia. Detrusor muscle hyperreflexia usually results from neurologic lesions that are located above the level of the micturition reflexes, whereas areflexia results from lesions at the level of the sacral micturition reflex or the peripheral autonomic innervation of the bladder. In addition to detrusor muscle disorders, disruption of micturition occurs when the neurologic control of external

sphincter function is impaired. Table 31-2 describes the characteristics of neurogenic bladder according to the level of the lesion.

Detrusor muscle hyperreflexia

The term reflex neurogenic bladder, sometimes called spastic neurogenic bladder, autonomic neurogenic bladder, cord bladder, or uninhibited bladder, is used to describe a neurogenic disorder that causes hyperreflexia of the detrusor muscle. It is caused by any neurologic lesion above the level of the voiding reflex arc. It involves the interruption of the sensory and voluntary control of micturition. Although both pathways are usually affected, the lesion may selectively involve either the sensory or the motor component, and it can occur at different levels of neural control. The most common cause of neurogenic bladder is spinal cord injury (Chap. 48).

Following the acute stage of spinal cord injury, the micturition response changes from a long-tract reflex to a segmental reflex.[7] Because the sacral reflex arc remains intact, stimuli generated by bladder stretch receptors during filling produce frequent spontaneous contractions of the detrusor muscle. This creates a small hyperactive bladder subject to high-pressure and short-duration uninhibited bladder contractions. Voiding is interrupted, involuntary, or incomplete. Hypertrophy of the trigone develops, often leading to vesicoureteral reflux and renal damage. Dilation of the internal sphincter and spasticity of the perineal muscles innervated by upper motor neurons occur, producing resistance to bladder emptying.

Bladder function during spinal shock.   The immediate and early effects of spinal cord injury on bladder function are quite different from those that follow recovery from the impact of the initial injury. During the period immediately following spinal cord injury (Chap. 48), a state of spinal shock develops during which all the reflexes, including the micturition reflex, are depressed. During this stage the bladder becomes atonic and cannot contract. Catheterization is necessary to prevent injury to urinary structures associated with overdistention of the bladder. Aseptic intermittent catheterization is the preferred method of catheterization. Depression of reflexes lasts for about 1 to 2 months, after which time the spinal reflexes return and become hyperactive.

Autonomic hyperreflexia.   Autonomic hyperreflexia is a life-threatening complication of spinal cord injuries above the level of T6.[7] Normally all viscerovascular reflexes are integrated at supraspinal levels so that a normal blood pressure is maintained. With spinal cord injury, this integration is lost. The condition is charac-

Table 31-2 Characteristics and Types of Neurogenic Bladder

Level of Lesion	Change in Bladder Function	Common Causes
Cortex or pyramidal tract	Loss of cortical ability to perceive bladder filling results in low volume; physiologically normal micturition occurs suddenly and is difficult to inhibit	Stroke and advanced age
Basal ganglia or extrapyramidal tract	Detrusor contractions are elicited suddenly without warning and are difficult to control; bladder contraction is shorter than normal and does not produce full bladder emptying	Parkinson's disease
Brain stem micturition center or communicating tracts in the spinal cord	Storage reflexes are provoked during filling, and external sphincter responses are heightened; uninhibited bladder contractions occur at a lower volume than normal and do not continue until the bladder is emptied; antagonistic activity occurs between the detrusor muscle and the external sphincter.	Spinal cord injury
Sacral cord or nerve roots	Areflexic bladder fills but does not contract; loss of external sphincter tone occurs when the lesion affects the alpha motor neurons or pudendal nerve.	Injury to sacral cord or spinal roots
Pelvic nerve	Increased filling and impaired sphincter control causes increased intravesicular pressure	Radical pelvic surgery
Autonomic peripheral sensory pathways	Bladder overfilling occurs with lack of appreciation of bladder events.	Diabetic neuropathies, multiple sclerosis

terized by excessive uninhibited autonomic reflexes triggered by stimuli such as overdistention of the viscera and visceral pain. The most common of these stimuli is an overdistended bladder. The manifestations of autonomic hyperreflexia include marked elevations in blood pressure, bradycardia, severe headache, flushing of the skin, diaphoresis below the level of spinal cord injury, blurred vision, nasal congestion, nausea, and spasm of the piloerector muscles (goose bumps). If untreated, the condition can lead to stroke or seizures. The treatment consists of immediate removal of the triggering event—catheterization in cases of bladder distention.

Uninhibited neurogenic bladder. A mild form of reflex neurogenic bladder, sometimes called the uninhibited bladder, can develop following a stroke, during the early stages of multiple sclerosis, or as a result of lesions located in the inhibitory centers of the cortex or the pyramidal tract. With this type of disorder the sacral reflex arc and sensation are retained, the urine stream is normal, and there is no residual urine. However, bladder capacity is diminished.

Detrusor–sphincter dyssynergy. Depending on the level of the lesion, the coordinated activity of the detrusor muscle and the external sphincter may be affected. Lesions that affect the micturition center in the brain stem or impair communication between this center and spinal cord centers interrupt the coordinated activity of the detrusor muscle and the external sphincter. This is called detrusor–sphincter dyssynergy. Instead of relaxing during micturition, the external sphincter becomes more constricted.

Detrusor muscle areflexia

Detrusor muscle areflexia, or flaccid neurogenic bladder, occurs when there is injury to the micturition center of the sacral cord, the cauda equina, or the sacral roots that supply the bladder. Atony of the detrusor muscle and loss of the perception of bladder fullness permit the overstretching of the detrusor muscle that contributes to weak and ineffective bladder contractions. External sphincter tone and perineal muscle tone are diminished. Voluntary urination does not occur, but fairly efficient emptying can be achieved by increased intra-abdominal pressure or manual suprapubic pressure. Among the causes of flaccid neurogenic bladder are myelomeningocele and spina bifida.

Bladder neuropathies.   In addition to central nervous system (CNS) conditions that disrupt bladder function, disorders of the peripheral (pelvic, pudendal, and hypogastric) neurons that supply the bladder can occur. These neuropathies can selectively interrupt sensory or motor pathways for the bladder or can involve both pathways. The most common causes of bladder neuropathies are diabetes mellitus and multiple sclerosis.

Epidemiologic studies indicate that diabetic bladder neuropathy occurs in 43% to 87% of insulin-dependent diabetics, with no age or sex difference.[8] Initially the disorder affects the sensory axons of the urinary bladder without involvement of the pudendal nerve. There is an insidious onset of bladder dysfunction during which time voidings gradually decrease until urine is passed only once or twice a day.[9] Frequently there is need for straining, accompanied by hesitation, weakness of the stream, dribbling, and a sensation of incomplete bladder emptying. The chief complication is infection, with development of vesicoureteral reflux and ascending pyelonephritis. Because persons with diabetes are at risk for developing glomerular disease (see Chap. 28), this can have serious effects on kidney function. Treatment consists of surgical methods to create a temporary urinary diversion, bladder training, and pharmacologic manipulation of bladder function with parasympathetic drugs.[10] As a means of compensating for the decreased contractile properties of the detrusor muscle, bladder neck resection may be done to decrease the resistance to outflow of urine from the bladder. Because the innervation of the external sphincter is not disturbed, continence is maintained.

Nonrelaxing external sphincter.   Another condition that affects the peripheral innervation of micturition is called *nonrelaxing external sphincter*.[11] This condition is usually related to a delay in maturation, developmental regress, psychomotor disorders, or locally irritative lesions. Inadequate relaxation of the external sphincter can be the result of anxiety or depression. Any local irritation can produce spasms of the sphincter by means of sensory input from the pudendal nerve; included are inflammation or irritation of the urethra, vaginitis, and perineal inflammation. In men, chronic prostatitis contributes to the impaired relaxation of the external sphincter.

Treatment

The goals of treatment for neurogenic bladder disorders focus on preventing bladder overdistention, urinary tract infections, and renal damage that can be life-threatening

and reducing the undesirable social and psychological effects of the disorder. The treatment is based on the type of neurologic lesion that is involved, information obtained through use of urodynamic studies, other health problems, and the ability of the individual to participate in the treatment. The treatment methods include catheterization, bladder training, pharmacologic manipulation of bladder function, and surgery.

Catheterization.   Catheterization involves the insertion of a small-diameter latex or silicon tube into the bladder through the urethra. The catheter may be inserted on a one-time basis to relieve temporary bladder distention, left indwelling (retention catheter), or inserted intermittently. With acute overdistention of the bladder, no more than 1000 ml of urine are removed from the bladder at one time. The theory behind this limitation is that removing more than this amount at one time releases pressure on the pelvic blood vessels and predisposes to shock.[5] Permanent indwelling catheters are used when there is urinary retention or incontinence in persons who are ill or debilitated or when conservative or surgical methods for the correction of incontinence are not feasible. The treatment of spinal cord injury patients with the use of permanent indwelling bladder catheters has been shown to produce a number of complications, including urinary tract infections, urethral irritation and injury, epididymo-orchitis, pyelonephritis, kidney stones, and bladder carcinoma.[12]

Intermittent catheterization is used to treat urinary retention or incomplete emptying secondary to various neurologic or obstructive disorders. Properly used, it prevents bladder overdistention and urethral irritation, allows for more freedom of activity, and provides for periodic distention of the bladder to prevent muscle atony. It is often used with pharmacologic manipulation to achieve continence; and when possible, it is learned and managed as a self-care procedure (intermittent self-catheterization). It may be carried out as either an aseptic (sterile) or a clean procedure. Aseptic intermittent catheterization is used in persons with spinal shock and in persons who need short-term catheterization. The clean procedure is usually for self-catheterization. It is performed at 3-hour to 4-hour intervals to prevent overdistention of the bladder. The best results are obtained if only 300 ml to 400 ml are allowed to collect in the bladder between catheterizations. The use of the clean as opposed to the sterile procedure has been defended on the basis that most urinary tract infections are due to some underlying abnormality of the urinary tract that leads to impaired tissue resistance to bacterial infection, the most common cause of which is decreased blood flow due to overdistention.[13] Overdistention has also been shown to decrease the mucin layer that protects the mucosal surface of the bladder.[14] Studies have shown up to a 48% decrease in bacteriuria after the institution of intermittent self-catheterization.[13] Intermittent self-catheterization has proved particularly effective in children with meningomyelocele.

Bladder training. Bladder training differs with the type of injury that is present. Training includes the use of body positions that facilitate micturition and the monitoring of fluid intake to prevent urinary tract infections and to control urine volume and osmolality.

Among the considerations when monitoring fluid intake is the need to insure adequate fluid intake to prevent an unduly concentrated urine that will stimulate afferent neurons of the micturition reflex. In hyperreflexive bladder or detrusor-sphincter dyssnergy, the stimulation of afferent nerve endings by irritating urine constituents results in increased vesicular pressures, vesicoureteral reflux, and overflow incontinence. On the other hand, fluid intake must be balanced to prevent bladder overdistention from occurring during the night. Adequate fluid intake is also needed to prevent urinary tract infections, the irritating effects of which increase bladder irritability and increase the risk of urinary incontinence and renal damage.

The methods used for bladder retraining depend on the type of lesion that is present. In spastic neurogenic bladder, methods designed to trigger the sacral micturition reflex are used; in flaccid neurogenic bladder, manual methods that increase intravesicular pressure are used. *Trigger voiding methods* include manual stimulation of the afferent loop of the micturition reflex through such maneuvers as tapping the suprapubic area, pulling on the pubic hairs, stroking the glans penis, or rubbing the thighs. *Credé's method,* which is done with the person in a sitting position, consists of applying pressure (with four fingers of one hand or both hands) to the suprapubic area as a means of increasing intravesicular pressure. Use of the Valsalva maneuver (bearing down by exhaling against a closed glottis) increases intra-abdominal pressure and aids in bladder emptying. This maneuver is repeated until the bladder is empty. For the best results, the patient must cooperate fully with the procedures or, if possible, learn to perform them independently.

Biofeedback methods have been useful for teaching some aspects of bladder control. Biofeedback involves the use of EMG or cystometry as a feedback signal for training a person to control the function of the external sphincter or raise intravesicular pressure enough to overcome outflow resistance.

Pharmacologic manipulation. Pharmacologic manipulation includes the use of drugs to increase the contractile properties of the bladder, decrease the outflow resistance of the internal sphincter, and relax the external sphincter. Often the usefulness of drug therapy is evaluated during cystometric studies. Bethanechol and methacholine may be used to increase detrusor muscle tone in spastic bladder. Methantheline and propantheline are used in spastic bladder to reduce vesicle tone and increase bladder capacity. Muscle relaxants such as diazepam (Valium) and baclofen (Lioresal) may be used to decrease the tone of the external sphincter. Table 31-1 describes the drugs that affect bladder function.

Surgical procedures. Among the surgical procedures used in the management of neurogenic bladder are sphincterectomy or transurethral resection of the bladder neck in men with prostatic hypertrophy, reconstruction of the sphincter, nerve resection (the sacral reflex nerves that cause spasticity or the pudendal nerve that controls the external sphincter), and urinary diversion. Extensive work is now being done to find a feasible means of implanting a stimulating electrode in the sacral canal around one or more of the sacral roots to control detrusor activity in persons with flaccid neurogenic bladder.[6]

Urinary diversion can be done by creating an ileal or a colon loop into which the ureters are anastomosed; the distal end of the loop is brought out and attached to the abdominal wall. Other procedures include the attachment of the ureters to the skin of the abdominal wall or the attachment of the ureters to the sigmoid colon with the rectum serving as a receptable for the urine.

Urinary Incontinence

The International Continence Society for Standardization of Terminology has defined incontinence as a condition in which involuntary loss of urine is a social or hygienic problem and is objectively demonstrable.[15] Incontinence occurs in all age groups. More than 90% of children are continent by 5 years of age. Many motor skills decline with age, and incontinence, although not a normal accompaniment of the aging process, is seen with increased frequency in the elderly. It has been reported that 10% of men and 17% of women over age 65 have problems with incontinence. The increase in health problems often seen in the elderly probably contributes to the greater frequency of incontinence.

Incontinence can be caused by a number of conditions. It can occur without the person's knowledge, and at other times the person may be aware of the condition but unable to prevent it. The International Continence Society for Standardization of Terminology has identified four categories of incontinence: stress incontinence, urgent incontinence, overflow incontinence, and reflex incontinence. Table 31-3 describes the mechanisms and characteristics of each of these types of incontinence. Other sources use other categories of incontinence, including a category called psychological incontinence.

Table 31-3   Types and Characteristics of Incontinence

Type of Incontinence	Characteristics
Stress incontinence	Involuntary loss of urine associated with activities, such as coughing, that increase intra-abdominal pressure
Urgency incontinence	Involuntary loss of urine associated with the desire to void
Overflow incontinence	Involuntary loss of urine when intravesicular pressure exceeds maximal urethral pressure in the absence of detrusor activity
Reflex incontinence	Involuntary loss of urine due to abnormal activity of the spinal cord reflex
Psychological incontinence	Awareness of need to urinate, but failure to respond appropriately due to conditions such as dementia or confusional state

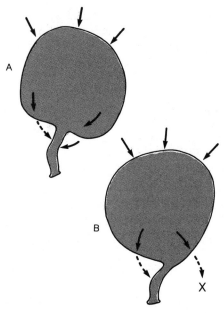

Figure 31-6   Importance of the posterior urethrovesical (PU-V) angle to the continence mechanism. (A) The presence of the normal PU-V angle permits maximal transmission (indicated by the arrows with dotted lines) on all sides of the proximal urethra of sudden changes in intra-abdominal pressure. In this way intraurethral pressure is maintained higher than the simultaneously elevated intravesicular pressure. This prevents loss of urine with sudden stress. (B) Loss of the PU-V angle results in displacement of the vesicle neck to the most dependent portion of the bladder, preventing the equal transmission of sudden increases in intra-abdominal pressure to the lumen of the proximal urethra. Thus, the pressure in the region of the vesical neck rises considerably more than the intraurethral pressure just beyond it, and stress incontinence occurs. (From Green JT, Jr: Obstet Gynecol Surv 23:603, 1968. Reprinted with permission.)

Stress incontinence.   Stress incontinence is the involuntary loss of urine that occurs when intravesicular (bladder) pressure exceeds maximal urethral pressure in the absence of detrusor activity.[15] Stress incontinence commonly occurs with the vesicular pressure changes instituted by coughing, laughing, lifting, or even climbing up and down stairs. It can result from weakness of the urethral sphincter and anatomic changes in the urethrovesical angle. In women, the angle between the bladder and the posterior proximal urethra (urethrovesical junction) is important to continence. Normally this angle is 90 to 100 degrees, with at least one-third of the bladder base contributing to the angle when not voiding (Fig. 31-6).[16] During the first stage of voiding this angle is lost as the bladder descends. In women, dimunition of muscle tone associated with normal aging, childbirth, or surgical procedures can cause weakness of the pelvic floor muscles and result in stress incontinence by obliterating the critical posterior urethrovesical angle. In these women loss of the posterior urethrovesical angle, descent and funneling of the bladder neck, and backward and downward rotation of the bladder occur, so that the bladder and urethra are already in an anatomic position for the first stage of voiding. Therefore, any activity that causes downward pressure on the bladder is sufficient to allow the urine to escape involuntarily.

Local urethral irritation caused by infection or a decreased estrogen effect can also precipitate incontinence. In men stress incontinence usually occurs only with urinary tract infection, radiation damage, or following surgical procedures such as a prostatectomy.

Urgency incontinence.   Urgency incontinence is the involuntary loss of urine associated with a strong desire to void. It can be subdivided into motor urgency incontinence associated with uninhibited detrusor contractions and sensory urgency incontinence that is not caused by uninhibited detrusor contractions.

Among the causes of urgency incontinence are those conditions in which a partial upper motor neuron lesion makes movement difficult, so that the interval between knowing the bladder needs to be emptied and the ability to stop it from emptying may be less than the time needed to reach the lavatory. Multiple sclerosis is a common cause of this type of incontinence. Musculoskeletal disorders such as arthritis or joint instability may also prevent an otherwise continent person from reaching the toilet in time.

Drugs such as hypnotics, tranquilizers, and sedatives can interfere with the conscious inhibition of voiding, leading to urgency incontinence. Diuretics, particularly in the elderly, increase the flow of urine and may contribute to incontinence, particularly in persons with diminished bladder capacity. Urinary infections, increased bladder irritability, urgency, and frequency occur in persons of all ages. In the elderly these conditions often precipitate incontinence.

Overflow incontinence. Overflow incontinence is an involuntary loss of urine that occurs when intravesicular pressure exceeds the maximal urethral pressure because of bladder distention in the absence of detrusor activity. It can occur with retention of urine due to nervous system lesions or obstruction of the bladder neck. With this type of incontinence the bladder is distended, and small amounts of urine are passed, particularly at night. In males, one of the most common causes of obstruction incontinence is enlargement of the prostate gland. Another cause that is often overlooked is fecal impaction (the presence of dry and hard feces in the rectum). When a large amount (bolus) of stool forms in the rectum it can push against the urethra and block the flow of urine. Medications such as beta-adrenergic blocking drugs can block the urine, leading to overflow incontinence.

Reflex incontinence. Reflex incontinence is due to abnormal activity in the spinal cord in the absence of sensation, usually associated with the desire to void. This occurs in persons with severe or complete upper or lower motor neuron lesions. It involves contraction of the bladder wall, with or without connection to the central nervous system, and is the basis for automatic micturition, previously described.

Psychological incontinence. The person with psychological incontinence may be aware of the need to urinate but make no effort to urinate in an appropriate setting. This occurs in dementia and confusional states. Because of the person's decreased mental acuity, it is often difficult to establish whether the need to urinate has not been sensed or the ability to act appropriately is impaired.

Diagnosis and treatment

Urinary incontinence is a frequent and major health problem. It increases social isolation, frequently leads to institutionalization, and predisposes to infections and skin breakdown.

Urinary incontinence is not a single disease but a symptom with many possible causes. As a symptom it requires full investigation to establish its cause. This is usually accomplished through a careful history and physical examination. Because many drugs affect bladder function, a full drug history is essential. Urodynamic studies may be needed to provide information about urinary pressures and urine flow rates.

The treatment or management depends on the type of incontinence that is present, accompanying health problems, and age. Exercises to strengthen the pelvic muscles and surgical correction of pelvic relaxation disorders are often used in women with stress incontinence. Noncatheter devices to obstruct urine flow or collect urine as it is passed may be used when urine flow cannot be controlled. Urinary incontinence is a major problem in the elderly, who have special treatment needs. Indwelling catheters (discussed earlier in the chapter), though a solution to the problem of urinary incontinence, are usually considered only after all other treatment methods have failed. In some types of incontinence, such as that associated with spinal cord injury or meningomyelocele, self-catheterization provides the means for controlling urine elimination.

Treatment of stress incontinence. Stress incontinence can be treated by physiotherapeutic measures, surgery, or a combination of the two. Surgical correction of cystocele and pelvic relaxation disorders in the female may be needed. Often, however, active muscle tensing exercises of the pelvic muscles may prove effective. These exercises were first advocated by Kegel, and hence they are often called *Kegel exercises*.[17] Two groups of muscles are strengthened: (1) those of the back part of the pelvic floor (these are the muscles used to contract the anus and control the passing of stool) and (2) the front muscles of the pelvic floor (these are the muscles used to stop the flow of urine during voiding). In learning the exercises, a woman concentrates on identifying the muscle groups and learning how to control contraction. Once this has been accomplished, she can start an exercise program that consists of slowly contracting the muscles, beginning at the front and working to the back while counting to four and then releasing. The exercises can be done while sitting or standing. Initially, doing four sets of exercises about once every hour is recommended.[18]

Noncatheter devices. Two types of noncatheter devices are commonly used in the management of urinary incontinence; one obstructs flow, and the other collects urine as it is passed. Obstruction of urine flow is achieved by compressing the urethra or stimulating the contraction of the pelvic floor muscles. Penile clamps are available that occlude the urethra without obstructing blood circulation to the penis. Because these devices obstruct blood flow if they are clamped too tightly, their usefulness is essentially limited to males with dribbling incontinence due to proximal urethral destruction, usually resulting from prostatic surgery. In females, compression of the urethra is usually accomplished by intravaginal devices. Surgically implanted artificial sphincters are available for use in both males and females.[19] These devices consist of an inflatable cuff that surrounds the proximal urethra. The cuff is connected by tubing to an implanted fluid reservoir and an inflation bulb. Pressing the bulb, which is placed in the scrotum in males, inflates the cuff. It is emptied in a similar manner. Another method of occluding the bladder outlet in both males and females is the use of battery-operated electrodes that cause contraction of the pelvic floor muscles. This treatment is most effective in women with stress incontinence due to weakness of the pelvic floor muscles. Implantable electrodes have largely been replaced by those that can be worn in the vagina or in the anus.

When urinary incontinence cannot be prevented, various types of urine collection devices or protective pads are used. Men can be fitted with collection devices (condom or sheath urinals) that are worn over the penis and attached to a container at the bedside or body. There are no effective external collection devices for women. Pants and pads are usually used. Dribbling bags (males) and pads (females) in which the urine turns to a nonpourable gel are available for occasional dribbling but are unsuitable for considerable wetting.

Special needs of the elderly.   Urinary incontinence is a common problem in the elderly. The incidence is reported to vary from 11% to 42%, depending on whether the survey is taken in the community or in the hospital.[20] Many factors contribute to incontinence in the elderly, many of which can be altered. Pelvic relaxation disorders occur more frequently in older than in younger females; and prostatic hypertrophy is more common in older than in younger males. Elderly persons often have difficulty in getting to the toilet on time. This can be caused by arthritis that makes walking or removing clothing difficult or by failing vision that makes trips to the bathroom precarious, especially in new and unfamiliar surroundings. Medication prescribed for other health problems may prevent a healthy bladder from functioning normally. Potent, fast-acting diuretics are known for their ability to cause urgency incontinence. Psychoactive drugs such as tranquilizers and sedatives may diminish normal attention to bladder clues. Impaired thirst or limited access to fluids predispose to constipation with urethral obstruction and overflow incontinence and to concentrated and infected urine, which increases bladder excitability.

According to Stanton, "there are two guiding principles in management of incontinence in the elderly. First, growing old does not imply becoming incontinent and, second, incontinence should not be left untreated just because the patient is old." Treatment may involve changes in the physical environment so that the older person can reach the bathroom more easily or remove clothing more quickly. It may require changes in the diet to prevent constipation or a plan for fluid intake that prevents urine from becoming concentrated and irritat-

ing to the bladder. Some of the common problems of elderly incontinent persons and suggested actions are described in Table 31-4.

In summary, alterations in bladder function include both urinary obstruction with retention of urine and urinary incontinence with involuntary loss of urine. Urinary retention occurs when the outflow of urine from the bladder is obstructed, because of either urethral obstruction or impaired bladder innervation. Urethral obstruction causes bladder irritability, detrusor muscle hypertrophy, trabeculation and the formation of diverticula, development of hydroureters, and eventual renal failure. Neurogenic bladder is caused by interruption in the innervation of the bladder. It can cause detrusor muscle hyperreflexia or areflexia, depending on the level of the lesion. Urinary incontinence occurs with involuntary loss of urine. It can present as stress incontinence, in which the loss of urine occurs with increases in bladder pressure such as that caused by coughing; urgency incontinence, in which there is a strong desire to void; overflow incontinence that results from bladder overdistention; reflex incontinence that is due to uncontrolled reflex activity of the sacral micturition reflex, such as occurs following spinal cord injury; or psychological incontinence, in which the person may be aware of the need to void but does not respond appropriately. The treatment of urinary obstruction, neurogenic bladder, and incontinence requires careful diagnosis to determine the cause and contributing factors.

■ Cancer of the Bladder

Bladder cancer is the most frequent form of urinary tract cancer, accounting for 37,000 new cases each year and 2.5% of cancer deaths in 1982.[21] It is seen most frequently in the 50- to 70-year age groups and occurs twice as frequently in men as in women.

Bladder cancers are described as papillary (characterized by polypoid lesions attached by stalks to the bladder mucosa), noninvasive (characterized by thickening of the mucosa but without penetration of the basement membrane), invasive (characterized by penetration into the mucosal basement membrane and possibly into other structures), and flat lesions that lack the well-defined structures of the papillary lesions. Flat lesions may be either *in situ* or invasive cancers and tend to be more anaplastic than the papillary tumors.[22] Almost 70% of bladder tumors are papillary, noninvasive, low-grade cancers and they have a good prognosis. Hematuria, obstruction, and infection are potential complications that require tumor removal. These tumors frequently recur; with each recurrence 10% to 20% will

**Table 31-4 Some Common Problems Found During Home
Assessments of Incontinent Patients**

Problem	Action
Toilet	
Outside, upstairs, or difficult to get to	Provide commode, grab rails, or personal urinal
Mobility and dexterity	
Impaired due to, *e.g.,* arthritis	Advise on use of walking and toilet aids and on suitable clothing
Vision	
Failing	May need to refer to a specialist
Constipation	Advise on diet; treatment with enemas may be necessary
Obesity	Start reducing diet
Fluid intake	
Often too low, leading to concentrated, possibly infected, and smelly urine	Increase fluid intake to 6–8 cups per day. Take MSU; antibiotic treatment may be required.
May be too high	Check amounts of fluid taken and restrict evening drinks
Medication	
May be on unnecessarily potent diuretics or on night-time sedatives, so sleeps through desire to void	Ask general practitioner to review medication
Depression	
Due to recent bereavement or loneliness	Show sympathy; suggest involvement in organized activities at day centers

Source: From Kennedy AP: Nursing and the incontinent patient. In Brocklehurst (ed): Urology in the Elderly. New York; Churchill Livingstone, 1984

have a higher cytologic grade, so that the prognosis for any person with papillary lesions may worsen with time.[23] Highly invasive bladder tumors constitute 25% to 30% of bladder cancers. These tumors may present as *in situ* lesions or progress rapidly to invasive lesions. The most common sites of metastasis are the pelvic lymph nodes, lungs, bones, and liver.

Although the cause of bladder cancer is unknown, evidence suggests that its origin is related to local influences such as carcinogens that are excreted in the urine and stored in the bladder. This includes the breakdown products of analine dyes used in the rubber and cable industry. Smoking also deserves attention. As many as 50% of cases of cancer in men and 33% in women may be attributed to this habit. It has been estimated that 3 mg of 2-naphthylamine, one of the first bladder carcinogens to be identified, is absorbed from the smoke of 20 unfiltered cigarettes.[24] Although earlier studies have suggested an association between bladder cancer and artificial sweeteners such as saccharin and cyclamates, this has not been proven. Chronic bladder infections and calculus disease also increase the risk of bladder cancer. Bladder cancer occurs among persons harboring the parasite *Schistosoma haematobium* in their bladders. It has been estimated that 85% of Egyptians are infected with the parasites, and bladder tumors represent 10% to 40% of all cancers in

Egypt.[22] It is not known whether the parasite excretes a carcinogen or produces its effects through irritation of the bladder.

Diagnosis and Treatment

The most common sign of bladder cancer is hematuria. Gross hematuria is a presenting sign in 75% of persons with the disease, and microscopic hematuria is present in most others. Occasionally frequency, urgency, and dysuria accompany the hematuria. Because hematuria is often intermittent, the diagnosis is often delayed. Periodic urine cytology is recommended for all persons who are at high risk for the development of bladder cancer because of exposure to urinary tract carcinogens.

The diagnostic methods include cytologic studies, excretory urograms, and cystoscopy and biopsy. High-grade cancers, including *in situ* lesions, are readily diagnosed in urinary samples using the Papanicolaou stain (Pap smear). Low-grade tumors are more difficult to detect by this method. Automated systems have been developed and are nearly ready for clinical use. They should be valuable in the detection and follow-up of persons with superficial cancers and may be adapted to the screening of select populations, such as persons with industrial exposure to carcinogenic agents. Ultrasonography and CT scans are used as an aid for staging of the tumor.

The treatment depends on the extent of the lesion and the health of the patient. Endoscopic resection is usually done for diagnostic purposes and may be used as a treatment for superficial lesions. Segmental surgical resection may be used for removing a large single lesion. Intravesicular instillation of chemotherapeutic drugs such as thiotepa, mitomycin C, and doxorubicin (Adriamycin) may be used in persons who present with cancer *in situ* or multiple superficial lesions.[23,24] When cancer is invasive, cystectomy with resection of the pelvic lymph nodes, prostate, seminal vesicles, and urethra in males is frequently the treatment of choice. Cystectomy requires urinary diversion. Preoperative radiotherapy appears to be beneficial for deeply infiltrating lesions.

In summary, cancer of the bladder is the most common form of urinary tract cancer, accounting for 37,000 new cases each year and 2.5% of all cancer deaths in the United States. Cancer of the bladder can present as low-grade papillary lesions and high-grade flat-type *in situ* or invasive lesions. The Pap smear is a useful screening test for high-grade carcinomas of the bladder. Although the cause of cancer of the bladder is unknown, evidence suggests that carcinogens excreted in the urine may play a role. Hematuria is the most common sign of bladder cancer, occurring in 75% of persons with the disease. Treatment of bladder cancer depends on the cytologic grade of the tumor and the extent of the invasiveness of the lesion.

■ Study Guide

After you have studied this chapter, you should be able to meet the following objectives:

☐ Cite the two functions of the bladder.

☐ Describe the structure of the bladder.

☐ Trace the innervation of the bladder from the afferent stretch receptors to reflex control of detrusor muscle contraction and voluntary control of the external sphincter.

☐ Explain the function of the parasympathetic and sympathetic nervous systems on bladder function.

☐ List five classes of autonomic drugs and explain their potential effect on bladder function.

☐ Describe at least three urodynamic studies that can be used to assess bladder function.

☐ State the signs of urinary retention.

☐ State the difference between bladder changes that occur during the spinal shock stage of spinal cord injury and those that occur following recovery of the spinal cord reflexes.

☐ Explain the common cause, symptoms, and dangers of autonomic hyperreflexia in a spinal cord injured patient.

☐ Differentiate between lesions that produce detrusor muscle hyperreflexia and those that produce detrusor muscle areflexia in terms of the level of the lesions and their effects on bladder function.

☐ Cite the pathology and causes of nonrelaxing external sphincter.

☐ Describe the symptoms of diabetic bladder neuropathy.

☐ State the rationale for the use of clean self-catheterization in terms of preventing bladder infections.

☐ Describe the difference between bladder training methods used for neurogenic bladder due to a lesion of the spinal cord micturition reflex center and to a lesion above the level of the reflex center.

☐ Define the four categories of incontinence recognized by the International Continence Society for Standardization of Terminology.

☐ Describe Kegel's exercises and explain their use in the control of stress incontinence.

☐ List at least four special problems of the elderly that contribute to the development of incontinence.

☐ State the most common sign of bladder cancer.

☐ Cite a possible mechanism responsible for the development of bladder cancer.

☐ Relate the use of the urine Pap smear to the detection of bladder cancer.

■ References

1. McGuire EJ: Physiology of the lower urinary tract. Am J Kidney Dis 2, No 4:402, 1983
2. McGuire EJ: Urinary dysfunction in the aged: Neurological considerations. Bull NY Acad Med 56:275, 1980
3. Berne RM, Levy MN: Physiology, p 890. St Louis, CV Mosby, 1983
4. Mahoney DT, Laferte RL, Blias DJ: Integral storage function and voiding reflexes. Urology 9:95, 1977
5. McConnell EA, Zimmerman MF: Care of Patients with Urologic Problems, pp 32. Philadelphia, JB Lippincott, 1983
6. Smith DR: General Urology, 11th ed, p 156. Los Altos, CA, Lange Medical Publishers, 1984

7. Krane RJ, Siroky MB: Clinical Neuro-Urology. Boston, Little, Brown, 1979

8. Fimodt-Moller C: Diabetic cystopathy: Epidemiology and related disorders. Ann Intern Med 92, P 2:318, 1980

9. Ellenberg M: Development of urinary bladder dysfunction in diabetes mellitus. Ann Intern Med 92, P 2:321, 1980

10. Frimodt-Moller C, Mortenson S: Treatment of diabetic cystopathy. Ann Intern Med 92, P 2:327, 1980

11. Thon W, Altwein JE: Voiding dysfunction. Urology 23:323, 1984

12. Jacobs SC, Kaufman JM: Complications of permanent bladder catheter drainage in spinal cord injury patients. J Urology 119:740, 1978

13. Lapides J, Diokno AC, Silber SJ: Clean, intermittent self-catheterization in treatment of urinary tract disease. Trans Am Assoc Genitourin Surg 63:92, 1971

14. Perlow DL, Gikas PW, Horwitz EM: Effects of vesicle overdistention on bladder mucin. Urology 18:380, 1981

15. Bates P, Bradley WE, Glen E et al: The standardization of terminology of lower urinary tract function. J Urology 121:551, 1979

16. Green TH: Urinary stress incontinence: Differential diagnosis, pathophysiology, and management. Am J Obstet Gynecol 122:368, 1975

17. Kegel AH: Progressive resistance exercises in the functional restoration of the perineal muscles. Am J Obstet Gynecol 56:238, 1948

18. Mandelstam D: Strengthening the pelvic floor muscles. Geriatrics Nurs 1:251, 1980

19. Brocklehurst JC: Noncatheter devices for urinary incontinence in the elderly. Med Instrum 16, No 3:167, 1982

20. Stanton SL: Surgical management of female incontinence. In Brocklehurst JC: Urology in the Elderly, p 93. New York, Churchill Livingstone, 1984

21. Frank IN, Keys HM, McCune CS: Urologic and male genital cancers. In Rubin P: Clinical Oncology, 6th ed, p 205. New York, American Cancer Society, 1983

22. Robbins SL, Cotran RS, Kumar V: Pathologic Basis of Disease, 2nd ed, p 1072. Philadelphia, WB Saunders, 1984

23. Murphy WM: Current topic in the pathology of bladder cancer. Pathol Annu 18, P 1:1, 1983

24. Wynder EL, Goldsmith K: The epidemiology of bladder cancer: A second look. Cancer 40:1246, 1977

deGroat WC, Booth AM: Physiology of the urinary bladder and urethra. Ann Intern Med 92, P2:312, 1980

Field MA: Urinary incontinence in the elderly: An overview. J Gerontol Nurs 5:12, 1979

Fossberg E, Beisland HO, Sander S: Urinary continence in old age. Ann Chir Gynaecol 71:228, 1982

Freed SZ: Urinary incontinence in the elderly. Hosp Pract 17:81, 1982

Gershon CR: Rebirth of an old technique—the use of clean, intermittent self-catheterization. J Med Assoc Ga 71:605, 1982

Helzer MJ, Bartone FF: Intermittent self-catheterization: A revolutionary breakthrough. Nebr Med J 4:73, 1982

Kaufman JM: Stress urinary incontinence: Current concepts of diagnosis and treatment. J SC Med Assoc 98:671, 1982

Keegan GT, McNichols DW: The evaluation and treatment of urinary incontinence in the elderly. Surg Clin North Am 62:261, 1982

Mastri AR: Neuropathology of diabetic neurogenic bladder. Ann Intern Med 92, P2:316, 1980

Mix LC: Occult neuropathic bladder. Urology 10:1, 1977

Murphy WM, Soloway MS: Developing carcinoma (dysplasia) of the urinary bladder. Pathol Annu 18, P1:197, 1983

Pierson CA: Urinary incontinence: New methods of diagnosis and treatment. JOGN Nursing 10:407, 1981

Rawl JC: Clean intermittent catheterization-an update. J SC Med Assoc 78:715, 1982

Sheperd A, Tribe E, Torrens MJ: Simple practical techniques in the management of urinary incontinence. Inter Rehabil Med 4:15, 1982

Soloway MS: Bladder cancer: Management of an increasingly common tumor. Postgrad Med 73:138, 1983

Weiss RM: Clinical correlations of ureteral physiology. Am J Kidney Dis 2:409, 1983

Wells T: Promoting urine control in older adults. Geriatric Nurs 1:236, 1980

Williams ME, Pannill FC: Urinary incontinence in the elderly. Ann Intern Med 97:895, 1982

Willington FL: Urinary incontinence: A practical approach. Geriatrics 6:41, 1980

■ Additional References

Abramson AS: Neurogenic bladder: A guide to evaluation and management. Arch Phys Med Rehabil 64:6, 1983

Bissada NK, Finkbeiner AE: Pharmacology of continence and micturition. AFP 20:128, 1979

Bradley WE: Autonomic neuropathy and the genitourinary system. J Urol 119:299, 1978

Bradley WE: Diagnosis of urinary bladder dysfunction in diabetes mellitus. Ann Intern Med 92, P2:323, 1980

Chapter 32

Structure and Function of the Male Genitourinary System

Stephanie MacLaughlin

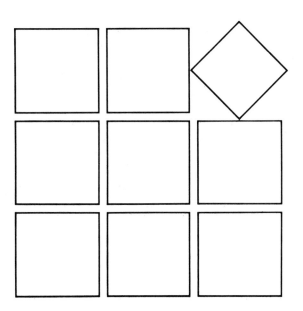

The male genitourinary system consists of a pair of gonads, the testes, a system of excretory ducts, and the accessory organs. The accessory organs include the penis, the bulbourethral glands, the prostate gland, and the seminal vesicles. This system has two basic functions—urine elimination and reproduction. The embryonic development of the male reproductive structures, structure of the male genitourinary system, spermatogenesis, sexual performance, hormonal regulation of reproductive function in the male, and changes in genitourinary function that occur at the time of puberty and as a result of the aging process are discussed in this chapter.

■ Genitourinary Structures

Embryonic Development

The sex of an individual is determined at the time of fertilization by the sex chromosomes. In the early stages of embryonic development the tissues from which the male and female reproductive organs develop are undifferentiated. Until approximately the seventh week of gestation, it is impossible to determine whether the embryo is male or female unless the chromosomes are studied. Until this time, the genital tracts of both the male and the female consist of two wolffian ducts, from which the male genitalia develop, and two müllerian ducts, from which the female genital structures develop. During this period of gestation, the gonads (ovaries and testes) are also undifferentiated.

In the seventh week of embryonic life a portion of the gonads differentiates into the testes in males. At this point, the gonadal ridge of an embryo with XY chromosomes develops into testes and that with XX chromosomes develops into ovaries. The fetal testes produce two hormones: one stimulates development of the wolffian ducts into structures that form seminal vesicles, vas deferens, and epididymis; the other suppresses the development of female genital structures from the müllerian ducts. Development of the external male genital structures begins during the twelfth week of embryonic life. It is the absence or presence of the androgen testosterone that determines whether an embryo will develop male or female genital structures. In the absence of testosterone, a male embryo with an XY chromosomal pattern will develop female genitalia. It has been hypothesized that the Y chromosome contains a gene that codes for a substance called the H-Y antigen. In the presence of the H-Y antigen, the embryonic gonads develop into testes and in its absence the gonads develop into ovaries.[1]

Testes and Scrotum

The testes, or male gonads, are two egg-shaped structures located outside the abdominal cavity in the scrotum, where they are suspended by the spermatic cord (Fig. 32-1). The spermatic cord is composed of the arteries, veins, lymphatics, and excretory ducts that supply the testes. The cremaster muscle that suspends the testes and forms the muscle of the scrotum is also contained in the spermatic cord. The testes are responsible for both testosterone and sperm production.

The scrotum, which houses the testes, is made up of an outer skin layer, which forms rugae or folds and is continuous with the perineum and outer skin of the thighs. Under the outer skin lies a thin layer of muscle and fascia, the *tunica dartos*. This layer contains a septum that separates the two testes.

A function of the scrotum is to *regulate the temperature of the testes*. The optimum temperature for sperm production is about 2 to 3 degrees below body temperature. If the testicular temperature is too low, the muscles within the scrotum contract, causing the testes to be brought up tight against the body. On the other hand, when the testicular temperature rises, the muscles relax, which allows the scrotal sac to fall away from the body. Some tight-fitting undergarments hold the testes against the body and are thought to contribute to infertility by interfering with the thermoregulatory function of the scrotum. Cryptorchidism, the failure of the testes to descend into the scrotum, also exposes the testes to the higher temperature of the body.

The testes and epididymis are enclosed in a double-layered membrane, the *tunica vaginalis*, which is derived embryonically from the abdominal peritoneum. An outer covering, the *tunica albuginea*, is a tough white fibrous sheath that resembles the sclera of the eye. The tunica albuginea protects the testes and gives them their ovoid shape.

Embryologically, the testes do not develop within the scrotal sac; they develop in the abdominal cavity and then descend through the inguinal canal into a long pouch of peritoneum (which becomes the tunica vaginalis) in the scrotum during the seventh to the ninth month of fetal life. The descent of the testes is thought to be caused by the male hormone, testosterone, which is very active during this stage of development. Just prior to birth, the inguinal canal closes almost completely. Failure of this canal to close predisposes to the development of an inguinal hernia later in life.

Duct system

Internally, the testes are composed of several hundred compartments or lobules (Fig. 32-2). Each lobule contains one or more coiled *seminiferous* tubules. These

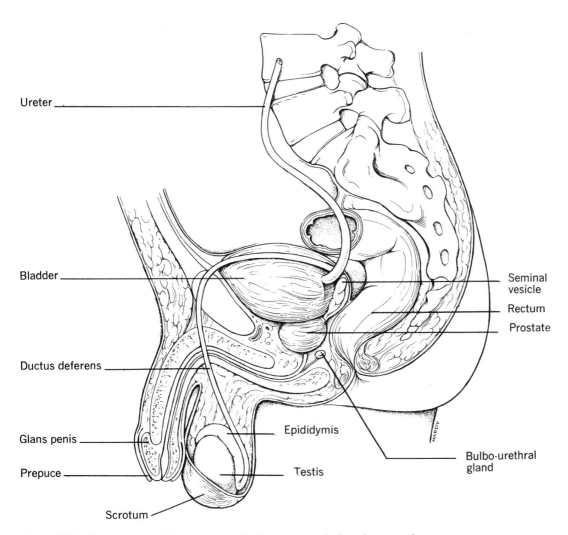

Figure 32-1 *The structures of the male reproductive system, including the testes, the scrotum, and the excretory ducts. (From Chaffee EE, Greisheimer EM: Basic Physiology and Anatomy, 3rd ed. Philadelphia, JB Lippincott, 1974)*

tubules are the site of sperm production. As the tubules lead into the *efferent ducts*, the seminiferous tubules become the *rete testis*. Ten thousand to 20,000 efferent ducts emerge from the rete testis to join the epididymis, which is the final site for sperm maturation. Interspersed in the connective tissue that fills the spaces between the seminiferous tubules are the epithelial cells—the *cells of Leydig*—which produce *testosterone*.

Accessory organs
Sperm are transported through the reproductive structures by movement of the seminal fluid, which is combined with secretions from the accessory sex glands, epididymis, seminal vesicles, prostate, and Cowper's glands. When sperm is combined with the seminal plasma it is called *semen*.

The sperm enters the epididymis from the efferent ductules in the testes. Because the sperm are not mobile at this stage of development, peristaltic movements of the ductal walls of the epididymis aid in sperm movement. The sperm continue their migration through the *ductus deferens*, or vas deferens, and enter the *ampulla*, where they are stored until they are released through ejaculation (Fig 32-3). Sperm can be stored in the genital ducts for as long as 42 days and still maintain their fertility. The ampulla joins with the *seminal vesicle*, which secretes a fluid containing fructose and other substances required to nourish the sperm. The seminal vesicle leads into the *ejaculatory duct*, which enters the posterior part of the prostate, and continues through this gland until it ends in the prostatic portion of the urethra. The *prostate* adds a thin, milky, alkaline fluid to the semen. The optimum *p*H

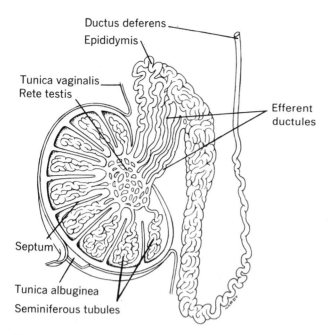

Figure 32-2 *The parts of the testes and epididymis. (From Chaffee EE, Lytle IM: Basic Physiology and Anatomy, 4th ed. Philadelphia, JB Lippincott, 1980)*

for sperm mobilization is 6.0 to 6.5. The alkaline nature of the prostatic fluid is necessary for successful fertilization of the ovum, because both the fluid from the vas deferens and the vaginal secretions of the female are strongly acid.

The *bulbourethral,* or *Cowper's glands,* lie on either side of the membranous urethra. These glands secrete an alkaline mucus which probably aids in neutralizing acids from urine that remains in the urethra.

A man usually ejaculates about 2 ml to 5 ml of semen. The ejaculate may vary with frequency of intercourse. It is less with frequent ejaculation and may increase two to four times its normal amount following periods of abstinence. The semen that is ejaculated is largely fluid—98% fluid and only about 2% sperm.

Penis

The penis is the external genital organ through which the urethra passes. Anatomically, the external penis consists of a shaft that ends in a tip called the *glans* (Fig. 32-4). The loose skin of the penis shaft folds to cover the glans, forming the *prepuce,* or *foreskin*. It is this cuff of skin that is removed during *circumcision.* In some situations, an adult who has not been circumcised as an infant may need to have the foreskin removed. For instance, the foreskin may become too tight and reduce blood flow or it may not be retractable for cleaning purposes. Usually circumcision is a religious (Moslem and Jewish) or social (United States) custom. Most male infants in the United States are circumcised shortly after birth. The value of the procedure is controversial. It has been proposed that uncircumcised males and their sexual partners may have a higher incidence of genital cancer that those who were circumcised. This may, however, have resulted from sexual habits or lack of hygiene, rather than lack of circumci-

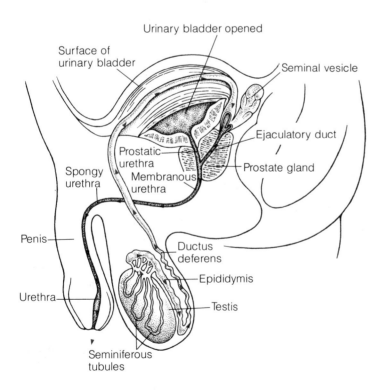

Figure 32-3 *The excretory ducts of the male reproductive system and the path that sperm follows as it leaves the testis and travels to the urethra. (From Chaffee EE, Gresheimer EM: Basic Physiology and Anatomy, 3rd ed. Philadelphia, JB Lippincott, 1974)*

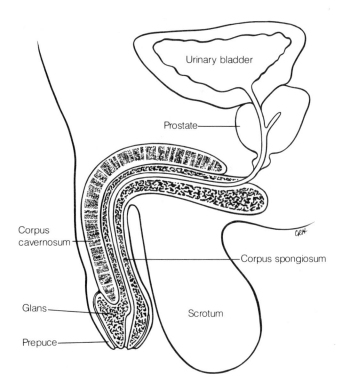

Figure 32-4   *Sagittal section of the penis, showing the prepuce, glans, corpus cavernosum, and corpus spongiosum.*

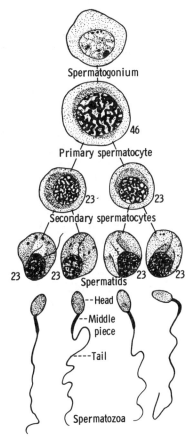

Figure 32-5   *The various stages of spermatogenesis. (From Chaffee EE, Lytle IM: Basic Physiology and Anatomy, 4th ed. Philadelphia, JB Lippincott, 1980)*

sion. One practical argument for circumcision is cleanliness. The uncircumcised male must retract his foreskin and remove any accumulation (smegma) produced by the oil glands in the foreskin. If this is not done, the resulting irritation may cause inflammation and infection. Should the inflammation become chronic, it may predispose to cancer of the penis.

The glans of the penis contains many sensory nerves, making this the most sensitive portion of the penile shaft. The cylindrical body or shaft of the penis is composed of three masses of erectile tissue held together by fibrous strands and covered with skin. The two lateral masses of tissue are called the *corpora cavernosa*. The third ventral mass is called the *corpus spongiosum*. The cavernous masses are erectile tissue that distends with blood during penile erection.

In its normal flaccid state, the penis hangs down loosely. The flaccid penis is 3 to 4 inches long; the erectile penis, 5 to 7 inches long. The penis may temporarily decrease in size in situations such as cold weather, failed intercourse, or extreme exhaustion. Aging may also cause it to decrease in size. Contrary to popular belief, the size of the penis has no relationship to race, body build, sexual prowess, or frequency of intercourse.

In summary, the male genitourinary system functions in both urine elimination and reproduction. The reproductive system consists of a pair of gonads (the testes), a

system of excretory ducts (seminiferous tubules and efferent ducts), the accessory organs (epididymis, seminal vesicles, prostate and Cowper's glands), and the penis. The sex of an individual is determined by the sex chromosomes at the time of fertilization. During the seventh week of gestation, the XY chromosome pattern in the male is responsible for the development of the testes with the subsequent production of testosterone and testosterone-stimulated development of the internal and external male genital structures. Prior to this period of embryonic development, the tissues from which the reproductive structures of the male and female develop are undifferentiated. In the absence of testosterone production, the male embryo with an XY chromosomal pattern will develop female genitalia.

■ Reproductive Function

Spermatogenesis

The *mature sperm cell,* or *spermatozoon,* is made up of an oval head, a neck, a middle piece, and a tail (Fig. 32-5). The *head* consists mainly of nuclear material with only a small amount of cytoplasm. The cytoplasm in the head is called the *acrosome* and is believed to contain the enzymes necessary for penetration and fertilization of the ovum. The *neck* connects the head to the middle piece, which is composed of a cylindrical fascicle called the axial filament. The middle piece is concerned with the metabolic activity, and the *tail* with the propulsion, of the sperm.

Spermatogenesis, as mentioned earlier, occurs in the seminiferous tubules of the testes. These tubules, if placed end to end, would measure about 750 feet. The outer layer of the seminiferous tubules is made up of connective tissue and smooth muscle; the inner lining is composed of Sertoli cells, within which are embedded the spermatogonia and sperm at various stages of maturation. The tubules are lined with sperm cells in various stages of development, and it is these cells that eventually become the mobile spermatozoa (Fig. 32-6).

The layer of cells that lie adjacent to the tubule wall are the small unspecialized germinal cells called the *spermatogonia*. These cells undergo rapid mitotic division, providing a continuous source of new germinal cells. As the cells multiply the more mature spermatogonia divide into two "daughter cells," which grow in size and become the *primary spermatocytes*. These large primary

spermatocytes divide by meiosis to form two smaller *secondary spermatocytes*. Each of the secondary spermatocytes, in turn, divides to form two *spermatids*, or infant sperm. These spermatids burrow into the Sertoli cells, which are dispersed throughout the seminiferous tubules, until they reach maturity. As the spermatids grow to full size and increase in maturity, they move into the epididymis for final maturation and storage. Each tubule contains germ cells in various stages of development, so that a continuous supply is readily available.

The entire process of spermatogenesis takes about 60 to 70 days. The sperm count in a normal ejaculate is about 100 million to 400 million. *Infertility* may occur when an insufficient number of motile, healthy sperm is present.

Hormonal Control of Male Reproductive Function

The male sex hormones are called androgens. Testosterone is the main androgen produced in the testes. The adrenal cortex also produces androgens, but in much smaller quantities than the testes. Over 95% of the tes-

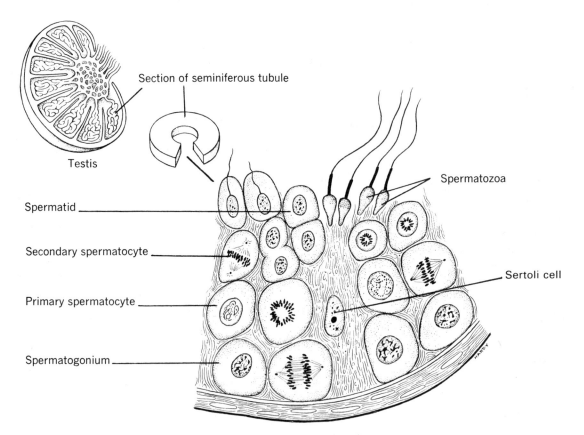

Figure 32-6   *A section of a seminiferous tubule, showing the various stages of spermatogenesis. (From Chaffee EE, Lytle IM: Basic Physiology and Anatomy, 4th ed. Philadelphia, JB Lippincott, 1980)*

tosterone is secreted by the testes; the remainder is secreted by the adrenals.

Testosterone is secreted by the interstitial cells of Leydig in the testes. It is metabolized in the liver and then excreted by the kidneys. In the bloodstream testosterone exists as a free or a bound form. The bound form is attached to plasma proteins, including albumin and the sex-hormone binding protein produced by the liver. About 2% is not bound and is able to enter the cell and exert its metabolic effects. Testosterone exerts a variety of biologic effects in the male (Table 32-1). In the male embryo, testosterone is essential for the appropriate differentiation of the internal and external genitalia. Testosterone is essential to the development of primary and secondary male sex characteristics during puberty and for the maintenance of these characteristics during adult life. In addition, androgens function as anabolic agents in both males and females to promote metabolism and musculoskeletal growth.

The hypothalamus and the anterior pituitary gland play an essential role in promoting spermatogenic activity in the testes and maintaining endocrine function of the testes by means of the gonadotropic hormones. The release of gonadotropic hormones from the pituitary gland is regulated by the gonadotropic-releasing factor (GnRH), which is synthesized by the hypothalamus and secreted into the hypothalamohypophyseal portal blood (Fig. 32-7). Two gonadotropic hormones are secreted by the pituitary gland: follicle-stimulating hormone (FSH) and luteinizing hormone (LH). In the male, LH is also called interstitial cell stimulating hormone (ICSH).

The production of testosterone by the interstitial cells of Leydig is regulated by LH (Fig. 32-7). FSH binds selectively to the Sertoli cells, where it functions in the initiation of spermatogenesis. Although FSH is necessary for the initiation of spermatogenesis, full maturation of the spermatozoa requires testosterone. The Sertoli cells produce an androgen-binding protein which binds testosterone; one of the major actions of FSH may be the regulation of androgen-binding protein production by the Sertoli cells as a means of maintaining high intratubular concentrations of testosterone.

Circulating levels of the gonadotropic hormones are regulated in a negative feedback manner by testosterone. High levels of testosterone produce a negative feedback suppression of LH secretion through a direct action on the pituitary and an inhibitory effect on the hypothalamus. FSH is thought to be inhibited by a substance called *inhibin*, which is produced by the Sertoli cells. Inhibin appears to act mainly at the level of the pituitary gland.[1] Unlike the cyclic hormonal pattern in the female, in the male FSH, LH, and testosterone secretion and spermatogenesis occur at relatively unchanging rates during adulthood.

Table 32-1   Main Actions of Testosterone

Differentiation of the male genital tract during fetal development
Development of primary and secondary sex characteristics
   Growth and maintenance of gonadal function
   External genitalia and accessory organs
   Male voice timbre
   Male skin characteristics
   Male hair distribution
Anabolic effects
   Protein metabolism
   Musculoskeletal growth
   Subcutaneous fat distribution
Spermatogenesis (in FSH-primed tubules)
   and maturation of sperm

Neural Control of Sexual Function

Erection and ejaculation are under the control of the autonomic nervous system. Erection can occur at all ages, even in infant boys a few hours after birth and quite elderly men. The capacity for voluntary erection usually develops with the onset of puberty.

Erection is initiated by parasympathetic fibers that originate in the second and fourth segments of the sacral cord and are transmitted by the nervi erigentes. The impulses cause dilatation of the penile arteries and compression of the penile veins. The increased blood supply to the penis and subsequent engorgement of the corpora cavernosa and the corpus spongiosum result in erection.

The process of *ejaculation* is initiated by peristaltic movements along the ductile pathways from the testes,

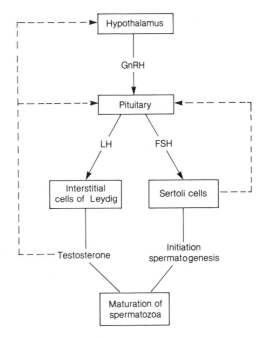

Figure 32-7 *Hypothalamic–pituitary feedback control of spermatogenesis and testosterone levels in the male.*

the epididymis, the seminal vesicles, and the prostate gland. Increased pressure causes expulsion of semen. The bulbourethral glands secrete additional fluid. *Emission* of semen is brought about by sympathetic impulses that leave the spinal cord at lumbar segments 1 and 2 and pass through the hypogastric plexus to the genitalia. Ejaculation is then caused by contraction of the muscles at the base of the penis, which are innervated by fibers of the pudendal nerve.

After ejaculation, sympathetic outflow causes vasoconstriction of the arteries of the penis, and as a result, the inflow of blood is decreased and *detumescence*, or decreased penile turgor, occurs. The man then passes through a refractory period during which he is unable to have an erection or ejaculation in response to sexual stimuli.

Pubertal Changes

At the time of puberty, the male gonads and testes begin to mature and begin to carry out spermatogenesis and hormone production. Sometime around the age of 10 or 11, the adenohypophysis, or anterior pituitary, begins to secrete the gonadotropins that stimulate testicular function and cause the interstitial cells to begin producing testosterone. About the same time, hormonal stimulation induces mitotic activity of the spermatogonia and primary spermatocytes. Once cell maturation has begun, the testes begin to enlarge rapidly as the individual tubules grow. Full maturity and spermatogenesis are usually attained by age 15 or 16.

Aging Changes

Like other body systems, the male reproductive system undergoes degenerative changes as a result of the aging process; it becomes less efficient with age. The declining physiologic efficiency of male reproductive function occurs gradually and involves the endocrine, circulatory, and neuromuscular systems. Compared with the marked physiologic change in aging females, the changes in the aging male are more gradual and less drastic. Gonadal and reproductive failure are not generally related directly to age, because a male remains fertile into advanced age. Eighty- and 90-year-olds have been known to father children.

Contrary to popular belief, many investigators negate a physiologic basis for what has been termed the male climacteric. Instead, they attribute its symptomatology to psychologic mechanisms. An aging man may experience midlife crisis with concomitant psychosomatic manifestations that mimic the menopausal symptomatology. Most experts agree that male sexual desire declines at a parallel rate with physical vigor and

represents the aging of all the body tissues and neural structures.

As the male ages, his reproductive system is measurably different in both structure and function from that of the younger male. The male sex hormones, particularly testosterone, decrease with age, starting later, on the average, than in women. The sex hormones play a part in the structure and function of the reproductive system and other body systems from conception to old age; they affect protein synthesis, salt and water balance, bone growth, and cardiovascular function. Decreasing levels of testosterone affect sexual energy, muscle strength, and the genital tissues. The testes become smaller and lose their firmness. The seminiferous tubules, which produce spermatozoa, thicken and begin a degenerative process which finally inhibits sperm production, resulting in a decrease of viable spermatozoa.[2] The prostate gland enlarges, and its contractions become weaker. The force of ejaculation decreases because of a reduction in the volume and viscosity of the seminal fluid. The seminal vesicle changes little from childhood to puberty. The pubertal increases in the fluid capacity of the gland remain throughout adulthood and then decline after age 60. After 60, the walls of the seminal vesicles thin, the epithelium decreases in height, and the muscle layer is replaced by connective tissue. Age-related changes in the penis consist of fibrotic changes in the trabeculae in the corpus spongiosum, with progressive sclerotic changes in both arteries and veins. Sclerotic changes also follow in the corpora cavernosa, the condition becoming generalized in the 55- to 60-year-old age group.[3]

As a sexual partner, the aging male exhibits some differences in responsiveness and activity from his younger counterpart. Masters and Johnson (1970) studied the significant aging changes in the physiology of the sex act.[4] They noted that frequency of intercourse, intensity of sensation, speed of attaining erection, and force of ejaculation are all reduced.

Many of our social and cultural practices do not support or encourage sexual activity in the elderly. Research, however, indicates that not only does sexual thought and feeling continue into old age but sexual activity also continues for most healthy older individuals.[5] Most gerontologists would agree that continued sexual interest and activity can be therapeutic for the elderly.

Sexual dysfunction in the elderly male is often directly related to the general physical condition of the individual. Diseases that accompany aging can have direct bearing on male reproductive organs. Various cardiovascular, respiratory, hormonal, neurologic, and hematologic disorders can be responsible for secondary impotence. For example, vascular disease affects male potency because it may impair blood flow to the pudendal arteries or their tributaries, resulting in loss of blood volume with subsequent poor distention of the vascular spaces of erectile tissue. Other diseases affecting potency include hypertension, diabetes, cardiac disease, and malignancies of the reproductive organs.[5]

In summary, the function of the male reproductive system is under the negative feedback control of the hypothalamus and the anterior pituitary gonadotropic hormones FSH and LH. Spermatogenesis is initiated by FSH, and the production of testosterone is regulated by LH. Testosterone, the major sex hormone in the male, is produced by the interstitial cells of Leydig in the testes. In addition to the differentiation of the internal and external genitalia in the male embryo, testosterone is essential for the development of secondary male characteristics during puberty, the maintenance of these characteristics during adult life, and spermatozoa maturation.

Like other body systems, the male reproductive system undergoes changes as a result of the aging process. The changes occur gradually and involve parallel changes in endocrine, circulatory, and neuromuscular function. Testosterone levels decrease, the size and firmness of the testes decrease, sperm production declines, and the prostate gland enlarges. There is usually a decrease in frequency of intercourse, intensity of sensation, speed of attaining erection, and force of ejaculation. However, sexual thought, interest, and activity usually continue into old age.

■ Study Guide

After you have studied this chapter, you should be able to meet the following objectives:

- ☐ Describe the anatomy of the testes and scrotum.
- ☐ Describe the anatomy of the duct system and accessory organs.
- ☐ Explain why circumcision might be considered a desirable practice.
- ☐ Describe the process of spermatogenesis.
- ☐ State the name of the testicular cells that produce testosterone.
- ☐ State the functions of testosterone.
- ☐ Draw a diagram illustrating the secretion, site of action, and feedback control of GnRH, LH, and FSH.
- ☐ Describe the function of FSH in terms of spermatogenesis.
- ☐ Describe the autonomic nervous system control of erection and ejaculation.
- ☐ Describe changes in the male reproductive system that occur with aging.

■ References

1. Greenspan FS, Forshan PH: Basic and Clinical Endocrinology. pp 339-343. Los Altos, CA, Lange Medical Publications, 1983
2. Weg, RB: Normal aging changes in the reproductive system. In Burnside, (ed): Nursing and the Aged, pp 362-374. New York, McGraw-Hill, 1981
3. Croft, LH: Physiology of aging. In Sexuality in Later Life, pp 47-65. Boston, John Wright, 1982
4. Masters WH, Johnson V: Human Sexual Inadequacy, pp 337-338. Boston, Little, Brown, 1970
5. Yeaworth RC, Friedman JS: Sexuality in later life. Nurs Clin North Am 10, No 3:565-575, September 1975

Chapter 33

Alterations in the Structure and Function of the Male Genitourinary System

Stephanie MacLaughlin

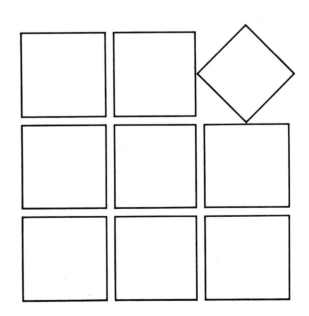

The male genitourinary system is subject to structural defects, inflammation, and neoplasms, with effects on urine elimination, sexual function, and fertility. This chapter discusses disorders of the penis, the scrotum and testes, and the prostate.

Disorders of the Penis

The penis houses the urethra and the erectile tissue, which becomes engorged with blood during sexual stimulation. Disorders of the penis include congenital and acquired defects, inflammatory conditions, and neoplasms.

Hypospadias and Epispadias

Hypospadias is a congenital defect present in about 1 out of every 400 to 500 male infants. In this disorder, the termination of the urethra is on the *ventral* surface of the penis. A less common defect is epispadias, in which the opening of the urethra is on the *dorsal* surface of the penis (Fig. 33-1). Both of these abnormalities are often accompanied by other congenital defects, such as undescended testicles and chordee, or ventral bowing, of the penis.

Surgery is required for the correction of both hypospadias and epispadias. Infants born with these disorders are not circumcised because the foreskin is required in the plastic surgery done to correct the defect. When

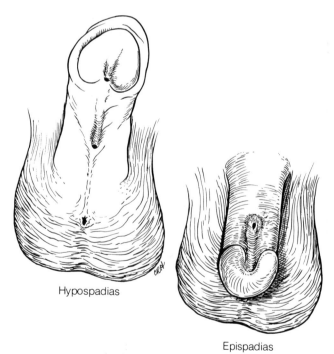

Hypospadias

Epispadias

Figure 33-1 Hypospadias and epispadias.

additional deformities such as chordee are present, the surgical repair procedure may be done in stages. Usually, it is suggested that surgical correction be done before the child enters school. The adult male who has not undergone surgery will not have problems with erection or sexual function, but his semen may run out of the vagina during intercourse and thus interfere with impregnation.

Phimosis

Phimosis is a tightening of the penile foreskin that prevents its retraction over the glans. Although phimosis is usually congenital, it may result from inflammation, with formation of scar tissue. When the foreskin is too tight to be retracted, excess oil gland secretions and smegma accumulate under the prepuce and may cause inflammation and infection. In the adult, phimosis can prevent erection. In both children and adults, circumcision is usually the treatment of choice.

In a related condition called *paraphimosis*, the foreskin is so tight and constricted that it cannot cover the glans. As with phimosis, accumulated secretions and microorganisms can cause inflammation and infection. A very tight foreskin can constrict the blood supply to the glans and lead to ischemia and necrosis.

Priapism

Priapism is a nonsexual, prolonged, painful erection that can persist for hours or days. The condition is caused by malfunction of the posterior venous valves with a resultant trapping of blood in the corpora cavernosa; this causes the cavernosa to remain hard while the rest of the penis becomes flaccid or relaxes. If the erection persists, there is danger of thrombosis with ischemia and necrosis.

The cause of priapism is uncertain. It is most common in the age group of 30 to 40 years and is seldom seen in children or in the elderly. Priapism is associated with tumors that encroach on the penile veins, injury to the penis, prolonged sexual stimulation, and diseases that impair venous drainage from the penis following erection. For instance, sickle cell disease is associated with increased incidence of priapism. Antihypertensive drugs, antianxiety medications, and testosterone have also been known to precipitate the condition.

The treatment includes application of ice packs to the penis and sedation. Hospitalization is usually required. When this less aggressive treatment does not correct the problem, shunt surgery to reroute the blood from the corpora cavernosa into veins in the corpus spongiosum may be done. Prolonged priapism often gives rise to partial or complete loss of the ability to achieve an erection.

Peyronie's Disease

Peyronie's disease involves a fibrous growth at the top of the penile shaft (Fig. 33-2) and is usually seen in middle-aged or elderly men. The fibrous tissue prevents lengthening of the involved area during erection, so the penis bends toward the affected area, making intercourse difficult. The treatment may consist of injecting hydrocortisone into the fibrous area, administering vitamin E, using ultrasound wave therapy, or administering fibrolytic agents, such as potassium para-aminobenzoate. The fibrous tissue can be removed surgically, although this may impair the ability to have an erection. Surgery is done when other treatment modalities fail.

Balanoposthitis

Balanoposthitis is an inflammation of the glans and prepuce due to the streptococcus, staphylococcus, coliform bacillus, or, less often, the gonococcus. It is often seen in the males whose foreskin is intact because desquamating epithelial cells, glandular secretions, and bacteria accumulate there. The surface of the glans becomes reddened, swollen, and itchy. As the condition progresses, a yellow exudate forms, with development of superficial ulcerations on the surface of the glans.

Most inflammations of the penis involve the glans and prepuce and may be due to any one of several pathogenic organisms. Sexually transmitted infections—one cause of penile infections—are discussed in Chapter 36.

Condyloma Acuminatum

Condyloma acuminatum is by far the most common form of benign penile growth. It is caused by a virus that can be transmitted to other parts of the body or to other persons and is characterized by the presence of tumors around the foreskin. These tumors range in size from minute sessile or pedunculated growths to large masses several centimeters in diameter, not unlike raspberries in appearance. The lesions are easily macerated and have a foul odor. If left untreated, they tend to become ulcerated and infected. In the absence of histologic examination, it is often difficult to distinguish these growths from carcinoma. They are usually treated by electrocautery or cryosurgery.

Leukoplakia of the Penis

Leukoplakia is a common complication of chronic irritation and inflammation of the penis. The skin on the affected area becomes indurated and assumes a bluish white appearance, and the foreskin is rigid and inelastic. It is considered a precancerous lesion and is significant because it can progress to squamous cell carcinoma. When histologic examination reveals bizarre cell types with marked cellular disarrangement, the leukoplakia is then termed Bowen's disease, or carcinoma *in situ*.

Cancer of the Penis

Squamous cell cancer of the penis accounts for approximately 1% of male genital tumors in the United States, and it is most common in the age group of 45 years to 60 years.[1] It is rare in the circumcised male; a predisposition to penile cancer appears to be linked to the irritation due to accumulated smegma under the foreskin. Many of these patients have a history of venereal disease.

The tumor is usually found on the prepuce, the glans, or the coronal sulcus. In most cases, it is a slow-growing squamous cell carcinoma, well differentiated and of low malignancy. Usually metastatic spread occurs by means of the lymphatics and involves the superficial and deep inguinal lymph nodes.[2] Distant metastases are rare and usually occur late in the disease.

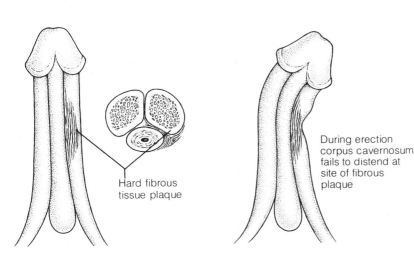

Hard fibrous tissue plaque

During erection corpus cavernosum fails to distend at site of fibrous plaque

Figure 33-2 *A hard, fibrous plaque occurs with Peyronie's disease. (Adapted from Blandy J: Lecture Notes on Urology, 2nd ed. Oxford, Blackwell Scientific Publications, 1977)*

The tumor begins as a small lump or ulcer on the penis. If phimosis is present, there may be painful swelling, purulent drainage, or difficulty in urinating. Palpable lymph nodes in the inguinal region and positive biopsy of the lesion will confirm the diagnosis. Lymphangiography may be done to assess the extent of lymphatic involvement.

Treatment methods include surgery and radiation therapy. If the lesion is confined to the prepuce, circumcision is the treatment of choice. More commonly, partial or complete penile amputation is required. Where there is no regional lymph involvement, radiation therapy is a less mutilating form of treatment.

In summary, disorders of the penis can be either congenital or acquired. Hypospadias and epispadias are congenital defects in which there is a malposition of the urethral opening; it is located on the ventral surface in hypospadias and on the dorsal surface in epispadias. Phimosis is the condition in which the opening of the foreskin is too tight to permit retraction over the glans. Prolonged, painful, and nonsexual erection that can lead to thrombosis with ischemia and necrosis is called priapism. Peyronie's disease is characterized by the growth of a band of fibrous tissue on top of the penile shaft. Cancer of the penis is relatively rare, accounting for only 1% of male genital cancers. Leukoplakia is a precancerous lesion caused by chronic irritation and inflammation of the penis.

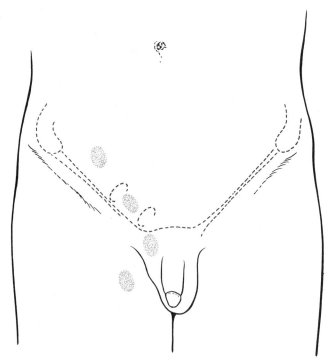

Figure 33-3 *Possible locations of undescended testicles.*

■ Disorders of the Scrotum and Testes

The tunica vaginalis is a serosa-lined sac containing the testicles and epididymis, both of which descend from the peritoneal cavity during fetal development. Defects of the scrotum and testes include cryptorchidism, disorders of the scrotal sac, vascular disorders, inflammation of the scrotum and testes, and neoplasms.

Cryptorchidism

The testes develop intra-abdominally in the fetus and usually descend into the scrotum through the inguinal canal during the eighth and ninth month of gestation. Cryptorchidism, or undescended testes, occurs when one or both of the testicles fail to move down into the scrotal sac. The undescended testes may remain within the lower abdomen or at a point of descent within the inguinal canal (Fig. 33-3). The cause of cryptorchidism is poorly understood. It may be related to some hormonal imbalance with incomplete sexual development, a short spermatic cord, a narrow inguinal ring, or fibrous adhesions in the pathway of descent.[3] In a small percentage of cases, it is believed to be hereditary. The incidence of cryptorchidism is directly related to birth weight and gestational age, smaller and shorter gestational age infants having a much greater incidence of the disorder. In most children with cryptorchidism, the testes descend into the scrotum within the first 3 to 6 months after birth because of the occurrence of a peak in plasma testosterone levels at the time. In 75% of full-term infants and 95% of premature infants born with cryptorchidism, spontaneous testicular descent occurs within the first year of life. Spontaneous descent rarely occurs after this age.

In children with cryptorchidism, histologic abnormalities of the testes occur secondarily to intrinsic defects in the testicle or to the adverse effects of the extrascrotal environment. Temperatures in the inguinal canal are 1 to 2 times higher than in the scrotum. This increased temperature may damage the undescended testicle; it may even produce morphologic changes in the contralateral testes, reflecting possible autosensitization through the production of antibodies against spermatozoa, germinal epithelium, or Sertoli's cells. These testicular changes may cause infertility and increase the risk of testicular cancer in later life.

Males with unilateral or bilateral cryptorchidism usually have decreased sperm counts in both the undescended testes and the contralateral testes. At age 3, the number of spermatogonia will have decreased and the seminiferous tubules will be underdeveloped; these changes will be irreversible even with late spontaneous descent or orchiopexy (surgical fixation of an undescended testis in the scrotum). Spermatogonia counts in males with cryptorchidism never reach the normal counts that are found in males whose testes have descended in the usual manner. Studies have shown abnormalities in the sperm density and hormonal levels of men who underwent orchiopexy between the ages of 4 and 12. The results of these studies indicate that with cryptorchidism both testes have an inherent defect and that often surgical correction does not bring about fertility correction.

The risk of testicular cancer in men with cryptorchidism is 20 to 50 times greater than it is in the control population.[4] This risk is not significantly affected by orchiopexy, hormonal therapy, or late spontaneous descent after the age of 2 years, indicating the importance of treatment before that age.[5]

In men with cryptorchidism, 15% to 20% have nonpalpable testes. Improved techniques for testicular localization include ultrasonography (visualization of the testes by recording the pulses of ultrasonic waves directed into the tissues), gonadal venography and arteriography (x-ray of the veins and arteries of the testes after the injection of a contrast medium), and laparoscopy (examination of the interior of the abdomen using a visualization instrument).

The treatment goals for the male with cryptorchidism include measures to (1) enhance fertility, (2) place the gonad in a favorable place for cancer detection, and (3) improve cosmetic appearance. Regardless of the type of treatment that is employed, it should be carried out before the child reaches 2 years of age.[5] Treatment modalities for children with unilateral or bilateral cryptorchidism include initial hormone therapy with human chorionic gonadotropin (HCG). The gonadotropin-releasing hormone (GnRH), a hypothalamic hormone that stimulates production of the gonadotropic hormones by the anterior pituitary gland, has been used with considerable success in Europe and has recently been released in the United States. For children who do not respond to hormonal treatment, orchiopexy has proved effective.

Hydrocele

The testes and epididymis are almost completely surrounded by the tunica vaginalis, a serous pouch derived from the peritoneum during the fetal descent of the testes from the abdomen into the scrotum. The tunica vaginalis has an outer parietal layer as well as a deeper visceral layer that adheres to the dense fibrous covering of the testes, the tunica albuginea. A scrotal hydrocele is a collection of fluid within the layers of the tunica vaginalis. Normally, the space between these two layers contains only a few milliliters of clear fluid.

A hydrocele can develop in the child as a result of a congenital defect or as a process secondary to injury or disorders of the scrotum. A patent processus vaginalis or potential indirect hernia are often associated with congenital hydroceles. The size of the hydrocele may be increased by crying or physical activity. A congenital hydrocele often corrects itself spontaneously during the first year of life. If the hydrocele persists beyond 18 months of age, surgical revision and high ligation of the processus vaginalis at the level of the internal ring is usually recommended.

In the adult, acute hydrocele may be a complication of an infectious process, such as gonorrhea, a neoplasm, or trauma to the scrotum that causes the visceral membrane to become more permeable, allowing fluid to accumulate. The tunica vaginalis may also become fluid filled under conditions such as heart failure, in which edema is widespread. The fluid is usually serous but may become a reddish brown with slight hemorrhage. Transillumination, which is done by shining a light through the scrotum for the purpose of visualizing its internal structures, may be used to reveal the translucent character of the excess fluid and outline the opaque testes within the scrotal sac. The fluid may be surgically drained to prevent scrotal overheating and consequent sterility.

Hematocele

A hematocele is an accumulation of blood in the tunica vaginalis, which in turn causes the scrotal skin to become dark red or purple. It may develop as a result of an abdominal surgical procedure, scrotal trauma, or a bleeding disorder.

Spermatocele

A spermatocele is a painless sperm-containing cyst that forms at the end of the epididymis. The usual cause is partial obstruction of the ducts that transport sperm from the testes to the urethra. If the cyst is bothersome, it can be evacuated with a hollow needle.

Testicular Torsion

Testicular torsion is a twisting of the spermatic cord that suspends the testicle. It is the most common acute scrotal disorder in the pediatric and young adult population. Testicular torsion can be divided into two distinct clinical entities: extravaginal and intravaginal torsion.

In extravaginal torsion, the testicle and the fascial tunicae that surround it rotate around the spermatic cord at a level well above the tunica vaginalis. Extravaginal torsion, the least common form of testicular torsion, occurs almost exclusively in neonates. The torsion probably occurs during fetal or neonatal descent of the testes before the tunica adheres to the scrotal wall. At birth or shortly thereafter a firm, smooth, painless scrotal mass is identified. The scrotal skin appears red, and some edema is present. Differential diagnosis is relatively easy, because testicular tumors, epididymitis, and orchitis are exceedingly rare in neonates, and a hydrocele is softer and can be transilluminated. A physical examination will exclude the presence of hernia. The treatment often includes elective unilateral surgical exploration and orchiectomy (removal of the testis). Contralateral fixation is not usually indicated with extravaginal torsion.

Intravaginal torsion (torsion of the testicle) is due to the absence of the posterior attachments of the testicle within the tunica vaginalis that normally prevent the testicle from twisting. It is considerably more common than extravaginal torsion. Although anomalies of suspension vary, in general the tunica vaginalis completely surrounds the testicle and epididymis, allowing the testicle to rotate freely within the tunica. In some instances, the epididymal attachment may be sufficiently loose to permit torsion between the testicle and the epididymis. More commonly, however, the testicle rotates about the distal spermatic cord. Because this abnormality is developmental, bilateral anomalies are quite common.

Intravaginal torsion occurs most frequently in those aged 8 to 18 years and is rarely seen after age 30. Males usually present in severe distress within hours of onset. Nausea, vomiting, and tachycardia are often present. The affected testicle is large and tender with pain radiating to the inguinal area. Extensive cremaster muscle contraction causes thickening of the spermatic cord. Radioscopic blood flow studies or Doppler ultrasound help to confirm the diagnosis.[6,7]

Testicular torsion is a true surgical emergency because the viability of testicular tissues diminishes rapidly with time. Surgical intervention involves correcting the abnormal rotation of the testicle and "fixing" it in the scrotal sac (orchiopexy). It is important that surgery be performed within 6 hours after the onset of symptoms. The longer the testes remain without blood flow, the lower the testicular salvage rate becomes. Subsequent torsion of the contralateral testicle is a well-recognized phenomenon; therefore, bilateral orchiopexy is the treatment of choice. When efforts to restore blood flow fail, orchiectomy is necessary.

Varicocele

Varicocele is characterized by varicosities of the pampiniform plexus, a network of veins supplying the testes. A varicocele is found more often on the left side because of the difference in the venous conformation between the right and left testes. The left internal spermatic vein inserts into the left renal vein at a right angle, while the right spermatic vein usually enters the inferior vena cava. Varicoceles are rarely found in men before puberty, the highest incidence being observed in men between 15 and 35 years of age.[7]

The possible etiologic mechanisms of varicocele include an insufficiency of the venous valve at the point where the spermatic vein joins the renal vein, causing a reflux of blood back into the veins of the pampiniform plexus. The force of gravity resulting from the upright position and the insertion of the left spermatic vein at a right angle with the renal vein contribute to venous dilatation. If the condition persists, a reduction of the elastic fibers and hypertrophy of the vein walls occur, as in the formation of leg varices. A hereditary weakness of the connective tissue in the vessel walls may contribute to a predisposition to develop varicocele.

The presence of a varicocele may be associated with male infertility. Although the exact mechanism whereby varicocele produces infertility is not fully understood, several theories of pathogenesis exist. One theory suggests that because a varicocele may be caused by a retrograde flow of blood down the internal spermatic vein, metabolites may be refluxed down the vein, producing adverse effects on both testes. Toxic substances from the renal or adrenal veins may also have an inhibiting effect on sperm production. The data on the role of metabolites in causing infertility are inconclusive at this time. A second theoretical mechanism involves the effect of heat on the testes. It proposes that a varicocele can cause an increase in scrotal temperature, a factor that is thought to impair spermatogenesis. A third theory links epididymal factors with infertility. Several factors in the epididymis determine the motility and maturation of the spermatozoa, including blood supply, tissue androgens, and electrolyte composition. The retrograde flow of blood in the pampiniform plexus could adversely affect environmental conditions in the epididymis and thereby impair the maturation of the spermatozoa, leading to disturbances in motility. It is also possible that occult epididymal obstruction accounts for impaired spermatogenesis and infertility. Each of these factors may interact and impair fertility in the presence of varicocele. The number and combination of these factors may explain why not all patients with varicocele are infertile.[8]

Symptoms of varicocele often include an abnormal feeling of heaviness in the left scrotum, although many varicoceles are asymptomatic. Usually the presence of varicocele is readily diagnosed on physical examination in both the standing and the recumbent positions. Classically, the varicocele will disappear in the lying position because of venous decompression into the renal vein. If the varicocele is secondary to a tumor in the renal vein, it will remain palpable. Scrotal palpation of a varicocele has been compared to feeling a "bag of worms." Small varicoceles may be accentuated by having the patient perform the Valsalva maneuver (forced expiration against a closed glottis) while standing. Diagnostic methods used to confirm varicocele include testicular biopsy, which classically shows germinal cell hypoplasia and premature sloughing of immature sperm forms within the lumen of the seminiferous tubules, venogram, scrotal thermography, and Doppler ultrasound.

Surgical treatment of varicocele is indicated in selected patients with infertility and in others with local symptomatology.[9] At present 60% to 80% of males who undergo surgical varicocelectomy will have improved semen characteristics, and 35% to 50% will accomplish impregnation.[10]

Inflammation of the Scrotum and Testes

Inflammation of the scrotum and testes can involve either the external scrotal sac or the intrascrotal contents, including the epididymis and testes.

Inflammation of the scrotum

Certain normal characteristics of the scrotum can be predisposing factors to inflammation of the sac. First, the scrotal rugae prevent air circulation and evaporation of moisture from the skin surface; together with the close proximity of the anus and the urethra, this provides a favorable environment for bacterial growth. Second, the loose scrotal skin reacts to inflammation by becoming highly edematous, which in turn decreases circulation and delays healing. Third, contact of the scrotum with the thighs can cause maceration of the skin surface and prolong healing.

A common infection of the scrotum and thighs is a type of *dermatosis* called tinea cruris or "jock itch." It is characterized by reddened patches with raised scaling edges. Pruritus is common, and repeated scratching often encourages secondary infections. Obesity, excessive perspiration, poor hygiene, and tight-fitting synthetic underwear that prevents air circulation are other predisposing factors in dermatosis. Treatment consists of improved hygiene, air-drying of underclothing, and use of an antifungal agent.

Epididymitis

Epididymitis is an inflammation of the epididymis, the elongated cordlike structure that lies along the posterior border of the testis, whose function is the storage, transport, and maturation of spermatozoa. It is commonly related to infections in the urinary tract that presumably reach the epididymis through either the vas deferens or the lymphatics of the spermatic cord. Rarely is the epididymis seeded through the bloodstream from other foci of infection. Epididymitis is the most common cause of intrascrotal pathology in postpubertal males.

A number of organisms are known to cause epididymitis. In men under 35 years of age, *Chlamydia trachomatis* is the major cause of nonspecific epididymitis, and the infection is considered a sexually transmitted disease.[11] In men over 35 years of age, epididymitis is usually related to urinary tract infections caused by gram-negative bacteria.

Epididymitis is characterized by unilateral pain and swelling, accompanied by erythema and edema of the overlying scrotal skin that develops over a period of 24 to 48 hours. Initially the swelling and induration are limited to the epididymis. However, the distinction between the testes and epididymis becomes less evident as the inflammation progresses. Fever and complaint of dysuria occur in about half of the affected individuals. The presence of urethral discharge is dependent on the organism causing the infection. A discharge usually occurs in gonorrheal infections, is common in chlamydial infections, and is less common in infections due to gram-negative organisms. Pyuria may be present, depending on the method of urine collection.

The treatment consists of bed rest during the acute phase (which usually lasts for 3 to 4 days), scrotal support, and antibiotics. Gonorrhea is usually treated with intramuscularly administered procaine penicillin and oral probenecid (see Chap. 36). Follow-up cultures are needed to ensure successful treatment. Chlamydial infections are treated with tetracycline. Because these infections are sexually transmitted diseases, treatment of the sexual partner is strongly recommended.

In older males with epididymitis, gram-negative bacteria are frequently the etiologic agents. Often, benign prostatic hypertrophy, neurogenic bladder, or urethral stricture is present concomitantly and must be considered in the treatment plan. Prostatitis may coexist; hence, antibiotics that are effective in treating chronic bacterial prostatitis are often used. Antibiotic choice can be adjusted when sensitivity testing is complete.

Orchitis

Orchitis, an infection of the testes, can be precipitated by a primary infection in the genitourinary tract, such as urethritis, cystitis, or seminal vesiculitis. Many infections from other parts of the body spread to the testes through the bloodstream or the lymphatics. Orchitis can develop as a complication of a systemic infection, such as mumps, scarlet fever, or pneumonia. Probably the best known of these is orchitis caused by the mumps virus. About 25% to 30% of males 10 years of age or older with parotitis (mumps) develop this form of orchitis.[3] The symptoms usually run their course in 7 to 10 days. Mumps orchitis causes painful enlargement of the testes, with small hemorrhages into the tunica albuginea. Microscopically, an acute inflammatory response is seen in the seminiferous tubules with proliferation of neutrophils, lymphocytes, and histiocytes, causing distention of the tubules. Mumps orchitis causes testicular damage in 30% of males who get the disease after puberty. The residual effects that are seen after the acute phase include hyalinization of the seminiferous tubules, atrophy of the testes, and elevation of FSH levels because of a lack of testosterone and negative feedback control of FSH. If bilateral involvement occurs, the male will be infertile.[2]

Neoplasms

Tumors can arise from either the scrotum or the testes. Benign scrotal tumors are quite common and often do not require treatment. Carcinoma of the scrotum is rare and is usually linked to exposure to carcinogenic agents. On the other hand, almost all solid tumors of the testes (96%) are malignant.[12] Although testicular tumors are rare, their virulence and the fact that they develop in relatively young men make them a significant health problem.

Cancer of the scrotum

Cancer of the scrotum is primarily an occupational disease linked to contact with petroleum products, such as tar, pitch, and soot. The malignancy often occurs after 20 to 30 years of exposure. In the early stages, it may appear as a small tumor or wartlike growth that eventually ulcerates. The thin scrotal wall lacks the tissue reactivity needed to block the malignant process; over half of the cases seen involve metastasis to the lymph nodes. The treatment includes wide local excision of the tumor with inguinal and femoral node dissection, because this tumor does not respond well to x-ray treatment.

Testicular cancer

Cancer of the testes accounts for about 1% of the cancers in males and about 3% of the cancers of the male urogenital system. The highest incidence of testicular cancer is found in the 20- to 40-year-old age group. It is the most common cancer in men between the ages of 29 and 35. With current treatment modalities, a large percentage of men who develop testicular cancer can be cured.

The etiology of testicular cancer is unknown. The risk is greatly increased in males with cryptorchidism. It has been estimated that 1 in 20 abdominal testes and 1 in 80 inguinal testes will develop a tumor.[1] Chronic irritation of the testes, from either infection or other inflammatory processes, is also thought to increase the risk of cancer formation.

Currently, there are several systems for the classification of testicular cancer. The Armed Forces Institute of Pathology (AFIP) classification system divides testicular cancer into germinal tumors arising from the spermatozoa and their derivatives and nongerminal cell tumors arising from other cellular components of the testes.[13] Germ cell tumors, which constitute about 95% of all testicular tumors, can be divided into two groups: seminoma and nonseminoma germ cell tumors. Seminomas are thought to arise from the seminiferous epithelium of the testes. They are the most common type of testicular cancer, accounting for approximately 40% of all germ cell tumors. The peak incidence of seminoma occurs in men between 30 and 40 years of age, whereas nonseminoma tumors are seen in men a decade younger.[14] Nonseminoma germ cell tumors can be divided into three histologic types: (1) embryonal carcinoma, (2) teratoma, and (3) choriocarcinoma.[15] Embryonal carcinomas represent about 15% to 20% of all germ cell tumors. They are less differentiated and more aggressive than seminomas. Teratomas are derived from totipotential cells that have the capacity to differentiate into tissues representing any of the three germ layers of the embryo—ectoderm, mesoderm, or endoderm. They constitute fewer than 10% of germ cell tumors and can occur at any age from infancy to old age. They usually behave like benign tumors in children; in adults they often contain minute foci of cancer cells. Choriocarcinoma is a highly malignant form of testicular cancer that is identical to tumors that arise in the placental tissue. Each of these basic histologic types can occur as a pure form or as a combination of cell types. Forty percent of testicular cancers are of mixed tissue types.[16] The most common mixture is teratocarcinoma, which contains both embryonal carcinoma and teratoma elements.

Often the first sign of testicular cancer is a slight painless enlargement of the testicle, occasionally accompanied by an ache in the abdomen or groin or a sensation of dragging or heaviness in the scrotum. Frank pain may be experienced in the later stages when the tumor is growing rapidly and hemorrhaging occurs. Testicular tumors often metastasize while the primary tumor is still small and only barely palpable, in which case the first indication of the disease is symptoms related to the organ or region to which the cancer has spread. Unfortunately, 80% to 90% of men with testicular cancer have metastatic disease by the time the diagnosis is made. This is because there are only a few early symptoms and, therefore, many men delay seeing a physician until the tumor has spread.[17]

The American Cancer Society strongly advocates that every young adult male examine his testes at least once a month as a means of early detection of testicular cancer. The examination should be done after a warm bath or shower when the scrotal skin is relaxed. This self-examination involves examining each testicle with the fingers of both hands by rolling it between the thumb and fingers to check for the presence of lumps. If any lump, nodule, or enlargement is noted, it should be brought immediately to the attention of a physician.

The initial diagnosis of testicular cancer is usually made by a physical examination. When a testicular tumor presents itself as a hard painless mass not involved with the scrotal wall or spermatic cord, surgical excision of the entire testicle through an inguinal incision is done to establish a diagnosis, including the histologic type of the tumor that is present. A biopsy, which is generally accepted as a diagnostic method with other types of cancer, is usually contraindicated in testicular cancer because of the danger of the tumor spreading.[18]

Treatment methods for testicular cancer are determined by the histologic type of the tumor that is present and the clinical stage of the disease. Two systems are generally used for the clinical staging of testicular cancers: the TNN classification system (see Chap. 5) and tumor dissemination according to whether the tumor is confined to the testes (stage I), has spread to the subdiaphragmatic lymph nodes (stage II), or has spread to more distant sites (stage III). Because of the embryonic origin of the testes, the testicular blood vessels and lymphatics originate high in the retroperitoneal cavity at the level of the kidneys. Hence, the primary spread of testicular cancers occurs through the retroperitoneal rather than the iliac or inguinal lymph nodes in the pelvis.[15] Because there is communication between the retroperitoneal and mediastinal lymph nodes, the extra-abdominal spread of testicular cancer generally involves the mediastinal and supraclavicular lymph nodes.

The development of tests for the detection of tumor-associated serum markers has assisted in the diagnosis, staging, and management of testicular tumors. Testicular germ cell tumors may produce alpha fetoprotein (AFP), a major serum protein produced in the early fetus, or human chorionic gonadotropin (HCG), a hormone normally synthesized and secreted by placental cells. Elevated levels of these markers are most often associated with nonseminomatous tumors.

Diagnostic methods used in the staging of testicular cancer include (1) physical examination (to detect lymphadenopathy or an abdominal mass), (2) chest radiography with tomography or computerized tomographic (CT) scans (to check for small mediastinal or lung lesions), (3) radioimmunoassay for AFP or HCG, (4) intravenous pyelogram (to assess renal function), (5) bipedal lymphangiography, (6) CT scan of the retroperitoneum, phlebography, and sonography (to assess for retroperitoneal lymph node involvement).[14]

By combining tests such as the CT scan, lymphangiogram, and tumor markers (such as AFP, HCG) one may detect almost 90% of the retroperitoneal masses in nonseminoma tumors.[19]

Testicular cancer may be treated with surgery (excision of the testicle with radical retroperitoneal lymph node resection), with radiotherapy, or with combination chemotherapy. Radiotherapy postorchiectomy is the treatment of choice for a pure seminoma. Because this tumor is extremely radiosensitive, there is a 90% to 95% cure rate with localized disease. Retroperitoneal node dissection is rarely indicated. Depending on the stage of the disease, nonseminoma germ cell tumors are treated with radical retroperitoneal lymph node resection and combination chemotherapy. A major advance in treating testicular cancer is combination chemotherapy using vinblastine and bleomycin. Cisplatin, the single most active agent used in testicular cancer, with relatively low myelosuppression, has been added to the vinblastine-bleomycin combinations with great success. The extent of metastatic disease present when chemotherapy is begun is the best predictor of success rate. An overall cure rate of 70% is projected using a combination of cisplatin, vinblastine, and bleomycin.[20]

In summary, disorders of the scrotum and testes include cryptorchidism or undescended testicles, hydrocele, testicular torsion, and varicocele. Inflammatory conditions can involve the scrotal sac, epididymis, or testes. Tumors can arise in either the scrotum or the testes. Scrotal cancers are usually associated with exposure to petroleum products such as tar, pitch, and soot. Testicular cancer accounts for about 3% of cancers of the male genitourinary system. With present treatment methods a large percentage of men with these tumors can be cured. Testicular self-examination is recommended as a means of early detection for this form of cancer.

■ Disorders of the Prostate

The prostate is a firm glandular structure that surrounds the urethra. It produces a thin, milky alkaline secretion that aids sperm motility by helping to maintain an optimum pH. The contraction of the smooth muscle in the gland promotes semen expulsion during ejaculation.

Prostatitis

Inflammation of the prostate gland is a common condition that can be traced to a number of organisms. It may occur spontaneously or as the result of catheterization or instrumentation or secondary to other diseases of the male genitourinary system. Prostatitis may be classified as acute or chronic. About 80% of the acute forms of prostatitis can be traced to strains of *E. coli* and the rest to klebsiella.[1] It is characterized by diffuse inflammation of the prostatic ducts and acini and may progress to abscess formation. Symptoms include fever, general malaise, frequency of urination, dysuria, and pain in the groin or perineal area. Hematuria, rectal pain, and pain on defecation may also be present. In younger men, erections are frequently painful. Rectal examination reveals a swollen and exquisitely tender prostate.

Chronic prostatitis is probably the most common cause of relapsing urinary tract infections in the male[21] and usually occurs in middle-aged or older men. It may give rise to vague perineal pain, dysuria, frequency of urination, low-back discomfort, and prostatic tenderness, as well as a slight early morning discharge or hematuria. The chronic form often is asymptomatic. Many times, cultures of midstream urine and prostatic fluid are sterile or contain only normal bacterial flora. It is thought that in some cases the prostatitis may be due to a viral infection such as herpes simplex II, a common sexually transmitted virus.[22] If no organisms are cultured, the treatment is usually symptomatic. Prostatic massage, warm baths, and avoidance of intercourse and alcohol may be suggested.

Benign Prostatic Hypertrophy

Benign prostatic hypertrophy (BPH), or hyperplasia, is a common disorder in men over 50 years of age. Postmortem examinations have shown that 50% to 60% of men ages 40 to 59 and 95% of men over age 70 have some degree of nodular hyperplasia of the prostate.[23] In about one-third of cases, the nodules can be detected on rectal examination, yet only 5% to 10% of these men have problems sufficient to warrant surgical intervention (Fig. 33-4).

BPH is characterized by the formation of large discrete lesions in the periurethral region. As they enlarge, these nodules tend to compress the urethra and cause partial or almost complete obstruction of urine flow. The etiology of BPH is uncertain, but the increasing incidence with advancing age suggests the possibility of an imbalance between male and female sex hormones. The nodules associated with BPH do not usually involve the posterior lobe of the prostate gland, which is a common site of prostatic cancer.

The resulting obstruction to urinary outflow can give rise to urinary tract infection, difficulty in voiding, hypertrophy, and eventually, destructive changes of the bladder wall, hydroureter, and hydronephrosis. Hypertrophy and changes in bladder-wall structure develop in stages. At first, the exaggerated crisscross fibers form trabeculations and then herniations, or sacculations; finally diverticula develop as the herniations extend through the bladder wall. These diverticula are readily infected, because urine is seldom completely emptied from them. Back pressure on the ureters promotes hydroureter and hydronephrosis, and, as a result, the kidney develops the physiologic sequelae of atrophy— failure to concentrate urine, to retain sodium, and to remove metabolic acids from the blood. There is danger of eventual renal failure.

The symptoms of BPH are related to the compression of the urethra with accompanying bladder distention and hypertrophy, urinary tract infection, and renal disease. The typical picture includes outflow obstruction with a decreased urinary stream. As the obstruction increases, acute retention with overdistention of the bladder may occur. The presence of residual urine in the bladder causes frequency of urination and a constant desire to empty the bladder, which becomes worse at night. With marked bladder distention, overflow incontinence may occur with the slightest increase in intra-

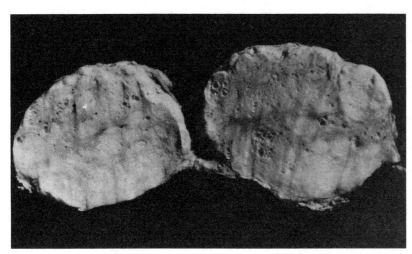

Figure 33-4 *Benign nodular hyperplasia of the prostate.*

abdominal pressure. Uremia, which occurs in the late stages of the disease, is discussed in Chapter 30.

Severe urinary obstruction is usually treated surgically. There are several surgical approaches. The preference of the surgeon, the severity of the disease, and the location of the nodules are usually determining factors in the type of procedure to be done. Prostate surgery for BPH does not usually cause loss of sexual function, because much of the gland remains. An occasional side effect of the surgery is retrograde ejaculation (into the bladder). When this happens, sensual pleasure will remain, but the man will be sterile.

Prostatic Cancer

Next to cancer of the lung, prostatic cancer is the most common type of cancer in men. It is estimated that each year approximately 73,000 new cases of prostate cancer are diagnosed and 23,000 deaths occur from this disease. It is one of the most common cancers in men over 50 years of age and is seldom seen in younger men.[24]

The etiology of prostatic cancer is unknown. Age, race, endocrine influences, and environmental agents have been suggested as possible contributing factors. The disease is extremely rare in Orientals and is more common among blacks than among whites in the United States.[2] In terms of environmental factors, it has been noted the incidence of this type of cancer among workers in the cadmium industries is increased. Evidence to support hormonal influences as causative factors in prostatic cancer are supported by the fact that tumor growth can often be arrested or retarded by castration or the administration of estrogen.[2]

Symptoms of prostatic cancer may be completely absent during the early stages of the disease. About 75% of men with prostatic cancer do not present with symptoms of the disease until the tumor has extended beyond the capsule of the prostate or when metastatic spread of the tumor has occurred. At this time there are usually urinary symptoms such as difficulty in stopping or starting the stream, dysuria, frequency of urination, or hematuria. Pain is a late symptom. Back pain may be caused by vertebral metastases.

Rectal examination is the primary method for diagnosing prostatic cancer. Palpation of a nodule or abnormal prostate during an examination is an indication for a needle biopsy of the gland. Prostate cancer spreads by both the lymph channels and the bloodstream with frequent metastases to the pelvic lymph nodes and distant bones. Direct spread to the seminal vesicles and bladder are often seen.

As in other types of cancer, the treatment methods for prostatic cancers are determined largely by the histologic characteristics of the tumor in terms of cell differentiation and the clinical stage of the disease, as determined by the size of the tumor and degree of spread. The radiologic techniques used to assess the stage of prostatic cancer include chest radiography, excretory urography, and radionuclide bone scintography (scans) in conjunction with selective skeletal radiography. When disseminated disease is not evident, lymphangiography may be used to search for lymph node metastases. Ultrasonography and CT scans have been introduced to further define the extent of the disease. Percutaneous biopsy of lesions in the lungs, bones, nodes, and other masses have also helped to stage the disease.

Both normal and malignant prostatic tissue produce acid phosphatase, which can be detected in the serum. For many years the diagnostic workup for prostatic cancer has included measurement of serum acid phosphatase levels. However, older laboratory methods were not able to distinguish between prostatic and nonprostatic sources of acid phosphatase, and elevated levels of the enzyme (a sign of prostatic cancer) were not detectable until the tumor had spread beyond the capsule or had metastasized. Recently, techniques have been developed that offer improved specificity for the acid phosphatase isoenzyme originating from the prostate. This allows for the detection of prostatic alkaline phosphatase (PAP) in the serum during the early localized stages of prostate cancer. Further diagnostic research is being done on methods for identifying prostatic cancer antigens and tumor receptors.

The availability of different treatment modalities and the lack of controlled comparisons have made the management of prostate cancer controversial. The treatment methods include surgery (radical prostatectomy), radiotherapy, and chemotherapy. For accurate staging, close attention is given to the pelvic lymph nodes. The treatment of choice for very early stage A_1 (three or fewer well-differentiated foci) is simply observation. The treatment during stage B_1, when the size of the tumor is less than 2 cm and involves only one lobe of the prostate, is radical retropubic prostatectomy. The treatment of well-advanced tumors is more controversial. Radical retropubic prostatectomy, pelvic irradiation, and iodine-125 implantation have been employed; however, their efficacy has not been thoroughly studied.[2] The primary treatment for patients with advanced prostatic cancer has centered on the suppression of androgenic hormones. This can be accomplished by bilateral orchiectomy or the administration of estrogens. The control of androgens is believed to be responsible for some symptomatic improvement in 80% to 90% of men with advanced disease.[12] Hormonal therapy is usually palliative. Although the therapy improves the quality of life, its effect on survival is questionable.

In summary, the prostate is a firm glandular structure that surrounds the urethra. Inflammation of the prostate occurs as either an acute or a chronic process. Chronic prostatitis is probably the most common cause of relapsing urinary tract infections in the male. Benign prostatic hypertrophy is a common disorder of men over 50 years of age. Because the prostate encircles the urethra, this condition tends to cause obstruction of urinary outflow from the bladder. Cancer of the prostate is the most common type of cancer of the male genitourinary system and is the third highest cause of cancer deaths in men 55 to 74 years of age.

Study Guide

After you have studied this chapter, you should be able to meet the following objectives:

☐ State the difference between hypospadias and epispadias.

☐ Cite the significance of phimosis.

☐ Describe the pathology of priapism.

☐ Describe the anatomic changes that occur with Peyronie's disease.

☐ Explain the relationship that may exist between circumcision and balanoposthitis.

☐ Explain the potential significance of condyloma acuminatum and penile leukoplakia.

☐ List the signs of penile cancer.

☐ State the cause of cryptorchidism.

☐ Describe potential risks associated with cryptorchidism.

☐ Differentiate hydrocele, hematocele, and spermatocele.

☐ State the difference between extravaginal and intravaginal testicular torsion.

☐ State why testicular torsion of the intravaginal type is a true surgical emergency.

☐ Explain the importance of early treatment for varicocele.

☐ Cite at least three factors that predispose to dermatosis.

☐ State the major cause of epididymitis in men under 35 years of age and those over 35 years of age.

☐ Describe the symptoms of epididymitis.

☐ State the risk associated with mumps orchitis.

☐ Relate environmental factors to scrotal cancer.

☐ State the age group that has the highest incidence of testicular cancer.

☐ Describe the testicular self-examination method recommended by the American Cancer Society.

☐ State a commonly used system for classifying testicular cancers.

☐ Relate the recent change in cure rate for testicular cancer to early detection, diagnostic, and treatment methods.

☐ State the clinical manifestations of prostatitis.

☐ Describe the physical dysfunction related to the presence of benign prostatic hypertrophy.

☐ State the treatment measures for prostatic cancer.

References

1. Robbins SL, Cotran RS: Pathologic Basis of Disease, pp 1220, 1223. Philadelphia, WB Saunders, 1979
2. Smith DR: General Urology, 11th ed, pp 368, 214, 342, 343, 350. Los Altos, CA, Lange Medical Publications, 1984
3. Robbins SL, Cotran RS, Kumar V: Pathologic Basis of Disease, pp 1087, 1089, 1092. Philadelphia, WB Saunders, 1984
4. Batata MA, Chu FCH, Hilaris BS et al: Testicular cancer in cryptorchidism. Cancer 49:1023, 1982
5. Kramer SA: Cryptorchidism: Current state of the art in diagnosis and treatment Continuing Education No 8:737, 1983
6. Thomas WE et al: Dynamic radionuclide scanning of the testes in acute scrotal conditions. Br J Surg 68:621, 1981
7. Rodriguez DD et al: Doppler ultra sound versus testicular scanning in evaluation of the acute scrotum. J Urol 125:346, 1981
8. Wirtz J: Epidemiology of idiopathic varicocele. In Jecht EW and Zietler E (eds): Varicocele and Male Infertility, pp 2-3. New York, Springer-Verlag, 1982
9. Bain J, Shell WB, Schwarzstein L: Treatment of Male Infertility. New York, Springer-Verlag, 1982
10. Lipschultz LI, Nagler H: Varicocele in Current Therapy of Infertility 1982-1983. St Louis, CV Mosby, 1982
11. Berger RE, Alexander ER, Harnich JP et al: Etiology, manifestations and therapy of acute epididymitis: Prospective study of 50 cases. J Urol 121:750, 1979
12. Frank IN, Keys HM, McCune CS: Urologic and male genital cancers. In Rubin P (ed): Clinical Oncology, 6th ed, pp 214, 213. New York, American Cancer Society, 1983
13. Yagoda A, Golbey RB (eds): Germ cell tumors. Semin Oncol 6:143, 1979
14. Catalona WJ: Current management of testicular cancer. Surg Clin North Am 62, No 6:1119, 1982
15. Hubbard SM, Jenkins J: An overview of current concepts

in the management of patients with testicular tumors of germ cell origin—Part I: Pathophysiology, diagnosis, and staging. Cancer Nurs 6:39, 1983

16. Mostofi FK: Testicular tumors. Cancer 32:1186, 1973
17. Drasgna RE, Eihorn LH, Williams SD: The chemotherapy of testicular cancer. CA 32, No 2:66, 1982
18. Fraley EF, Lange PH, Kennedy BJ: Germ cell testicular cancer in adults. N Engl J Med 301:1370, 1979
19. Murphy GP: Testicular cancer. CA 33, No 2:100, 1983
20. Einhorn L: Chemotherapy of testicular cancer. Med Times 110, No 9:32, 1982
21 Meres EM: Prostatitis. A review. Med Clin North Am 2:3, 1975
22. Blandy J: Urology, p 923. London, Blackwell Scientific Publications, 1976
23. Harbitz TB, Haugen OA: Histology of the prostate in elderly men. A study of autopsy series. Acta Pathol Microbiol Scand 80:756, 1972
24. Silverberg E: Cancer statistics. CA 31:1328, 1981

■ Additional References

Basso-Alise A: The prostate in the elderly male. Hosp Pract 12, No 10:117-123, 1977

Cohen S: Patient assessment: Examination of the male genitalia. Programmed instruction. Am J Nurs 79, No 4:689-712, 1979

Conklin M, Klint K, Morway A et al: Should health teaching include self-examination of the testes? Am J Nurs 78, No 12:207, 1978

Duckett JW: Epispadias. Urol Clin North Am 5, No 1:107-126, 1978

Dwoskin JY: Hypospadias. Urol Clin North Am 5, No 1:95-106, 1978

Fair WR: Carcinoma of the prostate: Current thoughts on diagnosis and staging. Surg Clin North Am 62, No 6, 1982

Hoppmann HJ, Fraley EE: Squamous cell carcinoma of the penis. J Urol 120, No 10:393-398, 1978

Hubbard SM, Jenkins J: An overview of current concepts in the management of patients with testicular tumors of germ cell origin—Part II: Treatment strategies by histology and stage. Cancer Nurs 6, No 2:125, 1983

Javadpour N: The National Cancer Institute experience with testicular cancer. J Urol 120, No 12:651-659, 1978

Kochen M, McCurdy S: Circumcision and the risk of cancer of the penis. Am Dis Child 134:484-486, 1980

McKenzie DJ: Peyronie's disease. J Med Assoc Ga 67:426-427, 1978

Murray BLS, Wilcox LJ: Testicular self-exam. Am J Nurs 78, No 12:2074-2075, 1978

Prostate Ca: Focus on early Dx and prognostic accuracy. Hosp Pract 14, No 9:129-131, 1979

Raifer J, Walsh P: Testicular descent. Urol Clin North Am 5, No 1:233-235, 1978

Sharer WC: Acute scrotal pathology. Surg Clin North Am 62, No 6, 1982

Tobiason SJ: Benign prostatic hypertrophy. Am J Nurs 79, No 2:286-290, 1979

Wilson JD: The pathogenesis of benign prostatic hyperplasia. Am J Med 68, No 5:745-756, 1980

Chapter 34

Structure and Function of the Female Reproductive System

Debbie L. Cook

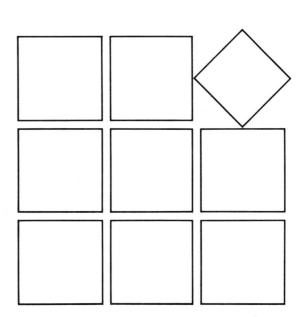

The female genitourinary system consists of the internal paired ovaries, the uterine tubes, the uterus, the vagina and the external mons pubis, the labia majora, the labia minora, the clitoris, the urethra, and the perineal body. Although the female urinary structures are anatomically separate from the genital structures, their anatomic proximity provides a means for cross-contamination and shared symptomatology between the two systems (Fig. 34-1). This chapter focuses on the internal and external genitalia. It includes a discussion of hormonal and physical changes that occur throughout the life cycle in response to the gonadotropic hormones. The reader is referred to a specialty text for a discussion of pregnancy.

■ Reproductive Structures

External Genitalia

The external genitalia are located at the base of the pelvis in the perineal area and include the mons pubis, labia majora, labia minora, clitoris, and perineal body. The urethra and anus, though not genital structures, are usually considered in a discussion of the external genitalia. The external genitalia, also known collectively as the vulva, are diagrammed in Figure 34-2.

Mons pubis

The mons pubis is a rounded eminence located anterior to the symphysis pubis of the bony pelvis. The mons is a fat pad covered with skin and hair. The amount of fat and hair of the mons pubis usually increases under the hormonal stimulus of puberty, and its color deepens. The skin, which has an abundance of sebaceous glands, may become infected because of changes in dietary habits, normal variations, or poor hygiene. The mons pubis is the most common site of pubic lice infestation in the female.

Labia majora

The labia majora (singular: labium majus) are analogous to the male scrotum. These structures are the outermost lips of the vulva, beginning anteriorly at the base of the mons pubis and ending posteriorly at the anus. The labia majora are composed of folds of skin and fat and become covered with hair at the onset of puberty. Prior to puberty, the labia majora have a skin covering similar to that covering the abdomen. With sufficient hormonal stimulation, the labia of a mature woman close over the urethral and vaginal openings; this can change following childbirth or surgery. The labia majora are rich in sebaceous glands. They are subject to the same types of problems as the mons pubis in regard to sebaceous cysts or lice infestations.

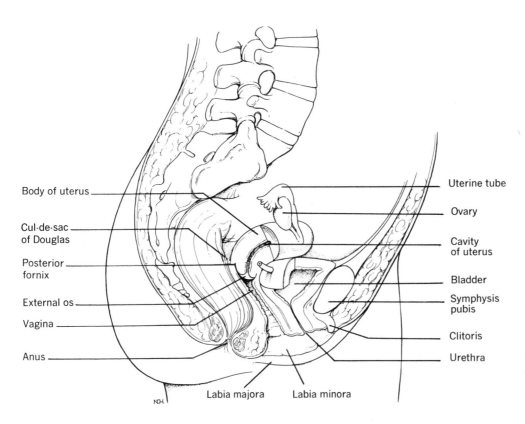

Body of uterus

Cul-de-sac of Douglas

Posterior fornix

External os

Vagina

Anus

Uterine tube

Ovary

Cavity of uterus

Bladder

Symphysis pubis

Clitoris

Urethra

Labia majora   Labia minora

Figure 34-1   *Female reproductive system as seen in sagittal section. (From Chaffee EE, Greisheimer EM: Basic Physiology and Anatomy, 3rd ed. Philadelphia, JB Lippincott, 1974)*

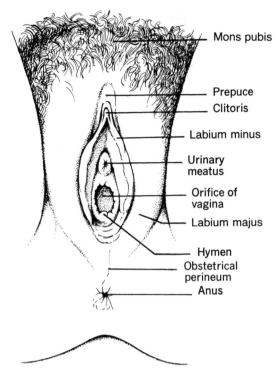

Figure 34-2 *External genitalia of the female. (From Chaffee EE, Lytle IM: Basic Physiology and Anatomy, 4th ed. Philadelphia, JB Lippincott, 1980)*

Labels in figure:
- Mons pubis
- Prepuce
- Clitoris
- Labium minus
- Urinary meatus
- Orifice of vagina
- Labium majus
- Hymen
- Obstetrical perineum
- Anus

Labia minora

The labia minora (singular: labium minus) are located between the labia majora. These delicate cutaneous structures are smaller than the labia majora and are made up of skin, fat, and some erectile tissue. Unlike the skin of the labia majora, that of the labia minora is hairless and usually light pink in color. The edges may be ragged or smooth and may protrude from the labia majora. This is particularly likely after childbearing. The labia minora begin anteriorly at the hood of the clitoris and end posteriorly at the base of the vagina. The area between them is called the vestibule. Within the vestibule are located the urethral and vaginal openings (introitus), as well as the Bartholin's lubricating glands. During sexual arousal, the labia minora become distended with blood and enlarged; with resolution, the labia throb, then return to normal size. The sebaceous glands secrete odoriferous fluid, in both the presence and absence of sexual arousal. The labia majora and labia minora are the most common sites of inflammation and structural changes as the result of certain sexually transmitted diseases.

Clitoris

The clitoris is located below the clitoral hood, or prepuce, which is formed by the joining of the two labia minora. The female clitoris is an erectile organ, rich in blood and nerve supply. Analogous to the male penis, it is a highly sensitive organ that becomes distended during sexual stimulation.

Urethra

The urethra, or urinary meatus, is the external opening of the internal urinary bladder. The urethra is posterior to the clitoris and is usually closer to the vaginal opening than to the clitoris. The urethra, the vaginal opening, and the Bartholin glands lie within the vestibule.

The urethral opening is the site of the Skene's glands, which have a lubricating function. When infected, these glands or the meatus may become inflamed and painful. An isolated urethral infection is most commonly caused by gonococci. Inflammation may occur secondary to trauma, increased sexual activity, or structural defects such as diverticula. Secretions indicating infections may be discharged during urination or gynecologic examination. Vigorous or frequent stimulation of the clitoris may cause irritation of the urethra. Cystitis may develop as a result of contamination with bacteria from the vagina or rectum during intercourse or foreplay or if the bladder is emptied infrequently or only partially.

Introitus and hymen

The vaginal orifice is commonly known as the introitus. The vaginal introitus is the opening between the external and internal genitalia. The opening may be oval, circular, or sievelike and may be partially or completely occluded. Occlusion may occur because of the presence of an intact or partially intact hymen. The hymen is composed of connective tissue. Contrary to a popular notion, an intact hymen may or may not indicate virginity, as this tissue can be stretched without tearing. At puberty, an intact hymen may require surgical intervention to permit discharge of menstrual fluids.

Bartholin glands

Between the hymenal opening and the posterior labia minora are the ducts of the Bartholin glands. These bilaterally located glands lubricate the vestibular area. Bacterial infection of the Bartholin ducts may cause bilateral or unilateral labial swelling and pain that may become so severe as to inhibit ambulation. Purulent discharge is suggestive of gonococcal infection, and a culture of the discharge is necessary to rule this out. Infection may progress to abscess formation, which requires excision and drainage. Once incised, the Bartholin gland cysts or infections commonly become recurrent. Therefore, perineal hygiene should be emphasized. Bartholin cysts can develop without evidence of infection and are palpable without tenderness.

Perineal body

The perineal body is that tissue located posterior to the vaginal opening and anterior to the anus. The perineal body is composed of fibrous connective tissue and is the site of insertion of several perineal muscles. To facilitate childbirth, it is sometimes necessary to make an incision, called an episiotomy, in this tissue, as well as in vaginal tissue.

Internal Genitalia

Vagina

The vagina is a fibromuscular tube lined with mucus-secreting stratified squamous epithelial cells. It connects the internal and external genitalia and is located behind the urinary bladder and urethra and anterior to the rectum. The vagina is essentially devoid of nerve-sensation fibers. The vagina is about 7.5 cm to 10 cm in length and functions as a route for the discharge of the menses and other secretions. It also serves as an organ of sexual fulfillment and reproduction.

The membranous vaginal wall forms two longitudinal folds and several transverse folds, or rugae. Vaginal tissue is usually moist, with a pH maintained within the bacteriostatic range of 3.8 to 4.2. The epithelial cells of the vagina, like other tissues of the reproductive system, respond to changing levels of the ovarian sex hormones. Estrogen stimulates the proliferation and maturation of the vaginal mucosa; this results in a thickening of the vaginal mucosa and an increased glycogen content of the epithelial cells. The glycogen is fermented to lactic acid by the lactobacilli (Döderlein's bacilli) that are part of the normal vaginal flora, accounting for the mildly acid pH of vaginal fluid. The vaginal ecology can be disrupted at many levels, rendering it susceptible to infection. Pregnancy and the use of oral contraceptive agents increase the amount of estrogen within the system. Diabetes or a prediabetic state may increase the glycogen content of the cells. The use of systemic antibiotics may decrease the number of lactobacilli within the vagina. During a routine pelvic exam, the estrogen level can be estimated by examining the cellular structure and configuration of the vaginal epithelial cells. This test is known as the maturation index.

Uterus and cervix

The uterus is a thick-walled muscular organ. This pear-shaped hollow structure is located between the bladder and the rectum. The uterus can be divided into three parts: the top, called the fundus, the lower constricted part, called the cervix, and the portion between the fundus and the cervix, called the body of the uterus (Fig. 34-3). The uterus is supported on both sides principally by the broad and round ligaments.

In most women, the uterus is found in a forward-lying or anteverted position, in which the uterine fundus and body rest on top of the urinary bladder. The uterus may assume other positions such as anteflexion, retroflexion, or retroversion without causing problems. Uterine position may change in response to many factors.

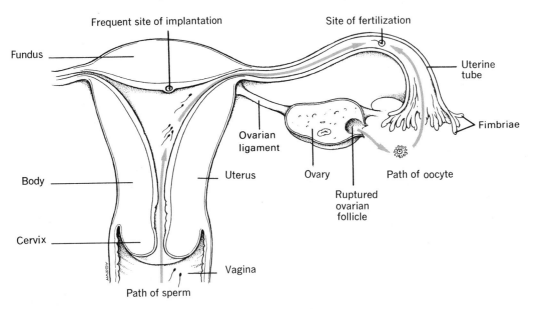

Figure 34-3 *Schematic drawing of female reproductive organs, showing the path of the oocyte as it moves from the ovary into the fallopian (uterine) tube; the path of sperm is also shown, as is the usual site of fertilization. (From Chaffee EE, Lytle IM: Basic Physiology and Anatomy, 4th ed. Philadelphia, JB Lippincott, 1980)*

The wall of the uterus is composed of three layers: the perimetrium, the myometrium, and the endometrium. The *perimetrium* is the outer serous covering that is derived from the abdominal peritoneum. This outer layer merges with the peritoneum that covers the broad ligaments. Anteriorly, the perimetrium is reflected over the bladder wall, forming the vesicouterine pouch, and posteriorly it extends to form the *cul-de-sac*, or *pouch, of Douglas*. Because of the proximity of the perimetrium to the urinary bladder, infection of this organ often causes uterine symptoms, particularly during pregnancy.

The middle muscle layer, the *myometrium,* forms the major portion of the uterine wall. The myometrium has the amazing capacity to change in length during pregnancy and labor. The *endometrium,* the inner layer of the uterus, is continuous with the lining of the fallopian tubes and vagina. The endometrium is made up of a basal and a superficial layer. The superficial layer is shed during menstruation and regenerated by cells of the basal layer. Ciliated cells promote the movement of tubal–uterine secretions out of the uterine cavity into the vagina.

The round cervix is the neck of the uterus that projects into the vagina. The cervix is composed of a connective tissue matrix of glands and muscular tissue elements, forming a firm, fibrous structure that becomes soft and pliable under the influence of hormones produced during pregnancy. Glandular tissue provides a rich supply of protective mucus that changes in character and quantity during the menstrual cycle as well as during pregnancy. The cervix is richly supplied with blood from the uterine artery and can be a site of significant blood loss during delivery.

The opening of the cervix, the *os*, forms a pathway between the uterus and the vagina. The vaginal opening is called the external os and the uterine opening, the internal os. The space between these two openings is the endocervical canal. Endocervical secretions protect the uterus from infection, alter receptivity to sperm, and form a mucoid "plug" during pregnancy. The endocervical canal provides a route for menstrual discharge and sperm entrance. Pelvic infection may ascend or descend through the cervix.

Fallopian tubes

The fallopian, or uterine, tubes are slender cylindrical structures attached bilaterally to the uterus and supported by the upper folds of the broad ligament. The end of the fallopian tube that is near the ovary forms a funnel-shaped opening with fringed projections called fimbriae (see Fig. 34-3). The fallopian tubes are formed of smooth muscle and lined with a ciliated mucus-producing epithelial layer. The beating of the cilia, along with the contractile movements of the smooth muscle, propel the nonmobile ova toward the uterus. If coitus has been recent, the ovum may encounter a sperm in the fallopian tube, and fertilization may occur. The fallopian tube is the normal site of fertilization. Besides providing a passageway for ova and sperm, the fallopian tubes also provide for drainage of tubal secretions into the uterus. Infection and inflammation may disrupt fallopian tube patency and impair their function.

Ovaries

By the third month of fetal life, the ovaries of the female have fully developed and have descended to their permanent pelvic position. Remnants of the primitive genital system provide lateral supporting attachments to the uterus, and in the mature female, these supporting structures evolve into the round and suspensory ligaments. Remnants that do not evolve may also form cysts, which may become symptomatic later in life.

Oogenesis is the process of generation of ova by mitotic division that begins at the sixth week of fetal life. These primitive germ cells will ultimately provide the 1 million or so oocytes that are present in each ovary at birth.[1] At puberty this number is reduced through cell death to about 250,000.

The newborn's ovaries are smooth, pale, and elongated. They become shorter, thicker, and heavier before the onset of menarche, which is initiated by pituitary influence. The initial hormonal stimulus for this development is believed to come from ovarian rather than systemic estrogen.

In the adult, the ovaries are flat almond-shaped structures measuring 4 cm to 5 cm in length and weighing approximately 2 gm to 3 gm. They are located on either side of the uterus below the fimbriated ends of the two oviducts, or fallopian tubes. The ovaries are attached to the posterior surface of the broad ligament and to the uterus by the ovarian ligament. They are covered with a thin layer of surface epithelium, which is continuous with the lining of the peritoneum. The integrity of this covering is periodically broken at the time of ovulation.

The ovaries, like the male testes, have a dual function: they store the female germ cells, or ova, and produce the female sex hormones estrogen and progesterone. Unlike the male gonads, which produce sperm throughout the man's reproductive life, the female gonads contain a fixed number of ova at birth that diminishes throughout the woman's life.

Structurally, the mature ovary is composed of an inner medulla, which contains the supportive connective tissue, and an outer cortex of germinal tissue. The germinal epithelium contains the primary oocytes that are present at birth and that become the graafian follicles under the influence of the pituitary and ovarian hormones. A graafian follicle is a fully developed follicle. Usually only one follicle develops during each ovulatory cycle throughout the reproductive years. The extruded ovum is engulfed by the fallopian tube fimbriae and propelled toward the uterus (see Fig. 34-3).

In summary, the female genitourinary system consists of the external and internal genitalia. The genitourinary system as a whole serves both sexual and reproductive functions throughout the life cycle. The gonads, or ovaries, which are internal in the female (unlike the testes in the male) have the dual function of storing the female germ cells, or ova, and producing the female sex hormones. Through the regulation and release of sex hormones the ovaries influence the development of secondary sexual characteristics, the regulation of menstrual cycles, the maintenance of pregnancy, and the advent of menopause.

■ The Menstrual Cycle

Between menarche (first menstrual bleeding) and menopause (last menstrual bleeding), the female reproductive system undergoes cyclic changes termed the menstrual cycle. This includes the maturation and release of oocytes from the ovary during ovulation and periodic vaginal bleeding resulting from the shedding of the endometrial lining. However, it is not necessary for a woman to ovulate in order to menstruate; anovulatory cycles do occur. Normal menstrual function results from an interaction between the central nervous system, hypothalamus, anterior pituitary, ovaries, and associated target tissues. Although each part of the system is essential to normal function, the ovaries are primarily responsible for controlling the cyclic changes and the length of the menstrual cycle. In most women in the middle reproductive years, menstrual bleeding occurs every 25 to 35 days, with a median length of 28 days.[2]

The menstrual cycle produces changes in the breasts, uterus, skin, ovaries, and perhaps other unidentified tissues. The maintenance of the cycle affects biologic and sociologic aspects of a woman's life, including fertility, reproduction, sexuality, and femaleness.

Hypothalamic and Pituitary Hormones

The growth, prepuberteral maturation, reproductive cycle, and sex hormone secretion in both males and females are regulated by the follicle-stimulating hormone (FSH) and the luteinizing hormone (LH) from the anterior pituitary gland (Fig. 34-4). Because these hormones promote the growth of cells in the ovaries and testes as a means of stimulating the production of sex hormones, they are called the gonadotropic hormones. The secretion of both LH and FSH is stimulated by a single hormone from the hypothalamus called gonadotropic-releasing hormone (GnRH).

In addition to LH and FSH, the anterior pituitary secretes a third hormone—prolactin. The exact function of prolactin in regulating ovarian function is complex and not fully understood; its main effect may involve the suppression of FSH and LH.[2] Its primary function is the stimulation of lactation in the postpartum period. During pregnancy prolactin, along with other hormones (estrogen, progesterone, insulin, and cortisol), contributes to breast development in preparation for lactation. Although prolactin does not appear to play a physiologic role in ovarian function, hyperprolactinemia leads to hypogonadism. There is usually an initial shortening of the luteal phase with subsequent anovulation, oligomenorrhea or amenorrhea, and infertility. One possible cause of hyperprolactinemia is treatment with the phenothiazine derivatives (antipsychotic drugs), in which hyperprolactinemia may occur as a side-effect. These drugs are thought to act at the level of the hypothalamus to increase prolactin release by the pituitary.

The hormonal control of the menstrual cycle is complex. For example, the biosynthesis of estrogens that occurs in adipose tissue may be a significant source of the hormone. There is evidence that a certain minimum amount of body fat content is necessary for menarche to occur and for the menstrual cycle to be maintained. This

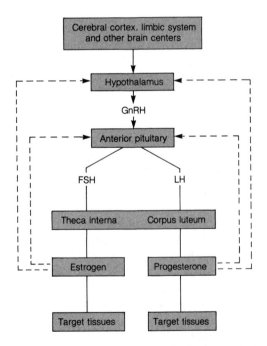

Figure 34-4 *Hypothalamic–pituitary feedback control of estrogen and progesterone levels in the female.*

is supported by the observation of amenorrhea in women with anorexia nervosa, chronic disease, and malnutrition, and women who are long-distance runners. In women with anorexia nervosa, gonadotropin and estriol secretion, including LH release and responsiveness to GnRH, can revert to prepubertal levels.[3] With resumption of weight gain and attainment of sufficient body mass, the normal prepubertal hormone pattern is usually reinstated.

Ovarian Hormones

The ovaries produce estrogens, progesterone, and androgens. Ovarian hormones are secreted in a cyclic pattern as a result of the interaction between the hypothalamic-releasing factors and the pituitary gonadotropic hormones.

The steroid sex hormones enter cells by passive diffusion, bind to specific receptor proteins in the cytoplasm, and then move to the nucleus where they bind to specific sites on the chromosomes (Chap. 37). These hormones exert their effects through gene–hormone interactions, which stimulate the synthesis of specific messenger RNA (Chap. 1). The number of hormonal receptor sites on a cell is not fixed; the evidence suggests that they are constantly being removed and replaced. An increase or decrease in the number of receptors can serve as a mechanism for regulating hormone activity. For example, estrogen may induce the development of an increased number of estrogen receptors in some tissues and may also stimulate the synthesis of progesterone receptors. In contrast, progesterone may cause a reduction in the number of estrogen and progesterone receptors.

Although the ovarian hormones produce many of their effects through mobile intercellular receptors, there is evidence of additional mechanisms. For example, the stimulatory effect that the estrogens have on uterine blood flow suggests that these hormones may also exert some of their effects at the level of the cell membrane.

Estrogens

Estrogens are a family of structurally related female sex hormones synthesized and secreted by the cells in the ovaries and in small amounts by cells in the adrenal cortex. In addition, androgens can be converted to estrogens peripherally, especially in fat tissue. Three estrogens occur naturally in humans: estrone (E_1), estradiol (E_2), and estriol (E_3). Of these, estradiol is the most biologically potent and the most abundantly secreted product of the ovary. Estrogens are secreted throughout the menstrual cycle; two peaks occur—one before ovulation and one in the middle of the luteal phase. Estrogens are transported in the blood bound to specific plasma globulins, which can also bind testoster-

one, inactivated and conjugated in the liver and then excreted in the bile.

Estrogens are necessary for the normal physical maturation of the female. In concert with other hormones, estrogens provide for the reproductive processes of ovulation, implantation, pregnancy, parturition, and lactation by stimulating the development and maintaining the growth of the accessory organs. In the absence of androgens, estrogens stimulate the intrauterine development of the vagina, uterus, and uterine tubes from the embryonic müllerian system. They also stimulate the stromal development and ductal growth of the breasts at puberty, are responsible for the accelerated pubertal skeletal growth phase and for closure of the epiphysis of the long bones, contribute to the growth of axillary and pubic hair, and alter the distribution of body fat to produce the typical female body contours, including the accumulation of body fat around the hips and breasts. Larger quantities also stimulate pigmentation of the skin in the nipple, areolar, and genital regions.

In addition to their effects on the growth of uterine muscle, estrogens also play an important role in the development of the endometrial lining. During anovulatory cycles, continued exposure to estrogens for prolonged periods of time leads to abnormal hyperplasia of the endometrium accompanied by abnormal bleeding patterns. When estrogen production is poorly coordinated during the normal menstrual period, inappropriate bleeding and shedding of the endometrium can also occur.

A number of important extragenital metabolic effects are caused by estrogens. Estrogens are responsible for maintaining the normal structure of skin and blood vessels in women. Because estrogens decrease the rate of bone resorption by antagonizing the effects of parathyroid hormone on bone, osteoporosis is a common problem in estrogen-deficient postmenopausal women. In the liver, estrogens increase the synthesis of transport proteins for thyroxin, estrogen, testosterone, and other hormones. Estrogens affect the composition of the plasma lipoproteins; they produce an increase in high-density lipoproteins (HDL), a slight reduction in low-density lipoproteins (LDL), and a reduction in cholesterol levels. Plasma triglyceride levels are increased. Estrogens enhance the coagulability of blood by effecting increased circulating levels of plasminogen and factors II, VII, IX, and X.

The estrogens cause moderate retention of sodium and water. Most women retain salt and water and gain weight just before menstruation. This occurs because the estrogens facilitate the loss of intravascular fluids into the extracellular spaces, producing edema and increased sodium and water retention by the kidneys because of the decreased plasma volume. The actions of estrogens are summarized in Table 34-1.

Table 34-1 Actions of Estrogens

General Function	Specific Actions
Growth and Development	
Reproductive organs	Stimulate embryonic development of vagina, uterus, and fallopian tubes and secondary sex characteristics during puberty
Skeleton	Accelerates growth of long bones and closure of epiphysis at puberty
Reproductive Processes	
Ovulation	Participates in growth of ovarian follicles
Fertilization	Alters the cervical secretions to favor survival and transport of sperm
	Promotes motility of sperm within the fallopian tubes by decreasing mucus viscosity
Implantation	Promotes development of endometrial lining in the event of pregnancy
Vagina	Proliferates and cornifices vaginal mucosa
Cervix	Increases mucus consistency
Breasts	Stimulate stromal development and ductal growth
General Metabolic Effects	
Bone resorption	Decreases rate of bone resorption
Plasma proteins	Increase production of thyroid and other binding globulins
Lipoproteins	Increase HDL

Progesterone

Although the term progesterone refers to a substance that maintains pregnancy, progesterone is secreted as a part of the normal menstrual cycle. The corpus luteum of the ovary secretes large amounts of progesterone after ovulation and the adrenal cortex secretes very small amounts. The hormone circulates in the blood attached to a specific plasma protein. It is metabolized in the liver and conjugated for excretion in the bile.

The local effects of progesterone on reproductive organs include the glandular development of the breasts and the cyclic glandular development of the endometrium. Progesterone can also compete with aldosterone at the level of the renal tubule, causing a decrease in sodium reabsorption with a resultant increase in secretion of aldosterone by the adrenal cortex (such as occurs in pregnancy).[2] Although the mechanism is uncertain, progesterone is known to increase the body temperature.

Progesterone's reputed ability to quiet uterine contractions makes it important in maintaining pregnancy. Vascular relaxation under the influence of progesterone is responsible for many of the common discomforts of pregnancy, such as edema, constipation, flatulence, and headaches. The increased progesterone present during pregnancy and the luteal phase of the menstrual cycle enhances the ventilatory response to carbon dioxide, leading to a measurable change in arterial and alveolar PCO_2.

Androgens

The normal female produces androgens as well as estrogens and progesterone. About 25% of these androgens are secreted from the ovaries, 25% from the adrenal cortex, and 50% from either ovarian or adrenal precursors. In the female, androgens contribute to normal hair growth at puberty and may have other important metabolic effects.

Ovarian Follicle Development and Ovulation

The tissues of the adult ovary can be conveniently divided into four compartments, or units: (1) the stroma, or supporting tissue, (2) the interstitial cells, (3) the follicles, and (4) the corpus luteum. The stroma is the connective tissue substance of the ovary in which the follicles are distributed. The interstitial cells are estrogen-secreting cells that resemble the Leydig cells, or interstitial cells, of the testes.

Beginning at puberty, a cyclic rise in anterior pituitary gonadotropic hormones, follicle-stimulating hormone (FSH), and luteinizing hormone (LH), stimulate the development of several graafian, or mature, follicles. Follicles at all stages of development can be found in both ovaries, except in menopausal women (Fig. 34-5). The vast majority of follicles exist as primary follicles, each of which consists of a round oocyte surrounded by a single layer of flattened epithelial-derived granulosa cells and a basement membrane. The primary follicles constitute an inactive pool of follicles from which all the ovulating follicles develop. Under the influence of endocrine stimulation, 6 to 12 primary follicles develop into secondary follicles once every ovulatory cycle. During the development of the secondary follicle, the primary oocyte increases in size, and the granulosa cells proliferate to form a multilayered wall around it. During this time a membrane called the zona pellucida develops and surrounds the oocyte, and small pockets of fluid begin to appear between the granulosa cells. Blood vessels, however, do not penetrate the basement membrane; the granulosa cell layer remains avascular until after ovulation has occurred.[3] Usually, only the most mature follicle will develop fully, whereas others will continue to produce hormone but will atrophy, or become atretic. As the follicles mature, FSH stimulates the development of the cell layers. Cells from the surrounding stromal tissue align themselves to form a cellular wall called the theca. The cells of the theca become differentiated into two layers, an inner theca interna, which lies adjacent to the follicular cells, and an outer theca externa. As the follicle enlarges, a single large cavity, or antrum, is formed and a portion of the granulosa cells and the oocytes are displaced to one side of the follicle by the fluid that accumulates. The secondary oocyte remains surrounded by a crown of granulosa cells, the corona radiata. As the follicle ripens, ovarian estrogen is produced by the granulosa cells. High levels of estrogen exert a negative feedback on FSH, inhibiting multiple follicular development and causing an increase in LH levels. This represents the follicular stage of the menstrual cycle. As estrogen suppresses FSH, the actions of LH predominate and the mature follicle (measuring approximately 23 mm) bursts; the oocyte, along with the corona radiata, is ejected from the follicle.[4] Normally, the ovum is then transported through the fallopian tube toward the uterus.

Following ovulation, the follicle collapses, and the luteal stage of the menstrual cycle occurs. The granulosa cells are invaded by blood vessels and yellow lipochrome-bearing cells from the theca layer. A rapid accumulation of blood and fluid forms a mass called the *corpus luteum*. Leakage of this blood onto the peritoneal surface that surrounds the ovary is thought to contribute to the *mittelschmerz* (middle, or intermenstrual, pain) of ovulation. During the luteal stage, progesterone is secreted

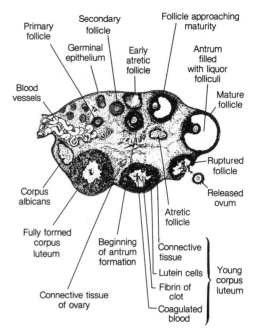

Figure 34-5 *Schematic diagram of an ovary, showing the sequence of events in the origin, growth, and rupture of an ovarian follicle, and the formation and retrogression of a corpus luteum. The atretic follicles are those that show signs of degeneration and death. (Patten BM: Human Embryology, New York, Blakiston, McGraw-Hill)*

from the corpus luteum. If fertilization does not take place, the corpus luteum atrophies and is replaced by white scar tissue (corpus albicans); the hormonal support of the myometrium is withdrawn, and menstruation occurs. In the event of fertilization, human chorionic gonadotropin (HCG) is produced by the trophoblastic cells within the blastocyst. The corpus luteum remains functional for 3 months and provides hormonal support for pregnancy until the placenta is fully functional. Figure 34-6 illustrates the hormonal changes that occur during the development of the ovarian follicle and ovulation.

Endometrial Changes

The endometrium consists of two distinct layers, or zones, that are responsive to hormonal stimulation: a basal layer and a functional layer. The basal layer lies adjacent to the myometrium and is not sloughed during menstruation. The functional layer arises from the basal layer and undergoes proliferative changes and menstrual sloughing. It can be subdivided into two components: a thin, superficial, compact layer and a deeper spongiosa layer that makes up most of the secretory and fully developed endometrium. The endometrial cycle can be divided into three phases: (1) the proliferative, or pre-

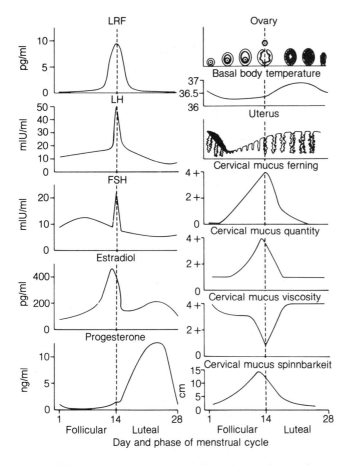

Figure 34-6 *Hormonal and morphologic changes during the normal menstrual cycle. (From Hershman JM: Endocrine Pathophysiology, 2nd ed. Philadelphia, Lea & Febiger, 1982)*

ovulatory phase, during which the glands and stroma of the superficial layer grow rapidly; (2) the secretory, or postovulatory phase, during which glandular dilatation, active mucus secretion, and highly vascular and edematous endometrium are present; and (3) the menstrual phase, during which the superficial layer degenerates and sloughs off.

Cervical Mucus

Cervical mucus is a complex heterogeneous secretion produced by the glands of the endocervix. It is composed of 92% to 98% water and 1% inorganic salts, mainly sodium chloride. The mucus also contains simple sugars, polysaccharides, proteins, and glycoproteins. Its pH is usually alkaline, ranging from 6.5 to 9.0.[2] Its characteristics are strongly influenced by serum estrogen and progesterone levels. Estrogen stimulates the production of large amounts of clear, watery mucus through which sperm can penetrate most easily. Progesterone, even in the presence of estrogen, reduces the secretion of mucus.

During the luteal phase of the menstrual cycle, mucus is scant, viscous, and cellular (Fig. 34-6).

Two methods are used to examine the properties of cervical mucus and correlate them with hormonal activity. Spinnbarkeit is the property that allows cervical mucus to be stretched or drawn into a thread. Spinnbarkeit can be estimated by stretching a sample of cervical mucus between two glass slides and measuring the maximum length of the thread before it breaks. At midcycle, spinnbarkeit usually exceeds 10 cm.[2] A second method of estimating hormonal levels is ferning, or arborization. Ferning refers to the characteristic microscopic pattern that results from the crystalization of the inorganic salts in the cervical mucus when it is dried. As the estrogen levels increase, the composition of the cervical mucus changes, so that dried mucus begins to demonstrate ferning in the latter part of the follicular phase. The absence of ferning can indicate inadequate estrogen stimulation of the endocervical glands or inhibition of the endocervical glands by increased secretion of progesterone. Persistent ferning throughout the menstrual cycle suggests anovulatory cycles or insufficient progesterone secretion.

Menopause

Menopause is the cessation of menstrual cycles. It is as much a process as menstruation—not an event. At first the process takes the form of less frequent and lighter menses; it then goes on to culminate in total cessation of menses. This process, also known as the climacteric, may go on for one to several years. The usual age of a menopausal woman is 45 to 50 years. However, with improved nutrition, menopause may occur later in life, so that a woman may have a longer reproductive period. A woman who has not menstruated for a full year is said to have completed menopause.

Menopause is due to the gradual cessation of ovarian function and the resultant diminished levels of estrogen. Although estrogens derived from the adrenal cortex continue to circulate in a woman's body, they are insufficient to maintain the secondary sexual characteristics in the same manner as ovarian estrogens. As a result, breast tissue, body hair, skin elasticity, and subcutaneous fat decrease as the ovaries and uterus diminish in size and the cervix and vagina become pale and friable. The woman may find intercourse painful and traumatic, though some type of vaginal lubrication may be helpful.

Systemically, a woman may experience significant vasomotor instability secondary to the decrease in estrogens and the relative increase in pituitary FSH. This instability may give rise to "hot flashes," palpitations, dizziness, and headaches as the blood vessels dilate. A woman may feel anxious or depressed about these uncontrollable and unpredictable events.

Societal mores influence behaviors. A society that emphasizes youthfulness, fitness, and vigor does not look on aging as a positive process, and menopause is regarded as a hallmark of advancing age. A woman who focuses her energy on beauty and youth may feel frustrated or depressed by the natural aging process. On the other hand, a woman who values her other, nonphysical attributes may welcome advancing age as a time when she may more fully develop as a person.

In summary, between the menarche and menopause, the female reproductive system undergoes cyclic changes in the breasts, uterus, skin, and ovaries termed the menstrual cycle. Normal menstrual function results from complex interactions between the hypothalamus, anterior pituitary gland, ovaries, and associated target tissues such as the endometrium and vaginal mucosa. Although each component of the system is essential for normal function, the ovaries are largely responsible for controlling the cyclic changes and length of the menstrual cycle.

■ The Breast

Although anatomically separate, the breasts are functionally related to the female genitourinary system, in that they respond to the cyclic changes in sex hormones and produce milk for infant nourishment. The breast is also important for its sexual function and for cosmetic appearance. Breast cancer represents one-fifth of all female malignancies. The high rate of breast cancer has drawn even greater attention to the importance of the breast throughout the life span.

Structure

The breast, or mammary tissue, is located between the third and seventh ribs of the anterior chest wall, supported by the pectoral muscles and superficial fascia. Breasts are specialized glandular structures that have an abundant shared nerve, vascular, and lymphatic supply (Fig. 34-7). What we commonly call breasts are actually two parts of a single anatomical breast. It is this contiguous nature of breast tissue that is important in both health and illness. Men and women alike are born with rudimentary breast tissue, the ducts lined with epithelium. In women, the pituitary release of FSH, LH, and prolactin at puberty stimulates the ovary to produce and release estrogen. This estrogen stimulates the growth and proliferation of the ductile system. With the onset of ovulatory cycles, progesterone release stimulates the growth and development of ductile and alveolar secretory epithelium. By adolescence the breasts have developed characteristic fat deposition and contours.

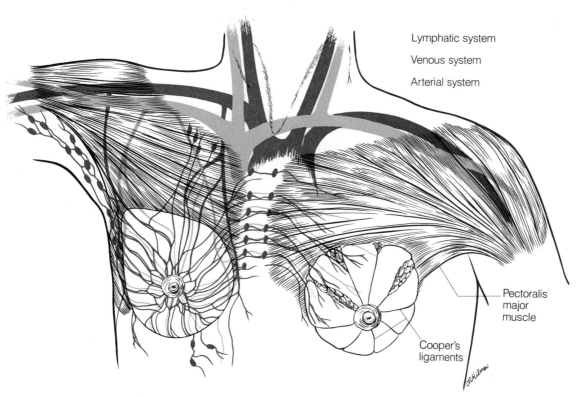

Lymphatic system
Venous system
Arterial system

Pectoralis major muscle

Cooper's ligaments

Figure 34-7   *The breasts, showing the shared vascular and lymphatic supply, as well as the pectoral muscles.*

Structurally, the breast consists of fat, fibrous connective tissue, and glandular tissue. The superficial fibrous connective tissue is attached to the skin, a fact that is important in the visual observation of skin movement over the breast during breast self-examination. The breast mass is supported by the fascia of the pectoralis major and minor muscles and by the fibrous connective tissue of the breast. Fibrous tissue ligaments, called Cooper's ligaments, extend from the outer boundaries of the breast to the nipple area in a radial fashion, like the spokes on a wheel (see Fig. 34-7). These ligaments further support the breast and form septa that divide the breast into 15 to 25 lobes. Each lobe consists of grapelike lobules, or alveoli or glands, which are interconnected by ducts. The alveoli are lined with secretory cells capable of producing milk or fluid under the proper hormonal conditions (Fig. 34-8). The route of descent of milk and other breast secretions is from alveoli to duct, to intralobar duct, to lactiferous duct and reservoir, to nipple. Breast milk is produced secondary to complex hormonal changes associated with pregnancy. Fluid is produced and reabsorbed during the menstrual cycle. The breast responds to the cyclic changes in the menstrual cycle with fullness and discomfort.

The nipple is made up of epithelial, glandular, erectile, and nervous tissue. Areolar tissue surrounds the nipple and is recognized as the darker smooth skin between the nipple and the breast. The small bumps or projections on the areolar surface are Montgomery's tubercles, sebaceous glands that keep the nipple area soft and elastic. At puberty and during pregnancy, increased levels of estrogen and progesterone cause the areola and nipple to become darker and more prominent and Montgomery's glands to become more active. The erectile tissue of the nipple is responsive to psychological and tactile stimuli, which contributes to the sexual function of the breast.

There are many individual variations in breast size and shape. The shape and texture vary with hormonal, genetic, nutritional, and endocrine factors, as well as with muscle tone, age, and pregnancy. A well-developed set of pectoralis muscles will support the breast mass higher on the chest wall. Poor posture, significant weight loss, and lack of support may cause the breasts to droop.

Pregnancy

During pregnancy the breast is significantly altered by increased levels of both estrogen and progesterone. Estrogen stimulates increased vascularity of the breast as well as growth and extension of the ductile structures, causing "heaviness" of the breast. Progesterone causes marked budding and growth of the alveolar structures. The alveolar epithelium assumes a secretory state in preparation for lactation. The progesterone-induced changes that occur during pregnancy may confer some protection against cancer. Cellular changes that occur within the alveolar lining are thought to change the susceptibility of these cells to estrogen-mediated changes later in life.

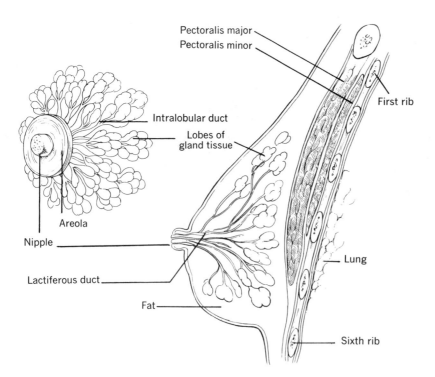

Pectoralis major
Pectoralis minor
First rib
Intralobular duct
Lobes of gland tissue
Areola
Nipple
Lactiferous duct
Fat
Lung
Sixth rib

Figure 34-8   The breast, showing the glandular tissue and ducts of the mammary glands. (From Chaffee EE, Lytle IM: Basic Physiology and Anatomy, 4th ed. Philadelphia, JB Lippincott, 1980)

Lactation

During lactation, milk is *secreted* by alveolar cells, which are under the influence of the anterior pituitary hormone prolactin. Milk ejection from the ductile system occurs in response to the release of posterior pituitary oxytocin. The stimulus for milk ejection occurs with the suckling of the infant. Suckling produces feedback to the hypothalamus, stimulating the release of oxytocin from the posterior pituitary. Oxytocin in turn causes contractile ejection of milk from the alveoli. A woman may have breast leakage for 3 months to a year after the termination of breast feeding as breast tissue and hormones regress to the nonlactating state. Overzealous breast stimulation with or without pregnancy can likewise cause breast leakage.

Changes with Menopause

At the onset of menopause, the levels of estrogen and progesterone are gradually reduced, and the breasts regress secondary to the loss of glandular tissue. The lobular–alveolar structures disappear, leaving fat, connective tissue, and ducts. The breast generally becomes pendulous with the decrease in tissue mass.

In summary, the breast is a complex structure of variable size, consistency, and composition. Although anatomically distinct, the breasts are functionally related to the female genitourinary system in that they respond to cyclic changes in sex hormones and produce milk for infant nourishment. Breast tissue is not static but changes throughout the life cycle.

■ Study Guide

After you have studied this chapter, you should be able to meet the following objectives:

☐ Describe the anatomic relationship of the structures of the external genitalia.

☐ Cite the location of the Skene's and Bartholin's glands.

☐ Cite the location of the ovaries in relation to the uterus, fallopian tubes, broad ligaments, and ovarian ligaments.

☐ Explain the function of the fallopian tubes.

☐ Describe the anatomic features of the uterine wall.

☐ State the function of endocervical secretions.

☐ Describe the anatomy of the ovaries.

☐ Describe the feedback control of estrogen and progesterone levels by means of GnRH, LH, FSH, and ovarian follicle function.

☐ List the actions of estrogen and progesterone.

☐ Describe the metabolism and peripheral sources of estrogen.

☐ Cite the function of androgens in the female.

☐ Describe the four functional compartments of the ovary.

☐ Relate FSH and LH levels to the stages of follicle development and to estrogen and progesterone production.

☐ Describe the endometrial changes that occur during the menstrual cycle.

☐ Describe the composition of normal cervical mucus and relate the changes that occur during the menstrual cycle.

☐ Describe the physiology of normal menopause.

☐ Describe the anatomy of the female breast.

☐ Describe the influence of hormones on breast development.

☐ Explain the effect of estrogen and progesterone on breast changes that occur during pregnancy.

■ References

1. Hadley ME: Endocrinology, p 422. Englewood Cliffs, NJ, Prentice-Hall, 1984
2. Greenspan FS, Forsham PH: Basic and Clinical Endocrinology, pp 41, 374, 377, 381, 383. Los Altos, CA, Lange Medical Publications, 1983
3. Hershman JM: Endocrine Pathophysiology, 2nd ed, p 146. Philadelphia, Lea & Febiger, 1982
4. Austin CR, Short RV: Hormonal Control of Reproduction, 2nd ed, p 107. New York, Cambridge Press, 1984

Chapter 35

Alterations in Structure and Function of the Female Reproductive System

Debbie L. Cook

Stephanie MacLaughlin

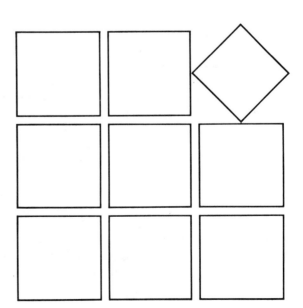

Disorders of the female genitourinary system have widespread effects on both physical and psychological function. Dysfunction of these organs may have a significant impact on sexuality and reproductive function. The reproductive structures are located very close to other pelvic structures, particularly those of the urinary system. Therefore, disorders of the reproductive system commonly affect the urinary system. The discussion in this chapter has been divided into four parts: (1) menstrual disorders, (2) disorders of the genitalia and uterus, (3) diseases of the ovary, and (4) diseases of the breast.

Menstrual Disorders

Dysfunctional Menstrual Cycles

Although unexplained uterine bleeding can occur for many reasons, such as pregnancy, abortion, blood dyscrasias, and neoplasms, the most frequent cause in the nonpregnant female is what is commonly referred to as dysfunctional menstrual cycles or bleeding. Dysfunctional cycles may take the form of *amenorrhea* (absence of menstruation), *oligomenorrhea* (scanty menstruation), *menorrhagia* (excessive menstruation), or *metrorrhagia* (bleeding between periods). *Menometrorrhagia* is heavy bleeding both during and between menstrual periods.

Dysfunctional menstrual cycles occur when the hormonal support of the normal cyclic endometrial changes is altered. Estrogen deprivation causes retrogression of a previously built-up endometrium and bleeding. Such bleeding is often irregular in amount and duration, the flow varying with the time and degree of estrogen stimulation, as well as the degree of estrogen withdrawal. A lack of progesterone can cause abnormal menstrual bleeding; in its absence, estrogen induces development of a much thicker endometrial layer with a richer blood supply. The absence of progesterone results from the failure of any of the developing ovarian follicles to mature to the point of ovulation with the subsequent formation of the corpus luteum and production and secretion of progesterone. Periodic bleeding episodes alternating with amenorrhea are caused by variations in the number of functioning ovarian follicles present. If a number are present and active, and if new follicles assume functional capacity, high levels of estrogen will develop, causing the endometrium to proliferate for weeks or even months. In time, however, estrogen withdrawal and bleeding will develop. This occurs for two reasons: (1) an absolute estrogen deficiency may develop when several follicles simultaneously degenerate or (2) a relative deficiency may develop as the needs of the enlarged endometrial tissue mass exceed the capabilities of the existing follicles even though estrogen levels remain constant. Both estrogen and progesterone deficiency are associated with the absence of ovulation, hence the term anovulatory bleeding. Because progesterone causes vasoconstriction and myometrial contractions at the time of menstruation, anovulatory bleeding is seldom accompanied by cramps, and the flow is frequently heavy.

Dysfunctional menstrual cycles can originate as a primary disorder of the ovaries or as a secondary defect in ovarian function related to hypothalamic-pituitary stimulation. The latter can be initiated by emotional stress, marked variation in weight (sudden gain or loss), or nonspecific endocrine or metabolic disturbances.

Dysmenorrhea

Dysmenorrhea is pain or discomfort with menstruation. Although not usually a serious medical disorder, dysmenorrhea causes some degree of monthly disability for a significant number of women. There are two forms of dysmenorrhea—primary and secondary.

Primary dysmenorrhea begins at the time of menarche or within several years of its onset. It is not associated with physical abnormality or pathology. The pain may be spasmodic or congestive in nature. Spasmodic dysmenorrhea, as the name implies, refers to spasmodic pain in the lower abdomen or back that is relieved with menses. Spasmodic dysmenorrhea diminishes following pregnancy, with use of oral contraceptives, and with the passage of the years. *Congestive dysmenorrhea* causes back, abdominal, and leg pains and is associated with premenstrual tension.

Secondary dysmenorrhea is the dysmenorrhea experienced by women whose menses previously were painless. The triggering event may be cervical stenosis related to surgical procedures such as cervical conization or cauterization, infections, or childbirth.

Treatment of dysmenorrhea is directed at symptom control. Diuretics may be prescribed for relief of the edema. Analgesic agents such as aspirin and acetaminophen (Tylenol) may relieve uterine cramping and back pain. Indomethacin (Indocin) and ibuprofen (Motrin), which are prostaglandin inhibitors, may be prescribed to treat primary dysmenorrhea. These drugs are taken several days before the start of menses. Ovulation may be suppressed and primary dysmenorrhea treated by any of the oral contraceptive drugs. Relief of secondary dysmenorrhea depends on identifying the cause of the problem.

Premenstrual Syndrome

The premenstrual syndrome (PMS) is a distinct clinical entity characterized by a cluster of physical and psychological symptoms that are limited to the week or so preceding menstruation and are relieved by onset of the menses. According to recent surveys, 30% to 40% of the adult female population in the United States experience some monthly symptoms that they attribute to PMS.[1] Just how many of these women have symptoms severe enough to warrant treatment is unknown. The incidence of PMS increases with age and body weight. It is an uncommon problem in women in their teens and twenties. There is clinical dispute about whether it occurs more frequently in women who have not had children or in those who have had children. The disorder is not culturally distinct; it affects non-Westerners as well as Westerners.

The physical symptoms of PMS include painful and swollen breasts, bloating, abdominal pain, headache, and backache. Psychologically there may be depression, anxiety, irritability, and behavioral changes. In some cases there are puzzling alterations in motor function, for example, clumsiness and altered handwriting. Women with PMS may report one or several symptoms, which may vary from woman to woman and from month to month in the same patient.[1] The signs and symptoms of the disorder are summarized in Table 35-1.

The effects of PMS can be significant in terms of a woman's ability to perform at normal levels. There may be time lost or inability to function effectively at work. Family responsibilities and relationships may suffer. Students have been known to have lower grades during PMS. More crimes are committed by females during the premenstrual phase of the cycle and more lives are lost to suicide during this period.

Though the causes of PMS are poorly documented, they are probably multifactorial. Like dysmenorrhea, PMS has only recently been recognized as a bona fide disease rather than merely a psychosomatic illness. In recent years, there has been a tendency to link the disorder with endocrine imbalances such as hyperprolactinemia, estrogen excess, and imbalance of the estrogen to progesterone ratio.[2] The role of hormonal factors in the etiology of PMS is supported by two well-established phenomena: first, women who have undergone a hysterectomy but not an oophorectomy may have cyclic symptoms resembling PMS; second, PMS symptoms are unknown in postmenopausal women. There is also evidence that learned beliefs about menstruation can contribute to the production of PMS or at least affect the woman's response to the symtoms.

In the past, treatment of PMS has been largely symptomatic. Attempts have been made to effect weight loss and reduce fluid retention through the use of diuretics. Tranquilizer drugs were used to treat mood changes, and pain was treated with mild analgesics. The current treatment is, to some extent, directed toward somatic complaints. Relief of somatic pain does not, however, totally resolve PMS suffering. The latest approach is to recommend an integrated program of personal assessment by diary, sometimes including physiologic measurement, a program of regular sleep and exercise, avoidance of caffeine, a diet low in simple sugars and high in lean proteins, and analgesics with an anti-prostaglandin action.

In summary, menstrual disorders include dysfunctional menstrual cycles, dysmenorrhea, and premenstrual syndrome. Dysfunctional menstrual cycles occur when the hormonal support of the endometrium is altered. These cycles produce amenorrhea, oligomenorrhea, metrorrhagia, or menorrhagia. Dysmenorrhea is characterized by pain or discomfort during menstruation. It can occur as a primary or secondary disorder. Primary dysmenorrhea is not associated with other disorders and begins soon after menarche. Secondary dysmenorrhea is usually associated with cervical injury or stenosis. It occurs in women who previously had painless menses. Premenstrual syndrome represents a cluster of physical and psychological symptoms that precede menstruation by a

Table 35-1   Symptoms of Premenstrual Syndrome (PMS) by System

Body System	Symptom
Cerebral	Irritability, nervousness, fatigue, and exhaustion; increased physical and mental activity; lability; crying spells; depression; inability to concentrate
Gastrointestinal	Craving for sweets or salt, lower abdominal pain, bloating, nausea, vomiting, diarrhea, constipation
Vascular	Headache, edema, weakness, or fainting
Reproductive	Swelling and tenderness of the breasts, pelvic congestion, ovarian pain
Neuromuscular	Trembling of the extremities, changes in coordination, clumsiness, backache, leg aches
General	Weight gain, insomnia

week or so. The true incidence and nature of PMS has only recently been recognized, and its true cause and methods of treatment are now being studied.

■ Alterations in Uterine Position and Pelvic Support

The uterus and the pelvic structures are maintained in proper position by the uterosacral ligaments, the round ligaments, the broad ligament, and the cardinal ligaments. The two cardinal ligaments maintain the cervix in its normal position. The uterosacral ligaments normally hold the uterus in a forward position (Fig. 35-1). The broad ligament suspends the uterus, fallopian tubes, and ovaries within the pelvis. The vagina is encased in the semirigid structure of the strong investing fascia. The muscular floor of the pelvis is a strong slinglike structure that supports the uterus, vagina, urinary bladder, and rectum.

Variations in the postion of the uterus are common. Some variations are innocuous; others, which may be a result of the weakness and relaxation of the perineum, give rise to various problems that compromise the structural integrity of the pelvic floor, particularly after childbirth.

Variations in Uterine Position

Usually the uterus is flexed about 45 degrees anteriorly, with the cervix positioned posteriorly and downward in the anteverted position. When the female is standing, the angle of the uterus is such that it lies practically horizon-

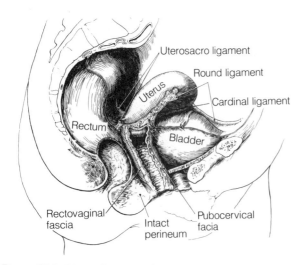

Figure 35-1 *Normal support of the uterus and vagina. (From Mattingly RF: TeLinde's Operative Gynecology, 5th ed, p 487. Philadelphia, JB Lippincott, 1977)*

tal, resting lightly on the bladder. Usually there are asymptomatic normal minor variations in the axis of the uterus in relation to the cervix and some physiologic displacements that arise during pregnancy. The displacements include anteflexion, retroflexion, and retroversion; anteflexion is the most common. An anteflexed uterus is flexed forward on itself. Retroversion is the condition in which the uterus remains tilted posteriorly while the cervix is tilted forward. Simple retroversion of the uterus is an asymptomatic disorder found in 20% of normal women. It is a congenital condition resulting from the shortness of the anterior vaginal wall and relaxed uterosacral ligaments; together these force the uterus to fall back into the cul-de-sac of Douglas. Retroversion can also follow certain diseases such as endometriosis or pelvic inflammatory disease, which produces fibrous tissue adherence with retraction of the fundus posteriorly. Large fibroids may also cause the uterus to move into a posterior position. Surgical treatment may be required to remove the fibroids if they interfere with function or cause significant discomfort or bleeding.

Pelvic Relaxation Disorders

In the female anatomy, nature is faced with the problems of supporting the pelvic viscera against the force of gravity and increases in intra-abdominal pressure associated with coughing, sneezing, defecation, laughing, and so on, while at the same time allowing for urination, defecation, and normal reproductive tract function (in particular, the delivery of a baby).

Three supporting structures are provided for the abdominal pelvic organs: the ilia, the peritoneum, and the pelvic diaphragm (Fig. 35-2). The bony pelvis provides support and protection for parts of the digestive tract and genitourinary structures, and the peritoneum holds the pelvic viscera in place. The main support for the viscera is, however, the pelvic diaphragm, made up of muscles and connective tissue that stretch across the bones of the pelvic outlet. An inherent weakness in the pelvic diaphragm is caused by the openings that must exist for the urethra, the rectum, and the vagina. During pregnancy and childbirth, the muscles of the pelvic diaphragm, or perineum, may become stretched and strained. After numerous pregnancies, the organs may begin to slide out, or prolapse.

Relaxation of the pelvic outlet usually comes about because of overstretching of the perineal supporting tissues during pregnancy and childbirth. Although the tissues may be stretched only during these times, there may be no difficulty until later in life, such as the fifth or sixth decade, when further loss of elasticity and muscle tone occurs. Even in a woman who has not borne children, the combination of aging and postmenopausal changes may give rise to problems related to relaxation of

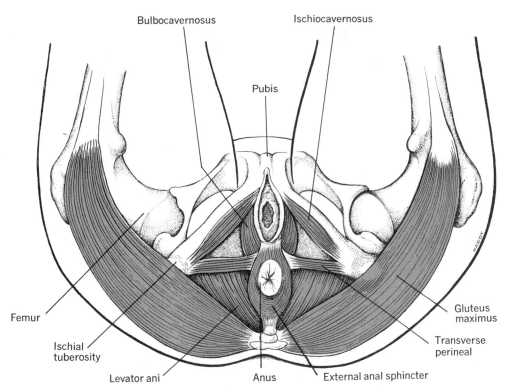

Figure 35-2 *Muscles of the pelvic floor (female perineum). (From Chaffee EE, Lytle IM: Basic Physiology and Anatomy, 4th ed. Philadelphia, JB Lippincott, 1980)*

the pelvic support structures. The three most common conditions associated with this relaxation are cystocele, rectocele, and uterine prolapse. These may occur separately or in association with one another.

Cystocele

Cystocele is a herniation of the bladder into the vagina. It occurs when the normal muscle support for the bladder is weakened, so that the bladder sags below the uterus. The vaginal wall stretches and bulges downward because of the force of gravity and the pressure from coughing, lifting, straining at stool, and so on. Finally, the bladder herniates through the anterior vaginal wall, and a cystocele forms (Fig. 35-3). The symptoms include an annoying bearing-down sensation, difficulty in emptying the bladder, frequency and urgency of urination, and cystitis. Stress incontinence may occur at these times (Chap. 31).

Rectocele and enterocele

Rectocele is the herniation of the rectum into the vagina. It occurs when the posterior vaginal wall and underlying rectum bulge forward, ultimately protruding through the introitus as the pelvic floor and perineal muscles are weakened. The symptoms include discomfort because of the protrusion of the rectum and difficulty in defecation (Fig. 35-3).

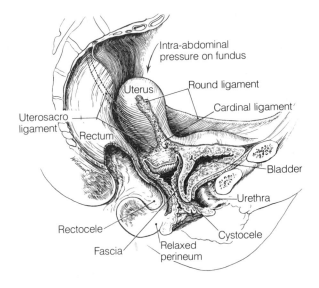

Figure 35-3 *Relaxation of pelvic support structures with descent of the uterus, as well as cystocele and rectocele. (From Mattingly RF: TeLinde's Operative Gynecology, 5th ed, p 488. Philadelphia, JB Lippincott, 1977)*

The area between the uterosacral ligaments just posterior to the cervix may weaken and a hernial sac form, into which the small bowel falls when the woman is standing. This defect, an *enterocele*, may extend into the rectovaginal septum. It may be congenital or acquired through birth trauma.

Uterine prolapse

Uterine prolapse is the bulging of the uterus into the vagina. Prolapse is ranked as *first, second,* or *third degree* depending on how far the uterus protrudes through the introitus.

The symptoms are due to irritation of the exposed mucous membranes of the cervix and vagina and the discomfort of the protruding mass. Prolapse is often accompanied by perineal relaxation, cystocele, or rectocele. Like cystocele, rectocele, and enterocele it occurs most commonly in multiparous women as a result of childbirth injuries to pelvic structures and ligaments that support the uterus. It may also result from pelvic tumors and neurologic conditions, such as spina bifida and diabetic neuropathy, which interrupt the innervation of pelvic muscles. A pessary may be inserted to hold the uterus in place and may stave off surgical intervention in women who want to have children and in older women for whom the surgery might pose a risk.

Treatment

Many of the disorders of pelvic relaxation require surgical correction. These are elective surgeries and are usually deferred until after the childbearing years. Often the symptoms associated with the disorders are not severe enough to warrant surgical correction. In other cases, the stress of surgery is contraindicated because of other physical disorders; this is particularly true of older women in whom many of these disorders occur.

There are a number of surgical procedures for the conditions resulting from relaxation of pelvic support structures. Removal of the uterus through the vagina (vaginal hysterectomy) with appropriate repair of the vaginal wall (colporrhaphy) is often done in uterine prolapse accompanied by cystocele or rectocele. A vesicourethral suspension may be done to alleviate the symptoms of stress incontinence. Finally, repair may involve abdominal hysterectomy along with anterior-posterior repair.

In summary, alterations in uterine position or pelvic support frequently occur as the result of weaknesses and relaxation of the pelvic floor and perineum. Retroversion of the uterus is a condition in which the uterus is tilted posteriorly; it is usually asymptomatic and is found in about 20% of women. Cystocele and rectocele involve herniation of the bladder and rectum into the vagina.

Uterine prolapse occurs when the uterus bulges into the vagina. Pelvic relaxation disorders frequently result from overstretching of the perineal supporting muscles during pregnancy and childbirth. The loss of elasticity of these structures, which is a normal accompaniment of aging, contributes to these problems.

■ Inflammation and Infection

Inflammations of the lower genitourinary tract (vulva, vagina, and cervix) are relatively common because these structures are readily accessible to infectious organisms, and the moisture and warmth of these tissues provide an excellent environment for the growth of pathogens. The upper genitourinary tract (uterus, fallopian tubes, and ovaries) is less accessible to infectious organisms because a natural barrier is provided by the mouth of the cervix. Although infections of the upper genitourinary tract are less common, the sequelae are much more severe because of proximity to the peritoneal cavity and possible effects on fertility. Sexually transmitted infections are discussed in Chapter 36.

Vaginal Infections

The normal vaginal ecology depends on the delicate balance of hormones and bacterial flora. Normal estrogen levels maintain a thick protective squamous epithelium that contains glycogen. Döderlein's bacilli, a part of the normal vaginal flora, metabolize glycogen and in the process produce the lactic acid that normally maintains the vaginal pH within a range that is usually less than 4.5. Disruptions in these normal environmental conditions predispose to infection.

Vaginitis is an inflammation of the vagina; it is characterized by vaginal discharge and burning, itching, redness, and swelling of vaginal tissues. Pain often occurs on urination and with sexual intercourse. Vaginitis may be caused by chemical irritants, foreign bodies, and infectious agents. The causes of vaginitis differ in various age groups. *Candida albicans, Trichomonas vaginalis,* and *Gardnerella (Hemophilus) vaginalis* are the most common causes of vaginal infections in the childbearing age. In postmenopausal women, atrophic vaginitis is the most common. In premenarchal girls, most vaginal infections are due to nonspecific causes such as poor hygiene, intestinal parasites, or the presence of foreign bodies. Vaginal infections due to *C. albicans, T. vaginalis,* and *G. vaginalis* (nonspecific vaginitis) are discussed in Chapter 36.

Atrophic vaginitis is an inflammation of the vagina that occurs after menopause or removal of the ovaries and their estrogen supply. Estrogen deficiency results in a lack of regenerative growth of the vaginal epithelium, rendering these tissues more susceptible to infection and irritation. Furthermore, Döderlein's bacilli disappear, so that the vaginal secretions become less acid. The symptoms of atrophic vaginitis include itching, burning, and painful intercourse. These symptoms can usually be reversed by local application of estrogen creams or vaginal suppositories.

Diagnosis and treatment

Every woman has a normal vaginal discharge during the menstrual cycle, but it should not cause burning or itching or have an unpleasant odor. These symptoms are suggestive of inflammation or infection. Because these symptoms are common to the different types of vaginitis, precise identification of the organism is essential for proper treatment. A careful history should include information about systemic disease conditions, the use of drugs, such as antibiotics, that foster the growth of yeast, dietary habits, stress, and other factors that alter the resistance of vaginal tissue to infections. A physical examination is usually done to evaluate the nature of the discharge and its effects on the genital structures. Microscopic examinations of a saline wet mount smear (prepared by dipping a cotton-tipped applicator into a test tube of saline solution and transferring a small amount to a slide) are the primary means of identifying the organism responsible for the infection. A small amount of potassium hydroxide (KOH) is added to the solution on the slide to aid in the identification of the *C. albicans*. Culture methods may be needed when the organism is not apparent on the wet-mount preparation.

The prevention and treatment of vaginal infections depend on proper health habits and accurate diagnosis and treatment of ongoing infections. Measures to prevent infection include dietary measures that avoid a predominance of simple carbohydrates, attention to hygiene, maintenance of normal vaginal flora and healthy vaginal mucosa, and avoidance of contact with organisms known to cause vaginal infections. Many feminine deodorants and douches are irritating and alter the normal vaginal flora. Tight clothing prevents the dissipation of body heat and evaporation of skin moisture and thus promotes favorable conditions for the growth of pathogens, as well as irritation. Nylon and other synthetic undergarments, panty hose, and swimsuits tend to hold body moisture next to the skin and to harbor infectious organisms, even after they have been washed. Cotton undergarments that withstand hot water and bleach (a fungicide) may be preferable for women to prevent such infections. Swimsuits and other garments that do not withstand hot water or bleaching should be hung in the sunlight to dry.

Cervicitis

Cervicitis is an acute or chronic inflammation of the cervix. Acute cervicitis may result from the direct infection of the cervix or may be secondary to a vaginal or uterine infection. It may be caused by a variety of infections including candidiasis, gardnerella vaginitis, gonorrhea, or chlamydial infections. It may also be caused by the herpes simplex virus. Chronic cervicitis represents a low-grade inflammatory process. It is common in parous women and may be a sequela to lacerations that occur during childbirth. The organisms are usually of a nonspecific type, often staphylococcus, streptococcus, or coliform bacteria.

With acute cervicitis, the cervix becomes reddened and edematous. Irritation from the infection results in copious drainage and leukorrhea. The symptoms of chronic cervicitis are less well defined. The cervix may be ulcerated or normal in appearance; nodules that result from the obstruction of the cervical glands, called nabothian cysts, may be present in the endocervix; mucopurulent discharge may also be present.*

Untreated cervicitis may extend to include the development of pelvic cellulitis, giving rise to back pain, painful intercourse, dysmenorrhea, and infection of the uterus, fallopian tubes, and ovaries. Depending on the causative agent, acute cervicitis is treated with appropriate antibiotic therapy. Diagnosis of chronic cervicitis is based on vaginal examination, colposcopy, cytologic smears, and biopsy to rule out malignant changes. The treatment usually involves cryosurgery or cauterization, which causes the tissues to slough and thus leads to eradication of the infection.

Vulvitis

Vulvitis, or inflammation of the vulva, is not generally considered a specific disease but tends to develop subsequent to other local and systemic disorders. The vulva is usually involved secondary to irritating vaginal discharge. With diabetes mellitus, the glycogen content of vaginal tissue is often increased, favoring the growth of *C. albicans*, which may be a normal inhabitant of vaginal tissue. Vulvitis may also be a component of venereal disease or local dermatitis. Finally, vulvar itching may be due to atrophy that is part of the normal aging process. The treatment of vulvitis focuses on measures to relieve the irritation, such as keeping the area clean and dry, using warm sitz baths with baking soda, and applying hydrocortisone cream for the immediate relief of symptoms.

---

*Nabothian cysts also occur without evidence of inflammation with metaplasia of the cervix.

Bartholin's Cyst/Bartholin's Abscess

Bartholin's cyst occurs secondary to the occlusion of the duct system within Bartholin's gland. When a cyst becomes infected, the content becomes purulent, and a Bartholin's abscess is formed. The obstruction that causes cyst and abscess formation most commonly follows a bacterial or gonorrheal infection, but it can occur with atrophic vaginitis. Cysts can attain the size of an orange and frequently recur (Fig. 35-4). Abscesses are extremely tender and painful. The treatment consists of the administration of appropriate antibiotics, local application of moist heat, and incision and drainage. Asymptomatic cysts require no treatment. Cysts that are frequently abscessed or are large enough to cause blockage of the introitus may require surgical intervention.

Pelvic Inflammatory Disease

Pelvic inflammatory disease (PID) is an inflammation of the upper reproductive tract involving the uterus (endometritis), the fallopian tubes (salpingitis), and the ovaries (oophoritis). The most common cause of PID is untreated gonorrhea; the organisms ascend through the endocervical canal to the endometrial cavity and then to the

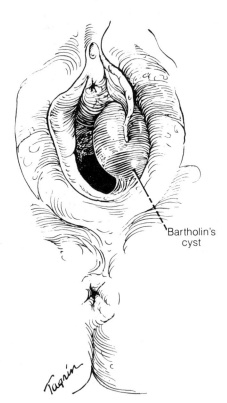

Figure 35-4 *Bartholin's cyst. (From Green TH, Jr: Gynecology: Essentials of Clinical Practice, 3rd ed. Boston, Little, Brown & Co, 1977)*

tubes and ovaries. Chlamydial infections are rapidly becoming an important cause of PID. The endocervical canal is slightly dilated during menstruation; thus, bacteria can gain entrance to the uterus and other pelvic structures. Once inside the uterus, the gonococci multiply rapidly in the favorable environment of the sloughing endometrium.

The symptoms of PID include vaginal discharge followed by fever and abdominal pain during or just after a menstrual period. Pelvic tenderness and an exquisitely painful cervix are present. Fever (102-103°F) and an elevated white blood cell count (20,000 to 30,000 per mm³) are seen, even though the woman may not appear acutely ill. Treatment may involve hospitalization with intravenous administration of antibiotics. Bed rest in Fowler's position (head and knees elevated) facilitates pelvic drainage.

Acute postabortal or puerperal infection accounts for some 15% to 20% of all cases of PID. This type of PID differs from gonorrheal infection in its course, complications, and clinical manifestations, all of which are more serious and may be life threatening. This is because the gravid (pregnant) or postpartal uterus is extremely susceptible to infection, and the site of placental attachment with its rich vascular channels offers little protection against bacterial invasion, affording direct tissue penetration. Thus, it is not uncommon for diffuse cellulitis (inflammation) and peritonitis to develop. Postabortal or puerperal PID is most often due to a mixed bacterial invasion, frequently by gram-negative bacteria (*e.g.,* E. coli, *Pseudomonas, Proteus,* and *Klebsiella*). These highly virulent pathogens liberate their toxins in massive quantities, and absorption of the endotoxins results in generalized vasoconstriction, with pale, cold, and clammy skin, even though marked fever is present. Hemodynamic changes may eventually give rise to endotoxic shock with progressive renal, cardiac, hepatic, and pulmonary failure—possibly death. Clinically, high fever, rapid pulse, and shaking chills occur; the woman appears extremely ill. Pelvic pain is extreme and there is a purulent discharge from the cervix. The treatment of endotoxic (septic) shock is discussed in Chapter 21.

In summary, infection and inflammation can affect the female genitourinary tract. Vaginitis is an inflammation of the vagina caused by chemical irritants, the presence of foreign bodies, or infectious agents. The most common types of vaginal infection are trichomonas, candidiasis, and *Gardnerella vaginalis*. Atrophic vaginitis results from an estrogen deficiency and occurs after menopause or removal of the ovaries. Cervicitis can occur as a primary infection with vaginitis, or secondarily from long-term infection following laceration of the cervix during childbirth. Vulvitis is an inflammation of the vulva, usually localized and sometimes developing as a secondary disorder in systemic diseases, such as diabetes. Pelvic inflammatory disease is a serious infection of the upper genitourinary system. It can result from a gonorrheal infection or occur acutely following childbirth or abortion.

Benign Growths and Aberrant Tissue

In endometriosis, tissue closely resembling endometrial tissue occurs aberrantly—outside the uterus; in *adenomyosis*, islands of endometrial and stromal tissue are found inside the myometrium. In either case, the aberrant tissue undergoes cyclic proliferative and secretory changes similar to those of the normal endometrium. A *leiomyoma* is a benign tumor of smooth muscle of the uterine wall.

Endometriosis

Endometriosis is the condition in which functional endometrial tissue is found in ectopic sites outside the uterus. The site may be the ovaries, the broad ligaments, the pouch of Douglas (cul-de-sac), the pelvis, the vagina, the vulva, the perineum, or the intestines. Rarely, endometrial implants have been found in the nostrils, umbilicus, lungs, and limbs.

The cause of endometriosis is not known. There appears to have been an increase in its incidence in the developed Western countries during the past four to five decades. It is more common in women who have postponed childbearing and is consistent with the Western trend of postponing childbearing and limiting family size. There are several theories that attempt to account for endometriosis. One theory suggests that menstrual blood containing fragments of endometrium is forced upward through the fallopian tubes into the peritoneal cavity. Another postulates that dormant, immature cellular elements are spread over a wide area, persisting into adult life, and the ensuing metaplasia accounts for the endometrial tissue. Yet another theory suggests that the endometrial tissue may metastasize through the lymphatics or the vascular system.

The gross pathologic changes that occur in endometriosis differ with location and duration. In the ovary, the endometrial tissue may form cysts that rupture, causing peritonitis and adhesions. Elsewhere in the pelvis, the tissue may take the form of small lesions, called "mulberry spots," which are surrounded by scar tissue and cause intermittent bleeding into the gastrointestinal tract or urinary tract at the time of menses. If extensive, this fibrotic tissue may occasionally mimic carcinoma and can cause bowel obstruction.

Endometriosis may be difficult to diagnose because its symptoms mimic those of other pelvic disorders. Furthermore, the severity of symptoms does not always reflect the extent of the disease. The most common symptoms are infertility, abnormal bleeding, and pain prior to and during menstruation or during intercourse. Accurate diagnosis can be accomplished only through laparoscopy.

The treatment centers on three aspects: (1) pain relief, (2) hormone therapy, and (3) surgery. In young unmarried women, simple observation and analgesics may be the sole treatment. The use of hormones to induce physiologic amenorrhea is based on the observation that pregnancy affords temporary relief by inducing atrophy of the endometrial tissue. This is accomplished through administration of estrogen or progesterone preparations, which inhibit the pituitary gonadotropins and suppress ovulation. Surgical treatment involves total hysterectomy (removal of the uterus) and bilateral salpingo-oophorectomy (removal of the fallopian tubes and ovaries).

Adenomyosis

Adenomyosis is the condition in which endometrial glands and stroma are found within the myometrium interspersed between the smooth muscle fibers. In contrast to endometriosis, which is usually a problem of young, infertile women, adenomyosis is generally found in multiparous women in their late thirties or forties. It is thought that events associated with repeated pregnancies, deliveries, and uterine involution may cause the endometrium to be displaced throughout the myometrium. Adenomyosis has also been associated with vigorous and deep curettage (surgical scraping of the uterine cavity). Adenomyosis may be associated with fibroids, endometrial polyps, and endometrial carcinoma.

The two common symptoms of adenomyosis are menorrhagia and dysmenorrhea, which become progressively more severe. An enlarged uterus is also common. In addition, dyspareunia, metrorrhagia, and a sensation of pelvic pressure or diffuse pelvic and lower abdominal pain may occur.

For younger women who desire to preserve their childbearing potential, surgical resection of the affected areas with preservation of the uterus is a feasible treatment modality. For older women who have completed their family and have severe symptoms, total hysterectomy (with preservation of the ovaries if they are premenopausal) is the treatment preferred.

Leiomyomas

Leiomyomas are benign neoplasms of smooth muscle origin. They are also known as myomas or, colloquially, as "fibroids." These are the most common form of pelvic tumor and are believed to occur in one out of every four or five women above the age of 35. They are seen more often and their rate of growth is more rapid in black women than in white women. Leiomyomas usually develop in the corpus of the uterus; they may be submucosal, subserosal, or intramural (Fig. 35-5). *Intramural* fibroids are embedded within the myometrium. They are the most common type of fibroids, taking the form of a symmetrical enlargement of the nonpregnant uterus. *Subserosal* tumors are located beneath the perimetrium of the uterus. These tumors are recognized as irregular projections on the uterine surface; they may become pedunculated, displacing or impinging on other genitourinary sructures and causing hydroureter or bladder problems. *Submucosal* fibroids displace endometrial tissue and are more likely to cause bleeding, necrosis, and infection than either of the other types.

   Leiomyomas may be manifested as follows: they may be asymptomatic and be discovered during a routine pelvic examination, or they may cause bleeding, particularly at the time of the menstrual period. Their rate of growth is variable, often with a rapid increase in size during pregnancy. However, interference with pregnancy is rare, unless the tumor is submucosal or obstructs the cervical outlet. These tumors may outgrow

their blood supply, become infarcted, and undergo degenerative changes. Most fibroids regress with menopause, but if bleeding or other problems persist, hysterectomy may be required. Malignant transformations are rare.

In summary, a number of benign conditions other than structural changes and infections affect the female genitourinary system. Endometriosis and adenomyosis are disorders of displaced endometrial tissue. In endometriosis the displaced tissue is located outside the uterus, and in adenomyosis it is located within the uterine wall. Leiomyomas are benign smooth muscle tumors. They are often called fibroids when they are located in the uterine wall.

■ Cancer of the Genital Structures

Significant changes in the frequencies of common gynecologic cancers have occurred in the United States between 1970 and 1980. Endometrial cancer is now the most commonly reported gynecologic cancer, with ovarian cancer reported second. Cervical cancer, ranked first until 1970, now ranks third. Clear-cell adenocarcinoma of the vagina, which was practically unheard of until the late 1960s, has been reported with increasing frequency, most often associatd with *in utero* exposure to diethylstilbestrol. Demographic changes, namely, an increased survival rate of elderly women, have brought about increases in the incidence of some forms of cancer, while advances in chemotherapy and radiation therapy have brought improvement in the cure rates of some gynecologic cancers.

Cancer of the Vulva

Carcinoma of the vulva has accounted for 3% to 5% of all malignancies of the female genitourinary system in the past; it now accounts for 8%. This type of cancer is seen most frequently in women who are 60 years of age or older; almost one-half are over 70 years of age.[3] Certain venereal diseases, such as condyloma accuminatum, predispose to vulvar cancer.

   More than 95% of cancers of the vulva are squamous cell carcinomas. The initial lesion often appears as an inconspicuous thickening of the skin, a small raised area or lump, or an ulceration that fails to heal. These lesions often resemble eczema or dermatitis and may produce few symptoms other than pruritus, local discomfort, and exudation. A recurrent, persistent, pruritic vulvitis may be the only complaint. Therefore, the symptoms are frequently treated with various home remedies before

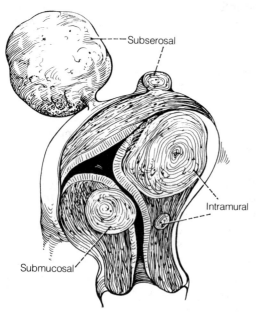

Figure 35-5 *Submucosal, intramural, and subserosal leiomyomas. (From Green TH, Jr: Gynecology: Essentials of Clinical Practice, 3rd ed. Boston, Little, Brown & Co, 1977)*

medical attention is sought. The lesion often becomes secondarily infected, and this causes pain and discomfort. Gradually the malignant lesion spreads superficially or as a deep furrow involving all of one labial side. Because there are many lymph channels around the vulva, the cancer metastasizes freely to the regional lymph nodes. It seems to make little difference whether the tumor is well differentiated or undifferentiated; lymph node metastases can occur in either case. The most common extension is to the superficial inguinal and femoral regions.

Early diagnosis is important in the treatment of vulvar carcinoma. Because the lesion is often mistaken for other conditions, such as dermatitis, biopsy and treatment are often delayed. The 5-year survival rate for women whose lesions are less than 3 cm in diameter is 60% to 80% following surgical treatment.[4] The 5-year survival rate for those whose lesions are larger is only 10% following surgical treatment. Once pelvic lymphadenopathy is established, the prognosis is poor.

Cancer of the Vagina

In general, primary cancers of the vagina are extremely rare. They account for about 1% of all malignancies of the female reproductive system. Like vulvar carcinoma, carcinoma of the cervix is largely a disease of older women, with a peak incidence between 50 and 70 years of age. Vaginal cancers may result from local extension of cervical cancer.[3,5] Vaginal cancer is also associated with local irritation, such as occurs with prolonged use of a pessary.

More than 90% of vaginal cancers are squamous cell carcinomas.[5] A second type of vaginal cancer, adenocarcinoma, has recently been associated with maternal use of diethylstilbestrol (DES) to prevent abortion; this was common practice during a period of time beginning in the 1940s.

In the late 1960s, eight cases of vaginal adenocarcinoma were reported in adolescents.[6] Investigation disclosed that the mothers of seven of the eight girls had taken DES, a nonsteroidal synthetic estrogen, during pregnancy.[7] A tumor registry of clear-cell adenocarcinoma of the genital tract in young women was established, and by 1979 close to 400 cases had been reported. About 60% of these women had definite prenatal exposure to DES. At the time of the banning of DES, an estimated 4 million American women had taken the drug.

The incidence of clear-cell adenocarcinoma of the vagina is quite low, approximately 0.1% in young women who were exposed *in utero* to maternal synthetic estrogen. Although only a small percentage of girls exposed to estrogen actually develop clear-cell adenocar-

cinoma, 75% to 90% of them do develop benign adenosis of the vagina. Adenosis may predispose to cancer. Thus, the really significant damage stemming from DES exposure may not be vaginal adenocarcinoma, but rather another form of carcinoma in daughters of women exposed to DES or in the women themselves.

Although many women with vaginal adenocarcinoma have abnormal bleeding, 20% are asymptomatic, with the cancer being discovered during a routine pelvic examination. The tumor is most often detected on the upper anterior wall of the vagina, although it may be found at any cervical or vaginal site. Any girl exposed to DES should be encouraged to have semiannual gynecologic examinations beginning at age 14 or at menarche. Examination should include careful inspection of the cervix and the vagina.

Treatment of vaginal adenocarcinoma must take into consideration the size, location, and spread of the lesion, and the patient's age. Radical surgery and radiation are both curative. In upper vaginal involvement, radical surgery includes a radical hysterectomy, pelvic lymph node dissection, and placement of a graft from the buttock to the area from which the vagina was excised. The ovaries are usually preserved unless they are diseased. Extensive lesions and those located in the middle or lower vaginal area are usually treated by radiation therapy. The prognosis depends on the stage of the disease, the involvement of lymph nodes, and the degree of mitotic activity of the tumor. With radiotherapy or radical surgery, the 5-year survival rate for cancer not related to DES is 20% to 30%; for DES-related cancers the survival rate is about 80%.[4]

Cancer of the Cervix

Fortunately, cervical cancer is the most readily detected and the most easily cured of all the female reproductive system cancers if detected early. Survival depends on, in order of priority, (1) the stage of the disease, (2) age at diagnosis, and (3) health status. Survival in stage-I carcinoma of the cervix is 80% to 90%; in stage IV it is 30% to 40%, with a cure rate of 60%.[8] Detection and cure are associated with more sensitive and readily available screening methods (Pap smear), consistent use of a standardized grading system that guides treatment, and effective treatment methods. Effective treatment, and thus survival outcome, is affected by health conditions such as obesity or illness, which may preclude the use of the most effective treatment.

Women who develop cervical carcinoma often have a history of frequent intercourse in their teens with multiple sexual partners. Cervical carcinoma is also more common when the male sex partner is uncircumcised and does not practice regular penile hygiene. The foreskin may harbor organisms that can cause cervical irritation. A relationship between herpes virus II and cancer of the cervix has been suggested.[9] In one study, 23% of women with herpes II infection had either cervical dysplasia or cancer of the cervix.[10] Because this virus is spread by sexual contact, its association with cervical cancer provides a tempting hypothesis to explain the possible relationship between sexual practices and cervical cancer.

One of the most important advances in the early diagnosis and treatment of cancer of the cervix was made possible by the observation that this cancer arises from precursor cell changes, which begin with the development of atypical cervical cells, with progression to cancer *in situ* and finally to invasive cancer of the cervix. Atypical cells differ from normal cervical squamous epithelium. There are changes in the nuclear and cytoplasmic parts of the cell, and more variation in cell size and shape (dysplasia). Cancer *in situ* is localized to the immediate area, whereas invasive cancer of the cervix is a cancer that spreads beyond the epithelial layer of the cervix. A system of grading and specific terminology has been devised to describe the dysplastic changes of cancer precursors.[11] This system involves the use of the term cervical intraepithelial neoplasia (CIN). The CIN system grades according to changes in the epithelial thickness of the cervix: grade I involves one-third of the epithelial layer; grade II, one-third to two-thirds; and grade III, two-thirds to full thickness changes. Once cancer has been diagnosed, the current preference is to use the International Federation of Gynecology and Obstetrics (FIGO) classification system to describe the histologic and clinical extent of the disease. The development of internationally acceptable grading criteria has significantly increased the data base concerning cervical cancer and the consistency of that data base.

The atypical cellular changes that precede frank neoplasia can be recognized by a number of direct and microscopic techniques, including the Pap smear. The precursor lesions can exist in a reversible form, which sometimes regresses spontaneously, or they may progress and undergo malignant change. Cancers of the cervix have a long latent period; the natural history of the disease indicates an average latent period of 8 to 30 years before it becomes invasive.[12] After the preinvasive period, growth is rapid, and, if the cancer is untreated, death follows within 2 to 5 years.

Diagnosis: The Pap smear

The Pap smear was discussed in Chapter 5. The purpose of the Pap smear or test is to diagnose and detect the presence of any abnormal cells on the surface of the cervix or within the endocervix. This test detects both precancerous and cancerous lesions. Although some clinicians suggest that the Pap test need not be done annually if several normal tests have been done in succession, other clinicians maintain that performing an annual test is the safest procedure to follow. If the woman has had a herpes infection, is a "DES daughter," or has a strong family history of cervical cancer, it has been suggested that yearly Pap smears be done.[12] There are several methods for classifying the Pap smear. One method divides the results into five classes:

Class I: Normal, or no abnormal cells
Class II: Atypical cells below the level of neoplasia
Class III: Abnormal cells typical of dysplasia
Class IV: Cells consistent with cancer *in situ*
Class V: Abnormal cells consistent with invasive squamous cell carcinoma

If the Pap smear shows atypical cells, a colposcopy is usually done. This is a vaginal examination with the colposcope, an instrument that affords a well-lighted and magnified stereoscopic view of the cervix. During colposcopy, staining of the cervical tissue with an iodine solution (Schiller's test) or other preparations may be done; and a biopsy, or removal of a tissue sample, may be made to evaluate changes in the layer structure of the tissue that covers the cervix.

Treatment

Early treatment of cervical cancer involves removal of the lesion by one of various techniques. Biopsy or local cautery may be therapeutic in and of itself. If the biopsy reveals severe dysplasia, a conization may be performed. For this procedure, the woman is hospitalized and given a general anesthetic; a cone-shaped section of tissue is removed from the cervical opening. Many physicians, trained in the use of the colposcope express the belief that conization is too radical a procedure. These physicians suggest that the scarring associated with this procedure can interfere with the ability to conceive and bear children, and they recommend the use of electrocautery, cryosurgery, or laser beam. If, under the view of the colposcope, the anterior edge of dysplasia cannot be seen because it is within the cervical canal, conization is usually performed for diagnostic purposes. Depending on the stage of involvement of the cervix, invasive cancer is treated with radiation, surgery, or both radiation and surgery. Both external beam irradiation and intracavitary cesium irradiation (insertion of a closed metal cylinder containing cesium) can be used in the treatment of cervical cancer. Intracavitary radiation is most effective when the tumor is small. The larger the tumor, the greater the reliance on external-beam radiation to shrink the tumor to a size at which it can be effectively irradiated by intracavitary irradiation. The choice of treatment may depend on age and health status.

Endometrial Cancer

Endometrial cancer is now becoming more common. There are two possible reasons for this increase in incidence. One is that endometrial cancer is primarily a disease of older women (peak age 55 to 65 years), and the increase in incidence reflects a demographic shift, that is, an increase in the elderly population. A second factor is the circumstantial evidence that excessive estrogen stimulation causes endometrial cancer. Recently, a sharp rise in endometrial cancer has been reported in middle-aged women who have received estrogen therapy for menopausal symptoms. In fact, the majority of women who develop endometrial cancer have a history of circumstances consistent with exposure to abnormal hormone levels. These women often are obese or have diabetes and other evidence of endocrine disturbances, are hypertensive, have the Stein-Leventhal syndrome, or have a history of previous use of sequential birth control pills. Some are mothers who took DES during pregnancy; others took estrogen for menopausal symptoms, are nulliparous and infertile, have had menstrual irregularities and ovulation failure, or have had breast cancer and been treated with hormone therapy.

As with cervical cancer, it is believed that precancerous abnormalities in the endometrium precede endometrial cancer. These precancerous changes include endometrial hyperplasia or an abnormal pattern of growth in the cells that line the uterus. These cellular changes may be spontaneous or they may be linked to excessive exposure to exogenous estrogens. Hyperplasia often causes abnormal bleeding and spotting and is usually diagnosed upon dilatation and curettage (D and C), which consists of dilating the cervix and scraping the uterine cavity.

The major initial symptom of endometrial cancer is abnormal painless bleeding. *Any postmenopausal bleeding is abnormal* and may indicate endometrial cancer or its precursor stages. Because bleeding is such an early warning sign of the disease and because endometrial cancer tends to be rather slow-growing, particularly in its early stages, the chances of cure are good if prompt medical attention is sought. Later signs of uterine cancer include cramping, pelvic discomfort, postcoital bleeding, lower abdominal pressure, and enlarged lymph nodes. Although the Pap test is useful in detecting endometrial cancer, it is negative in approximately 40% to 50% of women with endometrial cancer. Endometrial smears, obtained by direct aspiration of the uterine cavity, are far more accurate, with abnormal findings reported in about 73% of women with endometrial cancer.[5] Endometrial biopsy, which can be done in the physician's office, is another method of diagnosis, as is the D and C.

There is a disagreement concerning the treatment of endometrial cancer. The treatment usually consists of some form of combination therapy that involves irradiation and surgery. Controversy exists over which is the most appropriate form of irradiation therapy. The treatment usually involves a short course of external beam or internal irradiation followed by total abdominal hysterectomy and bilateral salpingo-oophorectomy. Surgery usually follows a four- to six-week rest period after irradiation therapy. In cases of advanced disease, surgery is followed by external beam irradiation. Once the disease has metastasized to the para-aortic and abdominal lymph nodes, the survival rate decreases.

In summary, significant changes in the frequency of the various gynecologic cancers have occurred during the past 10 years. The incidence of endometrial cancer has increased. This form of cancer affects older women and is associated with excessive estrogen stimulation of the endometrium, either from hormone therapy or as the result of endogenously produced estrogens. Vaginal cancer, which was practically unheard of before the 1960s, has been reported with increasing frequency, most often associated with *in utero* exposure to diethylstilbestrol. Cervical cancer is the most easily detected of the gynecologic cancers. It follows a predictable course of development involving precursor cell changes that can be identified through the Pap smear. If detected early, almost all cases of cervical cancer can be cured.

■ Diseases of the Ovary

Benign Ovarian Tumors

The ovaries have a dual function: they produce germ cells, or ova, and they synthesize the female sex hormones. Therefore, disorders of the ovaries frequently cause menstrual and fertility problems. Benign conditions of the ovaries can present as primary lesions of the ovarian structures or as secondary disorders related to hypothalamic, pituitary, or adrenal dysfunction. Included in the latter group are functioning ovarian tumors, benign ovarian cysts, and the Stein-Leventhal syndrome.

Functioning ovarian tumors

Functioning ovarian tumors are of three types: estrogen secreting, androgen secreting, and mixed estrogen–androgen secreting. These tumors may be either benign or malignant. One such tumor, the *granulosa cell* tumor, is associated with *excess estrogen production*. When it develops during the reproductive period, the persistent and uncontrolled production of estrogen interferes with the normal menstrual cycle, causing irregular and excessive bleeding or amenorrhea and fertility problems. When it develops after menopause, it causes post-menopausal bleeding, stimulation of the glandular tissues of the breast, and other signs of renewed estrogen production. *Androgen-secreting tumors* inhibit ovulation and estrogen production. They tend to cause hirsutism and development of masculine characteristics, such as baldness, acne, oily skin, breast atrophy, and deepening of the voice. The treatment is surgical removal of the tumor.

Benign ovarian cysts

Cysts are the most common form of ovarian tumor. Many are benign. A follicular cyst is one that results from occlusion of the duct of the follicle. Each month several follicles begin to develop and are blighted at various stages of development. These follicles may form cavities that fill with fluid, producing a cyst. There may be bleeding into the cyst. This causes considerable discomfort, a dull aching sensation on the affected side. The cyst may become twisted or may rupture into the intra-abdominal cavity. These cysts usually regress spontaneously.

Stein-Leventhal Syndrome

Ovarian dysfunction associated with infrequent or absent menses in obese infertile women was first reported in the 1930s by Stein and Leventhal, for whom the syndrome was named. It is relatively rare and is sometimes called *polycystic ovarian disease*. However, the word *ovarian* is misleading, in that the hypothalamic-pituitary hormones and the adrenal gland may be involved.

The syndrome is characterized by hirsutism, obesity, and infertility. It is usually recognized at puberty or soon after as the genitalia develop and the menses become irregular or are absent. There is bilateral ovarian enlargement. The condition is usually treated successfully by bilateral wedge resection of the ovaries. In other cases, fertility has been achieved by administration of the hypothalamic-pituitary-stimulating drug clomiphene (Clomid). This drug is used with utmost caution because it can induce extreme enlargement of the ovaries.

Ovarian Cancer

Ovarian cancer is the fourth most common cause of cancer of the female genitourinary system. In 1983, 18,000 new cases of ovarian cancer were reported, two-thirds of which were in advanced stages of the disease. Most of these women die of the disease.[5] The incidence of ovarian cancer increases with age, being greatest in the 50- to 59-year age group. Ovarian cancer is difficult to diagnose, and 60% to 70% of women have metastatic disease prior to the time of diagnosis. Unfortunately, there are no screening or other early methods of detection for this form of cancer. The lack of accurate diagnostic tools and previously inconsistent staging techniques have contributed to incomplete knowledge and treatment of the disease. In addition, the resistant nature of ovarian cancers is a significant factor in the success of treatment and thus survival.

Cancers of the ovary are frequently asymptomatic, or the symptoms are so vague that the woman rarely consults her physician until the disease is far advanced. These vague discomforts include abdominal distress, flatulence, and bloating (especially after ingesting food). These gastrointestinal manifestations may precede other symptoms by months. Many women will take antacids or bicarbonate of soda for a time before consulting a physician. The physician may also dismiss the woman's complaints as being due to other conditions, causing a further delay in diagnosis and treatment. It is not fully understood why the initial symptoms of ovarian cancer are manifested by gastrointestinal disturbances. It is thought that biochemical changes in the peritoneal fluids may irritate the bowel or that pain originating in the ovary may be referred to the abdomen and be interpreted as a gastrointestinal disturbance.

Cancer of the ovary is complex because of the diversity of tissue types originating in the ovary. As a result, there are a number of different types of ovarian cancers. These different cancers display various degrees of virulence depending on the type of tumor involved. A well-differentiated cancer of the ovary may have produced symptoms for many months and still be found operable at the time of surgery. On the other hand, a poorly differentiated tumor may have been clinically evident for only a few days but found to be widespread and inoperable. Often, no correlation exists between the duration of symptoms and the extent of the disease.

Clinically evident ascites (fluid in the peritoneal cavity) is seen in about one-fourth of women with malignant ovarian tumors and is associated with worsened prognosis. The old treatment of ovarian cancer consisted of homogeneous surgery, assessment of response, and subsequent chemotherapy. The latest treatment methods include cytoreductive and debulking surgery to reduce the size of the tumor, followed by immediate radiation or chemotherapy. Chemotherapy may be given prior to surgery. At the time of surgery, the uterus, fallopian tubes, ovaries, and omentum are removed; the liver, diaphragm, retroperitoneal and aortic lymph nodes, and peritoneal surface are commonly examined. Cytologic washings are commonly done to test for cancerous cells in the peritoneal fluid. Women who respond to postoperative radiation usually have a better prognosis than those requiring chemotherapy.

In summary, ovarian tumors are frequently functional, producing either female or male sex hormones. Benign ovarian cysts can result from accumulation of fluid within a follicle. The Stein-Leventhal syndrome is sometimes called polycystic ovarian disease. It is characterized by hirsutism, obesity, and infertility. Ovarian cancer, which produces few early symptoms, is the fourth leading cause of cancer deaths in women. At present, there are no screening tests for ovarian cancer.

■ Diseases of the Breast

Most breast disease may be described as either benign or malignant. Breast tissue is never static; the breast is constantly responding to changes in hormonal, nutritional, psychological, and environmental stimuli that cause continual cellular changes. Some forms of benign disease increase the risk of malignant disease. In light of this, strict adherence to a dichotomy of benign-malignant disease may not always be appropriate. However, this dichotomy is useful for the sake of simplicity and clarity.

Benign Conditions

Benign breast conditions are nonprogressive. The specific conditions discussed in this chapter are mastitis, galactorrhea, ductal ectasia, intraductal papilloma, fibroadenoma, and fibrocystic disease. Certain forms of fibrocystic disease may be part of a precancerous continuum.

Mastitis

Mastitis is an inflammation of the breast. It most frequently occurs during lactation, but may also result from other conditions.

In the lactating woman, inflammation results from an ascending infection that travels from the nipple to the ductile structures. The offending organisms originate from either the suckling infant's nasopharynx or the hands of the mother. During the early weeks of nursing, the breast is particularly vulnerable to bacterial invasion because of minor cracks and fissures that occur with vigorous suckling. Infection and inflammation cause obstruction of the ductile system; the breast area becomes hard, inflamed, and tender if not treated early. Without treatment, the area becomes walled off and may abscess, requiring incision and drainage. It is advisable for the mother to continue breast feeding during antibiotic therapy to prevent this. Mastitis is not confined to the postpartum period, however; it can occur as a result of hormonal fluctuations, tumors, trauma, or skin infection. Cyclic inflammation of the breast occurs most frequently in adolescents, who commonly have a fluctuating hormone level. Tumors may cause mastitis secondary to skin involvement or lymphatic obstruction. Local trauma or infection may develop into mastitis because of ductal blockage of trapped blood, cellular debris, or the extension of superficial inflammation.

The treatment for mastitis symptoms may include application of heat or cold, excision, aspiration, mild analgesics, antibiotics, and a well-supporting brassiere or breast binder.

Galactorrhea

Galactorrhea is the secretion of breast milk in a nonlactating breast. Galactorrhea may result from vigorous lovemaking, exogenous hormones, internal hormonal imbalance, or local chest infection or trauma. A pituitary tumor may produce large amounts of prolactin and cause galactorrhea. Galactorrhea occurs in both men and women and is usually benign. Observation is usually continued for 6 months prior to diagnostic hormonal screening.

Ductal ectasia

Ductal ectasia presents in older women as a spontaneous, intermittent, usually unilateral grayish green nipple discharge. Palpation of the breast increases the discharge. Ectasia occurs during or after menopause and is symptomatically associated with burning, itching, pain, and a pulling sensation of the nipple and areola. The disease results in inflammation of the ducts with subsequent thickening. The treatment requires removal of the involved ductal mass.

Intraductal papilloma

Intraductal papillomas are benign epithelial tissue tumors that range in size from 2 cm to 5 cm. Papillomas usually present with a bloody nipple discharge. The tumor may be palpated in the areolar area. The papilloma is probed through the nipple, and the involved duct thus removed.

Fibroadenoma

Fibroadenoma is seen in younger, premenopausal women. The clinical findings include a firm, rubbery, sharply defined round mass. On palpation the mass "slides" between the fingers and is easily movable. These masses are usually singular; only 15% are multiple or bilateral. Fibroadenoma is asymptomatic and usually found by accident. Fibroadenoma is not believed to be precancerous. The treatment involves simple excision.

Fibrocystic disease

Fibrocystic breast disease is a condition typified by the development of fibrosis and cystic tissue formation. It is the single most common disorder of the breast and accounts for more than half of the surgical procedures on the female breast.[4] The term *fibrocystic disease* has become a catchall for breast irregularities that occur bilaterally, change cyclically, and in younger women are accompanied by dull aching pain and heaviness. Some clinicians believe that the term is overused and that the breast changes representative of the disorder are nothing more than the result of years of wear and tear. On the other hand, some clinicians believe that fibrocystic disease is a part of a continuum of breast pathology related to cancer. This is particularly true when the fibrocystic disease includes epithelial hyperplasia and papillomatous or demonstrable calcifications. Precancerous potential, or risk, is related to the size of the initial benign mass and the bilateral as opposed to unilateral involvement.[13]

Fibrocystic disease usually presents as nodular ("shotty"), granular breast masses that are more prominent and painful during the luteal or progesterone-dominant portion of the menstrual cycle. Discomfort ranges from heaviness to exquisite tenderness, depending on the degree of vascular engorgement and cystic distention. Diagnosis is made by physical examination, biopsy (either aspiration or tissue sample), and mammography. The use of mammography for diagnosis in high-risk groups under 35 years of age on a routine basis is still controversial.

The treatment for fibrocystic breast disease is usually symptomatic. Aspirin, mild analgesics, and local heat or cold may be recommended. Some physicians attempt to aspirate prominent or persistent cysts and send any fluid obtained to the laboratory for cytologic analysis. Women are advised to avoid foods containing the xanthines (coffee and tea) in their daily diets, particularly premenstrually.

There is controversy regarding the relationship between fibrocystic disease and cancer of the breast. It appears that the catchall term of fibrocystic disease encompasses several different disorders, some of which have a greater tendency to undergo malignant changes. Suffice it to say that any mass or lump on the breast should be viewed as possible carcinoma, and malignancy should be ruled out before the conservative measures used to treat fibrocystic disease are employed.

Cancer

Cancer of the breast is the leading cause of death in women 40 to 44 years of age. One in 11 women in the United States will have breast cancer in her lifetime. Breast cancer strikes 114,000 American women every year and kills almost 36,000 women annually.[14]

Almost all breast cancers (90%) are found by women themselves, often through breast self-examination. Cancer may present clinically as a mass, a puckering, nipple retraction, or an unusual discharge. Some women identify cancer when only a thickening or subtle change in breast contour is noted. The various symptoms as well as the self-discovery rate of cancer support the need for regular, systematic self-examination.

Breast self-examination (BSE) should be done routinely by everyone at risk. In the premenopausal woman, examination should be done right after the cessation of menses. This time is most appropriate in relation to the cyclic breast changes in response to hormone levels. In postmenopausal women and in men, examination should be done at the same time, on the same day of every month. A woman can choose a day relative to her past menstrual history. Examination may conveniently be done in the shower or bath or at bedtime. The most important thing is to devise a regular, systematic, convenient, and consistent method of examination.

Diagnosis and treatment

Diagnostic procedures used in breast cancer include physical examination, mammography, thermography, percutaneous needle aspiration, and excisional biopsy. Tumors are classified histologically according to tissue characteristics and staged clinically according to tumor size, nodal involvement, and the presence of metastasis. It is recommended that estrogen receptor analysis be performed on surgical specimens. These receptors are found in approximately 60% of breast cancers in women under 50 years of age and in approximately 75% of tumors in women over 55 years of age.[14] Information regarding the presence or absence of estrogen (and sometimes progesterone) receptors can be used in predicting tumor responsiveness to hormonal manipulation methods.

At present, the treatment methods for breast cancer are controversial. The treatment may include surgery, chemotherapy, radiation, and hormonal manipulation. Radical mastectomy has, in general, fallen into disfavor as a primary surgical therapy for breast cancer. Modified surgical techniques accompanied by chemotherapy or radiation have achieved improved outcomes comparable to radical surgical methods. Prognosis is related more to the extent of nodal involvement than just to breast involvement. Greater nodal involvement requires more aggressive postsurgical treatment; therefore, many cancer specialists believe that a diagnosis of breast cancer is not complete until dissection and testing of the axillary lymph nodes have been accomplished.

Paget's disease

Paget's disease accounts for 2% to 3% of all breast cancers. The disease presents as an eczemoid lesion localized to the nipple and areola. Paget's disease is treated locally but may indicate systemic disease. Systematic breast examination is therefore done in cases of Paget's disease, including a mammogram and possibly biopsy.

In summary, the breasts are subject to both benign and malignant disease. Mastitis is inflammation of the breast, occurring most frequently during lactation. Galactorrhea is an abnormal secretion of milk that may occur as a symptom of increased prolactin secretion. Both ductal ectasia and intraductal papilloma cause abnormal drainage from the nipple. Fibroadenoma and fibrocystic disease are characterized by abnormal masses in the breast that are benign. By far the most important disease of the breast is breast cancer, which is the leading cause of death in women. At present, breast self-examination affords a woman the best protection against breast cancer. It provides the means for early detection of breast cancer and in many cases allows for early treatment and cure.

■ Study Guide

After you have studied this chapter, you should be able to meet the following objectives:

☐ State a physiologic reason for uterine bleeding due to estrogen withdrawal.

☐ Compare the symptoms of primary dysmenorrhea with those of secondary dysmenorrhea.

☐ Define PMS.

☐ List at least ten symptoms of PMS.

☐ Explain how uterine anterversion, retroflexion, and retroversion differ from normal uterine position.

☐ Describe three types of dysfunction that may result from pelvic relaxation.

☐ Describe conditions that predispose to the development of vaginal infections.

☐ List the most common causes of vaginal infections in women of childbearing age, premenarchal girls, and menopausal women.

☐ State measures to prevent vaginal infections that a health professional should convey to a client.

☐ List the triad of organs involved in PID.

☐ Describe the pathology involved in endometriosis on the basis of its location.

☐ List the symptoms by which the health professional would be able to identify adenomyosis.

☐ Compare intramural and subserosal leiomyomas.

☐ State the underlying cause of functioning ovarian tumors.

☐ Differentiate benign ovarian cyst from the Stein-Leventhal syndrome.

☐ State one important prophylactic measure related to vulvar carcinoma.

☐ Relate the association between the use of diethylstilbestrol and vaginal carcinoma.

☐ State a possible relationship between sexual practices and cervical cancer.

☐ State the purpose of the Pap smear.

☐ State the single most important factor in early detection of endometrial cancer.

☐ State one reason an ovarian cancer may be difficult to detect in an early stage.

☐ Name and describe four or more benign disorders of the female breast.

☐ Explain the importance of breast self-examination.

☐ List some contributory factors in the development of breast cancer.

■ References

1. Rose RM, Abplanalp JM: The premenstrual syndrome. Hosp Pract 18, No 6:129, 1983

2. Abplanalp JM, Haskett MB, Rose RM: The premenstrual syndrome. Psych Clin North Am 3, No 2:336, 1980

3. DiSaia PJ, Creasman WT: Clinical Gynecology Oncology, pp 57, 185. St Louis, CV Mosby, 1981

4. Robbins SL, Cotran RS, Kumar V: Pathologic Basis of Disease, 3rd ed, pp 1118, 1121. Philadelphia, WB Saunders, 1984

5. Beechman JB, Hemkamp BF, Rubin P: Tumors of the female reproductive organs. In Rubin P (ed): Clinical Oncology, 6th ed, 6, pp 467, 468, 446, 429. New York, American Cancer Society, 1983

6. Herbst AL, Alfelder H, Poskanzer D: Adenocarcinoma of the vagina: Association with maternal stilbesterol therapy with tumor appearance in young women. N Engl J Med 284:873, 1971

7. Welch WR et al: Pathology of prenatal diethylstilbesterol exposure. Pathol Annu 13, Part 1:305, 1983

8. Kapp DS, Fischer D, Gueirrez E et al: Pretreatment prognostic factors in carcinoma of the uterine cervix: A multivariate analysis of the effect of age, stage, history, and blood counts on survival. Int J Radiat Oncol Biol Phys 9, No 4:445, 1983

9. Wilbanks GD: The role of herpes virus in cancer of the cervix. Obstet Gynecol Annu 5:305, 1976

10. Nahimas AJ, Roizman B: Infections with herpes simplex I and II. N Engl J Med 289:667, 719, 781, 1973

11. Richart RM: Cervical intraepithelial neoplasia. Pathol Annu 8:301, 1973

12. Behrman SJ: The annual Pap smear: Justifiable. Hosp Pract 16, No 3:10, 1981

13. Hutchinson WB, Thomas DB, Hamlin WB: Risk of breast cancer in benign breast disease. JNCI 165, No 1:13, 1980

14. Keys HM, Bakemeier RF, Savolov ED: Breast cancer. In Rubin P (ed): Clinical Oncology, 6th ed, p. 120. New York, American Cancer Society, 1983

■ Additional References

Abraham GE: Nutritional factors in the etiology of premenstrual tension syndromes. J Reprod Health 28:446, 1983

Briggs RM: High prevalence of cervical dysplasia in STD clinic patients warrants routine cytologic screening. Am J Public Health 70:1212-1214, 1980

Cervical cancer screening: The Pap smear. Consensus Development Conference Summaries 3:27-31, 1970

Cooperman AM, Esselstyn CB: Breast cancer: An overview. Surg Clin North Am 58, No 4:659, 1978

Crile G: Axioms on cysts and benign tumors of the breast. Hosp Med 13, No 5:56, 1977

Dingfelder JR: Primary dysmenorrhea treatment with prostaglandin inhibition: A review. Am J Obstet Gynecol 140:874, 1981

Dunlay J: Premenstrual syndrome. J Fam Pract 17 (July):29, 1983

Gambrell RD: The menopause: Benefits and risks of estrogen-proestrogen replacement therapy. Fertil Steril 37:457, 1982

Gelms J: Vulvar carcinoma: Pre-, intra- and post-operative care. Point View 17:14–16, 1980

Gerbie MV: Malignant tumors of the vagina: Classification and approach to treatment. Postgrad Med 73:272, 1983

Gever LN: From arthritis pain to dysmenorrhea: A new indication for prostaglandin inhibitors. Nursing '80, 101:81, 1981

Gorline LL, Stegbauer CC: What every nurse should know about vaginitis. Am J Nurs 82:1851, 1982

Gollober M: Cervical cancer screening. Nurse Pract 4:17-18, 1979

Greenblatt RB: Estrogen replacement therapy? Yes. Patient Care 13:23-25, 1979

Hassey KM, Bloom LS, Burgess SL: Radiation: Alternative to mastectomy. Am J Nurs 83:1567, 1983

Henderson IC, Cancellos GP: Cancer of the breast: The past decade. N Engl J Med 302:17, 1980

Herbst AL: Diethylstilbesterol exposure—1984. N Engl J Med 311:1433, 1984

Hutchinson WB, Thomas DB, Hamlin WB et al: Risk of breast cancer in women with benign breast disease. JNCI 65:13, 1980

Jick H et al: The epidemic of endometrial cancer: A commentary. Am J Public Health 70:264-267, 1980

Kapp D, Schwartz P: Gynecologic oncology: Cancer update II. Conn Med 44, No 9:557, 1980

Kopans DB, Meyer J, Sadowsky N: Breast imaging. N Engl J Med 310:960, 1984

Labrum AH: Hypothalamic, pineal, and pituitary factors in the premenstrual syndrome. J Reprod Health 28:438, 1983

Larson E: Epidemiologic correlates of breast, endometrial, and ovarian cancers. Cancer Nurs 6:295, 1983

A late treatment for dysmenorrhea prostaglandin inhibitors. Emergency Medicine 12:138, 1980

Latinis B: Women's health care update. Nurse Pract 4:36-37, 1979

Levine RM, Lippman ME: Breast cancer management: Recent advances and recommendations. Adv Intern Med 29:215, 1984

Manni A: Hormone receptors and breast cancer. N Engl J Med 309:1383, 1983

McCann J: New fine needle aspiration use: Pelvic diagnosis. Medical News and International Report 5, No 4, 1981

McGowan L: Ovarian cancer: Improving survival. Hosp Med 15:6-7, 1979

Prilook ME (ed): Hysterectomy: For whom, when, how? Patient Care 14:16-17 +, 1980

Read RL, Yen SSC: Premenstrual syndrome. Am J Obstet Gynecol 139:85, 1981

Roberts SJ: Dysmenorrhea. Nurse Pract 5:9-10, 1980

Schwartz P, Kapp P: Gynecologic encology: Cancer update. Conn Med 44, No 8, 1980

Singer A: Further evidence for high risk male and female groups in the development of cervical cancer. Obstet Gynecol Surv 34:867-878, 1979

Stromberg M: Screening for early detection. Am J Nurs 81:1652, 1981

Vaitukaitis: Premenstrual syndrome. N Engl J Med 311:1371, 1984

Wilcox PM: Benign breast disorders. Am J Nurs 81:1644, 1981

Wilhelm-Hass E: Premenstrual syndrome: Its nature, evaluation, and mangement. JOGN Nurs 13:233, 1984

Winter WK: Laser treatment of cervical neoplasia: Am J Nurs 82:1384, 1982

Woods NF, Most A, Dery GK: Prevalence of perimenstrual symptoms. Am J Public Health 72:1257, 1982

Chapter 36

Sexually Transmitted Diseases

Debbie L Cook

Carol Mattson Porth

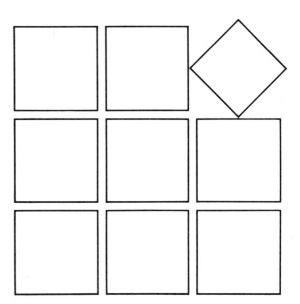

A number of diseases of the reproductive and associated structures affecting both the male and female are transmitted by intimate contact or sexual activity. The traditional venereal diseases such as gonorrhea, syphilis, and chancroid account for only a few of these diseases. For purposes of discussion in this chapter, sexual contact includes intimate contact, such as skin-to-skin contact that may be separate from or part of sexual activity.

The incidence and types of sexually transmitted diseases (STDs), as reported in the professional literature and public health statistics, are increasing. It must be recognized, however, that the incidence of disease is based on clinical reports, and many STDs are either not reportable or not reported. The agents of transmission include bacteria, chlamydiae, viruses, fungi, protozoa, parasites, and unidentified microorganisms (Chap. 7). Portals of entry include the mouth, genitalia, urinary meatus, rectum, and skin. All STDs are more common in sexually promiscuous persons, and it is not uncommon for an individual to be concurrently infected with more than one type of STD.

For purposes of discussion, the content in this chapter has been arbitrarily divided into major and minor sexually transmitted diseases based on the potential compromise of and complications affecting genital and extragenital structures. Other diseases, such as hepatitis, shigellosis, amebiasis, and giardiasis, which are normally spread by contaminated food and drink or by contact with the feces of infected persons can also be transmitted during sexual contact. Transmission of these diseases is possible in populations in which anal intercourse is practiced.

■ Major Sexually Transmitted Diseases

Gonorrhea

Gonorrhea (colloquially called clap, drip, gleet, strain, and whites) is a reportable disease that is caused by the bacterium *Neisseria gonorrhea*. In 1982, 960,633 cases of gonorrhea were reported in the United States.[1] Twenty-five percent of the persons involved were teenagers, and 38% were young adults (ages 20 to 24 years). Although the incidence of gonorrhea has continued to decline since the early 1970s, there has been an increase in infections caused by penicillinase-producing *Neisseria gonorrhea* that are resistant to all forms of penicillin treatment.[1]

The gonococcus is a pyogenic (pus-forming) diplococcus that evokes inflammatory reactions characterized by purulent exudates. The organism grows best in warm mucus-secreting epithelia. The portal of entry can be the genitourinary tract, eyes, oropharynx, anorectum, or skin. Transmission of the disease is usually by sexual intercourse, either heterosexual or homosexual. Auto-inoculation of the organism to the conjunctiva is possible. When a pregnant woman is infected, the infant is in danger of developing gonorrheal conjunctivitis (with resultant blindness unless treated promptly) as a result of transmission of the infection during passage through the birth canal. Because the organism can survive for 24 hours on household articles, infections can be transmitted to family members through the use of washcloths and towels containing the organism. However, when cases of genital gonorrhea are documented in young children, the possibility of sexual abuse should be considered.

The infection commonly becomes manifest 2 to 7 days after exposure. It usually begins in the anterior urethra, accessory urethral glands, Bartholin's and Skene's glands, and the cervix. If untreated, gonorrhea spreads from its initial sites upward into the genital tract. In males, it spreads to the prostate and epididymis, and in females, it commonly moves to the fallopian tubes. Pharyngitis may follow oral sexual contact. The organism can also invade the bloodstream, causing serious sequelae such as bacteremic involvement of joint spaces, heart valves, meninges, and other body organs and tissues.[2]

Persons with gonorrhea may be asymptomatic and thus spread the disease to their sexual partners unknowingly. Men are more likely to be symptomatic than women. In men, the initial symptoms include urethral pain with creamy yellow, sometimes bloody, discharge. The disorder may become chronic and affect the prostate, epididymis, and periurethral glands. Rectal infections are common in homosexual men. In women, recognizable symptoms include unusual genital or urinary discharge, dysuria, dyspareunia, pelvic pain or tenderness, unusual vaginal bleeding including bleeding after intercourse, fever, and proctitis. The symptoms may occur or increase during or immediately after menses because the bacterium is an intercellular diplococcus that thrives in menstrual blood but cannot survive for long outside the human body. Infections of the uterus may be present, and acute or chronic infection of the fallopian tubes (salpingitis) may develop, with ultimate scarring and sterility.

Diagnosis is based on the history of sexual exposure and symptoms. It is confirmed by identification of the organism on Gram stain or culture. A Gram stain is usually an effective means of diagnosis in symptomatic males (*i.e.*, those with discharge). In women and asymptomatic men, a culture is usually preferred, because the Gram stains are often unreliable. As in other significant sexually transmissible diseases in a given population, screening for other diseases, notably syphilis, is done at the time of the initial examination. Pregnant women are routinely screened because gonorrhea can cause blindness in the newborn. Newborns are routinely treated with various antibacterial agents applied to the conjunctiva within an hour of birth in order to protect against undiagnosed gonorrhea as well as other ocular infections.

Gonorrhea is usually treated with injectable penicillin and oral probenecid, a drug which delays the renal excretion of penicillin. Treatment with oral tetracycline for seven days may be used in the event of a penicillin allergy. In the presence of symptoms, particularly in the male partner, it is common practice to treat both partners before the culture results are available because of the potential loss of reproductive capacity. Persons with the disease, particularly pregnant women, are usually followed with repeat cultures to determine the effectiveness of treatment. Persons with gonorrhea are instructed to refrain from intercourse or use condoms until negative cultures are obtained. Because of the growing concern over concomitant chlamydial infection in women with gonococcal pelvic inflammatory disease, the Centers For Disease Control (CDC) are now recommending a treatment regimen for gonorrhea which treats both infections. The combination regimen supplements the penicillin/probenecid treatment with a 7-day treatment of oral tetracycline. Another alternative is a single dose of oral ampicillin or amoxicillin and probenecid and a 7-day treatment with tetracycline.[3]

Syphilis

Syphilis (colloquially called lues, old Joe, the sore, great poc, las bubas, and bad blood) is a reportable disease caused by a spirochete, *Treponema pallidum*. In 1983, 33,613 new cases of syphilis were reported in the United States.[1]

T. pallidum is readily killed by soap and ordinary disinfectant agents; hence, the disease is usually spread through sexual intercourse.[2] However, bacteria-laden secretions may transfer the organism during kissing or intimate contact. A skin abrasion provides another possible portal of entry. Because rapid transplacental transmission of the organism from the mother to the fetus occurs after 16 weeks gestation, active disease in the mother during pregnancy can produce congenital syphilis in the fetus. Untreated syphilis can cause congenital defects as well as active infection in the infant. Once treated for syphilis, a pregnant woman is usually followed throughout pregnancy by repeat serum titers.

The clinical disease is divided into three stages: primary, secondary, and tertiary syphilis. The first stage, primary syphilis, is characterized by the appearance of a chancre at the site of exposure. Even before the chancre

appears, however, the spirochete is seeded to other tissues through the bloodstream, producing later dissemination of the disease.[2] Chancres usually appear within 3 weeks of exposure but may incubate for a week to 3 months. The primary chancre begins as a single, indurated, buttonlike papule, up to several centimeters in diameter, which erodes to create a clean-based ulcerated lesion on an elevated base. These lesions are usually painless and located at the site of sexual contact. There is usually an accompanying regional lymphadenopathy. The disease is very contagious at this stage, but because of the mild symptoms, it frequently goes unnoticed. The chancre usually heals within 3 to 12 weeks, with or without treatment.

The timing of the second stage of syphilis varies even more than that of the first, ranging in duration from 1 week to 6 months. The symptoms of a rash (especially on the palms of the hands and soles of the feet), fever, sore throat, stomatitis, nausea, loss of appetite, and inflamed eyes may come and go for a year but usually last 3 to 6 months. Secondary manifestations may include alopecia and genital condylomata lata. Condylomata lata are elevated red-brown lesions that may ulcerate and produce a foul discharge. They vary in size up to 2 cm to 3 cm in diameter, contain many spirochetes, and are highly contagious.

Tertiary syphilis is a delayed response of the untreated disease. It can occur as long as 20 years after the initial infection. Not all persons with untreated syphilis progress to the tertiary stage of the disease. About one-third of persons with untreated syphilis progress to this stage, and only about half of these persons develop symptoms. About one-third undergo spontaneous cure, and the remaining one-third continue to have positive serologic tests but do not develop structural lesions.[2] When syphilis does progress to the symptomatic tertiary stage, it usually takes one of three forms: the development of (1) localized destructive lesions called gummas, (2) cardiovascular lesions, or (3) central nervous system lesions. The syphilitic gumma is a peculiar rubbery type of necrotic lesion caused by noninflammatory tissue necrosis. Gummas can occur singly or multiply and vary in size from microscopic lesions to large tumorous masses. They are most commonly found in the liver, testes, and bone. Central nervous system lesions can produce dementia, blindness, or injury to the spinal cord with ataxia and sensory loss (tabes dorsalis). Cardiovascular manifestations usually result from scarring of the medial layer of the thoracic aorta with aneurysm formation (Chap. 15). These aneurysms produce enlargement of the aortic valve ring with aortic valve insufficiency.

T. pallidum does not produce endotoxins or exotoxins but evokes a humoral immune response that provides the basis for serologic tests. Two types of antibodies—nonspecific and specific—are produced. The nonspecific antibodies can be detected by flocculation (VDRL) tests and complement fixation (Wasserman and Kahn) tests. Because these tests are nonspecific, positive results can also occur with diseases other than syphilis. The VDRL is easy, rapid, and inexpensive to perform and is frequently used as a screening test for syphilis. It generally becomes positive 4 to 6 weeks after infection or 1 to 3 weeks after the appearance of the primary lesion. The VDRL titer is usually high during the secondary stage of the disease and decreases during the tertiary stage. A falling titer during treatment suggests a favorable response. A specific test called the fluorescent treponemal antibody absorption (FTA-ABS) test is used as a test for specific antibodies to *T. pallidum*. It is used in determining whether a positive nonspecific test such as the VDRL is due to syphilis.

T. pallidum cannot be cultured. Therefore, diagnosis of syphilis is based on serologic tests or dark-field microscopic examination with identification of the spirochete in specimens collected from lesions. Because the disease's incubation period may delay test sensitivity, repeat serologic tests are usually done after 6 weeks when the initial test results are negative.

The treatment of choice for syphilis is penicillin. Because of the spirochetes' long generation time, effective tissue levels of penicillin must be maintained for several weeks. For this reason, long-acting injectable forms of penicillin are used. Tetracycline or erythromycin is used for treatment in persons who are sensitive to penicillin.

Genital Herpes

Genital herpes is a sexually transmitted disease caused by the herpes simplex virus. It may well become known as the sexual scourge of the eighties. Just as gonorrheal, staphylococcal, and streptococcal organisms have been past foci of medical conern, the herpes virus is today's. Because herpes virus infection is not a reportable infection in all states, reliable data on its true incidence and prevalence are lacking. Estimates indicate that about 400,000 to 600,000 new cases may occur each year.[3]

There are five types of herpesviruses that cause infections in humans: two types of herpes simplex virus (HSV-I and HSV-II)—type I (cold sores) and type II (genital)—varicella-zoster virus (chickenpox, shingles), Epstein-Barr virus (infectious mononucleosis, Burkitt's lymphoma), and cytomegalovirus (cytomegalic inclusion disease). Herpesviruses are neurotropic, that is, they grow within neurons and share the biologic property of latency.[4] Latency refers to the ability to maintain disease potential in the absence of clinical signs and symptoms (Chap. 7). In genital herpes the virus ascends through the peripheral nerves to the sacral dorsal root ganglia. There the virus can remain latent for a period of time, or it can become active, in which case viral particles are transported down the nerve root to the skin where they multiply and a lesion develops. It is not known what activates the virus. It may be that the body's defense mechanisms are altered.

Both HSV-I and HSV-II can cause genital lesions. The herpes simplex virus is shed from active lesions, and it is usually transmitted by close physical contact. With HSV-I the virus is often transmitted among family members by kissing. When one has a cold sore on the mouth, HSV-I may be spread to the genital area by autoinoculation secondary to poor handwashing or through oral intercourse. HSV-II is usually transmitted by sexual contact or to an infant during birth.

Genital herpes lesions usually begin as small blisters. They become excruciatingly painful to touch and crust over once the blister has broken. The initial, or primary, infection of the virus usually lasts longer and is more severe than recurrent infections. The symptoms may include fever, malaise, muscle ache, lymphadenopathy, dysuria, dyspareunia, and urinary infection. Primary infections may be significantly debilitating and may require hospitalization, particularly in females. First infections are usually self-limiting and last about 2 to 4 weeks. Except for the greater tendency of HSV-II to recur, the manifestations of HSV-I and HSV-II are similar.[5]

No method has been found to prevent the acquisition of genital herpes. The disease is spread through contact with infectious lesions or genital secretions. A recent retrospective study of source contacts of persons having first episodes of genital herpes indicated that 60% of new infections were acquired when lesions were present in the sexual partner.[6] Asymptomatic lesions may also be a source of viral spread, but usually the quantity of virus shed is small.

Recurrent infections result from reactivation of the virus, which is stored in the dorsal root ganglia of the infected dermatomes, and are usually less severe than primary infections. Actual outbreaks may be preceded by itching, burning, or tingling at the site of the future outbreaks. These symptoms indicating onset of an outbreak are referred to as a prodrome.

Diagnosis of genital herpes is based on the symptoms, the appearance of the lesions, and identification of the virus from a Tzanck smear or cultures taken from the lesions. Depending on the laboratory, cultures take about 3 days for a preliminary report and a week for a final report. The stability of the virus in transport media is excellent, making it suitable for mailing. Generally the likelihood of obtaining a positive culture decreases with each day after a lesion develops. The chances of obtaining a positive culture from a crusted lesion is slight, and persons suspected of having genital herpes are usually instructed to return for culture within 24 hours of developing new lesions.[7] A Tzanck smear is done by scraping a debrided lesion with a cytology spatula and smearing the exudate on a slide, allowing the slide to dry, and sending it to a laboratory for microscopic identification of multinucleated giant cells. About 50% of Tzanck smear results are falsely negative. They are, however, available in 24 to 48 hours as opposed to the 3 to 7 days required for a culture. It is anticipated that antibody tests for HSV-I and HSV-II will soon be available and will serve as a basis for more rapid diagnosis of lesions or as an adjunct to culture studies.

At present there is no cure for genital herpes; treatment is largely symptomatic. The antiviral drug acyclovir has recently been proposed as a treatment, along with antibacterial soaps, lotions, dyes, ultrasound, and ultraviolet light. Early studies show that although acyclovir does not prevent recurrences, it does shorten the duration of the lesions, and also reduces the number of new lesions formed and decreases viral shedding in primary cases. It is most useful in persons with depressed immune systems and in those experiencing an initial outbreak.

Good hygiene must be maintained to prevent secondary infection of the lesions. Fastidious handwashing is recommended to avoid hand-to-eye spread of the infection. To prevent spread of the disease, intimate contact should be avoided for 10 days after lesions heal. Because up to 50% of infected newborns will die if they contract herpes infections during vaginal delivery, active infection during pregnancy may necessitate cesarean delivery. Finally, because women with cervical herpes appear to be at increased risk for developing cervical cancer, it is recommended that they obtain annual Pap smears.

Chancroid

Chancroid (soft chancre) is a disease of the external genitalia and lymph nodes. The causative organism is the Gram-negative bacterium *Hemophilus ducreyi*, which causes acute ulcerative lesions with profuse discharge. This disease is somewhat uncommon in the United States, although in 1981 an outbreak of the disease occurred among Hispanic men in Orange County, California.[7] The disease is more prevalent in the Orient, West Indies, and North Africa. It is usually transmitted by sexual intercourse or through skin and mucous membrane abrasions. It is highly infectious, and autoinoculation may lead to multiple chancres.

The lesion begins as a macule, progresses to a pustule, and then ruptures. The ruptured lesion has a necrotic base and jagged edges. Subsequent discharge can lead to further infection of self or others. Upon physical examination, lesions and regional lymphadenopathy may be found. Secondary infection may cause significant tissue destruction. The diagnosis is confirmed through use of Gram stain and culture. The organism has shown resistance to treatment with sulfamethoxazole alone and to tetracycline. The CDC currently recommend treatment with erythromycin or an alternative regimen of sulfamethoxazole and trimethoprim.[7]

Granuloma Inguinale

Granuloma inguinale (granuloma venereum) is caused by *Calymmatobacterium donovani*, a tiny, encapsulated, intracellular bacillus sometimes referred to as a Donovan body. The incidence of this disease is decreasing in Western populations. It is, however, frequently found in New Guinea and India. Granuloma inguinale causes ulceration of the genitalia beginning with an innocuous papule. The papule progresses through nodular or vesicular stages until it begins to break down as pink granulomatous tissue. At this final stage, the tissue becomes thin and friable and bleeds easily. There are complaints of swelling, pain, and itching. Extensive inflammatory scarring may cause late sequelae such as lymphatic obstruction with the development of enlarged and elephantoid external genitalia. The liver, bladder, bone, joint, lung, and bowel tissue may become involved. Genital complications include tubo-ovarian abscesses, possible fistula, vaginal stenosis, and occlusion of vaginal or anal orifices. The lesions may become neoplastic. Diagnosis is made through the identification of Donovan bodies in tissue smears, biopsy, and/or culture. The antibiotics tetracycline, streptomycin, and gentamicin are used in the treatment of the disorder.

Chlamydial Infections

The *Chlamydia trachomatis* is an obligate intracellular bacterial pathogen that is closely related to Gram-negative bacteria. It resembles a virus in that it requires tissue culture for isolation, but like bacteria it has RNA and DNA and is susceptible to some antibiotics. The organism causes a wide variety of genitourinary infections, including nongonococcal urethritis in men and pelvic inflammatory disease in women. Chlamydial infection can cause significant ocular disease in the newborn and is a major health problem in underdeveloped countries where it is a leading cause of blindness. In these countries the organism is spread primarily by flies, fomites, and nonsexual personal contact. In industrial countries, however, the organism is spread almost entirely by sexual contact and therefore affects primarily the genitourinary structures. Although chlamydial infections are not reportable, their incidence has been estimated as probably twice that of gonorrhea.[3]

The signs and symptoms of chlamydial infections are similar to those produced by gonorrhea. In women chlamydial infections may cause frequency of urination, dysuria, and vaginal discharge. The most common sign is a mucopurulent cervical discharge. The cervix itself frequently hypertrophies and becomes erythematous, edematous, and extremely friable. The organism may cause pelvic inflammatory disease with its frequent sequelae of infertility or ectopic pregnancy. Ocular disease (inclusion conjunctivitis) develops in approximately 25% of infants born to mothers with cervical chlamydial infections, and chlamydial pneumonitis occurs in 10% of infants.

In men chlamydial infections cause urethritis, including meatal erythema and tenderness, urethral discharge, dysuria, and urethral itching. Prostatitis and epididymitis may develop. The most serious complication that develops with nongonococcal urethritis is Reiter's disease (Chap. 53). Two-thirds of men with untreated acute Reiter's disease had a demonstrated chlamydial urethral infection.[8]

Diagnosis of chlamydial infections is a problem because the two serologic tests available can be misleading. Complement fixation tests are positive in only 40% of women with proven genital infection.[9] Tissue cultures are definitive but slow (requiring at least 3 days), costly, and not always available. If culturing for *Chlamydia* among sexually active and pregnant women is shown to be cost-effective in terms of preventing morbidity, public health departments may be encouraged to increase the availability of low-cost tissue cultures. A new enzyme-linked immunosorbent assay, which utilizes antibodies against an antigen present in the *Chlamydia* cell wall, is being developed. If its development is successful, the test will provide an accurate and rapid (less than 4 hours) means for diagnosing chlamydial infections.

The CDC recommend the use of tetracycline or doxycycline in the treatment of chlamydial infection; penicillin is ineffective. Antibiotic treatment of both sexual partners simultaneously is recommended. Abstinence from sexual activity is encouraged to facilitate cure.

Lymphogranuloma venereum

Lymphogranuloma venereum is an acute and chronic venereal disease caused by *C. trachomatis* (types L-I and L-III). The disease, although worldwide, has a low incidence.

The lesions of lymphogranuloma can incubate for a few days to several weeks and thereafter cause a small painless genital lesion of variable appearance. An important characteristic of the disease is the early development of large, tender, and sometimes fluctuant inguinal lymph nodes called bubos. Flulike symptoms may occur, with joint pain, rash, weight loss, pneumonitis, tachycardia, splenomegaly, and proctitis. In the later stages of the disease, a small percentage of persons develop elephantiasis of the external genitalia; this is due to lymphatic obstruction or fibrous strictures of the rectum or urethra caused by inflammation and scarring.[2] Urethral involvement may cause pyuria and dysuria. The anorectal structures may be compromised to the point of causing incontinence. Complications of lymphogranuloma infection may be minor or extensive, involving the compromise of whole systems or progression to a cancerous state. The treatment involves use of the sulfa drugs or tetracycline, and surgery may be required.

In summary, the major sexually transmitted diseases—gonorrhea, syphilis, genital herpes, chancroid, granuloma inguinale, and chlamydial infections—afford the potential for relatively severe involvement of genital and extragenital structures. Portals of entry for the organisms causing these infections include the mouth, genitalia, urinary meatus, rectum, and skin. They are seen most commonly in the sexually promiscuous population, and it is not uncommon for a person to be concurrently infected with more than one disease. Although most STDs can be treated successfully with antibiotics, the treatment methods for genital herpes have been largely unsuccessful.

■ Minor Sexually Transmitted Diseases

Candidiasis

Candidiasis, yeast infection, thrush, and moniliasis are all names for the vaginal infection caused by the fungus *Candida albicans*. These organisms are often present in healthy people, and the decision whether or not to classify candidiasis as an STD is controversial. This is because candidiasis will not grow, regardless of sexual contact, unless there is a favorable vaginal environment for its growth. Causes for the overgrowth of *C. albicans* include (1) antibiotic therapy, which suppresses the normal protective bacterial flora, (2) high hormone levels due to pregnancy or the use of oral contraceptives, which cause an increase in vaginal glycogen stores, and (3) diabetes mellitus or a high dietary intake of simple sugars, which increase the sugar levels in the vaginal mucosa and thus become a predisposing factor in the overgrowth of the organism. In obese individuals, *Candida* may grow in the skin folds underneath the breast tissue, the abdominal flap, and the inguinal folds. The symptoms include a thick, cheesy, odorless vaginal discharge, and inflammation that causes intense itching and burning.

Accurate diagnosis is made by identification of budding yeast filaments or spores, using a potassium hydroxide (KOH) or wet-mount slide preparation. Fungicidal creams, ointments, and tablets such as clotrimazole, miconazole, nystatin, and candicidin are effective in treating *candidiasis*. Tepid sodium bicarbonate baths, clothing that allows adequate ventilation, and the application of dry talcum powder or corn starch will greatly increase comfort.

Trichomonas

Trichomonas vaginalis is a parasitic protozoan that can be transmitted sexually; it is shaped like a turnip and has three or four anterior flagella. Trichomonas infections can affect the vagina, Skene's glands, and lower genitourinary tract in women. The organism feeds on the vaginal mucosa and ingests bacteria and leukocytes. The organism can be harbored in the genital tract as well as the urinary tract without causing symptoms until some imbalance allows the protozoan to proliferate. The infection causes a copious frothy and malodorous discharge and occasional itching and irritation. Typically, there is spotty reddening and edema of the affected mucosa, sometimes with small blisters or granules referred to as strawberry mucosa.[2]

The diagnosis is made microscopically by identifying the protozoan on a wet-mount slide preparation. The treatment of choice is metronidazole (Flagyl), an oral medication with antabuse properties. Antabuse causes a severe reaction (nausea, vomiting, flushing of the skin, headache, palpitations, and lowering of the blood pressure) with alcohol ingestion. Metronidazole has many side effects and, like any drug, should be used with appropriate caution. The drug has not been proven safe in pregnancy and is used only after the first trimester for fear of potential teratogenic effects. Flagyl is known to cause leukopenia in some individuals. Trichomoniasis may be treated alternatively and effectively with acidification of the environment through dietary and topical treatment. In resistant cases or when the decision is made to use Flagyl, both partners are treated simultaneously in order to decrease the incidence of recurrence through cross infestation.

Nonspecific Vaginitis

Considerable controversy exists regarding the organism(s) responsible for a vaginal infection that produces a characteristic fishy or ammonia-smelling discharge, yet fails to produce an inflammatory response, which is characteristic of most infections. A number of terms (*Hemophilus vaginalis* vaginitis, *Corynebacterium vaginale* vaginitis, *Gardnerella vaginalis* vaginitis, and bacterial vaginosis) have been used to describe the nonspecific vaginitis that cannot be attributed to one of the accepted pathogenic organisms such as *Trichomonas vaginalis, Candida albicans,* or *Neisseria gonorrhea.* In 1955 Gardner and Dukes isolated an organism from women with vaginitis and proposed the name *H. vaginalis,* seemingly because the organism was gram negative and required blood for growth.[10] In 1963, gram-positive isolates were found and the organism was renamed *C. vaginale.* Because the organism did not meet all of the criteria of *Corynebacteria,* it was renamed *Gardnerella vaginalis* in 1980, after its original discoverer, and admitted to a taxonomic genus of its own.[11] Recently, it has been suggested that certain anaerobes act with *G. vaginalis* as causes of nonspecific vaginitis.[12] *Gardnerella vaginalis* grows poorly in the normal vaginal *p*H, which is usually below 4.5. It has been suggested that the presence of the anaerobes, which produce ammonia or amines from amino acids, favors the growth of the *G. vaginalis* organism by raising the vaginal *p*H. Because of the finding of a wide variety of anaerobic bacteria in addition to *G. vaginalis* among women with nonspecific vaginitis and because of the lack of an inflammatory response, a new term, *bacterial vaginosis,* has recently been proposed.[13]

Nonspecific vaginitis, or *G. vaginalis* vaginitis, is thought to be sexually transmissible and may be carried asymptomatically by both males and females. Reinfection is common and is greatly affected by vaginal *p*H in women. The symptoms of this type of vaginitis include a grayish discharge that has an intense fishy odor. Burning, itching, and erythema are usually absent because the bacteria have only minimal inflammatory potential.

The diagnosis is made on the basis of character of the discharge, a fishy amine odor, vaginal *p*H above 4.5, saline wet smear, Gram stain, and culture. In *Gardnerella* vaginitis, characteristic "clue cells" are found on wet-mount microscopic studies. These are squamous epithelial cells covered with masses of coccobacilli, often with large clumps of organisms floating free from the cell. Lactobacilli are absent on Gram stain. A wide spectrum of systemic antibiotics and topical creams are used in the treatment of the disease, most commonly metronidazole, ampicillin, or vaginal sulfonamides.

Nonspecific Urogenital Infection

Nonspecific urogenital infection is chiefly a disease of the male urethra but may involve the cervix, urethra, Bartholin's glands, vagina, and fallopian tubes in the female. Fifty percent of these infections are secondary to chlamydial infection. As was discussed earlier, chlamydia is a formidable pathogen because of its long-term effects and ability to affect the newborn. This disease entity, like nonspecific vaginitis, will most likely be more specifically named as the causative agents are identified. Diagnosis is made through the use of cultures. The treatment is by various antibiotic regimens and is dictated by the organism and antibiotic sensitivity.

Condylomata Acuminata

Condylomata acuminata (venereal warts, genital warts) are papillomavirus-induced soft, pink growths that occur singly or in clusters on the penis, scrotum, vulva, vagina, cervix, or rectum. They are one of the most prevalent STDs in the United States.[14] In 1981 there were 946,270 physician consultations for genital warts. Unlike the situation with gonorrhea, syphilis, and genital herpes, little is known about the epidemiology, microbiology, and complications of genital warts. They are sexually transmissible, occurring 1 to 3 months after exposure. The lesions tend to proliferate when moist or during pregnancy in the female. Diagnosis is made on the basis of appearance or biopsy. The treatment should be simultaneous for both partners and involves topically applied podophyllin. This is not considered safe during pregnancy. Occlusive or functionally compromising lesions may require surgical removal.

Molluscum Contagiosum

Molluscum contagiosum is a common viral disease of the skin and mucous membranes that gives rise to multiple umbilicated papules.[13] The disease is mildly contagious, since it can be transmitted by both direct and indirect contact. The lesions are domelike and have a dimpled appearance, resembling a localized neoplastic lesion. A curdlike material can be expressed from the center of the lesion. Necrosis and secondary infection are possible. Diagnosis is made by appearance and the microscopic identification of molluscum bodies. The treatment consists of manual expression of the contents of each lesion and the application of trichloroacetic acid to the cavity. The trichloroacetic acid destroys the epidermal cells in which the virus lives.

In summary, minor STDs include candidiasis, trichomonas, nonspecific vaginitis, nonspecific urethritis, condylomata acuminata, and molluscum contagiosum. These infections exert their main effects through local involvement of genital structures. Although the minor STDs may cause considerable discomfort, they seldom cause permanent dysfunction.

■ Study Guide

After you have studied this chapter, you should be able to meet the following objectives:

☐ Define STDs.

☐ Cite a reason why the reported incidences of STDs may not accurately reflect the true incidence.

☐ List the common portals of entry for STDs.

☐ Name the organisms responsible for gonorrhea, syphilis, genital herpes, chancroid, *Chlamydia* vaginitis, *Trichomonas*, nonspecific vaginitis, condylomata acuminata, and molluscum contagiosum.

☐ List the STDs that pose a threat to the unborn child either *in utero* or during the childbirth process.

☐ State the difference between the wet-mount slide method and culture method used in the diagnosis of STDs.

☐ Compare the signs and symptoms of gonorrhea in the male and the female.

☐ Describe the three stages of syphilis.

☐ Explain the recurrent infections in genital herpes.

☐ Compare the signs and symptoms of vaginitis due to *Chlamydia trachomatis*, *Candida albicans*, *Trichomonas vaginalis*, and *Gardnerella vaginalis*.

■ References

1. Centers for Disease Control: Annual Summary. MMWR 34, No 54:29, 77, 1983
2. Robbins SL, Cotran RS, Kumar V: Pathologic Basis of Disease, 3rd ed, pp 310, 335, 432. Philadelphia, WB Saunders, 1984
3. Centers for Disease Control: Sexually transmitted diseases treatment guidelines 1982. MMWR 31, No 2S, 1982
4. Tummon JS, Dudley DKL, Walters JH: Genital herpes simplex. CMAJ 125, No 1:23–29, 1981
5. Vontver LA, Reeves WC, Rattray M: Clinical course and diagnosis of genital herpes simplex virus infection and evaluation of topical surfactant therapy. Am J Obstet Gynecol 133:548, 1979
6. Mertz GJ, Jourdan J, Winter C et al: Sexual transmission of initial genital herpes (HSV): Implications for prevention. In Program and Abstracts of 21st Interscience Conference on Antimicrobial Agents and Chemotherapy. Abstract 622, Washington DC, American Society of Microbiology, 1981
7. Centers for Disease Control: Chancroid—California. MMWR 31, No 14, 1982
8. Holmes KK, Stamm WE: Chlamydial genital infections: A growing problem. Hosp Pract 14 No 10:107, 1979
9. Clues to chlamydia. Emerg Med 15, No 11:210, 1983

10. Gardner HL, Dukes CD: *Haemophilus vaginalis* vaginitis. Am J Obstet Gynecol 69:962, 1955
11. Jones BM: Gardnerella vaginitis. Med Lab Sci 40:53, 1983
12. Spiegel CA, Amsel R, Eschenbach D et al: Anaerobic bacteria in nonspecific vaginitis. N Engl J Med 303:601, 1980
13. Eschenbach DA: Diagnosis of bacterial vaginosis (nonspecific vaginitis): Role of the laboratory. Clin Microbiol Newsletter 6:18, 1984
14. Centers for Disease Control: Condyloma acuminatum—United States 1966-1981. MMWR 32, No 23:306, 1983

■ Additional References

Alexander FR: Chlamydia: The organism and neonatal infection. Hosp Pract 14 No 7:63, 1979

Amsel R, Totten PA, Spiegel CA: Nonspecific vaginitis. Am J Med 74:14, 1983

Bettoli EJ: Herpes: Facts and fallacies. Am J Nurs 82:924, 1982

Blackwell A, Barlow D: Clinical diagnosis of anaerobic vaginosis (non-specific vaginitis). Br J Vener Dis 58:387, 1982

Campbell CE, Herten RJ: VD to STD: Redefining venereal disease. Am J Nurs 81:1629, 1981

Corey L: The diagnosis and treatment of genital herpes. JAMA 248:1041, 1982

Corey L, Holmes KK: Genital herpes simplex virus infections: Current concepts in diagnosis, therapy, and prevention. Ann Intern Med 98:973, 1983

Fitzgerald FT: The classic venereal diseases. Postgrad Med 75, No. 8:91, 1984

Galasso GJ, Myers MW: The five human herpesviruses: Infection, prevention, and treatment. Adv Intern Med 29:25, 1984

Handsfield HH: Sexually transmitted diseases. Hosp Pract 17, No 1:99, 1982

Johnson AP: The pathogenesis of gonorrhea. J Infect 3:299, 1981

Kaufman RH: The origin and diagnosis of "nonspecific vaginitis." N Engl J Med 303:637, 1980

Novotny T: Vaginal disease: Venereal and nonvenereal types. Postgrad Med 73, No. 5:303, 1983

Peter JB, Bryson Y, Lovett MA: Genital herpes: Urgent questions, elusive answers. Diagn Med (March/April):1, 1983

Sacks SL, Bowie WR, Stayner M: Education and public awareness of sexually transmitted diseases. Can J Public Health 74:176, 1983

Schneider GT: Vaginal infections. Postgrad Med 73, No. 2:255, 1983

Unit VI

Alterations in Endocrine Function, Metabolism, and Nutrition

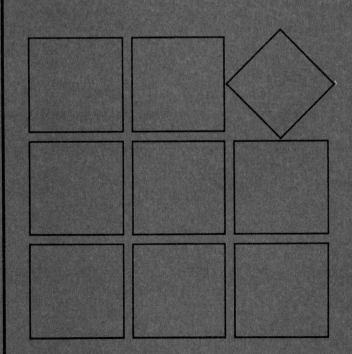

Chapter 37

Mechanisms of Endocrine Control

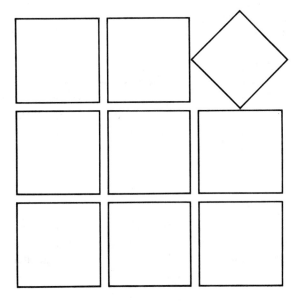

The endocrine system is involved in all of the integrative aspects of life, including growth, sex differentiation, metabolism, and adaptation to an ever-changing environment. This chapter focuses on general aspects of endocrine function, organization of the endocrine system, hormone receptors and hormone actions, and regulation of hormone levels.

■ The Endocrine System

Hormones

Hormones are generally thought of as *chemical messengers* that are transported in body fluids. Although the endocrine system was once thought to consist solely of discrete *endocrine glands* and their hormones, termed the *classic endocrine system,* it is now known that a number of other chemical messengers modulate the body processes.

Hormones of the classic endocrine system are synthesized by endocrine glands, secreted into the bloodstream, and then transported to distant sites, or target cells, where they exert their action. The neuromediators (neurohormones), such as the catecholamines (epinephrine, norepinephrine, and dopamine), are also chemical mediators that are synthesized by nerve cells and released from nerve endings.

A number of hormonal peptides have now been identified; these peptides are produced by what is sometimes referred to as the *diffuse endocrine system.* Unlike the well-defined glands of the classic endocrine system, the diffuse endocrine system is dispersed throughout various organs and cells and is intermingled with nonendocrine cells.[1] A great deal of mystery still surrounds these hormonal peptides. A number of them have been found in both brain and peripheral tissues, and their wide range of actions suggests that they act locally in a number of ways, depending on the tissues that they serve. Perhaps the most interesting of these peptides are the endorphins and enkephalins (Chap. 49).

Structural classification
Hormones have diverse structures ranging from single modified amino acids (epinephrine and thyroxin), polypeptides (growth hormone and insulin), and glycoproteins (follicle-stimulating hormone and luteinizing hormone) to lipids (steroid hormones such as cortisol). Table 37-1 presents a listing of hormones according to structure.

Function
Hormones do not initiate reactions; rather they are modulators of body and cellular responses. Most hormones are present in the blood at all times—but in greater or lesser amounts depending on the needs of the body. Hormones can produce either a generalized or a localized effect. For example, antidiuretic hormone (ADH) acts selectively on the distal tubules and collecting ducts of the kidney, whereas epinephrine affects the function of many body systems. Table 37-2 lists the major functions and sources of body hormones. These hormones are discussed more fully in other sections of the text.

Synthesis
The mechanisms for hormone synthesis vary with hormone structure. Protein and peptide hormones are synthesized and stored in granules or vesicles within the cytoplasm of the cell until secretion is required. The lipid-soluble steroid hormones are released as they are synthesized.

Protein and peptide hormones are synthesized in the rough endoplasmic reticulum in a manner similar to the synthesis of other proteins (see Chap. 1). The appropriate amino acid sequence is dictated by messenger RNAs from the nucleus. Usually synthesis involves the production of a prehormone, which is modified by the addition of peptides or sugar units. These prehormones often contain extra peptide units that ensure proper folding of the molecule and insertion of essential linkages. If extra amino acids are present, as in insulin, the hormone is called a *prohormone.* Following synthesis and sequestration in the endoplasmic reticulum, the protein and peptide hormones move into the Golgi complex where they are packaged in granules or vesicles. It is in the Golgi complex that prohormones are converted into hormones.

Steroid hormones are synthesized within the smooth endoplasmic reticulum, and steroid-secreting cells can be identified by their large amounts of smooth endoplasmic reticulum. Certain steroids serve as precursors for the production of other hormones. In the adrenal cortex, for example, progesterone and other steroid intermediates are enzymatically converted into either aldosterone, cortisol, or androgens (Chap. 39).

Transport
Hormones are delivered from cells of the endocrine gland to target cells by one of four mechanisms: (1) blood-borne delivery in which hormones that are synthesized by classic endocrine glands are released into the bloodstream; (2) neurocrine, in which the neuron contacts its target cells by axonal extensions, such as those that connect the hypothalamus with the posterior pituitary gland; (3) neuroendocrine, in which hormones, such as epinephrine, are released from neurons into the bloodstream; and (4) paracrine, in which the released chemical messenger diffuses to its target cell through the

Table 37-1   Classes of Hormones Based on Structure

Peptides and Proteins		Steroids	Amines
Glycoprotein	*Polypeptides*		
Follicle-stimulating hormone (FSH)	Adrenocorticotropic hormone (ACTH)	Aldosterone	Epinephrine
Human chorionic gonadotropin (hCG)	Angiotensin	Cortisol	Norepinephrine
Luteinizing hormone (LH)	Calcitonin	Estradiol	Thyroxine (T_4)
Thyroid-stimulating hormone (TSH)	Cholecystokinin	Progesterone	Triiodothyronine (T_3)
	Erythropoietin	Testosterone	
	Gastrin	Vitamin D	
	Glucagon		
	Growth hormone		
	Insulin		
	Insulinlike growth peptides (somatomedins)		
	Melanocyte-stimulating hormone (MSH)		
	Nerve growth factor		
	Oxytocin		
	Parathyroid hormone		
	Prolactin		
	Relaxin		
	Secretin		
	Somatostatin		
	Vasopressin (ADH)		

(From Greenspan FS, Forsham PH: Basic and Clinical Endocrinology, p 1. Los Altos, CA, Lange Medical Publications, 1983)

Table 37-2   Functional Classification of Hormones

Function	Hormone	Major Source
Control of water and electrolyte metabolism	Aldosterone	Adrenal cortex
	Antidiuretic hormone (ADH)	Posterior pituitary
	Calcitonin	C cells, thyroid
	Parathyroid hormone	Parathyroid
	Angiotensin	Kidney
Control of gastrointestinal function	Cholecystokinin	Gastrointestinal tract
	Gastrin	Gastrointestinal tract
	Secretin	Gastrointestinal tract
Regulation of energy, metabolism, and growth	Glucagon	α cells, pancreatic islets
	Insulin	β cells, pancreatic islets
	Growth hormone	Anterior pituitary
	Somatomedin	Liver
	Somatostatin	Hypothalamus, CNS, pancreatic islets
	Thyroid hormones	Thyroid gland
Neurotransmitters	Dopamine	CNS
	Epinephrine	Adrenal medulla
	Norepinephrine	Adrenal medulla and CNS
Reproductive function	Chorionic gonadotropins	Placenta
	Estrogens	Ovary
	Oxytocin	Posterior pituitary
	Progesterone	Ovary
	Prolactin	Anterior pituitary
	Testosterone	Testes
Stress and control of inflammation	Glucocorticoids	Adrenal cortex
Tropic hormones (regulation of other hormone levels)	Adrenocorticotropic hormone (ACTH)	Anterior pituitary
	Follicle-stimulating hormone (FSH)	Anterior pituitary
	Luteinizing hormone (LH)	Anterior pituitary
	Thyroid-stimulating hormone (TSH)	Anterior pituitary

interstitial fluid, such as occurs in the diffuse endocrine system.[2]

Hormones that are released into the bloodstream circulate either as free molecules or as hormones attached to transport carriers. Peptide hormones and protein hormones generally circulate unbound in the blood. Steroid hormones and thyroid hormone are carried by specific proteins synthesized in the liver. The extent of carrier binding influences the rate at which hormones leave the blood and enter the cells. The half-life of a hormone—the time it takes for the body to reduce the concentration of the hormone by one-half—is positively correlated with its percentage of protein binding. Thyroxin, which is more than 99% protein bound, has a half-life of 6 days. Aldosterone, which is only 15% bound, has a half-life of only 25 minutes.[3] Drugs that compete with a hormone for binding with the transport carrier molecules increase hormone action by increasing the availability of the active unbound hormone. For example, aspirin competes with thyroid hormone for binding to transport proteins;

this can produce serious effects during thyroid crisis, when affected individuals are already suffering from the effects of excessive hormone levels.

Metabolism

Hormones secreted by endocrine cells must be continuously inactivated to prevent their accumulation. Both intracellular and extracellular mechanisms participate in the termination of hormone function. Some hormones are enzymatically inactivated at receptor sites where they exert their action. Peptide hormones have a short life span and are inactivated by enzymes that split peptide bonds. They are inactivated mainly in the liver and kidneys. As was previously mentioned, steroid hormones are bound to protein carriers for transport and are inactive in the bound state. Their activity depends on the availability of transport hormones. Unbound adrenal and gonadal steroid hormones are conjugated in the liver, which renders them inactive, and then excreted in the bile or urine. Thyroid hormones are also transported by carrier molecules. The free hormone is rendered inactive by the removal of amino acids (deamination) in the tissues and is also conjugated in the liver and eliminated in the bile.

Rate of reaction

Hormones react at different rates. The neurotransmitters, such as epinephrine, have a reaction time of milliseconds. Thyroid hormone, on the other hand, requires days for its effect to occur. Hormones are continually being metabolized or inactivated and removed from the body.

Mechanisms of action

Hormones exert their action by binding to specific receptor sites that are located on the surfaces of the target cells. The function of these receptors is to recognize a specific hormone and translate the hormonal signal into a cellular response. The structure of these receptors varies in a manner that allows target cells to respond to one hormone and not to others. For example, receptors in the thyroid are specific for the thyroid-stimulating hormone, whereas receptors on the gonads respond to the gonadotropic hormones.

The response of a target cell to the action of a hormone will vary with the *number* of receptors that are present and with the *affinity* of these receptors for hormone binding. A variety of factors influence the number of receptors that are present on target cells and their affinity for hormone binding (Fig. 37-1).

There are generally 2000 to 10,000 hormone receptor molecules per cell.[3] The number of hormone receptors on a cell may be altered for any of several reasons.

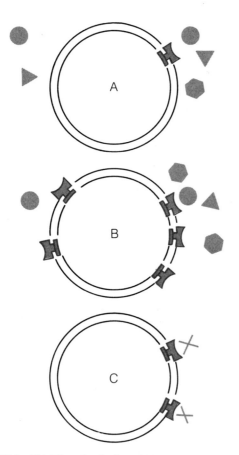

Figure 37-1 (A) *The role of cell-surface receptors in mediating the action of hormones. Hormone action is affected by* (B) *the number of receptors that are present and by* (C) *the affinity of these receptors for hormone binding.*

Antibodies may destroy the receptor proteins. Sustained levels of excess hormone may decrease the number of receptors per cell in a process called *down regulation*. This acts to modify the effect of chronic exposure to a given hormone. In some instances, the reverse effect occurs, and an increase in hormone levels appears to recruit its own receptors *(up regulation),* increasing the sensitivity of the cell to the hormone. Obesity has been shown to cause a decrease in the number of insulin receptors that are present on fat cells, and it is speculated that this may influence impaired glucose tolerance in the obese noninsulin-dependent diabetic. On the other hand, it has been shown that the oral hypoglycemic drugs, the sulfonylureas, cause an increase in the number of insulin receptors on body cells.

The affinity of receptors for binding hormones is also affected by a number of conditions. For example, the *p*H of the body fluids plays an important role in the affinity of insulin receptors. In ketoacidosis, the lowering of the *p*H from 7.4 to 7.0 reduces insulin binding by about one-half.[4]

Hormone–receptor interactions go about the process of modulating cell activity in two ways. One type of response occurs with the peptide hormones, which circulate in the blood in their free state. These hormones interact with fixed membrane receptors in a manner that incites the release of a *second messenger* (usually cyclic AMP), which in turn activates a series of enzyme reactions that serve to alter cell function (Fig. 37-2). Glucagon, for example, incites glycogen breakdown by way of the second messenger system.

A second type of receptor mechanism is involved in mediating the action of hormones, such as the steroid and the thyroid hormones, which are transported in body fluids attached to carrier proteins (Fig. 37-2). These hormones, being lipid soluble, pass freely through the cell membrane and then attach to an intracellular *mobile receptor* in the cytoplasm of the cell. This hormone–receptor complex moves through the cytoplasm, becomes activated, and enters the nucleus where it causes activation or repression of gene activity with subsequent production of messenger RNA and protein synthesis. Table 37-3 lists hormones that act by the two types of receptors.

Control of Hormone Levels

Hormone secretion varies widely over a 24-hour period. Some hormones, such as growth hormone and adrenocorticotropic hormone (ACTH), have diurnal fluctuations that vary with the sleep–awakening cycle. Others, such as the female sex hormones, are secreted in a complicated cyclic manner. The levels of hormones like insulin and antidiuretic hormone (ADH) are regulated by the amount of organic and inorganic substances present in the body. The levels of many of the hormones are regulated by feedback mechanisms that involve the hypothalamic–pituitary–target cell system.

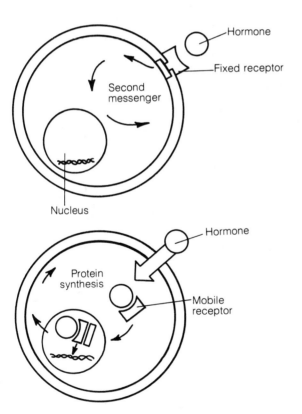

Figure 37-2 *The two types of hormone–receptor interactions: the fixed membrane receptor on the* top *and the intracellular mobile receptor on the* bottom.

Table 37-3 Hormone–Receptor Interactions

Fixed Messenger Interactions
 Glucagon
 Insulin
 Epinephrine
 Parathyroid hormone
 Thyroid-stimulating hormone
 Adrenocorticotropic hormone
 Follicle-stimulating hormone
 Luteinizing hormone
 Antidiuretic hormone
 Secretin
Mobile Hormone–Receptor–Nuclear Interactions
 Estrogen
 Testosterone
 Progesterone
 Adrenal cortical hormones
 Thyroid hormone

Hypothalamic–pituitary regulation

Because the integration of body function relies on input from both the nervous system and the endocrine system, it seems logical that input from the nervous system would participate in the regulation of hormone levels. In this respect, the hypothalamus and the pituitary (hypophysis) act as an integrative link between the central nervous system and the many endocrine-mediated functions of the body. These two structures are connected by blood flow in the hypophyseal portal system, which begins in the hypothalamus and drains into the anterior pituitary gland, and by the nerve axons that connect the supraoptic and paraventricular nuclei of the hypothalamus with the posterior pituitary gland (Fig. 37-3).

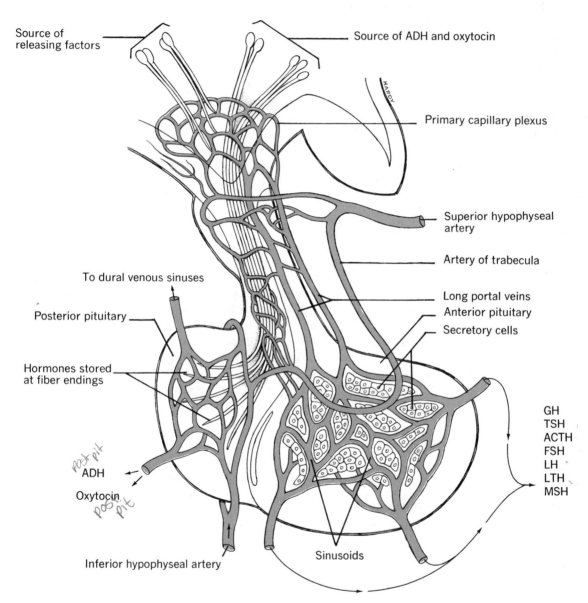

Figure 37-3   *The hypothalamus and the anterior and posterior pituitary. Hypothalamus releasing or inhibiting hormones are transported to the anterior pituitary via the portal vessels. ADH and oxytocin are produced by nerve cells in the supraoptic and paraventricular nuclei of the hypothalamus and then transported through the nerve axon to the posterior pituitary where they are released into the circulation. (From Chaffee EE, Greisheimer EM: Basic Physiology and Anatomy, 3rd ed. Philadelphia, JB Lippincott, 1974)*

Embryologically, the anterior pituitary gland developed from glandular tissue and the posterior pituitary from neural tissue.

The endocrine hypothalamus. The synthesis and release of anterior pituitary hormones is largely regulated by the action of releasing or inhibiting hormones from the hypothalamus, which is the coordinating center of the brain for endocrine, behavioral, and autonomic nervous system function. It is at the level of the hypothalamus that emotion, pain, body temperature, and other neural input are communicated to the endocrine system. The posterior pituitary hormones, ADH and oxytocin, are synthesized in the cell bodies of the nerve axons that travel to the posterior pituitary. The release and function of ADH are discussed in Chapter 25.

Anterior pituitary gland. The pituitary gland has been called the "master gland" because its hormones control the function of a number of target glands or cells. Hormones produced by the anterior pituitary control body growth and metabolism (growth hormone), function of the thyroid gland (thyroid-stimulating hormone), glucocorticoid hormone levels (adrenocorticotropic hormone), function of the gonads (follicle-stimulating and luteinizing hormones), and breast growth and milk production (prolactin). Melanocyte-stimulating hormone, which controls pigmentation of the skin, is produced by the pars intermedia of the pituitary.

Feedback mechanisms

The level of many of the hormones in the body is regulated by negative feedback mechanisms. The function of this type of system is similar to that of the thermostat in a heating system. In the endocrine system, sensors detect a change in the hormone level and adjust hormone secretion so that body levels are maintained within an appropriate range. When the sensors detect a decrease in hormone levels, they initiate changes that cause an increase in hormone production; and when hormone levels rise above the setpoint of the system, the sensors cause hormone production and release to decrease. For example, an increase in thyroid hormone is detected by sensors in the hypothalamus or anterior pituitary gland, and this causes a reduction in the secretion of thyroid-stimulating hormone with a subsequent decrease in the output of thyroid hormone from the thyroid gland. The feedback loops for the hypothalamic–pituitary feedback mechanisms are illustrated in Figure 37-4. Exogenous forms of hormones (given as drug preparations) can influence the normal feedback control of hormone production and release. One of the most common examples of this influence occurs with the administration of the

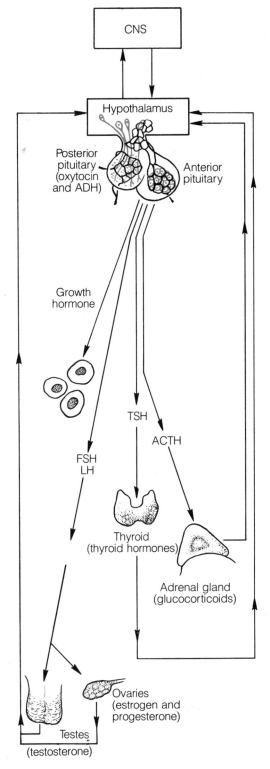

Figure 37-4 *Control of hormone production by hypothalamic–pituitary–target cell feedback mechanism. Hormone levels from the target glands regulate the release of hormones from the anterior pituitary by means of a negative feedback system.*

adrenal cortical hormones, which cause suppression of the hypothalamic–pituitary–target cell system that regulates the production of these hormones.

Although the levels of most hormones are regulated by negative feedback mechanisms, a small number are under positive feedback control in which rising levels of a hormone cause another gland to release a hormone that is stimulating to the first. There must, however, be a mechanism for shutting off the release of the first hormone, or its production would continue unabated. An example of such a system is that of the female ovarian hormone estradiol. Increased estradiol production during the follicular stage of the menstrual cycle produces increased gonadotropin (FSH) production by the anterior pituitary gland. This stimulates further increases in estradiol levels until the demise of the follicle, which is the source of estradiol, results in a fall in gonadotropin levels.

In summary, the endocrine system acts as a communications system that uses chemical messengers, or hormones, for the transmission of information from cell to cell and from organ to organ. Hormones act at the level of the cell membrane, which has surface receptors that are specific for the different types of hormones. Many of the endocrine glands are under the regulatory control of other parts of the endocrine system. The hypothalamus and the pituitary gland form a complex integrative network that joins the nervous system and the endocrine system, and it is this central network that controls the output from many of the other glands in the body.

■ General Aspects of Altered Endocrine Function

Hypofunction and Hyperfunction

Disturbances of endocrine function can usually be divided into two categories: hypofunction and hyperfunction.

Hypofunction of an endocrine gland can occur for a variety of reasons. Congenital defects can result in the absence or impaired development of the gland or the absence of an enzyme needed for hormone synthesis. Destruction of the gland may occur because of disruption in blood flow, infection or inflammation, autoimmune responses, or neoplastic growth. There may be a decline in function with aging, or the gland may atrophy as the result of drug therapy or for unknown reasons. Some endocrine-deficient states are associated with receptor defects: hormone receptors may be absent; the receptor binding of hormones may be defective; or the cellular responsiveness to the hormone may be impaired.

It is suspected that in some cases a gland may produce a biologically inactive hormone, or an active hormone may be destroyed by circulating antibodies before it can exert its action.

Hyperfunction is generally associated with excessive hormone production. This can result from excessive stimulation and hyperplasia of the endocrine gland or from a hormone-producing tumor of the gland. Sometimes an ectopic tumor will produce hormones; for example, certain bronchogenic tumors produce hormones such as antidiuretic hormone (ADH) and adrenocorticotropic hormone (ACTH).

Primary and Secondary Disorders

Endocrine disorders can generally be divided into two groups—primary and secondary. *Primary defects* in endocrine function originate within the target gland responsible for producing the hormone. In *secondary disorders* of endocrine function, the target gland is essentially normal, but its function is altered by defective levels of stimulating hormones or releasing factors from the hypothalamic–pituitary system. For example, adrenalectomy produces a primary deficiency of adrenal corticosteroid hormones. Removal or destruction of the pituitary gland, on the other hand, eliminates ACTH stimulation of the adrenal cortex and brings about a secondary deficiency.

Diagnostic Methods

There are a number of techniques for assessing endocrine function and hormone levels. One technique measures the effect of a hormone on body function. Measurement of blood glucose, for example, reflects insulin levels and is an indirect method of assessing insulin availability. Another technique, the *bioassay*, measures the effect of a hormone on animal function. A bioassay can be done using the intact animal or a portion of tissue from the animal. At one time, female rats or male frogs were used to test women's urine for the presence of human chorionic gonadotropin, which is produced by the placenta during pregnancy. Today, the most widely used technique for measuring hormone levels is the *radioimmunoassay*. This method uses a radiolabeled form of the hormone and a hormone antibody that has been prepared by injecting an appropriate animal with a purified form of the hormone. The unlabeled hormone in the sample being tested competes with the radiolabeled hormone for attachment to the binding sites of the antibody. Measurement of the radiolabeled hormone–antibody complex then provides a means of arriving at a measure of hormone level in the sample. Because hormone binding is competitive, the amount of radiolabeled hormone–antibody complex that is formed will decrease as the amount of unlabeled hormone in the sample is increased.

In summary, endocrine disorders are the result of hypo- or hyperfunction of an endocrine gland. They can occur as a primary defect in hormone production by a target gland or as a secondary disorder resulting from a defect in the hypothalamic–pituitary system that controls a target gland's function. Laboratory tests that measure hormone levels or assess the effect of a hormone on body function (*e.g.*, assessment of insulin function through blood sugar levels) are used in the diagnosis of endocrine disorders.

■ Study Guide

After you have studied this chapter, you should be able to meet the following objectives:

☐ Compare the classic endocrine system with the diffuse endocrine system.

☐ State a general definition of hormone function.

☐ State a difference between the synthesis of protein hormones and that of steroid hormones.

☐ Describe four mechanisms of hormone delivery to target cells.

☐ State three ways in which hormones are inactivated or metabolized.

☐ State the function of a hormone receptor.

☐ Describe two alterations in hormone receptors that could be used to explain changes in hormone action.

☐ State the difference between fixed hormone receptor interactions and mobile hormone receptor interactions.

☐ Describe the role of the hypothalamus in regulating pituitary control of endocrine function.

☐ State the major difference between positive and negative feedback control mechanisms.

☐ Compare endocrine hypofunction and endocrine hyperfunction.

☐ Describe the radioimmunoassay method of measuring hormone levels.

■ References

1. Polak JM, Path MRC, Bloom SR: Neuropeptides of the gut: A newly discovered major control system. World J Surg 3:393, 1979
2. Hadeley ME: Endocrinology, p 32. Englewood Cliffs, NJ, Prentice-Hall, 1984
3. Berne RM, Levy MN: Physiology. pp 901, 909. St Louis, CV Mosby, 1983
4. Kahn CR: Probing receptor activity in cell control. Patient Care 13, No 1:84, 1984

Chapter 38

Control of Metabolism

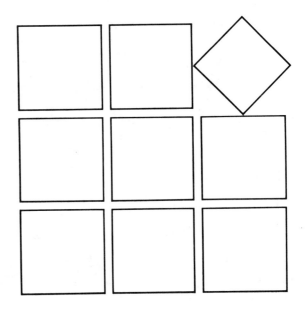

All body activities require energy whether they involve an individual cell, a single organ, or the entire body. Metabolism is the organized process through which carbohydrates, fats, and proteins from ingested food are broken down, transformed, or otherwise converted into cellular energy. This chapter focuses on glucose, fat, and protein metabolism and the hormonal regulation of this process.

Metabolism

The process of metabolism is unique in that it not only allows for the continuous release of energy, but it couples this energy release with physiologic functioning. For example, the energy used for muscle contraction is derived largely from energy sources that are stored in the muscle cells. This energy is then released as the muscle contracts. Because most of our energy sources come from the three to four meals that we eat each day, the ability to store energy and control its release is important.

Anabolism and Catabolism

There are two phases of metabolism—anabolism and catabolism. *Anabolism* is the phase of metabolic storage and synthesis of cell constituents. Anabolism does not

provide energy for the body; rather, it requires energy. *Catabolism*, on the other hand, involves the breakdown of complex molecules into substances that can be used in the production of energy. The chemical intermediates for anabolism and catabolism are called *metabolites*—for example, lactic acid is one of the metabolites formed when glucose is broken down in the absence of oxygen.

Both anabolism and catabolism are catalyzed by *enzyme systems* that are located within body cells. A *substrate* is a substance on which an enzyme acts. Enzyme systems selectively transform fuel substrates into cellular energy and facilitate the use of energy in the process of assembling molecules to form energy substrates and storage forms of energy.

Because body energy cannot be stored as heat, the cellular oxidative processes that release energy are flameless and have low temperature reactions. Instead of releasing only heat—as occurs when the same fuel is burned in the environment—the free energy that is released from the oxidation of foods is converted to chemical energy that can be stored. The body transforms carbohydrates, fats, and proteins into the intermediary compound, adenosine triphosphate (ATP). Adenosine triphosphate is often called the energy currency of the cell because almost all body cells use ATP as their energy source (Chap. 1). The metabolic events involved in ATP formation allow cellular energy to be stored, used, and then replenished.

Glucose Metabolism

Glucose is an efficient fuel which, when metabolized in the presence of oxygen, breaks down to form carbon dioxide and water. Although many tissues and organ systems are able to use other forms of fuel, such as fatty acids and ketones, the brain and nervous system rely almost exclusively on glucose as a fuel source. The nervous system can neither store nor synthesize glucose; rather, it relies on the minute-by-minute extraction of glucose from the blood as a means of meeting its energy needs. In the fed and early fasting state, the nervous system requires about 100 gm to 115 gm of glucose per day to meet its metabolic needs.[1,2]

The liver regulates the entry of glucose into the blood. Glucose ingested in the diet is transported from the gastrointestinal tract, through the portal vein, to the liver before it gains access to the circulatory system (Fig. 38-1). The liver both stores and synthesizes glucose. When blood sugar is increased, the liver removes glucose from the blood and stores it for future use. Conversely, the liver releases its glucose stores when blood sugar drops. In this way, the liver acts as a buffer system to regulate blood sugar levels. Generally speaking, it can be said that blood sugar levels reflect the difference between the amount of glucose that is released into the circulation

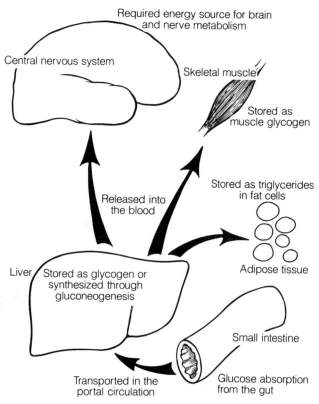

Figure 38-1 *Regulation of blood glucose by the liver.*

Required energy source for brain and nerve metabolism

Central nervous system

Skeletal muscle

Stored as muscle glycogen

Released into the blood

Stored as triglycerides in fat cells

Adipose tissue

Liver / Stored as glycogen or synthesized through gluconeogenesis

Small intestine

Transported in the portal circulation

Glucose absorption from the gut

by the liver and the amount of glucose that is removed from the blood by body cells.

Excess glucose is stored in two forms: (1) it can be converted to fatty acids and then stored in *fat cells as triglycerides*, or (2) it can be stored in the *liver and skeletal muscle as glycogen*. Small amounts of glycogen are also stored in the skin and in some of the glandular tissues.

Glycogenolysis

Glycogenolysis, or the breakdown of glycogen, is controlled by the action of two hormones: *glucagon* and *epinephrine*. Epinephrine is more effective in stimulating glycogen breakdown in muscle. The liver, on the other hand, is more responsive to glucagon. The synthesis and degradation of glycogen is important because it helps maintain blood sugar levels during periods of fasting and strenuous exercise. Only the liver, in contrast with other tissues that store glycogen, is able to release its glucose stores into the blood for use by other tissues, such as the brain and nervous system. This is because glycogen breaks down to form a phosphorylated glucose molecule. Glucose is too large, in its phosphorylated form, to pass through the cell membrane. The liver, but not skeletal muscle, has the enzyme glucose-6-phosphatase that is needed to remove the phosphate group and to allow the glucose molecule to enter the bloodstream.

Although they are rare, a number of genetic disorders exist in which glycogen breakdown is impaired. All of these disorders result in excessive accumulation of abnormal forms of glycogen. *Von Gierke's disease* involves a genetic *deficiency of glucose-6-phosphatase*. Children with this disease have stunted growth, liver enlargement, hypoglycemia, and hyperlipidemia resulting from mobilization of fatty acids. *McArdle's disease* is characterized by a deficiency in skeletal muscle glycogen; as a result of this deficiency, the disease causes extreme muscle weakness.

Gluconeogenesis

The synthesis of glucose is referred to as *gluconeogenesis*, or the building of glucose from new sources. The process of gluconeogenesis converts amino acids, lactate, and glycerol into glucose. Most of the gluconeogenesis occurs in the liver. Although fatty acids can be used as fuel by many body cells, they cannot be converted to glucose.

Glucose produced through the process of gluconeogenesis is either stored in the liver as glycogen or released into the general circulation. During periods of food deprivation or when the diet is low in carbohydrates, gluconeogenesis provides the glucose to meet the metabolic needs of the brain and other glucose-dependent tissues.

Several hormones stimulate gluconeogenesis, including *glucagon*, *glucocorticoid hormones* from the adrenal cortex, and *thyroid hormone*.

Alcohol ingestion interferes with the liver's ability to produce glucose. This is because the metabolism of alcohol competes for the use of the same hydrogen carrier, nicotinamide-adenine dinucleotide (NAD), that is needed for glucose production. Although probably not a common occurrence, alcohol-induced hypoglycemia can occur after a period of fasting. Because glucose stimulates insulin release, this tends to occur more readily when alcohol is drunk in combination with sugar-containing mixers.

Fat Metabolism

The average American diet provides 40% to 50% of calories in the form of fats. In contrast to glucose which yields only 4 calories per gram, each gram of fat yields 9 calories. Additionally, another 30% to 50% of the carbohydrates that are consumed in the diet are converted to triglycerides for storage.

A *triglyceride* contains *three fatty acids* that are linked by a *glycerol* molecule (Fig. 38-2). Fatty acids and triglycerides can be derived from dietary sources, they can be synthesized in the body, or they can be mobilized from fat depots. Excess carbohydrate is converted to triglyceride and is then transported by lipoproteins in the blood to adipose cells for storage. *One gram of anhydrous (water-free) fat stores more than six times as much energy as one hydrated gram of glycogen.* One reason weight loss is greatest at the beginning of a fast or weight-loss program is that this is when the body uses its glycogen stores. Later, when the body begins to use energy stored as

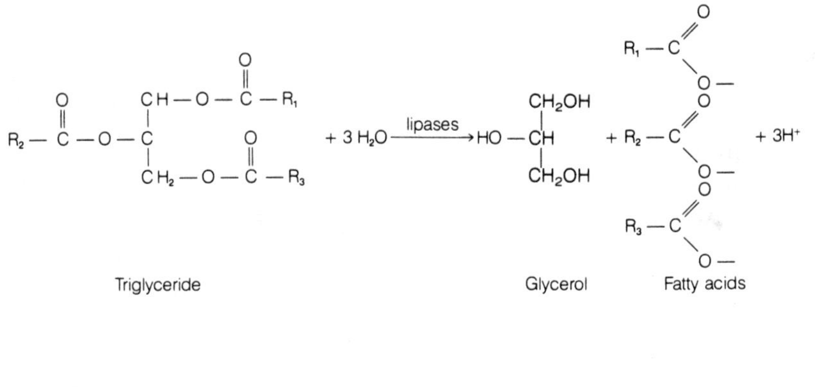

Figure 38-2 *Mobilization of fatty acids from triglycerides.*

triglycerides, water losses are decreased and weight loss tends to plateau.

The mobilization of fat for use in energy production is facilitated by the action of enzymes, or lipases, that break the triglycerides into three fatty acids and a glycerol molecule. Following triglyceride breakdown, both the fatty acids and the glycerol molecule leave the fat cell and enter the circulation. Once in the circulation, many of the fatty acids are transported to the liver, where they are removed from the blood and are then either used by liver cells as a source of energy or converted to ketones.

The efficient burning of fatty acids requires a balance between carbohydrate and fat metabolism. The ratio of fatty acid and carbohydrate utilization is altered in situations that favor fat breakdown, such as diabetes mellitus and fasting. In these situations, the liver produces more ketones than it can use; this excess is then released into the bloodstream. Ketones can be an important source of energy, since even the brain adapts to the use of ketones during prolonged periods of starvation. A problem arises, however, when fat breakdown is accelerated and the production of ketones exceeds tissue utilization. Because ketone bodies are organic acids they cause *ketoacidosis* when they are present in excessive amounts. The activation of lipases and the subsequent mobilization of fatty acids are stimulated by epinephrine, glucocorticoid hormones, growth hormones, and glucagon.

Protein Metabolism

About three-fourths of body solids are proteins. Proteins are essential for the formation of all body structures, including genes, enzymes, contractile proteins in muscle, matrix of bone, and hemoglobin of red blood cells.

Amino acids are the building blocks of proteins. Unlike glucose and fatty acids, there is only a limited facility for the storage of excess amino acids in the body. Most of the stored amino acids are contained in body proteins. Amino acids in excess of those needed for protein synthesis are converted to fatty acids, ketone bodies, or glucose and are then stored or used as metabolic fuel. Each gram of protein yields 4 calories. Because fatty acids cannot be converted to glucose, the body must break down proteins and use the amino acids as a major source of substrate for gluconeogenesis during periods when metabolic needs exceed food intake. The liver has the enzymes and transfer mechanisms needed to deaminate and to convert the amino groups (NH_2) from the amino acid to urea. Thus, the breakdown or degradation of proteins and amino acids occurs primarily in the liver, which is also the site of gluconeogenesis.

In summary, glucose, fats, and proteins serve as fuel sources for cellular metabolism. These fuel sources are ingested during meals and are then stored for future use. When sufficient insulin is present, glucose enters liver or muscle cells and is stored as glycogen or enters fat cells for storage as triglycerides. Glycogen provides for the short-term energy needs of the body. Storage forms of fat are mobilized during periods of food deprivation or in conditions such as diabetes mellitus in which glucose entry into body cells is impaired.

The brain relies almost exclusively on glucose as a fuel source; when glucose stores have been depleted, the liver synthesizes glucose from amino acids, lactate, and glycerol in a process called gluconeogenesis. It is important to note that although glucose can be converted to fatty acids for storage, there is no pathway for converting fatty acids to glucose. Instead, fatty acids are used directly as a fuel source or are converted to ketones by the liver. When ketone production exceeds utilization, ketoacidosis develops.

■ Hormonal Control of Metabolism

Metabolism is controlled by neural and endocrine influences. Neural stimuli influence the release of hormones that are concerned with metabolism. The autonomic nervous system has a direct effect on many metabolic functions through the release of *epinephrine* and *norepinephrine*.

Although the respiratory and circulatory systems combine efforts to furnish the body with oxygen needed for metabolic purposes, it is the liver, in concert with the pancreatic hormones insulin and glucagon, that controls the body's fuel supply (Fig. 38-3). Secretion of both insulin and glucagon is regulated by blood sugar levels. *Insulin* is released in response to an *increase in blood sugar levels*, and *glucagon release* occurs when *blood sugar levels drop*. Both insulin and glucagon are transported from the pancreas, through the *portal circulation*, to the liver where they exert an almost instantaneous effect on blood glucose levels.

Insulin

Insulin is produced by the pancreatic cells in the islets of Langerhans. The active form of the hormone is composed of two polypeptide chains—an A chain and a B chain (Fig. 38-4). Before 1967, it was assumed that each chain was formed separately and then joined. It is now known that the chains emerge with the appropriate linkage required for biologic activity from a single chain

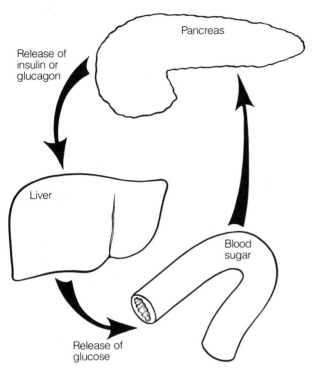

Figure 38-3 *Effect of the pancreatic hormones insulin and glucagon on the regulation of blood sugar by the liver. An increase in blood sugar produces an insulin-mediated decrease in glucose release from the liver; a decrease in blood glucose produces a glucagon-mediated increase in glucose release.*

called *proinsulin*. In converting proinsulin to insulin, enzymes in the beta cell cleave proinsulin at specific sites to form two substances, active *insulin* and a *C-peptide* chain (the link that served to join the A and B chains before they were separated). Both active insulin and the C-peptide chain are released simultaneously from the beta cell (Fig. 38-5). The C-peptide chains can be measured, and this measurement can be used as a means to study beta-cell activity. For example, injected insulin in the mature-onset diabetic would provide few, if any, C-peptide chains, whereas insulin secreted by the beta cells would be accompanied by secretion of C-peptide chains.

Insulin secreted by the beta cells enters the portal circulation and travels directly to the liver where about 50% is either utilized or degraded. Once it has been released into the general circulation, insulin has a half-life of about 15 minutes. This is because circulating insulin is rapidly bound to peripheral tissues or is destroyed by the liver or kidneys. There is much similarity in the structure of insulin among the different species; this has permitted the use of insulin extracted from beef and pork sources in the treatment of human diabetes mellitus.

The actions of insulin are threefold: (1) it provides for glucose storage, (2) it prevents fat breakdown, and (3) it increases protein synthesis. Although several hormones are known to increase blood sugar, *insulin is the only hormone that is currently known to have a direct effect in*

insulin
① provide for glucose storage
② prevents fat breakdown
③ ↑ protein synthesis

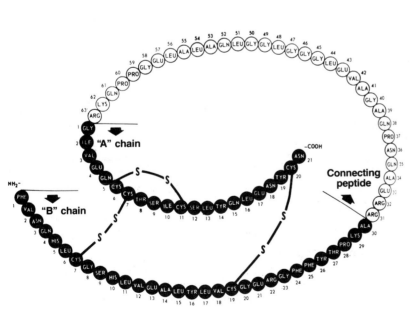

Figure 38-4 *Amino-acid sequence of porcine proinsulin showing the A chain, the B chain, and the C-peptide link. (From Shaw WN, Chance RE: Diabetes 17, No 12:738, 1968)*

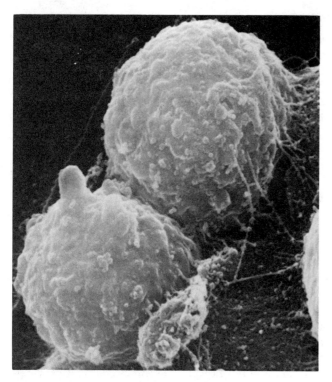

Figure 38-5 *A scanning electron micrograph of an insulin-secreting beta cell from the islets of Langerhans in the pancreas. (Courtesy of Kenneth Siegesmund, Ph.D., Anatomy Department, Medical College of Wisconsin)*

periods of food intake, insulin levels remain low and sources of stored glucose and amino acids are mobilized to supply the energy needs of glucose-dependent tissues. The glucose tolerance test, which is described in Chapter 40, uses a glucose challenge as an indirect measure of the body's ability to secrete insulin and to remove glucose from the blood.

Glucagon

Glucagon is a small protein molecule that is produced by the pancreatic alpha cells of the islets of Langerhans. Like insulin, glucagon travels by way of the portal vein to the liver where it exerts its main action.

The actions of glucagon are diametrically opposed to those of insulin. Glucagon stimulates *glycogenolysis* and *gluconeogenesis*, increases *lipolysis*, and enhances the *breakdown of proteins*. The actions of glucagon are summarized in Table 38-2.

lowering blood sugar. The actions of insulin are summarized in Table 38-1.

Insulin lowers blood sugar by *facilitating its transport into skeletal muscle and adipose tissue.* Although liver cells do not require insulin for glucose transport, a rise in insulin levels does cause an increase in hepatic uptake of glucose, presumably by increasing the intracellular trapping of glucose through the attachment of a phosphate group. Insulin also *decreases the breakdown of glucose and fat stores and stimulates both glycogen and triglyceride synthesis.* In relation to body proteins, insulin both *inhibits protein breakdown* and *increases protein synthesis.* When sufficient glucose and insulin are present, protein breakdown is inhibited because the body is able to use glucose and fatty acids as a fuel source. Insulin also increases the *active transport of amino acids into body cells and accelerates protein synthesis within the cell.* In the child and the adolescent, insulin is needed for normal growth and development.

Insulin is regulated by blood glucose levels, increasing as blood sugar levels rise and decreasing when blood sugar declines. Serum insulin levels begin to rise within minutes after a meal, reach a peak in about 30 minutes, and then return to baseline levels within 3 hours. Between

Table 38-1   Actions of Insulin on Glucose, Fats, and Proteins

Glucose
Increases glucose transport into skeletal muscle and adipose tissue
Increases glycogen synthesis
Decreases gluconeogenesis

Fats
Increases glucose transport into fat cells
Increases fatty acid transport into adipose cells
Increases triglyceride synthesis

Proteins
Increases active transport of amino acids into cells
Increases protein synthesis by accelerating translation of RNA by ribosomes and increases transcription of DNA in the nucleus to form increased amounts of RNA
Decreases protein breakdown by enhancing the use of glucose and fatty acids as a fuel source

Table 38-2   Actions of Glucagon on Glucose, Fats, and Proteins

Glucose
Promotes the breakdown of glycogen into glucose-6-phosphate
Increases gluconeogenesis

Fats
Enhances lipolysis in adipose tissue, liberating glycerol for use in gluconeogenesis

Proteins
Increases breakdown of proteins into amino acids for use in gluconeogenesis
Increases transport of amino acids in hepatic cells
Increases conversion of amino acids into glucose precursors

Table 38-3 Actions of Epinephrine on Metabolism

Mobilizes glycogen stores
Decreases movement of glucose into body cells
Inhibits insulin release from beta cells
Mobilizes fatty acids from adipose tissue

It has been suggested that abnormalities in glucagon secretion contribute to the elevation in blood sugar that is observed in diabetes mellitus. Unger suggests that it is the ratio of insulin to glucagon, rather than the absolute amount of either hormone, that determines blood sugar levels.[3] According to theory, glucagon secretion is unopposed in the diabetic because of the lack of insulin, which therefore leads to increased production of glucose by the liver.

Catecholamines

The catecholamines, epinephrine and norepinephrine, help maintain blood sugar levels during periods of stress. The actions of epinephrine are summarized in Table 38-3. Epinephrine inhibits insulin release and promotes glycogenolysis by stimulating the conversion of muscle and liver glycogen to glucose. It is important to recall that muscle glycogen cannot be released into the blood; nevertheless, the mobilization of these stores for muscle use conserves blood sugar for use by other tissues such as the brain and the nervous system. During periods of exercise and other types of stress, epinephrine inhibits insulin release from the beta cells and thereby decreases the movement of glucose into muscle cells. The catecholamines also increase *lipase activity* and thereby cause *increased mobilization of fatty acids;* this also serves to conserve glucose. The blood sugar elevating effect of epinephrine is an important *homeostatic mechanism in hypoglycemia.*

Somatostatin

Somatostatin is also produced in the pancreas; it is secreted by the delta cells in the islets of Langerhans. Somatostatin inhibits the secretion of insulin, glucagon, and growth hormone. At present, the physiologic significance of somatostatin is largely unknown.

Growth Hormone

Increased growth hormone tends to cause a state of insulin insensitivity. Growth hormone decreases both the cellular utilization and the uptake of glucose; therefore, increased levels of growth hormone tend to cause an increase in blood glucose levels. In turn, this increase in blood sugar increases the stimulus for insulin secretion by the beta cells. Growth hormone also has a direct stimulatory effect on the beta cells; thus, these two combined effects can literally cause the beta cells to "burn out." When this occurs, as it can in persons with increased levels of growth hormone (acromegaly), diabetes develops. In persons who already have diabetes mellitus, an increase in growth hormone tends to cause problems in the control of blood sugar levels.

Glucocorticoid Hormones

Cortisol and other glucocorticoid hormones stimulate gluconeogenesis by the liver, sometimes increasing the rate of hepatic glucose production sixfold to tenfold. These hormones also cause a moderate decrease in tissue utilization of glucose. In predisposed persons, the prolonged elevation of the adrenal cortical hormones can lead to hyperglycemia and the development of diabetes mellitus.

In summary, energy metabolism is controlled by a number of hormones, including insulin, glucagon, epinephrine, growth hormone, and the glucocorticoids. Of these hormones, only insulin has the effect of lowering blood sugar. Insulin's blood-lowering action results from its ability to increase the transport of glucose into body cells and to decrease hepatic production and release of glucose into the bloodstream. Other hormones—glucagon, epinephrine, growth hormone, and the glucocorticoids—serve to maintain or increase blood sugar. Glucagon and epinephrine promote glycogenolysis. Glucagon and the glucocorticoids increase gluconeogenesis. Growth hormone decreases the peripheral utilization of glucose. Whereas insulin has the effect of decreasing lipolysis and utilization of fats as a fuel source, both glucagon and epinephrine increase fat utilization. The actions of insulin, glucagon, and growth hormone are inhibited by somatostatin.

■ Study Guide

After you have studied this chapter, you should be able to meet the following objectives:

☐ Differentiate anabolism and catabolism.
☐ Name the compound that serves as the cellular energy source.
☐ Describe glucose regulation by the liver.
☐ Describe the role of glucagon in glycogenolysis.
☐ State the purpose of gluconeogenesis.

☐ Explain how fat is mobilized for use in energy production.

☐ Describe the role of the liver in protein metabolism.

☐ State the sequence of events in insulin production.

☐ Describe the actions of insulin with reference to glucose, fats, and proteins.

☐ Compare the actions of insulin with those of glucagon.

☐ Describe the role of epinephrine in glycogenolysis.

☐ Explain the relationship between growth hormone and diabetes mellitus.

☐ Explain the role of the adrenal cortical hormones in gluconeogenesis.

■ References

1. Sauded C, Felig P: The metabolic events of starvation. Am J Med 60:117, 1976
2. Cahill CF Jr: Starvation in man. Clin Endocrinol Metab 5, No 2:405, 1976
3. Unger RH: The essential role of glucagon in the pathogenesis of diabetes mellitus. Lancet 14, 1975

Chapter 39

Alterations in Endocrine Control of Growth and Metabolism

Linda S. Hurwitz

Carol Mattson Porth

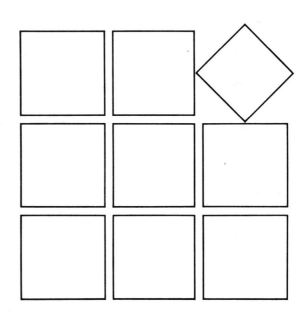

The endocrine system affects all aspects of body function, including growth and development, body appearance, and metabolism. In terms of body image, it is the endocrine system that determines the size, shape, texture, and sexual characteristics of the body. In this chapter, disorders of growth and growth hormone and alterations in thyroid and adrenocortical function will be discussed.

■ Growth and Growth Hormone Disorders

A number of hormones are essential for normal body growth. Pituitary growth hormone, one of the most important hormones, produces its growth effects through a group of polypeptide hormones called somatomedins. Insulin, thyroid hormone, and androgens are also essential for normal growth and maturation. In addition to its actions on carbohydrate and fat metabolism, insulin plays an essential role in growth processes. Children with diabetes, particularly those with poor control, often fail to grow normally even though growth hormone levels are normal. When levels of thyroid hormone are lower than normal, bone growth and epiphyseal closure are delayed. Androgens such as

testosterone and dihydrotestosterone exert anabolic growth effects through their actions on protein synthesis. Glucocorticoids, at excessive levels, are inhibitory to growth, apparently because of their antagonistic effect on growth hormone secretion.

Growth Hormone

Growth hormone (GH), also called somatotropin, is a 191-amino-acid polypeptide hormone synthesized and secreted by special cells in the anterior pituitary called somatotropes. It is carried unbound in the plasma and has a half-life of about 20 to 50 minutes. The secretion of GH is regulated by two hypothalamic hormones: GH-releasing factor and GH-inhibiting hormone. These hypothalamic influences are tightly regulated by neural, metabolic, and hormonal factors. The secretion of GH fluctuates over a 24-hour period, with peak levels occurring 1 hour to 4 hours after the onset of sleep (during sleep stages 3 and 4). The nocturnal sleep bursts, which account for 70% of daily GH secretion, are greater in children than in adults.[1] Growth hormone secretion is stimulated by hypoglycemia and starvation, increased blood levels of amino acids (particularly arginine), and stress conditions such as trauma, excitement, and heavy exercise. Growth hormone levels are also affected by emotional stress. Impairment of secretion, leading to growth retardation, is not uncommon in children with severe emotional deprivation.

Short Stature

Short stature is a condition in which the attained height is well below the fifth percentile or linear growth is below normal for age and sex. Short stature, or growth retardation, has a variety of causes, including abnormalities such as Turner's syndrome (Chap. 4), growth hormone deficiency, hypothyroidism, and panhypopituitarism. Other conditions known to cause short stature include protein-calorie malnutrition, chronic diseases such as renal failure and poorly controlled diabetes mellitus, certain therapies such as exogenous corticosteroid administration, and malabsorption syndromes. Emotional disturbances can lead to functional endocrine disorders causing psychosocial dwarfism. The causes of short stature are summarized in Table 39-1.

Two forms of short stature, genetic short stature and constitutional short stature, are not disease states but variations from population norms. Genetically short children tend to have a height close to the mean height of their parents. Constitutional short stature is a term used to describe children (particularly boys) who have moderately short statures, thin build, delayed skeletal and sexual

---

Table 39-1 Causes of Short Stature

Variants of Normal
  Genetic short stature
  Constitutional short stature
Endocrine Disorders
  Growth hormone deficiency
    Primary growth hormone deficiency
      Idiopathic growth hormone deficiency
      Pituitary agenesis
    Secondary growth hormone deficiency
      Hypothalamic–pituitary tumors
      Postcranial radiation
      Head injuries
      Brain infections
      Hydrocephalus
    Biologically inactive growth hormone production
  Hypothyroidism
  Diabetes mellitus in poor control
  Glucocorticoid excess
    Endogenous (Cushing's disease)
    Exogenous glucocorticoid drug treatment
Chronic Illness
Malnutrition
  Nutritional deprivation
  Malabsorption syndrome
Functional Endocrine Disorders
  Psychosocial dwarfism
Chromosomal Disorders
  Turner's syndrome

maturation, and absence of other causes of decreased growth.

Catch-up growth is a term used to describe an abnormally high growth rate that occurs as a child approaches normal height for age. It occurs after the initiation of therapy for GH deficiency and hypothyroidism and the correction of chronic diseases.

Psychosocial dwarfism involves a functional hypopituitarism and is seen in some emotionally deprived children. These children usually present with poor growth, potbelly, and poor eating and drinking habits. Typically, there is a history of disturbed family relationships in which the child has been severely neglected or disciplined. Often the neglect is confined to one child in the family. Growth hormone function usually returns to normal after the child is removed from the home. The diagnosis is dependent on improvement in behavior and catch-up growth. Family therapy is usually indicated, and foster care may be necessary.

Accurate measurement of height is an extremely important part of the physical examination of children. Completion of the developmental history and growth charts is essential. Growth curves and growth velocity studies are also needed. Diagnosis of short stature is not made on a single measurement but is based on actual height as well as velocity of growth and parental height. Children are considered short-statured when their height and linear growth velocity are below normal for their age and sex. Genetically short children generally have a well-proportioned stature.

The diagnostic procedures for short stature include tests to rule out nonendocrine causes. If the cause is hormonal, extensive hormonal testing procedures are initiated. Usually both GH and somatomedin levels are determined. Tests can be performed using insulin (to induce hypoglycemia), levodopa, and arginine, all of which stimulate and evaluate GH reserve. If a prompt rise in GH is realized, the child is considered normal. Radiologic films are used to assess bone age, which is most often delayed. The size and shape of the sella turcica is studied to determine if a pituitary tumor exists. Once the cause of short stature has been determined, treatment can be initiated.

Growth hormone deficiency

There are several forms of GH deficiency. Children with idiopathic GH deficiency lack GH-releasing factor but have adequate somatotropes, whereas children with pituitary tumors or agenesis of the pituitary lack somatotropes. The term panhypopituitarism refers to conditions that cause a deficiency of all the anterior pituitary hormones. In a rare condition called Laron's dwarfism, GH levels are normal or elevated but there is a hereditary defect in somatomedin production.

When short stature is caused by a growth hormone deficiency, growth hormone replacement therapy is the treatment of choice. Growth hormone is species specific, and only primate GH is effective in humans. Until now, human growth hormone (HGH) was derived solely from human cadavers, and the treatment of one child required one and one-half to two human pituitary glands a week. Recently, recombinant DNA (rDNA) technology has provided the means for producing relatively large amounts of HGH. The hormone produced by this method is a 192-amino-acid molecule that contains all 191 amino acids of HGH plus an additional methionyl molecule. For this reason the rDNA-derived hormone is commonly called *methionyl HGH*. Clinical trials of methionyl HGH were begun in the United States in 1981. The hormone is administered subcutaneously three times weekly during the period of active growth. Clinical studies are also being conducted on children with constitutional short stature and Turner's syndrome. It is still too early to predict the outcome of treatment for these children. There are concerns over misuse of the drug to produce additional growth in children with normal GH function who are of near-normal height. Guidelines for use of the hormone are being developed.[2] Methods for synthesis of HGH-releasing factor have recently been developed and it has become available for use in clinical research.[3]

Tall Stature

Just as there are children who are short for their age and sex, there are also children who are tall for their age and sex. Normal variants of tall stature include genetic tall stature and constitutional tall stature. As with short stature, children with exceptionally tall parents tend to be taller than children with short parents. The term *constitutional tall stature* is used to describe a child who is taller than his or her peers and is growing at a velocity that is within the normal range for bone age. Other causes of tall stature are genetic or chromosomal disorders such as Marfan's syndrome or XYY syndrome (Chap. 4). Endocrine causes of tall stature include excessive GH, sexual precocity because of early onset of estrogen and androgen secretion, and thyrotoxicosis. With sexual precocity linear growth during childhood is increased but stature in adulthood is decreased because of premature epiphyseal closure.

Exceptionally tall children (genetic tall stature and constitutional tall stature) can be treated with sex hormones (estrogens in girls and testosterone in boys) to effect early epiphyseal closure. Such treatment is undertaken only after full consideration of the risks involved. To be effective, such treatment must be instituted 3 to 4 years before epiphyseal fusion.

Isosexual Precocious Puberty

Precocious sexual development may be idiopathic or may be caused by gonadal, adrenal, or hypothalamic tumors. Isosexual precocious puberty is defined as early activation of the hypothalamic-pituitary-gonadal axis, resulting in the development of appropriate sexual characteristics and fertility.[4,5] Sexual development is considered precocious and warrants investigation when it occurs before 8 years of age for girls and before 10 years of age for boys. In girls, about 90% of cases are idiopathic. In boys, about 40% to 60% are related to central nervous system disease.

Diagnosis of precocious puberty is based on physical findings of early thelarche, adrenarche, and menarche. Radiologic findings may indicate advanced bone age. Individuals with precocious puberty are usually tall for their age as children, but are short as adults because of the early closure of the epiphyses. The most common sign in boys is early genital enlargement.

Depending on the cause of precocious puberty, the treatment may involve surgery, medication, or no treatment. In females, medroxyprogesterone can be given to arrest menstruation in the very young child. Parents often need education, support, and anticipatory guidance in dealing with their feelings and the child's physical needs and in relating to a child that appears older than his or her years.

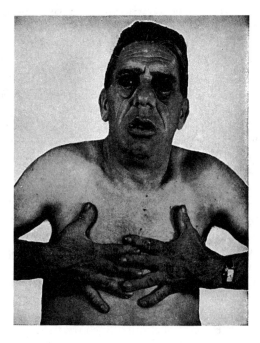

Figure 39-1 *Acromegaly, showing protrusion of the lower jaw, heavy lips, and "spade" hands. (From Chaffee EE, Lytle IM: Basic Physiology and Anatomy, 4th ed, p 527. Philadelphia, JB Lippincott, 1980)*

Growth Hormone Excess

Growth hormone excess occurring before puberty and before the fusion of the epiphyses for the long bones has occurred results in gigantism. When GH excess occurs in adulthood or after the epiphyses of the long bones have fused, a condition known as acromegaly develops.

Gigantism

Excessive secretion of GH by somatotrope adenomas causes gigantism in the prepubertal child. It occurs when the epiphyses are not fused and high levels of somatomedins stimulate excessive skeletal growth. Fortunately, the condition is now very rare because of early recognition and treatment of the adenoma.

Acromegaly

Acromegaly is a chronic and debilitating disease caused by excessive levels of GH. Most of the deleterious effects of excess GH are caused by excessive amounts of somatomedins. The growth-producing effects of the somatomedins lead to the proliferation of bone, cartilage, and soft tissue and hence to the changes in skeletal form that are characteristic of the disease. Enlargement of the small bones in the hands and feet and in the membranous bones of the face and skull results in a pronounced enlargement of the hands and feet, a broad and bulbous nose, a protruding lower jaw, and a slanting forehead (Fig. 39-1). The teeth become splayed, causing a disturbed bite and difficulty in chewing. The cartilaginous structures in the larynx and respiratory tract also become enlarged, resulting in a deepening of the voice and tendency to develop bronchitis. Vertebral changes often lead to kyphosis or hunched back.

The skeletal and soft tissue effects of GH excess are accompanied by systemic manifestations that include excessive sweating, heat intolerance, moderate weight gain, lethargy, and fatigue. Hypertension is relatively common. Bone overgrowth often leads to arthralgias and degenerative arthritis of the spine, hips, and knees.

The metabolic effects of GH include alterations in fat and carbohydrate metabolism. Increased levels of GH have a diabetogenic effect. The increase in mobilization of fatty acids predisposes to *ketoacidosis*, and the decrease in peripheral utilization of glucose tends to *elevate blood sugar*. The increase in blood sugar, in turn, stimulates the beta cells of the islets of Langerhans to produce additional insulin. Growth hormone also has a direct stimulatory effect on the beta cells.[6] Long-term elevation of GH results in overstimulation of the beta cells, literally causing them to "burn out," which predisposes the individual to diabetes.

The pituitary gland is located in the pituitary fossa, or sella turcica (Turkish saddle), which lies directly below the optic nerve. Almost all persons with acromegaly have a recognizable adenohypophyseal tumor.[7] Enlargement of the pituitary gland eventually causes erosion of the surrounding bone, and because of its location, this leads to visual complications resulting from compression of the optic nerve.

The present methods of diagnosis usually permit identification and treatment of the problem before damage to vision has occurred and before changes in the bony structures become permanent. This can be done by measuring growth hormone levels and using skull x-ray studies and computerized axial tomography (CAT scan). Pituitary tumors can be removed surgically or treated with radiation or chemotherapy or other forms of drug therapy.

In summary, a number of hormones are essential for normal body growth and maturation, including growth hormone, insulin, thyroid hormone, and androgens. Growth hormone exerts its growth effects through a group of polypeptide hormones called somatomedins. Growth hormone also exerts an effect on metabolism and is excreted in the adult as well as in the child. Its metabolic effects include a decrease in peripheral utilization of carbohydrates and an increased mobilization and utilization of fatty acids. In children, alterations in growth include short stature, isosexual precocious puberty, and tall stature. Short stature is a condition in which the attained height is well below the fifth percentile or the linear growth velocity is below normal for a child's age or sex. Short stature can occur as a variant of normal growth (genetic short stature and constitutional short stature) or as the result of endocrine disorders, chronic illness, malnutrition, emotional disturbances, or chromosomal disorders. Short stature resulting from growth hormone deficiency can now be treated with human growth hormone preparations. Isosexual precocious puberty defines a condition of early activation of hypothalamic-pituitary-gonadal axis (before 8 years of age in girls and 10 years of age in boys) resulting in the development of appropriate sexual characteristics and fertility. It causes tall stature during childhood but results in short stature in adulthood because of the early closure of the epiphyses. Tall stature describes the condition in which children are tall for their age and sex. It can occur as a variant of normal (genetic or constitutional tall stature) or as the result of a chromosomal abnormality or growth hormone excess. Growth hormone excess in adults results in acromegaly, which involves proliferation of bone, cartilage, and soft tissue along with the metabolic effects of excessive hormone levels.

■ Thyroid Disorders

The thyroid gland is a shield-shaped structure located immediately below the larynx in the anterior middle portion of the neck. The thyroid gland is composed of a large number of tiny saclike structures called follicles (Fig. 39-2). These are the functional cells of the thyroid. Each follicle is formed by a single layer of epithelial

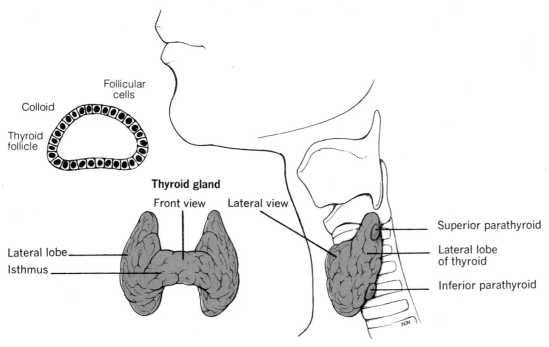

Figure 39-2 *The thyroid gland and the follicular structure. (From Chaffee EE, Lytle IM: Basic Physiology and Anatomy, 4th ed, p 434. Philadelphia, JB Lippincott, 1980)*

(follicular) cells and is filled with a secretory substance called colloid, which consists largely of a glycoprotein-iodine complex, thyroglobulin.

Control of Thyroid Function

The thyroglobulin that fills the thyroid follicles is a large glycoprotein molecule that contains 140 tyrosine amino acids. In the process of thyroid synthesis, iodine is attached to these tyrosine amino acids. Both thyroglobulin and iodide (I⁻) are secreted into the colloid of the follicle by the follicular cells.

The thyroid is remarkably efficient in its utilization of iodine. A daily absorption of 100 µg to 200 µg of dietary iodine is sufficient to form normal quantities of thyroid hormone. In the process of removing iodine from the blood and storing it for future use, iodine is pumped into the follicular cells against a concentration gradient. As a result, the concentration of iodide within the normal thyroid gland is about 40 times that in the blood. Once inside the follicle, most of the iodide is oxidized by the enzyme peroxidase in a reaction that facilitates combination with a tyrosine molecule to form *monoiodotyrosine* and then *diiodotyrosine* (Fig. 39-3). In time, two diiodotyrosine residues become coupled to form *thyroxine* (T_4); or a monoiodotyrosine and a diiodotyrosine become coupled to form *triiodothyronine*(T_3). Only T_4 (90%) and T_3 (10%) are secreted into the circulation. Thyroid hormones are bound to thyroid-binding globulin and other plasma proteins for transport in the blood. There is evidence that T_3 is the active form of the hormone and that T_4 is converted to T_3 before it becomes active.

The secretion of thyroid hormone is regulated by the *hypothalamic-pituitary-thyroid* feedback system (Fig. 39-4). In this system, *thyrotropin-releasing hormone* (TRH), which is produced by the hypothalamus, con-

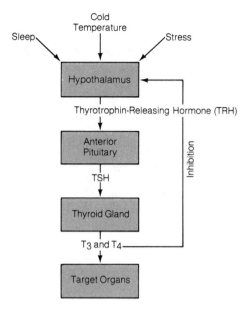

Figure 39-4 *The hypothalamic–pituitary–thyroid feedback system, which regulates the body levels of thyroid hormone.*

trols the release of *thyroid-stimulating hormone* (TSH) from the anterior pituitary gland. TSH increases the overall activity of the thyroid gland by (1) increasing the thyroglobulin breakdown and release of thyroid hormone from follicles into the bloodstream, (2) activating the iodide pump, (3) increasing the oxidation of iodide and coupling of iodide to tyrosine, and (4) increasing the number of follicle cells and the size of the follicles. The effect of TSH on the release of thyroid hormones occurs within about 30 minutes, whereas the other effects require days or weeks. Increased levels of thyroid hormone act in the feedback mechanism by inhibiting TRH. High levels of iodide cause a temporary decrease in thyroid activity that lasts for several weeks, probably

Tyrosine

Monoiodotyrosine

Diiodotyrosine

Triiodothyronine (T_3)

Thyroxine (T_4).

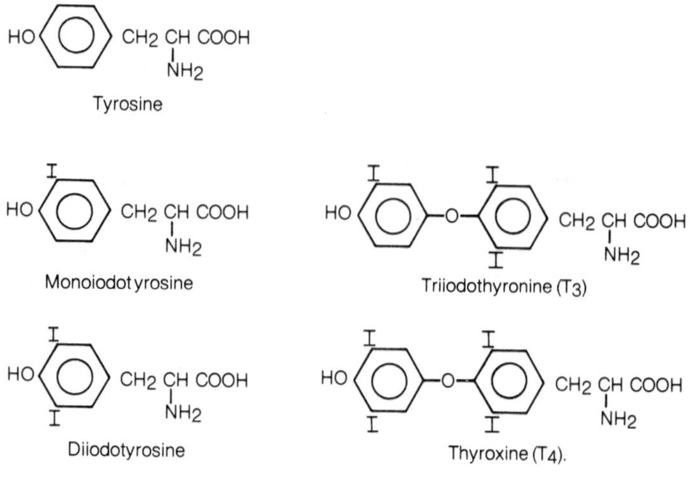

Figure 39-3 *Chemistry of thyroid hormone production.*

through a direct inhibition of TSH on the thyroid. Lugol's solution, which is an iodide preparation, is sometimes given to hyperthyroid patients in preparation for surgery as a means of decreasing thyroid function. Cold exposure is one of the strongest stimuli for increased thyroid hormone production and is probably mediated through TRH from the hypothalamus.

Actions of thyroid hormone

All the major organs in the body are affected by altered levels of thyroid hormone. Thyroid hormone has two major effects: (1) it increases metabolism and (2) it is necessary for growth and development in children, including mental development and attainment of sexual maturity.

Metabolic rate. Thyroid hormone increases the metabolism of all body tissues except the retina, spleen, testes, and lungs. The basal metabolic rate (BMR) can increase by 60% to 100% above normal when large amounts of thyroxine are secreted.[6] As a result of this higher metabolism, the rate of glucose, fat, and protein utilization increases. Lipids are mobilized from adipose tissue, and the catabolism of cholesterol by the liver is increased. As a result, blood levels of cholesterol are decreased in hyperthyroidism and increased in hypothyroidism. Muscle proteins are broken down and used as fuel, probably accounting for some of the muscle fatigue that occurs with hyperthyroidism. The absorption of glucose from the gastrointestinal tract is increased. Since vitamins are essential parts of metabolic enzymes and coenzymes, an increase in metabolic rate "speeds up the use" of vitamins and tends to cause vitamin deficiency.

Cardiovascular function. Cardiovascular and respiratory functions are strongly affected by thyroid function. With an increase in metabolism, there is a rise in oxygen consumption and production of metabolic end products with an accompanying increase in vasodilatation. Blood flow to the skin, in particular, is augmented as a means of dissipating the body heat that results from the higher metabolism. Blood volume, cardiac output, and ventilation are all increased as a means of maintaining blood flow and oxygen delivery to body tissues. Heart rate and cardiac contractility are enhanced as a means of maintaining the needed cardiac output. Blood pressure, on the other hand, is apt to change very little, because the increase in vasodilatation tends to offset the increase in cardiac output.

Gastrointestinal tract function. Thyroid hormone enhances gastrointestinal function with an increase in both motility and production of gastrointestinal secretions. An increase in appetite and food intake accompanies the higher metabolic rate. At the same time weight loss occurs because of the increased utilization of calories.

Neuromuscular effects. Thyroid hormone produces marked effects on muscle function and tone. Slight elevations in hormone levels cause skeletal muscles to react more vigorously, and a drop in hormone levels causes muscles to react more sluggishly. In the hyperthyroid state, a fine muscle tremor is present. The cause of this tremor is unknown, but it may represent an increase sensitivity of the neural synapses in the spinal cord that control muscle tone.

In the infant, thyroid hormone is necessary for normal brain development. The hormone enhances cerebration; in the hyperstate, it causes extreme nervousness, anxiety, and difficulty in sleeping.

Evidence suggests a strong interaction between thyroid hormone and the sympathetic nervous system. As will be discussed later, many of the signs and symptoms of hyperthyroidism suggest overactivity of the sympathetic division of the autonomic nervous system, for example, tachycardia, palpitations, and sweating. In addition, tremor, restlessness, anxiety, and diarrhea may reflect autonomic nervous system imbalances. Drugs that block sympathetic activity have proved to be valuable adjuncts in the treatment of hyperthyroidism because of their ability to relieve some of these undesirable symptoms.

Tests of thyroid function

There are various tests that aid in diagnosing thyroid disorders. *Direct measures* of T_3, T_4, TSH, and thyroid-binding globulin have been made through *radioimmunoassay methods*. The *resin uptake test* for T_3 and T_4 measures the unsaturated binding sites of the thyroid hormones. The *TSH-stimulating test* differentiates primary and secondary thyroid disorders. The *radioactive iodine uptake test* measures the abiity of the thyroid gland to remove and concentrate iodine from the blood. The *thyrotropin-releasng hormone (TRH) test* is used to differentiate between hypothalamic and pituitary causes of secondary hypothyroidism. A test dose of TRH is given, and serum levels of TSH are measured. The *thyroid scan* detects thyroid nodules and active thyroid tissue. *Ultrasonography* can be used to differentiate between cystic and solid thyroid lesions. *Protein-bound iodine* (PBI) measures the organic iodine that is bound to plasma proteins. This test is easily influenced by medications that contain iodine and by conditions that affect binding of thyroid hormone; therefore, it is not used as frequently as it was in the past.

The *basal metabolic rate* (BMR) is an indirect measure of thyroid function, and it, too, has been largely replaced by more accurate and quantitative tests. The *photomotogram* is a test that measures the speed of relaxation of the Achilles tendon. This test is done with the person kneeling on a chair with the foot positioned in such a way as to interrupt a photoelectric light beam. In this way, a timer is initiated when the Achilles tendon is tapped with a reflex hammer and is stopped when the foot returns to its normal position. The reflex time is increased in hypothyroidism and decreased in hyperthyroidism.

Alterations in Thyroid Function

An alteration in thyroid function can represent either a hypofunctional or a hyperfunctional state. The manifestations of these two altered states are summarized in Table 39-2. Disorders of the thyroid may represent a congenital defect in thyroid development or they may develop later in life, with a gradual or a sudden onset.

Goiter is an increase in the size of the thyroid gland. It can occur in hypothyroid, euthyroid, and hyperthyroid states. Goiters may be diffuse, involving the entire gland without evidence or nodularity, or they may contain nodules. Diffuse goiters usually become nodular. Goiters may be toxic, producing signs of extreme hyperthyroidism, or *thyrotoxicosis*, or they may be nontoxic. Diffuse nontoxic and multinodular goiters are the result of compensatory hypertrophy and hyperplasia of follicular epithelium secondary to some derangement that impairs thyroid hormone output. The degree of thyroid enlargement is usually proportional to the extent and duration of thyroid deficiency. The increased thyroid mass usually achieves a normal, or *euthyroid*, state eventually. Multinodular goiters produce the largest thyroid enlargements and are often associated with thyrotoxicosis. When sufficiently enlarged they may compress the esophagus and trachea, causing difficulty in swallowing, a choking sensation, and inspiratory stridor. Such lesions may also compress the superior vena cava, producing distention of the veins of the neck and upper extremities, edema of the eyelids and conjunctiva, and syncope with coughing.

Hypothyroidism

Hypothyroidism can occur as a congenital or an acquired defect. The absence of thyroid function at birth is called *cretinism*. When the condition occurs later in life it is called *myxedema*. Currently the term *cretin* hardly seems appropriate for describing the normally developing infant in whom replacement thyroid hormone therapy was instituted shortly after birth.

Congenital hypothyroidism. Congenital hypothyroidism is perhaps one of the most common causes of preventable mental retardation. It affects about 1 out of 5000 infants. Hypothyroidism in the infant may result from a congenital lack of the thyroid gland or from abnormal biosynthesis of thyroid hormone or deficient TSH secretion. With congenital lack of the thyroid gland, the infant usually appears normal and functions

Table 39-2 Manifestations of Hypothyroid and Hyperthyroid States

Level of Organization	Hypostate	Hyperstate
Basal metabolic rate	Decreased	Increased
Sensitivity to catecholamines	Decreased	Increased
General features	Myxedematous features	Exophthalmos
	Deep voice	Lid lag
	Impaired growth (child)	Decreased blinking
Blood cholesterol levels	Increased	Decreased
General behavior	Mental retardation (infant)	Restlessness, irritability, anxiety
	Mental and physical sluggishness	Hyperkinesis
	Somnolence	Wakefulness
Cardiovascular function	Decreased cardiac output	Increased cardiac output
	Bradycardia	Tachycardia and palpitations
Gastrointestinal function	Constipation	Diarrhea
	Decreased appetite	Increased appetite
Respiratory function	Hypoventilation	Dyspnea
Muscle tone and reflexes	Decreased	Increased, with tremor and fibrillatory twitching
Temperature tolerance	Cold intolerance	Heat intolerance
Skin and hair	Decreased sweating	Increased sweating
	Coarse and dry skin and hair	Thin and silky skin and hair
Weight	Gain	Loss

normally at birth because hormones have been supplied *in utero* by the mother.

Thyroid hormone is essential for normal brain development and growth, almost half of which occurs during the first 6 months of life. If untreated, congenital hypothyroidism causes mental retardation and impairment of growth. In hypothyroid infants treated before 3 months of age, 70% will have an IQ higher than 85. However, if treatment is delayed to between 3 months and 7 months, 85% of these infants will have definite retardation.[8]

Fortunately, neonatal screening tests have been instituted to detect congenital hypothyroidism during early infancy. Screening is usually done in the hospital nursery between the first and the fifth days of life. In this test, a drop of blood is taken from the infant's heel and analyzed for T_4 and TSH. In 1977, the cost of the screening test was but 60¢ per infant (testing for TSH added slightly to this cost).[9] Clearly, the cost of detecting congenital hypothyroidism is far less than the cost of institutionalization would be were mental retardation to occur because of a delay in diagnosis and treatment.

Myxedema (acquired hypothyroidism). When hypothyroidism occurs in older children or adults it is called *myxedema*. The term myxedema implies the presence of a nonpitting mucus-type edema caused by an accumulation of a hydrophilic mucopolysaccharide substance in the connective tissues throughout the body. The hypothyroid state may be mild, with only a few signs and symptoms, or it may progress to a life-threatening condition called *myxedematous coma*. It can result from destruction or dysfunction of the thyroid gland (primary hypothyroidism) or as a secondary disorder caused by impaired hypothalamic or pituitary function.

Primary hypothyroidism is much more common than secondary hypothyroidism. It may result from thyroidectomy (surgical removal) or ablation of the gland with radiation. Certain goitrogenic agents, such as lithium carbonate (used in the treatment of manic-depressive states) and the antithyroid drugs propylthiouracil and methimazole in continuous dosage, can block hormone synthesis and produce hypothyroidism with goiter. Large amounts of iodine (ingestion of kelp tablets or iodide-containing cough syrups or administration of iodide-containing radiographic contrast media) can also block thyroid hormone production and cause goiter, particularly in persons with autoimmune thyroid disease. Iodine deficiency, which can cause goiter and hypothyroidism, is rare in the United States because of the widespread use of iodized salt and other iodide sources. Probably the most common cause of hypothyroidism is Hashimoto's thyroiditis, an autoimmune disorder in which the thyroid gland may be totally destroyed by an immunologic process. It is the major cause of goiter and hypothyroidism in children. Hashimoto's thyroiditis is predominantly a disease of women, with a female to male ratio of 10:1.[10] The course of the disease varies. At the onset only a goiter may be present. In time, hypothyroidism usually becomes evident. Although the disorder generally causes hypothyroidism, a hyperthyroid state may develop midcourse in the disease. The transient hyperthyroid state is due to leakage of preformed thyroid hormone from damaged cells of the gland.

Myxedema affects almost all of the organ systems in the body. The manifestations of the disorder are largely related to two factors: (1) the hypometabolic state resulting from thyroid hormone deficiency and (2) myxedematous involvement of body tissues. Although the myxedema is most obvious in the face and other superficial parts, it also affects many of the body organs and is responsible for many of the manifestations of the hypothyroid state (Fig. 39-5).

The hypometabolic state associated with myxedema is characterized by a gradual onset of fatigue, a tendency to gain weight despite a loss in appetite, and cold intolerance. As the condition progresses, the skin becomes dry and rough and acquires a pale yellowish cast that is due primarily to carotene deposition. Gastrointestinal motility is decreased, giving rise to constipation,

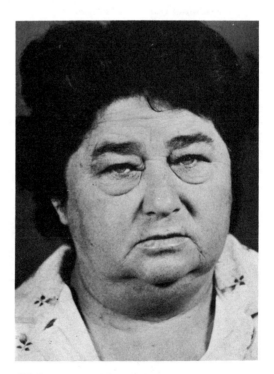

Figure 39-5 *Patient with myxedema. (Courtesy of Dr. Herbert Langford. From Guyton A: Medical Physiology, 6th ed, p 941. Philadelphia, WB Saunders, 1981. Reprinted by permission.)*

flatulence, and abdominal distention. Nervous system involvement is manifested in mental dullness, lethargy, and impaired memory.

As a result of fluid accumulation, the face takes on a characteristic puffy look, especially around the eyes. The tongue is enlarged, and the voice is hoarse and husky. Myxedematous fluid can collect in the interstitial spaces of almost any organ system. Pericardial or pleural effusion may develop. Mucopolysaccharide deposits in the heart cause generalized cardiac dilatation, bradycardia, and other signs of altered cardiac function. The signs and symptoms of hypothyroidism are summarized in Table 39-2.

Diagnosis of hypothyroidism is based on history, physical examination, and laboratory tests. A low serum T_4, low resin T_3, and elevated TSH are characteristic of primary hypothyroidism. The tests for antithyroid antibodies may be done when Hashimoto's thyroiditis is suspected. In secondary hypothyroidism, a TRH test is helpful in differentiating between pituitary and hypothalamic disease. Hypothyroidism is treated by replacement therapy with purified thyroid hormones obtained from domestic animals such as cows, pigs, and sheep, or with synthetic preparations.

Myxedematous coma. *Myxedematous coma* is a life-threatening end-stage expression of hypothyroidism. It is characterized by coma, hypothermia, cardiovascular collapse, hypoventilation, and severe metabolic disorders that include hyponatremia, hypoglycemia, and lactic acidosis. It occurs most often in the elderly and is seldom seen in persons under age 50.[11] The fact that it occurs more frequently in winter months suggests that cold exposure may be a precipitating factor. The severely hypothyroid person is unable to metabolize sedatives, analgesics, and anesthetic drugs, and these agents may precipitate coma.

Hyperthyroidism

Hyperthyroidism, or *thyrotoxicosis*, results from excessive delivery of thyroid hormone to the peripheral tissue. It is seen most frequently in women 20 to 40 years of age. It is commonly associated with hyperplasia of the thyroid gland, multinodular goiter, and adenoma of the thyroid. Occasionally it develops as the result of the ingestion of an overdose of thyroid hormone. When the condition is accompanied by exophthalmos (bulging of the eyeballs) and goiter, it is called Graves' disease. Thyroid crisis, or storm, is an acutely exaggerated manifestation of the hyperthyroid state.

Many of the manifestations of hyperthyroidism are related to the increase in oxygen consumption and increased utilization of metabolic fuels associated with the *hypermetabolic state* as well as the *increase in sym-pathetic nervous system activity* that occurs. The fact that many of the signs and symptoms of hyperthyroidism resemble those of excessive sympathetic activity suggests that the thyroid hormone may heighten the sensitivity of the body to the catecholamines or that thyroid hormone itself may act as a pseudocatecholamine. With the hypermetabolic state, there are frequent complaints of nervousness, irritability, and fatigability. Weight loss is common despite a large appetite. Other manifestations include tachycardia, palpitations, shortness of breath, excessive sweating, and heat intolerance. The person appears restless and has a fine muscle tremor. Even in persons without exophthalmos there is an abnormal retraction of the eyelids and infrequent blinking so that they appear to be staring. The hair and skin are usually thin and have a silky appearance. The signs and symptoms of hyperthyroidism are summarized in Table 39-2.

Graves' disease. *Graves' disease* is a state of *hyperthyroidism*, *goiter*, and *exophthalmos*. The cause of Graves' disease and the development of the exophthalmos, which results from edema and cellular infiltration of the orbital structures and muscle, is poorly understood. Current evidence suggests that it is an immune disorder characterized by abnormal stimulation of the thyroid gland by thyroid-stimulating antibodies that act through the normal TSH receptors. The exophthalmos is thought to result from an exophthalmos-producing factor whose action is enhanced by antibodies. The ophthalmopathy of Graves' disease can cause severe eye problems, including paralysis of the extraocular muscles, involvement of the optic nerve with some visual loss, and corneal ulceration because the lids do not close over the protruding eyeball. The exophthalmos usually tends to stabilize following treatment of the hyperthyroidism. Unfortunately, not all of the ocular changes are reversible. Figure 39-6 depicts a woman with Graves' disease.

Thyroid storm. *Thyroid storm* (crisis) is an extreme and life-threatening form of thyrotoxicosis, rarely seen today because of improved diagnosis and treatment methods. When it does occur, it is seen most often in undiagnosed cases or in persons with hyperthyroidism who have not been adequately treated. It is often precipitated by stress, such as an infection (usually respiratory), by diabetic ketoacidosis, by physical or emotional trauma, or by manipulation of a hyperactive thyroid gland during thyroidectomy. Thyroid storm is manifested by a very high fever, extreme cardiovascular effects (tachycardia, congestive failure, and angina), and severe central nervous system effects (agitation, restlessness, and delirium). The mortality is high.

The *treatment* of hyperthyroidism is directed toward reducing the level of thyroid hormone. This can

In summary, thyroid hormones play a role in the metabolic process of almost all body cells and are necesary for normal physical and mental growth in the infant and small child. Alterations in thyroid function can present as either a hypostate or a hyperstate. Hypothyroidism can occur as either a congenital or an acquired defect. When it is present at birth, it is called cretinism; when it occurs later in life, it is termed myxedema. Congenital hypothyroidism leads to mental retardation and impaired physical growth unless treatment is initiated during the first months of life. Hypothyroidism leads to a decrease in metabolic rate and an accumulation of a mucopolysaccharide substance within the intercellular spaces; this substance attracts water and causes a mucus-type of edema called myxedema. Hyperthyroidism causes an increase in metabolic rate and alterations in body function that are similar to those produced by enhanced sympathetic nervous system activity. Graves' disease is characterized by the triad of hyperthyroidism, goiter, and exophthalmos.

■ Disorders of Adrenal Cortical Function

Control of Adrenal Cortical Function

The adrenal glands are small, bilateral structures that weigh about 5 gm each and lie retroperitoneally at the apex of each kidney (Fig. 39-7). The medulla, or inner, portion of the gland secretes epinephrine and norepinephrine and is an extension of the sympathetic nervous system. The cortex forms the bulk of the adrenal gland and is responsible for secreting three types of hormones: the glucocorticoids, the mineralocorticoids, and the adrenal sex hormones. Because the sympathetic nervous system secretes catecholamines, adrenal medul-

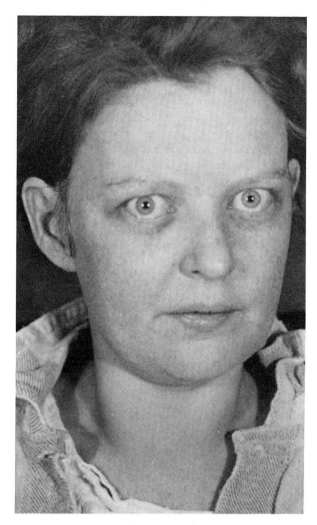

Figure 39-6 *Woman with Graves' disease. Note the exopthalmos and enlarged thryoid gland. (From Chaffee EE, Lytle IM: Basic Physiology and Anatomy, 4th ed. Philadelphia, JB Lippincott, 1980)*

be accomplished through *surgical removal* of part or all of the thyroid gland, *eradication* of the gland with *radioactive iodine*, or the use of drugs that decrease thyroid function and thereby the effect of the thyroid hormone on the peripheral tissues. The beta-adrenergic blocking drug *propranolol* is often administered to block the effects of the hyperthyroid state on sympathetic nervous system function. It is given in conjunction with other antithyroid drugs such as *propylthiouracil* and *methimazole*. These drugs prevent the thyroid gland from converting iodine to its organic (hormonal) form in the thyroid and block the conversion of T_4 to T_3 in the tissues. *Lugol's solution* (iodide) may be given to depress the thyroid gland in preparation for surgery. Unfortunately, this action is short-lived, and in a few weeks the symptoms reappear and may be intensified.

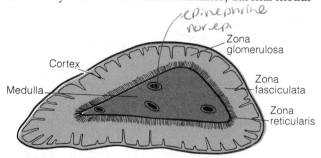

Figure 39-7 *The adrenal gland, showing the medulla and the three layers of the cortex. The zona glomerulosa is the outer layer of the cortex and is primarily responsible for mineralocorticoid production. The middle layer, the zona fasciculata, and the inner layer, the zona reticularis, produce the glucocorticoids and the adrenal sex hormones.*

lary function is not essential for life, but adrenal cortical function is. The total loss of adrenal cortical function is fatal in 3 to 10 days if untreated.[8] This section of the chapter describes the synthesis and function of the adrenal cortical hormones and the effects of adrenal cortical insufficiency and excess.

Biosynthesis of adrenal cortical hormones

More than 30 hormones are produced by the adrenal gland. Of these hormones, *aldosterone* is the principal *mineralocorticoid*, cortisol (hydrocortisone) the major glucocorticoid, and androgens the chief sex hormones. All of the adrenal cortical hormones have a similar structure in that all are steroids and are synthesized from acetate and cholesterol; thus, the glucocorticoid drugs are often called steroids. Each of the steps involved in the synthesis of the various hormones requires a specific enzyme (Fig. 39-8).

Actions of adrenal cortical hormones

Adrenal sex hormones. The adrenal sex hormones are synthesized primarily by the zona reticularis and the zona fasciculata of the cortex (see Fig. 39-7). These sex hormones probably exert little effect on normal sexual function. There is evidence, however, that the adrenal sex hormones contribute to the pubertal growth of body hair, particularly pubic and axillary hair in women. They may also play a role in the steroid hormone economy of the pregnant woman and the fetal-placental unit.[12]

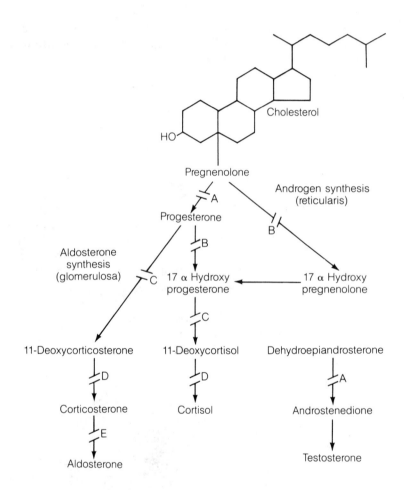

Figure 39-8 *Predominant biosynthetic pathways of the adrenal cortex. Critical enzymes in the biosynthetic process include 11-beta-hydroxylase and 21-hydroxylase. A deficiency in one of these enzymes blocks the synthesis of these hormones dependent on that enzyme and routes the precursors into alternative pathways.*

Site of enzyme action

A) 3-beta-dehydrogenase
B) 17-hydroxylase
C) 21-hydroxylase
D) 11-beta-hydroxylase
E) 18-hydroxylase

Mineralocorticoids. The mineralocorticoids play an essential role in regulating potassium and sodium levels and water balance. They are produced in the zona glomerulosa, the outer layer of cells of the adrenal cortex. Aldosterone is regulated by the renin-angiotensin mechanism and by blood levels of potassium. Adrenocorticotropic hormone (ACTH) is relatively unimportant in the day-to-day regulation of aldosterone. Increased levels of aldosterone promote sodium retention by the distal tubules of the kidney while increasing urinary losses of potassium. The influence of aldosterone on fluid and electrolyte balance is discussed in Chapter 25.

Glucocorticoids. The glucocorticoid hormones are synthesized in the zona fasciculata and the zona reticularis. The blood levels of these hormones are regulated by negative feedback mechanisms of the hypothalamic-pituitary-adrenal (HPA) system (Fig. 39-9). In this system, cortisol levels increase as ACTH levels rise. There is considerable diurnal variation in ACTH levels, which reach their peak in the early morning (around 6 AM to 8 AM) and decline as the day progresses. As will be discussed later, one of the earliest signs of Cushing's syndrome is loss of this diurnal variation. Increased plasma cortisol levels act in a negative feedback manner on receptors in the hypothalamus to decrease corticotropin-releasing factor and on the anterior pituitary to decrease ACTH. The stimulation of hypothalamic receptors and the release of cortisone-releasing factor (CRF) serve to integrate neural influences with the function of the adrenal cortex.

The glucocorticoids perform a necessary function in response to stress and are essential for survival. When produced as part of the stress response, these hormones aid in *regulating the metabolic functions* of the body and in *controlling the inflammatory response*. The actions of cortisol are summarized in Table 39-3. The reader will note that many of the anti-inflammatory actions attributed to cortisol result from the administration of pharmacologic levels of the hormone.

Metabolic effects. Cortisol stimulates glucose production by the liver, promotes protein breakdown, and causes mobilization of fatty acids. As body proteins are

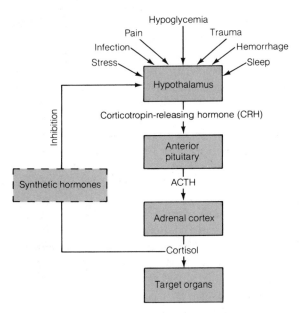

Figure 39-9 *The hypothalamic–pituitary–adrenal (HPA) feedback system that regulates glucocorticoid (cortisol) levels. Cortisol release is regulated by ACTH. Stress exerts its effects on cortisol release through the HLA system and the corticotropin-releasing factor (CRF), which controls the release of ACTH from the anterior pituitary gland. Increased cortisol levels incite a negative feedback inhibition of ACTH release. Pharmacologic doses of synthetic steroids inhibit ACTH release by way of the hypothalamic CRF. (Modified from Tepperman J: Metabolic and Endocrine Physiology, 4th ed, p 173. Chicago, Year Book Medical Publishers, 1980)*

Table 39-3   Actions of Cortisol

Major Influence	Effect on Body
Glucose metabolism	Stimulates gluconeogenesis
	Decreases glucose utilization by the tissues
Protein metabolism	Increases breakdown of proteins
	Increases plasma protein levels
Fat metabolism	Increases mobilization of fatty acids
	Increases utilization of fatty acids
Anti-inflammatory action (pharmacologic levels)	Stabilizes lysosomal membranes of the inflammatory cells, preventing the release of inflammatory mediators
	Decreases capillary permeability to prevent inflammatory edema
	Depresses phagocytosis by white blood cells to reduce the release of inflammatory mediators
	Suppresses the immune response
	Causes atrophy of lymphoid tissue
	Decreases eosinophils
	Decreases antibody formation
	Decreases the development of cell-mediated immunity
	Reduces fever
	Inhibits fibroblast activity
Psychic effect	Tends to contribute to emotional stability
Permissive effect	Facilitates the response of the tissues to humoral and neural influences, such as that of the catecholamines, during trauma and extreme stress

broken down, amino acids are mobilized and transported to the liver, where they are used in the production of glucose. The mobilization of fatty acids serves to convert cell metabolism from the utilization of glucose for energy to the utilization of fatty acids instead.

As glucose production by the liver rises and peripheral glucose utilization falls, there is moderate insulin resistance. In diabetics and persons who are diabetes-prone, this has the effect of raising the blood sugar.

Psychic effects. The glucocorticoid hormones appear to be involved either directly or indirectly in emotional disturbances. Receptors for these hormones have been identified in brain tissue, which suggests that they play a role in the regulation of behavior.[13] It has been noted that persons treated with adrenal cortical hormones have displayed behavior ranging from mildly aberrant to psychotic.

Anti-inflammatory effects. Large quantities of cortisol are required for an effective anti-inflammatory action. This is achieved by the administration of pharmacologic doses of synthetic cortisol. The increased cortisol blocks inflammation at an early stage by decreasing capillary permeability and stabilizing the lysosomal membranes so that inflammatory mediators are not released. Cortisol suppresses the immune response by reducing antibody and cell-mediated immunity. With this lessened inflammation comes a reduction in fever. During the healing phase, cortisol suppresses fibroblast activity and thereby lessens scar formation. A recently described attribute of cortisol is its ability to inhibit prostaglandin synthesis, which may account in large part for its anti-inflammatory actions.[12]

Suppression of adrenal function
A highly significant aspect of long-term therapy with pharmacologic preparations of the adrenal cortical hormones is adrenal insufficiency on withdrawal of the drugs. The deficiency is due to suppression of the HPA axis. Chronic suppression causes atrophy of the entire system, and abrupt withdrawal of drugs can cause acute adrenal insufficiency. Furthermore, recovery to a state of normal adrenal function may be prolonged, requiring up to 12 months.[12]

Tests of adrenal function
There are a number of diagnostic tests by which adrenal cortical funtion and the hypothalamic-pituitary axis may be evaluated. Blood levels of cortisol and ACTH can be measured using radioimmunoassay methods. A *24-hour urine specimen* measures the excretion of *17-ketosteroids, 17-ketogenic steroids,* and *17-hydroxycorticosteroids.* These

metabolic end products of the adrenal hormones and the male androgens provide information about alterations in the biosynthesis of the adrenal cortical hormones. *Suppression and stimulation tests* afford a means of assessing the state of the *hypothalamic-pituitary-adrenal feedback system.* For example, a test dose of ACTH may be given to assess the response of the adrenal cortex to pituitary stimulation. Similarly, administration of dexamethasone (a synthetic glucocorticoid drug) provides a means of measuring negative feedback suppression of ACTH. Adrenal tumors and ectopic ACTH-producing tumors are generally unresponsive to ACTH suppression by dexamethasone. Metyrapone (Metopirone) blocks the final step in cortisol synthesis, producing 11-dehydroxycortisol, which does not inhibit ACTH. This test measures the ability of the pituitary to release ACTH.

Congenital Adrenal Hyperplasia (Adrenogenital Syndrome)
Congenital adrenal hyperplasia (CAH) describes a congenital disorder caused by an autosomal recessive trait in which a deficiency exists in any of the five enzymes necessary for the synthesis of cortisol. A common characteristic of all types is a defect in the synthesis of cortisol that results in increased levels of ACTH and adrenal hyperplasia. The increased levels of ACTH overstimulate the pathways of steroid hormone production, particularly those involving the production of adrenal androgens. Mineralocorticoids may be produced in excessive or insufficient amounts, depending on the precise enzyme deficiency. Both males and females are affected. Males are seldom diagnosed at birth unless they have enlarged genitalia or lose salt and manifest adrenal crisis; in female infants, an increase in androgens is responsible for creating the virilization syndrome of ambiguous genitalia.

The two most common enzyme deficiencies are the 21-hydroxylase and 11-beta-hydroxylase deficiencies. The clinical manifestations of both deficiencies are largely determined by the functional properties of the steroid intermediates and the completeness of the block in the cortisol pathway.

A spectrum of 21-hydroxylase deficiency states exists, which ranges from simple virilizing CAH to a complete salt-losing enzyme deficiency. Simple virilizing CAH impairs the synthesis of cortisol, and steroid synthesis is shunted to androgen production. Persons with these deficiencies usually produce sufficient aldosterone or aldosterone intermediates to prevent signs and symptoms of mineralocorticoid deficiency. The salt-losing form is accompanied by deficient production of aldosterone and its intermediates. This results in fluid and electrolyte disorders after the fifth day of life, including hyponatremia, hyperkalemia, vomiting, dehydration, and shock.

The 11-beta-hydroxylase deficiency also manifests a spectrum of clinical severity. There is not only excessive androgen production but also impaired conversion of 11-deoxycorticosterone to corticosterone. 11-deoxy-corticosterone has mineralocorticoid activity, and its overproduction is responsible for the hypertension that accompanies this deficiency.

Diagnosis of adrenogenital syndrome depends on the precise biochemical evaluation of metabolites in the cortisol pathway as well as on clinical signs and symptoms. The signs and symptoms of the salt-losing form of 21-hydroxylase deficiency include dehydration, shock, vomiting, decreased sodium levels, and increased potassium levels. In both 11-beta-hydroxylase and 21-hydroxylase deficiencies, virilization of the female genitalia is evident. In the female one may see an enlarged clitoris, fused labia, and urogenital sinus (Fig. 39-10). Males may have no outward features that are noticeable at birth. In both males and females other secondary sex characteristics are normal, and fertility is unaffected if appropriate therapy is instituted.

Medical treatment of adrenogenital syndrome includes oral or parenteral cortisol replacement. Desoxy-corticosterone acetate (DOCA) pellets may be implanted in the skin of the scapula as a mineralocorticoid replacement. Fludrocortisone acetate may also be given to children who are salt losers. Depending on the degree of virilization, reconstructive surgery during the first 2 years of life is indicated to reduce the size of the clitoris, separate the labia, and exteriorize the vagina. Surgery has provided excellent results and does not impair sexual function.

Adrenal Insufficiency

There are two forms of adrenal insufficiency: primary and secondary. Primary adrenal insufficiency, or Addison's disease, is due to the destruction of the adrenal gland. Secondary adrenal insufficiency is due to a disorder of the HPA system.

Primary adrenal insufficiency (Addison's disease)

In 1855, Thomas Addison, an English physician, provided the first detailed clinical description of primary adrenal insufficiency. Addison's disease is a relatively rare disorder in which all the layers of the adrenal cortex are destroyed. Most often the underlying problem is idiopathic adrenal atrophy, which probably has an autoimmune basis. Tuberculosis is an infrequent cause, as is amyloidosis, or a fungal infection (particularly histoplasmosis). Bilateral adrenalectomy, sometimes done in

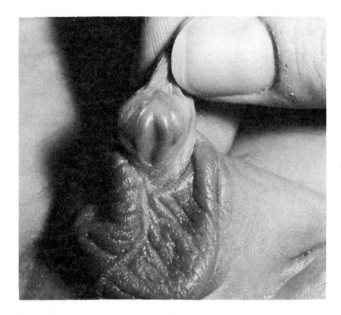

Figure 39-10 *Female infant with congenital adrenal hyperplasia demonstrating virilization of the genitalia. Note the enlarged clitoris and the fused labia, which resembles a scrotal sac. (Hurwitz LS: Nursing implications of selected endocrine disorders. Nurs Clin North Am 15, No. 3:528, 1980. Reprinted with permission)*

the past for breast cancer, is an obvious cause of primary adrenal insufficiency.

Addison's disease, like insulin-dependent diabetes mellitus, is a *chronic metabolic disorder that requires lifetime hormone replacement therapy.* The adrenal cortex has a large reserve capacity, and the manifestations of adrenal insufficiency do not usually become apparent until about 90% of the gland has been destroyed.[10] These manifestations are primarily related to (1) hyperpigmentation resulting from elevated ACTH levels, (2) mineralocorticoid deficiency, and (3) glucocorticoid deficiency. Although lack of the adrenal androgens exerts few effects in men because the testes produce these hormones, women will have sparse axillary and pubic hair. The manifestations of adrenal insufficiency are summarized in Table 39-4.

Hyperpigmentation. In Addison's disease, ACTH levels are elevated in respone to the fall in cortisol. At this point it is important to note that the amino acid sequence of ACTH is strikingly similar to that of melanocyte-stimulating hormone (MSH); thus, *hyperpigmentation* is seen in about 98% of persons with Addison's disease and is *helpful in distinguishing the primary and secondary forms.* The skin looks bronzed or suntanned in both exposed and unexposed areas, and the normal creases and pressure points tend to become especially dark. The gums

Table 39-4   Manifestations of Adrenal Cortical Insufficiency and Excess

Parameter	Adrenal Cortical Insufficiency	Glucocorticoid Excess
Electrolytes	Hyponatremia* Hyperkalemia*	Hypokalemia
Fluids	Dehydration* (elevated BUN, others)	Edema
Blood pressure	Hypotension* Shock* Orthostatic hypotension	Hypertension
Musculoskeletal	Muscle weakness* Fatigue*	Muscle wasting Fatigue
Hair and skin	Skin pigmentation Loss of hair (axillary and pubic)	Easy bruisability Hirsuitism, acne, and striae (abdomen and thighs)
Inflammatory response	Low resistance to trauma, infection, and stress	Decrease in eosinophils Lymphocytopenia
Gastrointestinal	Nausea, vomiting* Abdominal pain*	Possible gastrointestinal bleeding
Glucose metabolism	Hypoglycemia*	Impaired glucose tolerance Glycosuria Elevated blood sugar
Emotional	Depression and irritability	Emotional lability to psychosis
Other	Menstrual irregularity Decreased axillary and pubic hair in women	Oligomenorrhea Impotence in the male Centripetal obesity (moon face and buffalo hump)

*Present in acute adrenal insufficiency.

and oral mucous membranes may become bluish black in color. This hyperpigmentation becomes more pronounced during periods of stress.

Mineralocorticoid deficiency.   Mineralocorticoid deficiency causes increased urinary losses of sodium, chloride, and water along with decreased excretion of potassium. The result is hyponatremia, loss of extracellular fluid, decreased cardiac output, and hyperkalemia. There may be an abnormal appetite for salt. Orthostatic hypotension is common. Dehydration, weakness, and fatigue are often present as early symptoms. If loss of sodium and water is extreme, cardiovascular collapse and shock will ensue.

Glucocorticoid deficiency.   Because of a lack of glucocorticoids, the patient has poor tolerance to stress. This deficiency causes hypoglycemia, lethargy, weakness, fever, and gastrointestinal symptoms such as anorexia, nausea, vomiting, and weight loss.

Secondary adrenal insufficiency

Secondary adrenal insufficiency can occur as the result of hypopituitarism or because the pituitary gland has been surgically removed. However, a far more common cause than either of these is the rapid withdrawal of glucocorticoids that have been administered therapeutically.

These drugs suppress the HPA system, with resulting adrenal cortical atrophy and lack of cortisol. It is important to note that this suppression continues long after drug therapy has been discontinued and could be critical during periods of stress or when surgery is done. It has been suggested that a person receiving pharmacologic doses of the glucocorticoids for more than 1 to 4 weeks may have suppression of the HPA system for up to a year after the drugs have been discontinued.[14]

Acute adrenal crisis

Acute adrenal crisis is a life-threatening situation. If Addison's disease is the underlying problem, exposure to even a minor illness or stress can precipitate nausea, vomiting, muscular weakness, hypotension, dehydration, and vascular collapse. The onset of adrenal crisis may be sudden, or it may progress over a period of several days. The symptoms may also occur suddenly in children with salt-losing forms of the adrenogenital syndrome. Massive bilateral adrenal hemorrhage causes an acute fulminating form of adrenal insufficiency. Hemorrhage can be caused by meningococcal septicemia (called *Waterhouse–Friderichsen syndrome*), adrenal trauma, anticoagulant therapy, adrenal vein thrombosis, or adrenal metastases.

Adrenal insufficiency is treated with replacement glucocorticoid therapy. In acute adrenal insufficiency, cortisol is given intravenously followed by rapid infusion of saline and glucose. The day-to-day regulation of the chronic phase of Addison's is usually accomplished with oral cortisol, and higher doses are given during periods of stress. Because these patients are likely to have episodes of hyponatremia and hypoglycemia, they need to have a regular schedule for meals and exercise.

Glucocorticoid Hormone Excess (Cushing's Syndrome)

Cushing's syndrome is characterized by a chronic elevation in glucocorticoid (and adrenal androgen) hormones. Because the condition is most frequently caused by increased ACTH production, the mineralocorticoids are usually not involved in the syndrome.

Cushing's syndrome can result from either overproduction of hormones by the body or long-term therapy with one of the potent pharmacologic preparations of glucocorticoids (*iatrogenic Cushing's syndrome*). Three important forms of Cushing's syndrome result from excess glucocorticoids production by the body. One is a *pituitary form*, which results from excessive production of ACTH by a tumor of the pituitary gland; it accounts for about two-thirds of the disease cases, and because this form of the disease was the one originally described by Cushing, it is called Cushing's disease. The other forms of excess glucocorticoid levels are referred to as Cushing's syndrome.* The second form is the *adrenal form*, caused by an adrenal tumor. The third is the *ectopic* Cushing's, due to an ACTH-producing tumor such as occurs in some bronchogenic cancers.

The major manifestations of Cushing's syndrome represent an exaggeration of the normal effects of cortisol. Altered *fat metabolism* causes a peculiar deposition of fat characterized by a protruding abdomen, subclavicular fat pads or "buffalo hump" on the back, and a round, plethoric "moon face." There is muscle weakness and the extremities are thin because of *protein breakdown* and muscle wasting. In advanced cases, the skin over the forearms and legs becomes thin, having the appearance of parchment. Purple striae (stretch marks), from stretching of the catabolically weakened skin and subcutaneous tissues, are distributed on the abdomen and hips. *Osteoporosis* results from destruction of bone proteins and alterations in calcium metabolism. With osteoporosis there may be back pain, compression fractures of the vertebrae, and rib fractures. As calcium is mobilized from bone, renal calculi may develop. Derangements in glucose metabolism are found in some 90% of patients, with clinically overt *diabetes mellitus* occurring in about

*In this text the term Cushing's syndrome designates both Cushing's disease and Cushing's syndrome.

20%.[10] The glucocorticoids possess mineralocorticoid properties; this causes hypokalemia as a result of excessive potassium excretion and hypertension resulting from sodium retention. *Inflammatory and immune responses are inhibited*, resulting in increased susceptibility to infection. Cortisol increases gastric acid secretion, and this may provoke gastric ulceration and bleeding. An accompanying *increase in androgen* levels causes hirsutism, mild acne, and menstrual irregularities in women.

Excess levels of the glucocorticoids may give rise to extreme emotional lability, ranging from mild euphoria and absence of normal fatigue to grossly psychotic behavior. The manifestations of glucocorticoid excess are summarized in Table 39-4.

Diagnosis of Cushing's syndrome depends on the finding of elevated plasma levels of cortisol. As was mentioned, one of the prominent features of Cushing's syndrome is loss of the diurnal pattern of cortisol secretion. Therefore, cortisol determinations are often made on three blood samples: one taken in the morning, one in late afternoon or early evening, and a third drawn the following morning after a midnight dose of dexamethasone. Measurement of plasma ACTH, 24-hour urinary 17-ketosteroids, 17-ketogenic steroids, and 17-hydroxycorticosteroids, and suppression or stimulation tests of the HPA system are often made. Skull x-ray films and intravenous pyelograms, which outline the shadows of the kidneys and adrenal glands, may be done. Computerized tomograms (CT) afford a means for locating adrenal or pituitary tumors.

The *treatment of Cushing's syndrome*, whether by surgery, irradiation, or drugs, is largely determined by the etiology. Adrenalectomy may be done if an adrenal tumor is present. With the recent development of the transsphenoidal approach for removal of a pituitary tumor using microsurgical techniques, surgical treatment today is far more efficient than in the past. In children and in adults with mild clinical symptoms, cobalt radiation is often the preferred method for treating pituitary Cushing's. One drawback of radiation therapy is the long time lag (18 months in some cases) before complete remission occurs.[15] Adrenolytic agents are administered in persons with inoperable tumors, in those whose tumors have not been fully treated, and in those in whom irradiation has not yet taken effect. Two such agents are cyproheptadine and *O,p'*-dichlorodiphenyl dichloroethane.

In summary, the adrenal cortex produces three types of hormones: mineralocorticoids, glucocorticoids, and adrenal sex hormones. The mineralocorticoids along with the renin-angiotensin mechanism aid in controlling body levels of sodium and potassium. The glucocorticoids have anti-inflammatory actions and aid in regulating glucose, protein, and fat metabolism during periods of stress. These hormones are under the control of the hypothalamic-pituitary-adrenal (HPA) system. The adrenal sex hormones exert little effect on the day-to-day control of body function, but probably contribute to the development of body hair in women. The adrenal genital syndrome describes a genetic defect in the cortisol pathway resulting from a deficiency of one of the enzymes needed for its synthesis. Depending on the enzyme involved, the disorder causes virilization of female infants and in some instances fluid and electrolyte disturbances because of impaired mineralocorticoid synthesis. Chronic adrenal insufficiency is called Addison's disease. It can be caused by destruction of the adrenal gland or by dysfunction of the HPA system. Adrenal insufficiency requires replacement therapy with cortical hormones. Acute adrenal insufficiency is a life-threatening situation. Cushing's syndrome exists when the glucocorticoid level is abnormally high. This syndrome may be a result of pharmacologic doses of cortisol, a pituitary or adrenal tumor, or an ectopic tumor that produces ACTH. The clinical manifestations of Cushing's syndrome reflect the very high level of cortisol that is present.

■ Study Guide

After you have studied this chapter, you should be able to meet the following objectives:

☐ State the general functions of growth hormone and the somatomedins.

☐ State the effects of a deficiency in growth hormone.

☐ Define short stature.

☐ Define constitutional short stature.

☐ State the mechanisms of short stature in hypothyroidism, poorly controlled diabetes mellitus, treatment with adrenal glucocorticosteroid hormones, malnutrition, and psychosocial dwarfism.

☐ List three causes of tall stature.

☐ Explain why children with isosexual precocious puberty are tall statured as children, but short statured as adults.

☐ Describe the conditions predisposing to acromegaly.

☐ Explain the potential relationship between growth hormone and diabetes.

☐ Describe the synthesis of thyroid hormones.

☐ Describe the hypothalamic-pituitary-thyroid feedback system.

☐ Explain why blood cholesterol levels are decreased in hyperthyroidism.

☐ State the relationship between cardiovascular function and thyroid function.

☐ Describe the general effects of thyroid hormone on the muscular system.

☐ Name three tests of thyroid function.

☐ List the signs and symptoms of hyperthyroidism the health professional should be able to recognize.

☐ State the manifestations of thyroid storm.

☐ State the triad of conditions that constitute Graves' disease.

☐ Describe the effects of congenital hypothyroidism.

☐ Describe the manifestations of the condition known as myxedema.

☐ State the underlying cause of the adrenogenital syndrome.

☐ State the role of the adrenal sex hormones and the mineralocorticoids.

☐ Explain the regulation of the glucocorticoids by negative feedback mechanisms.

☐ Explain the influence of cortisol on body metabolism.

☐ Describe the action of cortisol on inflammation.

☐ State the purpose of the 24-hour urine specimen with reference to adrenal cortical function.

☐ State the underlying cause or causes of Cushing's syndrome.

☐ Describe the clinical manifestations of Cushing's syndrome.

☐ Explain the underlying pathology that is present in Addison's disease.

☐ Compare the manifestations of Addison's disease with those of secondary adrenal insufficiency.

☐ Describe the overall treatment of adrenal insufficiency.

■ References

1. Findling JW, Tyrell BJ: Anterior pituitary and somatomedins: 1. Anterior pituitary. In Greenspan FS, Forsham PH (eds.): Basic and Clinical Endocrinology, p 45. Los Altos, Lange Medical Publishers, 1983
2. Underwood LE: Report on the conference on uses and possible abuses of biosynthetic human growth hormone. N Engl J Med 311:606, 1984

3. Thorner MO, Reschke J, Chitwood J et al: Acceleration of growth in two children treated with human growth hormone-releasing factor. N Engl J Med 312:4, 1985

4. Tichy AM, Malasanos LG: The physiological role of hormones in puberty. Am J Matern Child Nurs 1:384, 1976

5. Williams RH (ed): Textbook of Endocrinology. Philadelphia, WB Saunders, 1974

6. Guyton A: Textbook of Medical Physiology, 6th ed, pp 924, 936, 944. Philadelphia, WB Saunders, 1981

7. Daughaday WH, Cryer P: Growth hormone hypersecretion and acromegaly. Hosp Pract 13, No 8:76, 1978

8. Klein AH et al: Improved prognosis in congenital hypothyroidism treated before age three months. J Pediatr 81:912, 1972

9. Fisher D: Screening for congenital hypothyroidism. Hosp Pract 12, No 12:77, 1977

10. Robbins SL, Cotran RS, Kumar V: Pathologic Basis of Disease, 3rd ed, pp 1207, 1235, 1238. Philadelphia, WB Saunders, 1984

11. Meek JC: Myxedema coma. Crit Care Q 3:131, 1980

12. Tepperman J: Metabolic and Endocrine Physiology, 4th ed, pp 173, 189, 187. Chicago, Year Book Medical Publishers, 1980

13. McEwan BS: Influences of the adrenocortical hormone on pituitary and brain function. Monogr Endocrinol 12:467–492, 1978

14. Axelrod L: Glucocorticoid therapy. Medicine 55, No 1:49, 1976

15. Gold EM: Cushing's syndrome. Hosp Pract 14, No 6:75, 1979

■ Additional References

Hurwitz LS: Nursing implications of selected pediatric endocrine disorders. Nurs Clin North Am 15, No 3, 1980

Leigh H, Kramer SI: The psychiatric manifestations of endocrine disease. Adv Intern Med 29:413, 1984

Nasr H: Endocrine disorders in the elderly. Med Clin North Am 67, No 2:481, 1983

Sowers DK, Sowers JR: Pituitary emergencies. Crit Care Q 3:45-54, 1980

Vinicor F, Cooper J: Early recognition of endocrine disorders. Hosp Med 15, No 9:38, 1979

Volpe R: The role of autoimmunity in hypoendocrine and hyperendocrine function. Ann Intern Med 87, No 1:86-99, 1977

Adrenal

Crapo L: Cushing's disease: A review of diagnostic tests. Metabolism 28:955, 1979

Fredlund PN, Mecklenburg RS: Acute adrenal insufficiency: Diagnosis and management. Hosp Med 15, No 6:28-47, 1979

Gold EM: The Cushing's syndromes: Changing views of diagnosis and treatment. Ann Intern Med 90:829, 1979

Hall RCW, Popkin MK, Stickney SK, Gardner ER: Presentation of the steroid psychoses. J Nerv Ment Dis 167, No 4:229, 1979

Hardy J: Cushing's disease some 50 years later. Can J Neurol Sci 9:375, 1982

McEwen BS: Influences of adrenocorticol hormones on pituitary and brain function. Monogr Endocrinol 12:467, 1978

Mininberg DT, Levine LS, New MI: Current concepts in congenital adrenal hyperplasia. Ann Pathol 17, Part 2:179, 1982

Sanford SJ: Dysfunction of the adrenal gland: Physiologic considerations and nursing problems. Nurs Clin North Am 15, No 3:481, 1980

Schimke RN: Adrenal insufficiency. Crit Care Q 3:19, 1980

Styne DM, Grumbach MM, Kaplan SL et al: Treatment of Cushing's disease in childhood and adolescence with transsphenoidal microadenomectomy. N Engl J Med 310:889, 1984

Tzagournis M: Acute adrenal insufficiency. Heart Lung 7, No 4:603, 1978

Wachter-Shikora N: ACTH—A review of anatomy, physiology, and structure related to neuroendocrine effects. Neurosur Nur 11, No 2:105, 1979

Wilson KS, Parker A: Adrenal suppression after short-term corticosteroid therapy. Lancet 1030, 1979

Growth and growth hormone

Baxter JD: Mechanisms of glucocorticoid inhibition of growth. Kidney Int 14:330, 1978

Frazer T, Gavin JR, Daughaday WH et al: Growth-hormone dependent growth failure. J Pediatr 101:12, 1982

Hintz RL, Rosenfeld RG: Clinical uses of synthetic growth hormone. Hosp Pract 18, No 10:115, 1983

Rimoin DL, Horton WA: Short stature. Part I and Part II. J Pediatr 92:523, 697, 1978

Vliet GV, Styne DM, Kaplan SL et al: Growth hormone treatment of short stature. N Engl J Med 309:1016, 1983

Whitehead EM, Shalet SM, Davies D et al: Pituitary gigantism: A disabling condition. Clin Endocrinol 17:271, 1982

Zachmann M: Diagnosis of treatable types of short and tall stature. Postgrad Med 54:121, 1978

Thyroid

Chopra IJ, Solomon DH: Pathogenesis of hyperthyroidism. Annu Rev Med 34:267, 1983

Cooper DS: Antithyroid drugs. N Engl J Med 311:1353, 1984

Dussault JH, Morissette J, Letarte J et al: Modification of a screening program for neonatal hypothyroidism. J Pediatr 92, No 2:274, 1978

Evangelisti JT, Thorpe CJ: Thyroid storm—A nursing crisis. Heart Lung 12:184, 1983

Gorman G: Ophthalmopathy of Graves' disease. N Engl J Med 308:453, 1983

Fisher DA, Klein AH: Thyroid development and disorders of thyroid function in the newborn. N Engl J Med 304, No 12:702, 1981

Hurley JR: Thyroid disease in the elderly. Med Clin North Am 67:497, 1983

Jackson IMD: Thyrotropin-releasing hormone. N Engl J Med 306:145, 1982

Larsen PR: Thyroid-pituitary interaction. N Engl J Med 306:23, 1982

Lyon J, Spence DA: Congenital thyroid disease detected by screening program. Alaska Med 20, No 4:56, 1978

Mazzaferri EL: Thyroid storm. Hosp Med 15, No 11:7, 1979

Mazzaferri EL: Thyrotoxicosis. Postgrad Med 73, No 4:85, 1983

McClung MR, Greer MA: Treatment of hyperthyroidism. Annu Rev Med 31:385, 1980

Oppenheimer JH, Surks MI: The peripheral action of the thyroid hormones. Med Clin North Am 59, No 5:1055, 1975

Safrit HF: Diagnosis and management of Graves' disease. Hosp Med 15, No 10:74, 1979

Sakamoto A, Salamoto G, Sugano H: History of cervical radiation and incidence of carcinoma of the pharynx, larynx and thyroid. Cancer 44:718, 1979

Sawin CT, Herman T, Molitch ME et al: Aging and the thyroid. Am J Med 75:206, 1983

Spaulding SW, Noth RH: Thyroid-catecholamine interactions. Med Clin North Am 59, No 5:1123, 1975

Strakosch C, Wenzel B, Row VV et al: Immunology of auto-immune thyroid disease. N Engl J Med 307:1499, 1983

Utiger RD: Beta-adrenergic-antagonist therapy for hyperthyroid Graves' disease. N Engl J Med 310:1597, 1984

Verebey K, Volavka J, Clouet D: Endorphins in psychiatry: An overview and a hypothesis. Arch Gen Psychiatry 35:877, 1978

Vope R: Thyroiditis: Current views of pathogenesis. Med Clin North Am 59, No 5:1163, 1975

Wake MM, Brensinger JF: The nurse's role in hypothyroidism. Nurs Clin North Am 15, No 3:453, 1980

Chapter 40

Diabetes Mellitus

Linda S. Hurwitz

Carol Mattson Porth

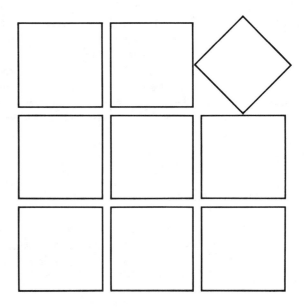

Diabetes mellitus is a chronic alteration in health that currently affects more than 12 million persons in the United States. Each year the incidence of diabetes increases by 6%; this is evidenced by the fact that 600,000 Americans are diagnosed annually as having the disease. If the present trend continues, the number of persons with diabetes in the United States can be expected to double every 15 years. This means that every baby born today has a one-in-five chance of developing diabetes in its lifetime.[1]

Diabetes affects persons in all age groups and from all walks of life. Among both young and old, diabetes increases the risk of vascular problems, blindness, peripheral neuropathies, and kidney disease. Diabetes increases the risk of maternal complications during pregnancy, and infants of diabetic mothers have a greater than normal incidence of congenital anomalies; they are also more prone to develop neonatal complications, such as respiratory distress syndrome and hypoglycemia.

The term diabetes mellitus means "the running through of sugar." In spite of its recent increase, the disease did not originate in the twentieth century. Reports of the disorder can be traced back to the first century A.D. when Aretaeus the Cappadocian described the disorder as a chronic affection that was characterized by intense thirst and voluminous honey-sweet urine— "the melting down of flesh into urine."[2] It was the discovery of insulin by Banting and Best in 1921 that transformed the once-fatal disease into a chronic health problem.

Diabetes can be defined as a disorder of carbohydrate, protein, and fat metabolism resulting from an imbalance between insulin availability and insulin need. It can represent an absolute insulin deficiency, a condition in which insulin production is insufficient because of decreased tissue sensitivity, or a condition in which the insulin that is produced is not active or is destroyed before it can carry out its action. The person with uncontrolled diabetes is unable to transport glucose into fat and muscle cells, and as a result breakdown of fat and protein is increased. Diabetes is accompanied by a predisposition to vascular changes in the vessels of both the microcirculation and the macrocirculation. Some believe that the vascular disorders are a complication of diabetes, and others believe that diabetes is an accompaniment of vascular disorders.

■ Types of Diabetes

Although diabetes mellitus is clearly a disorder of insulin availability, it is probably not a single disease. A classification system that divides diabetes into *insulin-dependent* and *noninsulin-dependent* forms was developed by an international workshop sponsored by the National Diabetes Data Group of NIH (Table 40-1).[3] The system has been endorsed by the American Diabetes Association. The group also proposed a classification of *gestational diabetes* (diabetes that develops during pregnancy), *impaired glucose tolerance* (abnormal glucose tolerance test without other signs of diabetes), and *diabetes caused by other conditions* (*e.g.*, Cushing's disease).

Type I Insulin-Dependent Diabetes Mellitus (IDDM)

Insulin-dependent diabetes is characterized by an absolute insulin deficiency state. This form of diabetes was formerly called juvenile diabetes, but the term has proved to be inaccurate because it can occur at any age. Persons with IDDM often experience marked alterations in blood sugar and are frequently referred to as "brittle diabetics." Because of their absolute lack of insulin, persons with this form of diabetes are particularly prone to develop ketoacidosis.

Type II Noninsulin-Dependent Diabetes Mellitus (NIDDM)

This form of diabetes has been called maturity-onset diabetes and is associated with a lack of insulin availability or effectiveness rather than an absolute insulin deficiency. This relative insulin deficiency has been reported to arise because (1) inadequate amounts of insulin are produced in relation to need, (2) insulin is destroyed before it can exert its effect, (3) insulin release is out of phase with food intake and blood sugar levels, or (4) the number of insulin receptors on the cells decreases. Individuals with NIDDM are usually older and frequently overweight and have fewer problems with control than juvenile-onset diabetics. Often this form of diabetes can be controlled by diet alone. Noninsulin-dependent diabetes is said to be ketosis resistant, meaning that persons with this form of diabetes do not readily develop ketoacidosis. Evidence suggests that more insulin is needed to transport glucose into fat cells than is required to prevent lipolysis (fat breakdown) and the release of fatty acids. It is these fatty acids that are converted to ketone bodies by the liver during ketoacidosis. In NIDDM insulin is usually sufficient to prevent lipolysis and the development of ketosis but not to lower blood sugar by effecting the transport of excess glucose into fat cells.

Other Types

In other types of diabetes, formerly known as secondary diabetes, the relationship between the etiologic agent and glucose intolerance is known. Diabetes can occur

Table 40-1 Classification of Diabetes and Glucose Intolerance States

Classification	Former Terminology	Characteristics
Diabetes Mellitus (DM)		
Type I		
Insulin-dependent diabetes mellitus (IDDM)	Juvenile-onset diabetes	Persons in this subclass are dependent upon injected insulin Ketosis prone
Type II		

Noninsulin-dependent diabetes mellitus (NIDDM)
    1. Nonobese NIDDM
    2. Obese NIDDM (60%–90%)
	Adult-onset, maturity-onset diabetes	Persons in this subclass are not insulin dependent, but they may use insulin
		Not ketosis prone
		Frequently obese

Other Types		
Pancreatic disease	Secondary diabetes	Presence of diabetes and associated condition

Hormonal
  Drug- or chemical-induced insulin receptor abnormalities
  Certain genetic defects
  Other types		

Impaired Glucose Tolerance (IGT)		
Nonobese IGT	Asymptomatic, chemical, subclinical, borderline, latent diabetes	Based on nondiagnostic fasting glucose levels and glucose tolerance test between normal and diabetic
Obese IGT IGT associated with other conditions, including (1) pancreatic disease, (2) hormonal, (3) drug or chemical, (4) insulin-receptor abnormalities, or (5) genetic syndromes		
Gestational Diabetes Mellitus (GDM)	Gestational diabetes	Glucose intolerance that developed during pregnancy Increased risk of perinatal complications Increased risk of developing diabetes within 5 to 10 years after parturition

(Adapted from National Diabetes Data Group: Classification and diagnosis of diabetes mellitus and other categories of glucose intolerance. Diabetes 28:1042, 1979. Reprinted with permission of the American Diabetic Association.)

secondary to pancreatic disease or the removal of pancreatic tissue; endocrine diseases, such as acromegaly, Cushing's syndrome, or pheochromocytoma. Endocrine disorders that produce hyperglycemia do so by either increasing the hepatic production of glucose or decreasing the cellular utilization of glucose.

Several diuretics—thiazides, furosemide, and ethycrynic acid—tend to elevate blood sugar. These diuretics increase potassium loss, which is thought to impair insulin release. Other drugs known to cause hyperglycemia include the following: diazoxide, glucocorticoids, levodopa, oral contraceptives, sympathomimetics, phenothiazines, phenytoin, and total parenteral nutrition (hyperalimentation). Drug-related increases in blood sugar are usually reversed once the drug has been discontinued.

Impaired glucose tolerance

The diagnosis *impaired glucose tolerance* describes an individual with plasma glucose levels between those considered normal and those considered diabetic. Calorie restriction and weight reduction are important for overweight individuals in this class.

Gestational diabetes

Gestational diabetes refers to glucose intolerance that occurs during pregnancy. Indications for the use of glucose tolerance tests during pregnancy are a family history of diabetes, glycosuria, a history of stillbirth or spontaneous abortion, the presence of fetal anomalies in previous pregnancy, a previous large or heavy-for-date baby, obesity in the mother, advanced maternal age, or five or more pregnancies. The presence of more than one of these risk factors is particularly indicative of increased risk. Diagnosis and careful medical management are essential because these women are at higher risk for complications of pregnancy, fetal abnormalities and mortality, and the development of diabetes 5 to 10 years after delivery. After pregnancy, the woman must be reclassified as either a person with diabetes mellitus or one with impaired glucose tolerance. In most women, glucose tolerance returns to normal, and a classification of previously abnormal glucose tolerance is made.[3]

Etiology

Because diabetes is apparently not a single disorder, it probably does not have a single cause. A number of etiologic factors, including inheritance, have been implicated in the development of diabetes. Inheritance is thought to be autosomal recessive, with variable penetrance of the genes that determine the expression of diabetes. Studies suggest that heredity plays a greater role in the development of NIDDM than it does in the development of IDDM.[4,5] Of particular interest is a new approach to the study of genetics that uses antigens detected on the cell surface of nucleated cells—histocompatibility antigens (HLA antigens, Chap. 9). Insulin-dependent diabetes is associated with an increased or decreased frequency of certain HLA types.

Although their role is not clearly understood, viruses and beta-cell toxins have also been suspected as causative factors in diabetes. The onset of insulin-dependent diabetes has been observed to rise in later summer and winter; this corresponds with the prevalence of common viral infections in the community.[6,7] Mumps,[8] Coxsackievirus-group B, type A,[9] and congenital rubella[10,11] have been associated with the development of insulin-dependent diabetes.

Fortunately, not all predisposed individuals—those with a family history of diabetes or known exposure to beta toxic agents—develop diabetes. This suggests that other environmental or risk factors contribute to the development of clinical diabetes. A significant risk factor for the development of diabetes in predisposed individuals is obesity. Most individuals with NIDDM (80%) are overweight.[12] Obese individuals have been shown to have increased resistance to the action of insulin and impaired suppression of glucose production by the liver, resulting in both hyperglycemia and hyperinsulinemia (Fig. 40-1). The increased insulin resistance has been attributed to either a decreased number of insulin receptors in the peripheral tissues or the impairment of insulin receptor function. Insulin resistance usually decreases with weight loss, to the extent than many obese individuals with NIDDM can be managed with a weight reduction diet and exercise.

In summary, diabetes mellitus is a disorder of carbohydrate, protein, and fat metabolism resulting from an imbalance between insulin availability and insulin need. The disease can be classified as insulin-dependent diabetes mellitus (IDDM), in which there is an absolute insulin deficiency, or noninsulin-dependent diabetes mellitus (NIDDM), in which there is a lack of insulin availability or effectiveness. At present the etiology of IDDM and NIDDM is unknown. Other types of diabetes include secondary forms of carbohydrate intolerance which occur secondary to some other condition, such as pancreatic disorders, which destroy beta cells, or endocrine diseases such as Cushing's disease, which causes increased production of glucose by the liver and decreased utilization of glucose by the tissues. Gestational diabetes develops during pregnancy, and although glucose tolerance often returns to normal after childbirth, it indicates increased risk of developing diabetes.

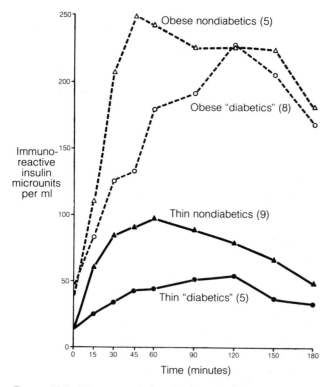

Figure 40-1 *The mean absolute insulin responses in thin and obese diabetic subjects during a 3-hour (100-G) oral glucose tolerance curve. (From Bagdade JD, Biermann EL, Porter D: The significance of basal insulin levels in evaluation of the insulin response to glucose in diabetic and nondiabetic subjects. J Clin Invest 46, No 10:1553, 1967)*

■ Manifestations

Diabetes mellitus may have a rapid or insidious onset. In IDDM, signs and symptoms are often acute and of sudden origin. On the other hand, NIDDM often develops more insidiously; its presence may be detected during a routine medical examination or when a patient seeks medical care for other reasons.

The most commonly identified signs and symptoms of diabetes are those which are often referred to as the three "polys"—*polyuria* (excessive urination), *polydipsia* (excessive thirst), and *polyphagia* (excessive hunger). These three symptoms are closely related to the hyperglycemia (elevated blood sugar) and glycosuria (sugar in the urine) that are present in diabetes. Glucose is a small, osmotically active molecule. When blood sugar is sufficiently elevated, the amount of glucose that is filtered by the glomeruli of the kidney will exceed the amount that can be reabsorbed by the renal tubules; this results in *glycosuria* and large accompanying losses of water in the urine. Thirst results from intracellular dehydration that occurs as blood-sugar levels rise and water is pulled out of body cells, including those in the thirst center. Cellular dehydration also causes dryness of the mouth. This early symptom may be easily overlooked in NIDDM, in which there is a gradual increase in blood sugar without accompanying signs of ketoacidosis. Polyphagia is usually not present in persons with NIDDM. In IDDM, it probably results from cellular starvation and the depletion of cellular stores of carbohydrates, fats, and proteins.

Weight loss is a common occurrence in the person with uncontrolled insulin-dependent diabetes. The cause of weight loss is twofold. First, loss of body fluids results from osmotic diuresis. Vomiting may exaggerate the fluid loss in ketoacidosis. Second, body tissue is lost as the lack of insulin forces the body to use its fat stores and cellular proteins as sources of energy. In terms of weight loss, there is often a marked difference between NIDDM and IDDM. Weight loss is an almost universal phenomenon in the person with uncontrolled insulin-dependent diabetes, whereas the individual with uncomplicated NIDDM often has problems with obesity.

There are other signs and symptoms related to hyperglycemia, including recurrent blurring of vision, fatigue, paresthesias, and increased incidence of yeast infections. In NIDDM, these are often the symptoms that prompt an individual to seek medical attention. Blurred vision occurs at a time when blood sugar levels are being brought under control. This is because water is lost from the lens of the eye during the period of poor control; then, as blood sugar decreases with treatment, water moves back into the lens, making it difficult to focus. Both hyperglycemia and glycosuria favor the growth of yeast organisms. Pruritus and vulvovaginitis resulting from candidal infections are common initial complaints in women with NIDDM.

Acute Complications

The three major acute complications of diabetes are hypoglycemia, ketoacidosis, and hyperosmolar coma. It is important for the reader to recognize that *the body responds to acute changes in physiologic functioning with a series of predictable compensatory responses.* The acute complications of diabetes are no exception.

Hypoglycemia

Hypoglycemia, or an insulin reaction, usually occurs in insulin-treated diabetics. It occurs when blood sugar falls below 50 mg per 100 ml of blood and is characterized by sudden onset and rapid progression (see Table 40-2). The signs and symptoms of hypoglycemia can be divided into two categories, those caused by *altered cerebral function* and those related to *activation of the autonomic nervous system.* Because the brain relies on blood glucose as its main energy source, hypoglycemia causes behaviors related to altered cerebral function. Headache, difficulty in problem solving, disturbed or altered behavior, coma, and convulsions are common. At the onset of the hypoglycemic episode, activation of the *parasympathetic nervous system* causes hunger. The initial parasympathetic response is followed by activation of the *sympathetic nervous system;* this causes anxiety, sweating, and constriction of the skin vessels (the skin is cool and clammy). Although individuals respond differently in insulin reaction, each person usually has the same pattern of response during each insulin reaction. For this reason, it

Table 40-2 Signs and Symptoms of Insulin Reaction*

Onset—sudden
Laboratory findings
  Blood sugar less than 50 mg/100 ml
Impaired cerebral function (due to decreased glucose availability for brain metabolism)
  Feeling of vagueness
  Headache
  Difficulty in problem solving
  Slurred speech
  Impaired motor function
  Change in emotional behavior
  Convulsions
  Coma
Compensatory autonomic nervous system responses
  Parasympathetic responses
    Hunger
    Nausea
    Hypotension
    Bradycardia
  Sympathetic responses
    Anxiety
    Sweating
    Vasoconstriction of skin vessels (skin is pale and cool)
    Tachycardia

*There is a wide variation in manifestation of signs and symptoms among individuals, that is, not every person with diabetes will have all or even most of the symptoms.

is helpful if this response pattern can be identified during the early stages of treatment in the person with insulin-dependent diabetes.

The signs and symptoms of hypoglycemia are more variable in children and in the elderly. Elderly persons may not display the typical autonomic responses that are associated with hypoglycemia but frequently develop signs of impaired function of the central nervous system, including mental confusion and bizarre behavior.

Many factors tend to precipitate insulin reaction in the person with insulin-dependent diabetes: error in insulin dose, failure to eat, increased exercise, decreased insulin needs following removal of a stress situation, change in insulin site. Alcohol tends to decrease liver gluconeogenesis, and the person with diabetes needs to be cautioned about its potential for causing hypoglycemia, especially if it is consumed in large amounts or on an empty stomach.

The most effective treatment of an insulin reaction is the immediate ingestion of a concentrated carbohydrate source, such as sugar, honey, candy, or orange juice. Alternative methods for elevating blood sugar may be required when the diabetic is unconscious or unable to swallow. Glucagon may be given intravenously, intramuscularly, or subcutaneously. The liver contains only a limited amount of glycogen (about 75 gm); glucagon will be ineffective in persons whose glycogen stores have been depleted. A small amount of honey or glucose gel available in most pharmacies can be inserted into the buccal pouch (under the tongue) in situations in which swallowing is impaired. Monosaccharides such as glucose or fructose, which can be absorbed directly into the bloodstream, work best for this purpose. In situations of severe, life-threatening hypoglycemia, it may be necessary to administer glucose (20–50 ml of a 50% solution) intravenously. It is important not to overtreat hypoglycemia so as to cause hyperglycemia. Usually treatment consists of an initial administration of about 10 gm glucose, which can be repeated as necessary. Complex carbohydrates may be administered once the acute reaction has been controlled (see Diabetic Diet section).

Diabetic ketoacidosis

Ketoacidosis occurs when ketone production by the liver exceeds cellular utilization and renal excretion. In the person with insulin-dependent diabetes, lack of insulin leads to the mobilization of fatty acids and a subsequent increase in ketone production.

Compared with an insulin reaction, diabetic ketoacidosis is usually slower in onset, and recovery is more prolonged. Blood sugar levels are elevated and urine sugar is greater than 2%. Plasma pH and bicarbonate are decreased, and urine tests for acetone (Acetest or Ketostix) are positive. The signs and symptoms of ketoacidosis are summarized in Table 40-3.

There are two major metabolic derangements in diabetic ketoacidosis, *hyperglycemia* and *metabolic acidosis*. The hyperglycemia leads to osmotic diuresis, dehydration, and a critical loss of electrolytes. The metabolic acidosis is caused by the excess ketoacids that require buffering by the bicarbonate ion; this leads to a marked decrease in serum bicarbonate levels. The breath has a characteristic fruity smell because of the presence of the volatile ketoacids. A number of signs and symptoms that occur in diabetic ketoacidosis are related to compensatory mechanisms. The heart rate increases as the body compensates for a decrease in blood volume, and the rate and depth of respiration increase (Kussmaul breathing) as the body attempts to prevent further decreases in pH. Metabolic acidosis and its treatment are discussed in Chapter 27.

Diabetic ketoacidosis is seen most frequently in the insulin-dependent diabetic. It can occur at the onset of the disease, often before the disease has been diagnosed. For example, a mother may bring a child into the hospital with reports of lethargy, vomiting, and abdominal pain, unaware that the child has diabetes. Stress tends to increase the release of gluconeogenic hormones and predisposes the person to the development of ketoacidosis. Consequently, the development of ketoacidosis is often preceded by physical or emotional stress, for example, infection, pregnancy, or extreme anxiety.

The treatment of diabetic ketoacidosis focuses on correcting the fluid and electrolyte imbalances and

---

Table 40-3 Signs and Symptoms of Diabetic Ketoacidosis

Onset—(1–24 hours)

Laboratory findings
  Blood sugar greater than 250 mg/100 ml
  Urine sugar greater than 2%
  Ketonemia and presence of ketones in the urine
  Decreased plasma pH (less than 7.3) and
    bicarbonate (less than 24 mEq)

Dehydration due to hyperglycemia
  Warm, dry skin
  Dry mucous membranes
  Tachycardia
  Weak, thready pulse
  Acute weight loss
  Hypotension

Ketoacidosis
  Anorexia, nausea, and vomiting
  Odor of ketones on the breath
  Depression of the central nervous system
    Lethargy and fatigue
    Stupor
    Coma
  Abdominal pain

Compensatory responses
  Rapid, deep respirations (Kussmaul breathing)

returning blood *p*H to normal. Usually this is accomplished through the administration of insulin and intravenous fluid and electrolyte replacement solutions. Because insulin resistance accompanies severe acidosis, the current practice is to use smaller doses of insulin (added to the intravenous solution) than were used in the past. Frequent monitoring of laboratory tests of serum electrolytes is used as a guide for fluid and electrolyte replacement. The identification and treatment of the underlying cause, for example, infection, are also important.

Hyperosmolar coma

Hyperosmolar, hyperglycemic nonketotic coma (HHNK) is characterized by plasma osmolarity of 350 mOsm/liter or more, blood sugar in excess of 600 mg per 100 ml of blood, the absence of ketoacidosis, and depression of the sensorium.[13]

Hyperosmolar coma may occur in a variety of conditions, including NIDDM, acute pancreatitis, severe infections, myocardial infarction, hyperthyroidism, and treatment with oral or parenteral hyperalimentation solutions. Two factors appear to contribute to the hyperglycemia that precipitates the condition: an increased resistance to the effects of insulin and an excessive carbohydrate intake.

In hyperosmolar states, the increased serum osmolarity has the effect of pulling water out of body cells, including brain cells. The most prominent manifestations are dehydration, neurologic signs and symptoms, polyuria, and thirst (Table 40-4). One patient is reported to have consumed 9 quarts of skim milk in a single day. The neurologic signs include grand mal seizures, hemiparesis, Babinski reflexes, aphasia, muscle fasciculations, hyperthermia, hemianopia, nystagmus, visual hallucina-

tions, and others.[14] Blood glucose levels of 4800 mg per 100 ml of blood have been reported. The onset of hyperosmolar coma is often insidious; and because it occurs most frequently in older individuals, it may be mistaken for a stroke.

Treatment of hyperosmolar coma requires judicious medical observation and care. This is because water moves back into brain cells during treatment, posing a threat of cerebral edema. Extensive potassium losses that have also occurred during the diuretic phase of the disorder require correction. Because of the problems encountered in the treatment and the serious nature of the disease conditions that cause hyperosmolar coma, the prognosis for this disorder is less favorable than that for ketoacidosis; the mortality rate has been reported to be 40% to 70%.[14]

Somogyi phenomenon

The Somogyi phenomenon describes a cycle of insulin-induced posthypoglycemic episodes. In 1924, Joslin and his associates noted that hypoglycemia was associated with alternate episodes of hyperglycemia.[15] It was not until 1959, however, that Somogyi presented the results of his 20 years of studies, which confirmed the observation that "hypoglycemia begets hyperglycemia."[16] In a diabetic with the Somogyi mechanisms designed to elevate blood sugar, there is an increase in blood levels of catecholamines, glucagon, cortisol, and growth hormone. These hormones, sometimes called *counter-regulatory hormones,* cause blood sugar to become elevated and produce some degree of insulin resistance. A vicious circle begins when the increase in blood sugar and insulin resistance are treated with larger insulin doses. Often the hypoglycemic episode occurs during the night or at a time when it is not recognized, rendering the diagnosis of the phenomenon more difficult. Figure 40-2 illustrates the events that occur with the Somogyi phenomenon.

Recent research suggests that even rather mild insulin-associated hypoglycemia, which may be

---

Table 40-4 Signs and Symptoms of Hyperosmolar Coma

Onset—insidious; 24 hours to 2 weeks
Laboratory findings
    Blood sugar greater than 600 mg/100 ml
    Serum osmolarity 350 mOsm/liter or greater
Severe dehydration
    Dry skin and mucous membranes
    Extreme thirst
Neurologic manifestations
    Depressed sensorium
        lethargy to coma
    Neurologic deficits
        positive Babinski sign
        paresis or paralysis
        sensory impairment
        hyperthermia
        hemianopia
Seizures

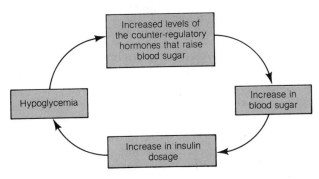

Figure 40-2 *The cycle of events that occur with the Somogyi phenomenon.*

asymptomatic, can cause hyperglycemia in IDDM through the recruitment of counterregulatory mechanisms, although the insulin action does not wane. A concomitant waning of the effect of insulin (end of the duration of action), when it occurs, exacerbates posthypoglycemic hyperglycemia and accelerates its development. It was suggested that these research findings may explain the brittleness of the disease in some persons with diabetes. Measures to prevent hypoglycemia and the subsequent activation of counterregulatory mechanisms include a redistribution of dietary carbohydrates and an alteration in insulin dose or method of administration.[17]

Chronic Complications

The chronic complications of diabetes include neuropathies, nephropathies, and other vascular lesions. Interestingly, these disorders occur in the insulin-independent tissues of the body—those tissues that do not require insulin for glucose entry into the cell. This probably means that intracellular glucose concentrations in these tissues approach or equal those in the blood.

Theories of pathogenesis
The interest among researchers in explaining the causes and development of chronic lesions in the person with diabetes has led to a number of theories. Several of these theories have been summarized to prepare the reader for understanding specific chronic complications.

Polyol pathway. A polyol is an organic compound that contains three or more hydroxyl groups. The polyol pathway refers to the intracellular enzymes and mechanisms responsible for changing the number of hydroxyl units on a sugar. In the sorbitol pathway, glucose is transformed to sorbitol, and sorbitol is then converted to fructose. The rate at which sorbitol can be converted to fructose and then metabolized is limited. Sorbitol is osmotically active, and it has been hypothesized that the presence of excess amounts may alter cell function in those tissues that use this pathway.

Formation of abnormal glycoproteins. Glycoproteins, or what might be termed sugar proteins, are normal components of the basement membrane in smaller blood vessels and capillaries. It has been suggested that the increased intracellular concentration of glucose associated with diabetes favors the formation of abnormal glycoproteins. These abnormal glycoproteins are thought to produce structural defects in the basement membrane of these vessels.

Problems with tissue oxygenation. Proponents of the tissue oxygenation theories suggest that many of the chronic complications of diabetes arise because of a decrease in oxygen delivery in the small vessels of the microcirculation. Among the factors believed to contribute to this inadequate oxygen delivery is a defect in red cell function that interferes with the release of oxygen from the hemoglobin molecule. In support of this theory is the finding of a twofold to threefold increase in glycosylated hemoglobin (HbA_{1a} + HbA_{1b} + HbA_{1c}) in persons with diabetes. In glycosylated hemoglobin, a glycoprotein is substituted for valine in the beta chain, causing a high affinity for oxygen.[18] There is a reported decline in red cell 2,3-diphosphoglycerate (2,3-DPG) during the acidotic and recovery phases of diabetic ketoacidosis. The glycolytic intermediate 2,3-DPG reduces the hemoglobin affinity for oxygen. Both an increase in glycosylated hemoglobin and a decrease in 2,3-DPG tend to increase the hemoglobin's affinity for oxygen, and less oxygen is released for tissue use.

Peripheral neuropathies
Although the incidence of peripheral neuropathies is known to be high among people with diabetes, it is difficult to document exactly how many individuals are affected by these disorders. This is because of the diversity in clinical manifestations and because the condition is often far advanced before it is recognized.

Two types of pathologic changes have been observed in connection with diabetic peripheral neuropathies. The first is a thickening of the walls of the nutrient vessels that supply the nerve, leading to the assumption that vessel ischemia plays a major role in the development of these neural changes. The second and more recent finding has been a segmental demyelinization process that affects the Schwann cell. This demyelinization process is accompanied by a slowing of nerve conduction. Recent research on the sorbitol pathway suggests that the formation and accumulation of sorbitol within nerve cells may lead to injury and impair nerve conduction.

It now appears that the diabetic peripheral neuropathies are not a single entity. The clinical manifestations of these disorders vary with the location of the lesion(s). Although there are several methods for classifying the diabetic peripheral neuropathies, a simplified system divides them into somatic and autonomic disturbances (Table 40-5).

In addition to the actual discomforts associated with the loss of sensory or motor function, lesions in either the somatic or peripheral nervous system predispose the person with diabetes to additional complications. Loss of feeling, touch, and position sense increases the risk of falling. Impairment of temperature and pain

Table 40-5   Classification of Diabetic Peripheral Neuropathies

Somatic
　Polyneuropathies, bilateral sensory
　　Paresthesias, including numbness and tingling
　　Impaired pain, temperature, light touch, two-point
　　　discrimination, and vibratory sensation
　　Decreased ankle and knee-jerk reflexes
　Mononeuropathies
　　Involvement of a mixed nerve trunk that includes loss of
　　　sensation, pain, and motor weakness
　Amyotrophia
　Associated with muscle weakness, wasting, and severe pain of
　　muscles in the pelvic girdle and thigh
Autonomic
　Impaired vasomotor function
　　Postural hypotension
　Impaired gastrointestinal function
　　Gastric atony
　　Diarrhea, often postprandial and nocturnal
　Impaired genitourinary function
　　Paralytic bladder
　　Incomplete voiding
　　Impotence
　　Retrograde ejaculation
　Cranial nerve involvement
　　Extraocular nerve paralysis
　　Impaired pupillary responses
　　Impaired special senses

sensation increases the risk of serious burns and injuries to the feet. Defects in vasomotor reflexes can lead to dizziness and syncope when the person moves from the supine to the standing position. Incomplete emptying of the bladder due to vesicle dysfunction predispose the person to urinary stasis and bladder infection and increases the risk of renal complications (see Chap. 31).

Nephropathies

The person with diabetes is predisposed to several types of renal disease, including pyelonephritis and nephropathies. Pyelonephritis occurs in the nondiabetic person as well as in the diabetic (discussed in Chap. 29). Nephropathies refer to chronic renal vascular complications and are a common cause of death in long-term diabetic patients.

The basement membrane of the glomerulus is composed of complex glycoproteins. It has been suggested that the increased intracellular concentration of glucose in the person with diabetes contributes to the formation of abnormal glycoproteins and glycoprotein linkage in the basement membrane of the glomerulus. Kimmelstiel–Wilson's disease is a form of glomerulosclerosis that involves the development of nodular lesions in the glomerular capillary of the kidney. The accompanying arteriolar lesions impair blood flow. There is a pro-

gressive loss of kidney function and eventual renal failure. Kimmelstiel–Wilson lesions are thought to occur only in people with diabetes. Diffuse glomerulosclerosis, which is a linear thickening of the glomerular membrane, is found in both diabetics and nondiabetics. Changes in the basement membrane in Kimmelstiel–Wilson's disease and diffuse glomerulosclerosis allow plasma proteins to escape in the urine, causing proteinuria, the development of hypoproteinemia (decreased levels of plasma proteins), and edema.

Retinopathies

Diabetes is the leading cause of acquired blindness in the United States. Although the person with diabetes is at increased risk for developing cataracts and glaucoma, retinopathy is the most common pattern of disease in the eye. It has been estimated that 20% to 50% of persons with diabetes may have retinopathy, and 10% of those may be at risk for visual loss.[19]

There are two types of diabetic retinopathy: (1) background, or nonproliferative, retinopathy and (2) proliferative retinopathy (Fig. 40-3). Nonproliferative, or background, retinopathy is characterized by microaneurysms, or fusiform outpouchings, that protrude from one side of the capillary. These microaneurysms form weakened spots in the capillary wall that tend to leak fluid or to rupture, giving rise to retinal edema and hemorrhage. Hard waxy exudates form as pockets of protein, and lipids leak through the wall of the weakened capillary. Usually old hemorrhages and exudate are constantly reabsorbed as new hemorrhages are formed. The retinopathies are discussed further in Chapter 46.

Proliferative retinopathy differs from background retinopathy in that new blood vessels (neovascularization) develop on the surface of the retina and extend into the area between the retina and vitreous. These new vessels, like the background microaneurysms, are very fragile and tend to rupture easily. When hemorrhage occurs, blood from these lesions flows into the vitreous, obstructing the flow of light from the lens to the retina. As the condition progresses, scar tissue and adhesions develop between the vitreous and the retina. When the scar tissue contracts, it can cause vitreous hemorrhage or retinal detachment.

The retinal vessels can be viewed by means of an ophthalmoscope. This allows for early diagnosis and follow-up observation of retinal lesions. The intravenous injection of fluorescein dye provides a method for outlining the retinal vasculature and detecting sites of obstruction and leakage. Normally, the retinal capillary endothelial cells are tightly joined, so that the dye does not escape into the vitreous.

Methods used in the treatment of diabetic retinopathy include the destruction and scarring of the pro-

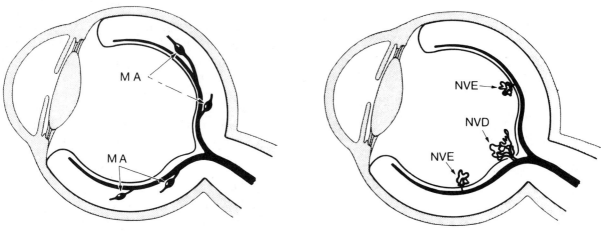

Figure 40-3 *Proliferative and nonproliferative lesions in retinopathy of the person with diabetes.* Background retinopathy: *In background diabetic retinopathy, the blood vessel changes are contained within the retina. The microaneurysms (MA) are shown schematically within the substance of the retina.* Proliferative retinopathy: *In proliferative diabetic retinopathy, new vessel formation breaks through the surface of the retina to grow into the vitreous cavity. When the vessels are near the optic nerve or disk area, they are termed neovascularization of the disk (NVD); when the new vessel formation occurs elsewhere in the retina away from the disk, it is referred to as neovascularization elsewhere (NVE). (Copyright 1978 by the American Diabetes Association, Inc. Reprinted from Diabetes Forecast by permission.)*

liferative lesions with photocoagulation. The diabetic retinopathy study demonstrated that panretinal photocoagulation may delay or prevent visual loss in more than 50% of eyes with proliferative retinopathy.[20] Removal and replacement of the vitreous with a clear replacement solution (vitrectomy) may be used in those situations in which vitreal hemorrhage has caused blindness.

Vascular complications

There is little doubt that diabetes contributes to disease of both the microcirculation and the macrocirculation. Diabetic involvement of the small vessels in the retina is an example of disease of the microcirculation. It is also known that people with diabetes are at risk for developing lesions of vessels in the macrocirculation, including the coronaries, cerebral vessels, and peripheral arteries.

Studies suggest that diabetes is an important risk factor in the development of heart disease, including coronary artery disease, and other forms of myocardial dysfunction.[21] Autonomic innervation of the heart may also become impaired in the person with diabetes. With impaired autonomic function, the heart rate response to many stresses is lessened.

Vascular disorders also affect the cerebral circulation. Evidence suggests that cerebral artery atherosclerosis develops earlier and is more extensive in people with diabetes than in nondiabetic persons.

The effects of the disease on vessels in the lower extremities is evidenced by an increased frequency of peripheral vascular insufficiency and intermittent claudication in people with diabetes compared with nondiabetic persons. Impairment of the peripheral vascular circulation may become severe enough to cause ulceration, infection, and eventually gangrene of the feet. The need to amputate portions of the lower extremities because of complications arising from severe peripheral vascular disease is a threat to many older persons with diabetes.

There is much controversy about the cause(s) of vascular pathology in diabetes. Among the factors that are thought to contribute to the increased prevalence of atherosclerosis in people with diabetes are hypertension, hyperlipidemia, increased platelet adhesiveness, other alterations in blood coagulation factors, and accumulation of sorbitol within the walls of the larger vessels.

Infections

Although not specifically either an acute or a chronic complication, infections are common concerns of the person with diabetes. Certain types of infections occur with increased frequency in persons with diabetes: soft tissue infections of the extremities, osteomyelitis, urinary tract infections and pyelonephritis, candidal infections of skin and mucous surfaces, and tuberculosis. At present, there is a question whether or not the problem seems more prevalent because the infections are more serious in people with diabetes.

There are several known causes for the suboptimal response to infection in the person with diabetes. One is the presence of chronic complications, such as vascular disease and neuropathies; the other is the presence of hyperglycemia and altered neutrophil function. Sensory deficits may cause the person with diabetes to ignore minor trauma and infection, and vascular disease may impair circulation and delivery of blood cells and other substances needed to produce an adequate inflammatory response and effect healing. Pyelonephritis and urinary tract infections are relatively common in the person with diabetes, and it has been suggested that these infections may bear some relationship to the presence of a neurogenic bladder or nephrosclerotic changes in the kidney. Hyperglycemia and glycosuria may influence the growth of microorganisms and increase the severity of the infection. Recently, it has been shown that chemotaxis and phagocytosis are impaired in neutrophils that have been exposed to increased concentrations of glucose.

In summary, diabetes mellitus is a chronic disease characterized by a state of insulin deficiency. This insulin deficiency can be absolute, as in insulin-dependent diabetes mellitus, or it can be relative, as in noninsulin-dependent diabetes. The metabolic disturbances that are associated with diabetes affect almost every system in the body. The acute complications include diabetic ketoacidosis, hypoglycemia, and, in the person with noninsulin-dependent diabetes, nonketotic hyperosmolar coma. The chronic complications of diabetes affect the noninsulin-dependent tissues, including the retina, blood vessels, kidney, and peripheral nervous system.

■ Diagnosis and Management

There are various tests that measure blood and urine glucose levels. These tests are used to screen for diabetes and to follow the progress of persons with known diabetes. Tests that measure insulin levels usually involve the use of radioimmunoassay techniques. The treatment plan for diabetes usually involves diet, hypoglycemic agents, and exercise. Weight loss and dietary management may be sufficient to control blood sugar levels in persons with NIDDM. The continuous insulin pump has provided an alternative method for insulin administration, and beta-cell transplants are being studied as a possible future treatment for diabetes.

✓ *Blood Tests*

Glucose tolerance test

The glucose tolerance test is an important screening test for diabetes. The test measures the body's ability to store glucose by removing it from the blood. Using blood sugar levels, the test measures the response to a given amount of concentrated glucose at selected intervals, usually ½, 1, 1½, 2, and 3 hours (urine glucose is also measured at these times). Insulin levels may also be measured at these intervals. In the normal individual, blood sugars will return to normal within 3 hours after ingestion of a glucose load, in which case it can be assumed that sufficient insulin is present to allow glucose to leave the blood and enter body cells. Because the person with diabetes lacks the ability to respond to an increase in blood glucose by releasing adequate insulin to facilitate storage, blood sugar levels not only rise above those observed in normal individuals but remain elevated for longer periods of time (Fig. 40-4). The glucose tolerance test is a useful diagnostic measure for detecting subclinical forms of diabetes—the stage of the disease in which the fasting blood sugar may still be normal and other obvious signs of diabetes are not yet detectable. A variation of the glucose tolerance test is the cortisone glucose tolerance test. The administration of cortisone challenges the body's ability to metabolize glucose. Another form of the glucose tolerance test is used for screening purposes; this form of the test involves sampling blood sugar 2 hours following a glucose challenge.

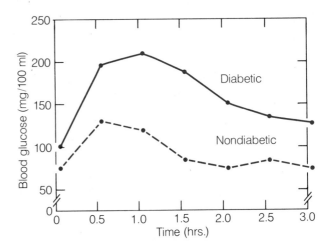

Figure 40-4 *Results of a glucose tolerance test for diabetics and nondiabetics. Blood samples are usually taken at half-hour intervals following ingestion of a glucose solution containing 1.75 g of glucose per kilogram of body weight. The test may be modified for use as a screening tool.*

Fasting blood sugar test

Fasting blood sugars measure blood sugar levels after food has been withheld for a period of 8 to 12 hours.

Capillary blood tests and self blood glucose monitoring

Technologic advances have provided the means for self blood glucose determination using a drop of capillary blood. This method has not only provided health professionals with a rapid and economical method for monitoring blood glucose but has given people with diabetes a means of maintaining near-normal blood glucose levels through self glucose monitoring techniques.[22] These methods use a drop of capillary blood obtained by pricking the finger with a special needle or small lancet. The drop of blood is placed on a reagent strip, and glucose levels are determined. New lancet types (*e.g.,* Autolet with a Monolet lancet) have made the technique virtually painless.

Several methods of self glucose monitoring are available, and new products are continually being developed. There are currently two types of reagent strip methods: a wash test and a dry test. Wash tests, such as Dextrostix and Visidex I, utilize a drop of blood on the reagent strip that is washed off with distilled water. After waiting a prescribed period of time, the result (in milligrams per deciliter) can be read by using either a color chart or an electronic meter. In the dry test method, the sample of blood is obtained in the same way, but the reagent strip is blotted with a cotton ball or cotton-tipped applicator. Tests such as Chemstrip BG, Visidex II, and Glucoscan GM utilize the dry method. As with the wash test results, the results of this test are read using a color chart or meter (Accu-check or Glucoscan). The ease, accuracy, and convenience of self blood glucose monitoring techniques have made urine testing a second choice in monitoring glucose levels. Urine tests provide only a reflection of blood glucose levels, whereas capillary blood glucose monitoring methods provide actual blood glucose levels. Self blood glucose monitoring has become a part of the standard care plan for people with labile or brittle diabetes and those on continuous subcutaneous insulin infusion and for pregnant women with diabetes mellitus. It is recommended for persons with both type I and type II diabetes mellitus who wish to maintain normal blood sugar levels. Capillary blood glucose monitoring is also the method of choice for testing and treating patients with diabetic ketoacidosis.

Insulin dose changes should be based on glucose levels rather than on urine test results. This change from the previous practice of titrating insulin dosages according to urine tests for glucose (sometimes called rainbow schedule) requires the reeducation of nurses and physicians involved in the care of people with diabetes. With the accuracy of self blood glucose monitoring techniques, the person with diabetes now has the means for adjusting insulin, food, and activity based on each day's blood glucose reading.

Glycosylated hemoglobin

This test measures the amount of glycosylated hemoglobin (hemoglobin into which glucose has been incorporated) present in the blood. Normally hemoglobin does not contain glucose when it is manufactured and released from the bone marrow. During its 120-day life span in the red blood cell, 5% to 10% of the hemoglobin normally becomes glycosylated.[23] Because glucose entry into the red blood cell is not insulin dependent, the rate at which glucose becomes attached to the hemoglobin molecule depends on blood sugar. Glycosylation is essentially irreversible; hence the level of glycosylated hemoglobin present in the blood provides an index of blood sugar levels over the previous 2 months or more.

Urine Tests

Two types of tests are used to measure glucose content in the urine—copper reduction and glucose oxidase tests. Clinitest uses a copper-reduction reagent that is responsive to a number of substances. Consequently, Clinitest may give false-positive results. The glucose oxidase tests (Tes-Tape, Clinistix, and Diastix) contain an enzyme that specifically reacts with glucose. Certain substances interfere with color changes in the glucose oxidase tests and in some situations may produce a false-negative result. The glucose oxidase tests are very sensitive to small amounts of glucose and are usually not recommended for use in children. The actual amount of glucose (milligram percent or milligrams/100 ml urine), represented by the results of the various tests as 1+, 2+, 3+, and 4+, also varies. For example, a 2+ result with Clinitest is representative of ¾ mg% glucose; with Diastix it represents ½ mg% glucose; and with TesTape, ¼ mg%. Because many factors affect the accuracy of both types of urine tests, the reader is referred to other literature sources, including the package insert that comes with the urine testing reagent. The pharmacist is a valuable resource when the effect of a specific drug on urine testing methods is under consideration.

Diabetic Diet

Diet therapy is usually prescribed to meet the specific needs of each person with diabetes. Goals and principles of diet therapy differ between type I and type II diabetes as well as between lean and obese individuals.

In the lean individual with type I diabetes the principles of diet therapy are (1) well-balanced and nutritious meals, (2) limitation of simple and concentrated sugars (monosaccharides are limited and polysaccharides are encouraged), (3) regulation of the percentage of carbohydrate (CHO), protein (PRO), and fat in the diet—usually 40% CHO, 40% PRO, and 20% fat or 60% CHO, 20% PRO, and 20% fat, (4) distribution of CHO, PRO, and fat content throughout the day to match insulin activity, and (5) provision of sufficient calories to maintain weight and satisfaction. In children, additional calories are included to provide for growth needs.

In the obese individual with type II diabetes, the principles of diet therapy are different. They include (1) well-balanced and nutritious meals, (2) control of calories for weight loss and achievement of ideal body weight, (3) control of monosaccharides, and (4) distribution of CHO, PRO, and fat according to individual taste and weight management.

Several methods of dietary control can be used. One is the free diet, which essentially allows the person to eat in a method that is satisfying but avoids concentrated sugars. A complete diet history should be taken before this method is suggested. For persons who have already established therapeutic eating habits, this method may be acceptable. A second method involves weighing food. This method is difficult for many people, but it is useful for those who have difficulty with portion control.

The third and most frequently prescribed meal plan is the exchange system.[24] In this system, foods are divided into six categories. Each food in a particular category (in the amount designated) has an equivalent amount of carbohydrate, protein, and fat. The six exchange categories are milk, meats, fruits, breads or grains, vegetables, and fats. The foods within each category are interchangeable in the prescribed amounts. For example, in the fruit list one-half cup of orange juice can be exchanged for one-fourth cup of grape juice or half a grapefruit. In the meat group one egg can be exchanged for 1 ounce of cheese or 1 ounce of chicken. Fats are included based on whether or not the meat choices are lean, medium, or high in fat content. Polyunsaturated fats are encouraged to avoid problems with hyperlipidemia. The exchange system is easy to learn and provides a highly nutritious, well-balanced diet.

Recently there has been much controversy over high-fiber and carbohydrate content in the diabetic diet. It is believed that high-fiber, complex-carbohydrate diets prevent large fluctuations in blood glucose levels, thereby providing better glucose control. For some persons with diabetes, pasta provides better glucose control curves than potatoes; rice may provide better control curves than bread. These concepts are particularly important

during pregnancy, in which the goal is to maintain glucose levels between 60 mg/dl and 120 mg/dl. Even mild hyperglycemia has been shown to be detrimental to the fetus; increased episodes of hyperglycemia have been shown to cause significant increases in congenital anomalies. The recommendation that pregnant women with diabetes avoid monosaccharides and include high-fiber complex carbohydrates in their diets is now widely accepted. In some instances, milk and other complex carbohydrate sources are used to treat hypoglycemia for the primary purpose of avoiding counterregulatory responses.

The reader is referred to the literature and the American Diabetes Association for more detailed information on diet therapy. Nutritionists are valuable resources to the nurse, physician, and patient and should be included in diet management.

Hypoglycemic Agents

There are two forms of hypoglycemic agents—the oral sulfonylureas and injectable insulin. Phenformin, a previously used oral hypoglycemic agent, was discontinued from general use in the United States in 1977 following a directive from the U.S. Department of Health, Education, and Welfare. This was because of a very toxic side effect, lactic acidosis.

Sulfonylureas

The sulfonylureas are thought to cause the release of insulin from the pancreas and to increase insulin binding and the number of insulin receptors. This means that these agents are effective only when some residual beta-cell function remains. They cannot be substituted for insulin in the person with insulin-dependent diabetes who has an absolute insulin deficiency. Both first- and second-generation sulfonylurea preparations are now available. The second-generation compounds are considered to be more potent than the first-generation agents. Glipizide is the newest of the second-generation drugs. This compound appears to be the most potent secretagogue of its generation, both for first-phase insulin secretion and in long-term sustained stimulation.[25] These preparations differ in dose and duration of action (Table 40-6). Because the sulfonylureas increase the rate at which glucose is removed from the blood, it is important to recognize that these drugs can cause hypoglycemic reactions.

Insulin

Insulin-dependent diabetes requires treatment with insulin. Insulin is destroyed in the gastrointestinal tract and must be administered by injection. All insulin is measured in units, the international unit of insulin being

Table 40-6   Sulfonylurea Preparations: Half-Life and Duration of Action

Sulfonylurea Preparations	Half-Life (hours)	Duration of Action (hours)
First Generation		
Tolbutamide (Orinase)	4–6	6–12
Tolazamide (Tolinase)	7	10–14
Acetohexamide (Dymelor)	5–7	12–14
Chlorpropamide (Diabinese)	36	Up to 60
Second Generation		
Glyburide (Micronase)	10	24
Glipizide (Glucotrol)	4	≤24

Table 40-7   Insulin: Activity Peak and Duration of Action

Type of Preparation	Activity Peak (hours)	Duration (hours)
Rapid-Acting		
Insulin injection (regular, crystalline zinc, Actrapid, Humulin R, Velosulin)	½–3	5–7
Prompt insulin zinc suspension (Semilente, Semitard)	1–4	12–16
Intermediate-Acting		
Isophane insulin suspension (NPH, Humulin, Protophane)	8–12	18–24
Insulin zinc suspension (Lente, Monotard, Lentard, Insulatard)	8–12	18–24
Combination of Rapid-Acting and Intermediate-Acting		
Insulin injection plus isophane insulin suspension (Mixtard 30:70)	½–3	18–24
Long-Acting		
Protamine zinc insulin suspension (PZI)	8–16	24–36
Insulin zinc suspension extended (Ultralente, Ultratard)	8–16	24–36

defined as the amount of insulin required to lower the blood sugar of a fasting 2-kg rabbit from 145 mg to 120 mg/100 ml blood. Insulin preparations are categorized according to onset, peak, and duration of action. There are three principal types of insulin: short, intermediate, and long acting (Table 40-7). Insulin is supplied in U100 (units per milliliter) strengths. Insulin regimens using two or three daily injections of regular insulin or regular mixed with intermediate-acting insulin are being used more often. These regimens provide a blood glucose level that is within a more normal physiologic range than that provided by the once-a-day injection.

In the last 5 years, many companies have entered the insulin-manufacturing market. To date 46 different types of insulin preparation are available.[26] After much research, human insulin has also become available. The current manufacture of human insulin uses recombinant DNA.[27] Because of this manufacturing method, human insulin is slightly more expensive than beef/pork mixtures or pure beef insulin but less expensive than pure pork insulin. Beef insulin differs from human insulin by three amino acids and pork insulin by one amino acid. Many people with diabetes develop antibodies to beef and pork insulin. The use of human insulin has the potential for eliminating these problems.

Continuous subcutaneous insulin infusion

Recent technologic advances have provided the means for improving control of diabetes through the use of continuous subcutaneous insulin infusion (CSII).[28,29] The method closely simulates the normal pattern of insulin secretion by the body. A basal insulin level is maintained, and bolus doses of regular insulin are delivered prior to meals. Multiple split-dose insulin injection management can also achieve this level of control. The choice of management is determined by the person with diabetes.

The CSII technique involves the subcutaneous insertion of a small needle into the abdomen. Tubing from the needle is connected to a syringe, which is set into a small infusion pump worn on a belt or in a jacket pocket. The computer-operated pump then delivers a set basal amount of insulin. In addition to the basal amount that is delivered by the pump, a bolus amount of insulin may be delivered when needed by pushing a button. Self blood glucose monitoring is a necessity when using this method of management. Each basal and bolus dose is determined individually and programmed into the computer of the infusion pump. Only those individuals who are highly motivated to do frequent blood glucose tests and to make daily insulin adjustments are candidates for this method of injection.

Examples of CSII pumps are the CPI, Minimed, and Autosyringe. Each pump is costly ($1100 to $2500), but because this method is no longer considered experimental, many health insurance companies cover the cost. Although the pump's safety has been proven, strict attention must be paid to signs of hypoglycemia. People with diabetes who do not sense hypoglycemia or whose counterregulatory response is impaired are not candidates for the CSII technique.

Artificial pancreas

Some institutions utilize the artificial pancreas (Biostator) to regulate individuals with diabetes who have extremely labile glucose levels or to study patients for new methods of glucose control. The artificial pancreas is a large machine that senses blood glucose levels and delivers the correct amount of insulin by means of computer analysis. Glucose levels can be documented as frequently as every 10 seconds, and insulin can be delivered at regular intervals. Two intravenous lines are maintained, one for glucose sampling and the other for insulin delivery. Approximately 2 ml of blood are removed every hour for glucose determination. As the artificial pancreas maintains blood glucose levels in a preestablished range, graphs are recorded and printed by the computer. Calculations are then produced that aid in glucose management after the person is disconnected from the machine and returns to normal activity. Although the artificial pancreas is large, research is being done to miniaturize the entire system so that it can be used for the management of persons with diabetes outside the hospital environment.

Islet cell transplantation

Much research is being directed toward the study of islet cell transplantation, which at present is experimental. Islet cell transplantation involves the separation of beta cells from pancreatic tissue. The possible sources of beta cells are (1) cadaver pancreases, (2) living relatives of people with diabetes who are willing to donate part of their pancreas, or (3) a controversial source, aborted fetuses. The results of transplantation up to this time have not been markedly effective. Rejection of cells or reversal to the diabetic state is problematic. Immunosuppressive therapy necessary for transplantation brings a greater risk of problems than does good control of diabetes and exogenous insulin therapy. Most candidates for islet cell transplantation are people with diabetes who are already immunosuppressed because of kidney transplantation.

Exercise

Exercise has long been credited with improving glucose tolerance and decreasing blood lipid levels. So important is exercise in the management of diabetes that a planned program of regular exercise is usually considered to be an integral part of the therapeutic regimen for every person with diabetes.

During short-term exercise, the uptake of glucose into the exercising muscle increases 7-fold to 20-fold. Blood levels of insulin tend to regulate glucose release by the liver. In the nondiabetic person, exercise is accompanied by an adrenergically induced decrease in insulin release from the beta cells and an increased breakdown of liver glycogen stores with the release of glucose into the bloodstream. When exercise is prolonged for more than 2 hours, the exercising muscles obtain the greater amount of their energy from fatty acids, and glucose release from the liver is derived from gluconeogenesis.

In the person with diabetes, the beneficial effects of exercise are accompanied by an increased risk of hypoglycemia. The reasons for a decrease in blood sugar levels during exercise in the person with insulin-dependent diabetes are twofold. First, there is often an increased absorption of insulin from the insulin injection site. This increased absorption is more pronounced when insulin is injected into the subcutaneous tissue of the exercised muscle, but it seems to occur even when insulin is injected into other body areas. Second, because the person with diabetes cannot reduce blood insulin levels, glucose release by the liver is reduced. However, for the person with IDDM who exercises during periods of poor control (when blood glucose levels are elevated and ketonemia is present), control of the diabetes will usually deteriorate further, and blood sugar and ketone levels will rise to higher levels. This is because the liver has already begun to produce glucose and ketones because of a preexisting insulin deficiency, and the additional stress of exercise causes a further increase.

In some persons with IDDM, the symptoms of hypoglycemia occur many hours after cessation of exercise. This may be because subsequent insulin doses (in persons using multiple daily insulin injections) are not adjusted to accommodate the exercise-induced decrease in blood sugars. The cause of hypoglycemia in persons who do not administer a second insulin dose is unclear. It may be related to the fact that skeletal muscles increase their uptake of glucose following exercise as a means of replenishing their glycogen stores or that the liver and skeletal muscles are more sensitive to insulin during this period of time. Persons with IDDM should be aware that delayed hypoglycemia may occur following exercise and that there may be a need to alter either their insulin dose and/or their carbohydrate intake.

In summary, the diagnosis of diabetes mellitus is based on clinical signs of the disease, including the presence of glucose in the urine and the blood. Blood insulin levels can be determined using radioimmunoassay methods. The glucose tolerance test is an important screening method for diabetes. It involves the body's response to a given amount of concentrated glucose, using blood sugar levels. In persons with insulin-dependent diabetes, the self-use of capillary glucose testing provides a means of maintaining near-normal blood sugar levels through frequent monitoring of blood glucose and adjustment of insulin dosage. Urine sugars provide an indirect method of monitoring glucose levels and may also be used in the management of diabetes. Glycosylation involves the attachment of glucose to the hemoglobin molecule; it is an irreversible process. The measurement of glycosylated hemoglobin provides an index of blood sugar levels over several months. The treatment of diabetes includes diet, exercise, and, in many cases, the use of a hypoglycemic agent. Dietary management focuses on maintaining a well-balanced diet, controlling calories to achieve and maintain an optimum weight, and regulating the distribution of carbohydrates, proteins, and fats. Two types of hypoglycemic agents are used in the management of diabetes: injectable insulin and the oral sulfonylurea drugs. Type I diabetes requires treatment with injectable insulin. The sulfonylurea agents increase insulin release from the pancreas, the number of insulin receptors, and the binding of insulin to these receptors. These drugs require a functioning pancreas and may be used in the treatment of non–insulin-dependent diabetes mellitus. Exercise improves glucose tolerance and reduces blood lipid levels. The presence of insulin in the blood impairs glucose release by the liver. Blood levels of injected insulin cannot be controlled by physiologic feedback mechanisms; therefore, the beneficial effects of exercise in persons with insulin-dependent diabetes is accompanied by an increased risk of hypoglycemia.

■ Study Guide

After you have studied this chapter, you should be able to meet the following objectives:

☐ Give a clinical description of diabetes mellitus.

☐ List the distinguishing characteristics of IDDM and NIDDM.

☐ Explain why IDDM predisposes to the development of ketoacidosis whereas NIDDM does not.

☐ List three causes of secondary diabetes.

☐ Cite at least three indications for the use of glucose tolerance tests during pregnancy.

☐ Describe the suspected role of two environmental factors in the etiology of diabetes mellitus.

☐ State the purpose of the glucose tolerance test.

☐ List the advantages of self blood glucose monitoring.

☐ Describe the possible relationship between obesity and the development of NIDDM.

☐ Explain the purpose of measuring the level of glycosylated hemoglobin in the blood.

☐ Describe the difference between the wash test and the dry test for self blood glucose monitoring.

☐ Name and describe two types of urinary tests for glucose.

☐ Describe the three "polys" that characterize diabetes mellitus.

☐ Describe the clinical manifestations of hypoglycemia that the health professional should be able to recognize.

☐ Cite the possible differences in symptoms of an insulin reaction in younger and in elderly persons.

☐ Describe measures used in the treatment of an insulin reaction.

☐ Describe the clinical manifestations of diabetic keto-acidosis and their physiologic significance.

☐ Explain how "hypoglycemia begets hyperglycemia."

☐ Describe the clinical condition resulting from the hyperosmolar state.

☐ Cite a common characteristic of tissues that are affected by the chronic complications of diabetes.

☐ Relate the possible mechanisms of the sorbitol pathway, formation of abnormal glycoproteins, and problems with tissue oxygenation to diabetes and the development of the chronic complications of the disease.

☐ Describe the pathologic changes that may occur with diabetic peripheral neuropathies.

☐ Describe the pathology underlying diabetic retinopathy.

☐ Describe the vascular complications that may occur with diabetes mellitus.

☐ Explain the relationship between diabetes mellitus and infection.

☐ List five principles for diet management in persons with diabetes.

☐ Explain the difference between the free, weighed, and exchange methods for diabetic diets.

☐ Explain the advantages of high-fiber and complex carbohydrates in the dietary management of diabetes.

☐ State the actions of the oral hypoglycemic agents in terms of the lowering of blood sugar.

☐ Name and describe the three types (according to duration of action) of insulin.

☐ Cite the advantages of human insulin versus pork or beef insulin.

☐ Explain how continuous subcutaneous insulin infusion systems function.

☐ Describe the present obstacles to the use of artificial pancreas and islet cell transplants.

☐ Explain why exercise is beneficial to diabetics.

☐ Explain the differences in blood sugar regulation during exercise in the nondiabetic person and the person with insulin-dependent diabetes and relate this to the increased risk for development of hypoglycemia in the person with diabetes during exercise.

■ References

1. Every sixty seconds. Diabetes Forecast, No 6, 1978, p 23
2. Waif SO (ed): Diabetes Mellitus. Indianapolis, Eli Lilly, 1980
3. National Diabetes Data Group: Classification and diagnosis of diabetes mellitus and other categories of glucose intolerance. Diabetes 28:1039, 1979
4. Tattersoll RB, Fajans SS: A difference between the inheritance of classical juvenile-onset and maturity-onset type of diabetes of young people. Diabetes 24:44, 1975
5. Cudworth AG, Woodrow JC: Evidence of HLA-linked genes in juvenile-onset diabetes. Br Med J 3:133, 1975
6. Gamble DR, Taylor KW: Seasonal incidence of diabetes mellitus. Br Med J 3:631, 1969
7. MacMillan DR, Kotoyan M, Zeidner D et al: Seasonal variations in the onset of diabetes in children. Pediatrics 59:113, 1977
8. Sulz HA, Hart BA, Zielezny M et al: Is mumps virus an etiologic factor in juvenile diabetes mellitus? Preliminary report. J Pediatr 86:654, 1975
9. Yoon JW, Onodera T, Jensen AB et al: Virus-induced diabetes mellitus, XI. Replication of Coxsackie B 3 virus in human pancreatic beta cell cultures. Diabetes 27:778, 1978
10. Johnson GM, Tudor RB: Diabetes mellitus and congenital rubella infection. Am J Dis Child 120:453, 1970
11. Plotkin SA, Kaye R: Diabetes mellitus and congenital rubella. Pediatrics 46:450, 1970
12. Defronzo RA, Ferrannini E, Koivisto V: New concepts in the pathogenesis and treatment of noninsulin-dependent diabetes mellitus. Am J Med 74, No 1:66, 1983
13. Whitehouse FW: Two minutes with diabetes: "My patient is not responding and is very dehydrated." Med Times 101:35, 1970
14. Podolsky S: Hyperosmolar nonketotic coma in the elderly diabetic. Med Clin North Am 62, No 4:816, 1978
15. Joslin EP, Gray H, Root HL: Insulin in hospital and home. J Metabol Res 2:651, 1924
16. Somogyi M: Exacerbation of diabetes in excess insulin action. Am J Med 26:169, 1957
17. Bolli GB, Gotterman IS, Campbell PJ: Glucose counter-regulation and waning of insulin in the Somogyi phenomenon (posthypoglycemic hyperglycemia). N Engl J Med 311:1214, 1984
18. Ditzel J, Standl E: The problem of tissue oxygenation in diabetes mellitus. Acta Med Scand (Suppl 578):49, 1975
19. Centers for Disease Control: Screening for Diabetic Eye Disease—Mississippi. MMWR 32, No 12:157, 1983
20. The Diabetic Retinopathy Study Research Group: Photocoagulation treatment of proliferative diabetic retinopathy. Clinical application of diabetic retinopathy study (DRS) findings (DRS report No 8). Ophthalmology 88:583, 1981
21. Sanderson JE: Diabetes and the heart. Chest Heart Stroke 3:35, 1978–79
22. Skyler JS: Patient self-monitoring of blood glucose. Clin Diabetes 1, No 4:12, 1983
23. Diabetic control measured by glycosylated Hb level. Hosp Pract 12, No 4:42, 1977
24. American Diabetes Association: Exchange Lists for Meal Planning. New York, 1976
25. Shuman CR: Glipizide: An overview. Am J Med 74:55, 1983
26. Karam JH, Etzwiler DD: Insulins: Overview and outlook. Clin Diabetes 1, No 4:1, 1983
27. Skyler JS (ed): Symposium on human insulin of recombinant DNA origin. Diabetes Care. 5 (Suppl 2):1, 1982
28. Felig P, Bergman M: Insulin pump treatment of diabetes. JAMA 250:1045, 1983
29. American Diabetes Association (Policy Statement): Indications for use of continuous insulin delivery systems and self-measurement of blood glucose. Diabetes Care 5:140, 1982

■ Additional References

Bantle JP, Laine DC, Castle GW: Postprandial glucose and insulin responses to meals containing different carbohydrates in normal and diabetic subjects. N Engl J Med 309:7, 1983

Bar RS: Factors that control insulin action at the receptor. Am J Med 74, No 1:18, 1983

Benson E, Metz R: Diabetic ketoacidosis. Hosp Med 15, No 5:26, 1979

Boden G, Master R, Gordon S et al: Monitoring metabolic control in diabetic outpatients with glycosylated hemoglobin. Ann Intern Med 92, No 3:357, 1980

Bolli GB, Dimitriadis GD, Pehling BA et al: Abnormal glucose counterregulation after subcutaneous insulin in insulin-dependent diabetes mellitus. N Engl J Med 310:1706, 1984

Bruce GL: The Somogyi phenomenon: Insulin-induced posthypoglycemic hyperglycemia. Heart Lung 7, No 3:463, 1978

Cahill GF: Hyperglycemic hyperosmolar coma. J Am Geriatric Soc 31:103, 1983

Cahill GF, McDevitt HO: Insulin-dependent diabetes mellitus: The initial lesion. N Engl J Med 304:1454, 1981

Clement RS, Vourganti B: Fatal ketoacidosis: Major causes and approaches to their prevention. Diabetes Care 1, No 5:314, 1978

Colwell JA, Halushka PV, Sarji KE et al: Platelet function and diabetes mellitus. Med Clin North Am 62, No 4:753, 1978

Colwell JA, Winocur PD, Lopes-Virella M et al: New concepts of the pathogenesis of atherosclerosis in diabetes mellitus. Am J Med 75, No 5:67, 1983

Crapo PA, Olefsky JM: Food fallacies and blood sugar. N Engl J Med 309:44, 1983

Cristiansen C, Sachse M: Home blood glucose monitoring. Diabetes Educator (Fall):13, 1980

Cryer PE: Hypoglycemic glucose counterregulation in patients with insulin-dependent diabetes mellitus. J Lab Clin Med 99:451, 1982

Duchen LW, Anjorin A, Watkins PJ et al: Pathology of autonomic neuropathy in diabetes mellitus. Ann Intern Med 92, Part 2:301, 1980

Ellenberg M: Sexual functioning in diabetic patients. Ann Intern Med 92, Part 2:331, 1980

Flood TM: Diet and diabetes mellitus. Hosp Pract 14, No 2:61, 1979

Foster DW, McGarry JD: The metabolic derangements and treatment of diabetic ketoacidosis. N Engl J Med 309:159, 1983

Fulop M: The treatment of severely uncontrolled diabetes mellitus. Adv Intern Med 29:327, 1984

Gale EAM, Kurtz AB, Tattersall RB: In search of the Somogyi effect. Lancet 279, 1980

Graighead JE: Current views on the etiology of insulin dependent diabetes mellitus. N Engl J Med 299, No 26:1439, 1978

Goldstein DE: Is glycosylated hemoglobin clinically useful. N Engl J Med 310:384, 1984

Hamburger SC: Diagnosis and management of diabetic keto-acidosis—Selected aspects. Crit Care Q 2:53, 1979

Hare JW, Rossini A: Diabetic comas: The overlap concept. Hosp Pract 14, No 5:95, 1979

Hilsted J: Pathophysiology of diabetic autonomic neuropathy. N Y State J Med (May):892, 1982

Holt WS, Wolf KP, Takach RJ: Diabetic retinopathy. J Maine Med Assoc 70, No 11:9, 1979

Horton ES: Role of environmental factors in development of noninsulin dependent diabetes mellitus. Am J Med 75, No 5:32, 1983

Hosking DJ, Bennett B, Hampton JR et al: Diabetic autonomic neuropathy. Diabetes 27, No 10:1043, 1978

Kiser D: The Somogyi effect. Am J Nurs 80, No 2:236, 1980

Kitabchi AE, Fisher JN, Matteri R: The use of continuous insulin delivery systems in treatment of diabetes mellitus. Adv Intern Med 28:49, 1983

Kroc Collaborative Study: Blood glucose control and the evolution of diabetic retinopathy and albuminuria. N Engl J Med 311:365, 1984

Kumar D: Insulin allergy: Differences in the binding of porcine, bovine, and human insulins with anti-insulin IgE. Diabetes Care 4:104, 1981

Kosel K, Gibb-Matas P, Seaborne L et al: Total pancreatectomy and islet cell autotransplantation. Am J Nurs 82:568, 1982

LoGero FW, Coffman JD: Vascular and microvascular disease of the foot in diabetes. N Engl J Med 311:1615, 1984

Mogensen CE, Christensen: Predicting diabetic nephropathy in insulin-dependent patients. N Engl J Med 311:89, 1984

Permutt MA, Rotwein P: Analysis of the insulin gene in noninsulin-dependent diabetes. Am J Med 75, No 5:1, 1983

Perrin ED: Laser therapy for diabetic retinopathy. Am J Nurs 80, No 4:664, 1980

Plasse NJ: Monitoring blood glucose at home: A comparison of three products. Am J Nurs 81:2018, 1981

Pollett RJ: Insulin receptors and action in clinical disorders of carbohydrate tolerance. Am J Med 75, No 5:15, 1983

Rayfield EJ, Ault MJ, Keusch GT: Infection and diabetes: The case of glucose control. Am J Med 72:439, 1982

Richter EA, Ruderman NB, Schneider SH: Diabetes and exercise. Am J Med 70:201, 1981

Robbins DC, Tager HS, Rubenstein AH: Biologic and clinical importance of proinsulin. N Engl J Med 310:1165, 1984

Rosenbloom AL: Primary and subspecialty care of diabetes mellitus in children and youth. Med Clin North Am 31, No 1:107, 1984

Roth J: Insulin receptors in diabetes. Hosp Pract 15, No 5:98, 1980

Rubenstein P, Suciu-Foca N, Nicholson JF: Genetics of juvenile diabetes mellitus. N Engl J Med 297, No 19:1036, 1977

Schade DS, Eaton RP: Pathogenesis of diabetic ketoacidosis: A reappraisal. Diabetes Care 3, No 2:296, 1979

Skyler JS: Counterregulatory hormones, rebound hyperglycemia, and diabetic control. Diabetes Care 6, No 2:526, 1979

Sonsken PH: Home monitoring of blood glucose in diabetic patients. Acta Endocrinol (Suppl 238) 94:145, 1980

Spratt IL: Seasonal increase in diabetes mellitus (Letter). N Engl J Med 308:775, 1983

Symposium on Human Insulin. Diabetes Care. 6 (Suppl 1, March–April), 1983

Teutsch SM, Herman WH, Dwyer DM: Mortality among diabetic patients using continuous subcutaneous insulin-infusion pumps. N Engl J Med 310:361, 1984

Tillerman DB, Miller ME, Pitchon HE: Infection and diabetes mellitus. West J Med 130, No 6:515, 1979

Transplants: The hope and the hurdles. Diabetes Forcast (Nov–Dec):24, 1984

Turkington RW: Depression masquerading as diabetic neuropathy. JAMA 243, No 11:1147, 1980

Unger RH: Nocturnal hypoglycemia in aggressively controlled diabetes (letter). N Engl J Med 306:1292, 1982

Ventura E: Foot care in diabetes. Am J Nurs 78, No 5:886, 1978

Vranic M, Berger M: Exercise and diabetes mellitus. Diabetes 78:147, 1979

West K, Erdreich L, Stober J: A detailed study of risk factors for retinopathy and nephropathy in diabetes. Diabetes 29:501, 1980

Wilson HK, Field JB: Understanding insulin: The old and new. Adv Intern Med 29:357, 1984

Wimberley D: When a pregnant woman is diabetic: Intrapartal care. Am J Nurs 79, No 3:451, 1979

Chapter 41

Control of Gastrointestinal Function

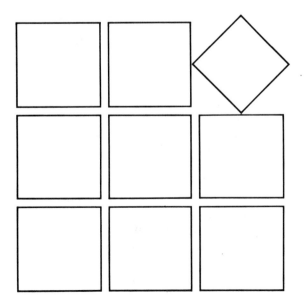

The process of digestion and absorption of nutrients requires an intact and healthy gastrointestinal tract epithelial lining that can resist the effects of its own digestive secretions. It involves the movement of materials through the gastrointestinal tract at a rate that facilitates absorption, and it requires the presence of enzymes for the digestion and absorption of nutrients. Structurally, the gastrointestinal tract is a long, hollow tube with its lumen inside the body and its wall acting as an interface between the internal and external environments. The wall does not normally allow harmful agents to enter the body, nor does it permit body fluids and other materials to escape.

The digestive system is truly an amazing structure. In this system, enzymes and hormones are produced, vitamins are synthesized and stored, and food is dismantled and then reassembled. Catalysts and reactants play a role, and some are recycled and used again. Finally, wastes are collected and eliminated efficiently. No doubt a man-made system designed to accomplish similar functions would require miles of space, elaborate equipment, and a huge expenditure of capital. Although this chapter cannot cover gastrointestinal function in its entirety, it is designed to provide the reader with an overview that is deemed essential to an understanding of subsequent chapters.

Nutrients, vitamins, minerals, electrolytes, and water enter the body through the gastrointestinal tract. As a matter of semantics, it should be pointed out that the gastrointestinal tract is also referred to as the digestive tract, the alimentary canal, and, at times, the gut. The intestinal portion may also be called the bowel. For our purposes, the salivary glands, the liver, and the pancreas, which produce secretions that aid in digestion, are considered accessory structures.

■ Structure and Organization of the Gastrointestinal Tract

In the digestive tract, food and other materials move slowly along its length as they are systematically broken down into ions and molecules that can be absorbed into the body itself. In the large intestine unabsorbed nutrients and wastes are collected for later elimination. What is important for the reader to recognize is that although the gastrointestinal tract is located within the body, it is really a long hollow tube the lumen of which is an extension of the external environment. Thus, nutrients do not become part of the internal environment until they have passed through the intestinal wall and have entered the blood or lymph channels.

For simplicity and understanding, the digestive system can be divided into four parts (Fig. 41-1). The *upper part*—the mouth, esophagus, and stomach—acts as an intake source and holding tank in which initial digestive processes take place. The *middle portion* consists of the small intestine—the duodenum, jejunum, and ileum. Most digestive and absorptive processes occur in the small intestine. The *lower segment*—the cecum, colon, and rectum—serves as a storage channel for the efficient elimination of waste. The *fourth part* consists of the accessory structures, the salivary glands, the liver, and the pancreas. These structures produce digestive secretions and help regulate the use and storage of nutrients. The discussion in this chapter focuses on the first three parts of the gastrointestinal tract. The liver and pancreas are discussed in Chapter 43.

Upper Gastrointestinal Tract

The mouth forms the entryway into the gastrointestinal tract for food; it contains the teeth, used in the mastication of food, and the tongue and other structures needed to direct food toward the pharyngeal structures and the esophagus.

The esophagus begins at the lower end of the pharynx. It receives food from the pharynx and with a series of peristaltic contractions, moves the food into the stomach. The esophagus is a muscular collapsible tube, about 25 cm (10 in.) long, that lies behind the trachea. The muscular walls of the upper third of the esophagus are striated muscle; these muscle fibers are gradually replaced by smooth muscle fibers until at the lower third of the esophagus it is entirely smooth muscle. The striated muscle of the upper esophagus, however, is not under voluntary control but is supplied by the autonomic fibers that travel in the vagus nerve and supply the smooth muscle. The upper and lower ends of the esophagus act as sphincters. The upper sphincter is formed by a thickening of the striated muscle. The lower sphincter, which is not identifiable anatomically, occurs at a point 1 cm to 2 cm from where the esophagus joins the stomach.

The stomach is a pouchlike structure that lies in the upper part of the abdomen and serves as a food storage reservoir during the early stages of digestion. Although the luminal volume of the stomach is only about 50 ml, it can increase its volume to almost 1000 ml before intraluminal pressure begins to rise. The esophagus opens into the stomach through an opening called the cardiac orifice, so named because of its proximity to the heart. The part of the stomach that lies above and to the left of the cardiac orifice is called the fundus, the central portion is called the body, and the orifice encircled by a ringlike muscle that opens into the small intestine is called the pylorus. The presence of a true pyloric sphincter is controversial. Whether or not an actual sphincter is present, contractions of the smooth muscle in the pyloric area control gastric emptying.

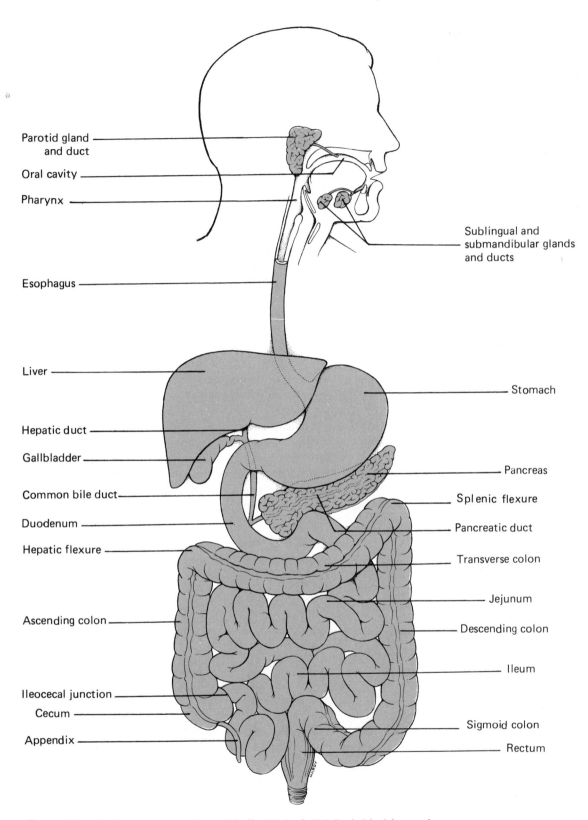

Parotid gland and duct
Oral cavity
Pharynx
Sublingual and submandibular glands and ducts
Esophagus
Liver
Stomach
Hepatic duct
Gallbladder
Pancreas
Common bile duct
Splenic flexure
Duodenum
Pancreatic duct
Hepatic flexure
Transverse colon
Jejunum
Ascending colon
Descending colon
Ileum
Ileocecal junction
Cecum
Appendix
Sigmoid colon
Rectum

Figure 41-1   *The digestive system. (From Chaffee EE, Lytle IM: Basic Physiology and Anatomy, 4th ed. Philadelphia, JB Lippincott, 1980)*

Middle Gastrointestinal Tract

The small intestines, which form the middle portion of the digestive tract, consist of three subdivisions: the duodenum, the jejunum, and the ileum. It is in the jejunum and ileum, which are about 7 m (23 ft) in length and must be folded on themselves, that food is digested and absorbed. The duodenum, which is about 22 cm (10 in.) in length, connects the stomach to the jejunum and contains the opening for the common bile duct and the main pancreatic duct. Bile and pancreatic juices enter the intestine through these ducts.

Lower Gastrointestinal Tract

The large intestine is about 1.5 m (4.5-5 ft) in length and 6 cm to 7 cm (2.5 in.) in diameter. It is divided into the cecum, colon, rectum, and anal canal. The cecum is a blind pouch that hangs down at the junction of the ileum and the colon. The ileocecal valve lies at the upper border of the cecum and prevents the return of feces from the cecum into the small intestine. The appendix arises from the cecum about 2.5 cm (1 in.) from the ileocecal valve. The colon is further divided into ascending, transverse, descending, and sigmoid portions. The ascending colon extends from the cecum to the undersurface of the liver, where it turns abruptly to form the right colic (hepatic) flexure. The transverse colon crosses the upper half of the abdominal cavity from right to left and then curves sharply downward beneath the lower end of the spleen, forming the left colic (splenic) flexure. The descending colon extends the colic flexure to the rectum. The rectum extends from the sigmoid colon to the anus. The anal canal passes between the two medial borders of the levator ani muscles. Powerful sphincter muscles guard against fecal incontinence.

Gastrointestinal Wall Structure

The digestive tract, once it leaves the upper third of the esophagus, is essentially a five-layered tube (Fig. 41-2). The inner luminal layer, or *mucosa*, is so named because its cells produce mucus that lubricates and protects the inner surface of the alimentary canal. The epithelial cells in this layer have a rapid turnover rate being replaced every 4 to 5 days. Approximately 250 gm of these cells are shed each day in the stool. Because of the regenerative capabilities of the mucosal layer, injury to this layer of tissue heals rapidly without leaving scar tissue. The *submucosal layer* is made up of connective tissue. This layer contains blood vessels, nerves, and structures responsible for secreting digestive enzymes. Movement in the gastrointestinal tract is facilitated by the *circular* and *longitudinal* smooth muscle layers. The fifth layer, the *peritoneum*, is loosely attached to the outer wall of the intestine.

The *peritoneum* is the largest serous membrane in the body, having a surface area about equal to that of the skin. The peritoneal membrane is composed of two layers, a thin layer of squamous cells resting on a layer of connective tissue. If the squamous layer is injured because of surgery or inflammation, there is danger that

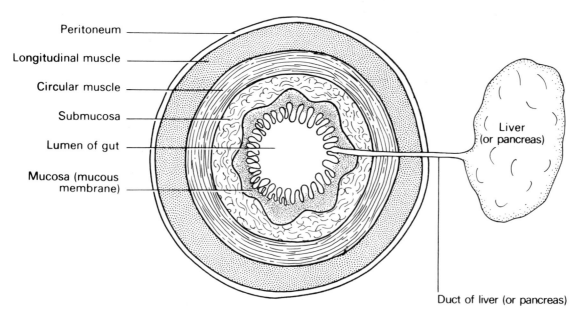

Peritoneum
Longitudinal muscle
Circular muscle
Submucosa
Lumen of gut
Mucosa (mucous membrane)

Liver (or pancreas)

Duct of liver (or pancreas)

Figure 41-2 *Transverse section of the digestive system. (From Thompson JS: Core Textbook of Anatomy. Philadelphia, JB Lippincott, 1977)*

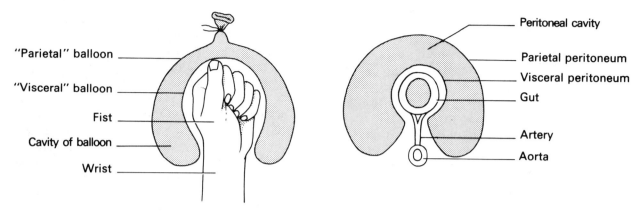

Figure 41-3 *Comparison of the peritoneal cavity with a balloon. (From Thompson JS: Core Textbook of Anatomy. Philadelphia, JB Lippincott, 1977)*

adhesions (fibrous scar-tissue bands) will form, causing sections of the viscera to heal together. Unfortunately, adhesions may alter the position and movement of the abdominal viscera.

The *peritoneal cavity* is potential space formed between what is called the *parietal peritoneum* and the *visceral peritoneum*. The parietal peritoneum comes in contact with and is loosely attached to the abdominal wall, whereas the abdominal organs are in contact with the visceral peritoneum. Thompson compares the two layers of the peritoneum to a deflated balloon.[1] If you make a fist into the balloon, the outer surface can be equated with the parietal peritoneum and the fist interface with the visceral peritoneum (Fig. 41-3). In this case, the area within the balloon would approximate the peritoneal cavity. The connective tissue layer of the peritoneum forms both the parietal and the visceral peritoneum, while the smooth squamous-cell layer of the membrane lines the cavity. The adjacent membrane layers within the peritoneal cavity are separated by a thin layer of serous fluid. This fluid prevents friction between continuously moving abdominal structures. In certain pathologic states the fluid in the potential space of the peritoneal cavity is increased, causing ascites.* The *mesentery* is a double fold of peritoneum that encloses and supports the abdominal organs (Fig. 41-4). The mesentery is no more than 20 cm to 25 cm deep, about 15 cm long in the small intestine, and 7 cm long in the large intestine.

In summary, the gastrointestinal tract is a long hollow tube the lumen of which is an extension of the external environment. The digestive tract can be divided into four parts: an upper part consisting of the mouth, esophagus,

and stomach; a middle part consisting of the small intestines; a lower part consisting of the cecum, colon, and rectum; and the accessory organs consisting of the salivary glands, the liver, and the pancreas. Throughout its length, except for the mouth, throat, and upper esophagus, the gastrointestinal tract is composed of five layers: an inner mucosal layer, a submucosal layer, a layer of circular smooth muscle fibers, a layer of longitudinal smooth muscle fibers, and an outer serosal layer that forms the peritoneum and is continuous with the mesentery.

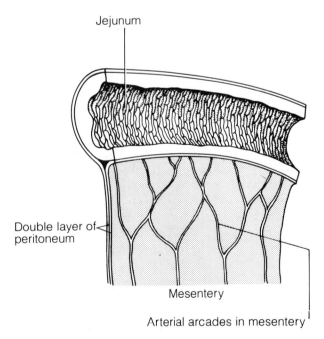

Figure 41-4 *The attachment of the mesentery to the portions of the small bowel. (From Thompson JS: Core Textbook of Anatomy. Philadelphia, JB Lippincott, 1977)*

*The reader is referred to Chapter 26 for a discussion of edema fluid.

■ Motility

The motility of the gastrointestinal tract moves food products and fluids along its length, from mouth to anus, in a manner that facilitates digestion and absorption. Except in the pharynx and upper third of the esophagus, smooth muscle provides the contractile force for gastrointestinal motility. The rhythmic movements of the digestive tract are self-perpetuating, much like the activity of the heart, and are influenced by local, humoral, and neural influences. The ability to initiate impulses is a property of the smooth muscle itself. Contractions occur in sheets or tubes of completely denervated muscle. Impulses are conducted from one muscle fiber to another.

The movements of the gastrointestinal tract are both tonic and rhythmic. The *tonic movements* are continuous movements that last for long periods of time—minutes or even hours. Tonic contractions *occur* at *sphincters*. The rhythmic movements consist of intermittent contractions that are responsible for mixing and moving food along the digestive tract. *Peristaltic movements* are *rhythmic propulsive* movements that occur when the smooth muscle layer constricts, forming a contractile band that forces the intraluminal contents forward. During peristalsis the segment that lies distal to, or ahead of, the contracted portion relaxes, so that the contents move forward with ease. Normal peristalsis always moves from the direction of the mouth toward the anus.

Neural Control Mechanisms

The neural control of gastrointestinal tract motility involves a plexus, or neural network, of ganglion cells located within the gastrointestinal wall. This intramural (within the wall) plexus extends along the length of the gastrointestinal tract and controls the activity of both longitudinal and circular smooth muscle fibers. In the intestines, the intramural plexus is located between the circular and longitudinal muscle layers and is called the *myenteric* plexus, or *Auerbach's* plexus. The activity of the neurons in the myenteric plexus is regulated by both local reflexes and the autonomic nervous system. These ganglionic cells are excited by acetylcholine and serotonin (5-hydroxytryptamine) released from presynaptic terminals on or near the nerve cells.

Nerves of the digestive tract contain many visceral afferent fibers, which can be divided into two classes: (1) those whose cell bodies are located in the nervous system and (2) those whose cell bodies are within the intramural plexuses. The first group has receptors in the mucosal epithelium and in the muscle layers; their fibers pass centrally in vagal and sympathetic fibers. The second group exerts local control over motility by means of the activity of the intramural plexus.

Efferent parasympathetic innervation to the stomach, small intestine, cecum, ascending colon, and transverse colon is by way of the vagus (Fig. 41-5). The rest of the colon is innervated by parasympathetic fibers in the pelvic nerve that exits from the sacral segments of the spinal cord. Preganglionic parasympathetic fibers synapse with intramural plexus neurons, or they can act directly on intestinal smooth muscle. Most parasympathetic fibers are excitatory. Numerous vagovagal reflexes, whose afferent and efferent fibers are both vagal nerves, influence motility as well as secretions of the digestive tract.

Efferent sympathetic innervation of the gastrointestinal tract is through the thoracic chain of sympathetic ganglia and the celiac, superior mesenteric, and inferior mesenteric ganglia. The sympathetic nervous system exerts several effects on gastrointestinal function. It controls the extent of mucus secretion by the mucosal glands, reduces motility by inhibiting the activity of intramural plexus neurons, enhances sphincter function, and increases vascular smooth muscle tone of the blood vessels that supply the gastrointestinal tract. The effect of the sympathetic stimulation and the release of the sympathetic neuromediators (epinephrine and norepinephrine) is to block the release of the excitatory neuromediators in the intramural plexuses, inhibiting gastrointestinal motility. The effect of sympathetic stimulation occurs when there is ongoing activity within the intramural plexuses. For example, in situations in which gastric motility is enhanced because of increased vagal activity, stimulation of sympathetic centers in the hypothalamus promptly and often completely inhibits motility. The sympathetic fibers that supply the lower esophageal, pyloric, and internal and external anal sphincters are largely excitatory, but their role in controlling these sphincters is poorly understood.[2]

Intramural plexus neurons also communicate with neurons from receptors in the mucosal and muscle layers. Mechanoreceptors monitor the stretch and distention of the gastrointestinal tract wall, and chemoreceptors monitor the chemical composition (osmolality, pH, and digestive products of protein and fat metabolism) of its contents. These receptors can communicate directly either with ganglionic cells in the intramural plexuses or with afferent fibers of the sympathetic or parasympathetic nervous system.

Chewing and Swallowing

Chewing begins the digestive process; it breaks the food into particles of a size that can be swallowed, lubricates it by mixing it with saliva, and mixes starch-containing

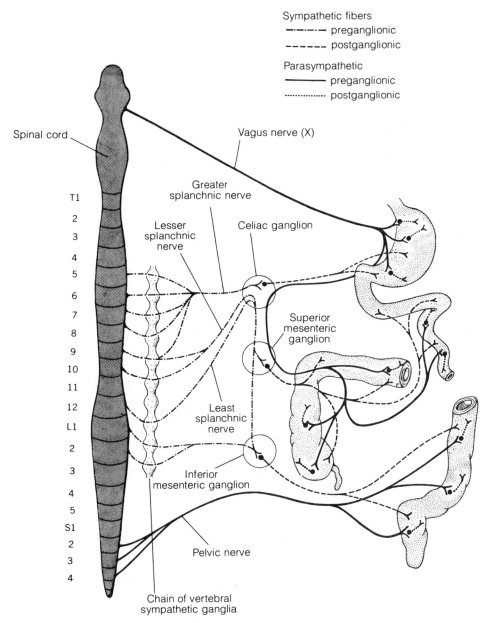

Figure 41-5 *The autonomic innervation of the gastrointestinal tract. (Drawing by Edith Tagrin reproduced from* Human Design *by William S. Beck, © 1971 by Harcourt Brace Jovanovich, Inc. by permission of the publisher.)*

food with salivary amylase. Although chewing is usually considered a voluntary act, it can be carried out involuntarily in the decerebrate patient.

The swallowing reflex is a rigidly ordered sequence of events that results in the propulsion of food from the mouth to the stomach via the esophagus. Although swallowing is initiated as a voluntary activity, it becomes involuntary. Sensory impulses for the reflex begin at tactile receptors in the pharynx and esophagus and are integrated in the reticular formation of the medulla and lower pons, producing the motor components of the

response. Diseases that disrupt these brain centers disrupt the coordination of swallowing and predispose an individual to the risk of food and fluid lodging in the trachea and bronchi, leading to asphyxiation or aspiration pneumonia.

Swallowing consists of three phases: an oral, or voluntary phase; a pharyngeal phase; and an esophageal phase. During the oral, or voluntary, phase the bolus is collected at the back of the mouth so that the tongue can lift the food upward until it touches the posterior wall of the pharynx. At this point, the second stage of swallowing is initiated: the soft palate is pulled upward, the palatopharyngeal folds are pulled together so that food does not enter the nasopharynx; the vocal cords are pulled together, and the epiglottis is moved so that it covers the larynx; respiration is inhibited; and the bolus is moved backward into the esophagus by constrictive movements of the pharynx. Although the striated muscles of the pharynx are involved in the second stage of swallowing, it is an involuntary stage.

The third stage of swallowing is the esophageal stage. As food enters the esophagus and stretches its walls, both local and central nervous system reflexes that initiate peristalsis are triggered. There are two types of peristalsis—primary and secondary. Primary peristalsis is controlled by the swallowing center in the brain stem and begins when food enters the esophagus. Secondary peristalsis is partially mediated by smooth muscle fibers in the esophagus and occurs when primary peristalsis is inadequate to move food through the esophagus.[3] Peristalsis begins at the site of distention and moves downward. Before the peristaltic wave reaches the stomach, the lower esophageal sphincter relaxes, to allow the bolus of food to enter the stomach. The pressure in the lower esophageal sphincter is always greater than that in the stomach, an important factor in preventing the reflux of gastric contents. The opening of the lower esophageal sphincter is mediated vagally. Increased levels of the parasympathetic neuromediator acetylcholine increase the constriction of the sphincter. The hormone gastrin also increases constriction of the sphincter. Gastrin provides the major stimulus for stomach acid production, and its action on the lower esophageal sphincter serves to protect the esophageal mucosa when gastric acid levels are elevated.

Gastric Motility

The stomach serves as a reservoir for ingested solids and liquids. Motility of the stomach results in the churning and grinding of solid foods and regulates the emptying of the gastric contents, or chyme, into the duodenum. Peristaltic mixing and churning contractions begin in a pacemaker area in the middle of the stomach and move toward the antrum (Fig. 41-6). They occur at a frequency of 3 to 5 contractions per minute, with a duration of 2 seconds to 20 seconds. As the peristaltic wave approaches the antrum, it speeds up, and the entire terminal 5 cm to 10 cm of the antrum contracts, occluding the pyloric opening. Contraction of the antrum reverses the movement of the chyme, returning the larger particles to the body of the stomach for further churning and kneading. Because the pylorus is contracted during antral contraction, the gastric contents are emptied into the duodenum between contractions.

Although the pylorus does not contain a true anatomic sphincter, it does function as a physiologic sphincter to prevent the backflow of gastric contents and allow them to flow into the duodenum at a rate commensurate with the ability of the duodenum to accept them. This is important because the regurgitation of bile salts and duodenal contents can damage the antrum and lead to gastric ulcers. Likewise, the duodenum can be damaged by the rapid influx of highly acid gastric contents.

Like other parts of the gastrointestinal tract, the stomach is richly innervated by both intrinsic and extrinsic nerves. Axons from the intramural plexuses innervate the smooth muscles and glands of the stomach. Extrinsic parasympathetic innervation is provided by the vagus, and sympathetic innervation by the celiac ganglia. The emptying of the stomach is regulated by both hormonal and neural mechanisms. The hormones cholecystokinin and gastric inhibitory peptide, which are thought to control gastric emptying, are released in response to the osmolar, *p*H, and fatty acid composition of the chyme. Both local and central circuitry are involved in the neural control of gastric emptying. Afferent receptor fibers either synapse with the neurons in the intramural plexus or trigger intrinsic reflexes by means of the vagus or sympathetic pathways to participate in extrinsic reflexes.[3]

Disorders of gastric motility can occur when the rate is too slow or too fast (see the discussion in Chap. 42). A rate that is too slow causes gastric retention. It can be caused by either obstruction or gastric atony. Obstruction can result from the formation of scar tissue follow-

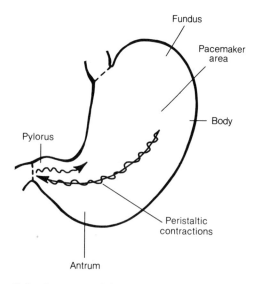

Figure 41-6 *Structures of the stomach, showing the pacemaker area and the direction of chyme movement resulting from peristaltic contractions.*

ing peptic ulcer. Another example of obstruction is hypertrophic pyloric stenosis. This can occur in infants with an abnormally thick muscularis layer in the terminal pylorus. Myotomy, or surgical incision of the muscular ring, is usually done to relieve the obstruction. Gastric atony can occur as a complication of visceral neuropathies in diabetes mellitus. Surgical procedures that disrupt vagal activity can also result in gastric atony. Abnormally fast emptying occurs in the dumping syndrome, which is a consequence of certain types of gastric surgeries. This condition is characterized by the rapid dumping of highly acidic and hyperosmotic gastric secretions into the duodenum.

Small Intestine Motility

The small intestine is the major site of the digestion and absorption of food; its movements are both mixing and propulsive. Regular peristaltic movements begin in the duodenum near the entry sites of the common duct and the main hepatic duct. A series of local pacemakers functions to maintain the frequency of intestinal contraction. The peristaltic movements (about 12 per minute in the jejunum) become less frequent as they move further from the pylorus, becoming about 9 per minute in the ileum. The contractions produce both segmentation waves and propulsive movements through the muscles of the small intestine. With segmentation waves, slow contractions of circular muscle occlude the lumen and drive the contents forward and backward. Most of the contractions that produce segmental waves are local events involving only 1 cm to 4 cm at a time. They function mainly to mix the chyme with the digestive enzymes from the pancreas and to ensure adequate exposure of all parts of the chyme to the mucosal surface of the intestine where absorption takes place. The frequency of segmenting activity increases after a meal. Presumably it is stimulated by receptors in the stomach and intestine, because the activity does not occur following denervation of the intestine. Propulsive movements occur with synchronized activity in a section 10 cm to 20 cm in length. They are accomplished by contraction of the proximal, or oral, portion of the intestine with the sequential relaxation of its distal, or anal, portion (Fig. 41-7). Once material has been propelled to the ileocecal junction by peristaltic movement, stretching of the distal ileum produces a local reflex that relaxes the sphincter and allows fluid to squirt into the cecum.

Motility disturbances of the small bowel are common, and auscultation of the abdomen can be used to assess bowel activity. Inflammatory changes increase motility. In many instances it is not certain whether changes in motility occur because of inflammation or secondary to toxins or secreted and unabsorbed mate-

Peristalsis

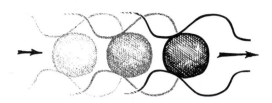

Figure 41-7 *Peristaltic movements in the intestine. Areas of contraction are preceded by areas of relaxation.*

rials. Delayed passage of materials in the small intestine can also be a problem. A condition called Hirschsprung's disease is characterized by a lack of neurons in the myenteric plexus in a segment of the intestine. Its correction requires surgical removal of the affected segment. Transient interruption of intestinal motility often occurs following gastrointestinal surgery. Intubation with suction is required to remove the accumulating intestinal contents and gases until activity is resumed.

Colonic Motility

As might be expected, the storage function of the *colon* dictates that movements within this section of the gut be different from those in the small intestine. Basically, movements in the colon are of two types. First are the segmental mixing movements, called *haustrations*, so named because they occur within the sacculations called haustra. These movements produce a local digging type of action which ensures that all portions of the fecal mass are exposed to the intestinal surface. Second are the *propulsive mass movements*, which may occur several times a day. Defecation is normally initiated by the mass movements.

Defecation

Defecation is controlled by the action of two sphincters, the *internal* and *external sphincters*. The internal sphincter is controlled by the autonomic nervous system, and the external sphincter is under the conscious control of the cerebral cortex.

The defecation reflex is integrated in the sacral segment of the spinal cord. In this reflex arc, afferent fibers from the rectum communicate with nerves in the sacral cord and with parasympathetic efferent fibers that move back to the bowel (see Fig. 41-5). The efferent signals from this reflex produce increased activity along the entire length of the large bowel. Other actions associated with defecation, such as abdominal pushing movements, are simultaneously integrated in the spinal cord. To prevent involuntary defecation from occurring, the external anal sphincter is under the conscious control of the cortex. Thus, as afferent impulses arrive at the sacral cord, signaling the presence of a distended rectum, messages are transmitted to the cortex. If defecation is inappropriate, the cortex initiates impulses that constrict the external sphincter and inhibit efferent parasympathetic activity. Normally, the afferent impulses in this reflex loop fatigue easily and the urge to defecate soon dies out. At a more convenient time, contraction of the abdominal muscles compresses the contents in the large bowel, reinitiating afferent impulses to the cord.

In summary, motility of the gastrointestinal tract moves food products and fluids along its length from mouth to anus. Although the activity of gastrointestinal smooth muscle is self-propagating and can continue without input from the nervous system, its rate and strength of contractions are regulated by a network of intramural neurons that receive input from the autonomic nervous system and local receptors that monitor wall stretch and the chemical composition of its luminal contents. Parasympathetic innervation occurs by means of the vagus and nerve fibers from sacral segments of the spinal cord; it serves to increase gastrointestinal motility. Sympathetic activity occurs by way of thoracolumbar output from the spinal cord, its paravertebral ganglia, and celiac, superior mesenteric, and inferior mesenteric ganglia. Sympathetic stimulation enhances sphincter function and reduces motility by inhibiting the activity of intramural plexus neurons.

■ Secretory Function

Each day about 7000 ml of fluid is secreted into the gastrointestinal tract (Table 41-1). Only about 50 ml to 200 ml of this fluid leaves the body in the stool; the remainder is reabsorbed in the small and large intestines. These secretions are mainly water and have a sodium and potassium concentration similar to that of extracellular fluid. Because water and electrolytes for digestive tract secretions are derived from the extracellular fluid compartment, excessive secretion or impaired absorption leads to extracellular fluid deficits.

Table 41-1   Secretions of the Gastrointestinal Tract

Secretions	Amount Daily (ml)
Salivary	1200
Gastric	2000
Pancreatic	1200
Biliary	700
Intestinal	2000
Total	7100

Control of Secretory Function

The secretory activity of the gut is influenced by local, humoral, and neural influences. Neural control of gastrointestinal secretory activity is mediated through the autonomic nervous system. As with motility, the parasympathetic nervous system increases secretory activity, whereas sympathetic activity has an inhibitory action. Many of the local influences, including pH, osmolality, and chyme, consistently act as stimuli for neural and humoral mechanisms.

Gastrointestinal Hormones

The gastrointestinal tract is the largest endocrine organ in the body. It produces hormones that pass from the portal circulation into the general circulation and then back to the digestive tract where they exert their action. Among the hormones produced by the gastrointestinal tract are *gastrin, secretin*, and *cholecystokinin*. These hormones influence motility and the secretion of electrolytes, enzymes, and other hormones. It has been observed that gastrin also influences the growth of the exocrine pancreas and the mucosa of the stomach and small intestine. It is reported that removal of the tissue that produces gastrin results in atrophy. This atrophy can be reversed by the administration of exogenous gastrin. The gastrointestinal tract hormones and their functions are summarized in Table 41-2.

Salivary Secretions

Saliva is secreted in the mouth. The salivary glands consist of the parotid, submaxillary, sublingual, and buccal glands. Saliva has three functions. The first of these is protection and lubrication. Saliva is rich in mucus, which serves to protect the oral mucosa and to coat the food as it passes through the mouth, pharynx, and esophagus. The sublingual and buccal glands produce only mucous types of secretions. The second function is its protective antimicrobial action. The saliva not only cleanses the mouth but contains the enzyme lysosome, which has an antibacterial action. Third, saliva contains ptyalin and amylase, which initiate the digestion of dietary starches. Of particular interest is the high potassium content in saliva—2 to 30 times that of plasma, depending on the rate of secretion. Secretions from the salivary glands are primarily regulated by the autonomic nervous system. Parasympathetic stimulation increases flow. The dry mouth that accompanies anxiety attests to the effects of sympathetic activity on salivary secretions.

Mumps, or *parotitis*, is an infection of the parotid glands. Although most of us associate mumps with the contagious viral form of the disease, inflammation of the

Table 41-2 Major Gastrointestinal Hormones and Their Actions

Hormone	Site of Secretion	Stimulus for Secretion	Action
Cholecystokinin	Duodenum, jejunum	Amino acids	Stimulation of contraction of gallbladder; stimulation of secretion of pancreatic enzymes; slowing of gastric emptying
Gastrin	Antrum of the stomach, duodenum	Vagal stimulation; epinephrine; neutral amino acids; solutions of calcium salts, including milk; alcohol *Release inhibited* by acid contents in the antrum of the stomach (below *p*H 2.5)	Stimulation of gastric acid and pepsinogen secretion; production of an increase in gastric blood flow; stimulation of gastric smooth muscle contraction; stimulation of growth of gastric mucosa, small intestine mucosa, and exocrine pancreas
Secretin	Duodenum	Acid *p*H of chyme entering duodenum (below *p*H 3.0)	Stimulation of secretion of bicarbonate-containing solution by pancreas and liver

parotid glands can occur in the seriously ill person who does not receive adequate oral hygiene and who is unable to take fluids orally. The drug potassium iodide increases the secretory activity of the salivary glands, including the parotid glands. In a small percentage of persons, parotid swelling may occur in the course of treatment with this drug.

Gastric Secretions

Three types of gastric glands in the stomach produce secretions: the cardiac, gastric, and pyloric glands. These glands are closely packed and oriented perpendicular to the mucosa, with one end opening into the surface epithelium. Both the cardiac glands (located in the vicinity of the esophageal orifice) and the pyloric glands (located in the distal 4 cm to 5 cm of the antrum) produce a protective mucus. The gastric glands, which are located in the fundic area of the stomach, contain chief cells, parietal cells, mucus-producing cells, and argentaffin cells. The parietal cells produce hydrochloric acid. There are about a billion parietal cells in the stomach; together they produce and secrete about 20 mEq of hydrochloric acid in several hundred milliliters of gastric juice each hour. The chief cells secrete pepsinogen, which is rapidly converted to pepsin because of the low *p*H of the gastric juices. Some of the argentaffin cells produce serotonin (5-hydroxytryptamine). Similar cells, located in the antrum, produce gastrin. Gastric intrinsic factor, which is produced by the parietal cells, is necessary for the absorption of vitamin B_{12}.

One of the important characteristics of the gastric mucosa is its resistance to the highly acid secretions that it produces, a property derived from the mucosa's imper-

meability to hydrogen ions. When the gastric mucosa is damaged by aspirin, indomethacin, ethyl alcohol, or bile salts, this impermeability is disrupted and the hydrogen ions move into the tissue. This is called breaking the mucosal barrier, and substances that alter the permeability are called barrier breakers. As the hydrogen ions accumulate in the mucosal cells, intracellular *p*H decreases, enzymatic reactions become impaired, and cellular structures are disrupted. The result is local ischemia, vascular stasis, hypoxia, and tissue necrosis. The mucosal surface is further protected by prostaglandins. Aspirin and indomethacin inhibit prostaglandin synthesis, which impairs the integrity of the mucosal surface.

Both parasympathetic stimulation (via the vagus) and gastrin increase gastric secretions. It has long been known that histamine increases gastric-acid secretions. Recent research and clinical use of the histamine-H_2 receptor antagonists suggest that histamine may be the final common pathway for gastric-acid production. Gastric-acid secretion and its relationship to peptic ulcer are discussed in Chapter 42.

Tests of gastric acid production

A laboratory procedure called gastric analysis is done to assess the hydrochloric acid content of gastric secretions. This procedure involves the withdrawal of samples of gastric secretions through a tube that has been inserted into the stomach. Histamine or its analog may be administered subcutaneously during the sampling procedure for the purpose of stimulating acid production. When pernicious anemia is present, such stimulation fails to increase acid levels. In this case, the observed achlorhydria is said to be histamine fast. A second means for assessing hydrochloric acid secretion is a method called *tubeless gastric analysis.* Tubeless gastric analysis is a screening test that involves the use of a cation resin dye. An acid *p*H of less than 3.5 is required so that the dye can be released and absorbed in the small intestine. The presence of dye in the urine is interpreted to mean that sufficient hydrochloric acid is in the stomach to maintain a *p*H that favors dye absorption.

Intestinal Secretions

The *small intestine* both secretes digestive juices and receives secretions from the liver and pancreas (Chap. 43). Mucus-producing glands are concentrated in the duodenum at the site where the contents from stomach and secretions from the liver and pancreas enter. These glands, called *Brunner's glands*, serve to protect the duodenum from the acid content in the gastric chyme and from the action of the digestive enzymes. The activity of Brunner's glands is strongly influenced by autonomic factors. For example, sympathetic stimulation causes a marked decrease in mucus production, leaving this area more susceptible to irritation. Interestingly, 50% of peptic ulcers occur at this site.

In addition to mucus, the intestinal mucosa produces two other types of secretions. The first is a secretion of a serous type of fluid (*p*H 6.5-7.5) by specialized cells (crypts of Lieberkühn) in the intestinal mucosal layer. This fluid, which is produced at the rate of 2000 ml/day, acts as a diluent for absorption. The second type consists of surface enzymes that aid absorption. These enzymes are the peptidases—enzymes that separate amino acids—and the disaccharidases—enzymes that split sugars.

The *large intestine* usually secretes only mucus. Autonomic nervous system activity strongly influences mucus production by the bowel, as in other parts of the digestive tract. During intense parasympthetic stimulation, mucus secretion may increase to the point at which the stool contains large amounts of obvious mucus. Although the bowel normally does not secrete water or electrolytes, these substances are lost in large quantities when the bowel becomes irritated or inflamed.

In summary, the secretions of the gastrointestinal tract include saliva, gastric juices, bile, and pancreatic and intestinal secretions. Each day more than 7000 ml of fluid are secreted into the digestive tract; all but 50 ml to 200 ml of these fluids are reabsorbed. Water, derived from the extracellular fluid compartment, is the major component of gastrointestinal tract secretions. Neural, humoral, and local mechanisms contribute to the control of these secretions. The parasympathetic nervous system increases secretion, whereas sympathetic activity exerts an inhibitory effect. In addition to secreting fluids containing digestive enzymes, the gastrointestinal tract produces and secretes hormones, such as gastrin, secretin, and cholecystokinin, that contribute to the control of gastrointestinal function.

■ Digestion and Absorption

Digestion is the process of dismantling foods into their constituent parts, which are small enough to be absorbed. Digestion requires hydrolysis, enzyme cleavage, and fat emulsification. Hydrolysis is the breakdown of a compound that involves a chemical reaction with water. The importance of hydrolysis to digestion is evidenced by the amount of water (7-8 liters) that is secreted into the gastrointestinal tract daily.

Absorption occurs mainly in the small intestine. The stomach is a poor absorptive structure, and only a few lipid-soluble substances, including alcohol, are absorbed from the stomach. The absorptive function of the large intestine focuses mainly on water reabsorption.

The mucosal surface of the small intestine is designed to facilitate absorption (Fig. 41-8). The mucosal folds, the villi, and the microvilli in the small intestine increase its absorptive capacity 600-fold, providing a total surface area of about 250 square meters.

Absorption for the intestine is accomplished by active transport and diffusion. A number of substances require a specific transport carrier or system. For example, vitamin B_{12} is not absorbed in the absence of intrinsic factor. Transport of amino acid and glucose occurs only in the presence of sodium. Water is absorbed passively, obeying the usual laws of osmosis.

The small intestine is involved primarily in the digestion and absorption of nutrients. The intestinal mucosa is impermeable to most large molecules. Therefore, most proteins, fats, and carbohydrates must be broken down into smaller particles before they can be absorbed. Although some digestion of carbohydrates and proteins begins in the stomach, digestion takes place mainly in the small intestine. The hydrolysis of fats to free fatty acids and monoglycerides takes place entirely in the small intestine. The liver, with its production of bile, and the pancreas, which supplies a number of digestive enzymes, also play important roles in digestion.

The distinguishing characteristics of the small intestine is its large surface area, which in the adult is estimated to be about 4500 m². Anatomic features that contribute to this enlarged surface area are the circular folds that extend into the lumen of the intestine and the villi, which are fingerlike projections of mucous membrane numbering as many as 25,000, that line the entire small intestine. Each villus is covered with cells called enterocytes that contribute to the absorptive and digestive functions of the small bowel and goblet cells that provide mucus. The crypts of Lieberkühn are glan-

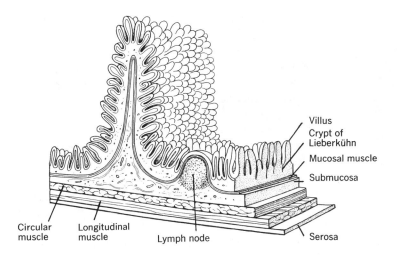

Figure 41-8 *The mucous membrane of the small intestine. Note the numerous villi on a circular fold. (Chaffee EE, Lytle IM: Basic Physiology and Anatomy, 4th ed. Philadelphia, JB Lippincott, 1980)*

dular structures that open into the spaces between the villi. The enterocytes have a life span of about 4 to 5 days, and it is believed that replacement cells differentiate from cells located in the area of the crypts. The maturing enterocytes migrate up the villus and are eventually extruded from the tip.

Each villus is equipped with an artery, vein, and lymph vessel (lacteal), which brings blood to the surface of the intestine and transports the nutrients and other materials that have passed into the blood from the lumen of the intestine (Fig. 41-9). Fats rely largely on the lymphatics for absorption. This means that a decrease in blood flow to the gut, which is caused by atherosclerosis or heart failure, may impair absorption of nutrients. Another cause of malabsorption is lymphatic obstruction resulting from lymphoma.

The enterocytes secrete a number of proteins, including enzymes that aid in the digestion of carbohydrates and proteins. These enzymes are called *brush border enzymes* because they adhere to the border of the villus structures. In this way they have access to the carbohydrates and protein molecules as they come in contact with the absorptive surface of the intestine. This mechanism of secretion places the enzymes where they are needed and eliminates the need to produce enough enzymes to mix with the entire contents that fill the lumen of the small bowel. The digested molecules either diffuse through the membrane or are actively transported across the mucosal surface to enter the blood or, in the case of fatty acids, the lacteal. These molecules are then transported through the portal vein or lymphatics into the systemic circulation.

Carbohydrate Absorption

Carbohydrates must be broken down into monosaccharides, or single sugars, before they can be absorbed from the small intestine. The average daily intake of

carbohydrate in the American diet is about 350 gm to 400 gm. Starch makes up about 50% of this total, sucrose (table sugar) about 30%, lactose (milk sugar) about 6%, and maltose about 1.5%.[4] Digestion of starch begins in the mouth with the action of amylase. Pancreatic secretions also contain an amylase. As a result of the action of amylase, starch is broken down into several disaccharides, including maltose, isomaltose, and α-dextrins. It is the brush border enzymes that convert the disaccharides into monosaccharides that can be absorbed (Table 41-3). Sucrose yields glucose and fructose, lactose is converted to glucose and galactose,

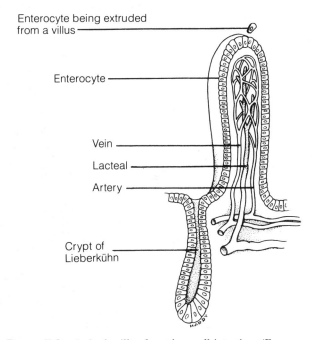

Figure 41-9 *A single villus from the small intestine. (From Chaffee EE, Lytle IM: Basic Physiology and Anatomy, 4th ed. Philadelphia, JB Lippincott, 1980)*

Table 41-3   Enzymes Used in Digestion of Carbohydrates

Dietary Carbohydrates	Enzyme	Monosaccharides Produced
Lactose	Lactase	Glucose and galactose
Sucrose	Sucrase	Fructose and glucose
Starch	Amylase	
Maltose and maltotriose	Maltase	Glucose and glucose
α-Dextrins	Isomaltase	Glucose and glucose

and maltose is changed to glucose. When the disaccharides are not broken down to monosaccharides, they cannot be absorbed but remain as osmotically active particles in the contents of the digestive system causing diarrhea.

Fructose is transported across the intestinal mucosa by facilitated diffusion, which does not require energy expenditure. In this case, fructose moves along a concentration gradient. Glucose and galactose, on the other hand, are transported by way of a sodium-dependent carrier system that utilizes ATP as an energy source (Fig. 41-10). Water absorption from the intestine is linked to absorption of osmotically active particles, such as glucose and sodium. It follows that an important consideration in facilitating the transport of water across the intestine (and decreasing diarrhea) following temporary disruption in bowel function is to include both sodium and glucose in the fluids that are taken. A number of carbonated soft drinks can be used for this purpose.

Lactase deficiency

The most common disaccharidase deficiency involves lactase. Although human infants have a high concentration of lactase following birth, this concentration falls rapidly in the first 4 to 5 years of life and may reach low levels in adolescence and adult life. It has been estimated that 3% to 19% of the adult white population, 70% of American blacks, and 90% of native Americans are deficient in lactase.[5] With a lactase deficiency, intolerance to milk occurs, manifested in bloating, flatulence, cramping abdominal pain, and diarrhea. These symptoms are usually relieved by avoiding lactose (milk) in the diet. Recently, yogurt has been shown to be a well-tolerated source of milk for lactase-deficient persons.[6]

The fact that lactase availability declines following childhood and may be rather limited in the adult may help to explain why milk is sometimes poorly tolerated following gastrointestinal tract "flu" or other disorders. One can assume that with a limited ability to produce lactase, any disruption in the regeneration of intestinal mucosa might reduce lactase levels to a point at which a temporary deficiency could occur.

Fat Absorption

The average adult eats about 60 gm to 100 gm of fat daily, principally as triglycerides containing long-chain fatty acids. These triglycerides are broken down by pancreatic lipase. Bile salts act as a carrier system for the fatty acids and fat-soluble vitamins A, D, E, and K by forming micelles, which transport these substances to the surface of intestinal villi where they are absorbed. The major site of fat absorption is the upper jejunum. Medium-chain triglycerides, with fatty acids of lengths C-6 to C-10, are absorbed better than longer chains of fatty acids because they are more completely hydrolyzed by pancreatic lipase and they form micelles more easily. Because they are easily absorbed, medium-chain triglycerides are often used in the treatment of persons with malabsorption syndrome. The absorption of vitamins A, D, E, and K, which are fat-soluble vitamins, requires bile salts.

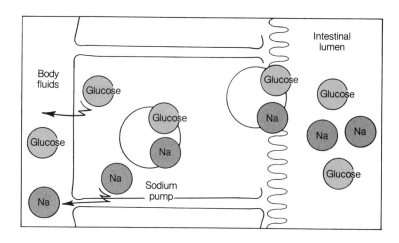

Figure 41-10 *The hypothetical sodium-dependent transport system for glucose. The concentration of glucose builds up within the intestinal cell until a diffusion gradient develops, causing glucose to move into the body fluids. Sodium is transported out of the cell by the energy-dependent (ATP) sodium pump. This creates the gradient needed to operate the transport system.*

Fat that is not absorbed in the intestine is excreted in the stool. *Steatorrhea* is the term used to describe fatty stools. It usually indicates that there are 20 gm or more fat in a 24-hour stool sample.[2] Normally, a chemical test is done on a 72-hour stool collection, during which time the diet is restricted to 80 gm to 100 gm of fat per day.

Protein Absorption

Proteins are broken down by pancreatic enzymes, such as trypsin, chymotrypsin, carboxypeptidase, and elastase. The amino acids are liberated either intramurally or on the surface of the villi by brush border enzymes that degrade proteins into one, two, and three amino acid particles. These amino acids are transported across the mucosal membrane in a sodium-linked process that utilizes ATP as an energy source.

In summary, the digestion and absorption of foodstuffs take place in the small intestine. Proteins, fats, carbohydrates, and other components of the diet are broken down into molecules that can be transported from the intestinal lumen into the body fluids.

■ Study Guide

After you have studied this chapter, you should be able to meet the following objectives:

☐ Describe the physiologic function of the four parts of the digestive system.

☐ Describe the function of the intramural plexuses in control of gastrointestinal function.

☐ Differentiate between sites of tonic and rhythmic contraction in the gastrointestinal tract.

☐ Compare the effect of parasympathetic and sympathetic activity on motility and secretory function of the gastrointestinal tract.

☐ Describe the physiology of peristalsis.

☐ List stimuli for gastrointestinal mechanoreceptors and chemoreceptors.

☐ Trace a bolus of food through the stages of swallowing.

☐ Describe at least two general disorders of gastric motility.

☐ Cite the pathology of Hirschsprung's disease.

☐ Describe the action of the internal and external sphincters in control of defecation.

☐ State the source of water and electrolytes in digestive secretions.

☐ Explain the protective function of saliva.

☐ Describe the function of the gastric secretions in the process of digestion.

☐ List three major gastrointestinal hormones and cite their function.

☐ Describe the site of gastric acid and pepsin production and secretion in the stomach.

☐ Relate the actions of aspirin and alcohol to the disruption of the integrity of the gastric mucosa.

☐ State the effect of sympathetic stimulation on mucus production by Brunner's glands.

☐ Name the secretions of the small and the large intestine.

☐ Describe the characteristics of the small intestine in relation to its absorptive function.

☐ Explain the function of intestinal brush border enzymes.

☐ Compare the absorption of carbohydrates, fats, and proteins.

■ References

1. Thompson JS: Core Textbook of Anatomy, p 292. Philadelphia, JP Lippincott, 1977
2. Davenport HW: Physiology of the Digestive Tract, ed 5, pp 4, 229. Chicago, Year Book Medical Publishers, 1982
3. Berne RM, Levy MN: Physiology, pp 755, 760. St Louis, CV Mosby, 1983
4. Castro GA: Digestion and absorption of specific nutrients. In Johnson LR (ed): Gastrointestinal Physiology, p 122. St Louis, CV Mosby, 1977
5. Kosek MS: Medical genetics. In Krupp MA, Chatton MJ (eds): Current Medical Diagnosis and Treatment, p 1045. Los Altos, Lange Medical Publications, 1984
6. Kolars JC, Levitt MD, Motafa A et al: Yogurt—An autodigesting source of lactose. N Engl J Med 310:1, 1984

Chapter 42

Alterations in Gastrointestinal Function

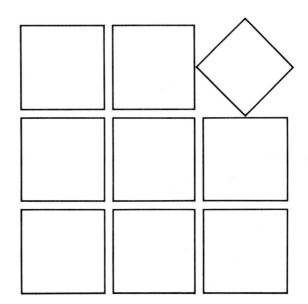

Gastrointestinal disorders are not cited as the leading cause of death in the United States, nor do they receive the same publicity as heart disease and cancer. Yet, according to government reports, digestive diseases rank third in the total economic burden of illness, causing considerable human suffering, personal expenditures for treatment, lost working hours, and a drain on the nation's economy. It has been estimated that 20 million Americans, one out of every nine persons in the United States, have digestive disease.[1] Even more important is the fact that proper nutrition or a change in health practices could prevent or minimize many of these disorders. The content of this chapter focuses on three types of gastrointestinal disorders: (1) disorders that result in alterations in the integrity of the gastrointestinal tract, (2) alterations in the digestive and absorptive functions of the gastrointestinal tract, and (3) altered motility of the gastrointestinal tract.

■ Manifestations of Gastrointestinal Tract Disorders

Several signs and symptoms are common to many types of gastrointestinal disorders. These include anorexia, nausea, vomiting, eating disorders, and gastrointestinal bleeding. Because they occur with so many of the disorders, they are discussed separately as an introduction to the content that follows.

Anorexia

Anorexia is loss of appetite. A number of factors influence appetite. One of these factors is hunger, which is stimulated by contractions of the empty stomach. The desire for food intake is also regulated by the hypothalamus and other associated centers in the brain. Smell plays an important role, as evidenced by the fact that appetite can be stimulated or suppressed by the smell of food. Loss of appetite is associated with emotional situations, such as fear, depression, frustration, and anxiety. Many drugs and disease states cause anorexia. In uremia, for example, the accumulation of nitrogenous wastes in the blood contributes to the development of anorexia. Anorexia is often a forerunner of nausea, and most conditions that cause nausea and vomiting also produce anorexia.

Nausea

Nausea is an ill-defined and unpleasant subjective sensation. It is basically a conscious recognition of stimulation of the medullary vomiting center. Nausea is usually preceded by anorexia, and stimuli such as foods and drugs that cause anorexia in small doses will usually produce nausea when given in larger doses. A common cause of nausea is distention of the duodenum, or upper small intestinal tract. Nausea is frequently accompanied by autonomic responses such as watery salivation and vasoconstriction with pallor, sweating, and tachycardia. Nausea may function as an early warning signal of pathology.

Vomiting

Vomiting is the sudden and forceful oral expulsion of the contents of the stomach. It is usually, but not always, preceded by nausea. The contents that are vomited are called *vomitus.*

The act of vomiting is integrated by the *vomiting center,* which is located in the dorsal portion of the reticular formation of the medulla near the sensory nucleus of the vagus. The act of vomiting consists of taking a deep breath, closing the airways, and producing a strong, forceful contraction of the diaphragm and abdominal muscles along with relaxation of the gastroesophageal sphincter. Respiration ceases during the act of vomiting. Vomiting may be accompanied by dizziness, light-headedness, decrease in blood pressure, and bradycardia.

The vomiting center may be stimulated directly or by impulses from the chemoreceptor trigger zone or afferent neurons of the autonomic nervous system. Many chemicals and drugs incite nausea and vomiting. These agents exert their effect by stimulating the medullary *chemoreceptor trigger zone,* which relays impulses to the vomiting center. The phenothiazine derivatives, such as chlorpromazine (Thorazine) and prochlorperazine (Compazine), depress vomiting caused by stimulation of the chemoreceptor trigger zone. *Hypoxemia* exerts a direct effect on the vomiting center, producing nausea and vomiting. This direct effect probably accounts for the vomiting that occurs during periods of decreased cardiac output, shock, environmental hypoxia, and brain ischemia caused by increased intracranial pressure. Inflammation of any of the intra-abdominal organs, including the liver, gallbladder, or urinary tract, can cause vomiting because of stimulation of the *visceral afferent pathways* that communicate with the vomiting center. Distention or irritation of the gastrointestinal tract also causes vomiting through stimulation of visceral afferent neurons. Vomiting, as a basic physiologic protective mechanism, limits the possibility of damage from ingested noxious agents by emptying the contents of the stomach and portions of the small intestine. Nausea and vomiting may represent a total-body response to drug overdosage, cumulative effects, toxicity, and side effects.

Eating Disorders

Eating disorders include the abnormal intake of food despite a normally functioning gastrointestinal tract and appetite, pica, anorexia nervosa, and bulimarexia and bulimia. Obesity, a common problem related to food intake in excess of that needed to maintain normal weight, is not included in this discussion.

Pica

Pica is the chronic ingestion of paint, clay, starch, ice, or other nonnutritive substances. There is usually no aversion to food or distorted perception of body image or weight, as in anorexia nervosa. Pica is most commonly seen in association with cultural beliefs (eating of white clay during pregnancy), deficiencies of minerals such as iron and zinc, and mental retardation. Its dangers include toxicity from the material ingested (lead poisoning from paint), malnutrition from lack of a balanced diet (starch or clay ingestion), and problems associated with untreated conditions such as iron-deficiency anemia.

Anorexia nervosa

Anorexia nervosa is a well-known eating disorder. Its diagnosis is based on the progressive loss of at least 25% of ideal weight, resulting in protein–calorie malnutrition. The disorder is almost 20 times more prevalent in young women than in men; the age of onset extends from midadolescence to the young adult years. The disorder is typically accompanied by grossly distorted attitudes about food, eating, and body weight. These attitudes perpetuate a state of intentional malnourishment despite hunger and threats and admonitions from others.[2]

Many organ systems are affected by the malnutrition that occurs in persons with anorexia nervosa. The severity of the abnormalities tends to be related to the degree of malnutrition and to be reversed with refeeding. Reduced gonadal function manifested by amenorrhea and the loss of secondary sex characteristics is typical of the disorder. Constipation, cold intolerance and failure to shiver in the cold, bradycardia and hypotension, decreased heart size and electrocardiographic changes, and dry skin with lanugo (increased amounts of fine hair) are common. Unexpected sudden deaths have been reported; the risk appears to increase as the weight drops to less than 35% to 40% of ideal weight. These deaths are believed to be due to myocardial degeneration and heart failure.[2]

Bulimarexia and bulimia

Bulimarexia is an eating disorder characterized by binge eating followed by self-induced vomiting or abuse of cathartic or diuretic drugs. It has been described both as a sequela of anorexia nervosa and a distinct eating disorder. The purging behaviors that accompany binge eating distinguish bulimarexia from bulimia, in which there is binge eating without purging. The exact incidence of bulimarexia is unknown. The disorder was found to be present in 19% of college students in one study.[3] The ages of onset and highest prevalence parallel those of anorexia nervosa. The complications of bulimarexia include those resulting from overeating, self-induced vomiting, and cathartic and diuretic abuse.[4]

Among the complications of self-induced vomiting are dental disorders, esophagitis, fluid and electrolyte disorders, and parotitis. Dental abnormalities such as sensitive teeth, increased dental caries, and periodontal disease occur with frequent self-induced vomiting. This is because the frequent presence of vomitus with its high acid content causes tooth enamel to dissolve. Esophagitis, dysphagia, and esophageal strictures are common. With frequent vomiting, gastric contents often reflux into the lower esophagus because of relaxation of the lower esophageal sphincter. The relaxation of the lower esophageal sphincter also allows reflux of gastric contents between vomiting episodes. Vomiting may lead to aspiration pneumonia, especially in intoxicated or debilitated persons. Potassium, chloride, and hydrogen are lost in the vomitus, and frequent vomiting also predisposes to metabolic alkalosis with hypokalemia (Chaps. 25 and 27). An unexplained physical response to bulimarexia is the development of benign, painless parotid gland enlargement.

The use of emetic drugs and cathartics is associated with problems of drug overdose and abuse. Excessive doses of syrup of ipecac, which is sometimes used to induce vomiting, can produce serious cardiac disorders, including conduction defects, dysrhythmias, and myocarditis. Chronic laxative use disrupts intestinal motility and normal bowel habits and poses a risk of serum electrolyte imbalance. The most common complication of diuretic abuse is potassium deficiency.

Gastrointestinal Tract Bleeding

Bleeding from the gastrointestinal tract can be evidenced by blood that appears in either the vomitus or the feces. It can result from disease or trauma to the gastrointestinal structures, as a result of primary diseases of the blood vessels (*i.e.*, esophageal varices or hemorrhoids), or because of disorders in blood clotting.

Hematemesis

The presence of blood in the stomach is usually irritating and causes vomiting. Hematemesis refers to blood in the vomitus. It may be bright red or have a "coffee ground" appearance because of the action of the digestive enzymes.

Melena

Blood that appears in the stool may range in color from bright red to tarry black. Bright-red blood usually indicates that the bleeding is from the lower bowel. When it coats the stool, it is often the result of bleeding hemorrhoids. The word *melena* means black and refers to the passage of black and tarry stools. These stools have a characteristic odor that is not easily forgotten. The presence of tarry stools usually indicates that the source of bleeding is above the level of the ileocecal valve, although this is not always the case. With hypermotility of the gastrointestinal tract, bright-red blood may be present in the stools even though the bleeding is from the upper gastrointestinal tract. Melena can occur when as little as 100 ml of blood enters the gastrointestinal tract.[5] Furthermore, tarry stools have been shown to continue for as long as 3 days to 5 days following administration of 1000 ml to 2000 ml of blood into the gastrointestinal tract, indicating that melena is not necessarily a good sign of continued bleeding.[6] *Occult* (hidden) blood that can only be detected by chemical means, may persist for 2 weeks to 3 weeks.[5]

Blood urea nitrogen (BUN) is frequently elevated following hematemesis or melena. This results from breakdown of the blood by the digestive enzymes and the absorption of the nitrogenous end products into the blood. The BUN usually reaches a peak within 24 hours following the gastrointestinal hemorrhage. It does not appear when the bleeding is in the colon, because digestion does not take place at this level of the digestive system. An elevation in body temperature also usually follows gastrointestinal hemorrhage. This also occurs within 24 hours and may last for a few days to a few weeks.

In summary, many gastrointestinal tract disorders are manifested by anorexia, nausea, and vomiting. Anorexia, or loss of appetite, may occur alone or may accompany nausea and vomiting. Nausea, which is an ill-defined, unpleasant sensation, signals the stimulation of the medullary vomiting center. It often precedes vomiting and is frequently accompanied by autonomic responses such as salivation and vasoconstriction with pallor, sweating, and tachycardia. The act of vomiting, which is integrated by the vomiting center, involves the forceful oral expulsion of the gastric contents. It is a basic physiologic mechanism that rids the gastrointestinal tract of noxious agents. Anorexia nervosa, bulimarexia, and bulemia are eating disorders. In anorexia nervosa distorted attitudes about eating lead to serious weight loss and malnutri-

tion. Bulemia is characterized by binge eating, and bulimarexia by binge eating and purging with self-induced vomiting, laxatives, or diuretics. Disorders that disrupt the integrity of the gastrointestinal tract often cause bleeding, which can be manifested as blood in the vomitus (hematemesis) or as blood in the stool (melena).

■ Alterations in the Integrity of the Gastrointestinal Tract Wall

Characteristic of the gastrointestinal tract is the mucous membrane that lines its entire length from mouth to anus. This mucosal layer varies somewhat in structure, depending on its location and function. In the upper part of the digestive tract (mouth and esophagus) the mucus produced by the goblet cells acts as a lubricant to facilitate passage of food particles. In the stomach and small intestine, the mucous membrane is required to withstand the corrosive effects of hydrochloric acid and digestive enzymes. The mucosal layer in the small intestine is designed to facilitate absorption of nutrients.

The mucus-producing cells of the epithelial layer of the gastrointestinal tract have a rapid turnover rate of about 4 to 5 days. During periods of irritation or injury, this turnover rate is increased and the cells are shed at a more rapid rate. When this occurs, the rate of replacement does not always keep pace with the rate of cell loss, and the area becomes denuded, reddened, and swollen. Fortunately, the mucosal surface heals rapidly, and the area usually regenerates within a few days once the irritating stimulus has been removed. Cell regeneration is impaired, however, when the injury is extensive or prolonged. Radiation, anticancer drugs, and other factors that impair the growth of rapidly proliferating cells interfere with regeneration of the gastrointestnal mucosal lining. Treatment with anticancer agents frequently causes such side effects as stomatitis, anorexia, nausea, vomiting, and diarrhea.

Smooth muscle of the gastrointestinal tract heals by scar tissue replacement. Thus, when the injury extends into the smooth muscle layer, regeneration of both the muscularis and the mucosal layers is impaired; this renders the area more susceptible to future irritation and injury.

Esophagus

The esophagus is a tube that connects the oropharynx with the stomach. It lies posterior to the trachea and larynx and extends through the mediastinum, intersecting the diaphragm at the level of the 11th thoracic vertebra. The esophagus functions primarily as a conduit for passage of food from the pharynx to the stomach, and the structures of its walls are designed for this purpose; the smooth muscle layers provide the peristaltic movements needed to move food along its length, while the epithelial layer secretes mucus, which protects its surface and aids in lubricating food.

Dysphagia

The act of swallowing is dependent on the coordinated action of the tongue and pharynx. These structures are innervated by the 5th, 9th, 10th, and 12th cranial nerves. *Dysphagia* refers to difficulty in deglutition (the act of swallowing). It can result from altered nerve function or from narrowing of the esophagus. Lesions of the central nervous system, such as a stroke, often involve the cranial nerves that control deglutition. Cancer of the esophagus and stenosis resulting from scarring reduce the size of the esophageal lumen and make swallowing difficult.

Achalasia

In achalasia the lower esophageal sphincter fails to relax. Food that has been swallowed has difficulty passing into the stomach, and the esophagus above the sphincter becomes enlarged. One or several meals may lodge in the esophagus and pass slowly into the stomach over a period of time. There is the risk of aspiration of esophageal contents into the lungs when the person lies down. Treatment is mechanical dilatation or surgical procedures to weaken the sphincter.

Esophagitis

Esophagitis refers to inflammation of the esophagus. Causative agents include chemical injury (lye, ammonia, and other caustic substances), infections, and trauma from repeated ingestion of irritating foods, such as hot liquids and spicy foods. The most common cause of esophagitis is the reflux of gastric secretions into the esophagus as the result of a hiatal hernia. Symptoms associated with esophagitis include heartburn and pain. The pain is usually located in the epigastric or retrosternal area and often radiates to the throat, shoulder, or back. As with inflammation of the mucosal layer in other parts of the gastrointestinal tract, esophagitis causes hyperemia, edema, and erosion of the luminal surface. When the damage is severe or prolonged, scarring occurs and the wall of the esophagus becomes thickened and fibrotic; this leads to difficulty in swallowing.

Hiatal hernia

A hiatal, or diaphragmatic, hernia is the herniation of the stomach through the diaphragm into the thorax. Because intra-abdominal pressure is greater than thoracic pressure, the main problem associated with a hiatal hernia is reflux of gastric secretions into the esophagus.

There are two types of hiatal hernias. The more common one is the sliding type in which the esophagogastric junction slides into the thoracic cavity when the person lies down, then moves back into the abdomen when the person assumes the upright position. The rolling, or paraesophageal, hernia is the condition in which the gastroesophageal junction remains in its normal anatomic position while the curvature of the stomach herniates through the diaphragmatic opening (Fig. 42-1).

Conditions that predispose to the development of a hiatal hernia and reflux of gastric contents into the esophagus include (1) congenital or acquired weakness of the hiatal muscle, (2) conditions that increase intra-

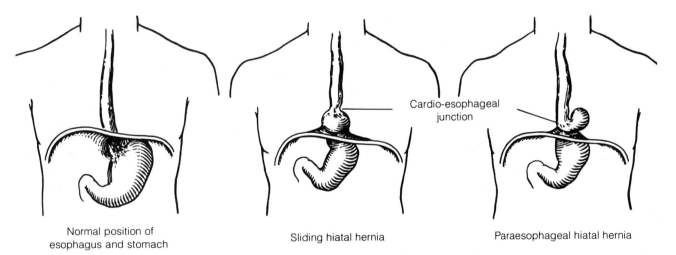

Normal position of esophagus and stomach

Sliding hiatal hernia

Cardio-esophageal junction

Paraesophageal hiatal hernia

Figure 42-1 *Normal position of the esophagus and stomach and positional changes that occur with a sliding and paraesophageal hernia. (From Brunner LS, Suddarth DS: Textbook of Medical Surgical Nursing, 3rd ed. Philadelphia, JB Lippincott, 1975)*

abdominal pressure (*e.g.,* obesity, pregnancy, tight-fitting clothes, and ascites), or (3) a congenital or acquired shortening of the esophagus. The latter can occur with extensive scarring of the esophagus or can result from reflex spasms.

The signs and symptoms of a hiatal hernia are related to the reflux of gastric contents into the esophagus. The most common manifestation is pain and heartburn, which occur about ½ hour to 1 hour following a meal. Heartburn is aggravated by any bodily position, such as the recumbent position, that increases the reflux. Often the heartburn occurs during the night. Because of its location, the pain may be confused with angina. Swelling or stenosis caused by scar tissue may cause dysphagia.

The treatment of a hiatal hernia generally focuses on conservative measures. These measures include avoidance of positions and conditions that increase gastric reflux. Frequent, small feedings are preferred to large meals because they prevent gastric distention. It is recommended that meals be eaten sitting up and that the recumbent position be avoided for several hours following a meal. Bending for long periods should be avoided, since it tends to increase intra-abdominal pressure and cause gastric reflux. Sleeping with several pillows helps to prevent reflux during the night. When esophagitis occurs, it may be necessary to institute treatment measures, such as the use of antacids, to reduce gastric secretions. Surgical treatment may become necessary when persistent gastric reflux causes damage to the esophageal wall and cannot be controlled by conservative means.

Esophageal diverticulum

A diverticulum of the esophagus is an outpouching of the esophageal wall caused by a weakness of the muscularis layer. An esophageal diverticulum tends to retain food. Complaints that the food stops before it reaches the stomach are very common, as are reports of gurgling, belching, coughing, and foul-smelling breath. Additionally, the trapped food may cause esophagitis and ulceration. Because the condition is usually progressive, correction of the defect requires surgical intervention.

Carcinoma of the esophagus

Carcinoma of the esophagus accounts for 2% of all cancer deaths in the United States. This disease is common in men over age 60.[3] It is reported that environmental factors contribute to the development of esophageal cancers. These environmental factors include (1) alterations in function that cause food or drink to remain in the esophagus for prolonged periods of time, (2) reflux esophagitis, and (3) continued exposure to irritants such as alcohol and tobacco. The incidence of esophageal cancer among heavy drinkers is 25 times greater than that of nondrinkers. In contrast to cancer of the lung,

esophageal cancer is seen more frequently among pipe and cigar smokers than cigarette smokers. Unfortunately, the outlook for persons with cancer of the esophagus is particularly grim, the 5-year survival rate being only about 4%.[8] This is because the tumor has usually spread to other areas before symptoms develop.

Stomach

The stomach is a large reservoir for the digestive tract; it lies in the upper abdomen, anterior to the pancreas, splenic vessels, and left kidney. Anteriorly, the stomach is bounded by the anterior abdominal wall and the left inferior lobe of the liver. While in the stomach, food is churned and mixed with hydrochloric acid and pepsin before being released into the small intestine.

Gastritis

Acute gastritis. Acute gastritis is a transient irritation of the gastric mucosa caused by local irritants such as bacterial endotoxins, caffeine, alcohol, and aspirin. Normally, the stomach lining is impermeable to the acid it secretes, a property that allows the stomach to contain acid and pepsin without having its wall digested. It is becoming increasingly evident that the production of prostaglandins is an important factor in protecting the gastrointestinal mucosa against the injurious effects of irritating luminal agents. The mechanism by which this works is unknown. Drugs such as aspirin and indomethacin inhibit prostaglandin production. Occult bleeding due to gastric irritation occurs in a significant number of persons who take aspirin on a regular basis (*e.g.,* as a treatment for arthritis).[9] Alcohol is also known to disrupt the mucosal barrier; and when aspirin and alcohol are taken in combination, as they often are, there is increased risk of gastric irritation.

The complaints of persons with acute gastritis vary. Often, persons with aspirin-related gastritis are totally unaware of the condition or may complain only of heartburn or sour stomach. Gastritis associated with excessive alcohol consumption is a different situation: it often causes transient gastric distress, which may lead to vomiting and in more severe situations, to bleeding and hematemesis. Gastritis caused by infectious organisms, such as the staphylococcus endotoxins, usually has an abrupt and violent onset, with gastric distress and vomiting, following the ingestion of a contaminated food source by about 5 hours. Acute gastritis is usually a self-limiting disorder; complete regeneration and healing usually occur within several days.

Chronic gastritis. Chronic gastritis is a separate entity from that of acute gastritis. This condition is characterized by progressive and irreversible atrophy of the glandular epithelium of the stomach. Atrophy of the epithelial layer involves the pepsin-producing chief cells and the acid-producing parietal cells. The parietal cells also produce intrinsic factor, which is required for vitamin B_{12} absorption. This means that both achlorhydria (lack of hydrochloric acid) and pernicious anemia occur when there is extensive atrophy of the gastric mucosa.

There appear to be two forms of chronic gastritis. The most common form is referred to as *simple atrophic gastritis*. Simple atrophic gastritis is seen most frequently in elderly persons and in heavy drinkers or cigarette smokers. A second form of the disorder, *autoimmune atrophic gastritis,* is thought to be caused by antibodies that destroy gastric mucosal cells. With the simple form of the disease there is usually only moderate impairment of acid and pepsin secretion, and vitamin B_{12} absorption remains unimpaired. This retention of acid production in a mucosal surface that has impaired defenses predisposes to peptic ulcer formation. Persons with autoimmune gastritis usually have severe impairment of acid and pepsin secretion, and about 20% of such persons have pernicious anemia.

The signs and symptoms of chronic gastritis are rather vague. Often the disorder produces no discernible symptoms. Symptoms, when they do occur, range from mild distress to complaints similar to those of peptic ulcer. In contrast to gastric ulcer pain, the discomfort associated with atrophic gastritis is not relieved by antacid therapy, nor does true gastritis pain occur during the night.

The clinical significance of atrophic gastritis resides not in its symptoms, but in its ability to produce more serious disorders—namely, pernicious anemia. Although chronic gastritis can occur without impairment of vitamin B_{12} absorption, pernicious anemia develops only in its presence. When pernicious anemia is present, there is an accompanying histamine-fast lack of hydrochloric acid.

Atrophic gastritis also predisposes to gastric ulcer, anemia, and cancer of the stomach. It has been estimated that 50% of persons with gastric ulcers have an associated chronic gastritis. A second problem that frequently occurs with chronic gastritis is a recurrent iron-deficiency anemia. The cause of this anemia is unclear, although there is evidence to suggest that a minimum level of hydrochloric acid is required for iron absorption. A more serious outcome is cancer of the stomach. Approximately 7% to 10% of persons with atrophic gastritis eventually develop gastric carcinoma.[9]

Peptic ulcers

Gastric and peptic ulcers, with their remissions and exacerbations, represent a chronic health problem. At present, 10% of the population has or will develop a peptic ulcer. As a health problem, ulcer disease accounts for 10% of hospital admissions. In terms of location, duodenal ulcers are five to ten times more common than gastric ulcers. Ulcers in the duodenum occur at any age and are frequently seen in early adulthood. Interestingly, duodenal ulcers seem to have a seasonal trend, with a higher incidence of recurrence in the spring and fall. Gastric ulcers, on the other hand, tend to affect the older age group with peak incidence in the sixth and seventh decades. Both types of ulcers affect men three to four times as frequently as they do women.

At present, there is considerable confusion regarding the terms *peptic ulcer* and *gastric ulcer*. A peptic ulcer can occur in any area of the gastrointestinal tract that is exposed to acid–pepsin secretions. For example, ulcerations in the esophagus caused by reflux of gastric secretions would be classified as a peptic ulcer. Peptic ulcers also occur in the stomach, in the duodenum, at the surgical junction where the stomach has been resected and joined to the jejunum (gastrojejunostomy), and in a Meckel's diverticulum that contains misplaced gastric tissue. A gastric ulcer, as the word implies, is an ulcer of the stomach. An ulcer of the stomach can be either a peptic gastric ulcer or a gastric ulcer associated with chronic gastritis. The remaining discussion of ulcers focuses on peptic ulcer, although the reader is reminded that not all stomach ulcers are peptic ulcers.

Predisposing factors. A peptic ulcer represents a break in the continuity of the mucosal layer. Generally speaking, it can be said that peptic ulcer formation reflects (1) an imbalance between acid and pepsin production or (2) an inability of the affected mucosal layer to resist the destructive action of these digestive agents. Evidence suggests that hydrochloric acid is an important causative agent in duodenal ulcers, whereas decreased tissue resistance plays a greater role in the development of gastric ulcers. Simple as this sounds, only in rare cases can ulcer development be traced to a single cause. It is more likely that both factors contribute to the development of a peptic ulcer. Nevertheless, it seems helpful, in terms of understanding ulcer development, to view these differences in causation in terms of the function that the mucosal surface affords the stomach and the duodenum.

Increased acid–pepsin production. Hydrochloric acid production is influenced by several factors, including neural and hormonal stimulation. The hormone gastrin, which is produced in the antrum of the stomach, is a potent stimulus for hydrochloric acid secretion. Increased levels of gastric acid have also been attributed to (1) increased numbers of acid–pepsin producing cells in the stomach, (2) increased sensitivity of the parietal cells to food and other stimuli (*e.g.,* both alcohol and caffeine are potent stimulators of hydrochloric acid secretion), (3) excessive vagal stimulation, and (4) impaired inhibition of gastric secretions as food moves into the intestine.

The intractable peptic ulcers observed in the *Zollinger–Ellison syndrome* are caused by a gastrin-secreting tumor of the pancreas. In persons with this disorder, gastric acid secretion reaches such levels that ulceration becomes inevitable.

Normally, gastrin secretion is inhibited as food moves into the intestine. It has been postulated that this reflex inhibition of gastrin may be impaired in certain types of ulcers. For example, *Cushing's ulcer* is a special type of stress ulcer that occurs in association with severe brain injury or neurosurgery. It results from increased central stimulation of the vagus nerve, which is unresponsive to reflex mechanisms that normally control gastric secretions.

Resistance of the mucosal surface. The defenses of the mucosal surface are dependent on an adequate blood flow and an intact mucosal barrier. It can be assumed that any disruption in the mucosal barrier reduces these defenses and renders the mucosal surface more susceptible to the destructive effects of the hydrogen ion.

It has been suggested that a basic abnormality in persons with gastric peptic ulcers is an increased permeability of the epithelial layer of the stomach to hydrogen ions, which causes injury to the mucosal surface and reduces its resistance to further injury. It also is possible that a chronically diseased mucosal membrane is unable to secrete sufficient mucus to form an effective barrier. Bile is known to disrupt the mucosal barrier, and reflux of bile from the intestine into the stomach has been implicated in peptic ulcer. In addition to bile, a number of drugs are recognized as "barrier breakers." Both aspirin and alcohol are known to damage this barrier.

The duodenum, which acts as a passageway for digestive enzymes and acid-laden chyme, is a common site of peptic ulcers. Brunner's glands, which are located between the pylorus and the site where bile and pancreatic enzymes enter the duodenum, produce a large amount of viscid mucus, which serves to protect this area. The activity of these glands is inhibited by sympathetic stimulation; this may help to explain why anxiety and stress contribute to duodenal ulcer development.

Ischemia or decreased blood flow impairs mucus secretion and tends to make the mucosal surface less resistant to the destructive effects of hydrochloric acid. *Curling's ulcer* is a stress ulcer that occurs following severe burns, trauma, or sepsis and is thought to result from local ischemia.

Of recent interest is the relationship between the incidence of duodenal ulcers and blood types. It has been observed that persons with duodenal ulcers have a higher-than-normal frequency of blood group O compared with an ulcer-free population. As a further explanation, it should be pointed out that about 75% of the general population secrete a water-soluble substance, similar to their blood type, into their saliva and gastric secretions. Persons with type O blood and certain other persons with a particular red cell antigen (Lewis a) are nonsecretors of a primary-blood-group antigen in their saliva. For reasons that are unclear, these persons appear to be more susceptible to duodenal ulcers than persons who secrete primary-blood-group antigens.

Clinical manifestations. The clinical manifestations of uncomplicated peptic ulcer focus on discomfort and pain. The pain, which is described as burning, gnawing, or cramplike, is usually rhythmic and frequently occurs when the stomach is empty—between meals and at 1 o'clock or 2 o'clock in the morning. Characteristically, the pain is relieved by food or antacids. A peptic ulcer can affect one or all of the layers of the stomach or duodenum. The ulcer may penetrate only the mucosal surface or it may extend into the smooth muscle layers. Occasionally, an ulcer will penetrate the outer wall of the stomach or duodenum. Healing of the muscularis layer involves replacement with scar tissue; although the mucosal layers that cover the scarred muscle layer regenerate, the regeneration is often less than perfect, which contributes to repeated episodes of ulceration and complications.

Complications. Complications of peptic ulcer include hemorrhage, obstruction, and perforation. *Hemorrhage* occurs in 10% to 15% of persons with ulcers. Evidence of bleeding may consist of hematemesis or melena. Bleeding may be sudden, severe, and without warning, or it may be insidious, producing only occult (hidden) blood in the stool. *Obstruction* is caused by edema, spasm, or contraction of scar tissue; it occurs with impairment of free passage of luminal contents through the pylorus or adjacent areas. *Perforation* occurs when the ulcer erodes all the layers of the wall of the stomach or duodenum. With perforation, gastrointestinal contents enter the peritoneum and cause peritonitis, or penetrate adjacent structures such as the pancreas. Peritonitis is discussed as a separate topic at the end of this chapter.

Treatment. Treatment of peptic ulcer focuses on measures to (1) decrease or neutralize the hydrochloric acid, (2) increase the resistance of the mucosal layer, and (3) promote healing.

Conservative treatment measures include (1) efforts to relieve stress and anxiety, (2) dietary management, (3) antacids, and (4) other medications that act to reduce gastric-acid secretion.

Although in the past the conservative treatment of peptic ulcers has usually included use of a bland diet, at present there is considerable controversy over its value. Most physicians would agree that coffee and alcoholic beverages should be avoided. Most physicians would agree, too, that the use of food as an antacid should also be avoided, because such feedings are generally accompanied by a rebound increase in gastric acid secretion. The value of the hourly milk-and-cream regimen, which has been used for years, has also come under question. There is evidence that the calcium in milk may act as a stimulus for gastrin release and thereby increase gastric acid secretion. The use of milk and cream is also associated with an increased risk of developing the milk-alkali syndrome.

Medications used in the treatment of peptic ulcers include the selective use of antacids, anticholinergic drugs, cimetidine, and sedatives or tranquilizers (Table 42-1). Anticholinergic drugs are less effective inhibitors of gastric acid secretions than antacids and histamine$_2$ receptor antagonists (cimetidine and ranitidine), and therefore they are usually used in combination with other methods of treatment. Sedatives and tranquilizers are individualized forms of treatment that are used for persons in whom stress is a large contributing factor.

Antacids. Antacids, either self-prescribed or physician prescribed, represent a large business in the United States; approximately $110 million are spent each year for these medications.[10] Essentially four types of antacids are used to relieve gastric acidity: sodium bicarbonate, calcium carbonate, aluminum hydroxide, and magnesium hydroxide. Because *sodium bicarbonate* is water soluble, it leaves the stomach rapidly and produces a very transient effect. It contains large amounts of sodium and tends to cause metabolic alkalosis. It is mainly used as a home remedy. *Calcium preparations* are constipating and may cause hypercalcemia and the milk-alkali syndrome. There is also evidence that oral calcium preparations increase gastric-acid secretion after their buffering effect has been utilized. *Magnesium hydroxide* is a potent antacid that acts as a laxative. Approximately 5% to 10% of the magnesium in this preparation is absorbed from the intestine; therefore, magnesium hydroxide should not be used in persons with renal failure, because magnesium must be excreted through the kidneys. *Aluminum hydroxide* reacts with hydrochloric acid to form aluminum chloride. It combines with phosphate in the intestine and is often used for treating the hyperphosphatemia that occurs with renal failure. The adsorptive effects of aluminum hydroxide may affect absorption of other substances, such as bile salts and tetracycline. Many antacids contain a combination of ingredients, such as magnesium aluminum hydroxide.

Histamine$_2$ antagonists. Cimetidine and ranitidine are histamine$_2$ antagonists that block the secretion of hydrochloric acid regardless of the stimulus for its secretion, suggesting that histamine is the final common mediator of gastric acid secretion. In 1977, when cimetidine was released for clinical use by the Food and Drug Administration, only two indications for its use were approved: short-term use in treatment of duodenal ulcer and hypersecretion of gastric acid, such as occurs with the Zollinger–Ellison syndrome. There is evidence that the histamine$_2$ antagonists are now being used for more diverse purposes.[11] Recently, reduction in liver blood flow accompanying treatment with cimetidine and decreased metabolism of drugs (propranolol) by the liver following its use have been reported.[12]

Surgical treatment. When the conservative management of peptic ulcer is ineffective, surgical intervention is often needed. Three types of surgical procedures are done: (1) subtotal gastrectomy, in which 75% to 80% of the stomach is removed and the remaining portion is attached to

Table 42-1 Drugs Used in Treatment of Peptic Ulcer

Drug	Mechanisms of Action
Anticholinergics	Block vagal stimulation of gastric acid secretion
	Decrease gastric motility, allowing antacids to remain in the stomach
Antacids	
Calcium carbonate	Neutralizes the gastric acid, but may cause rebound gastric acid secretion
	Can cause hypercalcemia associated with the milk-alkali syndrome
	Has a constipating effect
Magnesium hydroxide	Neutralizes gastric acid
	About 5% to 10% is absorbed in the intestine and may cause an increase in blood magnesium levels in persons with renal failure
	Has a laxative effect
Aluminum hydroxide	Neutralizes gastric acid
	Binds with phosphate in the intestine and may be used to treat hyperphosphatemia in renal failure
	May also bind with other substances and drugs, increasing their excretion in the stool
Histamine$_2$ antagonists	Block histamine$_2$ receptors, inhibiting gastric acid secretion
Sedatives and tranquilizers	Relieve anxiety and tension in persons in whom this is a problem

the jejunum; (2) truncal vagotomy and drainage, in which the vagus nerve trunks are cut and the outlet of the stomach is enlarged; and (3) truncal vagotomy and antrectomy, in which the vagus nerve trunks are cut and the distal 50% of the stomach is removed.

One of the complications following surgery for peptic ulcers is the *dumping syndrome*. It occurs to some extent in about 20% of persons who have this type of operation. It is believed to be caused by the rapid entry of hyperosmolar liquids into the intestine and is characterized by nausea, vomiting, diarrhea, diaphoresis, palpitations, tachycardia, lightheadedness, and flushing that occurs either while eating or shortly after. It is often followed (in about 2 hours) by an episode of hypoglycemia, resulting from the rapid absorption of glucose, which acts as a stimulus for insulin release by the beta cells of the pancreas. Treatment consists of limiting the diet to small, frequent feedings, which are taken without liquids and which are low in simple sugars (these are the most osmotically active parts of the diet). Symptoms usually diminish with time.

Cancer of the stomach

Cancer of the stomach strikes approximately 24,000 persons each year and accounts for 10% of cancer deaths.[7] Although its incidence has decreased about 40% in the last 30 years, it remains the seventh leading cause of death in the United States.[7] Among the factors that increase the risk of gastric cancer are a genetic predisposition, carcinogenic factors in the diet (*e.g.,* nitrates, smoked foods), atrophic gastritis, and gastric polyps. Fifty percent of gastric cancers occur in the pyloric region or adjacent to the antrum. Compared with a benign ulcer, which has smooth margins and is concentrically shaped, gastric cancers tend to be larger, are irregularly shaped, have irregular margins, and are usually located in the greater curvature of the stomach.

Unfortunately, stomach cancers are often asymptomatic until late in their course. Symptoms, when they do occur, are usually vague and include indigestion, anorexia, weight loss, vague epigastric pain, vomiting, and an abdominal mass. Diagnosis of gastric cancer is accomplished by means of a variety of techniques, including barium x-ray studies, gastroscopy studies with biopsy, and cytologic studies (Pap smear) of gastric secretions. Cytologic studies can prove particularly useful as a routine screening test in persons with atrophic gastritis or gastric polyps.

Surgery in the form of radical subtotal gastrectomy is usually the treatment of choice. Radiation and chemotherapy have not proved particularly useful as primary treatment modalities in stomach cancer. When these methods are used, it is usually for palliative purposes or to control metastatic spread of the disease.

Small and Large Intestines

There are many similarities in conditions that disrupt the integrity of the small and large bowels. The wall of both the small and large intestines consists of five layers (Chap. 41, Fig. 41-2): an outer serosal layer, a muscularis layer, which is divided into a layer of circular and a layer of longitudinal muscle fibers, a submucosal layer, and an inner mucosal layer, which lines the lumen of the intestine. Among the conditions that predispose to disruption of the integrity of the intestine are inflammatory bowel disease, diverticulitis, appendicitis, and cancer of the colon and rectum.

Inflammatory bowel disease

Inflammatory bowel disease, which includes Crohn's disease and ulcerative colitis, affects more than 100,000 persons in the United States.[13] Recent estimates indicate that 20,000 to 25,000 new cases of inflammatory bowel disease were seen in community hospitals in 1980.[14] There is evidence to suggest that the incidence of ulcerative colitis, which is an inflammatory disorder of the rectum and colon, has reached a plateau, whereas that of Crohn's disease, which can affect either the large or small bowel, has increased steadily over the past 20 years.

The causes of both Crohn's disease and ulcerative colitis are largely unknown. The diseases appear to have a familial occurrence that suggests a hereditary predisposition. One of the common beliefs is that hereditary factors increase the susceptibility to other etiologic factors, such as immune responses and viral infections. The Jewish population is especially susceptible to both Crohn's disease and ulcerative colitis. Although psychogenic factors may contribute to the severity and onset of both conditions, it seems unlikely that they are the primary cause.

Both Crohn's disease and ulcerative colitis are considered systemic diseases that affect organs other than the intestine. More than 100 complications have been identified in the two diseases, including erythema nodosum, arthritis, stomatitis, ankylosing spondylitis, autoimmune anemia, hypercoagulability of blood, iritis, myopericarditis, obstructive pulmonary disease, sclerosing cholangitis, and growth retardation in children.[14]

Crohn's disease. Crohn's disease is a recurrent granulomatous type of inflammatory response that can affect any area of the gastrointestinal tract. It is a slowly progressive, relentless, and often disabling disease. The disease usually strikes in early adulthood and affects both men and women equally. Its lesions are observed most frequently in the terminal ileum or ileocecal area of the bowel. The ileum is involved in about 80% of the cases. The colon is the second most common site of involvement, and the condition may be confused with ulcerative colitis. Crohn's disease is a multisystem disease that is often accompanied by other manifestations, such as arthritis, gallstones, skin disorders, iritis, and keratitis.

A characteristic feature of Crohn's disease is the sharply demarcated granulomatous lesions that occur and that are surrounded by normal-appearing mucosal tissue. When the lesions are multiple, they are often referred to as skip lesions because they are interspersed between what appear to be normal segments of the bowel. All the layers of the bowel are involved, the submucosal layer being affected to the greatest extent. The surface of the inflamed bowel usually has a characteristic "cobblestone" appearance resulting from the fissures and crevices that develop and surround areas of submucosal edema. There is usually a relative sparing of the smooth muscle layers of the bowel with marked inflammatory and fibrotic changes of the submucosal layer. The bowel wall, after a time, often becomes thickened and inflexible; its appearance has been likened to a lead pipe or rubber hose. The adjacent mesentery may become inflamed and the regional lymph nodes and channels enlarged. Fistulas are tubelike passages from a normal cavity or abscess that extend to a free surface of the body or another body cavity. In Crohn's disease, the inflammatory lesions may extend and penetrate the entire wall of the gut, causing abscess formation and the development of fistulous tracts. The characteristics of Crohn's disease are summarized in Table 42-2.

Clinical manifestations.   The clinical course of Crohn's disease is variable; often there are periods of exacerbations and remissions, with symptoms being related to the location of the lesions. The principal symptoms include intermittent diarrhea, colicky pain (usually in the lower right quadrant), weight loss, malaise, and low-grade fever. Perianal abscesses and fistula formation are com-

mon. Their occurrence is largely due to the severity of the diarrhea, which produces ulceration of the perianal skin. As the disease progresses, there may be bleeding and malabsorption. Complications include intestinal obstruction, abdominal abscess formation, and fistula formation. The overall mortality rate is about 18%. The majority of persons with Crohn's disease eventually develop complications that require surgery.

Diagnosis and treatment.   Diagnosis is usually made following x-ray studies of the gastrointestinal tract using barium as a radiopaque contrast medium. Proctosigmoidoscopy is often done to visualize the bowel and to obtain a biopsy.

Treatment methods focus on maintaining adequate nutrition, promoting healing, and preventing and treating complications. Nutritional deficiencies are common in Crohn's disease because of diarrhea, steatorrhea, and other malabsorption problems. A nutritious diet that is high in calories, vitamins, and proteins is recommended. Fats often aggravate the diarrhea, and it is generally recommended that they be avoided. Elemental diets, which are nutritionally balanced, yet are residue free and bulk free, may be given for a period of time during the acute phase of the illness. These diets are largely absorbed in the jejunum and allow the inflamed bowel to rest. Total parenteral nutrition (parenteral hyperalimentation) consists of intravenous administration of hypertonic glucose solutions to which amino acids and fats may be added. This form of nutritional therapy may be needed when food cannot be absorbed from the intestine. Because of the hypertonicity of these solutions, they must be administered through a large-diameter central vein.

In addition to nutritional therapy, salicylazosulfapyridine (Azulfidine), a poorly absorbed drug with

Table 42-2   Differentiating Characteristics of Crohn's Disease and Ulcerative Colitis

Characteristic	Crohn's Disease	Ulcerative Colitis
Type of inflammation	Granulomatous	Ulcerative and exudative
Type of lesion	Cobblestone	Crypt abscesses and pseudopolyps
Level of involvement	Primarily submucosal	Primarily mucosal
Extent of involvement	Skip lesions	Continuous
Areas of involvement	Primarily ileum Secondarily colon	Primarily rectum and left colon
Diarrhea	Common	Common
Rectal bleeding	Rare	Common
Fistulas	Common	Rare
Strictures	Common	Rare
Perianal abscesses	Common	Rare
Toxic megacolon	Rare	Common
Development of cancer	Rare	Relatively common

anti-inflammatory action, and the adrenocorticosteroid hormones are frequently prescribed to treat the acute disease. Surgery is usually reserved for treatment of complications.

Ulcerative colitis. Ulcerative colitis is a nonspecific inflammatory condition of the colon. It usually begins in the rectum and spreads to the left colon. It may involve the entire colon. Like Crohn's disease, the chronic form of the disease is often associated with systemic manifestations such as migratory polyarthritis, ankylosing spondylitis, uveitis, inflammatory liver disease, and various skin manifestations. There are many similarities between ulcerative colitis and Crohn's disease and, at present, it is questioned whether or not the two disorders might represent different manifestations of the same disease.

With ulcerative colitis, the inflammatory process tends to be confluent and continuous instead of skipping areas, as it does in Crohn's disease. Ulcerative colitis affects primarily the mucosal layer, although it can extend into the submucosal layer. Characteristic of the disease are the lesions that form in the crypts of Lieberkühn (see Fig. 41-8) in the base of the mucosal layer. The inflammatory process causes pinpoint mucosal hemorrhages to occur, which in time suppurate and develop into *crypt abscesses*. These inflammatory lesions become necrotic and ulcerate. Although the ulcerations are usually superficial, they often extend, causing large, denuded areas. As a result of the inflammatory process, the mucosal layer often develops tonguelike projections that resemble polyps and are therefore called *pseudopolyps*. Because ulcerative colitis affects the mucosal layer, bleeding is an almost constant manifestation, and bloody diarrhea is the most common complaint during the acute phase of the disease. With repeated episodes of colitis, there is thickening of the bowel wall. The pathologic features of Crohn's disease and ulcerative colitis are summarized in Table 42-2.

Clinical manifestations. Ulcerative colitis usually follows a course of remissions and exacerbations. The severity of the disease varies from mild to fulminating. Accordingly, the disease has been divided into three types depending on its severity: acute fulminating, chronic intermittent, and mild chronic. About 15% to 20% of persons with ulcerative colitis present with the *fulminating form* of the disease. This form presents with an acute episode of bloody diarrhea, fever, and acute abdominal pain. This is the most serious form of the disease, and it has been reported that as many as 35% of persons with severe attacks may die.[15] About 60% have a *mild* form of the disease, in which bleeding and diarrhea are mild and systemic signs are absent. This form of the disease can usually be managed by conservative means. The remainder of the persons with chronic ulcerative colitis

have a *chronic* form, which continues after the initial attack. Compared with the milder form, usually more of the colon surface is involved and the presence of systemic signs and complications is greater.

Diarrhea, which is the characteristic manifestation of ulcerative colitis, will vary according to the severity of the disease. There may be up to 30 to 40 bowel movements a day. Typically, the stools contain blood and mucus. Nocturnal diarrhea is usually present when daytime symptoms are severe. There may be mild abdominal cramping and incontinence of stools. Anorexia, weakness, and fatigability are common.

Complications. *Toxic megacolon* is an acute, life-threatening complication of ulcerative colitis. It is characterized by dilatation of the colon and signs of systemic toxicity. It results from extension of the inflammatory response, with involvement of neural and vascular components of the bowel. Contributing factors include use of laxatives, narcotics, and anticholinergic drugs and the presence of hypokalemia.

Cancer of the colon is one of the feared complications of ulcerative colitis. The risk of developing cancer among persons who have had the disease for 15 years is about 5% to 10%, and after 25 years the risk becomes 40% to 50%.[16]

Diagnosis and treatment. Diagnostic measures include colonoscopic examination, often with biopsy. Colon x-ray studies may be done using barium as a radiopaque contrast medium.

Measures used in treating ulcerative colitis vary with the severity of the disease. Hospitalization is required for persons with the acute, fulminating form of the disease. Sulfasalazine (an antimicrobial agent) may be used for both short-course and long-term therapy. The adrenocorticosteroid hormones are selectively used to lessen the inflammatory response. These drugs can be given by enema or in the form of a suppository. Surgical treatment (removal of the rectum and entire colon) with the creation of an ileostomy may be required for those persons who do not respond to conservative methods of treatment.

Diverticular disease

Diverticulosis is a condition in which herniation of the mucosal layer of the colon occurs through the muscularis layer. Diverticular disease is very common in the United States. It is thought to affect about 50% of persons over age 60.[17] Although the disorder is very prevalent in the developed countries of the world, it is almost nonexistent in many of the African nations and other underdeveloped countries. This suggests that dietary factors (lack of fiber content), a decrease in physical activity, and poor bowel habits (in which the urge to defecate is neglected), along with the effects of aging, contribute to the development of the disease.

Most diverticula occur in the sigmoid colon. In the colon, the longitudinal muscle does not form a continuous layer, as it does in the small bowel. Instead there are three separate longitudinal bands of muscle called the taeniae coli (Fig. 42-2). It is between these muscles, in the area where the blood vessels pierce the circular muscle layer to bring blood to the mucosal layer, that diverticula develop. An increase in intraluminal pressure provides the force for creating these herniations. The increase in pressure is thought to be related to the volume of the colonic contents. The more scanty the contents, the more vigorous the contractions and the greater the pressure. When the vigorous contractions continue over time, both the circular and longitudinal muscle layers hypertrophy. In many cases, the haustra may become so thick from the hypertrophy that they are approximated during contractions, causing a marked increase in the pressure within the isolated segment. According to the laws of physics, the pressure within a tube increases as its diameter decreases. The sigmoid colon, which is the segment most vulnerable to the development of diverticula, is the segment of the colon with the narrowest diameter.

The vast majority of persons with diverticular disease remain asymptomatic. The disease is often found when x-ray studies are done for other purposes. When symptoms do occur, they are often attributed to irritable bowel syndrome or other causes. Ill-defined lower abdominal discomfort, a change in bowel habits, such as diarrhea and constipation, bloating, and flatulence are often present. One of the most common complaints is pain in the lower left quadrant. When it is accompanied by other symptoms, it is often referred to as *left-sided appendicitis*. This left-sided appendicitis is often accompanied by nausea and vomiting, tenderness in the lower left quadrant, a slight fever, and elevation in white blood cell count. These symptoms usually last for several days, unless complications occur, and are usually caused by localized inflammation of the diverticula, with perforation and development of a small localized abscess. Complications include perforation with peritonitis, hemorrhage, and bowel obstruction.

The usual treatment for diverticular disease is to prevent symptoms and complications. This includes increasing the bulk in the diet and bowel retraining so that the person has at least one bowel movement a day. Surgical treatment is reserved for complications.

Appendicitis

Acute appendicitis is extremely common. It is seen most frequently in the 5-year to 30-year age group but can occur at any age. The appendix becomes inflamed, swollen, and gangrenous, and it eventually perforates if

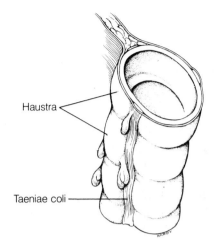

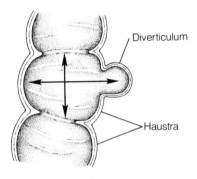

Figure 42-2   (Top) *A portion of the sigmoid colon, showing the haustra and taeniae coli; (bottom) a longitudinal section of the colon showing the changes that occur in diverticular disease. The muscle wall is hypertrophied, which causes the haustra to approximate during contractions of the colon. This causes a marked increase in pressure within that segment of the colon, which contributes to diverticulum formation.*

not treated. Although the cause of appendicitis is not known, it is thought to be related to intraluminal obstruction due to a fecalith (hard piece of stool) or twisting.

Appendicitis usually has an abrupt onset, with pain referred to the epigastric or periumbilical area. This pain is due to stretching of the appendix during the early inflammatory process. At about the same time that the pain appears, there are one or two episodes of nausea. Initially the pain is vague, but over a period of 2 hours to 12 hours it gradually increases and may become colicky in nature. When the inflammatory process has extended to involve the serosal layer of the appendix and the peritoneum, the pain becomes localized to the lower right quadrant. There is usually an elevation in temperature and a white blood cell count of over 10,000 per mm³ with 75% or more polymorphonuclear cells. Palpation of the abdomen usually reveals a deep tenderness in the lower right quadrant, which is confined to a small area about the size of the fingertip. It is usually located at about the site of the inflamed appendix. Many times the person with appendicitis will be able to place his or her finger directly over the tender area. Rebound tenderness, pain that occurs when pressure is applied to the area and then released, and spasm of the overlying abdominal muscles are common. Treatment consists of surgical removal of the appendix. Complications include peritonitis, localized periappendiceal abscess formation, and septicemia.

Colorectal cancer

More than 57,000 persons in the United States die each year of colorectal cancer. It is the second most common site of fatal cancer.[7] The main drawback to successful treatment is the fact that most lesions do not produce symptoms until late in the course of the disease.

Almost all cancers of the colon and rectum are carcinomas. Of these, about 16% occur in the cecum and ascending colon, 8% in the transverse and splenic flexures, 6% in the descending colon, 20% in the sigmoid colon, and 50% in the rectum.[7]

The cause of cancer of the colon and rectum is largely unknown. Its incidence increases with age, as evidenced by the fact that 95% of persons who develop this form of cancer are over age 50. Its incidence is increased in persons with a *family history of cancer,* in persons with *ulcerative colitis,* and in those with *familial multiple polyposis* of the colon.

Usually, cancer of the colon and rectum is present for a long period of time before it produces symptoms. *Bleeding* is a highly significant early symptom, and it is usually the one that causes people to seek medical care. Other symptoms include a *change in bowel habits,* either diarrhea or constipation, and sometimes a sense of urgency or incomplete emptying of the bowel. Pain is usually a late symptom.

The prognosis for persons with colorectal cancer depends largely on the extent of bowel involvement and on the presence of metastasis at the time of diagnosis. This form of cancer can be divided into four categories according to the classification system by Duke. The type A tumor is limited to invasion of the mucosal and submucosal layers of the colon and has a 5-year survival rate of almost 100%. Type B tumor involves the entire wall of the colon and has a 5-year survival rate of about 54% to 67%. With type C tumor, there is invasion of the serosal layer, with involvement of the regional lymph nodes. The 5-year survival rate is approximately 23%. Type D colorectal cancer involves far-advanced metastasis.[9]

Diagnosis and treatment. Among the methods used in the diagnosis of colorectal cancers are stool occult blood tests and digital rectal examination, usually done during routine physical examinations; x-ray studies using barium (barium enema); and proctosigmoidoscopy and colonoscopy. Digital rectal examinations are most helpful in detecting neoplasms of the rectum. Rectal examination should be considered a routine part of a good physical examination. Half of all colon and rectal cancers can be detected by digital examination.[7] The American Cancer Society recommends that all asymptomatic men and women over age 50 should have a stool occult blood test and digital rectal examination done every year and a proctosigmoidoscopy examination done every 3 to 5 years after two initial negative examinations done one year apart as a means of early detection of colorectal cancer.[18] Persons with positive stool occult blood tests should be referred to their physicians for further study. Usually a physical examination, rectal examination, barium enema, and proctosigmoidoscopy or colonoscopy are done.

Almost all cancers of the colon and rectum bleed intermittently even though the amount of blood is small and usually not apparent in the stools. It is therefore feasible to screen for colorectal cancers using commercially prepared tests for occult blood in the stool that are now available. This method utilizes a guaiac-impregnated filter paper. The technique involves preparing two slides per day from different portions of the same stool for 3 days to 4 days while the patient follows a high-fiber diet that is free of meat and ascorbic acid. Although the diet is not particularly appealing, this has been shown to be a relatively reliable and inexpensive method of screening for colorectal cancer. Proctosigmoidoscopy involves examination of the rectum and sigmoid colon with a hollow, lighted tube that is inserted through the rectum. Polyps can be removed or tissue obtained for biopsy during the procedure.

Colonoscopy provides a means for direct visualization of the rectum and colon. The colonoscope consists of a flexible 4-cm glass bundle that has some 250,000 glass fibers with a lens at either end to focus and magnify the image.[19] Light from an external source is transmitted by the fiberoptic viewing bundle. Instruments are available that afford direct examination of the sigmoid colon or the entire colon. This method is used for screening persons at high risk for developing cancer of the colon (*e.g.,* those with ulcerative colitis) and for those with symptoms. Colonoscopy is also useful for obtaining a biopsy and for removing polyps. Although this method is one of the most accurate for detecting early colorectal cancers, it is not suitable for mass screening because it is expensive and time-consuming and must be done by a person who is highly trained in the use of the instrument.

The only recognized *treatment* for cancer of the colon and rectum is surgical removal. Preoperative radiation may be used and has in some cases demonstrated increased 5-year survival rates. Postoperative adjuvant therapy with 5-fluorouracil (5-FU) has had some success. Both radiation and chemotherapy are palliative treatment methods.

Peritonitis

Peritonitis represents an inflammatory response of the serous membrane that lines the abdominal cavity and covers the visceral organs. It can be caused by either bacterial invasion or chemical irritation. Most commonly, enteric bacteria enter the peritoneum because of a defect in the wall of one of the abdominal organs. The most common causes of peritonitis are perforated peptic ulcer, ruptured appendix, perforated diverticulum, gangrenous bowel, pelvic inflammatory disease, and gangrenous gallbladder. Other causes are abdominal trauma and wounds. Generalized peritonitis, though no longer the overwhelming problem it once was, is still a leading cause of death following abdominal surgery.

The peritoneum has several characteristics that either increase its vulnerability to or protect it against the effects of peritonitis. One weakness of the peritoneal cavity is that it is a large, unbroken space that favors the dissemination of contaminants. For the same reason, it has a large surface that permits rapid absorption of bacterial toxins into the blood. On the other hand, the peritoneum is particularly well adapted for producing an inflammatory response as a means of controlling infection. It tends, for example, to exude a thick, sticky, and fibrinous substance that adheres to other structures, such as the mesentery and omentum, and that serves to seal off the perforated viscus and aid in localizing the process. Localization is further enhanced by sympathetic stimulation that inhibits peristalsis. Although the paralytic ileus that occurs tends to give rise to associated problems, it does inhibit the movement of contaminants throughout the peritoneal cavity.

One of the most important manifestations of peritonitis is the translocation of extracellular fluid into the peritoneal cavity (through weeping of serous fluid from the inflamed peritoneum) and into the bowel as a result of bowel obstruction. Nausea and vomiting cause further losses of fluid. The fluid loss may then encourage development of hypovolemia and shock.

The onset of peritonitis may be acute, as in a ruptured appendix, or it may have a more gradual onset such as occurs in progressive inflammatory disease. Pain and tenderness are common symptoms. The pain is usually more intense over the inflamed area. The person with peritonitis usually lies very still because any movement aggravates the pain. Breathing is often shallow, in order to prevent movement of the abdominal muscles. The abdomen is usually rigid and sometimes described as boardlike, because of reflex muscle guarding. Vomiting is common. Fever, elevation in white blood cell count, tachycardia, and frequently hypotension are present. Hiccoughs may develop because of irritation of the phrenic nerve. Paralytic ileus occurs shortly after the onset of widespread peritonitis and is accompanied by abdominal distention. Peritonitis that progresses and is untreated leads to toxemia and shock.

Treatment measures for peritonitis are directed toward (1) preventing the extension of the inflammatory response, (2) minimizing the effects of paralytic ileus and abdominal distention, and (3) correcting the fluid and electrolyte imbalances that develop. Surgical intervention may be needed to remove an acutely inflamed appendix or to close the opening in a perforated peptic ulcer. Oral fluids are forbidden. Nasogastric suction, which entails the insertion of a tube (placed through the nose) into the stomach or intestine, is employed to decompress the bowel and relieve the abdominal distention. Fluid and electrolyte replacement is essential. These fluids are prescribed on the basis of frequent blood chemistry determinations. Antibiotics are given to combat infection. Narcotics are often needed for pain relief.

A potential complication of peritonitis is abscess formation. Should it occur, the most desirable area for drainage is into the pelvis rather than into the area under the diaphragm. Therefore, the head of the bed is usually elevated about 60° to 70° (semi-Fowler's position) to encourage drainage of inflammatory exudate from the flank area into the pelvis.

In summary, the gastrointestinal tract is a five-layered tube that consists of an inner mucosal layer, a submucosal layer, a layer of circular and longitudinal smooth muscle, and an outer serosal layer. Disruption of the integrity of its wall can occur at any level, because of numerous pathologic processes, including injury to the mucosal barrier, inflammation, structural changes, and neoplasms. The manifestations of alterations in the integrity of the digestive system depend on the process involved, the extent of the injury, and the area of the gastrointestinal tract that is involved.

■ Alterations in Motility

The movement of contents through the gastrointestinal tract is controlled by neurons that are located in the submucosal and myenteric plexuses of the gut. The axons from the cell bodies in the myenteric plexus innervate both the circular and longitudinal smooth muscle layers of the gut. These neurons receive impulses from local receptors that are located in the mucosal and muscle layers of the gut and extrinsic input from the parasympathetic and sympathetic nervous systems. As a general rule, the parasympathetic nervous system tends to increase the motility of the bowel, whereas sympathetic stimulation tends to slow its activity.

The colon, which has sphincters at both ends—the ileocecal sphincter, which separates it from the small intestine, and the anal sphincter, which prevents the movement of feces to the outside of the body—acts as a reservoir for fecal material. Normally, about 400 ml of water, 55 mEq of sodium, 30 mEq of chloride, and 15 mEq of bicarbonate are absorbed each day in the colon. At the same time, about 5 mEq of potassium are secreted into the lumen of the colon. The amount of water and electrolytes that remain in the stool reflect the absorption or secretion that occurs in the colon. The average adult ingesting a "typical" American diet evacuates about 200 gm to 300 gm of stool each day.

Diarrhea

The usual definition of diarrhea is excessively frequent passage of unformed stools. The complaint of diarrhea is a general one and can be related to a number of factors, pathologic and otherwise. Diarrhea is usually divided into two types: large-volume and small-volume. Large-volume diarrhea results from an increase in the water content of the stool and small-volume diarrhea from an increase in the propulsive activity of the bowel. Some of the common causes of small- and large-volume diarrhea are summarized in Table 42-3. Often diarrhea is a combination of these two types.

Table 42-3 Causes of Large- and Small-Volume Diarrhea

Large-Volume Diarrhea
  Osmotic diarrhea
    Saline cathartics
    Dumping syndrome
    Lactase deficiency
  Secretory diarrhea
    Failure to absorb bile salts
    Fat malabsorption
    Chronic laxative abuse
    Carcinoid syndrome
    Zollinger–Ellison syndrome
    Fecal impaction
    Acute infectious diarrhea
Small-Volume Diarrhea
  Inflammatory bowel disease
    Crohn's disease
    Ulcerative colitis
  Infectious disease
    Shigellosis
    Salmonellosis
  Irritable colon

Large-volume diarrhea

Large-volume diarrhea can be classified as secretory or osmotic, according to the cause of the increased water content in the feces. Water is either pulled into the colon along an osmotic gradient or is secreted into the bowel by the mucosal cells. This form of diarrhea is usually a painless, watery type without blood or pus in the stools.

In *osmotic diarrhea,* water is pulled into the bowel by the hyperosmotic nature of its contents. It occurs when osmotically active particles are not absorbed. In lactase deficiency, the lactose that is present in milk cannot be broken down and absorbed. Magnesium salts, which are contained in milk of magnesium and many antacids, are poorly absorbed and cause diarrhea when taken in sufficient quantities. Another cause of osmotic diarrhea is decreased transit time, which interferes with absorption. This happens in the dumping syndrome, which was discussed earlier in relation to the surgical treatment of peptic ulcer. Osmotic diarrhea disappears with fasting.

Secretory diarrhea occurs when the secretory processes of the bowel are increased. Most acute infectious diarrheas are of this type. This type of diarrhea also occurs when excess bile salts or fatty acids are present in the gut contents as they enter the colon. This often happens with disease processes of the ileum, because bile salts are absorbed here. It may also occur when bacterial overgrowth occurs in the small bowel, which also interferes with bile absorption. Some tumors, such as Zollinger–Ellison syndrome and carcinoid syndrome, cause increased secretory activity of the bowel.

Fecal impaction (the retention of hard, dried stool in the rectum and colon) stimulates increased secretory activity of the portion of the bowel proximal to the impaction. In this case the watery stool flows around the fecal mass, representing the body's attempt to break up the mass so that it can be evacuated. This cause should be considered in any elderly or immobilized person who develops watery diarrhea. Digital examination of the rectum is done to assess the fecal mass. In some cases, the mass may need to be removed manually with a gloved finger.

Small-volume diarrhea

Small-volume diarrhea is usually evidenced by frequency and urgency and colicky abdominal pains. This form of diarrhea is commonly associated with intrinsic disease of the colon, such as ulcerative colitis or Crohn's disease. It is usually accompanied by tenesmus (painful straining at stool), fecal soiling of clothing, and awakening during the night with the urge to defecate.

Treatment

Diarrhea causes loss of fluid and electrolytes from the body. This can be particularly serious in infants and small children, persons with other illness, the elderly, and even previously healthy persons if it continues for any length of time. Fluid and electrolyte corrections are, therefore, considered to be a primary therapeutic goal in the treatment of diarrhea. Oral electrolyte replacement solutions can be given in situations of uncomplicated diarrhea that can be treated at home. Restricting oral foods and fluids may be helpful in acute diarrhea, because this decreases peristalsis. When intake is resumed following diarrhea, the diet should consist of bland foods that will not stimulate gastrointestinal motility. Cold liquids that move rapidly from the stomach to the small intestine and stimulate peristalsis should be avoided.

Drugs used in the treatment of diarrhea include camphorated tincture of opium (paregoric), diphenoxylate (Lomotil), and loperamide (Imodium), which are opiumlike drugs. Adsorbents, such as kaolin and pectin, are able to adsorb undesirable constituents from solutions. These ingredients are included in many over-the-counter antidiarrheal preparations because they adsorb toxins responsible for certain types of diarrhea.

Constipation

Constipation can be defined as the infrequent passage of stools. The difficulty with this definition arises from the many individual variations of a function that are normal. In other words, what might be considered normal for one person (two or three bowel movements per week) might well be considered evidence of constipation by another.

Some common causes of constipation are failure to respond to the urge to defecate, inadequate fiber in the diet, inadequate fluid intake, weakness of the abdominal muscles, inactivity and bed rest, pregnancy, hemorrhoids, and gastrointestinal disease. Drugs such as narcotics, belladonna derivatives, diuretics, calcium, iron and aluminum hydroxide, and phosphate gels tend to cause constipation. The sudden onset of constipation may indicate serious disease (*e.g.,* one sign of cancer of the colon and rectum is a change in bowel habits).

The treatment of constipation is usually directed toward relieving the cause. A conscious effort should be made to respond to the defecation urge. A time should be set aside after a meal, when mass movements in the colon are most apt to occur, for a bowel movement. An adequate fluid intake and bulk in the diet should be encouraged. Moderate exercise is essential, and persons on bed rest benefit from passive and active exercises. Laxatives and enemas should be used judiciously. They should not be used on a regular basis to treat simple constipation because they interfere with the defecation reflex and actually damage the rectal mucosa.

Intestinal Obstruction

Intestinal obstruction designates an impairment of movement of intestinal contents in a cephalocaudal direction. The causes of intestinal obstruction can be categorized under two headings: mechanical and reflex paralytic (adynamic).

Mechanical obstruction can result from a number of conditions, either intrinsic or extrinsic, which encroach on the patency of the bowel lumen. These conditions include adhesions of the peritoneum, hernias, twisting of the bowel (volvulus), telescoping of the bowel (intussusception), fecal impaction, strictures, and tumors. There are three types of mechanical obstruction: simple, strangulated, and closed. With a *simple* obstruction, there is no alteration in blood supply. The term *strangulated* implies impairment of blood flow. When the bowel is obstructed on both ends, it is called a *closed* obstruction.

Reflex paralysis usually affects the small bowel. Because the ileum has the narrowest lumen, it is the most prone to obstruction. *Paralytic ileus* is seen most commonly following abdominal surgery or trauma. It occurs early in the course of peritonitis and can result from chemical irritation caused by bile, bacterial toxins, electrolyte imbalances as in hypokalemia, and vascular insufficiency.

The major effects of both types of intestinal obstruction are intestinal distention and loss of fluids and electrolytes. Gases and fluids accumulate within the area. About 7 liters to 8 liters of electrolyte-rich extracellular fluid moves into the small bowel each day, and normally most of this is reabsorbed. Intestinal obstruction interferes with this reabsorption process and a small amount of this extracellular fluid remains in the bowel or is lost in the vomitus. A loss of 7 liters to 8 liters, which represents about half of the extracellular fluid volume of an average adult, can occur in 24 hours or less following acute intestinal obstruction.

If untreated, the distention resulting from bowel obstruction tends to perpetuate itself by causing atony of the bowel and further distention. Distention is further aggravated by the accumulation of gases. About 70% of these gases are estimated to be due to swallowed air. As the process continues, the distention moves proximally involving additional segments of bowel.

Either form of obstruction may eventually lead to strangulation, gangrenous changes, and ultimately perforation of the bowel. The increased pressure within the intestine tends to compromise mucosal blood flow, leading to necrosis and exudation of blood into the luminal fluids. This promotes rapid growth of bacteria within the obstructed bowel. Anaerobes grow rapidly in this favorable environment and produce a lethal endotoxin.

The manifestations of intestinal obstruction depend

on the degree of obstruction and its duration. With acute obstruction, the onset is usually sudden and dramatic. With chronic conditions, the onset is often more gradual. The cardinal symptoms of intestinal obstruction are pain, absolute constipation, abdominal distention, and vomiting. These symptoms are common to intestinal obstruction resulting from either mechanical obstruction or paralytic ileus. Electrolyte imbalances are also common to both.

With *mechanical obstruction,* there is development of hyperperistalsis as the body attempts to move the contents of the intestine around the occluded area. This causes severe colicky pain, in contrast with the continuous pain and silent abdomen seen with paralytic ileus. With mechanical obstruction, there is also borborygmus (rumbling sounds made by propulsion of gas in the intestine), audible high-pitched peristalsis, and peristaltic rushes. Visible peristalsis may appear along the course of the distended intestine. There is extreme restlessness and conscious awareness of intestinal movements. Weakness, perspiration, and anxiety are obvious. As the condition progresses, the vomitus may become fecal in nature and the peristaltic movements may decrease, and then disappear as the bowel fatigues.

Should *strangulation* occur, the symptoms change. The character of the pain shifts from the intermittent colicky pain caused by the hyperperistaltic movements of the intestine to a severe, unrelenting pain that is made worse by movement. Signs of *peritoneal irritation,* such as rigidity of the abdomen, become apparent. If bowel sounds had been present, they disappear because of the peritoneal irritation. Strangulation increases the risk of mortality by about 25%.

Diagnosis of intestinal obstruction is usually based on history and physical findings. Abdominal x-ray studies will reveal a gas-filled bowel.

The treatment consists of decompression of the bowel through nasogastric suction and correction of fluid and electrolyte imbalances. Strangulation and complete bowel obstruction require surgical intervention.

In summary, motility of the contents through the gastrointestinal tract relies on the activity of the myenteric plexus, which is located between the circular and longitudinal smooth muscle layers. Alterations in gastrointestinal motility can be evidenced by diarrhea, by constipation, or in acute situations by intestinal obstruction.

■ Malabsorption

Malabsorption is the failure to transport dietary constituents, such as fats, carbohydrates, proteins, vitamins, and minerals, from the lumen of the intestine to the body fluids. It can selectively affect a single constituent, such as vitamin B_{12} or lactose, or its effects can extend to all of the substances absorbed in a specific segment of the intestine. Malabsorption can occur because of a primary defect in the intestinal wall itself or because of impaired digestion such as occurs with deficiency of liver bile or pancreatic digestive enzymes. In selected cases, absorption of fats may be impaired by the obstruction of lymph flow from the intestine. Liver and pancreatic disorders are discussed in Chapter 43.

Malabsorption Syndrome

Malabsorption refers to impaired absorptive function. The term *syndrome* indicates a constellation of symptoms arising from multiple causes. Thus, the *malabsorption syndrome* can be caused by celiac disease, tropical sprue, Crohn's disease, resection of large segments of the small bowel, or other conditions that reduce the surface area or function of the small intestine. *Celiac disease* is a condition in which an intolerance to dietary gluten exists and which results in the loss of villi from the small intestine. The effects of celiac disease are reversed by the elimination of gluten from the diet. In tropical sprue, the changes that occur in the villi resemble those seen in celiac disease. The cause of this disorder is unclear, although administration of folic acid is known to be helpful in treatment.

The chief symptom of malabsorption syndrome is steatorrhea. The fat content causes bulky, yellow-gray, malodorous stools that float in the toilet and are difficult to dispose of by flushing the toilet. Weakness, weight loss, anorexia, and abdominal distention are often present. Along with loss of fat in the stools, there is failure to absorb the fat-soluble vitamins. This can lead to easy bruising and bleeding (vitamin K deficiency), bone pain, predisposition to develop fractures and tetany (vitamin D and calcium deficiency), macrocytic anemia, and glossitis (folic acid deficiency). Neuropathy, atrophy of the skin, and peripheral edema may be present. Table 42-4 describes the signs and symptoms of impaired absorption of dietary constituents.

In summary, the digestion and absorption of foodstuffs take place in the small intestine. Here proteins, fats, carbohydrates, and other components of the diet are broken down into molecules that can be transported from the intestinal lumen into the body fluids. Malabsorption results when this transport system becomes impaired. It can involve a single dietary constituent or extend to involve all of the substances that are absorbed in a particular part of the small intestine. Malabsorption can result from disease of the small bowel and disorders that impair digestion and can (in some cases) obstruct the lymph flow by which fats are transported to the general circulation.

Table 42-4 Sites of Absorption and Requirements for Absorption of Dietary Constituents

Dietary Constituent	Site of Absorption	Requirements	Manifestations
Water and electrolytes	Mainly small bowel	Osmotic gradient	Diarrhea Dehydration Cramps
Fat	Upper jejunum	Pancreatic lipase Bile salts Functioning lymphatic channels	Weight loss Steatorrhea Fat-soluble vitamin deficiency
Carbohydrates			
Starch	Small intestine	Amylase Maltase Isomaltase α-dextrins	Diarrhea Flatulence Abdominal discomfort
Sucrose	Small intestine	Sucrase	
Lactose	Small intestine	Lactase	
Maltose	Small intestine	Maltase	
Fructose	Small intestine	—	
Protein	Small intestine	Pancreatic enzymes (trypsin, chymotrypsin, elastin, etc.)	Loss in muscle mass Weakness Edema
Vitamins			
A	Upper jejunum	Bile salts	Night blindness Dry eyes Corneal irritation
Folic acid	Duodenum and jejunum	Absorptive; may be impaired by some drugs (*i.e.*, anticonvulsants)	Cheilosis Glossitis Megaloblastic anemia
B_{12}	Ileum	Intrinsic factor	Glossitis Neuropathy Megaloblastic anemia
D	Upper jejunum	Bile salts	Bone pain Fractures Tetany
E	Upper jejunum	Bile salts	Uncertain
K	Upper jejunum	Bile salts	Easy bruising and bleeding
Calcium	Duodenum	Vitamin D and parathyroid hormone	Bone pain Fractures Tetany
Iron	Duodenum and jejunum	Normal *p*H (hydrochloric acid secretion)	Iron-deficiency anemia Glossitis

■ Study Guide

After you have studied this chapter, you should be able to meet the following objectives:

☐ Describe four manifestations of gastrointestinal disorders.

☐ Explain the significance of melena.

☐ Define pica.

☐ Compare the eating disorders and complications associated with anorexia nervosa and bulimarexia.

☐ State the alteration in function that describes achalasia.

☐ Describe the symptoms of hiatal hernia that the health professional should be able to recognize.

☐ Explain why chronic gastritis is a more serious disorder than acute gastritis.

☐ Distinguish between gastric ulcer and peptic ulcer.

☐ State the factors that may influence hydrochloric acid production.

☐ Explain the conditions under which Cushing's ulcer and Curling's ulcer might occur.

☐ Describe the overall goals in treatment of peptic ulcer.

☐ Describe the symptoms and treatment of the dumping syndrome.

☐ List at least four systemic manifestations of inflammatory bowel disease.

☐ Describe the underlying pathology found in Crohn's disease.

☐ Summarize the pathology involved in ulcerative colitis.

☐ Characterize toxic megacolon.

☐ Explain why diverticular disease may be linked to environmental factors.

☐ Explain what is meant by the phrase *left-sided appendicitis*.

☐ Describe the symptoms of acute appendicitis.

☐ State the significant symptoms of colorectal cancer.

☐ Describe the American Cancer Society's colorectal cancer screening program recommendations.

☐ List five causes of peritonitis.

☐ Describe the chief symptoms of peritonitis.

☐ Explain how the villi are adapted to their function.

☐ Trace absorption of carbohydrates from the small intestine.

☐ Describe the possible result of a lactase deficiency.

☐ State the function of micelles in fat absorption.

☐ Describe the symptoms that may be associated with the presence of the malabsorption syndrome.

☐ Compare osmotic diarrhea, secretory diarrhea, and small-volume diarrhea.

☐ Explain why a failure to respond to the defecation urge may result in constipation.

☐ Explain why intestinal obstruction may ultimately result in strangulation.

■ References

1. Report of the Congress of the United States. National Commission on Digestive Disease, Vol 1. Findings and Long-Range Plans. National Institute of Health, Public Health Service, 1979. DHEW Publication No (NIH) 79–1878
2. Drossman DA: Anorexia Nervosa: A comprehensive approach. Adv Intern Med 28:339, 1983
3. Halmi KA, Falk JR, Schwartz E: Binge-eating and vomiting: A survey of college population. Psychol Med 11:697, 1981
4. Harris RT: Bulimarexia and related serious eating disorders with medical complications. Ann Intern Med 99:800, 1983
5. McBryde CM: Signs and Symptoms, p 400. Philadelphia, JB Lippincott, 1970
6. Schiff L, Stevens RJ, Shapiro N, Goodman S: Observation of oral administration of citrated blood in man. Am J Med Sci 203:409, 1942
7. Morton JH, Poulter CA, Pandya KJ: Alimentary tract cancer. In Rubin P (ed): Clinical Oncology, 6th ed, pp 154, 159, 167. New York, American Cancer Society, 1983
8. Facts About Stomach and Esophageal Cancer, p 13. New York, American Cancer Society, 1978
9. Robbins SL, Cotran RS, Kumar V: Pathologic Basis of Disease, 3rd ed, pp 810, 812, 873. Philadelphia, WB Saunders, 1984
10. Isenberg JI: Peptic ulcer medical treatment. In Beeson PB, McDermott W, Wyngaarden JB (eds): Cecil Textbook of Medicine, 15th ed, p 1513, Philadelphia, WB Saunders, 1979
11. Scade RR, Donaldson RM Jr: How physicians use cimetidine. N Engl J Med 304, No 21: 1283, 1981
12. Freely J, Wilkinson GR, Wood JJA: Reduction in liver blood flow and propranolol metabolism by cimetidine. N Engl J Med 304, No 12:692–695, 1981
13. Report of the Congress of the United States. National Commission on Digestive Diseases, Vol 4. Epidemiology and Impact. National Institute of Health, Public Health Service, 1979. DHEW Publication No (NIH) 79–1887
14. Kirsner JB, Shorter RG: Recent developments in "nonspecific" inflammatory bowel disease. N Engl J Med 306:775, 1982
15. Janowitz HD: Chronic inflammatory disease of the intestine. In Beeson PB, McDermott W, Wyngaarden JB (eds): Cecil Textbook of Medicine, 15th ed, p 1570. Philadelphia, WB Saunders, 1979
16. Hill MJ: Etiology of colon cancer. CRC Crit Rev Toxicol 4:31, 1975
17. Griffen WO: Management of diverticular disease of the colon. Hosp Med 14, No 11:108, 1978
18. Holleb AI (ed): Detecting colon and rectum cancer. CA 33, No. 3:5, 1983
19. Overholt BF: Colonoscopy. New York, American Cancer Society, 1975

■ Additional References

Alpers D, Avioli LV: Inflammatory bowel disease (ulcerative colitis). Arch Intern Med 138:286, 1978

Ballantine TVN: Appendicitis. Surg Clin North Am 6, No 5:1117, 1981

Bauer CL: Managing upper G.I. bleeding. Consultant 20:35, 1980

Bayless TM: Malabsorption in the elderly. Hosp Pract 14, No 8:57–63, 1979

Binder HJ: The pathophysiology of diarrhea. Hosp Pract 19:107, 1984

Borthistle BK: Managing lower G.I. bleeding in the elderly patient. Consultant 20, No 10:230, 1980

Brady PG: Small intestinal syndromes: A guide to diagnosis. Hosp Med 15, No 5:41, 1979

Code CF: Prostaglandins and gastric ulcer. Hosp Pract 15, No 7:62, 1980

Cohen S: Pathogenesis of coffee-induced gastrointestinal symptoms. N Engl J Med 303, No 3:122, 1980

Dworkin HJ: Crohn's disease. Ann Intern Med 101:258, 1984

Fazio VW: Early diagnosis of anorectal and colon carcinoma. Hosp Med 15, No 1:66–85, 1979

Fischer RS: Modern concepts of peptic ulcer disease: Advances in treatment. Med Times 111:111, 1983

Floch MH: Nutritional support in inflammatory bowel disease. Curr Concepts Gastroenterol 9:13, 1984

Fromm D: Stress ulcer. Hosp Med 14, No 11:58, 1978

Goldstein F: Inflammatory bowel disease—better prospects. Consultant 20, No 12:68, 1980

Greenburg JL: Constipation—"congestive bowel failure." Consultant 20, No 11:94, 1980

Gryboski J, Hillemeier C: Inflammatory bowel disease in children. Med Clin North Am 64:1185, 1980

Holt KM, Isenberg JI: Peptic ulcer disease: Physiology and pathophysiology. Hosp Pract 20, No 1:89, 1985

Kirsner JB, Hanauer SB: Crohn's disease: The problem and its management. Hosp Pract 19, No 7:121, 1984

Kolars JC, Levitt MD, Aouji M et al: Yogurt—an autodigesting source of lactose. N Engl J Med 310:1, 1984

Lanza FL, Royer GL, Nelson RS: Endoscopic evaluation of the effects of aspirin, buffered aspirin and entericcoated aspirin on gastric and duodenal mucosa. N Engl J Med 303, No 3:136, 1980

Lennard-Jones JE: Functional gastrointestinal disorders. N Engl J Med 308:431, 1983

Levitt MD: Intestinal gas production—recent advances in flatology. N Engl J Med 302, No 26:974, 1980

Lewicki LJ, Leeson MJ: The multisystem impact on physiologic processes of inflammatory bowel disease. Nurs Clin North Am 19:71, 1984

McCarthy DM: Peptic ulcer: Antacids or cimetidine? Hosp Pract 14, No 12:52, 1979

Menguy R: Gastric mucosal injury from common drugs. Postgrad Med 63, No 4:82, 1978

Mungas JE, Moossa AR, Block GE: Treatment of toxic megacolon. Surg Clin North Am 56, No 1:95, 1976

Myer SA: Overview of inflammatory bowel disease. Nurs Clin North Am 19:3, 1984

Nagamachi Y, Nakamura T: Role of gastric mucosal pepsin in the pathogenesis of acute stress ulceration. World J Surg 3:215, 1979

Newcomer AD, McGill DB: Clinical importance of lactase deficiency. N Engl J Med 310:42, 1984

Richter JE, Castell DO: Gastroesophageal reflux. Ann Intern Med 97:93, 1982

Rubin M, Battle WM, Snape WJ, Cohen S: The esophagus and dysphagia. Hosp Med 15, No 2:6, 1979

Sachar DB: Differentiating types of diarrhea. Consultant 20, No 3:29, 1980

Samborsky V: Drug therapy for peptic ulcer. Am J Nurs 78:2064, 1978

Sanger E, Cassino T: Eating disorders. Am J Nurs 84:31, 1984

Silverstein FE: Peptic ulcer: An overview of diagnosis. Hosp Pract 14, No 2:78, 1979

Steer ML, Silen W: Diagnostic procedures in gastrointestinal hemorrhage. N Engl J Med 309:646, 1983

Chapter 43

Alterations in Function of the Hepatobiliary System and Exocrine Pancreas

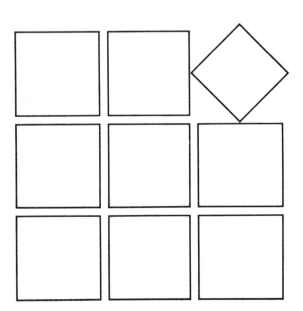

The liver, the gallbladder, and the exocrine pancreas are classified as accessory organs of the gastrointestinal tract. In addition to producing digestive secretions, both the liver and the pancreas have other important functions. The endocrine pancreas, for example, supplies the insulin and glucagon needed in cell metabolism, whereas the liver synthesizes glucose, plasma proteins, and blood-clotting factors and is responsible for the degradation and elimination of drugs and hormones, among other functions. The content of this chapter focuses on disorders of the liver, the biliary tract and gallbladder, and the exocrine pancreas.

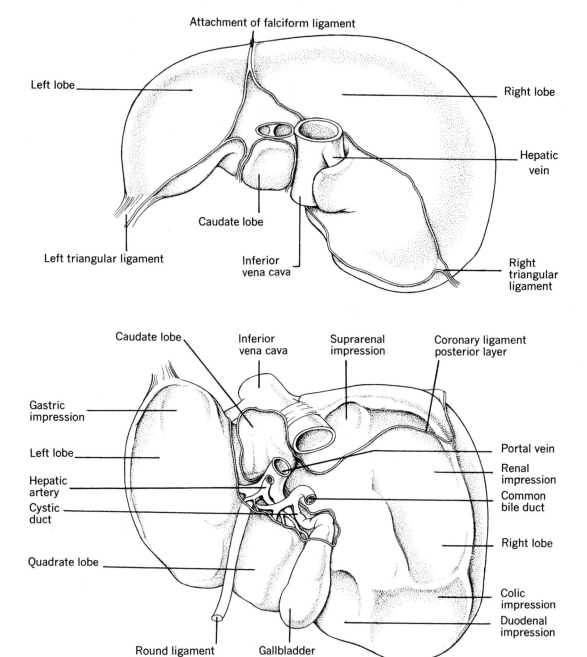

Figure 43-1 *Superior posterior view* (top) *and inferior view* (bottom) *of the liver. (Chaffee EE, Lytle IM: Basic Physiology and Anatomy, 4th ed. Philadelphia, JB Lippincott, 1980)*

■ Hepatobiliary Function

Liver

The liver is the largest organ in the body, weighing about 1.3 kg, or 3 lb, in the adult. It is located below the diaphragm and occupies much of the right hypochondrium. The falciform ligament, which extends from the peritoneal surface of the anterior abdominal wall between the umbilicus and diaphragm, divides the liver into two lobes, a large right lobe and a small left lobe (Fig. 43-1). There are two additional lobes on the visceral surface of the liver, the caudate and quadrate lobes.

Except for that portion which is in the epigastric area, the liver is contained within the rib cage and in healthy persons cannot normally be palpated. The liver is surrounded by a tough fibroelastic capsule called Glisson's capsule.

The liver is unique among the abdominal organs in having a dual blood supply—the hepatic artery and the portal vein. About 400 ml of blood enters the liver through the hepatic artery and another 1000 ml enters by way of the valveless portal vein, which carries blood from the stomach, the small and the large intestines, the pancreas, and the spleen (Fig. 43-2). Although the blood from the portal vein is incompletely saturated with oxy-

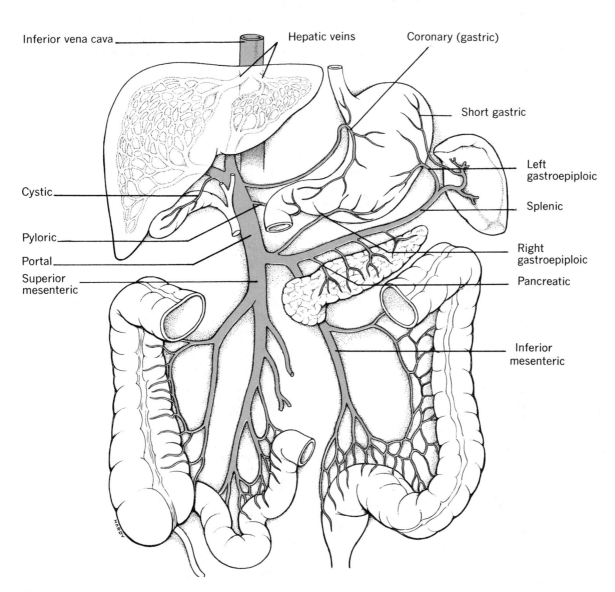

Figure 43-2 *The portal circulation. Blood from the gastrointestinal tract, spleen, and pancreas travels to the liver by way of the portal vein before moving into the vena cava for return to the heart. (From Chaffee EE, Lytle IM: Basic Physiology and Anatomy, 4th ed. Philadelphia, JB Lippincott, 1980)*

gen, it supplies about 60% to 70% of the oxygen needs of the liver.[1] The venous outflow from the liver is carried by the valveless hepatic veins, which empty into the inferior vena cava just below the level of the diaphragm. The pressure difference between the hepatic vein and the portal vein is normally such that the liver stores about 200 ml to 400 ml of blood. This blood can be shifted back into the general circulation during periods of hypotension and shock. In congestive heart failure, in which the pressure within the vena cava increases, blood backs up and accumulates in the liver.

The lobules are the functional units of the liver. Each lobule is a cylindrical structure that measures about 0.8 mm to 2 mm in diameter and is several millimeters in length. There are about 50,000 to 100,000 lobules in each of the two lobes. Each lobule is composed of cellular plates of hepatic cells arranged in spokelike fashion and encircling a central vein (Fig. 43-3). The central vein opens into the hepatic vein and then into the vena cava. The hepatic plates are usually two cells thick and are separated by canaliculi, which empty into the bile ducts. As bile is produced by the hepatic cells, it flows first into the canaliculi, then into the terminal bile ducts, and eventually into the one large bile duct that drains each lobe. Also, in the septa that separate the lobules are the smaller portal venules, which receive blood from the portal veins. The venules empty into the flat sinusoids that lie between the hepatic plates. Branches from the hepatic artery, which supplies the septal tissues, are also found in the intralobular septa, and blood from these arterioles empties into the sinusoids.

The venous sinusoids are lined with two types of cells: the typical endothelial cells and the Kupffer cells. The Kupffer cells are reticuloendothelial cells that are

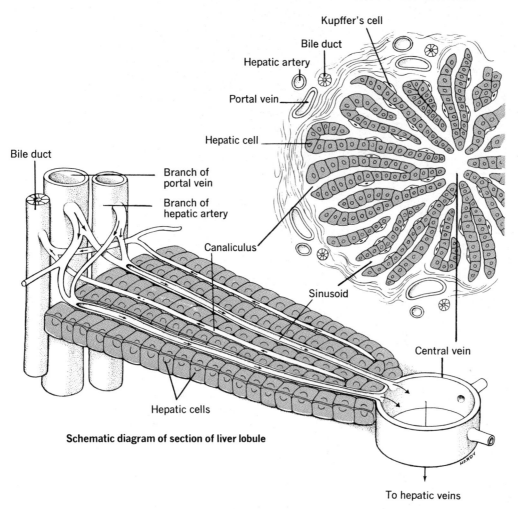

Cross section of liver lobule

Kupffer's cell

Bile duct

Hepatic artery

Portal vein

Hepatic cell

Bile duct

Branch of portal vein

Branch of hepatic artery

Canaliculus

Sinusoid

Central vein

Hepatic cells

Schematic diagram of section of liver lobule

To hepatic veins

Figure 43-3 *A section of liver lobule showing the location of the hepatic veins, hepatic cells, liver sinusoids, and branches of the portal vein and hepatic artery. (From Chaffee EE, Lytle IM: Basic Physiology and Anatomy, 4th ed. Philadelphia, JB Lippincott, 1980)*

capable of removing and phagocytizing old and defective blood cells, bacteria, and other foreign material from the portal blood as it flows through the sinusoid. This phagocytic action removes the colon bacilli and other harmful substances that filter into the blood from the intestine.

Functions of the liver

The liver is one of the most versatile and active organs in the body. It produces bile, metabolizes hormones and drugs, synthesizes proteins, glucose, and clotting factors, stores vitamins and minerals, and converts fatty acids to ketones—and has other functions as well. In this process, the liver degrades excess nutrients and converts them into substances essential to the body. It builds carbohydrates from proteins, converts sugars to fats that can be stored, and interchanges protein molecules so that they can be used for a number of purposes. In its capacity for metabolizing drugs and hormones, the liver serves as an excretory organ. In this respect, the bile, which carries the end products of substances metabolized by the liver, is much like the urine, which carries the body wastes that are filtered by the kidneys. The functions of the liver are summarized in Table 43-1. The liver's role in carbohydrate, fat, and protein metabolism is discussed in Chapter 39. The discussion in this chapter focuses on the function of the liver in alcohol metabolism, production of bile, and removal of bilirubin.

Alcohol metabolism

More than 90% of the alcohol a person drinks is metabolized by the liver. The rest is excreted through the lungs, kidneys, and skin. As a substance, alcohol fits somewhere between a food and a drug. It supplies calories, but cannot be broken down or stored as protein, fat, or carbohydrate. As a food, alcohol yields 7.1 kcal/gm compared with the 4.0 kcal produced by metabolism of an equal amount of carbohydrate. As a drug, it excites, hypnotizes, and then anesthetizes. (It is not a good anesthetic, however, because the euphoric stage lasts too long and the margin between the amount required for surgical anesthesia and that which will depress respiration is very narrow.)[2]

Alcohol is readily absorbed from the gastrointestinal tract, being one of the few substances that can be absorbed from the stomach. The overall metabolism of alcohol requires six oxidative steps and uses three molecules of oxygen to produce two molecules of carbon dioxide. In the process, it translocates 12 hydrogen ions and utilizes vital cofactors, particularly nicotinamide-adenine dinucleotide (NAD), that are needed for other metabolic processes, such as gluconeogenesis. At blood levels commonly obtained by drinking, the generation of hydrogen ions by the liver often exceeds hydrogen ion elimination.[3]

Table 43-1   Functions of the Liver and Manifestations of Altered Function

Function	Manifestations of Altered Function
Production of bile salts	Malabsorption of fat and fat-soluble vitamins
Elimination of bilirubin	Failure to eliminate bilirubin causes elevation in serum bilirubin and jaundice
Metabolism of steroid hormones	
Estrogens and progesterone	Disturbances in gonadal function, including gynecomastia in the male
Testosterone	
Glucocorticoids	Signs of Cushing's syndrome
Aldosterone	Sodium retention and edema; hypokalemia
Metabolism of drugs	Decreased plasma binding of drugs owing to a decrease in albumin production
	Decreased removal of drugs that are metabolized by the liver
Carbohydrate metabolism	Hypoglycemia may develop when glycogenolysis and gluconeogenesis are impaired
Stores glycogen	
Synthesizes glucose from	
Amino acids	Abnormal glucose tolerance curve may occur because of impaired uptake and release of glucose by the liver
Lactic acid	
Glycerol	
Fat metabolism	
Formation of lipoproteins	Impaired synthesis of lipoproteins
Conversion of carbohydrates and proteins to fat	
Synthesis of cholesterol	
Formation of ketones from fatty acids	
Protein metabolism	
Deamination of proteins	
Formation of urea from ammonia	Elevated blood ammonia levels
Synthesis of plasma proteins	Decreased levels of plasma proteins, particularly albumin, which contributes to edema formation
Synthesis of clotting factors	Bleeding tendency
Fibrinogen	
Prothrombin	
Factors V, VII, IX, X	
Storage of minerals and vitamins	Signs of deficiency of fat-soluble and other vitamins that are stored in the liver
Filtration of blood and removal of bacteria and particulate matter by Kupffer cells	Increased exposure of the body to colon bacilli and other foreign matter

The rate of alcohol metabolism is about the same for all persons, except the practicing alcoholic. The rate-limiting step in the process is the availability of the enzyme alcohol dehydrogenase, which is located in the cytosol of the liver cells. The average person can metabolize about 18 gm of alcohol per hour (it takes about 2 hours to metabolize one mixed drink). With prolonged and excessive ingestion of alcohol, the liver seems to develop a supplemental system for metabolizing alcohol and is able to almost double the rate at which it is metabolized. With cessation of drinking, the rate of alcohol metabolism rapidly returns to normal.

One of the main effects of alcohol is the accumulation of fat within the liver. When alcohol is present, it becomes the preferred fuel for the liver, displacing substrates such as fatty acids, which are normally used for this purpose. Triglycerides accumulate in the liver, probably as a result of increased production and because of increased trapping of fatty acids within the liver cells.

Because alcohol competes for utilization of cofactors normally needed by the liver for other metabolic processes, it tends to disrupt the other functions of the liver. An altered redox state (reduction and oxidation, with accumulation of hydrogen ions) and the preferential utilization of NAD for alcohol metabolism can result in increased production and accumulation of lactic acid in the blood. The increased lactate levels tend to impair uric acid excretion by the kidney, which probably explains why excessive alcohol consumption frequently aggravates or precipitates gout. By reducing the availability of the cofactor NAD, alcohol impairs the liver's ability to form glucose from amino acids and other glucose precursors. Thus, alcohol-induced hypoglycemia and alcoholic ketoacidosis can develop when excessive alcohol ingestion occurs during periods of depleted liver glycogen stores. This may become a particular problem for the alcoholic who has been vomiting and has not eaten for several days. Alcohol also increases the body's

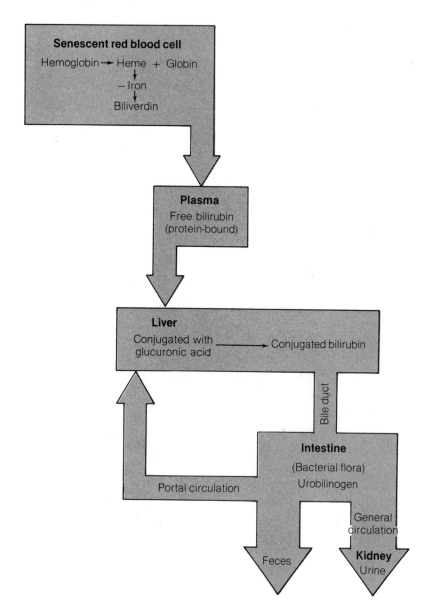

Figure 43-4 *The process of bilirubin formation, circulation, and elimination.*

requirements for the B vitamins and increases urinary losses of magnesium, potassium, and zinc.

There has been considerable controversy over the interaction of diet and liver changes observed with chronic alcoholism. In fact, one of the arguments that heavy drinkers often use to justify their habit is that with proper attention to diet, they can avoid the undesirable effects of alcohol on the liver. In the past, it has been difficult to study and document the influence of nutrition on liver changes that arise with chronic alcohol abuse. However, recent animal research has demonstrated that full-blown cirrhosis of the liver can develop even when the diet is adequate.[4] This suggests that the alcohol itself plays an important role in liver injury. Studies using alcohol-fed baboons led to the discovery of alcohol-related changes in one of the enzymes of protein metabolism, gamma-glutamyl transpeptidase transferase. Serum levels of this enzyme become elevated with prolonged heavy drinking, and this enzyme test has been used in rehabilitative and industrial settings to indicate active alcoholism.[4]

Production of bile

The liver produces about 600 ml to 800 ml of yellow-green bile daily. Bile contains water, bile salts, bilirubin, cholesterol, and various inorganic acids. Of these, only bile salts are important in digestion.

The liver forms about 0.5 gm of bile salts daily. Bile salts are formed from cholesterol, which is either supplied by the diet or synthesized by the liver. Bile salts serve an important function in digestion: they aid in *emulsifying dietary fats* and they are necessary for the *formation of the micelles* that transport fatty acids and fat-soluble vitamins to the surface of the intestinal mucosa for absorption. About 94% of bile salts that enter the intestine are reabsorbed into the portal circulation by an active transport process that takes place in the distal ileum. From the portal circulation, the bile salts pass into the liver where they are recycled. Normally, bile salts travel this entire circuit about 18 times before being expelled in the feces.[5] This system for recirculation of bile is called the *enterohepatic circulation*.

Excretion of bilirubin

Bilirubin is the substance that gives bile its color. It is formed from senescent red blood cells. In the process of degradation, the hemoglobin from the red blood cell is broken down to form biliverdin, which is rapidly converted to *free bilirubin* (Fig. 43-4). Free bilirubin, which is insoluble in plasma, is transported in the blood attached to plasma albumin. As blood passes through the liver, free bilirubin is absorbed by the hepatocytes and is released from the albumin-carrier molecule. Once inside

the hepatocyte, bilirubin is conjugated with either glucuronic acid or glucuronic sulfate, a process that enables the bilirubin to become soluble in bile. Conjugated bilirubin is then secreted into the canaliculi of the liver as a constituent of bile, and in this form it passes through the bile ducts into the small intestine. The bacterial flora in the intestine converts bilirubin to urobilinogen, which is highly soluble. Urobilinogen is either reabsorbed into the portal circulation or excreted in the feces. Most of the urobilinogen that is reabsorbed is returned to the liver to be reexcreted into the bile. A small amount of urobilinogen, about 5%, is reabsorbed into the general circulation and is then excreted by the kidneys.

Usually, only a small amount of bilirubin is found in the serum, the normal level of total serum bilirubin being 0.3 to 1.3 mg/dl. A simple test, the *van den Bergh test,* measures both the free and the conjugated bilirubin present in the total bilirubin. The *direct* van den Bergh test measures the conjugated bilirubin; the *indirect* test measures the free bilirubin.

Jaundice.   Jaundice (icterus) is due to an abnormally high accumulation of bilirubin in the blood, as a result of which there is a yellowish discoloration to the skin and deep tissues. Jaundice develops when the plasma contains about twice the normal amount of bilirubin. Normal skin has a yellow cast, and therefore early signs of jaundice are often difficult to detect. This is especially true in persons with dark skin. Because bilirubin has a special affinity for elastic tissue, the sclera of the eye, which contains considerable elastic fibers, is usually one of the first structures wherein jaundice can be detected. The four chief causes of jaundice are (1) excessive destruction of red blood cells, (2) decreased uptake of bilirubin by the liver cells, (3) decreased conjugation of bilirubin, and (4) obstruction of bile flow, either in the canaliculi of the liver or in the intra- or extrahepatic bile ducts (Table 43-2).

Hemolytic jaundice occurs when red blood cells are destroyed at a rate in excess of the liver's ability to remove the bilirubin from the blood. It may follow a hemolytic blood transfusion reaction or occur in diseases such as hereditary spherocytosis, in which the red cell membranes are defective, or in hemolytic disease of the newborn (Chap. 24). Kernicterus is a condition characterized by severe neurologic symptoms that are due to high blood levels of unconjugated bilirubin; because the unconjugated bilirubin is lipid soluble, it is able to enter nerve cells and cause brain damage. It is a common sequela in hemolytic disease of the newborn caused by the Rh factor. A physiologic jaundice may be seen in infants during the first week of extrauterine life and is related to the immaturity of the infant's liver and its

Table 43-2 Causes of Jaundice

Excessive red blood cell destruction
   Hemolytic blood transfusion reaction
   Hereditary disorders of the red blood cell
      Sickle cell anemia
      Thalassemia
      Spherocytosis
   Hemolytic disease of the newborn
Decreased uptake by the liver
   Gilbert's disease
Decreased conjugation of bilirubin
   Hepatocellular liver damage
      Hepatitis
      Cirrhosis
   Breast milk jaundice
Obstruction of bile flow
   Intrahepatic
      Drug-induced cholestasis
   Extrahepatic
      Structural disorders of the bile duct
      Cholelithiasis
      Tumors that obstruct bile duct
      Liver disease

inability to remove and conjugate sufficient amounts of bilirubin.

Another condition, called *breast milk jaundice,* occurs in a small percentage of breast-fed babies. These babies have significant levels of unconjugated bilirubin, which rises progressively from the fourth day of life and reaches a maximum in 10 to 15 days. It disappears if breast-feeding is discontinued. The disorder is thought to be due to enzymes in the mother's milk that liberate free fatty acids from the constituents of the breast milk.[6] An immaturity of the infant's intestinal tract allows these fatty acids to be absorbed into the portal circulation where they travel to the liver and inhibit bilirubin conjugation. Another possible mechanism for breast milk jaundice is some factor in the milk that increases the absorption of bilirubin in the duodenum. Preheating the milk to 56°C for 15 minutes has been reported to inactivate the factors that produce the jaundice, a point that should be considered for mothers who wish to continue breast-feeding or for those administering such milk to low-birth-weight infants.

In recent years it has become evident that sunlight breaks down bilirubin into products that can be excreted in stool and urine; this knowledge formed the basis of phototherapy for jaundiced newborns. Phototherapy can be used to treat babies with hemolytic jaundice caused by the Rh factor, physiologic jaundice, or breast milk jaundice. This simple and easily accomplished treatment is successful in many cases.

Gilbert's disease is inherited as a dominant trait and results in a reduced uptake of bilirubin. The disorder is benign and fairly common. Affected persons have no symptoms other than a slightly elevated unconjugated bilirubin, and hence jaundice. Conjugation of bilirubin is impaired whenever liver cells are damaged (hepatocellular jaundice), when transport of bilirubin into liver cells becomes deficient, or when the enzymes needed to conjugate the bile are lacking. Hepatitis and cirrhosis are the most common causes of this form of jaundice. Hepatocellular jaundice usually interferes with all phases of bilirubin metabolism—uptake, conjugation, and excretion.

Obstructive jaundice or *cholestatic jaundice* is seen when the flow of bile is obstructed. The obstruction may be of either intrahepatic or extrahepatic origin. In the *intrahepatic* form, both the conjugated and unconjugated serum bilirubin levels are abnormally high. Liver disease, drugs—especially the anesthetic halothane—oral contraceptives, estrogen, anabolic steroids, isoniazid, and chlorpromazine are all possible causative factors. *Extrahepatic cholestatic jaundice* is due to obstruction to bile flow between the liver and the intestine, with the obstruction located at any point between the junction of the right or left hepatic duct and the point where the bile duct opens into the intestine. With this form of jaundice, conjugated levels of bilirubin are elevated. Among the causes are strictures of the bile duct, gallstones, and tumors of the bile duct or the pancreas. Blood levels of bile acids are elevated in both intrahepatic and extrahepatic cholestatic jaundice. As the bile acids accumulate in the blood, pruritus develops. A history of pruritus preceding jaundice is common in obstructive jaundice of either intrahepatic or extrahepatic origin. The stools are usually clay colored because so little bile is entering the intestine, and, at the same time, the urinary bilirubin is increased. Also common to both intra- and extrahepatic jaundice is an abnormally high level of serum alkaline phosphatase. Alkaline phosphatase is produced by the liver and excreted with the bile, thus when bile flow is obstructed, the blood alkaline phosphatase becomes elevated.

Tests of liver function

The history and physical examination will, in most instances, provide clues about liver function. Diagnostic tests help to assess liver function and the extent of liver disease. A liver biopsy affords a means of examining liver tissue without necessitating surgery. Table 43-3 describes the common tests of liver function and their significance.

Gallbladder

The secretion of bile is essential for digestion of dietary fats and absorption of fats and fat-soluble vitamins from the intestine. Bile produced by the hepatocytes flows into

Table 43-3 Tests of Liver Function

Type of Test	Tests	Significance
Enzyme	Serum glutamic-oxaloacetic transaminase (SGOT)	Released into the serum when there is liver damage Elevated in hepatitis, cirrhosis, liver necrosis May also be elevated in myocardial infarction, skeletal muscle disease, and hematopoietic disorders
	Serum glutamic-pyruvic transaminase (SGPT)	Elevation indicates death of liver cells Elevated in hepatocellular disease, infectious hepatitis, liver injury, and liver congestion
	Alkaline phosphatase	Rises when excretion of the enzyme is impaired because of biliary obstruction Useful in differentiating hepatocellular and obstructive jaundice
	Lactic acid dehydrogenase (LDH)	The isoenzymes LDH_1 and LDH_2 are found primarily in liver, skeletal muscle, and lung; the test is sensitive enough to detect increased fractions in infectious hepatitis before jaundice appears
	Y-glutamyl transpeptidase transferase (YGT)	The liver is the main source of this enzyme; it facilitates the transport of amino acids across the cell membrane; used to detect alcoholic liver disease and alcohol consumption
Bilirubin	Total	Measures total serum bilirubin
	Direct	Measures conjugated bilirubin (an increase usually associated with liver disease or obstruction of bile duct)
	Indirect	Measures free bilirubin (an increase usually associated with increased destruction of red blood cells)
	Icterus index	Measures the degree of jaundice by comparing the yellowness of the serum with that of a standard yellow compound
	Tests for bilirubin in urine	Usually, there is no bilirubin in urine; when present it represents conjugated bilirubin because free bilirubin that is attached cannot be filtered in the glomerulus; presence suggests liver disease or obstructive jaundice
	Urinary and fecal urobilinogen	Absence of fecal urobilinogen indicates obstruction of biliary tract An increase in fecal urobilinogen indicates excessive bilirubin production An increase in urinary urobilinogen in absence of an increased fecal urobilinogen indicates liver disease
Blood ammonia		The liver normally removes ammonia from the blood and converts it to urea; blood ammonia levels are often elevated in severe liver disease
Blood coagulation	Prothrombin time	Liver disease causes impaired synthesis of clotting factors V, VII, IX, X, prothrombin (II), and fibrinogen; prothrombin time is affected by most of these factors; the test is used to assess the risk of bleeding
Dye clearance	Sodium sulfobromophthalein (Bromsulphalein, BSP)	Liver function test, which is based on the liver's ability to remove dye from the blood
	Indocyanine green (ICG)	Also measures ability of liver to remove dye from blood (used less frequently than BSP)
Plasma proteins	Total plasma proteins	Measures total plasma proteins, including albumin, globulins, and fibrinogen
	Albumin	Albumin is decreased in cirrhosis
	Globulins	Alpha and beta globulins are increased in infectious or obstructive jaundice and decreased in liver failure, which interferes with their synthesis
Liver scan	Blood vessel structural scan	Measures the size, shape, and filling defects of the liver after intravenous injection of a radioactive substance; a radioactive detector (or scanner) outlines the liver and spleen
	Liver cell function scan ^{99m}Tc IDAs ^{131}I rose bengal	Radioactive dye is cleared from the blood by the liver; the size, shape, and filling of the liver, gallbladder, and small intestine are determined by scanning following intravenous injection of the dye (Rose bengal is seldom used because of its effect on the thyroid)
	Ultrasound	Outlines hepatobiliary structures
	Computerized tomography	Outlines hepatobiliary structures

the canaliculi, and then to the periphery of the lobules, which drain into larger ducts, until it reaches the right and left hepatic ducts. These ducts unite to form the common duct (Fig. 43-5). The common duct, which is about 10 cm to 15 cm in length, descends and passes behind the pancreas and enters the descending duo-denum. The pancreatic duct joins the common duct in the ampulla of Vater, which empties into the duodenum through the duodenal papilla. Muscle tissue at the junction of the papilla, called the sphincter of Oddi, regulates the flow of bile into the duodenum. A second sphincter (sphincter of Boyden), which is just above the point

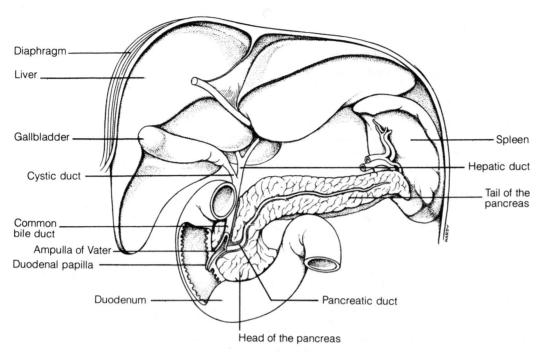

Figure 43-5 *The liver and biliary system, including the gall bladder and bile ducts. (From Chaffee EE, Lytle IM: Basic Physiology and Anatomy, 4th ed. Philadelphia, JB Lippincott, 1980)*

where the pancreatic duct fuses with the common duct, controls the flow of bile into this area of the common duct. When this sphincter is closed, bile moves back into the gallbladder.

The gallbladder is part of the biliary system. It is a distensible, pear-shaped muscular sac located on the ventral surface of the liver. It has a smooth muscle wall and is lined with a thin layer of absorptive cells. The cystic duct joins the gallbladder to the common duct. The function of the gallbladder is to store and concentrate bile. When full, it can hold 20 ml to 50 ml of bile. Entrance of food into the intestine causes contraction of the gallbladder and relaxation of the sphincter of Oddi. The stimulus for gallbladder contraction is primarily hormonal. Products of food digestion, particularly lipids, stimulate cholecystokinin release from the mucosa of the duodenum. The role of other gastrointestinal hormones in bile release is less clearly understood. Passage of bile into the intestine is largely regulated by the pressure within the common duct. Normally, the gallbladder serves to regulate this pressure: it collects and stores bile as the pressure increases and causes an increase in pressure when it contracts. Following gallbladder surgery, the pressure in the common duct changes, causing the common duct to dilate. The flow of bile is then regulated by the sphincters in the common duct.

In summary, the heptobiliary system consists of the liver, gallbladder, and bile ducts. The liver is the largest and, in function, one of the most versatile organs in the body. It is located between the gastrointestinal tract and the systemic circulation; venous blood from the intestine flows through the liver before it is returned to the heart. In this way, nutrients can be removed for processing and storage, and bacteria and other foreign matter can be removed by the Kupffer cells before the blood is returned to the systemic circulation. The liver synthesizes bile salts, fats, glucose, and plasma proteins. It metabolizes drugs and removes, conjugates, and secretes bilirubin into the bile. Jaundice occurs when bilirubin accumulates in the blood. Jaundice can occur because of excessive red blood cell destruction, failure of the liver to remove and conjugate the bilirubin, or obstructed biliary flow. The gallbladder and bile ducts serve as a passageway for the delivery of bile to the intestine, with the gallbladder storing and concentrating bile.

■ Alterations in Liver Function

Although the liver is among the organs most frequently damaged, only about 10% of hepatic tissue is required for the liver to remain functional.[1] Of the numerous pathologic processes to which the liver may be subject—including vascular disorders, inflammation, metabolic disorders, toxic injury, and neoplasms—three diseases have been selected for inclusion in this section: acute hepatitis, cirrhosis, and cancer.

Hepatitis

Hepatitis is an inflammation of the liver. It can be caused by a number of conditions, including reactions to drugs and toxins (alcoholic hepatitis) and infections such as malaria, mononucleosis, salmonellosis, and amebiasis, which cause a secondary hepatitis. One of the major infections in which the liver is the primary affected organ is viral hepatitis.

Viral hepatitis is an acute inflammatory disease usually caused by hepatitis virus A (HVA), hepatitis virus B (HVB), or other non-A, non-B virus(es) that have not yet been elucidated. Viruses such as cytomegalovirus, herpes simplex, and rubella virus may be rarely implicated. Table 43-4 describes the salient features of both hepatitis A and B.

Hepatitis A

Hepatitis A has a brief incubation period. It is usually spread by the fecal-oral route. Drinking contaminated milk or water and eating shellfish from infected waters are fairly common causes. Institutions housing large numbers of people (usually children) are sometimes striken by an epidemic of HVA. At special risk are persons

Table 43-4 Manifestations of Viral Hepatitis A and B

Features	Hepatitis A	Hepatitis B	Common Manifestations
Mode of transmission	Excreted in the stool 2 weeks prior to and for 1 week after onset of clinical disease; transmitted by fecal–oral route, contaminated water, milk, shellfish	Present in the serum; transmitted by blood transfusion and blood products, needles, and other inoculation equipment; can also be transmitted by intimate sexual partners or family members; mother-to-infant transmission	
Persons at risk	Young children and persons in institutions	Parenteral drug abusers; persons on hemodialysis; health care workers	
Carrier state	Not known to occur	Develops in about 5%–10% of persons who have the disease	
Incubation period*	15–40 days (average, 30–38 days)	43–160 days (average, 90 days)	Headache Nausea Vomiting
Preicterus period		Manifestations more severe, including Skin rash Arthralgia Test for HVB positive	3–12 days Fever Headache Epigastric distress Anorexia, nausea, vomiting Intolerance to fatty foods Diminished sense of smell Loss of taste for cigarettes Elevation of SGOT, SGPT, LDH$_1$, and LDH$_2$
Icterus period			2–6 weeks Jaundice Dark urine Clay-colored stool Elevated total bilirubin
Convalescent period			Abdominal pain and tenderness
Other		May progress to carrier state and chronicity Risk of later development of hepatocarcinoma in persons who develop chronic hepatitis	

*Developed from information in Richman A: Infectious hepatitis. Hosp Med 14, No 3:72, 1978

traveling abroad who have never previously been exposed to the virus. Hepatitis A is not usually transmitted by blood or plasma derivatives, presumably because its short period of viremia usually coincides with clinical illness, so that the disease is apparent and blood donations are not accepted.

Hepatitis B

Hepatitis B represents a more serious problem than hepatitis A; it has a longer incubation period and is more likely to cause serious illness and to become chronic. The sources of HVB are chronic carriers and persons with active hepatitis B. Infected blood or blood derivatives are also a source. Hepatitis B is associated with long periods of viremia, often years or even a lifetime. This means that infected blood or plasma donors may not even be aware that they are carriers. The risk of hepatitis associated with transfusions of blood derivatives results from the manufacture of these products from large pools of human plasma.[7]

Persons who habitually abuse certain drugs by injecting them directly into the bloodstream are also at special risk, because they frequently use needles contaminated by the blood of fellow addicts without first sterilizing the needles. It can also be transmitted by contaminated medical equipment. This is one reason why disposable needles and syringes are preferable. Persons on hemodialysis are also at high risk, in part because they often require blood transfusions and in part because their immune system is deficient. HVB has also been found in the saliva, urine, semen, menstrual blood, and other secretions of persons with the disease. Mother-to-infant transmission occurs, but whether transmission occurs *in utero* or during the birth process is not known.

Acute hepatitis

The injurious effects of both type A and type B hepatitis viruses are believed to arise because of an immune reaction in which the hepatitis virus in some way alters the antigenic properties of the hepatocytes. The extent of inflammation and necrosis, therefore, varies depending on the individual immune response.

The clinical manifestations of both hepatitis A and B have been divided into four phases: (1) the incubation period, (2) the preicterus period, (3) the icterus period, and (4) the convalescent period. Table 43-4 summarizes each of these phases.

Prevention and treatment

The treatment of hepatitis is largely symptomatic. Bed rest, which at one time was a mainstay in treatment, has now largely been replaced with a more liberal program that permits patients to pace their own activity. Most patients will elect to limit activity because of fatigue. Dietary restrictions are usually minimal. If oral intake becomes inadequate, glucose solutions may be administered intravenously. Patients are instructed to avoid strenuous exercise and alcohol and other hepatotoxic agents.

The most effective way to prevent hepatitis is to prevent opportunities for the transmission of the virus. Because *contamination* (of blood, needles, other equipment) affords the virus ready access to the body, as previously described, the health care worker should follow proper procedures when handling syringes and needles that have been used for drawing blood or injecting medications. Gloves should be worn when handling blood samples. Routine screening of blood donors has reduced the incidence of posttransfusion hepatitis B. There is increasing evidence, however, that other non-A, non-B viruses may be responsible for transfusion-induced hepatitis.

Gamma globulin is usually administered to close personal contacts of persons with hepatitis A. It may be advisable for persons traveling to countries where hepatitis A is endemic to receive a protective dose of gamma globulin within 2 weeks of arrival in that country and to receive booster doses if their stay is an extended one. The standard gamma globulin does not appear to afford protection against hepatitis B. However, hepatitis B immune globulin, which is not widely available, is effective if administered in a large dose within 10 days of exposure.

An inactivated subunit hepatitis B vaccine became available in the United States in 1982. Although the vaccine does not control the carrier state, it is an important step toward eventual control of the disease in this country.[8] At present, however, preparation of the vaccine is costly, and its availability may be limited in the immediate future. Questions about its long-term safety also need to be examined. Because of these factors, decisions are being made about who will benefit most from the vaccine.

Cirrhosis

The World Health Organization defines cirrhosis as "a diffuse process characterized by fibrosis and conversion of normal liver architecture into structurally abnormal nodules."[9] Although cirrhosis is usually associated with alcoholism, it can develop in the course of other disorders, including viral hepatitis, toxic reactions to drugs and chemicals, biliary obstruction, and cardiac disease. Cirrhosis also accompanies metabolic disorders that cause the deposition of minerals in the liver; two of these disorders are hemochromatosis (iron deposition) and Wilson's disease (copper deposition).

There are three types of cirrhosis: postnecrotic, biliary, and portal. Each of these has a different etiology; but in the end, each causes liver failure, and the ultimate outcome is much the same. Following a brief discussion of postnecrotic and biliary cirrhosis, we shall take portal (alcoholic) cirrhosis as our prototype.

Postnecrotic cirrhosis

This form of cirrhosis is characterized by the replacement of liver tissue with small to large nodules of fibrous tissue, with a resultant markedly deformed and nodular liver. Postnecrotic cirrhosis accounts for some 10% to 30% of cases of cirrhosis. It may follow viral hepatitis (type B or non-A, non-B type) or an autoimmune disease, or it may be a toxic response to drugs and other chemicals. It is a predisposing factor in hepatic cancer when it is caused by hepatitis type B.

Biliary cirrhosis

Biliary cirrhosis starts in the bile ducts, occurring as a primary or a secondary disorder and accounting for about 10% of cases of cirrhosis.[1] *Primary biliary cirrhosis* is seen most commonly in women 40 to 60 years of age. The cause is unknown. It is characterized by inflammation and scarring of the septal and intralobular bile ducts. The liver becomes enlarged and takes on a green hue. The earliest symptoms are pruritus, followed by dark urine and pale stools. Once symptoms become clinically evident, life expectancy is about 5 years.[10] As far as is known, in some persons the existence of the disease is detectable only through laboratory studies, because there are no symptoms. *Secondary biliary cirrhosis* develops as the result of prolonged obstruction of bile flow either within the liver or in the extrahepatic ducts. It is most commonly due to gallstones, stricture of the bile ducts, or neoplasms that obstruct bile flow. A secondary infection may develop and ascend, causing further liver damage.

Portal or alcoholic cirrhosis

Portal cirrhosis, often called alcoholic cirrhosis or Laennec's cirrhosis, is the fourth leading cause of death among adult Americans and the third leading cause of death among men 35 to 55 years of age. The most common cause of cirrhosis is excessive alcohol consumption. At least 75% of deaths attributable to alcoholism are caused by cirrhosis.[11] It is estimated that there are 10 million alcoholics in the United States. Interestingly, not all alcoholics develop cirrhosis, suggesting that other conditions such as genetic and environmental factors contribute to its occurrence. In fact, one-third of alcoholics never develop cirrhosis; in another one-third, fatty liver changes occur but not cirrhosis; the remaining one-third have cirrhosis.[12] Most deaths from alcoholic cirrhosis are attributable to liver failure, bleeding esophageal varices, or kidney failure.

Stages of development. Although the mechanism whereby alcohol exerts its toxic effects on liver structures is somewhat unclear, the changes that develop can be divided into three stages: (1) fatty changes, (2) alcoholic hepatitis, and (3) cirrhosis.

Fatty changes. During this stage, the liver enlarges because of excessive accumulation of fat within the liver cells. Alcohol replaces fat as a fuel for liver metabolism and impairs mitochondrial ability to oxidize fat. There is evidence that high ingestion of alcohol can cause fatty liver changes even in the presence of an adequate diet. For example, young nonalcoholic volunteers had fatty liver changes after 2 days of consuming 18 oz to 24 oz of alcohol, even though adequate carbohydrates, fats, and proteins were included in the diet.[13] The fatty changes that occur with ingestion of alcohol do not usually produce symptoms and are reversible once the alcohol intake has been discontinued.

Alcoholic hepatitis. Alcoholic hepatitis is the intermediate stage between fatty changes and cirrhosis. It is characterized by inflammation and necrosis of liver cells and thus is always serious and sometimes fatal. The necrotic lesions are generally patchy, but may involve an entire lobe. The cause is unknown. It is often seen after an abrupt increase in alcohol intake and is common in "spree" drinkers. "Ballooning" of hepatocytes and the toxic effects of the intermediates of alcohol metabolism, such as acetaldehyde, are believed to be contributory factors. This stage is usually characterized by hepatic tenderness, pain, anorexia, nausea, fever, jaundice, ascites, and liver failure; but some patients may be asymptomatic. There is a marked increase in the serum glutamic-oxaloacetic transaminase. Within 1 to 20 years, 80% of persons with alcoholic hepatitis who continue to drink will have liver changes consistent with cirrhosis.[12]

Cirrhosis. Cirrhosis is the direct result of liver injury caused by fatty changes and alcoholic hepatitis. The liver becomes yellow-orange, fatty, and diffusely scarred. Its normal structure is distorted by bands of fibrous tissue, which separate areas of regenerated cells. As the disease progresses, the liver shrinks. As normal tissue is replaced by scar tissue, blood flow through the liver is obstructed and extrahepatic shunts form, which serve as alternative routes for the return of portal blood to the heart.

Clinical manifestations. There may be no symptoms for long periods of time; when symptoms do appear, they are vague at first, with complaints of fatigability and weight loss. At this point, the liver is often palpable and hard. Diarrhea is frequently present, although some persons may complain of constipation. There may be abdominal pain because of liver enlargement or stretching of Glisson's capsule. This pain is located in the epigastric area or in the upper right quadrant and is described as dull and aching and causing a sensation of fullness. The late manifestations of cirrhosis are related to portal hypertension and liver cell failure. Portal hypertension causes complications such as esophageal varices and ascites; in hepatocellular failure, there are decreased production of bile, plasma proteins, and blood-clotting factors and interference with removal of bilirubin, ammonia, and other substances. The manifestations of cirrhosis are discussed in the section that follows and are summarized in Table 43-5.

Portal hypertension.   Portal hypertension describes a condition in which portal-vein pressure increases (10–12 mm Hg across the liver).[10] The presence of bands of fibrous tissue and fibrous nodules within the liver induces a gradual increase in portal-vein pressure with the development of (1) collateral channels between the portal and systemic veins, (2) splenomegaly, and (3) ascites.

Development of collateral channels.   With gradual obstruction of blood flow in the liver, the pressure in the portal vein increases and large collateral channels develop between the portal veins and the systemic veins in the esophagus and lower rectum and in the umbilical veins of the falciform ligament that attaches to the anterior abdominal wall. Splenomegaly occurs because of splenic vein congestion. The esophageal veins, being thin-walled, are vulnerable to the formation of varicosities (Fig. 43-6). These *esophageal varices* are subject to rupture, with massive and sometimes fatal hemorrhage. This acute bleeding is the most significant complication of

Table 43-5   Manifestations of Portal Cirrhosis

Primary Alteration in Function	Manifestation
Portal Hypertension	
Development of collateral vessels	Esophageal varices
	Hemorrhoids
	Caput medusae (dilated cutaneous veins around the umbilicus)
Increased pressure in the portal vein and decreased levels of serum albumin	Ascites
	Peripheral edema
Splenomegaly	Anemia
	Leukopenia
	Thrombocytopenia
Hepatorenal syndrome	Elevated serum creatinine
	Azotemia
	Oliguria
Portal–systemic shunting of blood	Hepatic-systemic encephalopathy
Hepatocellular Dysfunction	
Impaired metabolism of sex hormones	Female: menstrual disorders
	Male: testicular atrophy, gynecomastia, decrease in secondary sex characteristics
	Skin disorders: vascular spiders and palmer erythema
Impaired synthesis of plasma proteins	Decreased levels of serum albumin with development of edema and ascites
	Decreased synthesis of carrier proteins for hormones and drugs
Decreased synthesis of blood-clotting factors	Bleeding tendencies
Failure to remove and conjugate bilirubin from the blood	Jaundice
Impaired bile synthesis	Malabsorption of fats and fat-soluble vitamins
Impaired metabolism of drugs cleared by the liver	Risk of drug reactions and toxicities
Impaired gluconeogenesis	Abnormal glucose tolerance
Decreased ability to convert ammonia to urea	Elevated blood ammonia levels

portal hypertension. The presence of the collaterals between the inferior and internal iliac veins may give rise to *hemorrhoids*. In some persons, the fetal umbilical vein is not totally obliterated; it forms a channel between the portal vein and the vein on the anterior abdominal wall (Fig. 43-7). These dilated veins around the umbilicus are called *caput medusae*. Finally, portopulmonary shunts may arise, causing blood to bypass the pulmonary capillaries, thereby interfering with blood oxygenation and producing cyanosis.

Surgical treatment of portal hypertension consists of creating a portal–systemic shunt (an opening between the portal and a systemic vein). Although this procedure does not improve liver function, it does reduce the pressure within the esophageal veins and thus prevents esophageal hemorrhage. The two procedures that are done most frequently are portacaval shunt and splenorenal shunt. In a *portacaval* shunt, an opening is created between the portal vein and the vena cava. A *splenorenal* shunt involves removal of the spleen and anastomosis of the splenic vein to the left renal vein. It is often done when the spleen is enlarged and prevents further thrombocytopenia and leukopenia. One of the untoward sequelae that develop in some 10% of persons with a portal–systemic shunt is hepatic–systemic encephalopathy. As will be discussed, the neurologic manifestations of this disorder are believed to result from absorption of ammonia and other neurotoxic substances from the gut directly into the systemic circulation without going through the liver.

Splenomegaly. The splenomegaly observed in cirrhosis results from the shunting of blood into the splenic vein, which gives rise to such hematologic disorders as anemia, thrombocytopenia, and leukopenia.

Ascites and peripheral edema. Ascites is an accumulation of fluid within the peritoneal cavity. This fluid is a transudate of plasma, constantly being exchanged with fluid from the vascular compartment, and composed of electrolytes and albumin similar in composition to plasma. In cirrhosis, the two major factors contributing to ascites are (1) impaired synthesis of albumin by the liver, so that the plasma colloidal osmotic pressure falls, and (2) obstruction of venous flow through the liver. This obstruction causes increased production of lymph, with oozing of serous fluid from the liver surface. The decreased colloidal osmotic pressure causes fluid to leak out of the capillaries in the splanchnic (visceral) circulation. Added to these is a rise in aldosterone, which augments retention of sodium and water by the kidneys. Among the causes postulated to be responsible for the increased aldosterone levels are an impairment of aldosterone inactivation by the liver and production by the liver of a humoral substance that stimulates aldosterone secretion. The increased aldosterone leads to a potassium deficiency. Because of the fall in serum

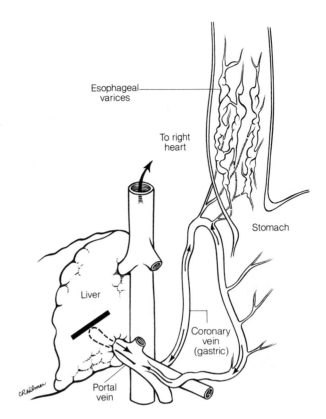

Figure 43-6 *Obstruction of blood flow in the portal circulation, with portal hypertension and diversion of blood flow to other venous channels, including the gastric and esophageal veins.*

albumin and the retention of sodium and water, peripheral edema develops, particularly in the dependent parts of the body, such as the feet.

Treatment of ascites usually focuses on dietary restriction of sodium and administration of diuretics. Water intake may also need to be restricted. To counteract the rise in aldosterone, an aldosterone-blocking diuretic along with one of the thiazide diuretics is usually prescribed. Oral potassium supplements are often given to prevent hypokalemia, because the potassium level probably has fallen before diuretic therapy is begun. Paracentesis may be done for diagnostic purposes but is seldom done to treat the ascites, because its effects are only temporary and it may cause a shift in fluid from the vascular compartment to the peritoneal cavity, along with complications such as infection and hemorrhage.

Hepatorenal syndrome. The hepatorenal syndrome refers to a functional state of renal failure that is sometimes seen during the terminal stages of cirrhosis and ascites. It is characterized by progressive azotemia, increased serum creatinine levels, and oliguria. Although the basic cause is not known, a decrease in renal blood flow is believed to play a part. Ultimately, when renal failure is superim-

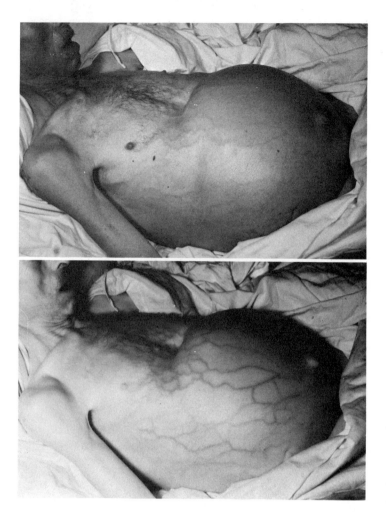

Figure 43-7 *Collateral abdominal veins on the anterior abdominal wall in a patient with alcoholic liver disease as recorded by black and white photography* (top) *and infrared photography* (bottom). *(From Schiff L: Diseases of the Liver, 5th ed, p 408. Philadelphia, JB Lippincott, 1982)*

posed on liver failure, elimination of bilirubin is impaired along with azotemia and elevated levels of blood ammonia; this often precipitates hepatic coma.

A surgical procedure called the *LaVeen* continuous peritoneal-jugular shunt has been devised; the peritoneal fluid is shunted from the abdominal cavity through a one-way pressure-sensitive valve into a silicone tube that empties into the superior vena cava. The procedure is reported to relieve refractory ascites in persons with cirrhosis and to reverse the pathophysiologic manifestations of the hepatorenal syndrome.[14]

Endocrine disorders.   Endocrine disorders are common accompaniments of cirrhosis, particularly disturbances in gonadal function. In women there may be menstrual irregularities (usually amenorrhea), loss of libido, and sterility. In men, the testosterone level usually falls, the testes atrophy, and loss of libido, impotence, and gynecomastia occur.

Skin disorders.   Liver failure brings on numerous skin disorders. These lesions, called variously *vascular spiders, telangiectasia, spider angiomas,* and *spider nevi,* most often

are seen in the upper half of the body. These lesions consist of a central pulsating arteriole from which smaller vessels radiate. (It should be kept in mind that spider angiomas may be seen in pregnancy even when liver function is normal.) *Palmar erythema* is redness of the palms, probably because of an increased blood flow resulting from higher cardiac output. Clubbing of the fingers may be seen in persons with cirrhosis. Jaundice is usually a late manifestation of liver failure.

Hematologic disorders.   Anemia, thrombocytopenia, coagulation defects, and leukopenia may arise in the presence of cirrhosis. *Anemia* may be due to blood loss, excessive red blood cell destruction, and impaired formation of red blood cells. A folic acid deficiency may lead to severe megaloblastic anemia. Changes in the lipid composition of the red cell membrane increase hemolysis. Because factors V, VII, IX, X, prothrombin, and fibrinogen are synthesized by the liver, their decline in liver disease contributes to bleeding disorders. Malabsorption of the fat-soluble vitamin K contributes further to the impaired synthesis of these clotting factors. Often a *thrombocytopenia* occurs as the result of splenomegaly.

Thus, the cirrhotic patient is subject to purpura, easy bruising, hematuria, and abnormal menstrual bleeding (women), and is vulnerable to bleeding from the esophagus and other segments of the gastrointestinal tract.

Fetor hepaticus refers to a characteristic musty, sweetish odor of the breath in the patient in advanced liver failure, resulting from the breakdown products of metabolism manufactured by intestinal bacteria.

Hepatic–systemic encephalopathy. Hepatic–systemic encephalopathy refers to the totality of central nervous system manifestations of cirrhosis. It is characterized by neural disturbances ranging from a lack of mental alertness to confusion, coma, and convulsions. A very early sign of hepatic encephalopathy is a flapping tremor called asterixis. Loss of memory of varying degrees may occur, coupled with personality changes, such as euphoria, irritability, anxiety, and lack of concern about personal appearance and self. There may also be impairment of speech and inability to perform certain purposeful movements. The encephalopathy may progress to decerebrate rigidity and finally to a terminal deep coma.

The essential cause of hepatic encephalopathy is not yet known. The presence of neurotoxins, which appear in the blood because the liver has lost its detoxifying capacity, is believed to be a related factor. As has been stated, hepatic encephalopathy develops in about 10% of persons having a portal–systemic shunt.

One of the suspected neurotoxins is ammonia. We may trace its development as follows: One function of the liver is to convert ammonia, a by-product of protein metabolism, to urea. Ammonia is also produced in the intestine. In the intestine, the bacterial flora converts proteins to ammonia, which normally diffuses back into the portal blood and thence to the liver, where it is converted to urea before entering the general circulation. This is the normal situation. However, should a pathologic process develop wherein blood from the intestine bypasses the liver, or the liver is no longer able to convert the ammonia to urea, the ammonia is able to reach the brain through the general circulation and there to exert its toxic effects. This is why hepatic encephalopathy is aggravated by a large protein meal, by bleeding from the gastrointestinal tract, and during periods of dehydration. When hypokalemic alkalosis is present, it causes increased renal production of ammonia. Narcotics and tranquilizers are poorly metabolized by the liver, and administration of these drugs may cause central nervous system depression and precipitate hepatic encephalopathy.

Treatment. The treatment is directed toward correcting fluid and electrolyte imbalances, particularly hypokalemia, and limiting ammonia production in the gastrointestinal tract by limiting protein intake. A non-absorbable antibiotic, such as neomycin, may be given to eradicate bacteria from the bowel and thus prevent this cause of ammonia production. Another drug that may be given is lactulose. It is not absorbed from the small intestine but moves directly to the large intestine where it is catabolized by the colon bacteria to small organic acids that cause production of large, loose stools with a low *p*H. The low *p*H is believed to convert ammonia to ammonium ions, which are not absorbed by the blood.[15]

Cancer of the Liver

Primary cancer of the liver, which accounts for 2% of all cancers, is relatively rare in the United States.[16] There are two primary types of cancer of the liver—hepatocarcinoma, which arises from the liver cells, and cholangiocarcinoma, which is a primary cancer of the bile duct cells. Sometimes cellular components of both types are present. Hepatocarcinoma is strongly associated with postnecrotic cirrhosis caused by hepatitis B and with hemochromatosis. A small number of cases have been reported to occur in women taking oral contraceptives. By far the most common basis of liver cancer is metastases, usually from the lung or the breast.

The initial symptoms are weakness, anorexia, fatigue, bloating, a sensation of abdominal fullness, and a dull, aching abdominal pain. Usually, the liver is enlarged at the time these symptoms appear, and there is a low fever without apparent cause. Serum-alpha fetoprotein, a serum protein present in fetal life, normally is barely detectable in the serum after the age of 2 years; but it is present in some 50% to 90% of cases of hepatocarcinoma.[1]

Primary cancers of the liver are usually far advanced at the time of diagnosis; the 5-year survival rate is about 1% and most patients die within 6 months. The treatment of choice is subtotal hepatectomy of 85% to 90% of the liver, if conditions permit.[16] The cancer is not radiosensitive. Chemotherapeutic drugs, among them methotrexate and 5-fluorouracil (5-FU) may be administered by cannula placed in the hepatic artery.

In summary, the liver is subject to most of the disease processes that affect other body structures, such as vascular disorders, inflammation, metabolic diseases, toxic injury, and neoplasms. Two of the most common liver diseases are hepatitis and cirrhosis. Acute viral hepatitis is caused by hepatitis A and hepatitis B viruses. Spread of hepatitis A occurs by oral-fecal transmission; it has a short incubation period and is usually followed by complete recovery. Hepatitis B has a longer incubation period and is spread through contact with contaminated blood, serum, instruments, and body secretions. Its symptoms are more severe and it may progress to the carrier or chronic state. Cirrhosis caused by hepatitis B is associated with increased risk of hepatocarcinoma. Cirrhosis is the fourth leading cause of death in the United States. It is characterized by fibrosis and conversion of the normal hepatic architecture into structurally abnormal nodules. There are three types of cirrhosis—postnecrotic, biliary, and portal, or alcoholic cirrhosis—of which the most common is alcoholic cirrhosis. Regardless of cause, the manifestations of end-stage cirrhosis are similar and result from portal hpertension and liver cell failure.

■ Alterations in Gallbladder Function

Two very common disorders of the biliary system are *cholelithiasis* (gallstones) and *cholecystitis* (inflammation of the gallbladder). Together, these diseases affect about 16 million persons living in the United States and account for some 16% to 18% of short-stay admissions to hospitals for treatment of digestive diseases.[11] Close to 400,000 cholecystectomies are performed in this country each year.[17]

Composition of Bile and Formation of Gallstones

Gallstones are due to the precipitation of substances contained in bile, mainly cholesterol and bilirubin. Bile contains bile salts, cholesterol, bilirubin, lecithin, fatty acids, and water as well as electrolytes normally found in the plasma. The cholesterol found in bile has no known function; it is assumed to be a by-product of bile salt formation, and its presence is linked to the excretory function of bile. Normally insoluble in water, cholesterol is rendered soluble by the action of bile salts, which combine with it to form micelles. In the gallbladder, water and electrolytes are absorbed from the liver bile, causing the bile to become more concentrated. Because neither lecithin nor bile salts are absorbed in the gallbladder, their concentration increases along with that of cholesterol, and in this way, the solubility of cholesterol is maintained.

The bile of which gallstones are formed is usually supersaturated with either cholesterol or bilirubinate. The majority of gallstones, about 75%, are composed primarily of cholesterol, and the other 25% are pigment, or calcium bilirubinate, stones. Many stones have a mixed composition. Three factors contribute to the formation of gallstones: (1) abnormalities in the composition of bile, (2) stasis of bile, and (3) inflammation of the gallbladder. The formation of cholesterol stones is associated with obesity and is seen more frequently in women, especially women who have had multiple pregnancies or who are taking oral contraceptives. All of these situations cause the liver to excrete more cholesterol into the bile. Drugs such as clofibrate, which lower serum cholesterol levels, also cause increased cholesterol excretion into the bile. Malabsorption disorders stemming from ileal disease or intestinal bypass surgery, for example, tend to interfere with the absorption of bile salts, which is needed to maintain the solubility of cholesterol. Inflammation of the gallbladder alters the absorptive characteristics of the mucosal layer, allowing for excessive absorption of water and bile salts. Cholesterol gallstones are extremely common among Native Americans, which suggests that a genetic component may have a role in gallstone formation. Pigment stones are seen in persons with hemolytic disease and hepatic cirrhosis.

Many persons with gallstones have no symptoms. Gallstones cause symptoms when they obstruct bile flow.[18] Small stones not more than 8 mm in diameter pass into the common duct, producing symptoms of indigestion and biliary colic. Larger stones are more likely to obstruct flow and cause jaundice.[19] The pain of biliary colic is generally abrupt in onset, increasing steadily in intensity until it reaches a climax in 30 to 60 minutes. The upper right quadrant, or epigastric area, is the usual location of the pain, often with referred pain to the back, above the waist, the right shoulder, and the right scapula or the midscapular region. A few persons will experience pain on the left side. The pain usually persists for 2 hours to 8 hours, and is followed by soreness in the upper right quadrant.

Cholecystitis and Cholelithiasis

Cholecystitis is inflammation of the gallbladder. It may be either acute or chronic, and both types are associated with cholelithiasis, or the formation of gallstones. Acute cholecystitis may be superimposed on chronic cholecystitis.

Acute cholecystitis is almost always associated with complete or partial obstruction of bile flow. It is believed that the inflammation is caused by chemical irritation from the concentrated bile, along with mucosal swelling and ischemia resulting from venous congestion and lymphatic stasis. The gallbladder is usually markedly distended. Bacterial infections may arise secondarily to the ischemia and chemical irritation. The bacteria reach the injured gallbladder through the blood, lymphatics, or bile ducts, or from adjacent organs. Among the common pathogens are staphylococci and enterococci. The wall of the gallbladder is most vulnerable to the effects of ischemia, as a result of which mucosal necrosis and sloughing occur. The process may lead to gangrenous changes and perforation of the gallbladder.

The symptoms of acute cholecystitis vary with the severity of obstruction and inflammation. It is often precipitated by a fatty meal and may be initiated with complaints of indigestion. Pain, initially similar to that of biliary colic, is characteristic of acute cholecystitis. It does not, however, subside spontaneously; it responds poorly or only temporarily to potent analgesics. When the inflammation progresses to involve the peritoneum, the pain becomes more pronounced in the right upper quadrant. The right subcostal region is tender, and there is spasm of the muscles that surround the area. *Vomiting* occurs in about 75% of patients and jaundice in some 25%. *Fever* and an abnormally high *white blood cell* count attest to the presence of inflammation. Total serum bilirubin, serum transaminase, and alkaline phosphatase are usually elevated.

The manifestations of chronic cholecystitis are more vague than those of acute cholecystitis. There may be intolerance to fatty foods, belching, and other indications of discomfort. Often there are episodes of colicky pain with obstruction of biliary flow caused by gallstones. The gallbladder, which in chronic cholecystitis usually contains stones, may be enlarged, shrunken, or of normal size. The passage of a stone into the common duct causes obstruction of bile flow and may contribute to carcinoma of the gallbladder.

Diagnosis and treatment

Radiologic techniques provide a means for visualizing the outline of the biliary tract. Ten percent to 15% of gallstones contain sufficient calcium to be visible on plain x-ray films. *Oral cholecystography* is effective when there are no symptoms of active gallbladder disease. The evening before the films are to be taken, tablets containing a contrast dye are administered orally. The dye is absorbed in the gut, excreted in the bile, and concenrated in the gallbladder. If stones are present, they will be outlined on the x-ray film. The gallbladder will not be outlined if the dye is not absorbed, if the common duct is obstructed, or if the gallbladder cannot concentrate the dye. *Intravenous cholangiography* involves the intravenous injection of a contrast dye, which is excreted by the liver. X-ray films are taken immediately following the injection and during a period of up to 4 hours, to afford sufficient time for the gallbladder to concentrate the dye. *Operative cholangiograms* are done at the time of gallbladder surgery to afford immediate visualization of the ductal system and detection of filling defects and the presence of stones in the hepatic and common duct. *T-tube cholangiography* can be done after gallbladder surgery when the T-tube is in place, in which case the dye is injected into the T-tube. *Transhepatic cholangiography* involves the inser-

tion of a needle through the eighth or ninth rib space into a bile duct in the center of the liver. A dye is injected into the duct for the purpose of visualizing the ductal structures and diagnosing strictures or neoplastic obstruction of the bile ducts. *Ultrasound* may be employed to demonstrate gallstones and biliary tract dilatation.

The usual treatment of choice for symptomatic cholelithiasis and cholecystitis is surgical removal of the gallbladder—*cholecystectomy*. If the inflammation is acute, the surgery is delayed, unless complications demand immediate surgery. This allows time for the inflammatory process to subside. Recently, there has been interest in administering *chenodeoxycholic acid* to dissolve radiolucent cholesterol stones. This drug causes bile to become unsaturated by reducing cholesterol production while increasing bile salt excretion. It dissolves most stones within a year or 2. However, it is not being administered to women of childbearing years for fear that it may adversely affect the fetal liver.

In summary, the biliary tract serves as a passageway for the delivery of bile from the liver to the intestine. This tract consists of the bile ducts and gallbladder. The most common causes of biliary tract disease are cholelithiasis and cholecystitis. Three factors contribute to the development of gallstones: (1) abnormalities in the composition of bile, (2) stasis of bile, and (3) inflammation of the gallbladder. Cholelithiasis predisposes to obstruction of bile flow, causing biliary colic and acute or chronic cholecystitis. Cholecystectomy is usually the treatment of choice for symptomatic cholelithiasis in persons who are good surgical risks. Chenodeoxycholic acid has recently become available for use in dissolving cholesterol gallstones. Its effect on the liver of the fetus has not been established, and therefore it is not being prescribed for women of childbearing years.

■ Exocrine Pancreas

The pancreas lies transversely in the posterior part of the upper abdomen. The head of the pancreas is at the right of the abdomen; it rests against the curve of the duodenum in the area of the ampulla of Vater and its entrance into the duodenum. The body of the pancreas lies beneath the stomach. The tail touches the spleen. The pancreas is virtually hidden because of its posterior position. Unlike many other organs, it cannot be palpated. Because of the position of the pancreas and its large functional reserve, symptoms of disease do not usually appear until the disorder is far advanced. This is particularly true of cancer of the pancreas.

The pancreas is both an endocrine and an exocrine organ. Its function as an endocrine organ was discussed in Chapter 40. The exocrine pancreas is made up of lobules that consist of acinar cells. These cells secrete digestive enzymes into a system of microscopic ducts. These ducts are terminal branches of larger ducts that drain into the main pancreatic duct, which extends from left to right through the substance of the pancreas (see Fig. 43-5). In most people, the main pancreatic duct empties into the ampulla of Vater, although in some persons it empties directly into the duodenum. The pancreatic ducts are lined with epithelial cells that secrete water and bicarbonate and thereby modify the fluid and electrolyte composition of the pancreatic secretions. The pancreatic secretions contain proteolytic enzymes that break down dietary proteins, including trypsin, chymotrypsin, carboxypolypeptidase, ribonuclease, and deoxyribonuclease. The pancreas also secretes pancreatic amylase, which breaks down starch, and lipase, which hydrolyzes neutral fats into glycerol and fatty acids. The pancreatic enzymes are secreted in the inactive form and become activated once in the intestine. This is important because the enzymes would digest the tissue of the pancreas itself were they to be secreted in the active form. The acinar cells secrete a trypsin inhibitor, which prevents trypsin activation. Since trypsin activates other proteolytic enzymes, the trypsin inhibitor prevents subsequent activation of those other enzymes. Two types of pancreatic disease are discussed in this chapter: acute and chronic pancreatitis and cancer of the pancreas.

Acute Hemorrhagic Pancreatitis

Acute pancreatitis is a severe and life-threatening disorder associated with the escape of activated pancreatic enzymes into the pancreas and surrounding tissues. These enzymes cause fat necrosis, or autodigestion, of the pancreas and produce fatty depots in the abdominal cavity with hemorrhage from the necrotic vessels. Although a number of factors are associated with the development of acute pancreatitis, the two most important are biliary tract disease with reflux of bile into the pancreas and alcoholism. Biliary reflux is believed to activate the pancreatic enzymes within the ductile system of the pancreas. Gallstones that obstruct the common duct account for approximately 60% of nonalcoholic acute pancreatitis.[20] The precise mechanisms whereby alcohol exerts its action are largely unknown. Alcohol is known to be a potent stimulator of pancreatic secretions, and at the same time it often causes partial obstruction of the sphincter of Oddi. Acute pancreatitis is also associated with hyperlipidemia, hyperparathyroidism, infections (particularly viral), abdominal and surgical trauma, and drugs such as steroids and thiazide diuretics.

An important disturbance related to acute pancreatitis is the loss of a large volume of fluid into the retroperitoneal and peripancreatic spaces and the abdominal cavity. The onset is usually abrupt and dramatic, and it may follow a heavy meal or an alcoholic binge. Severe epigastric and abdominal pain often radiates to the back. The pain is aggravated when the person is lying supine; it is less severe when the person is sitting and leaning forward. Abdominal distention accompanied by hypoactive bowel sounds is common. Tachycardia, hypotension, cool, clammy skin, and fever are often evident. Signs of hypocalcemia may develop, probably as a result of the precipitation of serum calcium in the areas of fat necrosis. Mild jaundice may appear after the first 24 hours because of biliary obstruction. The serum amylase becomes elevated within the first 24 hours, and serum lipase within 72 hours to 94 hours. Both enzymes remain elevated during the destructive stage of the disease and return to normal within 2 days to 5 days following the acute attack. Urinary clearance of amylase is increased. Because the serum amylase may be elevated as a result of the presence of other serious illnesses, the urinary amylase may be measured. Hyperglycemia and an elevated serum bilirubin may be present. About 5% of persons with acute pancreatitis die of the acute effects of peripheral vascular collapse. Serious complications include acute respiratory distress syndrome and acute tubular necrosis.

The treatment consists of measures directed at pain relief and restoration of lost plasma volume. Meperidine (Demerol) rather than morphine is usually given for pain relief because it causes fewer spasms of the sphincter of Oddi. Papaverine, nitroglycerin, barbiturates, or anticholinergic drugs may be given as supplements to provide smooth muscle relaxation. Oral foods and fluids are withheld, and gastric suction is instituted to treat distention of the bowel and prevent further stimulation of the secretion of pancreatic enzymes. Intravenous fluids and electrolytes are administered to replace those lost from the circulation and to combat the hypotension and shock. Intravenous colloid solutions are given to replace the fluid that has become sequestered in the abdomen and retroperitoneal space. Percutaneous peritoneal lavage has been tried as an early treatment of acute pancreatitis with encouraging results. Should a pancreatic abscess develop, it must be drained, usually through the flank. Pseudocysts that develop and persist must be treated surgically.

A *pseudocyst* is a collection of pancreatic fluid in the peritoneal cavity, enclosed in a layer of inflammatory tissue. Autodigestion of liquefaction of pancreatic tissue may be the cause. The pseudocyst is most often connected to a pancreatic duct, so that it continues to increase in mass. The symptoms depend on its location.

For example, jaundice may occur when a cyst develops near the head of the pancreas close to the common duct. Pseudocysts may resolve or may require surgical intervention.

Chronic Pancreatitis

Chronic pancreatitis is characterized by progressive destruction of the pancreas. It can be divided into two types: chronic calcifying pancreatitis and chronic obstructive pancreatitis. In *chronic calcifying pancreatitis,* calcified protein plugs (calculi) form in the pancreatic ducts. This form is seen most often in alcoholics. *Chronic obstructive pancreatitis* is associated with stenosis of the sphincter of Oddi. The lesions are prominent in the head of the pancreas. It is usually due to cholelithiasis and is sometimes relieved by removal of the sphincter of Oddi.

Chronic pancreatitis is manifested in episodes that are similar, albeit of lesser severity, to those of acute pancreatitis. There are persistent, recurring episodes of epigastric and upper left quadrant pain. Anorexia, nausea, vomiting, constipation, and flatulence are common. The attacks are often precipitated by alcohol abuse or overeating. Eventually, the disease progresses to the extent that both endocrine and exocrine pancreatic functions become deficient. At this point, signs of diabetes mellitus and the malabsorption syndrome become apparent. Pancreatic enzymes are given to treat the malabsorption, and the diabetes is treated with insulin. Narcotic addiction is a potential problem in persons with chronic pancreatitis.

Cancer of the Pancreas

The incidence of cancer of the pancreas has almost tripled in the past 40 years.[16] At present it is the fourth leading cause of cancer death in men and the fifth most common in women in the United States. Cancer of the pancreas is usually far advanced when diagnosed, and the 5-year survival rate is less than 9%. The cause of pancreatic cancer is unknown. Recently, an association between coffee and cancer of the pancreas was made. The relative risk associated with drinking two cups of coffee per day was 1.8 times normal; with three or more cups, it was reported to be 2.7 times normal.[21]

Cancer of the pancreas usually has an insidious onset, with symptoms of anorexia, weight loss, flatulence, and nausea. A dull, aching epigastric pain is present in about 70% to 80% of cases.[22] Overt diabetes mellitus is found in one-fifth of persons with pancreatic cancer, and almost all persons with the disease have an abnormal glucose tolerance.[22]

Because of the proximity of the pancreas to the common duct and the ampulla of Vater, cancer of the head of the pancreas tends to obstruct bile flow; this causes distention of the gallbladder and jaundice. The jaundice is frequently the presenting symptom in cancer of the head of the pancreas, and it is usually accompanied by complaints of pain and by pruritus. Cancer of the body of the pancreas generally impinges on the celiac ganglion, causing pain. The pain usually worsens with ingestion of food or with assumption of the supine position. Cancer of the tail of the pancreas has usually metastasized before symptoms appear.

Most cancers of the pancreas have metastasized by the time of diagnosis. Therefore, the treatment is usually palliative and consists of high-voltage irradiation and chemotherapy. Surgical resection of the tumor is done when the tumor is localized. The treatment results with use of single-agent or combination chemotherapy have shown steady improvement, providing some gains for survival.[16]

In summary, the pancreas is both an endocrine and an exocrine organ. Diabetes mellitus is the most common disorder of the endocrine pancreas, and it occurs independently of disease of the exocrine pancreas. The exocrine pancreas produces digestive enzymes that are secreted in an inactive form and transported to the small intestine through the main pancreatic duct, which usually empties into the ampulla of Vater and then into the duodenum through the sphincter of Oddi. The most common diseases of the exocrine pancreas are acute and chronic pancreatitis and cancer. Both acute and chronic pancreatitis are associated with biliary reflux and chronic alcoholism. Acute pancreatitis is a dramatic and life-threatening disorder in which there is autodigestion of pancreatic tissue. Chronic pancreatitis causes progressive destruction of both the endocrine and the exocrine pancreas. It is characterized by episodes of pain and epigastric distress that are similar to but less severe than that which occurs with acute pancreatitis. Cancer of the pancreas has shown a marked increase in incidence during the past 40 years. It is usually far advanced at the time of diagnosis, and as a result, the 5-year survival rate is less than 9%.

■ Study Guide

After you have studied this chapter, you should be able to meet the following objectives:

☐ Describe the anatomy of the liver.

☐ Describe the function of the liver as it relates to alcohol metabolism.

☐ Describe the enterohepatic circulation.

☐ Explain the formation and degradation of bilirubin.

☐ Compare hemolytic jaundice and obstructive jaundice with reference to their clinical manifestations.

☐ Summarize the salient features of hepatitis A and hepatitis B with which the health professional should be acquainted.

☐ Characterize postnecrotic cirrhosis and biliary cirrhosis.

☐ Summarize the three stages of alcoholic cirrhosis.

☐ Describe the clinical manifestations of alcoholic cirrhosis with reference to development of collateral channels.

☐ Explain the development of ascites in alcoholic cirrhosis.

☐ State a clinical definition of the hepatorenal syndrome.

☐ Explain the basis of bleeding disorders in alcoholic cirrhosis.

☐ Characterize hepatic–systemic encephalopathy.

☐ Explain the significance of the presence of serum-alpha fetoprotein in an adult.

☐ Describe the physiology of the gallbladder.

☐ Describe the formation of gallstones.

☐ Compare the symptoms of acute cholecystitis with those of chronic cholecystitis.

☐ Describe the exocrine function of the pancreas.

☐ Describe the clinical manifestations of acute pancreatitis.

☐ Compare chronic calcifying pancreatitis and chronic obstructive pancreatitis.

☐ State a significant statistic relating to pancreatic cancer.

7. Gerety RJ, Aronson DL: Plasma derivatives and viral hepatitis. Transfusion 22:347, 1982
8. Chin J: Use of hepatitis B virus vaccine. N Engl J Med 307:677, 1982
9. Anthony PP et al: The morphology of cirrhosis: Definition, nomenclature, and classification. Bull WHO 55, No 4:522, 1977
10. Jeffries GH: Diseases of the liver. In Beeson PB, McDermott W, Wyngaarden JB (eds): Cecil Textbook of Medicine, 15th ed, pp 1639, 1670. Philadelphia, WB Saunders, 1979
11. Report to the Congress of the United States of the National Commission on Digestive Diseases, Vol 2(A), p 305, and Vol 4(2A), p 395. National Institute of Health, Public Health Service. DHEW Publication No (NIH) 79–1884
12. Leevy CM, Kangasundororm N: Alcoholic hepatitis. Hosp Pract 13, No 10:115, 117, 1978
13. Rubin E, Lieber CS: Alcohol-induced hepatic injury in nonalcoholic volunteers. N Engl J Med 278:869, 1968
14. Wapnick S, Grosberg S, Kinney M, LaVeen HH: LaVeen continuous peritoneal-jugular shunt. JAMA 237, No 2:131, 1977
15. Hardison GM: Cirrhosis—treating the ascites and encephalopathy. Med Times 107, No 5:23, 1979
16. Adams JT, Poulter CA, Pondye KJ: Cancer of the digestive glands. In Rubin P (ed): Clinical Oncology, 6th ed, pp 178, 183. New York, American Cancer Society, 1983
17. Motson RW, Way LW: Differential diagnosis of gall bladder disease. Hosp Med 13, No 3:26, 1977
18. Gracie WA, Ranshoff DF: The natural history of silent gallstones. N Engl J Med 307:798, 1982
19. Iber FL: Axioms on biliary tract disease. Hosp Med 15, No 6:52, 1979
20. Ronson JHC: Etiologic and prognostic factors in human acute pancreatitis: A review. Am J Gastroenterol 77:633, 1982
21. MacMahon B et al: Coffee and cancer of the pancreas. N Engl J Med 304, No 11:630, 1981
22. Douglas HO, Karakousis C, Nava H: Guide to diagnosis of pancreatic cancer (part 2). Hosp Med 14, No 1:40, 1978

■ References

1. Robbins SL, Cotran RS, Kumar V: Pathologic Basis of Disease, 3rd ed, pp 884, 916, 938. Philadelphia, WB Saunders, 1984
2. Iber F: In alcoholism, the liver sets the pace. Nutrition Today 6, No 1:2, 1971
3. Lieber CS: Alcohol, protein metabolism, and liver injury. Gastroenterology 79, No 2:373, 1980
4. Lieber CS: Pathogenesis and early diagnosis of alcoholic liver injury. N Engl J Med 298, No 16:888, 889, 1978
5. Guyton AC: Textbook of Medical Physiology, 5th ed, p 872. Philadelphia, WB Saunders, 1981
6. Avery GB: Neonatology, 2nd ed, p 493. Philadelphia, JB Lippincott, 1981

■ Additional References

Altshuler A, Hilden D: The patient with portal hypertension. Nurs Clin North Am 12, No 12:317, 1977

Bennison LJ, Grundy MD: Risk factors for the development of cholelithiasis in man. Part I. N Engl J Med 299, No 21:1161, 1977

Bennison LJ, Grundy MD: Risk factors for the development of cholelithiasis in man. Part II. N Engl J Med 299, No 22:1221, 1977

Bouchier IAD: The medical treatment of gallstones. Annu Rev Med 31:59, 1980

Boyer CA, Oehlberg SM: Interpretation and clinical relevance of liver function tests. Nurs Clin North Am 12, No 2:275, 1977

Cello JP: Diagnostic approaches to jaundice. Hosp Pract 17, No 2:49, 1982

Douglass HO, Karakousis CP, Nava H: Guide to diagnosis of pancreatic cancer. Part 1. Hosp Med 13, No 12:8, 1977

Douglass HO, Karakousis CP, Nava H: Guide to diagnosis of pancreatic cancer. Part 2. Hosp Med 14, No 1:40, 1978

Gannon RB, Pickett K: Jaundice. Am J Nurs 83:404, 1983

Gelfand MD: Gallbladder disease: Diagnostic guide. Hosp Med 15, No 1:8, 1979

Gracie WA, Ransohoff DF: The innocent gallbladder is no myth. N Engl J Med 307:798, 1982

Gurevich I: Hepatitis precautions. Am J Nurs 83:572, 1983

Hardison GM: Cirrhosis: Treating the ascites and encephalopathy. Med Times 107, No 5:23, 1979

Hoyumpa AM Jr, Schenker S: Perspectives in hepatic encephalopathy. J Lab Clin Med 100:477, 1982

Kaplowitz N: Cholestatic liver disease. Hosp Pract 13, No 8:83, 1978

Katz J: How to manage the complications of chronic pancreatitis. Consultant 20, No 5:141, 1980

Klingenstein J, Dienstag JL: Viral hepatitis: The meaning of serologic markers. Consultant 20, No 10:53, 1980

McElroy DB: Nursing care of patients with viral hepatitis. Nurs Clin North Am 12, No 2:305, 1977

Moosa AR: Diagnostic tests and procedures in acute pancreatitis. N Engl J Med 311:639, 1984

Pierce L: Anatomy and physiology of the liver. Nurs Clin North Am 12, No 2:259, 1977

Ranson JH: Etiologic and prognostic factors in human acute pancreatitis: A review. Am J Gastroenterol 77:633, 1982

Regan PT, DiMagno EP: Acute pancreatitis: Diagnosis and treatment 15, No 8:30, 1979

Resnick RH: Treatment of bleeding varices: Controversy and opportunity. Hosp Pract 19, No 4:54A, 1984

Reynolds RB: What to do about esophageal varices. N Engl J Med 309:1575, 1983

Scharschmidt BF: Goldberg HI, Schmid R: Approach to the patient with cholestatic jaundice. N Engl J Med 308:1515, 1983

Schenker S, Hoyumpa AM Jr: Pathology of hepatic encephalitis. Hosp Pract 19, No 9:99, 1984

Schiff ER, Chiprut R: Chronic hepatitis: Guidelines for diagnosis and management. Hosp Med 14, No 9:59, 1978

Shahinpour N: The adult patient with bleeding esophageal varices. Nurs Clin North Am 12, No 2:331, 1977

Thistle JL, Cleary PA, Lachin JM et al: The natural history of cholelithiasis: The national cooperative gallstone study. Ann Intern Med 101:171, 1984

Williams RL: Drug administration in hepatic disease. N Engl J Med 309:1616, 1983

Willson RA: Acute fulminant liver failure. Hosp Med 13, No 10:8, 1977

Unit VII

Alterations in Neuromuscular Function

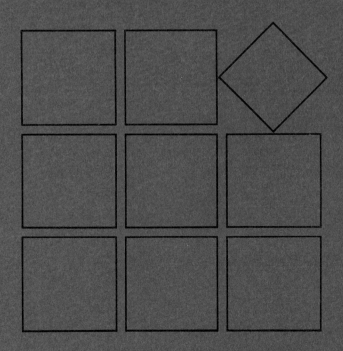

Chapter 44

Properties of Nervous Tissue

Robin L. Curtis

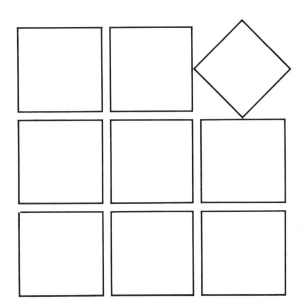

The nervous system in coordination with the endocrine system provides the means for all of the integrative aspects of life. It controls not only skeletal muscle movement but also the activity of cardiac and visceral smooth muscle. The nervous system makes possible the reception, integration, and perception of sensory information; it provides for memory and problem solving; and it facilitates adjustment to an ever-changing external environment. No part of the nervous system functions separately from other parts; and in the human, who is a

Free nerve endings in skin

Basement membrane

Schwann cell myelin

Axis cylinder

Node of Ranvier

Nucleolus   Nucleus

Nissl bodies   Cell body

↑ PNS
↓ CNS

Oligodendroglial cell myelin

Synapse

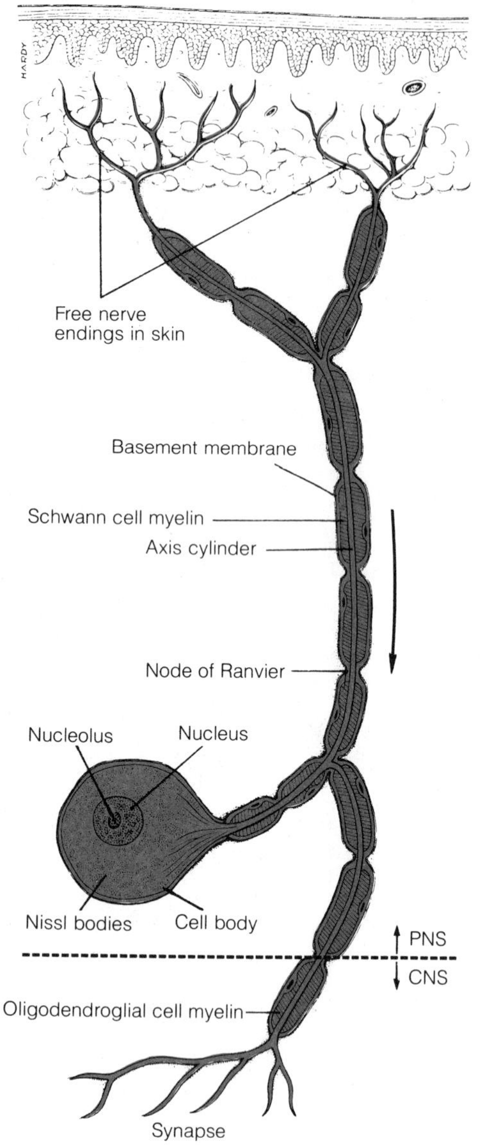

Figure 44-1 *A typical afferent neuron that carries information from surface receptors (in this case the skin) to the CNS. The cell body and axons are in the PNS, while the central axon penetrates into the CNS wherein myelin is provided by oligodendroglial cells. (From Chaffee EE, Lytle IM: Basic Physiology and Anatomy, 4th ed. Philadelphia, JB Lippincott, 1980)*

thinking and feeling creature, the effects of emotion can exert a strong influence on both neural and hormonal control of body function. On the other hand, alterations in both neural and endocrine function (particularly at the biochemical level) can exert a strong influence on psychological behavior.

To understand the brain and nervous system, we must understand how neurons are constructed, how they work, and how they communicate with one another. The human brain consists of several trillion cells, each of which must communicate with several thousand others. The average nerve cell ranges in size from 2/100 mm to 4/100 mm, and a synapse measures no more than 1/1000 mm.[1]

This chapter is divided into two parts: the first describes the cells of the nervous system and their response to injury, and the second describes the generation and transmission of nerve impulses.

Neurons have branching cytoplasm-filled processes, the dendrites and the axons, which project from the cell body and are unique to the nervous system. The axonal processes are particularly designed for rapid communication between other neurons and the many body structures that are innervated by the nervous system. *Afferent,* or *sensory,* neurons carry information from the peripheral nervous system (PNS) to the central nervous system (CNS), as shown in Figure 44-1. *Efferent,* or *motor,* neurons carry information away from the CNS (Fig. 44-2). Interspersed between the afferent and efferent neurons is a network of *interconnecting neurons,* which serve to modulate and control the body's response to changes in the internal and external environments. In the human, who is a thinking and feeling creature, these interconnecting networks facilitate the establishment of response patterns and allow for the storage of information on which learning and memory are based. Learning permits the modification of response patterns and allows for adaptation to an ever-changing environment. Complex neural networks provide the means for subjective experiences, such as perception and emotion. These also provide for intelligence, judgment, and anticipation of events.

■ Nervous Tissue Cells

Nervous tissue contains two types of cells—neurons and supporting cells. The neurons are the functional cells of the nervous system. Neurons exhibit membrane excitability and conductivity and secrete neuromediators and hormones, such as epinephrine and antidiuretic hormone. The *supporting cells,* such as the Schwann cells in the PNS and the glial cells in the CNS, function to *protect* the nervous system and *supply nourishment* for the neurons.

Neurons

Neurons have three distinct parts—the cell body and its cytoplasm-filled processes, the dendrites and the axons. These processes form the functional connections, or synapses, with other nerve cells, with receptor cells, or with effector cells.

The *cell body,* or *soma,* contains a large, vesicular nucleus, one or more distinct nucleoli, and a well-developed endoplasmic reticulum with ribosomes. The nucleus has the same DNA code content that is present in other cells of the body. The nucleoli, which are composed of both DNA and RNA, are associated with protein synthesis. There are large masses of ribosomes,

which are prominent in many neurons. These acidic RNA masses, which are involved in protein synthesis, stain as dark *Nissl* bodies with basic histologic stains (see Fig. 44-2).

The *dendrites* (treelike) are multiple, branched extensions of the nerve body; they are afferent and conduct information *toward* the cell body. The dendrites and cell body are studded with *synaptic terminals* from axons and dendrites of other neurons (Fig. 44-3).

The *axon* is a long efferent process that projects from the cell body and carries impulses away from the cell. There is usually only one axon to a nerve cell. Most axons undergo multiple branching, resulting in many axonal terminals. The cytoplasm of the cell body extends to fill both the dendrites and the axon (see Figs. 44-1 and 44-2). The reader will note that there are no Nissl bodies in the *axon hillock,* which is the point where the axon leaves the cell body. The proteins and other materials that are used by the axon are synthesized in the cell body and then flow down the axon through its cytoplasm.

The cell body of the neuron is equipped for a high level of metabolic activity. This is necessary because the cell body must synthesize the cytoplasmic and membrane constituents required to maintain the function of the axon and its terminals. Some of these axons extend for a distance of 1 m to 1.5 m and have a volume that is sometimes 200 to 500 times greater than the cell body itself. An active process, called axonal transport, serves as a transport and communication system between the various parts of the axon and cell body. It moves amino acids, polypeptides, and other substances through the axon. A reverse axonal transport also exists and serves to move materials from the axonal terminals back to the cell body. It is believed that the process of axonal transport not only facilitates the movement of metabolites between the cell body and the axonal terminals but also serves as an internal communication system between the two parts of the neuron. In secretory neurons, such as those in the hypothalamic pituitary stalk, axonal transport carries antidiuretic hormone or oxytocin from the cell body to terminals in the posterior pituitary, where these hormones are released.

Supporting Cells

Supporting cells of the nervous system, the Schwann cells of the PNS and the several types of glial cells of the CNS, provide the neurons with protection and nourishment. The supporting cells segregate the neurons into isolated metabolic compartments, which are required for normal neural function. Together with the tightly joined endothelial cells of the capillaries in the CNS, these supporting cells may contribute to what is called the blood–brain barrier. This term is used to emphasize the impermeability of the nervous system to large and poten-

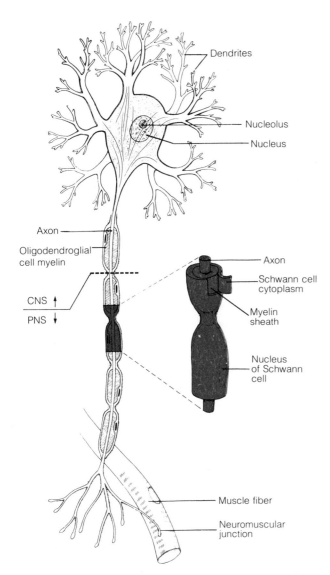

Figure 44-2 *Myelinated efferent neuron, with axon entering the PNS to innervate skeletal muscle cells. (From Chaffee EE, Lytle IM: Basic Physiology and Anatomy, 4th ed. Philadelphia, JB Lippincott, 1980)*

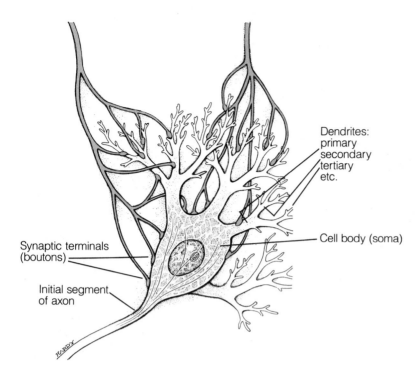

Dendrites:
primary
secondary
tertiary
etc.

Cell body (soma)

Synaptic terminals
(boutons)

Initial segment
of axon

Figure 44-3 *Synaptic terminals in contact with the dendrites and cell body of an efferent neuron. (From Chaffee EE, Lytle IM: Basic Physiology and Anatomy, 4th ed. Philadelphia, JB Lippincott, 1980)*

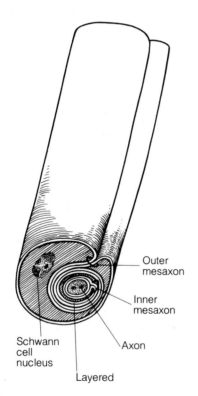

Outer
mesaxon

Inner
mesaxon

Schwann
cell
nucleus

Axon

Layered

Figure 44-4 *The Schwann cell migrates down a larger axon to a bare region, and then settles down and encloses the axon in a fold of its plasma membrane. It then rotates around and around, wrapping the axon in many layers of plasma membrane, with most of the Schwann cell cytoplasm squeezed out. The resultant thick, multiple-layered coating around the axon is called myelin.*

tially harmful molecules. In addition, the many-layered myelin wrappings of the Schwann cells of the PNS and the oligodendroglia of the CNS provide the myelin sheath segments that serve to increase the velocity of nerve impulse conduction in axons having larger diameters.

Normally, the nerve cell bodies in the peripheral nervous system are collected into *ganglia,* such as the dorsal root and autonomic ganglia. Each of the cell bodies and processes of the peripheral nerves is surrounded, or enclosed, in cellular sheaths of supporting cells. The cells that surround the ganglion cells are called *satellite cells.* The satellite cells secrete a basement membrane that apparently protects the cell body from the diffusion of large molecules. Collagen, secreted by fibroblasts, protects the nerve from mechanical forces. Thus, in the PNS, all parts of a neuron and its supporting cells are surrounded by an *endoneural sheath* made up of continuous basement membrane surrounded by layers of collagen. Finally, the entire ganglion is protected by a heavy collagenous layer that also surrounds the large bundles of neural processes in the PNS.

The processes of the larger nerves, the axons of both the afferent and efferent neurons, are surrounded by the plasma membrane and cytoplasm of the Schwann cells, which are close relatives of the satellite cells. The Schwann cell surrounds the nerve process and then twists many times in jelly-roll fashion (Fig. 44-4). The Schwann cells line up along the neuronal process; and each of these cells, in turn, forms its own discrete *myelin segment*. The end of each myelin segment attaches to the plasma membrane of the neuronal process by means of sealed junctions. Successive Schwann cells are separated by short gaps, the *nodes of Ranvier*, where the myelin is missing. The nodes of Ranvier serve to increase nerve conduction by allowing the impulse to jump from node to node in a process called *saltatory conduction*. In this way, the impulse can travel more rapidly through the extracellular fluid than it could if it were required to move systematically along the entire nerve process. This increased conduction velocity greatly reduces reaction time, or time between the application of a stimulus and the subsequent motor response. The short reaction time that occurs when there is a rapid conduction velocity is of particular importance in peripheral nerves with long distances (sometimes 1–2 m) for conduction between the CNS and distal effector organs (Fig. 44-5).

In addition to its role in increasing conduction velocity, the myelin sheath aids in nourishing the neuronal process. Because there are essentially no glycogen stores within the cytoplasm of the neuron, the major source of energy for the membrane of the neuronal process must be supplied by the supporting cells, in this case the myelin sheath, or from the vascular system at the nodes of Ranvier. In some pathologic conditions, the myelin may degenerate or be destroyed, leaving a section of bare axonal process that eventually dies unless remyelination takes place. Thus, the metabolic intervention of the supporting cells is essential for the long-term survival of the neuron and its processes.

Each of the end-to-end series of Schwann cells is enclosed within a continuous tube of basement membrane, which is surrounded by a multiple-layered collagen-rich *endoneurial tube* (Fig. 44-6). These endoneurial tubes are bundled together with blood vessels and lymphatics into nerve *fascicles*, which are surrounded

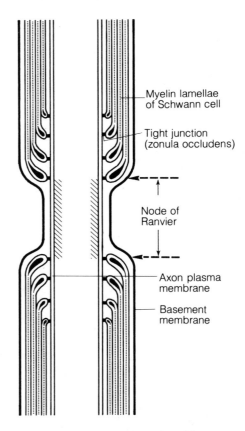

Figure 44-5 *Schematic drawing of a longitudinal section through a node of a myelinated axon of the PNS. Sealed junctions between myelin lamellae of the Schwann cell and the axon plasma membrane seal in the intracellular fluids within the internodal region. Extracellular fluids of the PNS communicate directly with the bare axon at the node. In the CNS there is no basement membrane in the internode and nodal regions.*

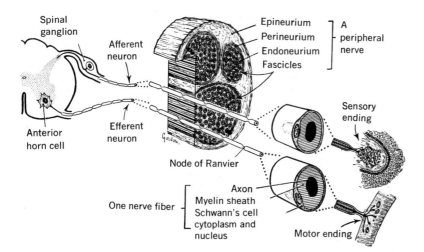

Figure 44-6 *Peripheral nerve sheaths. The heavy connective tissue epineurium sheathes the whole nerve trunk. The perineurium sheathes bundles of axons or fasciculi. A large fasciculus is enlarged and cut away to illustrate its internal structure and two smaller fasciculi at the bottom of the diagram. The innermost connective tissue layer, the endoneurium, is made up of several layers of connective tissue fibers and fibrocytes that surround each individual fiber or myelinated axon. Unmyelinated fibers are not visible at this magnification. (From Chaffee EE, Lytle IM: Basic Physiology and Anatomy, 4th ed. Philadelphia, JB Lippincott, 1980)*

by a collagenous *perineural sheath*. Usually, several fascicles are further surrounded by the heavy, protective *epineural sheath* of the peripheral nerve. The protective layers that surround the peripheral nerve processes are continuous with the connective tissue capsule of the sensory endings and the connective tissue that surrounds the effector structures, such as the skeletal muscle cell. Centrally, the connective tissue layers continue along the dorsal and ventral roots of the nerve and fuse with the meninges that surround the spinal cord and brain. The endoneurial tube does not penetrate the CNS. The absence of these tubular collagenous structures is thought to be a major factor in the less-effective axonal

regeneration that occurs within the CNS compared with the PNS.

The supporting cells of the CNS consist of the neuroglial cells—oligodendroglia, astroglia, and microglia—and the ependymal cells.

The *oligodendroglial cells* form the myelin for the CNS. Instead of forming a myelin covering for a single axon, these cells reach out with several processes, each wrapping around and forming a multilayered myelin segment around several different axons (Fig. 44-7). The coverings of the nerve processes in the CNS also function in speeding the velocity of nerve conduction in a manner similar to that of the peripheral myelinated fibers. Myelin has a high lipid content, which gives it a *whitish* color, and thus the name *white matter* is given to the masses of myelinated fibers of the spinal cord and brain.

A second type of glial cell, the *astroglia*, is particularly prominent in the *gray matter*, or more central portion of the brain. These large cells have many processes, some reaching to the surface of the capillaries, others reaching to the surface of the nerve cells, and still others filling most of the intercellular space of the CNS (see Fig. 44-7). The astrocytic linkage between the blood vessels and the neurons may provide a transport mechanism for the exchange of oxygen, carbon dioxide, metabolites, and so on. The astrocytes are capable of filling their cytoplasm with microfibrils, and masses of these cells form the special type of scar tissue that develops in the CNS when brain tissue is destroyed.

A third type of glial cell, the *microglia*, is really a *phagocytic cell* (histiocyte) that migrates into the CNS and is available for cleaning up debris following cellular damage and death.

The ependymal cells line the ventricular system and the choroid plexus. These cells are involved in the production of *cerebral spinal fluid*.

Metabolic Requirements

Nervous tissue has a high need for metabolic energy. Although the brain amounts to only 2% of the body's weight, it consumes 20% of its oxygen. Despite this high need, the brain cannot store oxygen nor can it engage in anaerobic metabolism. An interruption in the blood or oxygen supply to the brain leads to clinically observable signs and symptoms. In the absence of oxygen, brain cells continue to function for about 10 seconds. Unconsciousness occurs almost simultaneously when cardiac arrest occurs, and the death of brain cells begins within 4 to 6 minutes. Interruption of blood flow also leads to the accumulation of metabolic by-products that are toxic to neural tissue.

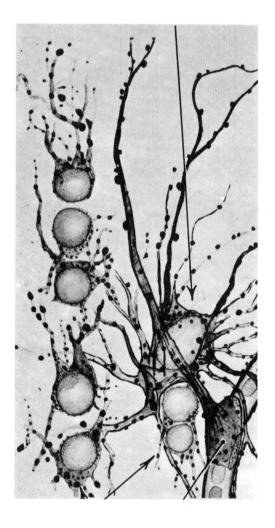

Figure 44-7 *The supporting cells of the nervous system: a row of oligodendroglial cells can be seen on the left, and a fibrous astrocyte on the right. (Modified from Penfield W: Brain 47:430, 1924. From Ham A, Cormack DH: Histology, 8th ed. Philadelphia, JB Lippincott, 1979)*

Glucose is the major fuel source for the nervous system, yet the nervous system has no provisions for storing glucose. Unlike muscle cells, it has no glycogen stores and must rely on glucose from the blood or the glycogen stores of supporting cells. Persons receiving insulin for diabetes may experience signs of neural dysfunction and unconsciousness (insulin reaction or shock) when blood glucose drops as a result of an insulin excess.

Nerve Injury and Regeneration

Neurons exemplify the general principle that the more specialized the function of a cell type, the less able it is to regenerate. In neurons, cell division ceases by the time of birth, and from then on the cell body of a neuron is unable to divide and replace itself. Although the entire neuron cannot be replaced, it is often possible for the axon of peripheral nerves to regenerate as long as the cell body remains viable.

When a peripheral nerve is destroyed by a crushing force or by a cut that penetrates the nerve, the portion of the nerve fiber that is separated from the cell body rapidly undergoes degenerative changes while the central stump and cell body of the nerve are able to survive (Fig. 44-8). Because the cell body synthesizes the material required for nourishing and maintaining the axon, it is likely that the loss of these materials results in the degeneration of the separated portion of the nerve fiber.

Following injury, the Schwann cells that are distal to the site of damage are also able to survive, but their myelin degenerates in a process called *wallerian degeneration*. The Schwann cells assist other phagocytic cells in the area in the cleanup of the debris caused by the degenerating axon and myelin. As they remove the debris, the Schwann cells multiply and fill the empty endoneurial tube. At this point, nothing further happens, unless a regenerating nerve fiber penetrates into the endoneurial tube, in which case, the Schwann cells reform the myelin segments around the fiber.

Meanwhile, the cell body of the neuron responds to the loss of part of its nerve fiber by shifting into a phase of greatly increased protein and lipid synthesis. It does this by dispersing the masses of ribosomes, which stain as Nissl granules. They cease to be stainable and disappear in a process called *chromatolysis*. In the process, the nucleus moves away from the axonal side of the cell body, as though displaced by the active synthetic apparatus of the cell. These changes reach their height within about 10 days of injury and continue until regrowth of the nerve fiber ceases.

In the process of regeneration, the injured nerve fiber develops one or more new branches from the proximal axon stump, which grow into the developing scar tissue. If a crushing injury has occurred and the endoneurial tube is intact through the trauma area, the outgrowing fiber will grow back down this tube to the structure that was originally innervated by the neuron. If, however, the injury involves the severing of a nerve, then the outgrowing branch must come in contact with its original endoneurial tube if it is to be reunited with its original target structure. The rate of outgrowth of regenerating nerve fibers is about 1 mm to 2 mm per day, so that the recovery of conduction to a target structure depends not only on regrowth into the proper endoneurial tube but also on the distance involved. It can take weeks or months for the regrowing fiber to reach the end organ and for communicative function to be reestablished. Further time is required for the Schwann cells to form new myelin segments and for the axon to recover its original diameter and conduction velocity.

The successful regeneration of a nerve fiber in the PNS depends on many factors. If a nerve fiber is

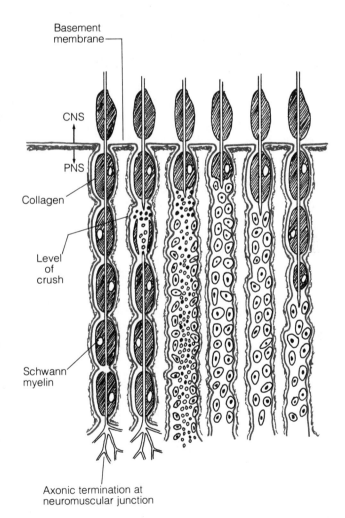

Figure 44-8 Changes that occur in an efferent nerve fiber that has been severed and then regenerates.

destroyed relatively close to the neuronal cell body, the chances are that the nerve cell will die, and if it does, it will not be replaced. If a crushing type of injury has occurred, partial and often full recovery of function occurs. A cutting type of trauma to a nerve is an entirely different matter. Connective tissue scar forms rapidly at the wound site, and when it does, only the most rapidly regenerating axonal branches are able to get through to the intact distal endoneurial tubes. A number of scar-inhibiting agents have been used in an effort to reduce this hazard but have met with only moderate success. In another attempt to improve nerve regeneration, various types of tubular implants have been placed to fill longer gaps in the endoneurial tube. The most successful of these has been a transplanted section of another peripheral nerve or a section of cadaver nerve. The latter is irradiated to destroy all cells in order to reduce the sources of tissue rejection. Perhaps the most difficult problem is the alignment of the proximal and distal endoneurial tubes so that a regenerating fiber can return down its former tube and innervate its former organ. This problem is similar to realigning a large telephone cable that has been cut in such fashion that all of the wires are reconnected exactly as before the separation. An efferent nerve fiber that formerly innervated a skeletal muscle, which regrows down an endoneurial tube formerly occupied by an afferent fiber, will stop growing, and eventually its cell body will die. Likewise, a sensory fiber that ends up growing down an endoneurial tube that connects with a skeletal muscle fiber will undergo the same fate. If, however, these fibers grow down endoneurial tubes that innervate the appropriate type of target organ, reinnervation and function may return, even though the fibers have changed places. Under the best of conditions, a 10% regeneration to the appropriate organ is considered a success once a peripheral nerve has been severed. Even so, considerable function will return with this amount of reinnervation.

In summary, nervous tissue is composed of two types of cells, neurons and supporting cells. Neurons are composed of three parts: a cell body, which controls cell activity, the dendrites, which conduct information toward the cell body, and the axon, which carries impulses from the cell body. The supporting cells consist of the Schwann cells of the PNS and the glial cells of the CNS. The supporting cells protect and nourish the neurons and aid in segregating them into isolated compartments, which is necessary for normal neuronal function. The function of the nervous system demands a high amount of metabolic energy. Glucose is the major fuel for the nervous system, and although the brain comprises only 2% of body weight, it consumes 20% of its oxygen supply. In general, neurons exemplify the principle that the more specialized the function of a cell type, the less its ability to regenerate. Although the entire neuron is unable to undergo mitosis and regenerate when injury occurs, it is often possible for the axons of the peripheral nervous system to regenerate, provided the cell body remains viable. Axonal regeneration and reinnervation of target structures is much more likely to be successful in the PNS where connective tissue of the endoneurial tube provides a conduit to the target structures. The absence of connective tissue in the CNS decreases the likelihood of successful regeneration. Scar tissue, whether glial (CNS) or connective tissue (PNS), is a major deterrent to successful regeneration to the former target structures.

■ Excitable Properties of Nervous Tissue

Neurons are classified as excitable tissue. This means that they are able to initiate and conduct electrical impulses. Basic to an understanding of nerve function is an appreciation of the events that occur during the excitation and initiation of an action potential in a nerve or muscle cell (see Chap. 1). The discussion in this chapter focuses on action potentials that occur in nerves; the reader is asked to remember that many of the same types of phenomena occur in other types of excitable tissue, such as muscle.

An impulse, or action potential, represents the lateral, or lengthwise, movement of electrical charge along the plasma membrane. This phenomenon is based on the rapid flow, sometimes called *conductance,* of charged ions through the membrane in a progressive manner along the length of the neuron's axon. In excitable tissue, ions such as sodium, potassium, chloride, and calcium carry the electrical charges that are involved in the initiation and transmission of such impulses.

Impulse Conduction

During the depolarization process, the rapid flow of sodium ions induces local currents that travel through the adjacent cell membrane and this, in turn, causes the sodium channels in this part of the membrane to open, and depolarization occurs. Thus, the impulse moves progressively along the nerve, depolarizing the membrane ahead of the action potential. The impulse is conducted longitudinally along the membrane from one part of the axon to other parts. In unmyelinated fibers, this sequence of events moves the impulse progressively along the axon. Conduction in myelinated fibers follows a similar pattern, but because of the high resistance in the myelinated segments, the current flow jumps from node to node (saltatory conduction) as was described earlier. This is a more rapid process, and myelinated axons conduct up to 50 times faster than unmyelinated fibers.

Neurotransmitters

Neurotransmitters, or neuromediators, are chemical messengers of the nervous system. These transmitters are synthesized in the cell body of the neuron or its axon terminals and released from the latter on arrival of an action potential. They exert their effect as they attach to *transmitter-specific membrane receptors* on other cells, particularly those of other neurons.

The distinction between the neurons and endocrine cells is somewhat blurred. Many neurons, such as those of the adrenal medulla, secrete neuromediators into the bloodstream just as endocrine cells do.

The neurotransmitters are rapidly removed from the synaptic cleft following their release (Fig. 44-9). Some transmitters, such as acetylcholine, are hydrolyzed by enzymes, in this case, acetylcholinesterase. Other mediators, such as epinephrine, are largely taken up into the presynaptic nerve terminals and are reused or diffuse away.

Neuromediators exert their action through membrane receptors that are similar to those discussed for hormones in Chapter 37. The action of a neurotransmitter is determined by the receptor site. For example, the neuromediator acetylcholine is excitatory when it is released at a myoneural junction and it is inhibitory when it is released into the sinoatrial node of the heart. Some neuromediators act as modulators rather than initiators (or inhibitors) of a neural action.

Recently, it has been found that neurons possess receptor sites for many *hormones*. Receptors, for example, which mediate indirect steroid effects have been characterized in brain and pituitary tissue for four out of the five classes of steroid hormones: estrogens, androgens, progestin, and glucocorticoids.[1] These receptors are similar to those that have been identified on nonneuronal cells.

Although neurons respond to circulating neuromediators, communication between neurons has particular advantages over communication with the endocrine system. This is because neurons have axonal processes that extend and secrete neurotransmitters directly on the surface of a target cell. In this way, selected neurons are stimulated and others with the same type of receptor sites remain unstimulated. This discreteness in location of neural secretion is quite different from the diffuse action of the endocrine hormones, which are released into the bloodstream and which have contact with *all* the cells of the body with the appropriate receptors that are perfused with blood containing the hor-

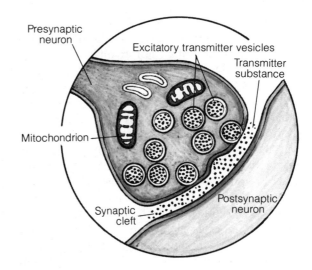

Figure 44-9 *Synapse, showing the pre- and postsynaptic neuron. (From Chaffee EE, Lytle IM: Basic Physiology and Anatomy, 4th ed. Philadelphia, JB Lippincott, 1980)*

mone; it allows for much more complex circuitry to be established in the nervous system than could occur without this specificity.

Sensory Receptors

Information from the internal and external environment reaches the nervous system through a variety of sensory receptors. Receptors from the *special senses* provide the body with vision, hearing, smell, and taste. Other types of receptors provide input needed for maintaining normal levels of blood gases, blood pressure, position sense, muscle tone, and others.

These receptors receive and transform energy from the environment into an action potential in an afferent neuron, which carries the impulse to the CNS. There are two types of impulses that contribute to sensory input to the CNS. One is the *local potential* of the receptor and the other is the *propagated afferent nerve impulse*.

For an impulse to be generated in a receptor, the stimulus must be appropriate: the adequate stimulus is the appropriate form of energy which, at its lowest intensity, will result in a change in membrane potential (*e.g.*, light for photoreceptors and sound for audioreceptors) of sufficient intensity to trigger propagated action potentials in an afferent neuron. Sensory receptors may be the terminal part of the neuron (naked nerve endings of pain fibers), or they may be associated with nonneural tissue, such as the connective tissue matrix of the pacinian corpuscle that surrounds the neuron, or they may be separate sensory cells that are innervated by the afferent neurons (glomus chemoreceptors of the carotid body, hair cells of the auditory apparatus, and so on). The sensory cells are very sensitive to a particular type of energy (adequate stimulus). For example, thermoreceptors respond to temperature changes; photoreceptors in the retina of the eye respond to light waves; mechanoreceptors, such as those in the skin and subcutaneous tissue, sense changes in pressure and touch; and chemoreceptors in the taste buds respond to changes in the chemical composition of food. The sensory input to the brain is influenced not only by the selective nature of the various receptors but by the number, frequency, and pattern of impulses. The intensity and pattern of stimulation provide a coding system whereby information about the internal and external environment is transmitted to the central nervous system. At high energy levels almost all receptors will respond to other forms of stimuli. Pressure on the eyeball, for example, is experienced as light.

Some receptors discharge continuously as long as the stimulus is applied; these are the *slowly adapting receptors*. Other receptors discharge only at the time the stimulus is initially applied and then cease to discharge even though the stimulus continues; these are the *rapidly adapting receptors*. Slowly adapting receptors provide information about steady-state conditions, whereas rapidly adapting receptors are designed for sensing changing conditions in the environment.

Synaptic Transmission

A chemical synapse serves as a *one-way* communication link between neurons. The *synapse* consists of *presynaptic* and *postsynaptic* terminals. The synaptic cleft separates the pre- and postsynaptic membranes. The presynaptic terminal secretes neurotransmitters into the synaptic cleft. Diffused transmitters unite with receptors on the postsynaptic membrane, and this causes either excitation or inhibition of the postsynaptic neuron by producing hypopolarization or hyperpolarization, respectively (see Fig. 44-9).

A neuron's cell body and dendrites are covered by thousands of synapses, any or many of which can be active at any moment in time. Because of this rich synaptic capability, each neuron resembles a little computer in which there are many circuits of neurons that interact with each other. It is the complexity of these interactions that gives the system its intelligence in terms of the subtle integrations involved in producing behavioral responses, and it is the complexity of these interactions that makes the prediction of stimulus-response relationships somewhat hazardous in the absence of a millisecond-to-millisecond knowledge of the excitatory and inhibitory activity that takes place on the surfaces of each neuron in a functional circuit. It is amazing, with billions of these little computers capable of becoming involved in such a

response, that predictions are possible at all. It is even more astounding that the basic microcircuitry involved in the nervous system is reliably reproduced during the development of each new organism. To put it more dramatically, humans produce human babies that behave like human babies—not like baby rabbits or baby eagles.

There are several types of synapses. Axonic terminals of an afferent neuron can develop in close apposition to the dendrites *(axodendritic synapse)*, to the cell body *(axosomatic synapse)*, or the axon *(axoaxonic synapse)* of a CNS neuron. The mechanism of communication between the *presynaptic* axonic terminal and the *postsynaptic* neuron is similar in all three types of synapses. In all three, the action potential sweeps into the axonic terminals of the afferent neuron and triggers rapid secretion of neurotransmitter molecules from the axonic, or presynaptic, surface. Conversion of action potentials into secretion is called coupling and, although it is not completely understood, it is believed that the release of calcium ions is involved.

The neuromediators are synthesized in the cytoplasm of the axonic terminal and are stored in small membrane-bound vesicles, the *synaptic vesicles*. Usually, the same transmitter compound is secreted from all axonic terminals of the same neuron. All afferent neurons do not, however, secrete the same neurotransmitter. Some neuromediators are rapidly inactivated by enzymes on the synaptic membranes. In synapses in which inactivating enzymes are not present, the messenger molecules diffuse away from synaptic terminals, and then portions of these transmitter molecules may reenter the presynaptic terminal to be reincorporated into a new transmitter.

During secretion, these vesicles of the presynaptic terminal move toward and fuse with the synaptic membrane and release their transmitter contents into the narrow *synaptic cleft*. The transmitter molecule diffuses through the intercellular fluid to the membrane of the postsynaptic neuron and unites with receptor sites that are specific for that particular transmitter. The combination of the neurotransmitter with the receptor sites causes partial depolarization of the postsynaptic membrane. This is called an *excitatory postsynaptic potential*, or *EPSP*. All afferent transmitters are excitatory to the CNS neurons with which they synapse.

The postsynaptic membrane region of any single dendrite-cell body synapse is not capable of inciting an action potential by itself. The inward depolarizing current of the EPSP neutralizes only part of the negative resting membrane potential. An action potential does not begin in the membrane adjacent to the synapse. Instead it begins in the initial segment of the axon (axon hillock), which is the most excitable part of the neuron (see Fig. 44-3). The currents resulting from any one EPSP (sometimes called a generator potential) are usually insufficient to pass threshold and thus cause depolarization in the axon's initial segment. However, if several EPSPs occur simultaneously, the area of depolarization can become large enough and the currents at the initial segment can become strong enough to exceed the threshold potential and initiate a conducted action potential. This summation of depolarized areas is called *spatial summation*. The EPSPs can also summate and cause an action potential if they come in close temporal relation to each other. This temporal aspect of the occurrence of two or more EPSPs is called *temporal summation*.

Many CNS neurons possess hundreds or thousands of synapses on their dendritic and soma surfaces. Some of these synapses are *inhibitory* in the sense that the combination of their transmitter with receptor sites causes the local membrane to become hyperpolarized and reduces the probability of an action potential by the postsynaptic neuron. This is called an *inhibitory postsynaptic potential,* or *IPSP*. The IPSPs can also undergo spatial and temporal summation with each other and with EPSPs, reducing the effectiveness of the latter by a roughly algebraic summation. If the sum of EPSPs and IPSPs keeps the depolarization at the initial segment below threshold levels, the generation of an action potential does not occur.

The *spatial* and *temporal* summation required in the distribution and timing of synaptic activity serves as a sensitive and very complicated switch, requiring just the right combination of incoming activity before it releases its own message in the form of the action potential. The frequency of action potentials in the axon, on the other hand, is an all-or-none language (digital language), which can vary only as to the presence or absence of such impulses and their frequency.

In summary, nervous tissue is able to initiate and conduct impulses, and is classified as excitable tissue. Receptors are special neuronal structures designed for providing the body with sensory input from the internal and external environments. Sensory receptors provide the body with hearing, vision, smell, and taste. Other receptors monitor blood gases, blood pressure, position sense, muscle tone, and other information. Neuromediators are chemical messengers that serve to control neuronal function; they selectively cause either excitation or inhibition of action potential generation. A synapse is a one-way communication link between neurons; it has both presynaptic and postsynaptic components. Neuromediators released from the presynaptic terminal of one neuron diffuse across the synaptic cleft and unite with receptor sites of the postsynaptic terminal of another neuron as a means of communicating information between the two neurons. Thus, the neuron integrates the ongoing synaptic activity on its dendritic and soma surface, resulting in

the production or nonproduction of an action potential. The latter travels rapidly along the cell's axon to trigger the release of transmitter substance on the postsynaptic surface of the next neuron in a circuit. This combination of integration of synaptic activity and rapid communication to discretely positioned sensory terminals permits the complex circuitry as well as rapid communication characteristic of neural tissue function.

Lastly, at present we have only scratched the surface compared to what we may ultimately learn about the details of neuronal circuitry: how it is formed and how it is modified by internal and external environmental factors during development and maturation. The alterations that must occur in neuronal circuitry during learning and forgetting also are not yet understood.

■ Study Guide

After you have studied this chapter, you should be able to meet the following objectives:

☐ Name and describe the anatomy of the three parts of a neuron.

☐ State the function of the supporting cells of the nervous system.

☐ Describe the function of the Schwann cells with reference to the nodes of Ranvier.

☐ State the purpose of saltatory conduction.

☐ Describe the function of the myelin sheath.

☐ Describe the consequences of an interruption to the brain's blood supply.

☐ State a general principle related to cell regeneration.

☐ Explain the sequence of events in chromatolysis.

☐ Explain the rationale underlying the use of scar-inhibiting agents and tubular implants in regeneration of nerve fibers.

☐ Define *conductance*.

☐ Describe the interaction of the presynaptic and the postsynaptic terminals.

☐ Explain the occurrence of both spatial and temporal summation.

■ Reference

1. Report on Convulsive and Neuromuscular Disorders to the National Advisory Neurological and Communicative Disorders and Stroke Council, p 103. National Institute of Health, National Institute on Communicative Disorders and Stroke, U.S. Department of Health, Education, and Welfare, Public Health Service, NIH Publication No 79–1913

Chapter 45

Control of Neuromuscular and Autonomic Nervous System Function

Robin L. Curtis

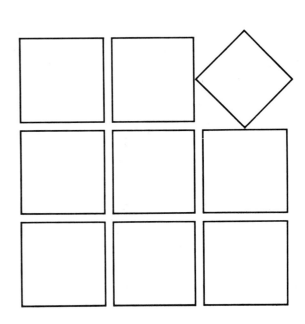

The nervous system is the most highly organized system in the body, regulating and controlling most of the other systems. Its functions are concerned with the reception of information from the internal and external environments, the transmission of information, and the integration of sensation and effector responses. No computer of human design is able to process such an immense amount and variety of information with the degree of precision, flexibility, and creativity found in the nervous system. Hundreds of billions of neurons are involved in these processes with all but a few million of them packed into the cavities of the cranium and spinal column.

The chapter discussion is organized in three basic parts: (1) the development and segmental organization of the nervous system, (2) the basic organization of the central nervous system (CNS), using somatic and autonomic systems as examples, and (3) a brief consideration of the complex, higher-order, functional organization of the brain.

■ Development and Segmental Organization of the Nervous System

Hierarchy of Control

The development of the nervous system can be traced far back into evolutionary history. In the course of its development, newer functional features were superimposed on more primitive ones. Greater complexity resulted from the modification and enlargement of older organization and structures. In a moving organism, rapid reaction to environmental danger, to potential food sources, or to a sexual partner was required for the survival of the species. Thus, the front, or rostral, end of the CNS became specialized as a means of sensing the external environment and controlling reactions to it. In time, the ancient organization, which is largely retained in the spinal cord segments, was expanded in the forward segments of the nervous system. Of these, the most forward have undergone the most radical modification and have developed into the forebrain: the diencephalon and the cerebral hemispheres. The dominance of the front end of the CNS is reflected in a hierarchy of control levels—brain stem over spinal cord, forebrain over brain stem. Because the newer functions were added onto the outside of older functional systems and because the newer functions became concentrated at the rostral end of the nervous system, they are much more vulnerable to injury. These three principles—(1) no part of the nervous system functions independently of the other parts, (2) newer systems control older systems, and (3) the newer systems are more vulnerable to injury—form a basis for understanding many of the manifestations that occur when the nervous system suffers injury or disease.

Organization

The nervous system can be divided into two parts—*the central nervous system* (CNS) and *the peripheral nervous system* (PNS). The CNS consists of the brain and spinal cord, which are located within the protected environment of the axial skeleton (cranium and spinal column). The PNS contains neurons and neuronal processes located outside the axial skeleton in the body wall (soma) and viscera. The basic design of the nervous system provides for the concentration of computational and control functions within the CNS. In this design, the PNS functions as an input-output system for relaying input to the CNS and for transmitting output messages that control effector organs, such as muscles and glands, in the periphery.

On cross section the body is organized into a soma and a viscera (Fig. 45-1). The soma, or body wall, includes all of the structures derived from the embryonic ectoderm, such as the epidermis of the skin and the CNS. A migrating ectodermal derivative called the *neural crest* is the source of many cell types, including the pigment cells of the dermis and afferent and autonomic ganglion neurons of the PNS. The mesodermal connective tissues of the soma include the dermis of the skin, skeletal muscle, bone, and the outer lining of the body cavity (somatic pleura and somatic peritoneum). For the

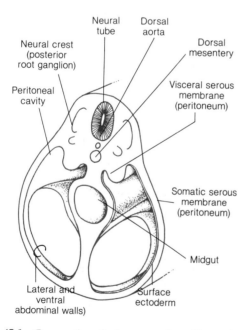

Figure 45-1 *Cross section of a human embryo, illustrating the development of somatic and visceral structures.*

nervous system, all of the more internal structures constitute the viscera, including the great vessels derived from the intermediate mesoderm, the urinary system, and the gonadal structures. The viscera also includes the inner lining of the body cavities, such as the visceral pleura and peritoneum, and the mesodermal tissues that surround the entoderm-lined gut and its derivative organs (lungs, liver, and pancreas).

There are both somatic and visceral nerves. The *somatic nerves* innervate the skeletal muscle and the smooth muscle and glands of the skin and body wall. The *visceral nerves* supply the visceral organs of the body, transmitting information through the autonomic nerves in the PNS to control the smooth and cardiac muscle as well as the glands of the visceral organs. This visceral system is largely of reflex, or involuntary, function.

Segmental Development

The central nervous system develops as a hollow tube, the cephalic portion of which becomes the brain and the more caudal part the spinal cord. In the process of development, the basic organizational pattern of the body is that of a longitudinal series of segments, each repeating the same fundamental organizational pattern. Although the early muscular, skeletal, vascular, and excretory systems and the nerves that supply these parts have this segmental pattern (Fig. 45-2), it is the nervous system that most clearly retains this organization in the adult. The CNS and its associated peripheral nerves are thus made up of 43 or so segments, 33 of which form the spinal cord and spinal nerves, and 10 the brain and its cranial nerves.

Each segment of the CNS is accompanied by a pair of dorsal root ganglia that contain the *afferent* neuron cell bodies. These ganglia have two axonlike processes: one process, which ends in receptor terminals, extends into either the soma or the viscera, and the other enters the central neural tube segment. Afferent neurons transmit sensory information from the body into the CNS, with somatic afferents transmitting information from the soma to the CNS and visceral afferents transmitting information from the viscera to the CNS.

On cross section, the hollow embryonic neural tube can be divided into a central canal, or ventricle, that contains the cerebrospinal fluid and the wall of the tube. The latter develops into the gray or cellular portion, and the white matter into the tract systems of the CNS (Fig. 45-3). The dorsal half of the gray matter is called the *dorsal horn*; it receives afferent nerve terminals and distributes and processes this incoming information. The ventral portion, or *ventral horn,* contains efferent neurons and is largely concerned with outward communication to the body segment and its effector organs, the

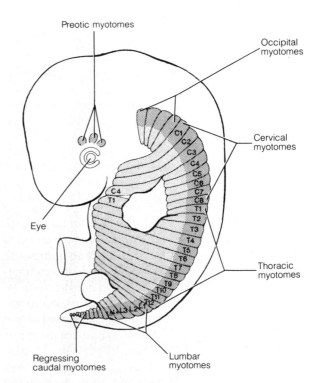

Figure 45-2 *The developing muscular system in a 6-week-old embryo. The segmental muscle masses, or myotomes, which give rise to most skeletal muscles, reflect the basic segmental organization of the body and head. Efferent cranial nerves innervating the myotomes of the head are as follows: preotic myotomes (nerves III, IV, and VI), and the occipital myotomes (XII). (Moore KL: The Developing Human, 2nd ed, p 317. Philadelphia, WB Saunders, 1977)*

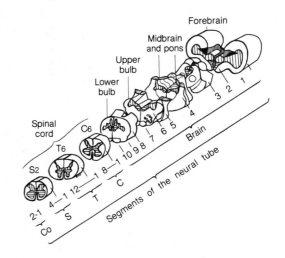

Figure 45-3 *The adult human CNS The dorsal* (vertical hatching) *and ventral* (horizontal hatching) *horns of the gray matter are surrounded by the white matter that contains the longitudinal tracts. Numbers indicate segmental divisions of the neural tube. (Adapted from Elliott HC: Neuroanatomy. Philadelphia, JB Lippincott, 1969)*

muscles and glands of the body segment reached by the axons of ventral horn neurons. Many of the CNS neurons develop as axons that grow longitudinally as tract systems that intercommunicate between neighboring and distal segments of the neural tube. As this developmental process occurs, the neural tube becomes segmented in a repeating pattern of entering *afferent neuron axons,* forming the *dorsal roots* of each succeeding segmental nerve, and exiting *efferent neuron axons,* forming the *ventral roots* of each succeeding segmental nerve.

The nerve cells in the gray matter are arranged longitudinally in *cell columns,* with nerve cells having similar functions grouped together. The axons of the cell column neurons can project out into the white matter of the CNS, forming the longitudinal tract systems. Both the cell columns and the longitudinal tracts extend along the entire length of the nervous system, through the brain and spinal cord (see Fig. 45-3).

Cell columns

The complexity of the organizational structure of the nervous system is somewhat simplified by a pattern in which PNS and CNS neurons are repeated as parallel cell columns running lengthwise along the nervous system. In this organizational pattern, afferent neurons, dorsal horn cells, ventral horn cells, and autonomic ganglion neurons are organized as a series of 12 cell columns. A box of 24 colored beverage straws (2 sets of 12 different colors) can be used as an analogy to represent the cell columns. In this model, each lateral half of the nervous system (right and left sides) is represented in mirror fashion by one set of 12 colored straws. If these straws were cut crosswise (equivalent to a transverse section through the nervous system) at several places along their length, the spacial relationship between these straws would be repeated in each section.

The 12 pairs of cell columns can be further grouped according to their location in the PNS: 4 in the dorsal root ganglia; 1 in the peripheral autonomic ganglia and their CNS components; 4 in the dorsal, or posterior, halves of the neural tube; and 3 in the ventral, or anterior, halves of the neural tube (Fig. 45-4). Each column of dorsal root ganglion cells projects to its particular column of input association (IA) neurons in the dorsal horn. These IA neurons distribute afferent information to reflex circuitry and to more rostral and elaborate segments of the CNS. The ventral horn contains both output association (OA) neurons and lower motor neurons (LMNs). The OA neurons provide the final circuitry for organizing efferent nerve activity. The efferent neurons of these cell columns send their axons into the body to innervate skeletal, smooth, or cardiac muscle and glandular cells.

Between the input association neurons and the output association neurons are chains of small internuncial neurons, which are arranged in complex circuits. It is the internuncial neurons that provide the discreteness, appropriateness, and intelligence of responses to stimuli. Most of the billions of CNS cells in the spinal cord and brain gray matter are internuncial neurons.

The effectiveness of a CNS-mediated response to changed environmental conditions depends on the functional integrity of the neurons and effector cells in the particular sequence called a *reflex.* A reflex is a highly predictable relationship between a stimulus and a response. It is mediated by the transmission of receptor-derived action potentials in the afferent neurons that stimulate activity in a network of CNS association neurons of the dorsal or ventral gray matter leading to action potentials in efferent neurons. These efferents, in turn, stimulate effector responses in structures such as skeletal, smooth, or cardiac muscle and glands. The activity of these effectors constitutes the reflex response.

The afferent dorsal root ganglion cells and the CNS dorsal horn input association cells are subdivided into two types of cell columns—general and special. The general somatic afferent (GSA) cell and its input association columns (GSIA) inervate somatic structures of the body wall, provide input for many reflexes, and project information about touch, vibration, temperature, pain, itch, and tickle to the forebrain. The special somatic afferent (SSA) cells and their input association columns (SSIA) transmit proprioceptive sensation information regarding the position of body parts and their relation to the gravitational field. These afferents are distributed in joints, tendons, muscles, and the auditory and vestibular sense organs of the inner ear. They are a source of spinal cord reflexes and project information to the cerebellum and forebrain. Because the inner ear organs are derived from a lateral groove on each side of the head in the embryo, these structures are often referred to as lateral line structures (see Fig. 45-4). General visceral afferent (GVA) cells and their input association columns (GVIA) provide sensory input from the viscera, which is distributed to vital visceral reflex circuits and relayed to the forebrain. These afferents are the source of sensations of fullness, pain, evacuation urgency, and sexual satisfaction. The special visceral afferent (SVA) cells and their input association columns (SVIA) are distributed to taste buds and olfactory sensory receptors. This information is transmitted to reflex circuits and to the forebrain as sensations of taste and smell.

The ventral horn contains three separate efferent cell and efferent output association columns: general visceral efferent (GVE) cells and their output association columns (GVOA), special visceral efferent (SVE) cells and

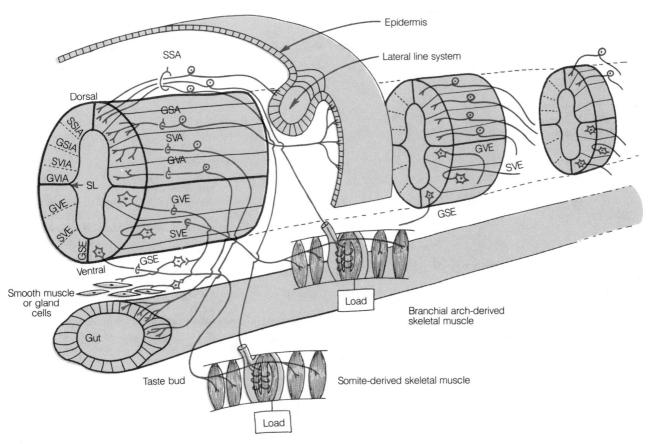

Figure 45-4 *Cell columns of the central nervous system. The columns in the dorsal horn contain input association neurons: special sensory (SSIA), general sensory (GSIA), special visceral (SVIA), and general visceral (GVIA). The ventral horn contains the efferent neurons: the general visceral efferent (GVE), special visceral efferent (SVE), and general somite efferent (GSE).*

their output association columns (SVOA), and general somite efferent (GSE) cells and their output association columns (GSOA). The GVE neurons transmit the efferent output of the autonomic nervous system and are called *preganglionic neurons.* Their axons project into the viscera where they innervate smooth and cardiac muscle and glandular cells of the body. The GVE cells of the autonomic nervous system are structurally and functionally divided into the sympathetic and parasympathetic systems (discussed later in this chapter). The SVE neurons leave the CNS laterally and innervate the branchial arch muscles: the muscles of mastication, facial expression, and head turning; the pharynx; and the larynx. The GSE neurons leave the CNS ventrally and supply the skeletal muscles of the body.

This chapter discussion focuses on the afferent cell columns of the GSA and GSIA (somatic sensation and reflexes), SSA and SSIA (postural reflexes and sensations of position), and GVA and GVIA (autonomic

reflexes and visceral sensations) and on the efferent cell columns of the GSE and GVE. The afferent and efferent cell columns of the PNS and CNS, their projections, and the type of information they transmit are summarized in Table 45-1.

Longitudinal tracts

The gray matter of the cell columns in the CNS is surrounded by bundles of myelinated and unmyelinated axons (white matter) that travel longitudinally along the length of the neural axis. This white matter can be divided into three layers—an inner, a middle, and an outer layer (Fig. 45-5). The inner, or *archi,* layer contains short fibers that project for a maximum of about five segments before reentering the gray matter. The middle, or *paleo,* layer projects six or more segments. Both the archi and the paleo layer fibers have many branches, or *collaterals,* that enter the gray matter of intervening segments. The outer, or *neo,* layer contains large-diameter

(Text continues on p. 734)

Table 45-1   The Segmental Nerves and Their Components

Segment	Segmental Nerve	GSA	GVA	GVE	GSE	Other	Innervation	Function
1	*Forebrain*							
	I. Olfactory					SVA	Olfactory mucosa	Smell
2								
3	*Midbrain*							
	V. Trigeminal—ophthalmic division					SSA	Extrinsic eye muscles; upper muscles of facial expression	Sensory input for control of eye movement
		X					Skin on forehead, upper face, and conjunctiva	Reflexes and somesthesia
	III. Oculomotor			X			Sphincter of iris; ciliary muscle	Pupillary constriction, accommodation
					X		Extrinsic eye muscles	Motor innervation of eye muscles and lid
4	*Pons*							
	V. Trigeminal—maxillary division					SSA	Muscles of facial expression	Sensory input for control of facial expression
		X					Skin, nose, upper jaw, nasal cavity	Somatic reflexes; somesthesia
	—mandibular					SSA	Muscles of mastication	Sensory input for control of mastication
		X					Skin of lower jaw, inside mouth, anterior ⅔ of tongue	Somatic reflexes; somesthesia
						SVE	Muscles of mastication, tensor, tympani	Mastication; protection of auditory apparatus
	IV. Trochlear				X		Extrinsic eye muscles	Control of superior oblique
5	*Caudal pons*							
	VIII. Vestibular, cochlear					SSA	Vestibular end organs; organ of Corti	Vestibular reflexes and sensation; auditory reflexes and hearing
	—int. intermedius	X						Somesthesia
						SVA	Taste buds; anterior ⅔ tongue; palate	Gustation
			X				Nasopharynx	Sneeze reflex; sensation
				X			Nasopharynx; lacrimal gland	Lacrimation
	VII. Facial					SVE	Muscles of facial expression; stapedius	Facial expression; protective reflex for auditory apparatus
	VI. Abducens				X		Extrinsic eye muscle	Control lateral eye movement
6	*Middle medulla*							
	IX. Glossopharyngeal					SSA	Pharyngeal muscle	Sensory input for movement control
		X					External ear; external acoustic meatus	Somesthesia
						SVA	Taste buds; posterior ⅓ tongue; oral pharynx	Gustation, particularly bitter
			X				Oral pharynx	Gag reflex; sensation
				X			Parotid salivary gland; pharyngeal mucosa	Salivation
						SVE	Pharyngeal muscle (stylopharyngeus)	Swallowing

Table 45-1　The Segmental Nerves and Their Components (continued)

Segment	Segmental Nerve	GSA	GVA	GVE	GSE	Other	Innervation	Function
7,8,9,10	*Caudal medulla*							
	X. Vagus					SSA	Pharyngeal, laryngeal muscles	Sensory input for movement control
		X					External ear; external acoustic meatus	Reflexes; somesthesia
						SVA	Taste buds: laryngeal pharynx, larynx	Gustation
			X				Laryngeal pharynx, larynx, trachea, bronchi, lung, esophagus, stomach, small intestine, ascending colon; ½ transverse colon	Input for reflexes; movement control of swallowing, phonation, emesis, peristalsis, and gastric gland secretion
				X			Heart, gallbladder, liver, pancreas, spleen, kidney, foregut, midgut	Autonomic parasympathetic control of smooth muscle, cardiac muscle, and glands of the viscera
						SVE	Pharyngeal, laryngeal muscles	Control of swallowing, phonation, other
	XII. Hypoglossal				X		Extrinsic, intrinsic muscles of tongue	Tongue reflexes and movements
Spinal Segmental								
C_1-C_4	*Upper cervical*							
	C_1-C_4					SSA	Neck muscles	Sensory input for movement control
		X					Neck and back of head	Reflexes, somesthesia
	IX. Spinal accessory					SVE	Sternocleidomastoid; trapezius	Control of head, shoulder movement
	C_1-C_4				X		Neck muscles	Control of head; shoulder movement
C_5-C_8	*Lower cervical*							
	C_5-C_8					SSA	Muscles of upper limb; pectoral muscles	Sensory input for movement control
		X					Upper limb	Reflexes; somesthesia
					X		Muscles of upper limb	Control of movement
T_1-L_2	*Thoracic, upper lumbar*					SSA	Muscles of thorax, abdomen, back	Sensory input for movement control
		X					Thorax, abdomen, back	Reflexes; somesthesia
			X				All of viscera	Input for visceral reflexes; sensation from stomach through transverse colon
				X			All of viscera; all of soma of body and head	Visceral reflexes; control of vasomotor, sweating, piloerection; all of body
					X		Muscles of thorax and back	Control of posture, movement
L_3-S_1	*Lower lumbar*							
	S_1					SSA	Muscles of lower back and abdomen, lower limb	Sensory input for movement control
		X					Lower back, abdomen, lower limb	Reflexes; somesthesia

(continued)

Table 45-1   The Segmental Nerves and Their Components (continued)

Segment	Segmental Nerve	GSA	GVA	GVE	GSE	Other	Innervation	Function
S₂-S₄	*Sacral 2–4*				X		Muscles of lower back and lower limb	Control of posture and movement
						SSA	Muscles: perineum, genitalia, pelvic diaphragm	Sensory input for movement control
		X					Perineum, genitalia, pelvic diaphragm	Reflexes; somesthesia
				X			Distal half transverse colon; descending colon; rectum; pelvic viscera, including bladder, uterus, prostate	Visceral reflexes; visceral sensation; autonomic control of lower visceral organs
					X		Skeletal muscles; perineum; genitalia; pelvic diaphragm	Reflex and movement control
S₅, Co₁, Co₂	*Lower sacral, coccygeal*					SSA	Muscles of sacrum	Sensory input for movement control
		X					Lower sacrum; anus	Reflexes; somesthesia
					X		Skeletal muscles; lower sacrum	Postural and movement control

axons that can travel the entire length of the nervous system (Table 45-2). The term *suprasegmental* refers to higher levels of the CNS, such as the brain stem and cerebrum. Both paleo and neo level fibers have suprasegmental projections.

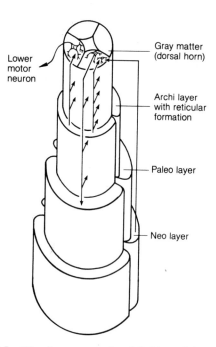

Figure 45-5   *The three concentric subdivisions of the tract systems of the white matter. Migration of neurons into the archi layer converts it into the reticular formation of the white matter.*

The longitudinal layers are arranged in bundles, or fiber tracts, which contain axons that have the same destination, origin, and function. These longitudinal tracts are named systematically to reflect their origin and destination, the site of origin being named first and the site of destination second. For example, the spinothalamic tract originates in the spinal cord and terminates in the thalamus. The corticospinal tract originates in the cerebral cortex and ends in the spinal cord.

Inner layer.   The inner layer of white matter contains the axons of neurons of the gray matter that interconnect with neighboring segments of the nervous system. The axons of this layer permit the pool of motor neurons of several segments to work together as a functional unit. They also allow the afferent neurons of one segment to trigger reflexes that activate motor units in neighboring as well as the same segments. In terms of evolution, this is the oldest of the three layers, and thus, it is sometimes referred to as the archi-level layer. It is the first of the longitudinal layers to become functional, and it appears to be limited to reflex types of movements. Reflex movements of the fetus (quickening) that begin during the fifth month of intrauterine life involve the inner archi-level layer.

The inner layer of the white matter differs from the other two layers in one important aspect. Many of the neurons in the embryonic gray matter migrate out into this layer, resulting in a rich mixture of gray and white fibers called the *reticular formation*. The circuitry of most

Table 45-2   Characteristics of the Concentric Subdivisions of the Longitudinal Tract System in White Matter of the Nervous System

Characteristics	Archi-Level tracts	Paleo-Level Tracts	Neo-Level Tracts
Segmental span	Intersegmental (less than five segments)	Suprasegmental (five or more segments)	Suprasegmental
Number of synapses	Multisynaptic	Multisynaptic but fewer than archi-level tracts	Monosynaptic with target structures
Conduction velocity	Very slow	Fast	Fastest
Examples of functional systems	Flexor withdrawal reflex circuitry	Spinothalamic tracts	Corticospinal tracts

reflexes is contained in the reticular formation. In the brain stem, the reticular formation becomes quite large and contains major portions of vital reflexes, such as those controlling respiration, cardiovascular function, swallowing, and vomiting, to mention a few.

A functional system called the *reticular activation system* (RAS) operates in the lateral portions of the reticular formation of the medulla, pons, and especially the midbrain. The convergence of information from all sensory modalities, including those of the somesthetic, auditory, visual, and visceral afferent nerves, bombards the neurons of this system. The RAS has both descending and ascending portions. The descending portion communicates with all spinal segmental levels through higher-level reticulospinal tracts and serves to facilitate many of the cord-level reflexes. For example, it speeds up reaction time and stabilizes postural reflexes. The ascending portion, sometimes called the *centroencephalic system,* accelerates brain activity, particularly thalamic and cortical activity. This is reflected by the appearance of awake brain-wave patterns. Thus, sudden stimuli not only result in protective and attentive postures but also increase awareness.

Middle layer. The middle layer of the white matter contains most of the major fiber tract systems required for sensation and movement. It contains the spinoreticular and spinothalamic tracts. This system consists of larger-diameter and longer suprasegmental fibers, which ascend to the brain stem and are largely functional at birth. In terms of evolutionary development, these tracts are quite old, and therefore this layer is sometimes called the paleo layer. It facilitates many of the primitive functions, such as the "auditory startle reflex," which occurs in response to loud noises. This reflex consists of turning the head and body toward the sound, dilating the pupils of the eyes, catching of the breath, and quickening of the pulse.

Outer layer. The outer layer of the tract systems is the newest of the three layers in terms of evolutionary development, and hence is sometimes called the neo layer. It becomes functional at about the second year of life, and it contains the pathways that are needed for bladder training. Myelination of the neo layer suprasegmental tracts, which include many of those required for the most delicate coordination and skill, is not complete until sometime around the 10th to the 12th year of life. This includes the development of tracts needed for fine manipulative skills, such as the finger–thumb coordination required for the use of many tools and the toe movements needed for acrobatics. Being the newest to evolve and being on the outside of the brain and spinal cord, these tracts are the most vulnerable to injury. When these outer tracts are damaged, the paleo and archi tracts often remain functional, and rehabilitation methods can result in quite effective use of the older systems. Delicacy and refinement may be gone, but basic function remains. For example, a very important outer system, or neo-system, the corticospinal system, permits the fine manipulative control required for writing. If this is lost, paleo-level systems remaining intact permit the grasping and holding of objects. Thus, the hand can still be used to perform its basic functions.

Collateral communication pathways. Axons in the archi and paleo layers characteristically possess many collateral branches, which move into the gray cell columns or synapse with the reticular formation as the axon passes each succeeding CNS segment. Should a major axon be destroyed at some point along its course, these collaterals provide multisynaptic alternative pathways that bypass the local damage. Neo-level tracts do not possess these collaterals but are instead highly discrete as to the target neurons with which they communicate. Because of their discreteness, damage to the neo tracts causes permanent loss of function. Damage to the archi or paleo systems, on the other hand, is usually followed by slow return of function, presumably through the use of these collateral connections. For example, the surgical section of pathways carrying pain impulses (spinothalamic paleo-level tracts) can be used for temporary relief of intractable pain. The pain experience usually returns after some weeks or months. When it does return, it is often poorly localized and sometimes more unpleasant than it was initially. Consequently, this surgical procedure, which is called a tractotomy, is usually reserved for persons who are not expected to survive for longer than a few months.

In summary, the nervous system can be divided into two parts: the CNS and the PNS. The CNS develops from the ectoderm of the early embryo by the formation of a hollow neural tube that closes and sinks below the surface of its longitudinal axis. The side walls of the neural tube develop to form the neural circuitry of the brain stem and spinal cord; it is subdivided into the dorsal horn, which receives and processes incoming or afferent information, and the ventral horn, which handles the final stages of output processing and contains the LMNs, which innervate the effector muscles and glands. The cavity of the neural tube develops to form the ventricles of the brain and the spinal canal.

The PNS is derived from neural crest ectodermal cells, which migrate into the soma and viscera during embryonic development to contribute to many structures and become the afferent neurons of the dorsal root ganglia and postganglionic efferent neurons of the autonomic ganglia.

The segmental pattern of early embryonic development is retained in the fully developed nervous system. Each of the 43 or more body segments is interconnected to corresponding CNS or neural tube segments by segmental afferent and efferent nerves. Afferent neurons of the dorsal root ganglion are of four types: GSA, which are the input source of somatic reflexes of somesthetic sensation; SSA, which send information to the cerebellum and motor control systems; GVA, which provide an input source for the autonomic and visceral afferents; and SVA, which are the sources of taste and smell. Efferent neurons of the ventral horn send their axons back into body segments to effector cells of the soma or viscera. The GVE preganglionic neurons send axons to the viscera, where they innervate postganglionic neurons of the peripheral autonomic nervous system. The SVE

neurons leave the neural column laterally and innervate the head and neck. The GSE neurons leave the neural tube ventromedially through the ventral roots and innervate the somite-derived muscles. The LMN that are located in the ventral horn innervate the skeletal muscles and supply the preganglionic sympathetic and parasympathetic neurons that innervate the smooth muscle, cardiac muscle, and glandular cells of the viscera and body walls. Input association neurons in the dorsal horn distribute information from the afferent neurons, and output association neurons provide the linkage between the efferent neurons and the LMN. This general pattern of afferent and efferent neurons, which is generally repeated in each segment of the body, forms parallel cell columns running lengthwise through the PNS and CNS.

Longitudinal communication between CNS segments is provided by neurons that send the axons into nearby segments by means of the innermost layer of the white matter, the ancient archi-level system of fibers; these cells provide for coordination between neighboring segments. Neurons have invaded this layer, and the mix of these cells and axons, called the reticular formation, is the location of much of the important reflex circuitry of the spinal cord and the brain stem. Paleo-level tracts, which are located outside this layer, provide the longitudinal communication between more distant segments of the nervous system; this layer includes most of the important ascending and descending tracts. The recently evolved neo-level systems, which become functional during infancy and childhood, travel on the outside of the white matter and provide the means for very delicate and discriminative function. The outside position of the neo tracts, as well as their lack of collateral and redundant pathways, makes them the most vulnerable to injury.

■ The Spinal Cord

In the adult, the spinal cord is located in the upper two-thirds of the vertebral canal of the body's vertebral column (Fig. 45-6). It extends from the foramen magnum at the base of the skull to a cone-shaped termination, the conus medullaris, which is usually located at the level of the first or second lumbar vertebra in the adult. The filum terminale, which is composed of nonneural tissues and pia mater, continues caudally and attaches to the second sacral vertebra.

Development of the Spinal Cord

The early embryo has three basic tissue layers: an outer ectoderm, a middle mesoderm, and an inner endoderm. The nervous system forms along the longitudinal axis of the early developing embryo as a thickening of the ecto-

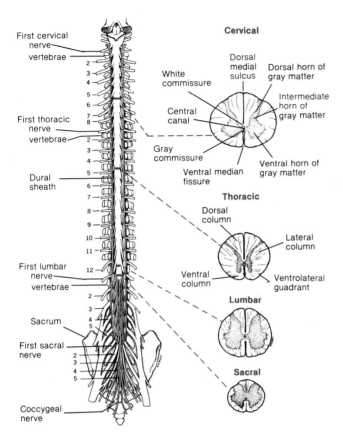

Figure 45-6 *The spinal cord within the vertebral canal. The spinal processes and meninges have been opened. The spinal nerves and vertebrae are numbered on the left. Cross (transverse) sections with regional variations in gray matter and increasing proportions of white matter as the cord is ascended appear on the right. (Adapted from Chaffee EE, Lytle IM: Basic Physiology and Anatomy, 4th ed. Philadelphia, JB Lippincott, 1980)*

derm, or outer cell layer; this layer of thickened epithelium has a midline groove with ridges on each side. The edges of these ridges fuse over the top, turning the groove into a tube called *the neural tube*. The neural tube extends the length of the embryo, the rostral portion becoming the brain, and the caudal end becoming the spinal cord. As the nervous system develops, the neural tube sinks below the surface, becomes surrounded by bony elements of the axial skeleton, and is then covered with skin. The fusion process that forms the neural tube begins at what becomes the high thoracic and cervical levels and proceeds like a zipper downward toward the sacral areas, while simultaneously "zippering" rostrally toward the brain end (Fig. 45-7). Eventually, the open ends of the tube close at the front end of the brain and at the caudal end of the spinal cord. The hollow cavity of the tube becomes the central canal in the spinal cord segments and the primitive ventricular system in the brain.

Closure defects

Various abnormalities of the fusion process can occur. They include (1) failure of the skeletal elements to close, called *spina bifida,* or split spine; (2) formation of a CSF-filled sac covered by meninges (spina bifida with meningocele); and (3) complete nonclosure of the neural tube and associated structures (spina bifida with myeloschisis or split marrow). If only a closure defect of the bony neural lamina occurs, called spina bifida occulta, the spinal cord develops normally, but the CNS is more vulnerable to trauma at that point. This defect often does not become apparent until an accident occurs with possible sensory or paralytic effects. The more severe defects must be repaired surgically shortly after birth in order to reduce the problems of repeated infection and damage to the CNS. If the neural tube does not close, the internal structures do not mature properly, and even following successful surgical repair, permanent flaccid paralysis results. In addition, nontransmission of sensory information, with a consequent anesthesia of the affected parts, often results from the defect.

Spinal Cord Structure

The spinal cord is oval or rounded and on transverse section is noted to have a gray interior portion shaped like a butterfly or letter H (Fig. 45-8). Some of the neurons that make up the gray matter of the cord have processes that leave the cord, enter the peripheral nerves, and supply tissues, such as autonomic ganglia. Other neurons in the gray portion of the cord are concerned with input or reflex mechanisms. The white matter of the cord contains fiber tracts that transmit information between segments of the cord or to higher levels of the central nervous system, such as the brain stem or cerebrum.

The horns of the cord that extend posteriorly are called the *dorsal* horns, and those that extend anteriorly are the *ventral* horns. The dorsal horns contain input association neurons that receive afferent nerve terminals through the dorsal roots and other interconnecting neurons. Examples include the GSIA and GVIA neurons that were described earlier. The ventral horns contain output association neurons of the GSOA type and efferent neurons of the GSE type. A central portion of the cord, which connects the dorsal and ventral horns and surrounds the central canal, is called the *intermediate gray*. In the thoracic area, the small, slender projections that emerge from the intermediate gray are called the *intermediolateral columns* or *horns*. These columns contain the output association (GVOA) and the efferent (GVE) neurons of the sympathetic nervous system.

The amount of gray matter that is present in the cord is largely determined by the amount of tissue that is innervated by a given segment of the cord. Increased

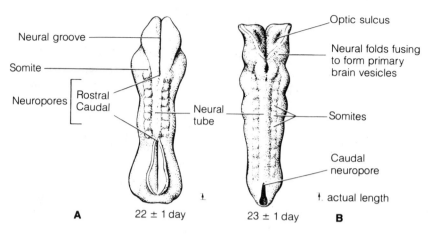

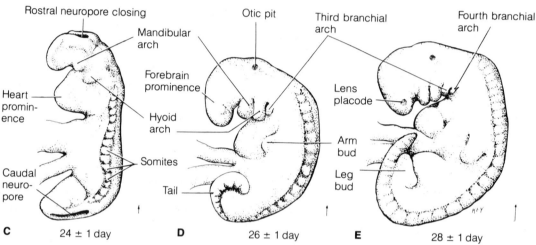

Figure 45-7 *A 4-week-old embryo: A and B dorsal views during stage 10 of development (22–23 days), showing 8 to 12 somites, respectively; C, D, and E, lateral views during stages 11, 12, and 13 (24–28 days), showing 16, 27, and 33 somites, respectively. (Moore KL: The Developing Human, 2nd ed, p 68. Philadelphia, WB Saunders, 1977)*

amounts of gray matter are present in the lower lumbar and upper sacral segments, which supply the lower extremities, and in cervical segment 5 to thoracic segment 1, where the innervation of the upper limbs occurs.

The volume of white matter in the spinal cord also increases progressively as it moves toward the brain because more and more ascending axons are added and because the mass of descending axons, many of which terminate in lower segments, is greater.

During the developmental process, the spinal cord stops growing in length before the spinal axial skeleton reaches its adult dimensions. This results in a disparity between the positions of each succeeding cord segment and the exit of its dorsal and ventral roots through the corresponding intervertebral foramen. This disparity becomes progressively more pronounced at the more caudal levels. In the adult, the sacral cord usually ends at

the level of the first or second lumbar segment. From this point, the dorsal and ventral roots angle downward from the cord, forming what is called the *cauda equina,* or horse's tail. The pia mater that covers the caudal end of the spinal cord continues as the filum terminale through the spinal canal and attaches to the coccygeal vertebrae. However, the arachnoid and its enclosed subarachnoid space, which is filled with cerebrospinal fluid (CSF), do not close down on the filum terminale until they reach the second sacral vertebra. This results in the formation of a pocket of CSF, the dural *cisterna spinalis,* which extends from about the second lumbar vertebra to the second sacral vertebra.

Because of the abundant supply of spinal fluid and the fact that the spinal cord does not extend this far, this area is often used for sampling the CSF. A procedure called a *spinal tap,* or *puncture,* can be done by inserting a

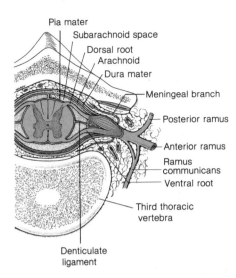

Figure 45-8   *Cross section of vertebral column at the level of the third thoracic vertebra, showing the meninges, the spinal cord, and the origin of a spinal nerve and its branches or rami. (Chaffee EE, Lytle IM: Basic Physiology and Anatomy, 4th ed, p 235. Philadelphia, JB Lippincott, 1980)*

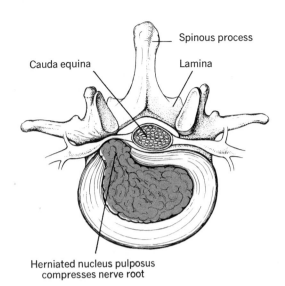

Figure 45-9   *A ruptured intervertebral disk. The soft central portion of the disk is protruding into the vertebral canal, where it exerts pressure on a spinal nerve root. (Chaffee EE, Lytle IM: Basic Physiology and Anatomy, 4th ed, p 103. Philadelphia, JB Lippincott, 1980)*

special type of needle into the dural sac at the level of L_3 and L_4. The spinal roots, which are covered with pia mater, are in relatively little danger of trauma from the needle used for this purpose.

Protective structures

The spinal cord and the dorsal and ventral roots are covered with a connective tissue sheath, the pia mater, which also carries the vascular supply to the white and gray matter of the cord (see Fig. 45-8). On the lateral sides of the spinal cord, extensions of the pia mater, the *denticulate ligaments,* attach the sides of the spinal cord to the bony wall of the spinal canal. Thus, the cord is suspended by both the denticulate ligaments and the segmental nerves. A fat- and vessel-filled epidural space intervenes between the spinal dura mater and the inner wall of the spinal canal. Each vertebral body has two *pedicles* that extend laterally and support the transverse processes of the neural laminae, which arch medially and fuse together to continue as the spinal process. The gaps between each of the vertebrae and its body parts are filled with tough ligaments. Thus, the spinal cord lives within the protective confines of this series of concentric flexible tissue and bony sheaths. A gap, the intervertebral foramen, occurs between each two succeeding pedicles, allowing for the exit of the segmental nerves and veins and the entrance of arteries.

The bony structure of the closely approximated vertebrae provides good protection for the spinal cord, nerve roots, and posterior root ganglia. Major weight bearing is accomplished through the column of vertebral bodies, and flexibility of the vertebral column is provided by fibrocartilaginous *intervertebral disks,* which lie between the centra of adjacent vertebrae. A firm, gelatinous structure called the nucleus pulposus gives substance to the disk. The nucleus pulposus is surrounded by a layer of fibrocartilage called the *annulus fibrosus.* The vertebral disks are held in place by a strong ventral longitudinal ligament and a weaker dorsal longitudinal ligament that interconnects neighboring vertebral bodies.

Herniation of the nucleus pulposus

If the dorsal ligament, which supports the vertebral column, becomes weakened, the nucleus pulposus can be squeezed out of place, and herniate through the annulus fibrosus, a condition often referred to as a herniated or slipped disk (Fig. 45-9). When this happens, the nucleus pulposus usually moves laterally and dorsally, causing irritation or crushing of a segmental nerve root. This irritation causes spontaneous firing of the afferent axons and severe pain along the peripheral distribution of the nerve. Crushing damage to the dorsal roots results in reduction or loss of sensation, and crushing of the ventral roots produces weakness. The signs and symptoms associated with a slipped disk are localized to the body segment that is innervated by the nerve roots. If the slipped disk moves straight back and compresses or destroys a part of the spinal cord, longitudinal communication along the ventral white matter of the cord is most likely to be blocked.

The level at which a slipped disk occurs is important. Usually, it occurs at the lower levels of the lumbar spine where both the mass being supported and the bending of the vertebral column are greatest. When the injury occurs in this area, only the cauda equina will be irritated or crushed. Because these elongated dorsal and ventral roots contain endoneurial tubes of connective tissue, regeneration of the nerve fibers is likely, although because of the distance to the innervated muscle or skin of the lower limbs, several weeks or months are required for full recovery to occur. A slipped disk into the spinal canal at higher levels can destroy the ventral white matter or can completely sever the cord. Here, regeneration is insignificant, and paralysis and anesthesia of the more caudal body regions may be permanent.

Spinal Nerve Roots and Peripheral (Spinal) Nerves

The segments of the spinal cord are grouped into five parts: 8 cervical, 12 thoracic, 5 lumbar, 5 sacral, and 2 to 3 coccygeal segments. Each segment communicates with its corresponding body segment through a pair of segmental nerves, one on each side (Fig. 45-10). The spinal nerve in the intervertebral foramen divides into two branches, or roots, one of which enters the dorsolateral surface of the cord (*the dorsal root*), carrying afferent neuron axons into the CNS. The other leaves the ventrolateral surface of the cord (*the ventral root*), carrying the axons of efferent neurons out to the periphery. These two roots fuse at the intervertebral foramen, forming the *mixed spinal nerve*—mixed because it has both afferent and efferent functions. Because the first cervical (C_1) spinal nerve exits the spinal canal just below the base of the skull, above the first cervical vertebra, in cervical segments the nerve is given the number of the bony vertebra just below it. The numbering was changed for all lower levels, however. Thus, an *extra* cervical nerve, the C_8 nerve, exists above the T_1 vertebra, and each subsequent nerve is numbered for the vertebra just above its point of exit.

A general organization plan is retained in all the segments. Using a thoracic-level segment as an example, the dorsal and ventral roots forming a peripheral nerve fuse at the *dorsal root ganglion* in a mixed spinal root, which contains both *afferent* and *efferent* neuronal processes (Fig. 45-11). Just outside the exit from the spinal cord, the spinal nerve divides into a *small dorsal primary ramus,* which carries efferent and afferent neuronal processes into the dorsal musculature and skin of the body, and a *larger ventral primary ramus,* which innervates the lateral and ventral parts of the body. Cutaneous branches of these rami innervate the skin and cutaneous fascia of the associated blood vessels and connective tissues. Other branches innervate the joints, the marrow cavities of the bones, and the meninges of the spinal canal. Branches from the anterior primary ramus interconnect with the peripheral nervous system, innervating the great vessels, genitourinary organs, and the gut and its derivatives.

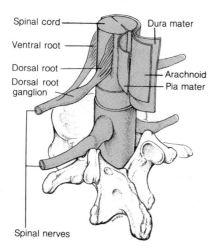

Figure 45-10 *Spinal cord and meninges. (Chaffee EE, Lytle IM: Basic Physiology and Anatomy, 4th ed, p 234. Philadelphia, JB Lippincott, 1980)*

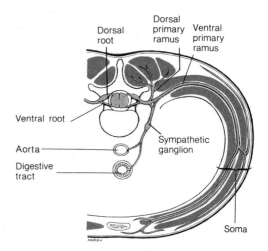

Figure 45-11 *Schematic cross section through the vertebral column and the left side of the trunk, showing anterior and posterior rami of one spinal nerve. Also shown are fibers leading to a sympathetic ganglion and to internal organs. (Chaffee EE, Lytle IM: Basic Physiology and Anatomy, 4th ed, p 235. Philadelphia, JB Lippincott, 1980)*

Spinal cord reflexes

Between 30,000 and 50,000 sensory or afferent neuron cell bodies lives in each of the pairs of connective tissue-enclosed colonies, or *dorsal root ganglia,* located on each side of the spinal cord in the openings (intervertebral foramina) between adjacent vertebrae. Each afferent neuron sends protoplasmic peripheral processes to receptors in the associated side of the body segment. If a skin receptor, such as that which responds to increased temperature, is stimulated by skin contact with a hot object, a series of events takes place in the nervous system (Fig. 45-12). First, a local change occurs in the receptor, which is converted to action potentials and transmitted through the peripheral nerve toward the cell body in the dorsal root ganglia and then through its axon into the spinal cord segment. At this point, internuncial or interconnecting neurons can trigger an action potential in a lower motor or efferent neuron that passes through a ventral root to a mixed (afferent and efferent) segmental nerve. Contraction of the muscles innervated by branches of this nerve results in movement of the skin surface away from the stimulus. This protective reflex is called the *flexor–withdrawal reflex.* It is an example of the many spinal cord reflexes that make standing, stepping, scratching, and walking possible.

Cutaneous distribution of spinal nerves (dermatomes)

Each segment of the body, with few exceptions, contains a pair of dorsal root ganglia within which the GSA neurons innervating the body wall, or soma, of that segment live. As a result, these stripes of segmental nerve-innervated regions, or *dermatomes,* occur in regular sequence from coccygeal 2, upward through the upper cervical segments. In the adult, these stripes overlap each other somewhat and also become distorted by the outgrowth of the limbs (Fig. 45-13). Yet these dermatomes reflect the basic segmental organization of the body and of the nervous system.

CNS distribution of input from spinal nerves

Primary afferent signals from receptors in the body wall are distributed to one or more dorsal horn association neuron cell columns. Each of these columns has characteristic patterns of central projections. The GSIA column relays afferent signals to (1) local reflex circuits, providing rapid, lower motor neuron responses; (2) more rostral parts of the reflex hierarchy, permitting more complex, organized response patterns; (3) the reticular activating system, contributing to general alerting of forebrain systems; and (4) the thalamus, where sensation and perceptive functions begin. A specialized

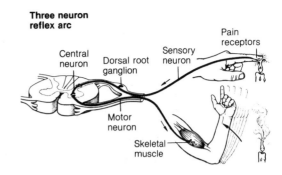

Figure 45-12 *The flexor–withdrawal reflex. (Adapted from Chaffee EE, Lytle IM: Basic Physiology and Anatomy, 4th ed, p 240. Philadelphia, JB Lippincott, 1980)*

association column (SSIA) provides a fifth projection to basic coordination systems.

The skin, fascial sheets, muscles, tendons, joint capsules, periosteum, marrow cavities, and parietal lining of the body cavities receive GSA neuron terminals. The peripheral axon of a GSA neuron branches many times before innervating a circumscribed arc of skin, for instance. Action potentials originating from receptors in any of these branches are conducted through the dorsal root into the spinal cord. This neuron, in a sense, cannot distinguish from which peripheral branch the impulse originated. Thus, it functions as a unit—the sensory unit. It is easy to fool such a mechanism. When the "funny bone" (ulnar nerve on the medial side of the elbow) is traumatized, the person experiences pain at the elbow and also tingling radiating from the palm and fingers. The CNS has interpreted the burst of impulses as coming from the GSA terminals in the hand. This referral to the innervated periphery explains why a pinched sacral nerve at the sacrum results in shooting pain down the back of the leg and foot, a condition called sciatica. Irritation of the stump of a nerve following limb amputation is interpreted as an annoying sensation in the nonexistent phantom limb.

The GSIA column neurons of the dorsal horn distribute the afferent signals to different reflex circuits—pain to the flexor–withdrawal circuit, deep pressure to a stepping reflex circuit, and so on. All the GSA input signals are projected by other central neurons to higher levels of the nervous system as necessary input to more complex reflex patterns. This spinoreticular projection, for instance, permits a fallen animal to regain its footing and depends on midbrain-level circuits. Stepping on a tack results not only in quick flexion of the injured limb but also in extension of the opposite limb to take over body weight support. The same information is projected by spinoreticular fibers to brain-stem levels, where the circuitry for catching the breath, sudden rise in blood

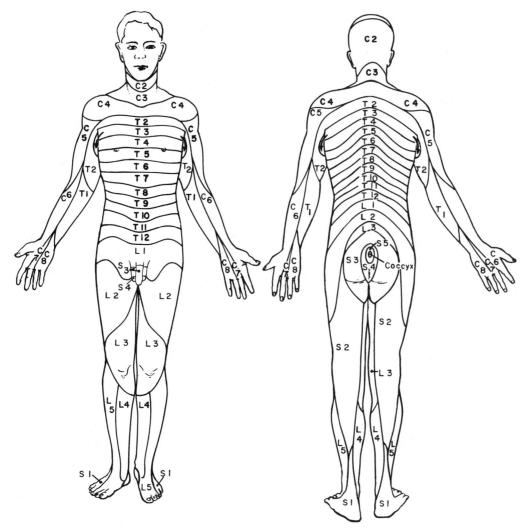

Figure 45-13 *Cutaneous distribution of spinal nerves (dermatomes). (Barr M: The Human Nervous System, p 253. New York, Harper & Row, 1979)*

pressure, and phonation (crying out) occur. This illustrates the concept of the hierarchy of reflexes in which the same afferent information contributes to more and more complex reaction patterns, each at a more rostral location and controlling various components organized at lower levels.

Stimulus discrimination

Discrimination of the location of a stimulus is based on the sensory field innervated by an afferent neuron. Intensity discrimination is based on the rate of impulses in the afferent neuron, and this is related to the intensity of the stimulus applied. Some afferent neurons maintain a more or less steady rate of firing to an uninterrupted stimulus. These slow-adapting afferent neurons contrast with rapid-adapting afferent neurons, which signal only

the onset and conclusion of a stimulus. Slow-adapting afferent neurons are required to maintain stable posture, for instance, whereas rapid-adapting afferent neurons are required to signal moving, brief, or vibrating stimuli.

The qualitative aspects of different types of stimuli are based on the differential sensitivity of the terminals of different afferent neurons. This is called the stimulus modality. Some afferent neurons are particularly sensitive to increased skin temperature, and these signals are interpreted as warm or hot. Others are particularly sensitive to slight indentations of the skin, and their signals are interpreted as touch. Cool–cold, sharp or bright pain, burning-aching pain, delicate touch, deep pressure, joint movement, joint position, muscle stretch, and tendon stretch sensations are based on the specific sensitivities of different GSA neurons. Each of these sensations is based on a different population of afferent neurons or on central integration of several modalities occurring at the same time.

Clinical assessment

Clinical neurologic examination of the patient uses the segmental sequence of afferent innervated zones to quickly test the integrity of the entire series of spinal nerves. A pinpoint pressed against the skin of the sole that results in a flexor–withdrawal reflex, and a complaint of pain confirms the functional integrity of the sacral dorsal root ganglion cell afferent terminals in the skin of the foot, the entire pathway of the afferent nerve neuron's peripheral axon to the S_1 dorsal root ganglion, and beyond the central axon through the S_1 dorsal root and into the spinal cord. It also means that the GSIA cells receiving this information are functioning, and the reflex circuitry of the cord segments (L_5-S_2) involved in functioning. Further, the GSE LMNs of the L_4-S_1 ventral horn are operational, and their axons conduct through the ventral roots, the mixed spinal nerve, and the muscle nerve to the muscles producing the withdrawal response. The communication between the lower motor neuron and the muscle cells is functional also. All of this information is obtained in a fraction of a second by pressing the pinpoint and observing the quick reflex response. If this is done at each segmental level, or dermatome, moving upward along the body and neck, and the reflexes are all in the normal range, the functional integrity of all of these spinal nerves, their roots, and the spinal gray matter of that side must be within normal limits—from coccygeal 2 through the high cervical levels. Similar dermatomes cover the face and scalp, and these, although innervated by cranial segmental nerves, are tested in the same manner.

Ascending afferent (sensory) pathways

Somesthetic afferents transmit the sensations of vibration and fine touch, as well as the more crude sensations of pain and temperature. The GSIA cell column is the indirect source of spinoreticular projections for these sensations to the reticular activating system. In addition, the cell column relays the afferent information to the forebrain, where sensation and perception occur. Two parallel pathways, the anterolateral and the discriminative, reach the thalamic level of sensation, each taking a different route. Many CNS lesions differentially damage these two pathways, and because their locations and routes are different, this helps in localizing the lesion.

Anterolateral pathway.   The anterolateral pathway processes information concerning temperature, touch, and pain. It includes a rapid monosynaptic neo-spinothalamic pathway associated with sharp, highly localized pain and a slower paleospinothalamic tract associated with burning, aching pain, and crude touch. The paleospinothalamic tract is, for the most part, a multisynaptic pathway by which local spinal afferent signals are relayed to both the lateral and the intermediate nuclei of the thalamus. For the sensation of pain, the axons travel almost exclusively up the opposite side of the nervous system. For the more crude aspects of touch, both sides of this anterolateral system are used. This is a slow-conducting pathway with many collateral branches feeding information into the reticular formation of segments along the way. Few fibers travel all the way to the thalamus. Most synapse on reticular formation neurons, which send their axons on toward the thalamus. The lateral nuclei of the thalamus receiving this information are capable of contributing a crude, poorly localized sensation to the body side opposite the thalamic nuclei receiving the information ("something touched my hand"). These same nuclei are in intimate communication with areas of the parietal cerebral cortex, and these communications are necessary for the sensation to be clear, well localizable, and graded in intensity. The spinothalamic tract system, or anterolateral pathway, also projects into the intermediate nuclei of the thalamus, which have close connections with the limbic cortical systems. It is this circuitry that gives sensation its affective or emotional aspects (*e.g.*, the hurtfulness of pain, the particular unpleasantness of itch or heavy pressure, and the peculiar pleasantness of tickle). For most sensations, the anterolateral pathway is multisynaptic and, therefore, slow and crudely graded.

Apparently most of the *perceptive* aspects of body sensation, or *somesthesia*, require the function of "associational" cortex neurons as well as other thalamic nuclei. The perceptive aspect or meaningfulness of a stimulus pattern involves the integration of present sensation with past learning. Your past learning plus present tactile sensation gives you the perception that you are sitting on a soft chair seat and not on a bicycle seat, for instance.

Discriminative pathway.   A more rapid pathway to the thalamus, which involves afferent axons traveling up the dorsal columns of white matter and synapsing in the GSIA nuclei in the medulla with further large-diameter projection through the brain stem without collateral branches, is called the *discriminative pathway*. The discriminative somesthetic pathway transmits accurate localization and delicate intensity discriminative information to the thalamus and the cerebral cortex. Sensory information arriving at the thalamus by this route is much more discretely localizable and more delicately analyzable in terms of intensity grades. This pathway has little projection into the intermediate thalamic nuclei, with a high dependency on parietal cortical function. This is the only pathway taken by sensations of joint movement (kinesthesis), body position (proprioception), vibration, and delicate, discriminative touch, such as is required to correctly differentiate between the touching of the skin at two neighboring points (two-point discrimination) versus only one point.

Alterations in somesthetic sensation. Abnormalities of somesthetic sensation can involve (1) reduced sensitivity: below normal (hypoesthesia); (2) increased sensitivity: beyond normal (hyperesthesia); disordered sensitivity (dysesthesia); or often very unpleasant sensitivity (paresthesia). These conditions can result from congenital, pharmacologic, traumatic, or metabolic modifications of peripheral nerve transmission and excitability or of the function of the CNS ascending systems. Congenital absence of pain (congenital analgesia) is a rare but dangerous disorder. An affected person is often unaware of minor infections or trauma, with resulting serious damage to body parts through lack of attention and care. Some forms of somesthetic sensation depend on input from multiple receptors. The sense of the shape and size of an object in the absence of visualization, called *stereognosis,* is based on afferent information from muscle, tendon, and joint receptors. A screwdriver has a different shape from a knife, not only in the texture of it parts (tactile sensibility), but also in its shape. This complex, interpretive perception requires not only proprioceptive input but also prior learning.

Abnormally high excitability, either centrally or peripherally, can result in sensation without obvious peripheral stimulation. The sensation of ringing in the ears (*tinnitus*) or sudden sharp and often painful somesthetic sensations are fairly common during local ischemia or during peripheral nerve regeneration (paresthesias). Direct trauma or irritation of the CNS portions of an ascending system can also result in sensations that are usually unpleasant and without any meaning or perception attached. Irritation of associational parts of the cerebrum can result in perceptual hallucinations. These hallucinations may indicate the presence and sometimes the location of irritative lesions. For example, repeated sensations of strong and extremely unpleasant odors not sensed by others in the room may be an early symptom of irritation of the olfactory association cortex by a meningeal tumor.

Postural Reflexes and Muscle Tone

Special soma afferent (SSA) neurons send branches of their central axons into the special soma input association (SSIA) cell column of the dorsal horn. These

SSAs include the afferent neurons from the vestibular and auditory end organs of the inner ear and also the primary afferent neurons innervating specialized muscle stretch receptors, called *muscle spindles.* These have in common the SSIA neuron projection of information to the cerebellum. The cerebellum is largely responsible for coordinating the timing of movement of various groups of muscles. Temporal smoothness in changing motor unit firing and, therefore, shifting the strength of muscle contraction in various muscles involved in a movement is an essential part of coordinated movement. The major function of this part of the CNS is the precise control of the sequential timing of motor unit firing during movement patterns.

In relation to an ongoing movement, muscles are classified into *agonists,* which promote the movement, *antagonists,* which resist it, and *synergists,* which assist the agonistic muscles by stabilizing a joint or contributing minor force to the movement. Keeping track of all of this during complex movements and smoothing the ongoing sequence of motor unit firing are the responsibilities of the cerebellar circuits. This is called the *synergistic aspect of coordination.*

A number of other sensory pathways project information to the cerebellum where it is integrated into the control of body and head movement. The vestibular nuclei, which receive information from the labyrinth system of the inner ear, are intimately concerned with cerebellar function. They provide input that makes adjustive changes in ongoing movements during alterations in head position possible. The auditory system, a specialized derivative of the vestibular system for sonic stimulus analysis, has a reduced projection to the cerebellum. Directional information about the location of sound is used during response patterns related to turning toward or away from the stimulus.

A necessary and major input to cerebellar function is required from muscle, tendon, and joint receptors. This feedback system provides the informational background for cerebellar control of ongoing movement. It is not surprising, therefore, to find that the SSIA column is present at all cord and brain-stem levels that receive muscle, tendon, and joint afferent neurons.

Muscle spindles

The stretch reflex is considered essential for the maintenance of normal muscle tone and posture. Most skeletal muscles contain large numbers of specialized stretch receptors, called *muscle spindles,* scattered throughout the muscle substance. These encapsulated receptor organs contain miniature skeletal muscle fibers that are surrounded at their middle by helical receptive terminals (annulospiral endings) of very-large-diameter afferent neurons (Group Ia). The muscle spindles are attached to the connective tissue within the skeletal muscle so that stretching a muscle stretches its muscle spindles, resulting in an increased impulse rate in the Ia afferent fibers. All of the miniature muscle fibers of one spindle are innervated by the same Ia afferent, and each Ia afferent innervates only one spindle. These SSA afferent neurons enter the spinal cord through the dorsal root and have several branches, one of which reaches the SSIA cell column for communication with the cerebellum. At the segment of entry, other large collateral branches make monosynaptic contact with each of the lower motor neurons that have motor units in the muscle containing the spindle source of input. Strong facilitory drive by the stretch afferent neurons on these lower motor neurons increases motor unit firing, opposing the stretch of the muscle. Axons from the spindle fibers also travel up the dorsal white columns to the medulla, and as they travel many collaterals are dropped into the dorsal horn of the succeeding segment, influencing reflex function at each level.

Joint position

The stretch reflex is useful in that it stabilizes joint position. A joint rotation will stretch one or more flexor, extensor, or rotator muscles, and this is immediately opposed by contraction of the stretched muscle. The greater the stretch, the greater the strength of motor unit response. This reflex is continuously available to all muscles in the body, neck, and head. It stabilizes posture against gravitational pull or against any other force that tends to move bones around joints.

Assessment

Clinically, the status of the stretch reflex is evaluated by asking a person to relax while supporting the limb, except at the joint being investigated. The distal part of the extremity is then moved passively around the joint. Normally, it is possible for the examiner to feel mild opposition to this movement. This is called *muscle tone* and can be less than normal (*hypotonia*) or absent (*flaccidity*). It can also be excessive (*hypertonia*) or extreme (*rigidity, spasticity,* or *tetany*). The latter three terms include extremes of hypertonia plus other distinguishing characteristics.

A second method for assessing stretch reflex excitability is to tap briskly with a reflex hammer on the tendon of a muscle, which is almost immediately followed by a sudden contraction or "muscle jerk" (Fig. 45-14). Here the stretch reflex has been "tricked" by the sudden tug on the tendon. A synchronous burst of Ia activity from spindles in the muscle results in essentially simultaneous firing of a large number of motor units. The stretch reflex was tricked into responding, as though the joint had been suddenly rotated. The knee with its

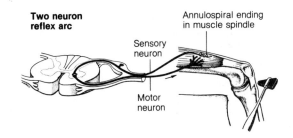

Figure 45-14 *Testing the stretch reflex with a reflex hammer. (Adapted from Chaffee EE, Lytle IM: Basic Physiology and Anatomy, 4th ed, p 240. Philadelphia, JB Lippincott, 1980)*

classic "knee jerk" is just one example of the many places where tendons can be reached and tested with a reflex hammer. These muscle jerk reflexes are called *deep tendon reflexes* (DTRs).

The DTRs can provide an amazing amount of information in a brief period of time. If a DTR is within normal range, you know that (1) the stretch afferent peripheral process in the peripheral muscle and nerves, is normal; (2) the dorsal root ganglion function is normal; (3) the dorsal root function is normal; and (4) the dorsal, intermediate, and ventral horns are functioning appropriately, as are the ventral root and lower motor neuron cell body and axon. It also means that the neuromuscular synapse is functioning normally and that the muscle fibers are capable of normal contraction. Using this method of assessment, it is possible to test the function of all the spinal nerves and spinal cord segments and most of the cranial nerves and brain stem segments in a short time. If abnormality of excitability is detected, further tests are required to determine the nature and location of the pathologic process.

Descending Efferent (Motor) Pathways

Lower motor neurons

The *GSE neurons* are found in the *ventral horns* of the gray matter of the spinal cord and brain stem. The axons of these LMNs pass through the segmental nerves to enter and innervate the skeletal muscle cells, including the limbs, back, abdominal muscles, and intercostals. Each LMN undergoes multiple branching before innervating single skeletal muscle cells. Thus, each LMN can innervate and control from 10 to 2000 individual muscle cells. In general, large muscles—those containing hundreds and thousands of muscle cells and providing gross motor movements—have large motor units. This is in sharp contrast with smaller muscles, such as those in the hand and the tongue and muscles that move the eye, in which the motor units are small and permit very discrete control. An LMN and the muscle fibers it innervates are called a *motor unit.*

The LMNs are surrounded by small internuncial neurons, which synapse with the cell body or dendrites of the efferent cells. Action potentials in the axons of these internuncial neurons exert either excitatory or inhibitory effects on the LMN. Although some CNS systems communicate directly with the LMN, almost all LMN activity is controlled by systems communicating through excitatory or inhibitory internuncial neurons. These internuncial GSOA neurons represent the final stage of communication between elaborate CNS neuronal circuits and the transmission of information to the skeletal muscle cells of the motor unit. Approximately 600,000 LMN-motor units provide the mechanism for all skeletal muscle movement. If movement, reflexes, or other behaviors are lost, evaluation of the function of the billions of CNS neurons becomes close to impossible.

Atrophy and hypertrophy. During early embryologic development, outgrowing GSE axons innervate partially mature muscle cells, which if not innervated, will not mature and will eventually die. Randomly contracting muscle cells become enslaved by the innervating neurons and from then on, the muscle cell will contract only when stimulated by that particular neuron. If the LMN dies or its axon is destroyed, the skeletal muscle cell is again free of neural domination. When this happens, it begins to have spontaneous contractions on its own. It also begins to lose its contractile proteins and, after several months, degenerates. This is called *denervation atrophy.*

If a peripheral nerve or muscle nerve is crushed and the endoneurial tubes remain intact, the outgrowing axonic branches may reinnervate the muscle cell. If the nerve is cut, however, the likelihood of axonic reinnervation by the original axon is slight, and muscle cell loss is likely to occur. If some intact LMN axons remain within the muscle, nearby denervated muscle cells apparently emit what is called a *trophic signal*, probably a chemical messenger, which signals intact axons to send outgrowing collaterals into the denervated area and capture control of some of the denervated muscle fibers. The degree of axonic regeneration that occurs after injury to an LMN depends on the amount of scar tissue that develops at the site of injury and how quickly reinnervation occurs. If reinnervation occurs after the muscle cell has degenerated, no recovery is possible. Thus, peripheral nerve section usually results in some loss of muscle cell function, which is experienced as weakness. Collateral sprout reinnervation results in enlarged motor units and, therefore, a reduction in the discreteness of muscle control following recovery.

If a normally innervated muscle is not used for long periods of time, the muscle cell diameter is reduced (*disuse atrophy*), and although the muscle cells do not die, they become weakened. With appropriate exercise, muscle strength will return. Exercise beyond the normal results in enlargement of the muscle fiber diameter with the addition of contractile substance, and muscle strength increases. There are limits, however, and when muscle *hypertrophy* becomes excessive, the largest of the muscle cells can undergo degeneration.

Effects of injury and infection. Infection or irritation of the cell body of the LMN or its axon can lead to hyperexcitability, which causes spontaneous contractions of the muscle units. These are often seen through the skin as twitching and squirming on the muscle surface. They are called *fasciculations*. Toxic agents, such as the tetanus toxin (*Clostridium tetani*), produce extreme hyperexcitability of the LMN, which results in firing at maximum rate. The resultant maximal contraction of the muscles is called *tetany*. Tetany of muscles on both sides of a joint produces immobility or tetanic paralysis. When the poliomyelitis virus attacks an LMN, it first irritates the LMN causing fasciculations to occur. These fasciculations are often followed by neuronal death. Weakness results. If muscles are totally denervated, total weakness, called *flaccid paralysis*, occurs. Abnormalities of the motor unit include problems such as myasthenia gravis, in which the transmission of impulses at the level of the myoneural junction is impaired, and disorders such as muscular dystrophy, in which pathology of skeletal muscle cells occurs (Chap. 48).

In summary, the spinal cord is supported and protected by connective tissue layers, the pia mater, arachnoid, and dura mater, with CSF filling the subarachnoid space. Outside the dura, the bony vertebrae provide a protective axial skeleton, and intervertebral disks of fibrocartilage provide flexibility to the vertebral column. The segmental nerves formed by fusion of the dorsal and ventral roots contain afferent and efferent neural processes directed dorsally (posterior primary ramus) or ventrally (anterior primary ramus) around the body wall. These have muscular, cutaneous, and visceral branches.

Afferent neurons of the dorsal root ganglia innervate a corresponding segment of the body as general somatic afferent (GSA) neurons or general visceral (GVA) neurons. The soma innervated by one set of dorsal root ganglia is called a dermatome. A sensory unit consists of a single dorsal root ganglion afferent neuron and its terminals in a small region of the periphery. Nociceptive GSA fibers terminate on dorsal horn association neurons. By means of a multisynaptic circuit, the GSIAs trigger a highly predictable flexor–withdrawal reflex by means of GSE-activated skeletal muscle contraction with inhibition of lower motor neurons (LMNs) of antagonistic muscles. Completion of this reflex arc requires the functional integrity of the afferent central circuit, the efferent motor neurons, and the effector organ.

Somesthetic afferents transmit the discriminative sensations of vibration and fine touch, as well as the more crude sensations of pain and temperature. Two parallel ascending pathways—the anterolateral and the discriminative—reach the thalamic level, each by its own route, and transmit sensation. The anterolateral system includes a rapid monosynaptic neospinothalamic pathway associated with sharp, highly localized pain and a multisynaptic, slower paleospinothalamic system associated with burning, aching pain. The rapid discriminative pathway is involved in sensations of joint movement and body position, vibration, and discriminative touch.

Muscle spindle afferents (SSA) include rapid conducting Ia neurons, which make contact with homonymous motor units, generating muscle tone or resistance to passive movement. This reflex provides the basis for all postural control. All skeletal muscle movement depends on the function of the motor unit, which consists of an LMN and the skeletal muscle fibers that it innervates.

■ The Brain

The brain is divided into three parts: the forebrain, which forms the two cerebral hemispheres, the thalamus and the hypothalamus; the midbrain; and the hindbrain, which is divided into the pons and the medulla. The structure and organization of the brain become clearer when considered in the context of embryonic development.

The important concept to keep in mind is that the more rostral, recently elaborated parts of the neural tube gain *domination,* or *control,* over regions and functions at lower levels. They *do not replace* the more ancient circuitry but merely dominate it. Thus, following damage to the more vulnerable parts of the forebrain, such as occurs in "brain death," a brain-stem organism remains capable of respiration and survival if environmental temperature is regulated and if nutrition and other aspects of care are provided. However, all aspects of intellectual function, including experience, perception, and memory, are usually permanently lost.

In the process of development, the most rostral part of the embryonic neural tube—in humans approximately ten segments—undergoes extensive modification and enlargement to form the brain. The brain stem is a modification of the neural tube segments. In the early embryo, three swellings, or primary vesicles, develop, subdividing these ten segments into the prosencephalon (forebrain), which contains the first two segments; the metencephalon, or midbrain, which develops from segment 3; and the rhombencephalon, or hindbrain, which develops from segments 4 to 10 (Fig. 45-15).

The central canal of the prosencepahalon develops two pairs of lateral outpouchings, which carry the neural tube with them: (1) the optic cup, which becomes the optic nerve and retina, and (2) the telencephalic vesicles, which become the cerebral hemispheres with their

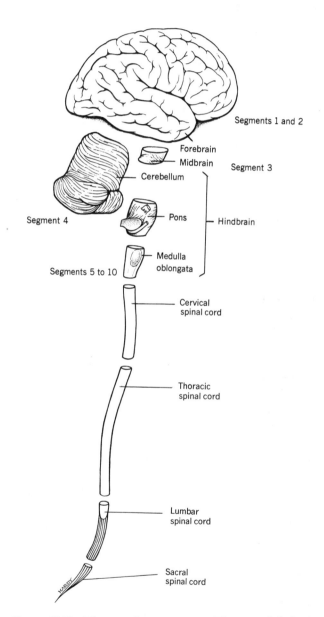

Figure 45-15 The central nervous system. The parts of the brain and the spinal cord have been separated. (Chaffee EE, Lytle IM: Basic Physiology and Anatomy, 4th ed, p 203. Philadelphia, JB Lippincott, 1980)

enlarged CSF-filled cavities, and the first and second, or lateral, ventricles. The remaining neural tube of these three segments is called the diencephalon ("between brain"); it becomes the adult thalamus and hypothalamus. The neurohypophysis (posterior pituitary) grows as a midline ventral outgrowth at the junctions of segments 1 and 2. A dorsal outgrowth, the pineal body, develops between segments 2 and 3, at the diencephalic–mesencephalic junction.

The ventral half of the neural tube gray matter, the basal lamina, becomes the ventral horn and remains relatively unchanged through the brain segments. Most of the brain, as seen grossly, represents tremendous enlargements, outpouchings, outgrowths, and cortex formation derived from the dorsal horns.

Both the central and the peripheral nervous systems differentiate very early in embryonic life and hold a critical position in providing a necessary stimulus for the differentiation of many other body tissues, particularly the skeletal muscles. By the end of the third month of gestation, the gross structure of the brain and spinal cord is established. The remaining period of intrauterine growth involves increases in cell numbers of both neurons and glial cells to a final neural-to-glial ratio of 1:20, as well as the development of the basic circuitry and myelination of the major tract systems of the spinal cord and brain stem. A phenomenal increase in brain weight occurs during the 3- to 5-month period of intrauterine life. At birth, the average brain weighs about 300 gm, approximately 12.5% of total body weight. During postuterine life, growth continues, but at a decreasing rate, while body growth continues. As a result, the adult human brain weight (1450–1500 gm in the male, and 1200–1300 gm in the female) is about five times that at birth and yet is only about 2.4% of total body weight. Maximum brain weight is reached between ages 20 and 29 and is then followed by a gradual decrease in weight with advancing years.

During the latter two-thirds of intrauterine life, the cerebral cortex increases its volume relative to that of deeper structures; this is achieved by a greatly increased surface area, which occurs with increasing development of the number and depth of infoldings. The ridge between these infoldings, or grooves, is called a gyrus; a groove is called a sulcus. The adult cerebral cortex, with its many gyri and sulci, is equivalent to an area of about 160,000 mm^2 and contains approximately 16.5 billion neurons.[2] The most recently enlarged parts of the neocortex develop later in postnatal life, particularly the portions of the frontal, parietal, and temporal cortex that grow out and cover the insula. The cerebellar cortex also undergoes a tremendous increase in area during the latter part of embryonic life and infancy, achieving an area of 84,000 mm^2, again with the development of many deep sulci and narrow gyri. The cerebellar cortex of the adult contains approximately 100 billion neurons.

The third neural tube segment, which forms the midbrain, retains its basic spinal segmentlike organization (see Fig.45-15). Segment 4, the rhombencephalon, becomes much enlarged and flattened laterally, giving the fourth ventricle its rhomboid shape. This segment, called the metencephalon, or pons, also grows up and over the fourth ventricle and is a major contributor to the adult cerebellum.

The remaining segments, 5 through 10, become the adult medulla oblongata, with the widened fourth ventricle narrowing to form a central canal, which continues through the spinal cord segments. The most rostral segment (5) of the medulla fuses with the pons and is often called the caudal pons. It also contributes to the caudal part of the cerebellum. The junction of segment 10 of the brain stem with the cervical spinal segments occurs at the foramen magnum, the large opening in the skull through which the neural tube passes.

Each of these brain-stem segments, except for segment 2, retains at least some portion of the basic segmental nerve organization. Our ancient ancestry is reflected in the cranial nerves and upper cervical segmental nerves because the original pattern was for many branches to occur directly from the neural tube, each containing a particular component, or functional grouping, of axons. Thus, one segment would have paired branches to somite muscles, another a set to gill arch muscles, and yet another a set to visceral structures, and so on. The classic pattern of the spinal nerve organization, which consists of a pair of dorsal and a pair of ventral roots, is a more recent evolutionary development that has not occurred in the cranial nerves. Consequently, the arbitrarily numbered 1 through 12 cranial nerves retain the ancient pattern, and more than one cranial nerve can branch from a single segment. The truly segmental nerve pattern of the cranial nerves is further clouded by the loss of all branches from segment 2 and most of the branches from segment 1. In segments 6 through 10, longitudinal fusions between segments and loss of components at some segments reflect the specialization of the head end of the organism through nearly a billion years of evolutionary history. It should also be noted that the classic second cranial nerve, the optic nerve, is not really a segmental nerve branch at all, but a brain tract connecting the retina (modified brain) with the first forebrain segment from which it developed.

Brain Stem

The adult brain stem is a distorted, enlarged, and elaborated version of the spinal cord. It contains the neuronal circuits required for the basic breathing, eating, and locomotive functions required for survival. It also is surrounded on the outside by the long tract systems that interconnect the forebrain with lower parts of the CNS (Fig. 45-16).

Medulla

The medulla oblongata represents the caudal 5 segments of the brain part of the neural tube, and thus the cranial nerve branches entering and leaving it have similar functions, as do the spinal segmental nerves. The ventral horn area in the medulla is quite small, but the dorsal horn is enlarged because of the great amount of information pouring through the cranial nerves. The segmental peripheral nerve components of the medulla can be divided into those that leave the neural tube ventromedially (hypoglossal and abducent cranial nerves), and those that exit dorsolaterally (vagus, spinal accessory, glossopharyngeal, and vestibulocochlear cranial nerves). Because the signs and symptoms reflect the spatial segregation of brain stem components, neurologic syndromes resulting from trauma, tumors, aneurysms, and cerebrovascular accidents are often classified as ventral or as dorsolateral syndromes.

Hypoglossal (XII) cranial nerve. The GSE LMNs of the lower segments of the medulla supply the extrinsic and intrinsic muscles of the tongue by means of the hypoglossal (XII) cranial nerve. Damage to the hypoglossal nerve results in partial or total denervation and, therefore, weakness or paralysis of tongue muscles.

When the tongue is protruded, it deviates or is pushed toward the weak side of the muscle by the unaffected side of the tongue. The axons of the hypoglossal nerve leave the medulla adjacent to two long, longitudinal ridges along the medial underspace of the medulla called the *pyramids*. The pyramids contain the corticospinal axons that provide for fine manipulative control for the spinal LMNs. Lesions of the ventral surface of the caudal medulla result in the syndrome of alternating *hypoglossal hemiplegia,* characterized by signs of ipsilateral (same side) denervation of the tongue and contralateral (opposite side) weakness or paralysis of both the upper and lower extremities.

Abducent (VI) cranial nerve. In the most rostral segment of the medulla, GSE LMNs send their axons out ventrally on either side of the pyramids and then forward into the orbit through the abducent (VI) cranial nerves to innervate the lateral rectus muscles of the eyes. As their name indicates, the abducent nerves abduct the eye (lateral or outward rotation); peripheral damage to them results in weakness or the loss of eye abduction.

Vagus (X) cranial nerve. The vagus (X) cranial nerve carries the innervation of the GVA, GVE, SVA, and SVE neurons. GVA and GVE fibers innervate the gastrointestinal tract (from the laryngeal pharynx to the midtransverse colon), the heart, and the lungs; SVA, the pharyngeal taste buds; and SVE, the branchial skeletal muscles of the pharynx and larynx. The fibers carried in

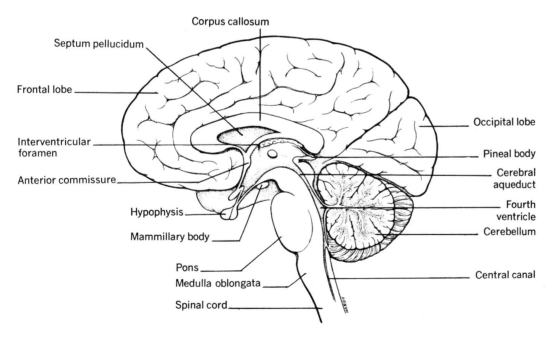

Figure 45-16 *Midsagittal section of the brain. (Chaffee EE, Lytle IM: Basic Physiology and Anatomy, 4th ed, p 214. Philadelphia, JB Lippincott, 1980)*

the vagus are responsible for the various innervations of these structures and for the initiation of reflexes. For example, SVE fibers are involved in swallowing and speech, and GVA fibers are involved in cough, hiccough, and vomiting reflexes. The unilateral loss of vagal function results in slowed gastrointestinal motility, a permanently husky voice, and deviation of the uvula away from the damaged side. Bilateral loss of vagal function seriously damages reflex maintenance of cardiovascular and respiratory reflexes. Swallowing becomes difficult and in some cases paralysis of laryngeal structures causes airway obstruction. Endotracheal intubation or tracheotomy is then necessary to prevent asphyxia.

Spinal accessory (XI) cranial nerve. The powerful head-turning muscle, the sternocleidomastoid, and the trapezius muscle, which elevates the shoulders, are also branchial arch (SVE)-derived skeletal muscles. They are innervated by the spinal accessory (XI) cranial nerve with lower motor neurons in the upper four cervical spine segments. Lateral rootlets from these segmental levels combine and enter the cranial cavity through the foramen magnum and then exit through the jugular foramen with the glossopharyngeal (IX) and vagus (X) cranial nerves. Loss of spinal accessory (XI) nerve function results in drooping of the shoulder on the damaged side and weakness when turning the head to the opposite side.

Glossopharyngeal (IX) cranial nerve. The dorsolateral glossopharyngeal (IX) cranial nerve contains the same components as does the vagus, but for a more rostral segment of the gut, the pharynx. This nerve provides the SVA innervation of the taste buds of the oral pharynx and the back of the tongue; GVA innervation of the oral pharynx and the baroreceptors of the carotid sinus; GVE innervation of the otic ganglion, which controls the major source of salivary secretion, the parotid gland; and SVE innervation of the stylopharyngeus muscle of the pharynx. This cranial nerve is seldom damaged, but when it is, anesthesia of the ipsilateral oral pharynx and dry mouth because of reduced salivation occur.

Vestibulocochlear (VIII) cranial nerve. Formerly called the auditory or acoustic nerve, the vestibulocochlear (VIII) cranial nerve is attached laterally at the junction of the medulla oblongata and the pons. It consists of two distinct fiber divisions, both of which are purely sensory (SSA): (1) the cochlear division, which arises from cell bodies in the cochlea in the inner ear and transmits impulses related to the sense of hearing, and (2) the vestibular division, which arises from cell bodies in the utricle, saccule, and semicircular canals and trans-mits impulses related to head position and movement of the body through space. Injury to the cochlear division results in deafness; injury to the vestibular division leads to dizziness and nystagmus (Chap. 46).

Pons

The pons, or bridge, developed from the fourth neural tube segment. The central canal of the spinal cord, which is greatly enlarged in the pons and rostral medulla, forms the fourth ventricle. An enlarged area on the ventral surface of the pons contains the pontine nuclei, which receive information from all parts of the cerebral cortex. The axons of these neurons form a massive bundle that swings around the lateral side of the fourth ventricle to enter the cerebellum. The trigeminal (V) and facial (VII) cranial nerves have their origin in the pons.

Trigeminal (V) cranial nerve. The trigeminal (V) cranial nerve is located laterally on the forward surface of the pons and has two subdivisions, sensory and motor. The GSA innervation of the front part of the head (forehead), the conjunctiva and orbit, the face, the paranasal sinuses, and the mouth, including the teeth and the anterior two-thirds of the tongue, is the major sensory component. The LMNs (SVE) in the pons send their axons through the motor component to innervate the muscles of mastication. The reticular formation of the pons is large and contains the circuitry for masticating food and manipulating the jaws during speech.

Facial (VII) cranial nerve. The facial nerve and its intermediate component (the intermedius) contain both afferent (GSA, SVA, GVA) and efferent (GVE) components. The intermedius nerve innervates the nasopharynx and taste buds of the palate, the forward two-thirds of the tongue, the submandibular and sublingual salivary glands, the lacrimal glands, and the mucous membranes of the nose and roof of the mouth. Loss of this branch of the facial nerve can lead to eye dryness with risk of corneal injury. The SVE LMNs of the facial nerve innervate the muscles that control head and neck facial expression: wrinkling of the brow, wiggling of the ears, smiling, movement of the scalp, and the forceful closure of the eyes, nose, and lips. Unilateral loss of the facial nerve function results in flaccid paralysis of the muscles for one-half of the head, a condition called Bell's palsy. The facial nerve passes through a bony canal at the back of the middle ear cavity, and Bell's palsy can develop as a complication of otitis media. Because such injuries result from pressure caused by edematous tissue, the endoneurial tube is retained and regeneration with full recovery of all muscles generally occurs within a period of several months.

Cerebellum

The cerebellum, or "little brain," sitting above the fourth ventricle, is a complicated computer necessary for inter-relating visual, auditory, somesthetic, and vestibular information with ongoing motor activity so that highly skilled movement can be smoothly performed.

Midbrain

The midbrain developed from the third segment of the neural tube, and its organization is not very different from that of a spinal cord segment. The central canal is reestablished as the cerebral aqueduct, interconnecting the fourth ventricle with the third ventricle, just rostral. The oculomotor (III) and trochlear (IV) nerves are located in the midbrain.

Massive fiber bundles of the cerebral peduncles pass from the forebrain to the pons along the ventral surface of the midbrain. On the dorsal surface, four "little hills," the superior and inferior colliculi, are areas of cortex formation. The inferior colliculus is involved in directional turning and, to some extent, the experiencing of the direction of sound sources. The superior colliculus is an essential part of the reflex mechanisms that control eye movements when the visual environment is being surveyed.

Oculomotor (III) cranial nerve. The central gray matter contains the LMNs that innervate most of the skeletal muscles that move the optic globe about and raise the eyelids. These axons leave the midbrain through the oculomotor (III) cranial nerve. This nerve also contains axons that control pupillary constriction and ciliary muscle focusing on the lens. Damage to the ventrally exiting cranial nerve III and to the adjacent cerebral peduncle, which includes the corticospinal axon system on one side, results in paralysis of eye movement combined with contralateral hemiplegia (discussed in Chap. 46).

Trochlear (IV) cranial nerve. A small compact group of cells in the ventral part of the central gray matter contains the LMNs that innervate the superior oblique eye muscles that tilt the upper part of the eye toward the face when it is abducted, or turned outward, and tilt it downward and away from the eye when the eye is adducted, or turned inward. These axons emerge dorsolaterally and caudally as the trochlear (VI) cranial nerve. They decussate (cross over) in the medulla before exiting the brain stem. Lesions involving the trochlear cranial nerve are unusual. The diplopia or double vision resulting from such lesions is vertical and affects downward gaze to the opposite side. Walking downstairs is particularly difficult.

Forebrain

The two forward-most brain stem segments form an enlarged dorsal horn–ventral horn structure with a narrow, deep, enlarged central canal—the third ventricle—separating the two sides. This region is called the *diencephalon*. The dorsal horn part of the diencephalon, the *thalamus*, is the location of the mechanisms that make experience or sensation possible (Fig. 45-17). Consequently, almost all afferent systems send information to the thalamus, and it is richly connected with all other forebrain areas.

The ventral horn portion of the diencephalon is subdivided into the medial *hypothalamus*, next to the third ventricle, and the more lateral *subthalamus*. The hypothalamus is the area of master-level integration of homeostatic control of the body's internal environment. Maintenance of blood gas concentrations, water balance, body temperature, food consumption, and major aspects of hormone level control, with the close tolerances necessary for normal function in a highly variable external environment, requires a functional hypothalamus. Many of the efferent functions integrated here involve the use of both autonomic and somatic motor systems. The subthalamic area is a part of movement control systems related to the basal ganglia.

The two *cerebral hemispheres* are lateral outgrowths of the diencephalon that become so massive that they

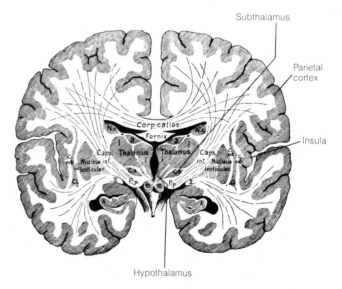

Figure 45-17   *Frontal section of the brain passing through the third ventricle showing the thalamus, subthalamus, hypothalamus, internal capsule* (caps int.), *external capsule* (c. ext.), *corpus callosum* (corp. callos.), *basal ganglia (caudate nucleus* [c.s.], *lenticular nucleus), insula, and parietal cortex. (From Villiger E, Addison WHF (eds): Brain and Spinal Cord. Philadelphia, JB Lippincott, 1931.)*

dominate the appearance of the forebrain. These hemispheres are hollow and contain the *lateral ventricles* (ventricles I and II), which are interconnected with the third ventricle of the diencephalon by a small opening, the interventricular foramen (of Munro).

The hemispheres are separated by the heavy longitudinal fold of the dura mater, called the *falx cerebri*. The falx cerebri carries the inferior sagittal venous sinus in its lower edge and the superior sagittal sinus at its junction with the outer dural lining of the cranial cavity. The corpus callosum is a massive commissure, or bridge, of myelinated axons interconnecting the cerebral cortex of the two sides of the brain. Two smaller commissures, the anterior and posterior commissures, connect the two sides of the more specialized regions of the cerebrum and diencephalon.

A section through the cerebral hemisphere will reveal a surface of *cerebral cortex,* a subcortical layer of *white matter* made up of masses of myelinated axons, and deep masses of gray matter, the *basal ganglia* (caudate, putamen, globus pallidus), which border on the internal, lateral ventricle.

The cerebral cortex exposed to view from the side is a recently evolved layered neocortex. It is arbitrarily divided into lobes named for the bones of the skull that cover them. The frontal lobe lies in front of the central sulcus and can be subdivided into the frontal pole (rostrally) and the *superior, middle,* and *inferior frontal gyri* (laterally), which continue on the undersurface over the eyes as the orbital cortex.

Primary motor cortex

The *precentral gyrus,* immediately bordering the central sulcus, is the *primary motor cortex* from which axons of large cortical neurons leave the cerebrum to reach the intermediate and ventral horns of all brain stem and spinal cord segments. These axons are known collectively as the *corticospinal system* and provide very discrete control of movement, particularly *fine manipulative movement.* For distal flexor muscles of the arm and leg, the corticospinal system makes monosynaptic contact with lower motor neurons. The corticospinal system is called the *upper motor neuron* (UMN) *system* because of its discrete control over lower motor neuron function during the initiation of highly skilled voluntary movements. Actually, corticospinal axons originate in all parts of the neocortex, but nearly 60% originate in the precentral gyrus and neighboring areas. The pattern of corticospinal origin in the cortex reflects the discreteness of control of lower motor neurons, innervating the *opposite side of the body.* Relatively less control of the trunk is reflected in a small trunk area of the cortex, and an extremely high level of control of the tongue, thumb, index finger, and large toe is reflected in larger areas. The

resultant distorted body "map" represented in the primary motor cortex is called the *motor homunculus* (Fig. 45-18). The lower limb of the opposite side is represented near the vertex, and the face is shown laterally at the edge of the lateral sulcus. Loss of a part of the primary motor cortex or of the large-diameter myelinated axons that pass through the cerebral white matter, down the ventral surface of the brain stem through the pyramids, and then down the opposite side of the spinal cord, results in a loss of the capacity to perform *delicate, refined movements,* particularly of the hands and fingers, of the toes, and of the laryngeal, tongue, and jaw movements required for speech.

Premotor area

The area of the superior, middle, and inferior frontal gyri just in front of the precentral gyrus is called the *premotor area* (areas 8,6) because it is involved in the organization of more complex movement patterns and is an important source of control for patterned activity of primary motor cortex neurons (see Fig. 45-17). Damage to premotor cortex results in *dyspraxia* or *apraxia.* Such patients can manipulate a screwdriver, for instance, but cannot use it to loosen a screw. They can handle a pencil well, but cannot use it to write with. Higher-order motor skills of the opposite side of the body are affected.

The major sources of input to the premotor and motor cortices are nuclei of the thalamus, which receive information from both the cerebellum and basal ganglia. The latter are masses of deep gray matter within the hemisphere, with complex interconnections with motor and premotor cortices, the thalamus, and the reticular formation of the brain stem. At present, their function is believed to be the organization of movement patterns characteristic of the species: swinging the arms during walking, following through with the arms and body in throwing a ball, or swinging a club.

Parietal lobe

The *parietal lobe* of the cerebrum lies behind the central sulcus and above the lateral sulcus. The strip of cortex bordering the central sulcus is called the *primary sensory cortex* because it receives very discrete projections of somesthetic information from the lateral nuclei of the thalamus. Again, the density of this input reflects the density of somesthetic receptors on the body surface and in the body wall. The tongue, the lips, and the palmar surface of the thumb, index finger, and large toe have the largest receptive areas. The *sensory homunculus* is organized with the leg at the vertex and the face laterally, next to the lateral sulcus (see Fig. 45-18). This cortical area must be functional for discrete, highly discriminative sensation to occur, originating from the opposite side of the body and face. If the area is damaged, sensation still

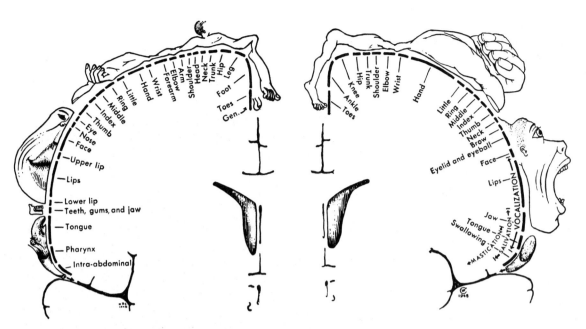

Figure 45-18   *Sensory* (left) *and motor* (right) *representations as determined by stimulation studies on the human cortex during surgery. Compare the sensory homunculcus* (left) *to the motor homunculcus* (right). *Note the relatively large area devoted to the lips, thumb, and fingers. (Penfield E, Rasmussen T: The Cerebral Cortex of Man. New York, Macmillan, 1955. Copyright © by Macmillan Publishing Co., Inc., renewed 1978 by Theodore Rasmussen.)*

occurs, probably at the thalamic level, but the delicacy of discrimination of location, intensity, and subtle aspects of the given situation are lost. Such a patient cannot tell the differences in texture between sandpaper and velvet or localize delicate touch other than to a vague, general area of the body. The sense of vibration is lost because this is really a delicate, temporal discrimination. The sense of the position or movement of body parts is also lost. This information is derived from joint, muscle, and tendon receptors and involves subtle discriminations involving joint movement and muscle tension.

A small secondary sensory cortical area just above the lateral sulcus and posterior to the primary somesthetic area seems to be involved in discrimination of the intensity and fine localization of *painful stimuli*. Electrical stimulation of this parietal cortex results only in a sharp, localized sensation but not of the painfulness or hurtfulness of a nociceptive stimulus. The latter aspects of experience involve the limbic areas of the cerebrum and thalamus.

Just behind the primary somesthetic cortex is a region of somesthetic association cortex (area 5, 7), which is interconnected with thalamic nuclei and the primary sensory area. This region is necessary to appreciate *perception* or meaningfulness. Lesions in this area lead to *somesthetic agnosia* (gnosis, perception). With this area

damaged, a patient can describe the size, shape, or texture of a screwdriver without seeing it but is unable to explain its use. However, if the patient can see the tool, he can then explain its function. So it is not the loss of meaning *per se* but of somesthetically derived meaning that is damaged.

Temporal lobe

The *temporal lobe* lies below the lateral sulcus and merges with the parietal and occipital lobes. It has a polar region and three primary gyri: superior, middle, and inferior (see Fig. 45-17). It is separated from limbic areas on the ventral surface by the collateral or rhinal sulcus. The *primary auditory* cortex (area 41) involves the part of the superior temporal gyrus that extends into the lateral sulcus. This is particularly important for fine discrimination of sound frequency. Octaves are represented at equal intervals along this cortex, and damage results in deficient but not lost pitch discrimination from sound entering the opposite ear. The more exposed part of the superior temporal gyrus involves the *auditory association,* or perception area (area 22). The gnostic aspects of hearing (*e.g.,* the meaningfulness of a certain sound pattern, such as that of water dripping or a fork dropped) require the function of this area. The remaining portion of the temporal cortex has a less well defined function, apparently important in long-term memory recall. Irritation or stimulation can result in vivid hallucinations of long-past events.

It should be noted that the cortices of the frontal, parietal, and temporal lobes surrounding the older cortex of the *insula,* deep in the lateral fissure, represent the most recently evolved parts of the cerebral cortex. These areas contain primary and associative functions for motor control and somesthesias for the lips and tongue and for audition; thus, they are particularly involved in *speech mechanisms,* which are discussed later.

Occipital lobe

The *occipital lobe,* is posterior to the temporal and parietal lobes and is only arbitrarily separated from them. The medial surface contains a deep sulcus extending from the limbic cortex to the occipital pole, the *calcarine sulcus,* which houses the *primary visual cortex* (area 17). Stimulation of this cortex causes the experiencing of bright lights in the visual field. Destruction results in "cortical blindness" in which the patient "sees nothing" yet has normal visual reflexes to bright light or moving objects. Just above and below and extending onto the lateral side of the occipital pole is the *association cortex for vision* (area 18 and 19). This area is closely connected with the primary visual cortex and with complex nuclei of the thalamus. Its integrity is required for the gnostic visual function—the meaningfulness of visual sensation (*e.g.,* is the streaking object a bird, a plane, or a ...?).

The neocortical areas of the parietal lobe, between the somesthetic and the visual cortices, have a function in interrelating the texture, or "feel," of an object with its visual image. Between the auditory and visual associa-tion areas, the parieto-occipital region is necessary for interrelating the sound and the image of an object or person.

Limbic lobe

The medial aspect of the cerebrum is organized as three concentric bands of cortex, the limbic lobe, surrounding the interconnection between the lateral and third ventricles (the interventricular foramen) (Fig. 45-19). The innermost band just above and below the cut surface of the corpus callosum is folded out of sight but is an ancient, three-layered cortex. Just outside that is a band of transitional cortex, which includes the cingulate and parahippocampal cortices. The neocortex, responsible for limbic function, includes the orbital cortex on the underside of the frontal lobe. Outside this is the neo-cortex of the hemisphere merging into the more specific areas briefly described earlier. This limbic lobe has intimate connections with the medial nuclei and the intra-laminar nuclei of the thalamus, with deep nuclei of the cerebrum (amygdaloid nuclei, septal nuclei), and with the hypothalamus. In general, this region of the brain is involved in *emotional experience* and in the control of emotion-related behavior. Stimulation of specific areas in this system can lead to feelings of dread, high anxiety, or exquisite pleasure.

The only cortical regions not discussed, the region of the *frontal pole* and that in front of the associative motor cortex, are called the *premotor* frontal cortices. These areas are associated with the medial thalamic nuclei, which also are related to the limbic system. In general terms, the prefrontal cortex appears to be involved in anticipation and prediction of the conse-

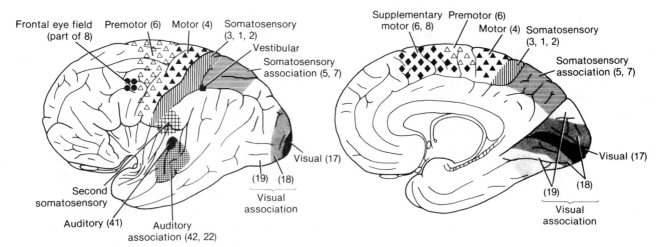

Figure 45-19 *Motor and sensory areas of the cerebral cortex. The lateral view (left) is drawn as though the lateral sulcus had been pried open, exposing the insula. The diagram on the right represents the areas in a brain that has been sectioned in the median plane. (Reproduced by permission from Nolte J: The Human Brain. St Louis, CV Mosby, 1981)*

quences of behavior. This "future-oriented" region is particularly depressed by many drugs, including a goodly dose of ethyl alcohol. Removal of the cortex leads to a less "worrying" personality, preoccupied with the present and giving little thought to the future.

In summary, the rostral ten segments of the neural tube become the brain by enlargement of the dorsal horn portion into elaborate outgrowths and outpouchings. The caudal five segments form the medulla oblongata, which includes within its reticular formation the circuitry of many life support reflexes, including basic vasomotor, respiratory, thermoregulatory, swallowing, vomiting, hiccoughing, coughing, gag, and gastrointestinal motility and secretory reflexes. The hypoglossal (XII), abducent (VI), spinal accessory (XI), vagus (X), and glossopharyngeal (IX) cranial nerves are located in the medulla. The pons develops from the fourth brain segment. It contains the circuitry for sensory innervation of the face and control of the mastication and facial expression muscles. It includes facial (VII) and trigeminal (V) cranial nerves. The third brain segment becomes the midbrain. It contains cranial nerves III and IV and the circuitry that controls locomotion and righting responses that protect one from falling, directional responses of the eyes and head, and the pupillary reflex and lens accommodation.

The cerebellum, which forms by enlargement over the roof of the fourth ventricle, provides important control of the sequencing and timing of motor unit activity required for coordinated motor skills. The first and second brain segments become the diencephalon, which consists of the thalamus, subthalamus, and hypothalamus. These regions of sensory experience are involved in the control of complex movements and the coordination of autonomic and life support reflexes. A paired outgrowth of the dorsal horn in the forward-most neural tube segment forms the optic cup from which the retina, iris, and optic nerve are derived. A second pair of lateral outpouchings from the dorsal horn develop into the cerebral hemispheres. The dorsal horn portion becomes the basal ganglia, the outer tract systems become the cerebral white matter, and neurons migrate through the latter to form the highly differentiated cerebral cortex.

The basal ganglia provide the major control patterns for graceful movements. The medial portion of the cerebral cortex retains its close relationship with the olfactory input and becomes the limbic lobe. The lateral portion of the cerebral cortex becomes the six-layered neocortex. The cortex and the dorsal horn portion of the neural tube or brain stem are intimately connected in the structure called the thalamus. The thalamocortical circuits of the neocortex of the frontal lobe are involved in the initiation of movement and anticipation of behavior and its consequences. Thalamocortical circuits of the parietal lobe are essential to the delicate analysis of somesthetic and proprioceptive sensation and perception. The occipital lobe interacts with thalamic nuclei to provide sensation and perception of visual stimuli. The temporal lobe–thalamic interaction provides discriminative analysis of auditory sensation and perception as well as long-term memory functions.

■ Supporting and Protective Structures

Skull and Vertebrae

Both the fragile and vital brain and the spinal cord are enclosed within the protective confines of rigid bony structures of the skull and vertebral column. Although these structures afford protection for the tissues of the CNS, they also afford the potential for the development of ischemic and traumatic nerve damage. This is because these structures cannot expand to accommodate the increase in volume that occurs when there is swelling within the nervous system or the expanded volume that occurs when there is bleeding within the confines of these structures. The bony structures themselves can also cause injury to the nervous system. Fractures of the skull and vertebral column can compress sections of the nervous system, or they can splinter and cause penetrating injuries. Surgical removal of the protective cover of the skull is called *craniotomy* and that of the arches of bone of each vertebra (neural laminae) covering the spinal cord is called *laminectomy*. This is done to relieve pressure on the CNS or to gain entrance for the removal of tumors, blood clots, or foreign objects around or within the CNS.

Meninges

Inside the skull and vertebral column, the brain and spinal cord are loosely suspended and further protected by several connective tissue sheaths called the meninges (Fig. 45-20). The surfaces of the spinal cord, brain, and segmental nerves are covered by a delicate connective-tissue layer called the *pia mater* (delicate mother). The surface blood vessels and those that penetrate the brain and spinal cord are also encased in this protective tissue layer. A second very delicate, nonvascular, and waterproof layer, called the *arachnoid* because of its spider-web appearance, encloses the entire CNS. The cerebrospinal fluid (CSF) is contained within the subarachnoid space. Immediately outside the arachnoid is a continuous sheath of strong connective tissue, the *dura mater* (tough mother), which provides the major protection for the brain and spinal cord. The cranial dura often splits into two layers, and the outer layer serves as the periosteum of the inner surface of the skull (Fig. 45-21).

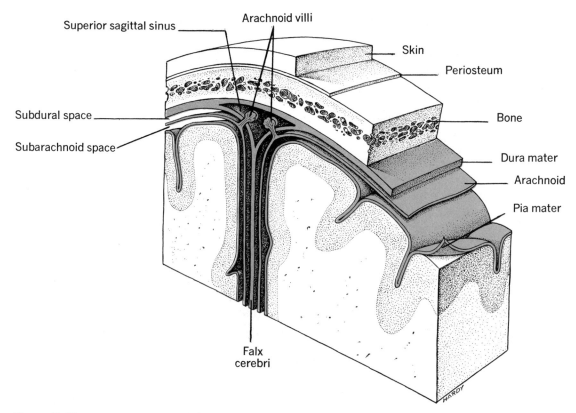

Figure 45-20 *The cranial meninges. Arachnoid villi shown within the superior sagittal sinus are one site of cerebrospinal fluid absorption into the blood. (Chaffee EE, Lytle IM: Basic Physiology and Anatomy, 4th ed. Philadelphia, JB Lippincott, 1980)*

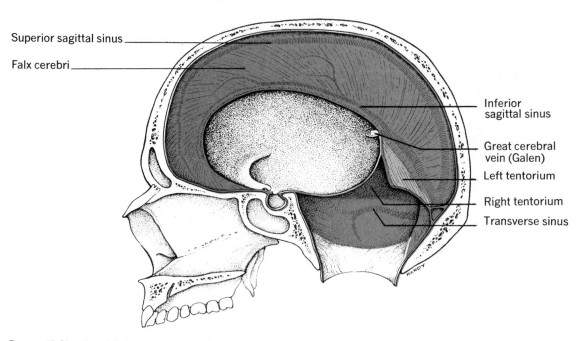

Figure 45-21 *Cranial dura mater. The skull is open to show the falx cerebri and the right and left portions of the tentorium cerebelli as well as some of the cranial venous sinuses. (Chaffee EE, Lytle IM: Basic Physiology and Anatomy, 4th ed, p 219. Philadelphia, JB Lippincott, 1980)*

The inner layer of the dura forms two folds. The first, a longitudinal fold, the *falx cerebri,* intervenes between the cerebral hemispheres and fuses with a second transverse fold, called the *tentorium cerebelli.* The latter acts as a hammock, supporting the occipital lobes above the cerebellum. The tentorium forms a tough septum, which divides the cranial cavity into the anterior and middle fossa, or hollow, which lies above the tentorium, and a posterior fossa, which lies below. The tentorium attaches to the petrous portion of the temporal bone and the dorsum sellae of the cranial floor, with a semicircular gap, or incisura, formed at the midline to permit the midbrain to pass forward from the posterior fossa. The resultant compartmentalization of the cranial cavity is the basis for the commonly used terms *supratentorial*—above the tentorium— and *infratentorial*—below the tentorium. The cerebral hemispheres and the diencephalon are supratentorial structures, and the pons, cerebellum, and medulla are infratentorial. The strong folds of the inner dura, the tentorium and the falx cerebri, support and protect the brain, which floats in cerebrospinal fluid within the enclosed space. During extreme trauma, however, the sharp edges of these folds can damage the brain as it floats inside the cranium. Space-occupying lesions such as enlarging tumors or hematomas can squeeze the brain against these edges or through the small opening of the tentorium, the incisura (herniation). As a result, brain tissue can be compressed, contused, or destroyed, often with permanent deficits (discussed in Chap. 48).

Ventricular System and Cerebrospinal Fluid

The lining of the embryonic neural tube undergoes multiple foldings in several areas to develop into structures called the choroid plexuses, which are present in the ventricular system and which secrete the cerebrospinal fluid (Fig.45-22). Although about 500 ml of CSF is secreted each day, the total volume in the spinal canal and

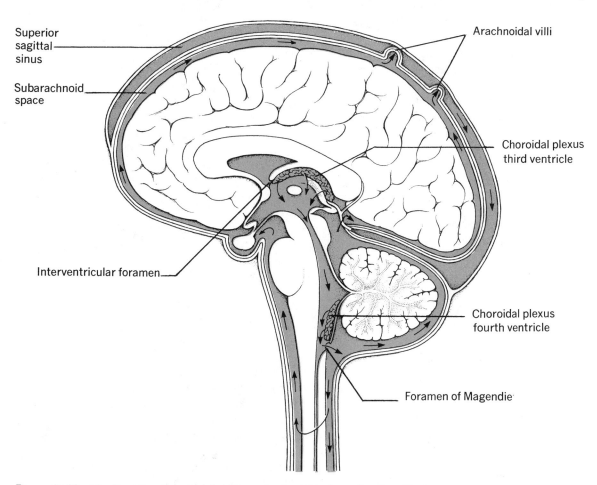

Superior sagittal sinus

Subarachnoid space

Interventricular foramen

Arachnoidal villi

Choroidal plexus third ventricle

Choroidal plexus fourth ventricle

Foramen of Magendie

Figure 45-22 *The flow of cerebrospinal fluid from the time of its formation from blood in the choroid plexuses until its return to the blood in the superior sagittal sinus. (Note: Plexuses in the lateral ventricles are not illustrated.) (Chaffee EE, Lytle IM: Basic Physiology and anatomy, 4th ed, p. 221. Philadelphia, JB Lippincott, 1980)*

ventricular system is only about 150 ml, so that the CSF is completely replaced about three times a day.

The CSF produced in the ventricles must flow through the interventricular foramen, the third ventricle, the cerebral aqueduct, and the midbrain and fourth ventricle to escape from the neural tube. Three other openings, or foramina, allow the CSF to flow into the subarachnoid space. Two of these, the foramina of Luschka, are located at the lateral corners of the fourth ventricle. The third, the medial foramen of Magendie, is located in the midline at the caudal end of the fourth ventricle. About 20% of the CSF passes down into the subarachnoid space that surrounds the spinal cord, mainly on its dorsal surface, and then moves back up to the brain along its ventral surface.

Reabsorption of the CSF into the vascular system occurs largely along the sides of the superior sagittal sinus in the anterior middle fossa. To reach this area, the CSF must pass along the sides of the medulla and pons, and then through the tentorial incisura that surrounds the midbrain. The major part of the flow continues along the sides of the hypothalamus to the region of the optic chiasma and then laterally and dorsally along the lateral fissure and over the parietal cortex to the superior sagittal sinus region. Here the waterproof arachnoid has protuberances, the *arachnoid villi,* which penetrate the inner dura and venous walls of the superior sagittal sinus.

The reabsorption of CSF into the vascular system occurs along a pressure gradient. The normal CSF pressure is about 150 mm H_2O throughout the system, whereas the venous pressure in the superior sagittal sinus is about 90 mm H_2O. The microstructures of the arachnoid villi are such that if the CSF pressure falls below approximately 50 mm H_2O, the passageways collapse and reverse flow is blocked. The villi, therefore, function as one-way valves, permitting CSF outflow into the blood but not allowing blood to pass into the subarachnoid spaces.

The cerebrospinal fluid is similar in many respects to the extracellular fluid (Table 45-3). The brain literally floats in CSF, and the CSF provides support for the

ventricular system. It may also be involved in a number of other control mechanisms. For example, blood glucose levels are reflected in the CSF, and hypothalamic centers have been shown to respond to these glucose levels, possibly contributing to hunger and eating behaviors.

When the CSF is removed from the ventricles or the subarachnoid spaces, as during a spinal puncture, the partially collapsed brain tugs on the meninges, stretching the free nerve endings in the inner dura, especially along its major vessels, and giving rise to a rather severe headache. The CSF refills fairly rapid, and the headache rarely lasts more than a day or so.

In summary, the central nervous system is enclosed within the bony confines of the vertebrae and the skull and within the protective tissue layers of the pia mater, arachnoid, and dura mater. The cranial dura mater is double layered, the inner layer forming the tough folds separating the cerebral hemispheres (falx cerebri). Within these folds, several venous sinuses allow venous outflow, thus providing protection from compression. The protective CSF in which the brain and spinal cord float, isolates them from minor and moderate trauma. Approximately 700 ml of CSF are produced each day by the choroid plexuses within the ventricles of the brain. The CSF has a composition similar to that of extracellular fluid and may be involved in many control systems, including the indirect monitoring of blood sugar levels in the hypothalamic receptors. The CSF flows through the third ventricle, cerebral aqueduct, and fourth ventricle and then escapes into the subarachnoid space. It also circulates dorsally down and ventrally up around the spinal cord, around the brain stem rostrally past the tentorial gap at the midbrain, and then around the cerebrum to the arachnoid villi, escaping into the superior sagittal sinus. The sagittal sinuses provide the major pathways for venous as well as CSF exit with eventual emptying into the internal jugular vein.

■ The Autonomic Nervous System

Control of the visceral functions of the body is largely vested in the autonomic nervous system, of which there are two divisions, the sympathetic and the parasympathetic nervous systems. Their functions differ. Generally, the functions of the sympathetic nervous system are designed to enable the body to deal with emergency or stress situations. The parasympathetic nervous system, on the other hand, is more concerned with the restorative functions of the body. Although the sympathetic system increases the heart rate and blood pressure needed for the "fight or flight" response, it is the parasympathetic sys-

Table 45-3	Composition of Cerebrospinal Fluid Compared with Plasma	
Substance	**Plasma**	**Cerebrospinal Fluid**
Protein mg/dl	7500.00	20.00
Na^+ mEq/liter	145.00	141.00
CL^- mEq/liter	101.00	124.00
K^+ mEq/liter	4.50	2.90
HCO^- mEq/l	25.00	24.00
*p*H	7.4	7.32
Glucose mg/dl	92.00	61.00

tem that controls the gut and the replenishment of the body's energy stores. The control of visceral function, like that of skeletal muscle contraction, requires both afferent (GVA) and efferent (GVE) neurons.

The innervation of visceral organs and the great vessels involves visceral afferent (GVA) neurons, dorsal root ganglion cells, and the efferent (GVE) autonomic nervous system. The role of the CNS in modulating the function of these organs and systems is different from the absolute control that lower motor neurons exert on skeletal muscle contraction. Therefore, the autonomic nervous system and its reflexes are considered separately. We will find that the distinction between autonomic and somatic function becomes blurred when the higher levels of integrated response mechanisms are considered. Indeed, almost all somatic reflexes have a visceral component and vice versa.

Afferent (GVA) Pathways

The visceral organs and great vessels are richly innervated by dorsal root ganglion cells. Many of these visceral afferent neurons terminate in specialized chemoreceptive organs, such as the carotid body and aortic bodies, or in pressure-sensitive endings in the carotid and aortic baroreceptors. Visceral afferent receptors are also present in the mucosal smooth muscle and connective tissue layers of the gastrointestinal tract. In the respiratory system, the trachea, bronchi, and lungs are richly innervated by afferent endings.

Visceral afferent neurons are located in the ganglia of the intermedius, the ninth and tenth cranial nerves, the thoracic and upper lumbar dorsal root ganglia, and the dorsal root ganglia of sacral levels 2, 3, and 4. Essentially, all visceral organs receive *dual* afferent innervation that travels with both sympathetic and parasympathetic portions of the autonomic nervous system.

The central axons of these GVA cells enter the dorsal horn gray matter or its equivalent in the medulla and synapse in the GVIA of the same segment or neighboring segments to those of entry. The association cells, utilizing multisynaptic pathways: (1) project into local reflex circuits; (2) project by way of spinoreticular projections to higher levels of the brain stem and contribute to hierarchical control mechanisms of visceral reflexes (the spinoreticular projection makes a moderate contribution to facilitating the ascending reticular system); and (3) project to the thalamus by way of the *anterolateral pathway,* the spinothalamic system of both sides of the cord and brain stem.

The contribution of visceral afferent endings to sensation is disproportionately small, considering the richness of afferent input from these regions. It reaches a sensation level in the thalamus that has a projection to a small parietal cortical area near the insula. Visceral sensation has a very strong emotional component, and the intermediate thalamic nuclei receive visceral signals and communicate with the limbic system. Sensations of fullness, pressure, and pain, and those associated with deep structure stimulation during evacuation and during sexual activity can have intensely unpleasant or pleasant aspects and can precipitate short-term as well as long-term behavioral consequences.

Despite the complete dual GVA innervation of the entire length of the gut, sensation from the viscera is separated into three parts: (1) input to the cranial nerves from the pharynx, larynx, and esophagus; (2) input to the thoracic–lumbar segments from the stomach, small intestine, and ascending and midtransverse colon; and (3) input to sacral segments 2 through 4 from the descending colon and rectum, bladder, and uterus. Although no explanation is available for this separation of GVA-derived sensation, it is useful to understanding. For example, pain and discomfort arising from the uterus and associated organs is experienced only by means of the GVA afferent neurons entering at sacral levels. Therefore, pharmacologic blockade of these roots or the spinal cord at low lumbar levels prevents pain information from being relayed through the anterolateral pathways from these levels, so that the pain associated with childbirth can be avoided. Visceral afferents also accompany the sympathetic innervation of the pelvic organs; GVA information from these same organs enters the cord through T^{10} to L^2 dorsal roots. These probably contribute to the normal vasomotor reflex control that is maintained by these organs during sacral afferent pain blockade.

Efferent (GVE) Pathways

General visceral efferent neurons of the ventral horn are called preganglionic neurons. These preganglionic neurons send their axons into the PNS to innervate a second postganglionic neuron located in the viscera. The axons of these postganglionic neurons innervate viscera, heart and vascular smooth muscles, and glandular structures throughout the body. The GVE consists of two subdivisions, the sympathetic and the parasympathetic nervous systems. Each system has the same preganglionic–postganglionic neural arrangement. These subdivisions differ in the location of outflow from the CNS, the relative length of the pre- and postganglionic axons, the predominant neurotransmitters secreted by the postganglionic neuron, and the nature of visceral function control (see Tables 45-1 and 45-4).

The GVE preganglionic neurons of the parasympathetic system originate in the cranial and sacral segments of the cell column, whereas the sympathetic

Table 45-4   General Characteristics of GVE Sympathetic and Parasympathetic Nervous Systems

Characteristic	Sympathetic Outflow	Parasympathetic Outflow
Location of preganglionic cell body in GVE column	Thoracic 1–12, lumbar 1 & 2	Cranial nerves: III, intermedius, IX and X, sacral segments 2, 3, 4
Relative length of preganglionic axon	Short; to sympathetic (paravertebral) chain of ganglia or to aortic (prevertebral) chain of ganglia	Long; to ganglion cells in ganglia near or in organ innervated
Transmitter between preganglionic terminals and postganglionic neuron	Acetylcholine (ACh)	Acetylcholine (ACh)
Transmitter of postganglionic neuron	ACh (sweat glands); NE (most synapses); NE and E (secreted by adrenal medulla)	ACh
General function	Mobilization of resources in anticipation of challenge to survival (preparation for "fight-or-flight")(catabolic)	Conservation of resources, renewal and recovery from mobilization (anabolic)
Specific examples:		
Iris	Dilation (radial muscle)	Constriction (sphincter muscle)
Salivation	Slight, viscid secretion	Fluid secretion
Gut	Reduced peristaltic activity and glandular secretion	Increased peristaltic activity, secretory activity
Sphincters of gut	Constriction	Relaxation
Heart rate	Increased rate	Decrease
Blood pressure	Increase	Decrease
Bronchi	Dilation of bronchial muscle	Constriction
Blood vessels:		
Skin	Constriction	None
Skeletal muscle	Dilation	None
Viscera	Constriction	None
Effect on adrenal medullary secretion	Secrete NE and E	None
Piloerector muscles	Erection of hair	None

preganglionic neurons have their origin in the thoracic and upper lumbar segments of the cell column. The relatively long parasympathetic preganglionic axons innervate the foregut, midgut, and associated visceral organs by way of cranial nerves III, and intermedius components of VII, IX, and X. The sacral parasympathetic outflow innervates the lower gut and related organs. Relatively short postganglionic neurons of this system lie in ganglionic clumps that are very near to or in the wall of the innervated organs. The transmitter at the ganglionic and postganglionic terminals is acetylcholine. This system is particularly involved in the innervation of smooth muscle and glandular cells of the visceral organs.

The sympathetic nervous system innervates the entire gut and viscera. Its preganglionic fibers are largely myelinated and relatively short. They exit the thoracolumbar cord segments in the spinal nerves and proceed toward viscera through branches called *white rami* (Fig. 45-23) to reach a chain of ganglia containing postganglionic sympathetic neurons. The axons of postganglionic sympathetic neurons proceed through visceral rami and spread longitudinally, especially along blood vessels. Some of the postganglionic neurons have migrated closer to the gut to form sympathetic ganglia

(celiac, superior mesenteric, aorticorenal, and inferior mesenteric) that are scattered along the dorsal aorta and its branches. Postganglionic axons also leave these prevertebral ganglia to innervate the smooth muscle and gland cells of the visceral organs. The adrenal medulla contains postganglionic sympathetic neurons that secrete the adrenergic neurotransmitters norepinephrine and epinephrine directly into the bloodstream.

The sympathetic nervous system, unlike the parasympathetic nervous system, innervates the smooth muscle and gland cells of the soma or body wall. This is accomplished by postganglionic sympathetic axons that are distributed along with peripheral nerves of the body wall to blood vessels of the skin and muscles. They also innervate the piloerector muscles of the hair follicles and the sweat glands of the skin.

As in the parasympathetic nervous system, the neurotransmitter at the preganglionic synapses of the sympathetic nervous system is acetylcholine. The responses at the postganglionic terminals are predominantly adrenergic, with the exception of the responses of the sweat glands and cholinergic vasodilator fibers in skeletal muscles, which are cholinergic. The effects of the transmitter substances are made more complex by the presence of

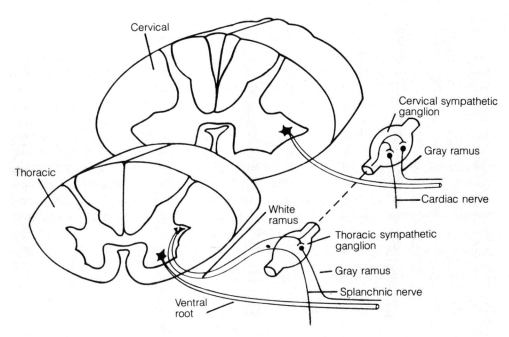

Figure 45-23 *Autonomic elements of the spinal nerves. In the thoracolumbar region, each ventral nerve root carries a contingent of efferent sympathetic fibers. These pass to the neighboring sympathetic trunk as a white ramus. Some of the fibers synapse in ganglia of corresponding levels, but others emerge from the trunk without synapsing. Fibers emerge from the ganglia to pass to plexuses or to rejoin the nerves as gray rami passing to peripheral or meningeal structures. In the cervical and sacral regions the ventral roots give off no white rami. Fibers from other levels synapse in the ganglia, however, and secondary fibers pass off as gray rami to join the nerve trunks. (Elliott HC: Neuroanatomy. Philadelphia, JB Lippincott, 1969)*

more than one class of adrenergic receptors, alpha and beta receptors (Chap. 16). Cholinergic receptors fall into two subcategories, nicotinic and muscarinic.

Functions of the Sympathetic Nervous System

In general, increased activity in the sympathetic nervous system shifts blood from the visceral organs into organs closely involved in meeting a challenge to survival (such as the skeletal muscles and the central nervous system). Thus, the sphincters of the stomach, intestine, anus, and bladder become constricted, and the rate of secretion of glands involved in digestion diminishes. One of the major functions of sympathetic innervation to these visceral organs is the control of vasoconstriction and, therefore, of blood flow. Sympathetic innervation of the SA node and particularly of the AV node of the heart provides strong acceleratory stimulation to heart rate.

This survival function of high sympathetic nervous system activity requires that postganglionic axons must also dilate the bronchial airway and increase the secretion

of the adrenal medulla, the cells of which are, in reality, postganglionic sympathetic neurons.

Emergency situations require the shunting of blood flow away from the skin and into the muscles and brain. This reduces the rate of bleeding should a wound occur and increases those particular resources required for either fighting or fleeing a threat to survival. Postganglionic sympathetic neurons of the sympathetic (paravertebral) ganglionic chain must therefore reach the body wall, or soma, and its organs; they do so by reentering the segmental nerve through the gray ramus to be distributed with the peripheral nerves to the blood vessels of the skin, muscles, and CNS (dilatory in skeletal muscles; constrictive in vessels of the skin). They also innervate the piloerector muscles which, when contracted, cause the hair to fluff—characteristic of an angry, challenging animal or of a cold animal—enhancing insulation by trapping air in the fur. Remnants of these functions in the human include "creeping" of hair, especially on the back of the neck during moments of fear or anger, and raising of "goose bumps" (short, thin hair shafts) when cold. Postganglionic axons of the autonomic system are unmyelinated and therefore have a gray cast; hence, the appellation gray ramus for the interconnecting link between the sympathetic chain ganglia and the segmental nerves traversed by these axons (Fig. 45-24).

The sympathetic outflow from the GVE cell column occurs only from the first thoracic to the second lumbar segments, yet the sympathetic innervation involves all regions of the viscera and soma. This innervation is accomplished by the longitudinal spread of preganglionic axons along the sympathetic chain of ganglia into cervical and sacral segments. Postganglionic sympathetic axons of the cervical and lower lumbar–sacral chain ganglia spread further through nerve plexuses along continuations of the great arteries. Thus, cranial structures, particularly blood vessels, are innervated by the spread of postganglionic axons along the internal and external carotid arteries into the face and the cranial cavity.

Functions of the Parasympathetic Nervous System

The parasympathetic portions of the GVE cell column are at the forward and caudal ends. Thus, parasympathetic preganglionic neurons of cranial nerve and sacral nerve distribution are located within the brain stem and sacral segments 2, 3, and 4 of the cord. Preganglionic neurons of these cells are distributed with the third, seventh, ninth, and tenth cranial nerves to the viscera of the head (salivary glands, lacrimal glands, mucosal glands, and smooth muscle of the nasal, oral, and laryngeal pharynx) and to the visceral organs of the thoracic and abdominal cavities (trachea and lungs, esophagus, heart, stomach, small intestine, and the ascending and transverse portions of the large bowel).

These preganglionic axons innervate postganglionic parasympathetic neurons, which lie in a series of autonomic ganglia of the head (ciliary, submandibular, pterygopalatine, and otic ganglia) on in the tissues of the thoracic and abdominal organs. Parasympathetic vagus (tenth cranial nerve) preganglionic axons innervate postganglionic parasympathetic neurons embedded in the wall of the heart near the AV and SA nodes, for example. The latter innervate the nearby nodal tissue and slow the heart rate. For most of these visceral organs, increased parasympathetic activity results in increased glandular secretion necessary for efficient digestive function or other anabolic and restorative activity, such as constriction of the pupil and the bronchi, increased salivary secretion, and opening of the sphincters of the gut. The preganglionic sacral axons of this system leave the sacral segmental nerves by gathering into the pelvic nerves, which lead to the autonomic plexuses along the great vessels. They spread to the hindgut and its deriva-

tives, the pelvic viscera (bladder, uterus, urethra, prostate, distal portion of the transverse colon, descending colon, and rectum). In the walls of these organs, postganglionic parasympathetic neurons send their axons to the smooth muscle and gland cells, facilitating digestive functions and urinary and fecal release.

Thus, the autonomic system dually innervates the visceral organs: the sympathetic system by spreading from the middle region of the neural tube (T_1–L_2 spinal segments) longitudinally to all parts of the foregut and middle and hindgut and associated organs. The parasympathetic system originates at the two ends (cranial nerves, sacral nerves) and spreads toward the middle. Both innervate the entire viscera but with somewhat opposing function: the parasympathetic system tends to facilitate anabolic recovery and regenerative functions of the unthreatened organism, and the sympathetic system facilitates preparation for encounters with survival-threatening challenges.

Recently, increased attention to the microcircuitry of the autonomic ganglia has revealed a much higher level of complexity than the above account might suggest. It has been demonstrated that within the sympathetic ganglia and within the parasympathetic ganglionic plexuses in the wall of the gut, the enteric plexuses, inhibitory and feedback circuits, and local afferent neurons continue to function as sources of local reflexes when isolated from the CNS. The peripheral autonomic system thus appears to have considerable computing capacity and autonomous function, with the CNS input via preganglionic axons as a modulating rather than a totally controlling influence on local function.

Hierarchy of Visceral Reflex Control

The basic hierarchical control of autonomic function is based on local circuits interrelating visceral afferent and autonomic efferent activity. Progressively greater complexity in the responses and greater precision in their control occurs at higher and higher levels of the brain stem. For much autonomic-mediated visceral function, the hypothalamus stands as the region of master control, even though it is under forebrain domination involving still more complex stimuli as well as the full effects of past learning. It should also be emphasized that most "visceral" reflexes also contain contributions from LMN-innervated striated muscle as part of the response pattern. In other words, the distinction between visceral and somatic reflex hierarchies becomes less and less meaningful at the higher levels of hierarchical control and behavioral integration.

Organization of many life-support reflexes occurs in the reticular formation of the medulla and pons. These areas of reflex circuitry, often called "centers," produce the complex combinations of autonomic and somatic

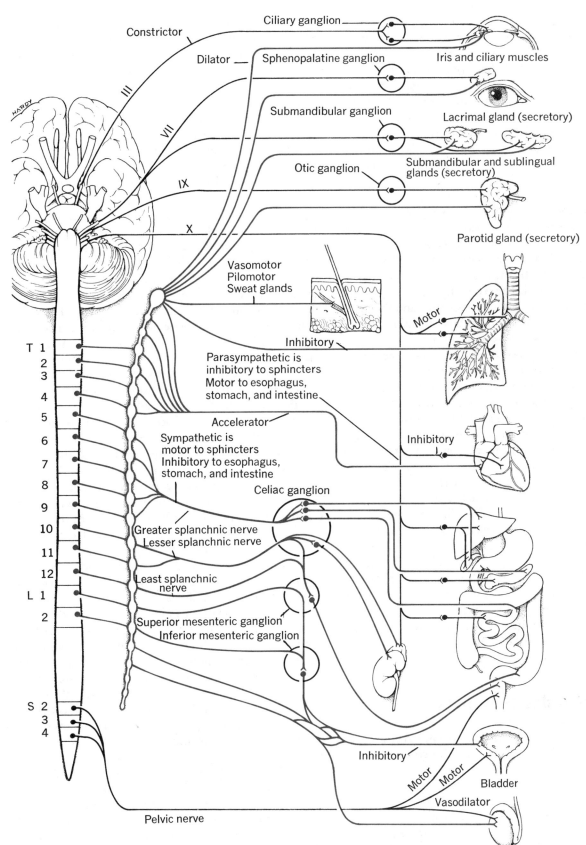

Figure 45-24 *The autonomic nervous system. The parasympathetic fibers are in black; the sympathetic fibers are in color. (Chaffee EE, Lytle IM: Basic Physiology and Anatomy, 4th ed, p 252. Philadelphia, JB Lippincott, 1980)*

efferent functions required for respiration, gag, cough, sneeze, swallow, and vomit reflexes as well as the more purely autonomic control of the cardiovascular system. At the hypothalamic level these reflexes are integrated into more general response patterns of rage, defense, eating, drinking, voiding, sexual mounting and copulation, and so on. Forebrain and especially limbic system control of these behaviors involves learning to inhibit or facilitate release of the behavior patterns according to social pressures or general emotion-provoking situations.

In summary, the autonomic nervous system, which is subdivided into the parasympathetic and sympathetic nervous systems, provides for the control of visceral function, including the activity of the gut and its secretory glands, the heart, blood vessels, and smooth muscle of the body wall. The sympathetic nervous system provides for the "fight or flight response" and the parasympathetic system for the restorative functions of the body. Both systems utilize a second neuron (postganglionic cell). These postganglionic cells make up the paravertebral sympathetic chain, which lies at the side of the axial skeleton, the prevertebral sympathetic ganglia, which are located near major vessels and somewhat distant from the effector organs, and the parasympathetic ganglia, which are located near or in the visceral organs. The two systems work in either a complementary or an opposing manner to provide balanced control of visceral, vascular, and secretory functions. The parasympathetic nervous system is particularly active in relatively non-challenging conditions and is specialized for the conservation of resources and renewal of anabolic activities. The sympathetic nervous system is particularly active in preparation for challenges to survival by mobilizing resources. The coordination of autonomic reflexes is based on a rich afferent visceral system and a hierarchy of reflex control regions culminating in the hypothalamus of the forebrain. This region is, in turn, under the control of cerebral circuits, particularly those of the limbic system.

■ Higher-Order Functions

The relationship between nervous system structure and specificity of function is the theme of this chapter. Yet, as more complex functions are considered, the reader should have noted that reference to areas or circuits became progressively more vague. This may be because of our current lack of knowledge or the nonspecificity of function of many forebrain regions. Attempts to interrelate neural structure and function, particularly in the forebrain, often fall into two schools: (1) The "lumper"

school tends to deny anything other than the most vague relationship. Emphasis here is on the vast redundancy of neuronal circuits and on the lack of highly specific functional loss with highly localized lesions, particularly of the associational cortex and basal ganglia. Theoretical frameworks here emphasize "field effects" and information storage or analysis based on interacting patterns of mass neuronal activity. (2) The other school, perhaps equally extreme, can be called the "splitters." They tend to seek minute correlations between structure and function often beyond the scientific data base. The truth may eventually be found to lie somewhere between these extremes. However, the more recent research using microelectrode studies of single neurons supports the concept of precisely localized functional circuitry in motor, sensory, and associational regions in the CNS.

One of the greatest dangers in making assumptions about the nervous system is to underestimate the complexity of neuronal circuits and networks. There are many examples of microcircuits between small populations of neurons that are now becoming evident.[3] Microcircuits involving dispersed groups or regions are also known for some neural systems. A radio set can be used as an analogy. You remove the transistor and the set does not function. Does the function of the set therefore reside in that transistor? Replace the transistor and remove another part, a condensor for instance. Again the set doesn't work. Now, is the function of the system residing in that condensor? The answer is that the different subcircuits of the set accomplish different aspects of the function of the set: feedback control systems maintain the current flow in one part of the set, or the overall voltage control regardless of temperature changes, or, in better sets, in spite of the aging of certain components. In the nervous system, the crispness and delicacy of function is the net result of many circuits, each containing redundant circuits for safety against local damage. Just as the function of the radio set cannot be adequately assessed with a hammer, neither can much of the neural circuitry of the brain be assessed with our present rather crude experimental methods. On the other hand, methods of assessing changes in function of an area of the nervous system as a result of localized cerebral vascular accident or tumor growth provide information about important components of the functional systems but do not tell us what all of the components of the system actually do.

In spite of these limitations, some evidence of localization of complex functions of the forebrain, for example, has accumulated. Lateral dominance, or the tendency to use one hand, eye, or foot over its contralateral competitor, is evidenced in humans, monkeys, and even mice. Studies of identical twins raised apart and of persons who have had the major side-by-side bridge of the neocortex or the corpus callosum removed for therapeutic purposes, generally confirm the biologic anatomic basis for side preference. In general, the left cerebral hemisphere tends to be dominant for speech and symbolic logic functions in the vast majority of persons.[4] In fact, the actual size of the two hemispheres differs; the speech dominant hemisphere possesses more mass of brain substance in the parieto-occipito-temporal region on the side of auditory speech analysis. This holds true for all but a small portion of extreme left-handed persons. In contrast to the sequential temporal logic functions of the dominant half of the forebrain, in most persons the nondominant half seems to be involved in the simultaneous integration of multiple modality sensory input, such as is required for the conceptualization of spatial relationships concerning the body or the surrounding environment. Map reading and sculpting exemplify classic nondominant hemisphere skills. Extensive destruction in the parieto-occipital-temporal cortex on the nondominant side results in astereognosis. When the left hand in these persons comes into view, it is treated as "a hand" but not "my hand." Because of this lack of recognition, these persons often neglect to shave, wash, and dress that side of the body. (This is called the hemineglect syndrome.) On the motor side of function, the assembly of words required for meaningful speech, called the *praxia of speech (phasia)*, appears to require the services of the opercular part of the premotor cortex, which is sometimes called Broca's area, usually located on the left side of the brain.

In spite of what is known about dominance, speech, and other areas of motor and sensory function, the anatomic–functional relationships of most important higher-order functions, such as memory and personality, remain mysterious. For example, different circuits in the limbic system are essential for the retrieval from storage of immediate memory, short-term memory, and, in the inferior portion of the temporal cortex, long-term memory. Just how or where information itself is stored is not yet known. Personality changes following major damage or multiple minor areas of damage are common.

In summary, traditionally two schools of thought—localization and nonlocalization—have competed in explaining higher order, complex functions related to brain structure. Recent microlevel neurophysiologic and neuroanatomic research strongly supports highly localized functional organization. It is likely that highly specific circuits can involve two and usually more brain structures; this premise is supported by the realization that many levels of organization are required for successful perception, skilled movement, spatial integration, planning, and memory functions. Studies have confirmed that the two cerebral hemispheres have some differential functions. The dominant, usually left, hemisphere is particularly involved in sequential logical functions, including the analysis as well as the production of speech. The nondominant (for speech) hemisphere is more involved in the integration of simultaneous and multimodality input and in the spatial aspects of complex motor functions. Extraction of stored data has been localized for immediate (medial thalamus and hypothalamus), intermediate (hippocampal formation), and long-term (inferior temporal cortex) memory. However, the mechanisms as well as the location of data storage have yet to be elucidated. The subtle personality characteristics are brain based, but these genetic and environmentally influenced traits have thus far escaped localization analysis.

■ Study Guide

After you have studied this chapter, you should be able to meet the following objectives:

☐ Compare the functions of the CNS with those of the PNS.

☐ Explain the hierarchy of control levels of the CNS.

☐ Explain the difference between the viscera and the soma of a body segment.

☐ Compare the location of afferent neurons with those of efferent neurons.

☐ State the purpose of a reflex.

☐ State the functions of GSA, GVA, SSA, GVE, SVE, and GSE neurons.

☐ Name the layers of the white matter.

☐ State the functions of input association and output association neurons.

☐ Explain the difference between skeletal muscle innervated by GSE neurons and that innervated by SVE neurons.

☐ Name the layer of white matter that is involved in the control of fine manipulative skills.

☐ Explain why a tractotomy may sometimes relieve intractable pain.

☐ Describe the protection of the brain afforded by the meninges.

☐ Trace the development of the spinal cord in the embryo.

☐ Describe the closure defect called spina bifida.

☐ Compare the functions of the dorsal and ventral horns of a spinal cord segment.

☐ Trace the steps involved in the development of the spinal cord.

☐ Explain how the spinal cord is protected.

☐ Describe the function of the denticulate ligaments.

☐ Explain why a lumbar puncture is performed below the level of the third lumbar vertebrae.

☐ Name the major branches of a typical spinal nerve.

☐ Describe the condition often called slipped disk.

☐ Name the reflex that causes the skin surface to be moved away from a noxious stimulus.

☐ State the significance of the dermatomes in a neurologic examination.

☐ Explain what is meant by the term stimulus modality within the general classification of somesthesis (GSA).

☐ Explain the meaning of the phrase *hierarchy of reflexes*.

☐ Compare the discriminative pathway with the anterolateral pathway and explain the clinical usefulness of this distinction.

☐ Define the following terms: hypoesthesia, hyperesthesia, dysesthesia, paresthesia, anesthesia, and stereognosis.

☐ Give an example of a perceptual hallucination.

☐ Explain the phrase *synergistic aspect of coordination*.

☐ Relate the function of the muscle spindle to muscle tone.

☐ By citing a clinical example, demonstrate why it is important for the health professional to understand the physiology of the stretch reflex.

☐ Explain why eliciting DTRs at specific segmental levels provides a rapid means of clinical assessment of the PNS and the functional integrity of the spinal cord.

☐ Explain the sequence of events involved in denervation atrophy.

☐ Describe the clinical condition called *tetany*, with reference to the underlying cause.

☐ Define a motor unit and explain why this is the smallest unit of motor function.

☐ Describe the organization of the brain on the basis of embryonic development.

☐ Describe the anatomy of the forebrain, the midbrain, the pons, cerebellum, and medulla oblongata.

☐ Explain the pathology associated with alternating hypoglossal hemiplegia and Bell's palsy.

☐ Describe the trigeminal (V) cranial nerve dermatomes of the head and how this somesthetic information reaches the pons.

☐ Explain the concept of the motor homunculus and sensory homunculus.

☐ Relate dyspraxia and apraxia to damage in particular cortical areas.

☐ Define somesthetic, auditory, and visual agnosias and relate them to abnormalities in a particular cortical area of the brain.

☐ Describe the limbic lobe and relate it to a general class of function.

☐ Cite one major function of the prefrontal cortex.

☐ Name the layers of the meninges.

☐ Trace the circulation of the CSF.

☐ Compare the functions of the sympathetic and parasympathetic divisions of the ANS.

☐ Explain a purpose of the dual afferent (GVA) innervation of the viscera.

☐ Compare the structural and functional differences between the two subdivisions of the autonomic nervous system (GVE): the sympathetic and parasympathetic systems.

☐ Explain the survival function of the sympathetic nervous system.

☐ Describe how postganglionic sympathetic axons reach blood vessels, sweat glands, and piloerector smooth muscles of the soma.

■ References

1. Head H, Holmes G: Sensory disturbances from cerebral lesions. Brain 34:1–51, 1911
2. Blinkov SM, Glezer II: The Human Brain in Figures and Tables, p 201. New York, Basic Books, 1968
3. Shepherd GM: The Synaptic Organization of the Brain. New York, Oxford University Press, 1979
4. Whitaker HA, Selnes OA: Anatomical variations in the cortex: Individual differences and the problem of localization of language function. Ann NY Acad Sci 280:844–854, 1976

Chapter 46

Alterations in Special Sensory Function

Robin L. Curtis

Carol Mattson Porth

Sheila M. Curtis

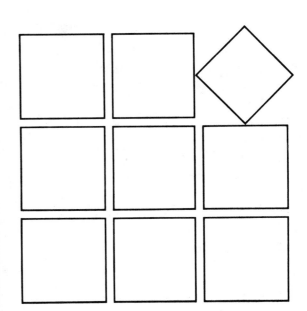

An essential aspect of meaningful brain function is the ability to respond appropriately to a constantly changing and challenging environment. The sensory systems sample the status of the internal and external world, coding, modulating, and transmitting this information to the central nervous system (CNS). Traditionally the senses have been divided into general and special senses. The general senses include touch, temperature, pressure, and position. The special senses include vision, hearing, balance, taste, and smell. The discussion in this chapter focuses on the special senses of vision, hearing, and vestibular function.

■ Vision

Nearly 11.5 million persons in the United States—1 in every 19—suffer from some degree of visual impairment. Of these, 12% are unable to see well enough to read ordinary newsprint, even with the aid of glasses, and another 4% are classified as legally blind.[1] More than 50% of blind people are over age 65, and the majority of these are over 85 years of age.

The optic globe, or eyeball, is a remarkably mobile, nearly spherical structure contained within a pyramidlike cavity of the skull called the *orbit*. The eyeball consists of an outer supporting fibrous layer (sclera), a vascular layer (uveal tract), and a neural layer (retina). The interior is filled with transparent media (the aqueous and vitreous humors), which allow the penetration and transmission of light to photoreceptors in the retina. The exposed surface of the eye is protected by the eyelid, a skin flap that provides a means for shutting out most light and pattern vision. Two eyes on the same horizontal plane, with extraocular muscles for directional rotation of the eyeball, provide different images of the same objects and the basis for depth perception of near objects. Alterations in vision can result from disorders of (1) the eyeball—its refractive power, its ability to transmit light, and the integrity of its photoreceptors, (2) the neural pathways and visual cortex, or (3) eye movements. This section of the chapter is divided into six parts: the optic globe and supporting structures, intraocular pressure, optics and lens function, retinal function, visual pathways and cortical centers, and eye movements.

Optic Globe and Supporting Structures

The optic globe, or eyeball, is protected posteriorly by the bony structures of the orbit and anteriorly by the eyelid (Fig. 46-1). Tears bathe its surface, protecting the eye from irritation by foreign objects, preventing friction between the eye and the lid, and maintaining the hydration of the cornea.

Orbit

The orbit is a pyramidal cavity with walls formed by the union of seven cranial and facial bones: the frontal, maxillary, zygomatic, lacrimal, sphenoid, ethmoid, and palatine bones (Fig. 46-2). The superior surface of the maxillary bone forms the main floor of the orbit. Tumors of the antrum may invade the orbit and cause the eyeball to protrude. The superior maxillary, lacrimal, and ethmoid bones form the medial wall of the orbit. This wall is very thin, and infections of the ethmoid sinus may invade

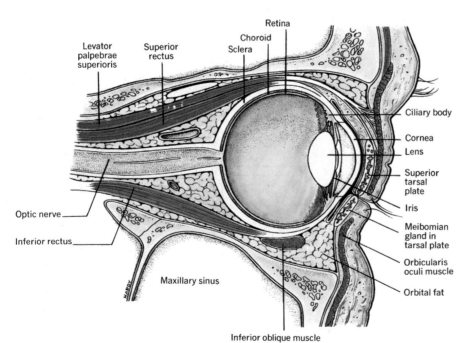

Figure 46-1 *The eye and its appendages, lateral view. (From Chaffee EE, Lytle IM: Basic Anatomy and Physiology, 4th ed. Philadelphia, JB Lippincott, 1980.)*

the orbit. The lateral wall is triangular in shape; it is formed anteriorly by zygomatic bone and posteriorly by sphenoid bone. It is the thickest wall, particularly at the orbital margin where the wall is most apt to be exposed to trauma. The apex of the orbital pyramid, located in the posterior medial part of the orbit, is pierced by an opening called the *optic foramen,* through which the optic nerve, ophthalmic artery, and sympathetic nerves from the carotid plexus pass. A larger opening, the superior orbital fissure, permits passage of branches of cranial nerves III, IV, V (ophthalmic division), and VI (ophthalmic division). The eyeball occupies only the anterior one-fifth of the orbit; the remainder is filled with muscles, nerves, the lacrimal glands, and adipose tissue that supports the normal position of the optic globe. A layer of fascia known as Tenon's capsule surrounds the globe of the eye from the cornea to the posterior segment and separates the eye from the orbital fat.

Exophthalmos.   Because the walls of the orbit are rigid, any space-occupying abnormality results in protrusion of the eyeball, a condition called *exophthalmos.* When the eyelid also protrudes, the condition is known as *proptosis.* Exophthalmos is associated with endocrine disorders of pituitary or hypothalamic origin. It is commonly seen in persons with hyperthyroidism (Chap. 39). The condition causes a delay in lid closure (lid lag) and, in severe cases, an inability of the lids to close completely, resulting in exposure and drying of the cornea. Because the optic nerve has sufficient length within the orbit, protrusion greater than 5 mm is required before nerve damage occurs.

Enophthalmos.   *Enophthalmos,* or deeply sunken eyes, may be an individual characteristic, but it also occurs with severe loss of orbital fat during malnutrition and starvation. Severe developmental defects during the first month of fetal life can result in the absence of one or both optic globes *(anophthalmos),* and growth defects during the last 3 months of gestation can result in abnormally small eyes *(microphthalmos).*

Eyelids

The eyelids are called the *palpebrae,* and the oval space between the upper and lower lids is the *palpebral fissure.* The angle where the upper and lower lids meet is referred to as a *canthus;* the lateral canthus is the outer, or temporal, angle and the medial canthus is the inner, or nasal, angle (Fig. 46-3). A line through the lateral and medial canthi defines the angle of the palpebral fissure and is usually horizontal. In children with Down's syndrome, this line slants upward laterally, giving the child a Mongolian appearance (Chap. 4). A fold of skin, the *epicanthal fold,* covers the medial canthus and is characteristic of the yellow race as well as persons with certain

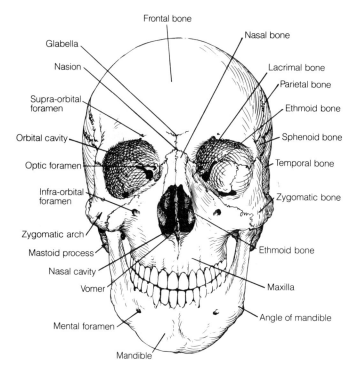

Figure 46-2   *Anterior view of skull. (From Chusid JG: Correlative Neuroanatomy and Functional Neurology, 19th ed. Los Altos, CA, Lange Medical Publications, © 1976. Reproduced with permission.)*

chromosomal abnormalities. The spacing between the two orbits is highly variable. The term *hypertelorism* is used if they are spaced abnormally far apart, and *hypotelorism* if they are abnormally close together.

In each lid a tarsus, or plate of dense connective tissue, gives the lid its shape (see Fig. 46-1). Each tarsus contains modified sebaceous glands (meibomian glands), the ducts of which open onto the eyelid margins. The sebaceous secretions enable airtight closure of the lids and prevent rapid evaporation of tears.

Infections and inflammatory conditions.   *Marginal blepharitis,* or inflammation of the eyelids, is the most common disorder of the eyelids. There are two main types: seborrheic and staphylococcal. The chief symptoms are irritation, burning, redness, and itching of the eyelid margins. The seborrheic form is usually associated with seborrhea (dandruff) of the scalp or brows. Treatment includes careful cleansing with a wet applicator or clean washcloth to remove the scales. A nonirritating baby shampoo can be used. When the disorder is associated with a microbial infection, an antibiotic ointment is prescribed.

A hordeolum (sty) is caused by infection of the sebaceous glands of the eyelid and can be either internal or external. The main symptoms are pain and redness. The treatment is similar to that for abscesses in other

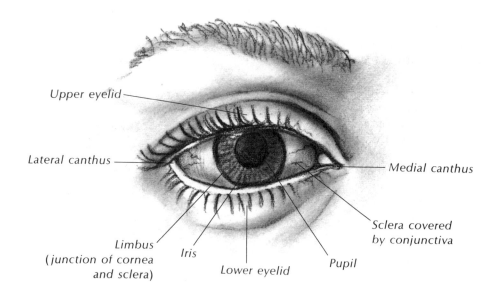

Upper eyelid

Lateral canthus

Medial canthus

Sclera covered
by conjunctiva

Limbus
(junction of cornea
and sclera)

Iris

Lower eyelid

Pupil

Figure 46-3   *Right eye. (From Bates B: Guide to Physical Examination, 3rd ed. Philadelphia, JB Lippincott, 1983)*

parts of the body: heat in the form of warm compresses is applied, and antibiotic ointment may be used. Incision or expression of the infectious contents of the abscess may be necessary. A *chalazion* is a small nodule that is formed when a meibomian gland is distended by accumulated secretions. It is treated by surgical excision.

Eyelid muscles.   The two striated muscles that provide movement of the eyelids are the levator palpebrae and the orbicularis oculi. The levator palpebrae, which is innervated by the oculomotor (III) cranial nerve, raises the upper lid. The orbicularis oculi, which is supplied by the facial (VII) cranial nerve, closes the lid. The palpebral portion of the muscle is used for gentle closure and the orbital portion for forcible closure of the lids.

Normally the edges of the eyelids are in such a position that the palpebral conjunctiva that lines the eyelids is not exposed and the eyelashes do not rub against the cornea. Turning in of the lid is called *entropion*. It is usually caused by scarring of the palpebral conjunctiva or degeneration of the fascial attachments to the lower lid that occurs with aging. Turning inward of the eyelashes causes corneal irritation. *Ectropion* refers to eversion of the lower lid. The condition is usually bilateral and caused by relaxation of the orbicularis oculi muscle because of seventh nerve palsy or the aging process. Ectropion causes tearing and ocular irritation and may lead to inflammation of the cornea. Both entropion and ectropion can be treated surgically. Electrocautery penetration of the lid conjunctiva can also be used to treat mild forms of ectropion. The scar tissue that follows tends to draw the lid up to its normal position.

Ptosis.   Drooping of the upper lid sufficient to interfere with the light path through the pupillary opening is called *ptosis*. It can result from extreme weakness of the

muscle that elevates the upper lid (levator palpebrae superioris) or of the circular ring of muscles (orbicularis oculi) that forcefully close the palpebral fissure. Severe weakness or flaccidity of the muscles can result from damage to the innervating cranial nerves or to the nerves' central nuclei in the midbrain and the caudal pons.

Facial nerve palsy.   The facial nerve reaches the orbicularis oculi after exiting the skull under the parotid gland and then traveling deep to the skin across the face. Thus, trauma to the zygomatic and buccal branches of the facial nerve with a resultant ptosis is relatively common. Weakness of the orbicularis oculi is tested by placement of the examiner's fingers on the muscular sphincter ring while the eye is open and then asking the person to close the eye. Movement of the eyelid is also affected in a condition called *Bell's palsy*, which involves paralysis of muscles on one side of the face because of a lesion of the facial nerve or its nucleus in the caudal pons.

Oculomotor palsy

Damage to the oculomotor nerve is much less common than damage to the facial nerve because the oculomotor nerve is protected by the skull throughout its path. However, ptosis resulting from third cranial nerve injury can occur in midbrain stroke and basal skull fractures and from tumors located deep in the orbit or in the cavernous sinus. Drooping of the eyelids because of generalized weakness of the extraocular muscles occurs in some forms of muscular dystrophy and is an early and common intermittent manifestation of myasthenia gravis (Chap. 48).

Horner's syndrome.   A third source of ptosis is the loss of sympathetic innervation to the smooth muscle on the inner surface of the upper lid, causing a droop of the inner lining of the upper lid over the pupil, one sign of a condition called Horner's syndrome. In addition to drooping of the inner lid lining, there are other manifestations of loss of sympathetic innervation, including a fixed and constricted pupil, loss of sweating (anhidrosis), and generalized vascular dilation over the affected half of the face. Postganglionic neurons of the superior cervical ganglion follow the internal carotid artery and then the ophthalmic artery into the orbit to innervate the blood vessels of the face, the dilator muscle of the iris, and the tarsal muscle of the eyelid (Fig. 46-4). Horner's syndrome is usually caused by damage to the sympathetic chain or the cervical ganglia located in the neck or internal carotid plexus. The most common causes are mediastinal tumors, particularly bronchiogenic carcinoma, Hodgkin's disease, and metastatic tumors.[2] Other causes are surgical or accidental trauma to the neck and CNS conditions, such as occlusion of the posterior inferior cerebellar artery and multiple sclerosis.

Conjunctiva and conjunctivitis

The inner surface of the eyelid is lined with a thin layer of mucous membrane, the palpebra conjunctiva. The conjunctiva folds back at the fornix and covers the optic globe to the junction of the cornea and sclera. When the eyes are closed, the conjunctiva lines the closed conjunctival sac. The conjunctiva is innervated by the ophthalmic division of the trigeminal (fifth cranial) nerve and is extremely sensitive to irritation and inflammation. The conjunctiva of the lower lid is supplied by the maxillary division of the trigeminal nerve.

Conjunctivitis, or inflammation of the conjunctiva, (sometimes called redeye or pinkeye) is one of the most common forms of eye disease. It varies in severity from mild hyperemia with tearing (hay fever conjunctivitis) to a severe necrotizing process (membranous conjunctivitis). Conjunctivitis may result from infection, allergens, chemical agents, physical irritants, or radiant energy. Infections may extend from areas adjacent to the conjunctiva or may be bloodborne, such as in measles or chickenpox.

The main symptoms of conjunctivitis are redness of the eye, ocular discomfort or foreign body sensation, gritty or burning sensation, and tearing. Severe pain suggests corneal rather than conjunctival disease. Itching is common in allergic conditions. A discharge, or exudate, is present with all types of conjunctivitis. It is usually watery when the conjunctivitis is caused by allergy, foreign body, or viral infection and mucopurulent in the presence of bacterial or fungal infection. A characteristic of many forms of conjunctivitis is papillary hypertrophy. This occurs because the conjunctiva is bound to the tarsus by fine fibrils. As a result, inflammation that accumulates between the fibrils causes the conjunctiva to be elevated in mounds called

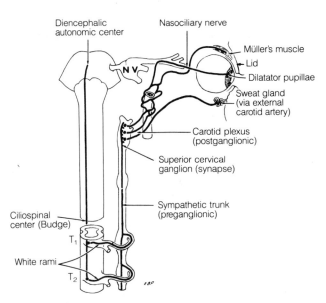

Figure 46-4 *Sympathetic nervous system of the eye. Efferent fibers synapse in the superior cervical ganglion. Postganglionic fibers then pass to the sweat glands of the face and eyelids along the external carotid artery. Other branches extend intracranially with the internal carotid artery and pass with the ophthalmic artery into the orbit. Vasomotor fibers are redistributed by the short ciliary nerves to blood vessels in the choroid. Fibers to the dilator pupillae muscle do not pass through the ciliary ganglion and are carried to the globe by the long ciliary branches of the nasociliary nerve (N V). (From Newell FW: Ophthalmology: Principles and Concepts, 5th ed. St Louis, CV Mosby, 1982)*

papillae. When the papillae are small, the conjunctiva has a smooth, velvety appearance. A red papillary conjunctivitis suggests bacterial or chlamydial conjunctivitis. In allergic conjunctivitis the papillae often becomes flat-topped, polygonal, and milky in color and have a cobblestone appearance. Edema of the conjunctiva is called *chemosis.* Among the more common types of conjunctivitis are allergic, bacterial, viral, and chlamydial conjunctivitis.

Allergic conjunctivitis. Allergic conjunctivitis (hay fever) is a common disorder associated with exposure to allergens such as pollen. It causes bilateral tearing, itching, and redness of the eyes. The treatment includes the use of cold compresses, antihistamines, and vasoconstrictor eyedrops. The local application of corticosteroids may be used on a short-term basis.

Bacterial conjunctivitis. Common agents of bacterial conjunctivitis are *Streptococcus pneumoniae, Staphylococcus aureus, Neisseria gonorrhoeae, Neissera meningitidis,* and *Hemophilus influenzae.* All of these organisms produce a copious purulent discharge. The eyelids are sticky, and there may be excoriation of the lid margins. There is usually no pain or blurring of vision. Treatment may include local application of antibiotics. The disease is usually self-limiting, lasting about 10 days to 14 days if untreated.

Viral conjunctivitis. One of the most common causes of viral conjunctivitis is adenovirus type 3, which is usually associated with pharyngitis, fever, and malaise. It causes generalized hyperemia, copious tearing, and minimal exudate. Children are affected more often than adults. Contaminated swimming pools are common sources of infection. There is no specific treatment for viral conjunctivitis; it usually lasts 7 days to 14 days.

Herpes simplex virus conjunctivitis can occur and is characterized by unilateral infection, irritation, mucoid discharge, pain, and mild photophobia. Herpetic vesicles may develop on the eyelids and lid margins. Although the infection is usually caused by the type 1 herpes virus, it can also be caused by the type 2 virus. It is often associated with herpes simplex virus keratitis, in which the cornea shows discrete epithelial lesions. Local corticosteroid preparations increase the activity of the herpes simplex virus, apparently by enhancing the destructive effect of collagenase on the collagen of the cornea. Therefore, the use of these medications should be avoided in persons suspected of having herpes simplex conjunctivitis or keratitis.

Chlamydial conjunctivitis. Inclusion conjunctivitis is a benign, self-limiting suppurative conjunctivitis transmitted by the *C. trachomatis* group that causes venereal infections (Chap. 36). It is spread by contaminated genital secretions and occurs in newborns of mothers having *C. trachomatis* birth canal infections. It can also be contracted through swimming in unchlorinated pools. The incubation period varies from 5 days to 12 days, and the disease may last for several months if untreated. The infection is usually treated with systemic erythromycin and topical tetracycline ointment.

A more serious form of infection is caused by a different group of *C. trachomatis*. This form of chlamydial infection not only affects the conjunctiva, but also causes ulceration and scarring of the cornea. It is the leading cause of blindness in many poorly developed countries with dry and sandy regions. In the United States, the infection is largely confined to the American Indians of the Southwest. It is transmitted by direct human contact, contaminated particles (fomites), and flies.

Diagnosis. Because a red eye may be the sign of several eye conditions, conjunctivitis must be differentiated from ciliary injection, glaucoma, subconjunctival hemorrhage, and blepharitis. The major causes of red eyes

and their diagnostic features are described in Table 46-1. The diagnosis of conjunctivitis is based on history, physical examination, and microscopic and culture studies to identify the cause. Infectious diseases are often bilateral and involve other family members. Unilateral disease suggests irritant sources, such as foreign bodies or chemical irritation.

Lacrimal apparatus

The lacrimal gland is the source of the serous secretions called tears. This gland lies in the orbit superior and lateral to the eyeball (Fig. 46-5). Approximately 12 small ducts connect the tear gland to the superior conjunctival fornix. Tears, which contain about 98% water, 1.5% sodium chloride, and the antibacterial enzyme lysozyme, are essential to the maintenance of vision because of their lubricant and possibly antibacterial properties. Lubrication between the two layers of conjunctiva permits comfortable eye movement. In addition, the thin layer of tears that covers the cornea is essential in preventing drying and damage to the outer layers of the cornea.

A reddish elevation, the lacrimal caruncle, is in the medial canthus. Minute openings, the lacrimal puncta, in the edge of the lids just above and below the caruncle, are the entrances of the superior and inferior canaliculi, which permit entrance of tears into the lacrimal sac and nasolacrimal duct (tear duct). The nasolacrimal duct empties into the nasal cavity.

Dry eyes. The tear film covering the eyes is composed of three layers: (1) the superficial lipid layer, derived from the meibomian glands and thought to retard evaporation of the aqueous layer, (2) the aqueous layer, secreted by the lacrimal glands, and (3) the mucinous layer that overlies the cornea and epithelial cells.[3] Because the epithelial cell membranes are relatively hydrophobic and cannot be wetted by aqueous solutions alone, the mucinous layer plays an essential role in wetting these surfaces. Periodic blinking of the eyes is needed to maintain a continuous tear film over the ocular surface. Disruption of any of the tear film components or the blinking action of the eyelids can lead to the breakup of the tear film and dry spots on the cornea. A number of conditions cause reduced function of the lacrimal glands. With aging, the lacrimal glands tend to diminish their secretion, and as a result, many older persons awaken from a night's sleep with highly irritated eyes. Dry eyes also result from loss of reflex lacrimal gland secretion due to congenital defects, infection, irradiation, damage to the parasympathetic innervation of the gland, and medications such as antihistamines, beta-adrenergic blocking drugs, and anticholinergic drugs (atropine and scopolamine). The wearing of contact lenses tends to contribute to eye dryness through decreased blinking.

Table 46-1 Red Eyes

	Conjunctival Injection	Ciliary Injection	Acute Glaucoma	Subconjunctival Hemorrhage	Blepharitis
Appearance					
Process	Dilatation of the conjunctival vessels	Dilatation of branches of the anterior ciliary artery, which supply the iris and related structures	Dilatation of branches of the anterior ciliary artery; may also show some conjunctival vessel dilatation	Blood outside the vessels between the conjunctiva and sclera	Inflammation of the eyelids
Location of Redness	Peripheral vessels of the conjunctiva, fading toward the iris	Central deeper vessels around the iris	Central deeper vessels around the iris; may also be peripheral	A homogeneous red patch, usually in an exposed part of the bulbar conjunctiva	Lid margins
Appearance of Vessels	Irregularly branched	May radiate regularly or appear as a diffuse flush around the iris	Radiating regularly around the iris; peripherally may be irregularly branching	Vessels themselves not visible	Conjunctival and ciliary vessels normal unless there is associated disease
Color	Vessels bright red	Vessels more violet or rose-colored	Vessels around iris violet or rose-colored	Patch is bright red, fading with time to yellow	Lid margins red, may have yellowish scales
Movability	Conjunctival vessels can be moved against the globe by pressure on the lower lid	Dilated vessels are deeper; cannot be moved by lid pressure	Dilated vessels around the iris are deep; cannot be moved by lid pressure	Not movable	Not relevant
Pupil Size and Shape	Normal	Normal or small and irregular	Dilated, often oval, seen through a steamy cornea	Normal	Normal
Visual Acuity	Not affected	Decreased	Decreased	Not affected	Not affected
Significance	Superficial conjunctival condition, as from irritation, infection, allergy, vasodilators	Disorder of cornea or inner eye. Requires prompt evaluation.	Sudden increase in intraocular pressure because of blocked drainage from the anterior chamber; an ocular emergency	Often none; may result from trauma, sudden increase in venous pressure (*e.g.*, cough), bleeding disorder	Often associated with seborrhea, staphylococcal infections

(From Bates B: A Guide to Physical Examination, 3rd ed. Philadelphia, JB Lippincott, 1983)

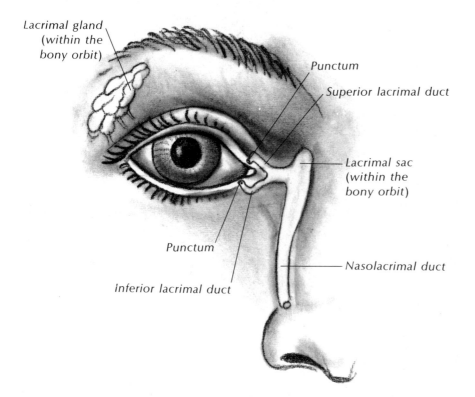

Lacrimal gland (within the bony orbit)

Punctum

Superior lacrimal duct

Lacrimal sac (within the bony orbit)

Punctum

Nasolacrimal duct

Inferior lacrimal duct

Figure 46-5 *Lacrimal apparatus. (From Bates B: A Guide to Physical Examination, 3rd ed. Philadelphia, JB Lippincott 1983)*

Sjörgren's syndrome is a systemic disorder in which there is lymphocytic and plasma cell infiltration of the lacrimal and parotid glands. The disorder is associated with diminished salivary and lacrimal secretions (sicca complex), resulting in keratoconjunctivitis sicca and xerostomia (dry mouth). The syndrome occurs mainly in women near menopause and is often associated with connective tissue disorders such as rheumatoid arthritis.

Persons with dry eyes complain of dry or gritty sensation in the eye, burning, itching, inability to produce tears, photosensitivity, redness, pain, and difficulty in moving the eyelids. Dry eyes and the absence of tears can cause keratinization of the cornea and conjunctival epithelium. In severe cases, corneal ulcerations can occur.

Assessment of tear formation can be done using the Schirmer filter paper test. With this test, a 35-mm by 5.0-mm strip of filter paper (Iso-Sol strips) is folded and placed in the lower conjunctival sac of both eyes for 5 minutes. Generally, tear formation is considered normal if the portion of the paper that is moistened measures 15 mm or more.

The treatment of dry eyes includes frequent irrigation of the conjunctival sac by artificial tear solutions. Recently, a slow-released artificial tear insert (Lactisert) has been made available. The insert, which contains hydroxypropyl cellulose, is inserted into the inferior cul-de-sac. Water is pulled into the insert from the capillaries and a hydroxypropyl cellulose tear solution is released over a 12-hour period.

Dacryocystitis. Dacryocystitis is an infection of the lacrimal sac. It occurs most often in infants or in persons over 40 years of age. It is usually unilateral and most often occurs secondary to obstruction of the nasolacrimal duct. Often the cause of the obstruction is unknown, although there may be a history of severe trauma to the midface. The symptoms include tearing and discharge, pain, swelling, and tenderness. The treatment includes application of heat (warm compresses) and antibiotic therapy. In chronic forms of the disorder, surgical repair of the tear duct may be necessary. In infants, dacryocystitis is usually due to failure of the nasolacrimal ducts to open spontaneously before birth. When one of the ducts fail to open, a secondary *Hemophilus influenzae* dacryocystitis develops. These infants are usually treated with forceful massage of the tear sac, instillation of antibiotic drops into the conjunctival sac, and if that fails, probing of the tear duct.

Sclera and cornea

The optic globe, or eyeball, is a spherical structure divided into two segments: an anterior segment that contains the aqueous humor and a posterior chamber that contains the vitreous humor (Fig. 46-6). The globe has three layers, each of which is further subdivided. The outer layer of the eyeball consists of a tough, opaque, white fibrous layer called the sclera. Its strong yet elastic properties maintain the shape of the globe. The sclera is homologous to the dermis of the facial skin and is con-

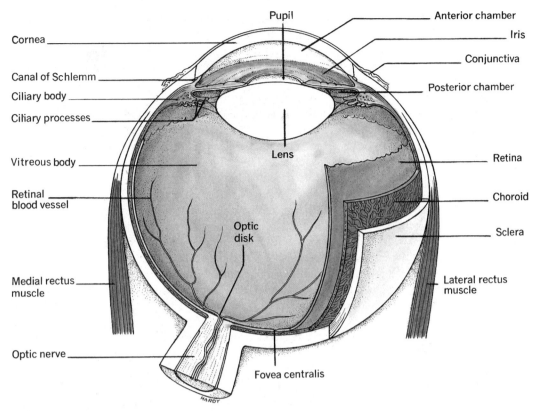

Figure 46-6 *Transverse section of the eyeball. (From Chaffee EE, Lytle IM: Basic Physiology and Anatomy, 4th ed. Philadelphia, JB Lippincott, 1980)*

tinuous except for a number of tiny holes at the optic disk, the lamina cribrosa sclera, through which the optic nerve axons exit the retina. In jaundice, the sclera appears yellow because of staining from excessive levels of circulating bilirubin. In an inherited collagen disease known as *osteogenesis imperfecta* (Chap. 52), the sclera is quite thin, and the pigmented choroid shows through, providing a bluish cast to the sclera. Subconjunctival hemorrhage frequently is associated with even light trauma to the head or optic globe.

At the anterior part of the eyeball, the scleral structure becomes the transparent cornea. The point at which the cornea joins the sclera is called the *limbus* (see Fig. 46-3). Because light passes from air into the liquid and solid transparent media of the eye at the corneal surface, the major part of refraction (bending) of light rays and focusing occurs at this point. The cornea has three layers: an extremely thin outer epithelial layer, which is continuous with the ocular conjunctiva, a middle stromal layer called the *substantia propria,* and an inner endothelial layer that lies adjacent to the aqueous humor of the anterior chamber. The thick substantia propria constitutes 90% of the cornea; its anterior condensation (Bowman's zone) is attached to the basement membrane of the epithelial layer. Descemet's membrane, the base-

ment membrane of the endothelium, separates the endothelium from the stromal layer. The substantia propria is composed of regularly arranged collagen bundles embedded in a mucopolysaccharide matrix. The regular organization of the collagen fibers, which makes the substantia propria transparent, is necessary for light transmission. Hydration within a limited range is necessary to maintain the spacing of the collagen fibers and transparency. The cornea is avascular and derives its nutrient and oxygen supply by means of diffusion from blood vessels of the adjacent conjunctiva, from the aqueous humor at its deep surface, and from tears. The corneal epithelium is heavily innervated by sensory neurons. Epithelial defects cause discomfort that ranges from a foreign body sensation and burning of the eyes to severe, incapacitating pain. Reflex lacrimation is common.

Trauma that causes abrasions of the cornea can be extremely painful, but, if minor, the abrasions usually heal in a few days. The epithelial layer is capable of regeneration, and small defects heal without scarring. If the stroma is damaged, healing occurs more slowly and the danger of infection is increased. Injuries to Bowman's zone and the stromal layer heal with scar formation and permanent opacification. Opacities of the cornea impair the transmission of light. A minor scar can severely distort vision because it disturbs the refractive surface.

The integrity of both the epithelium and the endothelium is necessary to maintain the cornea in its relatively dehydrated state. Damage to either structure leads to edema and loss of transparency. Among the causes of corneal edema are prolonged and uninterrupted wearing of hard contact lenses, which can deprive the epithelium of oxygen, disrupting its integrity. The edema disappears spontaneously when the cornea comes in contact with the atmosphere. Corneal edema also occurs when there is a sudden rise in intraocular pressure. If intraocular pressure rises rapidly above 50 mm Hg, as in acute glaucoma, subendothelial edema develops. With corneal edema, the cornea appears dull, uneven, and hazy. A decrease in visual acuity and iridescent vision (rainbows around lights) occur. Iridescent vision results from epithelial and subepithelial edema, which splits white light into its component parts with blue in the center and red on the outside.

Abnormal corneal deposits. The cornea is frequently the site of deposition of abnormal metabolic products. In hypercalcemia, calcium salts can precipitate within the cornea, producing a cloudy band keratopathy. Cystine crystals are deposited in cystinosis, cholesterol esters in hypercholesterolemia, and a golden ring of copper in hepatolenticular degeneration due to Wilson's disease (called a Kayser–Fleischer ring). Pharmacologic agents, such as chloroquine, can result in crystal deposits in the cornea. In corneal arcus, a grayish white infiltrate occurs at the periphery of the cornea. It represents an extracellular lipid infiltration and is seen in most persons over 60 years of age.

Keratitis. Keratitis refers to inflammation of the cornea. It can be caused by infections, hypersensitivity reactions, ischemia, defects in tearing, trauma, and interruption in sensory innervation, such as occurs with local anesthesia. Keratitis can be divided into two types: ulcerative, in which part of the epithelium, stroma, or both are destroyed, and nonulcerative, in which all the layers of the epithelium are affected by the inflammation but the epithelium remains intact. Causes of ulcerative keratitis include infectious agents such as those causing conjunctivitis (*e.g.,* staphylococcus, pneumococcus, chlamydia, and herpes virus) and exposure trauma. Exposure trauma may be due to deformities of the lid, paralysis of the lid muscles, or severe exophthalmos. Mooren's ulcer is a chronic, painful, indolent ulcer that occurs in the absence of infection. It is usually seen in older persons and may affect both eyes. Nonulcerative keratitis is associated with a number of diseases, including syphilis, tuberculosis, and lupus erythematosus. It

may also result from a viral infection entering through a small defect in the cornea.

Symptoms of keratitis include photophobia, discomfort, and lacrimation. The discomfort may range from foreign body sensation to severe pain. Defective vision results from the changes in transparency and curvature of the cornea that occur. If ulceration is present, it will stain green when a drop of fluorescein dye is instilled. Generally, peripheral involvement of the cornea is related to the same disorders that affect the conjunctiva (discussed earlier).

Advances in ophthalmologic surgery now permit corneal transplantation using a cadaver cornea. Unlike kidney or heart transplant procedures, which are associated with considerable risk of rejection of the transplanted organ, the use of cadaver corneas entails minimal danger of rejection, because this tissue is not exposed to the vascular and, therefore, immunologic defense system. Instead, the success of this type of transplant operation depends on the prevention of scar tissue formation, which would limit the transparency of the transplanted cornea.

Uveal tract

The middle vascular layer, or uveal tract, of the eye includes the choroid, the ciliary body, and the iris (see Figs. 46-1 and 46-6). The uveal tract is an incomplete ball with gaps at the pupil and at the optic disk, where it is continuous with the arachnoid and pial layers surrounding the optic nerve. The choroid is rich in dispersed melanocytes, which function to prevent the diffusion of light through the wall of the optic globe. The pigment of these cells absorbs light within the eyeball and light that penetrates the retina. The light absorptive function prevents the scattering of light and is important for visual acuity, particularly with high background illumination levels.

The ciliary body is an anterior continuation of the choroid layer. It has both smooth muscle and secretory functions. Its smooth muscle function contributes to alteration in lens shape, and its secretory function to production of aqueous humor.

The iris is an adjustable diaphragm that permits alteration in pupil size and in the amount of light entering the eye. The pupillary diameter can be varied from approximately 2 mm to 8 mm. The posterior surface of the iris is formed by a 2-layer epithelium continuous with those covering the ciliary body. The anterior layer contains the dilator, or radial muscles, of the iris (Fig. 46-7). Just anterior to these muscles is the loose, highly vascular connective tissue stroma. Embedded in this layer are concentric rings of smooth muscle cells that compose the sphincter muscle of the pupil. The anteriormost layer of the iris forms a highly irregular anterior surface and contains many fibroblasts and melanocytes.

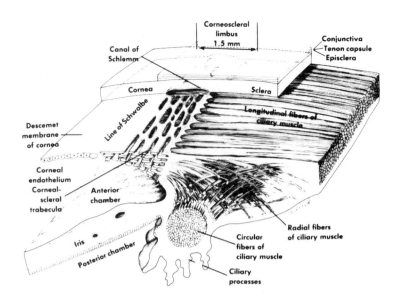

Figure 46-7 *Schematic construction of the ciliary body and angle recess in humans. Anteriorly the area is covered by the cornea and posteriorly by the sclera, which contains the canal of Schlemm. The termination of the corneal endothelium is marked by the line of Schwalbe. The ciliary muscle consists of longitudinal fibers, which are mainly parallel to the sclera; radial fibers, which are intermediate; and a circular muscle, which is, most internal. The corneoscleral trabecula provides a filtering area between the anterior chamber angle and the canal of Schlemm. (Redrawn from Von Mollendorf W, Bargmann W (eds): Handbuch der mikroskopischen Anatomie des Menschen, Berlin, Springer-Verlag, 1964. From Newell FW: Ophthalmology: Principles and Concepts, 5th ed. St Louis, CV Mosby, 1982)*

Eye color differences result from the density of the pigment. The amount of pigment decreases from dark brown eyes through shades of brown and gray to blue.

Several mutations affect the pigment of the uveal tract, including albinism. Albinism is a genetic (autosomal recessive trait) deficiency of tyrosinase, which is necessary for the synthesis of melanin by the melanocytes. Classic albinism is termed tyrosine-negative albinism, and the affected individual has white hair, pink skin, and light blue eyes. In these individuals, excessive light penetrates the unpigmented iris and to some extent the anterior sclera and unpigmented choroid. Their photoreceptors are flooded with excess light, and visual acuity is markedly reduced. In addition, excess stimulation of the photoreceptors at normal or high illumination levels is experienced as painful (photophobia). Tryrosine-positive albinism results from the genetic defects in which a reduced but variable amount of tyrosine is synthesized by the pigment cells. Hair and skin color vary among these persons. Reduced choroid and iris pigment result in variable acuity and photophobic abnormalities. A third type of hereditary defect involves the absence of pigment in the choroid and iris with normal pigmentation elsewhere. This is called ocular albinism and results from a chromosomal abnormality of the X chromosome. Other hereditary syndromes include reduced or absent choroid and iris pigment, as in phenlyketonuria. Persons with tyrosine-negative albinism or ocular albinism usually have nystagmus, which makes reading difficult. This may be the result of continuous reflex searching for improved visual acuity.

Uveitis. Inflammation of the entire uveal tract is termed uveitis. One of the serious consequences of the condition can be the involvement of the underlying ret-

ina. Parasitic invasion of the choroid can result in local atrophic changes that usually involve the retina; examples include toxoplasmosis and histoplasmosis. Sarcoid deposition in the form of small nodules results in irregularities of the underlying retinal surface.

In summary, the optic globe, or eyeball, is protected posteriorly by the bony structures of the orbit and anteriorly by the eyelids. It is continuously bathed by a protective layer of tears. Protrusion of the eyes is called exophthalmos, and deeply sunken eyes is called enophthalmos. The eyelids are called the palpebrae. Marginal blepharitis is the most common disorder of the eyelids. It is commonly caused by a staphylococcal infection or seborrhea (dandruff). The term ptosis refers to a drooping of the upper lid sufficient to interfere with the pupillary light opening. It can be caused by injury to the facial (VII) or oculomotor (III) cranial nerve, or by the loss of sympathetic innervation of the smooth muscle of the inner surface of the lid, causing the inner lining of the lid to droop over the pupil. The conjunctiva lines the inner surface of the eyelids and covers the optic globe to the junction of the cornea and sclera. Conjunctivitis (also called redeye or pinkeye) is a common eye disorder. It is important to differentiate between redness caused by conjunctivitis and that caused by more serious eye disorders, such as acute glaucoma or corneal lesions. Tears protect the cornea from drying and irritation. Impaired tear production or conditions that prevent blinking and the spread of tears produce drying of the eyes and predispose them to corneal irritation and injury. Trauma or disease that involves the stromal layer of the cornea heals with scar formation and permanent opacification. These opacities interfere with the transmission of light and impair vision. The uveal tract is the middle vascular layer of the eye. It contains melanocytes that prevent diffusion of light through the wall of the optic globe. Inflammation of the uveal tract (uveitis) can affect visual acuity; albinism, an inherited pigment defect, can cause photophobia.

Intraocular Pressure and Glaucoma

The fluid-filled anterior and posterior chambers of the anterior segment of the eye are divided by the iris and the closely adjacent lens into the posterior and anterior chambers, the pupil forming the only passageway between the two chambers (Fig. 46-8). The posterior chamber, which is the smaller chamber, is restricted by the gellike vitreous humor that fills the remaining space within the cavity of the globe.

The transparent aqueous humor, which fills the space between the cornea and lens, is secreted by the ciliary epithelium in the posterior chamber. The secreted aqueous humor flows slowly through the thin passageway between the lens and the iris and is then reabsorbed by a specialized region at the iridial angle. At the iridocorneal angle, the aqueous humor normally passes through a porous trabeculated region of the sclera (see Fig. 46-7) that permits entry into a circular venous ring called the *canal of Schlemm* and from there into the anterior ciliary veins. The anterior ciliary veins continue into the choroid and enter the ophthalmic veins at the back of the eye.

The aqueous humor helps to maintain the intraocular pressure and metabolism of the lens and posterior cornea. The interior pressure of the eye must exceed that

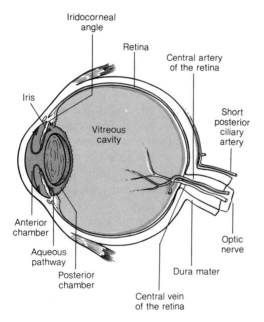

Figure 46-8 *Anterior and posterior chambers of the eye. Arrows indicate the pathway of aqueous flow.*

of the atmosphere to prevent the eyeball from collapsing. In addition, the aqueous humor serves a nutritive function for the lens and the posterior surface of the cornea. It contains a low protein concentration and a high concentration of ascorbic acid, glucose, and amino acids. It also mediates the exchange of respiratory gases.

The hydrostatic pressure of the aqueous humor results from a balance of several factors: (1) the rate of secretion, (2) the resistance to flow through the narrow opening between the lens and iris at the entrance into the anterior chamber, and (3) the resistance to resorption at the trabeculated region of the sclera at the iridocorneal angle. Normally the rate of aqueous production is equal to the rate of aqueous outflow, so that the intraocular pressure is maintained within a normal range of 12 mm Hg to 21 mm Hg. Abnormalities in the balance between these factors leads to increased pressure in the aqueous humor, a disease complex called glaucoma.

The secretion of aqueous humor is an active process that continues regardless of the pressure in the secreted fluid. The secretory activity of the ciliary epithelium requires the enzyme *carbonic anhydrase,* and medical management of excessive aqueous production often includes the use of the carbonic anhydrase inhibitor acetazolamide (Diamox). Rarely is increased intraocular pressure due to the overproduction of aqueous humor; instead, it usually results from interference with outflow anywhere along the outflow pathway (pupil, trabecular meshwork, or canal of Schlemm). Congenital deformities of the trabecular meshwork, clogging of the meshwork with cellular debris from various intraocular pathologies, and adhesions of the peripheral iris to the trabecular meshwork can all result in increased intraocular pressure. As intraocular pressure rises because of impaired outflow, the canal of Schlemm is compressed, causing a further reduction in aqueous outflow.

Types of glaucoma

Glaucoma includes a group of conditions in which the intraocular pressure increases sufficiently to cause degeneration of the optic nerve, leading to progressive blindness. An initial gradual loss of peripheral vision (Fig. 46-9) is followed by loss of central vision. Glaucoma can occur in any age group but is most prevalent in the elderly. It accounts for 13% of all cases of blindness and affects about 2% of people over 40 years of age.[1] The condition is often asymptomatic, and a significant loss of peripheral vision may occur before medical attention is sought, emphasizing the need for routine screening measurement of intraocular pressure in persons over age 40.

Glaucoma is commonly classified as closed-angle (narrow-angle) or open-angle (wide-angle) glaucoma depeding on the location of the compromised aqueous humor circulation and resorption. Glaucoma may occur

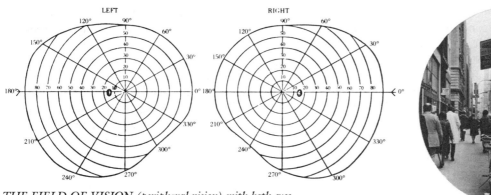

THE FIELD OF VISION (peripheral vision) with both eyes is 180° recorded on these charts.

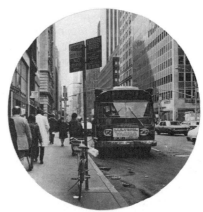

NORMAL VISION A person with normal or 20/20 vision sees this street scene.

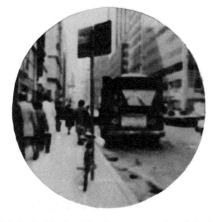

CATARACT diminished acuity from an opacity of the lens. The field of vision is **unaffected**. There is no scotoma, but the person has an overall haziness of the view, particularly in glaring light conditions.

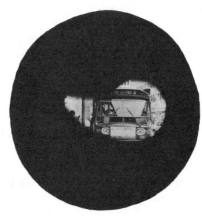

GLAUCOMA Advanced glaucoma involves loss of peripheral vision but the individual still retains most of his central vision.

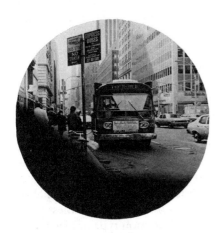

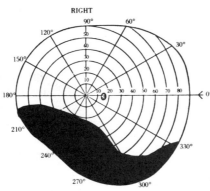

RETINAL DETACHMENT shown here in the active stage. There are many causes for detachment, but the hole or tear allows fluid to lift the retina from its normal position. This elevated retina causes a field or vision defect, seen as a dark shadow in the peripheral field. It may be above, or below as illustrated.

Figure 46-9   *Photographs representing the eye diseases, done as if the camera were the right eye. The accompanying visual-field chart showing the area of visual loss also represents the right eye. (Photo courtesy The Lighthouse, The New York Association for the Blind)*

as a congenital or an acquired condition, and it may present as a primary or secondary disorder. Primary glaucoma occurs without evidence of preexisting ocular or systemic disease. Secondary glaucoma can result from inflammatory processes that affect the eye, tumors that obstruct the outflow of aqueous humor, or hemorrhage caused by trauma.

Congenital (infantile) glaucoma. Congenital glaucoma is caused by a disorder in which the anterior chamber retains its fetal configuration, with the trabecular meshwork attached to the root of the iris, or is covered with a membrane. The earliest symptoms are excessive lacrimation and photophobia. Affected infants tend to be fussy, have poor eating habits, and rub their eyes frequently. Diffuse edema of the cornea is usually present, giving the eye a grayish white appearance. Chronic elevation of the intraocular pressure before the age of 3 years causes enlargement of the entire globe (buphthalmos). Early surgical treatment is necessary to prevent blindness.

Closed-angle glaucoma. In closed-angle (narrow-angle) glaucoma, the anterior chamber is narrow, and outflow becomes impaired when the iris thickens as the result of pupil dilatation. As the iris thickens, it restricts the circulation pathway between the base of the iris and the sclera, reducing or eliminating access to the angle where aqueous reabsorption occurs. Approximately 5% to 10% of all cases of glaucoma fall into this category.

The symptoms of closed-angle glaucoma are related to sudden intermittent increases in intraocular pressure.

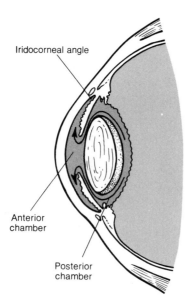

Figure 46-10 *Narrow anterior chamber and iridocorneal angle in closed-angle (narrow-angle) glaucoma.*

Iridocorneal angle

Anterior chamber

Posterior chamber

These occur after prolonged periods in the dark, emotional upset, and other conditions that cause extensive and prolonged pupil dilatation. Administration of pharmacologic agents such as atropine, which cause pupillary dilatation (mydriasis), can also precipitate an acute episode of increased intraocular pressure in persons with closed-angle glaucoma. Attacks of increased intraocular pressure are manifested by ocular pain and blurred or iridescent vision caused by corneal edema. The pupil may be enlarged and fixed. The symptoms are often spontaneously relieved by sleep and conditions that promote pupillary constriction. With repeated or prolonged attacks, the eye becomes reddened, and edema of the cornea may develop, giving the eye a hazy appearance. A unilateral, often excruciating, headache is common. Nausea and vomiting may be present, causing the headache to be confused with migraine.

Closed-angle glaucoma usually occurs as the result of an inherited anatomic defect that causes a shallow anterior chamber. This defect is exaggerated by the anterior displacement of the peripheral iris because of the increase in lens size that occurs with aging. Some persons with a congenitally narrow anterior chamber never develop symptoms, and others develop symptoms only when they are elderly. The depth of the anterior chamber can be evaluated by transillumination or by a technique called *gonioscopy* (to be discussed later). Because of the dangers of vision loss, persons with narrow anterior chambers should be warned, particularly concerning the occurrence of blurred vision, halos, and ocular pain.

The treatment of closed-angle glaucoma is primarily by surgical intervention. Removing the iris (iridectomy) or cutting a window through the base of the iris (iridotomy) by surgical incision or laser beam provides relief. The anatomic abnormalities responsible for closed-angle glaucoma are usually expressed bilaterally, but progression may not be symmetrical.

Open-angle glaucoma. With open-angle glaucoma, an abnormal increase in intraocular pressure occurs in the absence of an obstruction between the trabecular meshwork and the anterior chamber (Fig. 46-10). Instead, it usually occurs because of an abnormality of the trabecular meshwork that impairs the flow of aqueous humor between the anterior chamber and the canal of Schlemm. Open-angle glaucoma tends to manifest itself after age 35 and is the most common type of glaucoma, accounting for approximately 90% of all cases. The condition is usually asymptomatic, and chronic, causing progressive loss of visual field unless it is appropriately treated. Because it is usually asymptomatic, routine screening tonometry is the best means of detecting the disorder. In some persons, the use of moderate amounts of topical corticosteroid medications can cause an increase in intraocular pressure. Sensitive persons may also sustain an increase in intraocular pressure with the use of systemic corticosteroid drugs.

In contrast to closed-angle glaucoma, which can be treated surgically, open-angle glaucoma is usually treated medically. Among the drugs used in the treatment of open-angle glaucoma are miotics (drugs that cause pupillary constriction). These drugs increase the efficiency of the outflow channels, although the exact mechanism of their effect is unknown. Pilocarpine, a cholinergic-stimulating drug, is often used for this purpose. Other drugs that are used in the treatment of open-angle glaucoma are epinephrine, timolol, and acetazolamide. Epinephrine, an adrenergic neuromediator with both alpha and beta effects, reduces aqueous production by means of beta-receptor mechanisms (probably secondary to vasoconstriction in the ciliary processes) and increases aqueous outflow by means of alpha-receptor mechanisms. Timolol, a beta-adrenergic blocking drug, presumably lowers intraocular pressure by reducing aqueous production. Acetazolamide, a carbonic anhydrase inhibitor, reduces the secretion of aqueous humor by the ciliary epithelium. With the exception of acetazolamide, most drugs that are used in the treatment of glaucoma are applied topically.

When a reduction in intraocular pressure cannot be maintained through pharmacologic methods, surgical treatment may become necessary. Until recently, the main surgical treatment for open-angle glaucoma was a filtering procedure in which an opening is created between the anterior chamber and the subconjunctival space. A new argon laser technique, in which 100 spots are applied 360° around the trabecular meshwork, has now been developed.[4] The microburns resulting from the laser treatment scar rather than penetrate the trabecular meshwork, a process that is thought to enlarge the outflow channels by increasing the tension exerted on the trabecular meshwork. In another type of procedure, photocoagulation of the ciliary processes (cyclocryotherapy) may be used to destroy the ciliary epithelium and reduce aqueous humor production.

Diagnostic methods

Among the methods used in detecting and evaluating glaucoma are measurement of intraocular pressure, ophthalmoscopy, perimetry, transillumination technique, and gonioscopy. Perimetry, which is used to assess visual field loss, is discussed in the section on visual pathways.

Intraocular pressure measurements.   Intraocular pressure measurements are made indirectly by means of an instrument called a tonometer. There are two types of

tonometers: a contact tonometer, an instrument that is placed on the anesthetized eye, and a noncontact tonometer, in which an air pulse is used. The Schiotz tonometer (Fig. 46-11) is an indentation tonometer that measures the amount of corneal deformation produced by a given force. The noncontact tonometer flattens the cornea with an air blast, increasing the amount of light that is reflected from the cornea. The time required for complete flattening of the cornea is measured electronically and used as a measure of intraocular pressure. Although a single high measurement of intraocular pressure (24–32 mm Hg) is suggestive of glaucoma, repeated measurements are needed before a definite diagnosis can be made.[2]

Ophthalmoscopy.   Increased intraocular pressure causes damage to optic nerve structures (optic disk) that can be recognized on ophthalmoscopic examination. The normal optic disk has a centrally placed depression called the *optic cup*. With progressive atrophy of axons caused by glaucoma, pallor of the optic disk develops, and the size and depth of the optic cup increase. Regular ophthalmoscopic examination is important for detecting eye changes that occur with glaucoma, because changes in the optic cup precede the visual field loss.

Gonioscopy and transillumination.   Gonioscopy and transillumination are used to assess anterior chamber depth. Gonioscopy uses a special contact lens and either mirrors or prisms so that the angle of the anterior chamber can be seen and measured. The transillumination requires only a penlight. The light source is held at the

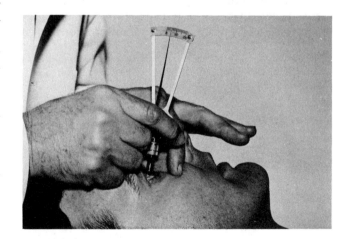

Figure 46-11   *After a local anesthetic is instilled into the eye, the Schiotz tonometer is gently rested on the eyeball; the indicator measures in millimeters of mercury the ocular tension. (Courtesy, F. H. Roy, M.D. From Brunner LS, Suddarth DS: Textbook of Medical-Surgical Nursing, 5th ed, Philadelphia, JB Lippincott, 1984)*

temporal side of the eye and directed horizontally across the iris.[5] In persons with a normal-sized anterior chamber, the light passes through the anterior chamber to illuminate both halves of the iris. In contrast, in a person with a narrow anterior chamber, only the half of the iris adjacent to the light source is illuminated (Fig. 46-12).

In summary, glaucoma is one of the leading causes of blindness in the United States. It is characterized by conditions that cause an increase in intraocular pressure, which leads to atrophy of the optic disk and progressive blindness. The aqueous humor is formed by the ciliary epithelium in the posterior chamber and flows through the pupil to the angle formed by the cornea and the iris. Here it filters through the trabecular meshwork and enters the canal of Schlemm for return to the venous circulation. Glaucoma results from the impeded outflow of aqueous humor from the anterior chamber of the eye. There are two major forms of glaucoma: closed-angle and open-angle. Closed-angle glaucoma is caused by a narrow anterior chamber and blockage of the outflow channels at the angle formed by the iris and the cornea. This occurs when the iris becomes thickened during pupillary dilatation. In open-angle glaucoma microscopic obstruction of the trabecular meshwork occurs. Open-angle glaucoma is usually asymptomatic, and considerable loss of the visual field often occurs before medical treatment is sought. Routine screening tonometry provides the means for early detection of glaucoma before vision loss has occurred.

Optics and Lens Function

The function of the eye is to transform light energy into nerve signals that can be transmitted to the brain for interpretation. Optically, the eye is similar to a camera. It contains a lens system, an aperture for controlling light exposure (the pupil), and a retina that corresponds to the film.

Refraction

When light passes from one medium to another, its velocity is either decreased or increased, and the direction of light movement is changed. The bending of light at an angulated surface is called *refraction*. When light rays pass through the center of a lens, their direction is not changed; however, rays passing laterally through a lens are bent (Fig. 46-13). Usually, the refractive power of a lens is described as the distance from its surface, at which the rays come into focus (focal length), or as the reciprocal of this distance in meters (diopters). With a fixed power lens, the closer an object is to the lens, the further behind the lens the focus point will be. The closer the object, the stronger as well as the more perfect the focusing system must be.

In the eye, the major refraction of light begins at the convex corneal surface. Further refraction occurs as light moves from the posterior corneal surface to the aqueous humor, from the aqueous humor to the anterior lens surface, and from the posterior lens surface to the vitreous humor. In the eye, the focusing surface, the retina, is at a fixed distance from the lens; thus, adjustability in the refractive power of the lens is needed to keep the image of close objects in sharp focus on the retina. This is called *accommodation*. The adjustable lens shape and the adjustable pupillary opening must be under the control of a feedback system that makes these adjustments while evaluating image sharpness. All of this is accomplished by accommodation and pupillary reflexes under the control of the visual acuity evaluation centers in the primary visual and association cortex. These areas project directly to the pretectal region and

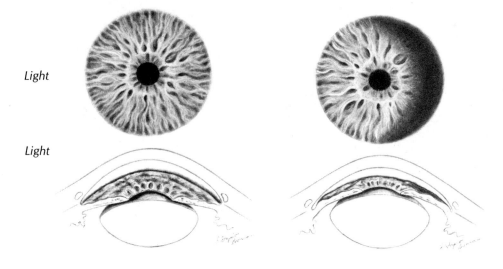

Light

Light

Figure 46-12   Transillumination of the iris. In the eye with a normal anterior chamber, the iris is evenly illuminated by light shining obliquely into the anterior chamber. In the eye with a narrow anterior chamber, the iris is unevenly illuminated and shadowed. (From Bates B: A Guide to Physical Examination, 3rd ed. Philadelphia, JB Lippincott, 1983)

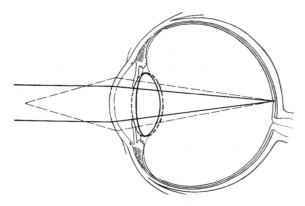

Figure 46-13 *Accommodation. The solid lines represent rays of light from a distant object, and the dotted lines represent rays from a near object. The lens is flatter for the former and more convex for the latter. In each case the rays of light are brought to a focus on the retina. (From Chaffee EE, Lytle IM: Basic Physiology and Anatomy, 4th ed. Philadelphia, JB Lippincott, 1980)*

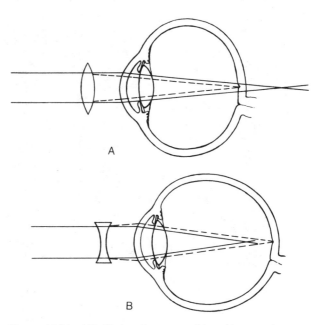

Figure 46-14 *(A) Hyperopia: corrected by a bioconvex lens, as shown by the dotted lines; (B) myopia: corrected by a bioconcave lens, shown by the dotted lines. (From Chaffee EE, Lytle IM: Basic Physiology and Anatomy, 4th ed. Philadelphia, JB Lippincott, 1980)*

provide feedback control of the lens shape and, therefore, of vision clarity.

A perfectly shaped optic globe and cornea result in optimal visual acuity, that is, a sharp image in focus at all points on the retinal surface in the posterior part, or fundus, of the eye (emmetropia). Unfortunately, individual differences in the formation and growth of the eyeball and cornea frequently result in inappropriate image focal formation. For distant vision, if the optic globe is too short, the image is focused posterior to (in back of) the retina. This is called *hyperopia*, or *farsightedness* (Fig. 46-14). In such cases, the accommodative changes of the lens cannot bring near objects into focus. This type of defect is corrected by appropriate biconvex lenses. If an infinitely distant target is focused anterior to (in front of) the retina, the eyeball is too long. This condition is called *myopia*, or *nearsightedness* (see Fig. 46-14). It can be corrected with an appropriate biconcave lens. Radial keratotomy, a form of refractive corneal surgery, can be performed to correct the defect. This surgical procedure involves the use of radial incisions to alter the corneal curvature.

Nonuniform curvature of the horizontal plane, in contrast with the vertical plane, of the refractive transparent media, usually of the cornea, is called *astigmatism* and must be corrected by a compensatory lens. Spherical aberration involves a cornea with a nonspherical surface. Correction can be made for this defect as well.

Accommodation

The lens is an avascular transparent biconvex body, whose posterior side is more convex than the anterior side. It measures about 9 mm to 10 mm in the transverse

diameter and about 4 mm in the anteroposterior diameter. A thin, homogeneous, and highly elastic carbohydrate-containing lens capsule is attached to the surrounding ciliary body by delicate suspensory ligaments called *zonules,* which hold the lens in place (Fig. 46-15). In providing for a change in lens shape, the tough and elastic sclera acts as a bow, and the zonules and lens capsule act as the bow string. Thus, the lens capsule is normally under tension, and the lens is flattened. Some of the smooth muscle fibers of the ciliary body are oriented parallel to the scleral surface and insert more anteriorly at the scleral–corneal junction. Many of the fibers are oriented radially as a sphincter around the eyeball (See Fig. 46-7). Contraction of the muscle fibers of the ciliary body results in a bending-in of the anterior sclera, relieving the tension on the zonules and thus on the lens capsule. Under these conditions, the rather elastic lens assumes a nearly spherical shape. Altering the normally flat lens shape to a more spherical shape increases the focusing power of the lens and has the effect of bringing the focused image of a near object forward to the retinal surface.

The lens consists of transparent fibers arranged in concentric layers, of which the external layers are the newest and softest. There is no loss of lens fibers with aging. Instead, additional fibers are added to the outermost portion of the lens. As the lens ages, it thickens and its fibers become less elastic, so that the range of focus is

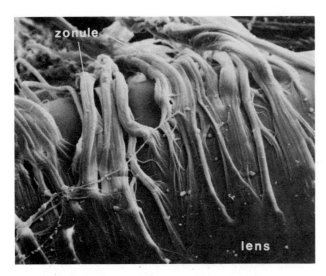

Figure 46-15 *Scanning micrograph of a portion of the zonule, attached to the periphery of the lens, from a monkey's eye. Note the large bundles of fibers attached to the capsule of the lens below. (Courtesy of P. Basu. From Ham AW, Cormack DH: Histology, 8th ed. Philadelphia, JB Lippincott, 1979)*

diminished to the point where reading glasses become necessary for near vision. This is called *presbyopia*.

Accommodation is the process whereby a clear image is maintained as the gaze is shifted from a far to a near object. It requires convergence of the eyes, pupillary constriction, and thickening of the lens through contraction of the ciliary muscle. Accommodation is under the control of the parasympathetic oculomotor (III) cranial nerve. The cell bodies of this nerve are contained in the oculomotor nuclear complex located in the midbrain, and its preganglionic axons synapse with postganglionic neurons of the ciliary ganglion in the orbit. The postganglionic axons enter the back of the eye and travel in the choroid layer to the ciliary muscle fibers. Visual function must be present to evaluate and adjust the clarity of the image. Thus, accommodation depends on the functional integrity of the entire visual system, including the forebrain and midbrain circuitry. Accommodation does not occur during sleep. An absolutely blind person cannot accommodate, nor can a person in a coma.

When a refractive defect of the corneal surface does not permit the formation of a sharp image, the accommodative reflex continues the unsuccessful attempts of ciliary muscle contraction to alter the lens shape. The discomfort or pain associated with continuous muscle contraction is experienced as eye strain.

Paralysis of the ciliary muscle, and thus of accommodation, is called *cycloplegia*. Pharmacologic paralysis is sometimes necessary to facilitate ophthalmoscope examination of the fundus of the eye, especially in small children who are unable to hold a steady fixation during the examination. The lens shape is totally under the control of the pretectal region and the parasympathetic pathway by way of the oculomotor nerve to the ciliary muscle. Accommodation is lost with the destruction of this pathway.

Pupillary reflexes

The pupillary reflex, which controls the size of the pupillary opening, is controlled by the autonomic nervous system. The sphincter muscle that produces pupillary constriction is innervated by postganglionic parasympathetic neurons of the ciliary ganglion and other scattered ganglion cells between the scleral and choroid layers (Fig. 46-16). The oculomotor (III) cranial nerve, located in the midbrain, provides the preganglionic innervation for these parasympathetic axons. Innervation for the dilator muscle is derived from thoracic sympathetic preganglionic neurons that send axons along the sympathetic chain to innervate the postganglionic neurons in the superior cervical ganglion. The postganglionic neurons send axons along the internal carotid and ophthalmic arteries to the posterior surface of the optic globe. These axons travel between the scleral and choroid layers to reach the dilator muscles of the iris. The pupillary reflex is controlled by a region in the midbrain called the pretectum. The pretectal areas on each side of the brain are interconnected, accounting for the binocular aspect of the light reflex. These areas project axons to nuclei of the midbrain called the *Edinger–Westphal nuclei*. These nuclei contain the parasympathetic preganglionic neurons, which innervate the ciliary ganglion and thus control the sphincters of the iris. Control of the pupillary opening by a brain level evaluation with feedback control provides an automatic brightness control mechanism. This represents a 16-fold range of brightness. The functional importance of this reflex mechanism is its rapidity, compared with the very slow light-and-dark-adaptive retinal mechanism.

Normal function of the pupillary reflex mechanism is tested by shining a bright light into one eye of the person being tested. A rapid constriction of the pupil exposed to light should occur (direct light reflex, or direct pupillary reflex). Because the reflex is normally bilateral, the contralateral pupil should also be constricted (consensual light reflex, or consensual pupillary reflex). By shining the light first into one eye and then into the other eye and noting the response of both pupils, considerable information can be gathered about the function of the central nervous system circuitry.

The circuitry of the light reflex is partially separated from the main visual pathway. This is illustrated by the fact that the pupillary reflex remains unaffected when lesions to the optic radiations or the visual cortex occur.

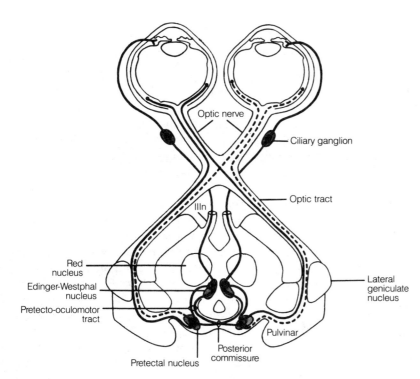

Figure 46-16   *Diagram of the path of the pupillary light reflex. (Reproduced, with permission, from Walsh FB, Hoyt WF: Clinical Neuro-ophthalmology, 3rd ed, Vol 1. Baltimore, Williams & Wilkins, © 1969)*

The cortically blind person retains direct and consensual light reflexes. The light reflex also functions under light anesthetic levels and is used to evaluate the depth of anesthesia. When the reflex is lost, the anesthesia level is approaching that which will depress the respiratory reflexes as well.

The function of the sympathetic and parasympathetic control of the iris (and pupillary size) is differentially affected by many pharmacologic agents. The integrity of the dual control of pupillary diameter is somewhat vulnerable to trauma, tumor enlargement, or vascular disease. Careful attention to inappropriate or unequal pupil diameters is diagnostically important. Reflex pupillary dilatation occurs more quickly in lightly pigmented eyes than in dark eyes. Damage to the oculomotor nucleus or nerve not only elimintes innervation of many of the extraocular muscles and the levator muscle of the upper lid but also results in permanent pupillary dilation *(mydriasis)* in the affected eye. Persons with mydriasis experience discomfort in normal or brightly lit environments because of loss of pupillary constriction in the affected eye. Lesions affecting the cervical spinal cord or the ascending sympathetic ganglionic chain in the neck or internal carotid artery (*e.g.,* Horner's syndrome) can interrupt the sympathetic control of the iris dilator muscle, resulting in permanent pupillary constriction *(miosis)*. Tumors of the orbit that compress structures behind the eye can eliminate all pupillary reflexes, usually before destroying the optic nerve. Inequality in pupillary size is called *anisocoria*.

Rarely is anisocoria present without pathologic significance.

Bilateral pupillary constriction is charcteristic of opiate usage. Bilateral pupillary dilation, being a sympathetic system function, is a part of general sympathetic activation, such as occurs during intense emotional responses associated with anger or fear. Unilateral pupillary dilation can be stimulated by a pinch to the lateral side of the neck, called the ciliospinal reflex. Pupillary dilation results when topical parasympathetic blocking agents such as atropine, homatropine, and scopolamine are applied and sympathetic pupillodilatory function is left unopposed. These medications are used by ophthalmologists to facilitate the examination of the transparent media and fundus of the eye. As was previously mentioned, pupillary dilation can increase the resistance to the flow of aqueous humor between the iris and lens, precipitating an increase in intraocular pressure in closed-angle glaucoma. Miotic drugs such as pilocarpine have the opposite effect, facilitating aqueous humor circulation.

Cataract

A cataract is a lens opacity that interferes with the transmission of light to the retina. It has been estimated that 5 million to 10 million persons in the United States are visually disabled because of cataracts.[1] A number of factors contribute to the development of cataracts, including genetic defects, environmental and metabolic influences, viruses, injury, and aging. Although there is no accepted method of classification, most cataracts can be described as congenital, senile, traumatic, or secondary to systemic or ocular disease.

Congenital cataract. Among the causes of congenital cataracts are genetic defects, toxic environmental agents, and viruses such as rubella. Active agents can damage lens differentiation during the second and third months of gestation and result in opacity, or primary cataract. Exposure of the embryo to ionizing radiation of levels as low as 50 rads, such as occurs during barium enema or fluoroscopy, can induce congenital cataract. Cataracts and other developmental defects of the ocular apparatus depend both on the total dose and the embryonic stage at the time of exposure. During the last trimester of fetal life, genetic or environmental malformation of the superficial lens fibers can occur. Most congenital cataracts are not progressive and are not dense enough to cause significant visual impairment. However, if the cataracts are bilateral, and significant opacity is present, lens extraction should be done on one eye by age 2 months, to permit the development of vision and prevent nystagmus. If the surgery is successful, the other eye should be done soon after.

Traumatic cataract. Traumatic cataracts are most often caused by foreign body injury to the lens or blunt trauma to the eye. Foreign body injury that interrupts the lens capsule allows aqueous and vitreous humor to enter the lens and initiate cataract formation. Other causes of traumatic cataract are overexposure to heat (glassblower's cataract) or to ionizing radiation. The radiation dose necessary to cause a cataract varies with energy and type; younger lenses are most vulnerable.

Senile cataract. With aging, both the nucleus and the cortex of the lens enlarge as new fibers are formed in the cortical zones of the lens. In the nucleus the old fibers become more compressed and dehydrated. In addition, metabolic changes occur. Lens proteins become more insoluble, and concentrations of calcium, sodium, potassium, and phosphate increase. During the early stages of cataract formation, a yellow pigment and vacuoles accumulate in the lens fibers. Unfolding of protein molecules, cross-linking of sulfhydryl groups, and conversion of soluble to insoluble proteins, leading to the loss of lens transparency occur.

Cataracts due to metabolic and toxic agents. Disorders of carbohydrate metabolism are the most common metabolic causes of cataract. Normally, glucose enters lens cells by diffusion and is then reduced to sorbitol (an alcohol) by the intracellular enzyme aldose reductase. Sorbitol diffuses out of the lens fibers very slowly, creating an osmotic gradient for the entry of water. In uncontrolled diabetes mellitus the entry of glucose into the lens fibers accelerates with increased production of osmotically active sorbitol. The lens fibers swell and change their refractive properties, causing myopic changes and blurring of vision. The condition is slowly reversible unless it is long-standing, in which case lens fiber destruction and permanent cataracts occur. The sugar galactose exerts the same effect in persons with galactosemia.

Cataract can result from a number of drugs. Dinitrophenol, a drug widely used for weight reduction during the 1930s, triparanol, chlorpromazine, and the adrenocorticosteroid drugs have all been implicated as causative agents in cataract formation. Busulfan, a cancer treatment drug, has been clearly linked to cataract formation. Frequent examination of lens transparency should accompany the use of these and any other substances with cataract-forming effects.

Signs and symptoms. The chief symptom of cataract is a gradual decline in visual acuity (see Fig. 46-9). Vision for far and near objects decreases. Dilation of the pupil in dim light improves vision. With nuclear cataracts (those involving the lens nucleus), the refractive power of the anterior segment often increases to produce an acquired myopia. Thus, persons with hyperopia may experience a second sight or improved reading acuity until increasing opacity reduces acuity. Central lens opacities may divide the visual axis and cause an optical defect in which two or more blurred images are seen. On ophthalmoscopic examination, cataracts may appear as a gross opacity filling the pupillary aperture or as an opacity silhouetted against the red background of the fundus.

Treatment. A partially opaque lens is termed an *immature cataract,* and a totally opaque lens is a *mature cataract.* Following the mature stage, leakage of protein from the degenerated cells results in shrinkage, and the lens is called *hypermature.* The treatment consists of surgical removal of the cataract (cataract extraction). Surgical removal is indicated when the opacity has advanced to the stage at which it produces a visual defect that interferes with normal activities or when the cataract threatens to cause other eye problems such as secondary glaucoma or uveitis. The absence of the lens is called *aphakia.* Following surgery to remove the lens, the loss of the refractive role of the lens can be compensated for by thick convex lenses, contact lenses, or an artificial lens implant. It has been estimated that 450,000 cataract extractions are performed annually in the United States, and an intraocular lens is used in approximately 150,000 of these.[6]

In summary, the refractive properties of the eye depend on the size and shape of the eyeball and the cornea and on the focusing abilities of the lens. In terms of visual function, refraction refers to the ability to focus an image on the retina. Errors in refraction occur when the visual image is not focused on the retina because of individual differences in the size or shape of the eyeball or cornea. In hyperopia, or farsightedness, the image falls in back of the retina. In myopia, or nearsightedness, the image falls in front of the retina. Because the focusing power of the eyeball and cornea is fixed, it is the lens that provides the means for the focusing of near images on the retina. The lens is a transparent and avascular biconvex structure suspended behind the iris and between the anterior chamber and the vitreous body that aids in visual focus. It is enclosed in an elastic capsule and attached to the ciliary body suspensory ligaments. When the ciliary muscle contracts, the ligaments relax and the lens becomes more nearly spherical, enabling the eye to focus on objects that are nearer to the eye. Relaxation of the ciliary muscle allows the eye to focus on distant objects. This mechanism is called accommodation and is controlled by the autonomic nervous system. Stimulation of the parasympathetic nervous system contracts the ciliary muscle and increases refractive power. With aging, the lens thickens and losses its ability to focus on near objects, a condition called presbyopia. A cataract is a lens opacity. It can occur as the result of congenital influences, metabolic disturbances, infection, injury, and aging. The most common type of cataract is the senile cataract that occurs with aging. The treatment for a totally opaque or mature cataract is surgical extraction. An intraocular lens transplant may be inserted during the surgical procedure to replace the lens that has been removed; otherwise, thick convex lenses or contact lenses are used to compensate for the loss of lens function.

Vitreous and Retinal Function

The posterior segment, which constitutes five-sixths of the eyeball, contains the transparent vitreous humor and the neural retina. It is this interior part of the posterior chamber, called the *fundus,* that is visualized through the pupil with an opthalmoscope.

Vitreous humor

The vitreous humor is a colorless, structureless gel that fills the posterior segment of the eye. It consists of about 99% water, some salts, glycoproteins, and dispersed collagen fibrils. The vitreous is attached to the ciliary body and the peripheral retina in the region of the ora serrata and to the periphery of the optic disk.

The vitreous is a biologic gel. Disease, aging, and injury can disturb the factors that maintain water in suspension, causing liquefaction to occur. With the loss of gel structure, fine fibers, membranes, and cellular debris develop. When this occurs, floaters (images), can often be noticed as these substances move within the vitreous cavity during head movement. In disease, blood vessels may grow from the surface of the retina or optic disk onto the posterior surface of the vitreous, and blood may fill the vitreous cavity.

The removal and replacement of the vitreous with a balanced saline solution (vitrectomy) can restore sight in some persons with vitreous opacities resulting from hemorrhage or vitreoretinal membrane formations that cause legal blindness. In this procedure, a small probe with a cutting tip is used to remove the opaque vitreous and membranes. The procedure is difficult and requires complex instrumentation. It is of no value if the retina is not functional.

Retina

The function of the retina is to receive visual images, partially analyze them, and transmit this modified information to the brain. Disorders of the retina and its function include (1) congenital photoreceptor abnormalities such as color blindness, (2) disturbances in blood vessels such as vascular retinopathies with hemorrhage and the development of opacities, (3) separation of the pigment and sensory layers of the retina (retinal detachment), (4) derangements of the pigment epithelium (retinitis pigmentosa), and (5) abnormalities of Bruch's membrane and choroid (macular degeneration). The retina has no pain fibers; therefore, most diseases of the retina are painless and do not cause redness of the eye.

The retina is composed of two parts: an outer pigmented layer and an inner neural layer. The neural retina covers the inner aspect of the posterior two-thirds of the eyeball. Posteriorly, the retina is continuous with the optic nerve; anteriorly, the neural retina ends a short distance behind the ciliary body in a wavy border called the *ora serrata.*

The single pigment layer is separated from the vascular portion of the choroid by a thin layer of elastic tissue (Bruch's membrane), which contains collagen fibrils in its superficial and deep portions. The cells of the pigmented layer receive their nourishment by diffusion from the choroid vessels. Its tight junctions (and those of the retinal blood vessels) provide the blood–retinal barrier. The neural retina is composed of three layers of neurons: a posterior layer of photoreceptors, a middle layer of bipolar and ganglion cells that converge with the photoreceptors, and a superficial marginal layer containing the axons of the ganglion cells as they collect and leave the eye via the optic nerve (Fig. 46-17). The interneurons, the horizontal and amacrine cells, have cell bodies in the bipolar layer, and they play an important

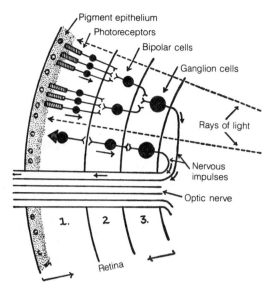

Figure 46-17 *Basic arrangement of the three orders of neurons in the nervous portion of the retina. Note that light rays and nerve impulses travel in opposite directions through the retina. (From Ham AW: Cormack DH: Histology, 8th ed. Philadelphia, JB Lippincott, 1979)*

role in modulating retinal function. Light must pass through the transparent inner layers of the sensory retina before it reaches the photoreceptors.

Photoreceptors.   There are two types of photoreceptors: rods, capable of black–white discrimination, and cones, capable of color discrimination. Both types of photoreceptors are thin, elongated, mitochondria-filled cells with a single highly modified cilium (Fig. 46-18). The cilium has a very short base, or inner segment, and a highly modified outer segment. The plasma membrane of the outer segment is highly folded to form membranous disks (rods) or conical shapes (cones) containing visual pigment. These disks are continuously synthesized at the base of the outer segment and shed at the distal end. The discarded membranes are phagocytized by the retinal pigment cells. If this phagocytosis is disrupted, as in retinitis pigmentosa, the sensory retina degenerates.

Rods.   Photoreception involves the transduction of light energy into an altered ionic membrane potential of the rod cell. Light passing through the eye penetrates the nearly transparent neural elements to produce decomposition of the photochemical substance (visual pigment) called *rhodopsin* in the outer segment of the rod. Light that is not trapped by a rhodopsin molecule is absorbed by either the retinal pigment melanin or the more superficial choroid melanin. Rhodopsin consists of a protein (opsin) and a vitamin A–derived pigment

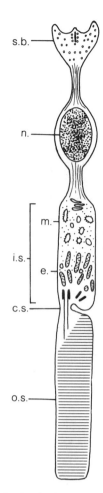

Figure 46-18 *Retinal rod, showing its component parts and the distribution of its organelles. Its outer segment (o.s.) contains the disks. The connecting structure between the outer and inner segments is labeled c.s. The inner segment is labeled i.s. In the outermost part of this there is a basal body, from which a modified cilium extends into the inner part of the outer segment. The inner segment is described as consisting of two parts, the ellipsoid portion (e) and the myoid portion (m). The former contains abundant mitochondria. The myoid portion contains rER, free ribosomes, and Golgi saccules. Farther in, the cell is constricted until it bulges to surround the nucleus (n). It then narrows again and ends in an expansion called the synaptic body (s.b.) because here the photoreceptor synapses with other nerve cells. (Courtesy of R. Young. From Ham AW, Cormack DH: Histology, 8th ed. Philadelphia, JB Lippincott, 1979)*

called *retinal*. During light stimulation, rhodopsin is broken down into its component parts (opsin and retinal), and retinal is converted into vitamin A. The reconstitution of rhodopsin occurs during total darkness; vitamin A is transformed into retinal and then opsin and retinal combine to form rhodopsin. Because there are considerable stores of vitamin A in the retinal pigment cells and in the liver, a vitamin A deficiency must exist for weeks or months to have an impact on the photoreceptive process. Reduced sensitivity to light, a symptom of vitamin A deficiency, first affects night vision and is quickly reversed by injection or ingestion of the vitamin.

A pattern of light on the retina falls on a massive array of photoreceptors. These photoreceptors communicate with bipolar and other interneurons before action potentials in ganglion cells relay the message to the brain. For rods, this microcircuitry involves the convergence of signals from many rods on a single ganglion cell. This arrangement maximizes spatial summation and the detection of stimulated (light versus dark) receptors. Rod-based vision is particularly sensitive to detecting light, and especially moving light, stimuli at the sacrifice of clear pattern discrimination. Thus, rod vision is particularly adapted for night and low-level illumination.

Dark adaptation is the process by which rod sensitivity increases to the optimum level. This requires approximately ½ hour in total or near-total darkness and involves only rod receptor (black-and-white) vision. During daylight, or high-intensity bombardment, the concentration of vitamin A increases and the concentration of the photopigment retinal decreases. During dark adaptation, increased synthesis of retinal from vitamin A results in a higher concentration of rhodopsin available to capture the light energy.

Cones and color sensitivity. Cone receptors that are selectively sensitive to different wavelengths of light provide the basis for color vision. Three types of cones, or cone-color systems, respond to the more blue, green, and red portions of the visible electromagnetic spectrum. This selectivity is due to the presence of one of three color-sensitive molecules to which the photochemical substance (visual pigment) is bound. The decomposition and reconstitution of the cone visual pigments is believed to be similar to that of the rods. The color a person senses depends on which set of cones or combination of sets of cones is stimulated in a given image.

Color vision vastly increases the richness of visual experience. The subjective experience of color can be analyzed according to three aspects: hue, saturation, and brightness. Hue is the experience of pure color. It is related to the proportion of involvement of each of the primary cone-color systems. Approximately 200 gradations of color dimension can be discriminated. Saturation refers to the purity of the color as contrasted with the amount of gray mixed with the color. The same red can be weak or strong (more saturated). Brightness experience refers to the total amount of light received from an object in relation to its background. Increased brightness turns brown into orange. Approximately 500 steps of brightness can be discriminated for each saturation of each hue. Brightness is shared by the black–white rod

system with gradations from black through grays to whites.

Cones do not have the dark adaptation of rods. Consequently, the dark-adapted eye is a rod receptor eye with only black–gray–white experience *(scotopic vision)*. The light-adapted eye *(photopic vision)* adds the capacity for color discrimination. Rhodopsin has its maximum sensitivity in the blue–green region of the spectrum. If red lenses are worn in daylight, only the red cones (and green cones to some extent) are in use; the rods (and blue cones) are essentially in the dark, and dark-adaptation proceeds. This method is used by military and night-duty airport control tower personnel to allow adaptation to take place before they go on duty in the dark.

Color blindness. Color blindness is a misnomer for a condition in which individuals appear to confuse, mismatch, or experience reduced acuity for color discrimination. Such people are often unaware of their defect until challenged by problems resulting from difficulties in discriminating a red from a green traffic light or mismatches of colors in an art class. Most often the result of genetic factors, the deficit can result from defective function of one or more of the three color-cone mechanisms. The deficiency is most often partial but can be complete. Rarely are two of the color mechanisms missing. When this does occur, usually red and green are missing. Extremely rare are persons with no color mechanisms (achromats). For such people, the world is experienced entirely as black, gray, and white.

The genetically color-blind person has never experienced the full range of normal color vision and is unaware of what he or she is missing. Color discrimination is necessary for everyday living, and color-blind people, knowingly or unknowingly, make color discriminations based on other criteria, such as brightness or position. For example, the red light of a traffic signal is always the upper light, and the green is the lower light. The color-blind individual gets into trouble when brightness differences are minimal and discrimination must be based on hue and saturation qualities.

The genes responsible for color blindness affect receptor mechanisms rather than central acuity. The gene for red and green mechanisms is sex-linked (on the X chromosomes), resulting in a much higher incidence among males (approximately 8% of males versus 0.5% of females). The gene affecting the blue mechanism is autosomal. Acquired color defects are more complex but tend to follow a general rule: disease of the outer retinal layer affects blue discrimination, and disease of the inner retinal layer affects red and green discrimination. This is because there are no blue cones in the central fovea.

The simplest test for color discrimination defects employs pseudoisochromatic plates that use numbers or letters buried in a matrix of colored dots. These plates are arranged so that common color-blindness defects result in misreading of the number or letter. Proper testing conditions require good lighting and the use of a control plate interpretable by the most color-blind individuals, in order to eliminate inability to read as a confounding factor.

Macula and fovea.   A minute area in the center of the retina, called the macula, is especially capable of acute and detailed vision. This area is composed entirely of cones. In the central portion of the macula, the *fovea centralis,* the blood vessels and innermost layers are displaced to one side instead of resting on top of the cones. This allows light to pass unimpeded to the cones without passing through several layers of retina. The density of cones drops off rapidly away from the fovea. There are no rods in the fovea, but their density increases as the cones decrease in density toward the periphery of the retina. Many cones are connected on a one-to-one basis with ganglion cells. In addition, retinal microcircuitry for cones emphasizes the detection of edges. This type of circuitry favors high acuity. A concentration of acuity favoring cones at the fovea supports the use of this part of the retina for fine analysis of focused central vision.

Disorders of the retina

Retinal blood supply.   The blood supply for the retina is derived from two sources: the choriocapillaries of the choroid and the branches of the central retinal artery. The nutritional needs of the retina, including oxygen supply to the pigment cells and rods and cones, involves diffusion from blood vessels in the choroid. Because the choriocapillaries provide the only blood supply for the fovea centralis, detachment of this part of the sensory retina from the pigment epithelium causes irreparable visual loss. The bipolar, horizontal, amacrine, and ganglionic cells as well as the ganglion cell axons that gather at the disk are supplied by the branches of the retinal artery. The central artery of the retina is a branch of the ophthalmic artery. It enters the globe through the optic disk. Branches of the artery radiate over the entire retina, except for the central fovea, which is surrounded but is not crossed by arterial branches. The retinal veins follow a distribution parallel to the arterial branches and bring venous blood to the central vein of the retina, which exits the back of the eye through the optic disk. Funduscopic examination of the eye with an ophthalmoscope provides an opportunity to examine the retinal blood vessels as well as other aspects of the retina (Fig. 46-19). Because the retina is an extension of the brain and the blood vessels are, to a considerable extent, representative of brain blood vessels, the ophthalmoscopic examination of the fundus of the eye provides an opportunity for the study and diagnosis of metabolic and vascular diseases of the brain, as well as pathologic processes that are specific to the retina itself.

The functioning of the retina, like that of other cellular portions of the central nervous system, is highly dependent on an oxygen supply from the vascular system. One of the earliest signs of decreased perfusion pressure in the head region is a graying-out or blackout of vision, which usually precedes loss of consciousness. This can occur with a large increase in intrathoracic pressure (*e.g.,* straining during defecation), which interferes with the return of venous blood to the heart, with systemic hypotension, and often during sudden postural movements under conditions of decreased vascular adaptability.

Ischemia of the retina occurs under general circulatory collapse. If a person survives cardiopulmonary arrest, for instance, permanent decreased visual acuity can occur as a result of edema and the ischemic death of retinal neurons. This is followed by primary optic nerve atrophy proportional to the extent of ganglionic cell death. The ophthalmic artery, the source of the central artery of the retina, takes its origin from the internal carotid artery. Intermittent retinal ischemia can accompany internal carotid or common carotid stenosis. In addition to ipsilateral intermittent blindness, contralateral hemiplegia or sensory deficits may accompany the episodes, depending on the competency of the circle of Willis in providing the brain with alternative arterial support. Treatment with anticoagulants or surgical endarterectomy may provide relief. Arteritis of the ophthalmic and central artery occurs more frequently in aged persons; if severe, it can result in occlusive disease and permanent visual deficits.

Papilledema.   The central retinal artery enters the eye through the optic papilla in the center of the optic nerve. Venous exit through the central vein of the retina follows the same path. The entrance and exit of the central artery and veins of the retina through the tough scleral tissue at the optic papilla can be compromised by any condition causing persistent increased intracranial pressure. The most common of these conditions are cerebral tumors, subdural hematomas, hydrocephalus, and malignant hypertension. The thin-walled, low-pressure veins are the first to collapse, with the consequent backup and slowing of arterial blood flow. Under these conditions, capillary permeability increases, and leakage of fluid results in edema of the optic papilla, called papilledema. The interior surface of the papilla is normally cup shaped and can be evaluated through an ophthalmoscope. With papilledema, sometimes called *choked disk,* the cup is distorted by protrusion into the interior of the eye. Because this sign does not occur until the intracranial

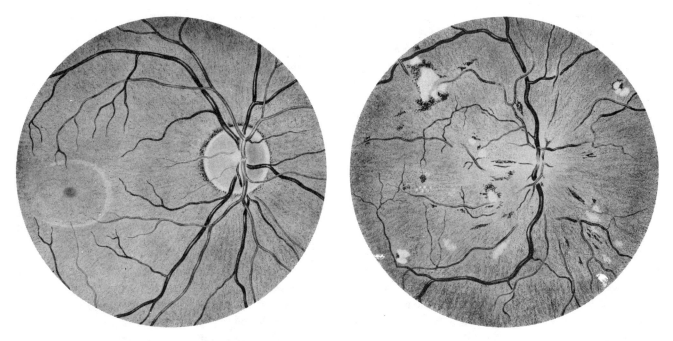

Figure 46-19 *Fundus of the eye as seen in retinal examination with an ophthalmoscope: (left) normal fundus; (right) pathologic fundus. The macula is not evident, but one can see flame-shaped hemorrhages and interrupted arteriovenous crossings. (From Chaffee EE, Lytle IM: Basic Physiology and Anatomy, 4th ed. Philadelphia, JB Lippincott, 1980)*

pressure is significantly elevated, compression damage to the optic nerve fibers passing through the lamina cribrosa may have begun. Thus, as a warning sign, papilledema occurs quite late. Unresolved papilledema will result in the destruction of the optic nerve axons and blindness.

Retrolental fibroplasia. Retrolental fibroplasia is a bilateral retinal disease of premature infants who must be given high concentrations of oxygen during the first 10 days of life to sustain life. Vascularization of the retina begins during the fourth month of gestation and moves from the optic nerve toward the ora serrata. The nasal periphery is completely vascularized by the eighth month and the temporal periphery only after full-term birth. During the period of blood vessel immaturity, the vessels respond to an increase in oxygen tension by vasoconstriction, obliteration, and suspension of normal vessel growth. This is followed by dilatation of the vessels that are present and growth of new vessels and supporting tissue (fibrovascular proliferation) into the vitreous. The disease often progresses rapidly to blindness. However, in many cases partial or complete regression may occur in one or both eyes. In some babies, photocoagulation of the ridge that forms between the vascular and avascular retina may be beneficial. Once blindness has developed, no treatment will restore sight.

Vascular retinopathies. Vascular disorders of the retina result in microaneurysms, neovascularization, hemorrhage, and formation of retinal opacities. *Microaneurysms* are outpouchings of the retinal vasculature. On ophthalmoscopic examination they appear as minute unchanging red dots associated with blood vessels. They tend to leak plasma and are often surrounded by edema, which gives the retina a hazy appearance. Microaneurysms can be identified with certainty using fluorescein angiography (the fluorescein dye is injected intravenously and the retinal vessels are subsequently photographed using a special ophthalmoscope and fundus camera). The microaneurysms may bleed. Areas of hemorrhage and edema tend to clear spontaneously; however, they reduce visual acuity if they encroach on the macula and cause degeneration before they are absorbed. Photocoagulation is often used to treat microaneurysms that involve the macula.

Neovascularization involves the formation of new blood vessels. They can develop from the choriocapillaries, extending between the pigment layer and the sensory layer, or from the retinal veins, extending between the sensory retina and the vitreous cavity and sometimes into the vitreous. These new blood vessels are fragile, leak protein, and tend to bleed. Neovascularization occurs in a number of conditions that impair retinal circulation, including stasis because of hyperviscosity of blood or decreased flow, vascular occlusion, sickle cell disease, sarcoidosis, diabetes mellitus, and retinopathy of prematurity (retrolental fibroplasia). The cause of new blood vessel formation is uncertain. The stimulus is presumably a diffusible factor that is released during impaired perfusion or oxygenation of retinal tissue. The vitreous humor is thought to contain a substance that normally inhibits neovascularization, and this is apparently inhibited under conditions in which the new blood vessels invade the vitreous cavity.

Hemorrhage can be preretinal, retinal, or subretinal. Preretinal hemorrhages occur between the retina and the vitreous. These hemorrhages tend to be large because the blood vessels are only loosely restricted; they may be associated with a subarachnoid or subdural hemorrhage and are usually regarded as a serious manifestation of the disorder. They usually reabsorb without complications unless they penetrate into the vitreous. Retinal hemorrhages occur because of abnormalities of the retinal vessels, diseases of the blood, increased pressure within the retinal vessels, or vitreous traction on the vessel. Systemic causes include diabetes mellitus, hypertension, and blood dyscrasias. Subretinal hemorrhages are those that develop between the choroid and pigment layer of the retina. A common cause of subretinal hemorrhage is neovascularization.

Light normally passes through the transparent inner portions of the sensory retina before reaching the photoreceptors. *Opacities* such as hemorrhages, exudate, cotton-wool patches, edema, and tissue proliferation produce a localized loss of transparency that can be observed with the use of an ophthalmoscope. *Exudates* are opacities resulting from inflammatory processes. The development of exudates often results in the destruction of the underlying retinal pigment and choroid layer. *Deposits* are localized opacities consisting of lipid-laden macrophages or accumulated cellular debris. *Cotton-wool patches* are retinal opacities with hazy, irregular outlines. They occur in the nerve fiber layer and contain cell organelles. Cotton-wool patches are associated with retinal trauma, severe anemia, papilledema, and diabetic retinopathy.

Atherosclerosis of retinal vessels.

In atherosclerosis, the lumen of the arterioles becomes narrowed. As a result, the retinal arteries and arterioles become tortuous and narrowed. At sites where the arteries cross and compress veins, the red cell column of the vein appears distended. Exudate accumulates on arteriolar walls as plaque or cytoid bodies. Deep and superficial hemorrhages are common. Atheromatous plaques of the central artery are associated with danger of stasis, thrombi of the central veins, and occlusion.

Retinal artery occlusion.

Complete occlusion of the central artery of the retina results in sudden unilateral blindness (anopsia). This is an uncommon disorder of older persons and is most often due to embolism or atherosclerosis. Because the retina has a dual blood supply, the survival of retinal structures is possible if blood flow can be reestablished within 2 hours.[3] If blood flow is not restored, the infarcted retina swells and opacifies. Because the receptors of the central fovea are supplied with blood from the choroid, they survive; a cherry-red spot (healthy fovea) is seen surrounded by the pale white opacified retina. Although the nerve fibers of the optic disks are adequately supplied by the choroid, the disk becomes pale because of the death of the optic fibers (optic atrophy) following the death of their ganglionic cells.

Occlusions of branches of the central artery, called branch arterial occlusions, are essentially retinal strokes. These occur mainly as a result of emboli and local infarction in the neural retina. The opacification that follows is often slowly resolved, and retinal transparency is restored. Local blind spots (scotomas) occur, however, because of the destruction of local elements of the retina. Loss of the axons of destroyed ganglion cells results in some optic nerve atrophy.

Central retinal vein occlusion.

Occlusion of the central retinal vein results in venous dilatation, stasis, and reduced flow through the retinal veins. It is usually monocular and causes rapid deterioration of visual acuity. Superficial and deep hemorrhages throughout the retina follow, because of the increased capillary wall fragility resulting from the decreased venous outflow as well as lack of arterial inflow. Among the causes of central retinal vein obstruction are hypertension, diabetes mellitus, and conditions such as sickle cell anemia, which slow the venous blood flow. The reduction in blood flow results in neovascularization with fibrovascular invasion of the space between the retina and the vitreous humor. In addition to obstructing normal visual function, the new vessels are fragile and prone to hemorrhage. Escaped blood may fill the space between the retina and vitreous, producing the appearance of a sudden veil over visual images. The blood can find its way into the aqueous humor (hemorrhagic glaucoma). Photocoagulation of the spreading new blood vessels with high-intensity light or laser beam is used to prevent blindness and eye pain. As the hemorrhage is resolved, degenerating blood products can produce contraction of the vitreous and formation of fibrous tissue within it, causing tears and detachment of the retina.

Much more common are local vein occlusions with regional and focal capillary microhemorrhages that produce the same but more restricted pathologic effects. These microhemorrhages result in the formation of rings of yellow exudate composed of lipid and lipoprotein blood-breakdown products. Microhemorrhages deep in the neural retina are somewhat restricted by the vertical organization of the neural elements and result in dot hemorrhages. Microhemorrhages in the layer of ganglionic cell axon bundles result in cotton-wool spots.

Diabetic retinopathy.

One of the complications of diabetes mellitus is the greatly increased fragility of the retinal capillaries (Chap. 40). Diabetic retinopathy is the third leading cause of new blindness, for all ages, in the United States. It ranks first as the cause of new blindness in persons between the ages of 20 and 74 years.[1] Diabetic retinopathy can be divided into two types: background and proliferative. Background retinopathy is confined to the retina. It involves thickening of the retinal capillary walls and microaneurysm formation. Ruptured capillaries cause small intraretinal hemorrhages, and microinfarcts may cause cotton-wool exudates. A sensation of glare (because of the scattering of light) is a common complaint.

Some diabetics with background retinopathy develop neovascularization on the back of the vitreous (proliferative retinopathy). New vessels with delicate supporting tissue grow from the retina. When this happens, the retina is still attached to the vitreous, and the neovascular tissue adheres to the posterior vitreous, forming a contractile vascular membrane. Repeated bleeding into the vitreous results from contraction of the vascular membrane, accompanied by retinal tears, detachment, and progressive blindness. Photocoagulation provides the only major direct treatment modality for the neovascularization that leads to microhemorrhage. It destroyes not only the proliferating vessels, but also the ischemic retina, and therefore reduces the stimulus for further neovascularization. Vitrectomy has proved effective in removing vitreous hemorrhage and severing vitreoretinal membranes that develop.

Hypertensive retinopathy.

Long-standing systemic hypertension results in the compensatory thickening of arteriolar walls, which effectively reduces capillary perfusion pressure. Ordinarily, retinal blood vessels are transparent and are seen as a red line; in venules, the red cells resemble a string of boxcars. The thickened arterioles in chronic hypertension become opaque and have a copperwiring appearance. Edema, microaneurysms, intraretinal hemorrhages, exudates, and cotton-wool spots are all observed. Malignant hypertension involves swelling of the optic disk as a result of the local edema produced by escaped fluid. If the condition is permitted to progress long enough, serious visual deficits result.

Sudden increases in blood pressure do not permit the protective thickening of arteriolar walls, and hemorrhage is likely to occur. Trauma to the optic globe or the head, sudden high blood pressure in eclampsia, and some types of renal disease are characteristically accompanied by edema of the retina and optic disk as well as an increased likelihood of hemorrhage.

Macular degeneration.

Macular degeneration is characterized by destructive changes of the macula resulting from vascular disorders. It is the leading cause of blindness in persons over 75 and of new blindness among persons over age 65 years.[1] Macular degeneration is characterized by the loss of central vision, usually in both eyes. The individual may find it difficult to see at long distances (*e.g.*, in driving), to do close work (*e.g.*, reading), to see faces clearly, or to distinguish colors. However, the person may not be severely incapacitated because the peripheral retinal function usually remains intact. With the help of low-vision aids, individuals can usually continue their normal activities.

The most common causes of macular degeneration are neovascularization and sclerosis of the choriocapillaries. Although rare, macular degeneration can occur as a hereditary condition in young people and sometimes in adults. With neovascularization there is growth of new vessels in the potential space between Bruch's membrane and the basement membrane of the pigment epithelium. It usually occurs in the posterior pole of the retina in areas where there is an abnormality of Bruch's membrane because of senile degeneration, choroidal scars, or high myopia. The new vessels cause serous and hemorrhagic detachment of the pigment epithelium and loss of vision. Sclerosis of the choriocapillaries, with irregular thickening of Bruch's membrane, is a frequent finding in the elderly. Loss of central vision may result from atrophy of the pigment epithelium, serous detachment, or development of new vessels with subsequent bleeding.

Retinal detachment.

Retinal detachment involves the separation of the sensory retina from the pigment epithelium (Fig. 46-20). It occurs when traction on the inner sensory layer or a tear in this layer allows fluid, usually vitreous, to accumulate between the two layers. Retinal detachment that occurs secondary to breaks in the sensory layer of the retina is termed rhegmatogenous detachment (rhegma in Greek meaning "rent" or "hole"). The vitreous is normally adherent to the retina at the optic disk, macula, and periphery of the retina. When the vitreous shrinks, it separates from the retina at the posterior pole of the eye (posterior vitreous detachment); but at the periphery, the vitreous pulls on the attached retina, which can lead to tearing of the retina. Sometimes flashing lights (photopsias) are experienced

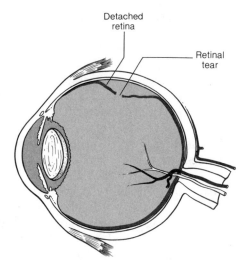

Figure 46-20   *Detached retina.*

when this occurs. Vitreous fluid can then enter the tear and add to the separation of the retina from its overlying pigment layer. Such tears can progress to retinal detachment. Detachment may also occur secondary to the presence of exudates that separate the two retinal layers. Exudative detachment may occur secondary to intraocular inflammations, intraocular tumors, or certain systemic diseases. Inflammatory processes include posterior scleritis, uveitis, or parasitic invasion. Leakage is most likely in vessels susceptible to damage, such as vessels of the retina (retina hemangioblastoma) and vessels of neoplasms of the choroid and retina.

Detachment of the neural retina from the retinal pigment layer (retinal detachment) separates the receptors from their major blood supply, the choroid. If detachment continues for some time, permanent destruction and therefore blindness of that part of the retina will occur. The bipolar and ganglion cells will survive because their blood supply, by way of the retinal arteries, remains intact. Without receptors, however, there is no visual function.

The primary symptom of retinal detachment is loss of vision. There is no pain. Because the process begins in the periphery and spreads circumferentially and posteriorly, initial visual disturbances may involve only one quadrant of the visual field. Large peripheral detachments may be present without involvement of the macula, so that visual acuity remains unaffected. The tendency, however, is for detachments to enlarge until all of the retina is detached.

Diagnosis is based on the ophthalmoscopic appearance of the retina. Surgical repair of extensive retinal detachment follows several strategies. One method, called scleral buckling, involves forcing infolds of the sclera so as to oppose the separated pigment and

retinal layers (Fig. 46-21). Another approach is used in severe cases. After the eyeball at the flat part of the ciliary body (pars plana) is surgically entered, the vitreous and retina are manipulated with instruments. When approximation of the two layers is accomplished, tiny laser beam burns are often made so that subsequent scar formation will weld the layers together.

Retinitis pigmentosa.   Retinitis pigmentosa is a group of hereditary diseases that cause slow degenerative changes in the retinal receptors. Slow destruction of the rods occurs, progressing from the peripheral to the central regions of the retina. Based on research with animal models, the probable mechanism of the disorder is a defect in phagocytic mechanisms of the pigment cells that cause membrane debris to accumulate and destroy the photoreceptors. The destruction results in dark lines and areas in which the pigment of the retinal pigment layer is unmasked by receptor loss. Night blindness, the first symptom of the disorder, often begins in early youth, with gross visual handicap occurring in the middle or advanced years. At present there is no effective treatment for this group of hereditary diseases.

Ultraviolet retinopathies.   Intense ultraviolet light is capable of destroying all the cells of the retina. Prolonged gazing at the sum is ordinarily prevented by the accompanying intense activity of the visual reflex mechanism. However, as a result of mental illness or drug-altered states some individuals may look at the sun for longer than a few seconds. This action results in focal burn of the macular retina (solar retinopathy), producing permanent damage to high-acuity vision. Direct viewing of a solar eclipse has similar effects because background light, and thus the protective reflexes, are reduced while direct and destructive ultraviolet light from the surface of the sun remains. Damage from arc welding without ultraviolet shielding and from electrical and lightning flash have the same basis.

Tests of retinal function

The diagnosis of retinal disease is based on history, tests of visual acuity, refraction, visual field tests, color vision tests, and often fluorescein angiography. Electroretinography (ERG) can be used to measure the electrical activity of the retina in response to a flash of light. The recorded ERG represents the difference in electrical potential between an electrode placed in a corneal contact lens and one placed on the forehead. The test can be used to evaluate retinal function in persons with an opaque lens or vitreous body. The electro-oculogram (EOG) records the electrical potentials between the front of the eye and the retina in the back of the eye. It is recorded from two electrodes placed on the forehead.

The EOG measures eye movement and is frequently used in sleep studies.

In summary, the retina covers the inner aspect of the posterior two-thirds of the eyeball and is continuous with the optic nerve. It contains the neural receptors for vision, and it is here that light energy of different frequencies and intensities is converted to graded action potentials and transmitted to visual centers in the brain. The retina is composed of an outer pigmented layer, which prevents the scattering of light stimuli and contains the enzymes for the synthesis of visual pigments. There are two types of photoreceptors: rods, capable of black and white discrimination, and cones, capable of color discrimination. Both rods and cones contain visual pigments. With exposure to light energy within a particular frequency, the visual pigment decomposes, causing nerve excitation. There is a maximal density of cones in an area of the posterior retina called the macula. The fovea centralis, the area of highest acuity, has no rods and contains the highest concentration of cones. The rods, which sense maximal spatial relationships, have their highest density toward the periphery of the eye. The photoreceptors normally shed portions of their outer segments. These segments are phagocytized by cells in the pigment epithelium. Failure of phagocytosis, as in retinitis pigmentosa, results in degeneration of the pigment layer and blindness. The retina receives its blood from two sources: the choriocapillaries, which supply the pigment layer and the outer portion of the sensory retina adjacent to the choroid, and the branches of the retinal artery, which supply the inner half of the retina. The retinal blood vessels are normally apparent through the ophthalmoscope. Disorders of retinal vessels can result from a number of local and systemic disorders, including diabetes mellitus, hypertension, sickle cell anemia, and vascular changes associated with aging. They cause vision loss through changes that result in hemorrhage and the production of opacities and separation of the pigment epithelium and sensory retina.

Visual Pathways and Cortical Centers

Full visual function requires normally developed brain-related functions of photoreception, visual sensation, and perception. These functions depend on the integrity of the retinal circuitry, optic nerve, forebrain, midbrain, and, to some extent, spinal cord.

Optic pathways

Visual information is carried to the brain by the axons of the retinal ganglion cells forming the optic nerve. Surrounded by pia mater, CSF, arachnoid, and dura mater,

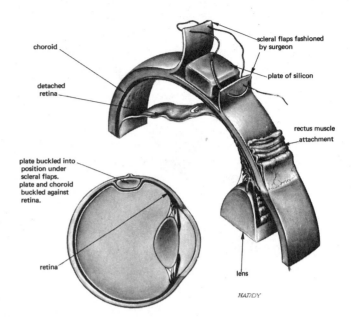

Figure 46-21 *Scleral buckling for detached retina (Ethicon, Inc.). (From Brunner LS , Suddarth DS: Textbook of Medical-Surgical Nursing, 5th ed. JB Lippincott, 1984)*

the optic nerve represents an outgrowth of the brain rather than a peripheral nerve. The optic nerve extends from the back of the optic globe through the orbit and the optic foramen, into the middle fossa, and on to the optic chiasm at the base of the brain—a distance of 40 mm to 50 mm in the adult (Fig. 46-22). Axons from the nasal half of the retina remain medial and those from the temporal retina remain lateral in the optic nerve.

The two optic nerves meet and fuse at the optic chiasm, located on the ventral and most rostral end of the brain stem, just in front of the infundibular stalk and pituitary gland. In the chiasm, axons from the nasal retina of the opposite side and axons from the temporal retina on the same side are organized to form the optic tracts. Thus, one optic tract contains fibers from both eyes that are transmitting information from the same visual field. The fibers of the optic tracts move laterally around the cerebral peduncles to synapse in the lateral geniculate nucleus (LGN) of the thalamus and from there pass through the optic radiation to the primary visual cortex in the calcarine area of the occipital lobe. The LGN receives input from the visual cortex, oculomotor centers in the brain stem, and the brain stem reticular formation. It is thought to modify the pattern and strength of the retinal input. Axons from cells located in the lateral geniculate form the optic radiations that travel to the visual cortex. The pattern for information transmission that was established in the optic tract is retained in the optic radiations. For example, the axons from the right visual field, represented by the nasal retina

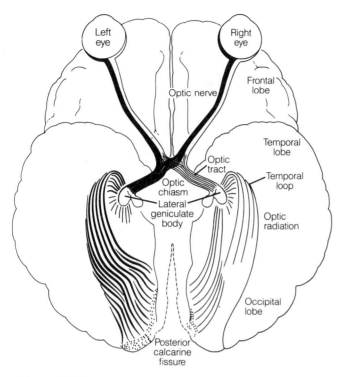

Figure 46-22   *Optic pathways. All of the nasal fibers of the right and left eye decussate (cross) at the optic chiasm. (From Newell FW: Ophthalmology: Principles and Concepts, 5th ed. St Louis CV Mosby, 1982)*

of the right eye and the left temporal retina of the left eye, are united at the chiasm and continue through the left optic tract and left optic radiation to the left visual cortex, where visual experience is first perceived. The left primary visual cortex thus receives two representations of the right visual field. The left LGN and the left primary

visual cortex retain physical separation of information from the left and right representations of the right visual field. At the cortical level, interaction between these slightly disparate representations occurs and provides the basis for the sensation of depth in the near visual field.

Visual cortex

The primary visual cortex (area 17) is located in the calcarine fissure of the occipital lobe; it is at this level that visual sensation is first experienced (Fig. 46-23). The immediately neighboring associational visual cortex (areas 18 and 19), together with their thalamic nuclei, must be functional for added meaningfulness of visual perception. This higher-order aspect of the visual experience depends on previous learning.

Approximately 1 million retinal ganglion cell axons pass through the optic nerve and tract to reach the LGN in the thalamus, and more than 100 million geniculate neuron axons provide the input to the billions of neurons in the visual cortex. Here the spatial representation of the visual field is retained in a distorted retinal map. The proportion of cells of the LGN and of the primary visual area devoted to analysis of the central visual field is greatly expanded, compared with that of the peripheral retina. From 80% to 90% of the cellular mass and area of the primary visual cortex is concerned with central vision. This accounts for the greatly increased visual acuity of central vision, not only at the retina but also at all levels of the visual pathway.

Circuitry in both the primary visual cortex and the associational visual areas is extremely discrete with respect to the location of retinal stimulation. For example, specific neurons respond to the moving edge of a particular inclination, specific colors, or familar shapes.

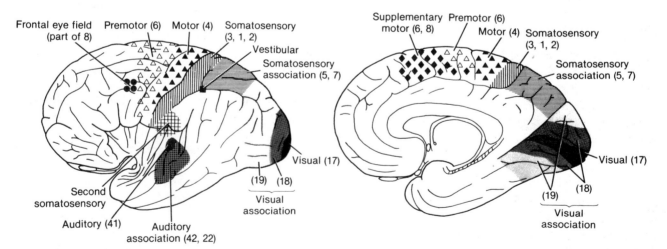

Figure 46-23   *Lateral view of the cortex with the lateral sulcus pried open to expose the insula (left) and medial section of the cortex (right), illustrating the location of the visual, visual association, auditory, and auditory association areas. (From Nolte J: The Human Brain, p 271. St Louis, CV Mosby, 1981. Reproduced with permission.)*

This fine-grained organization of the visual cortex with functionally separate and multiple representations of the same visual field provides the major basis for visual sensation and perception. Because of this discrete circuitry, lesions of the visual cortex must be large to be detected clinically.

A flash of light delivered to the retina will evoke potentials that can be measured and recorded by placing electrodes on the scalp over the occipital lobes. The waves of the evoked potentials have proven to be a useful tool for clinical evaluation of the functional integrity of the successive levels of the visual pathway.

Visual fields

The visual field refers to that area that is visible during fixation of vision in one direction. Because the visual system is organized with reference to the visual fields rather than to direct measures of neural function, the terminology for normal and abnormal visual characteristics is usually based on visual field orientation.

Most of the visual field is binocular, or seen by both eyes. This binocular field is subdivided into central and peripheral portions. The central portion provides high visual acuity and corresponds to the field focused on the central fovea; the peripheral and surrounding portion provides the capacity to detect objects, particularly moving objects. Beyond the visual field shared by both eyes, the left lateral periphery of the visual field is seen exclusively by the left nasal retina, and the right peripheral field by the right nasal retina.

As with a camera, the simple lens system of the eye inverts the image of the external world on each retina. The right and left sides of the visual field are also reversed. The right binocular visual field is seen by the left retinal halves of each eye: the nasal half of the right eye and the temporal half of the left eye.

Once the level of the retina is reached, the nervous system plays a consistent game. The upper half of the visual field is received by the lower half of the retinas of both eyes, and the representations of this upper half of the field are carried in the lower half of each optic nerve to synapse in the lower half of the LGN of each side of the brain. Neurons in this part of the LGN send their axons through the inferior half of the optic radiation to the lower half of the primary visual cortex on each side of the brain.

Because of the lateral separation of the two eyes, the visual field as viewed by the two eyes results in a slightly different view of the world by each eye, called *binocular disparity*. Disparity between the laterally displaced images seen by the two eyes provides a powerful source of three-dimensional depth perception for objects within a distance of 30 m. Beyond that distance, the difference in the two images becomes insignificant, and depth perception is based on other cues such as the superimposi-

tion of the image of near objects over that of far objects, or the relatively faster movement of near objects than of far objects.

Visual field defects. Visual field defects occur as a result of damage to the visual pathways or the visual cortex. Visual field testing or perimetry is used to identify defects and determine the location of lesions.

Retinal defects. All of us possess a hole, or scotoma, in our visual field of which we are unaware. Because the optic nerve does not contain photoreceptors, a corresponding location in the visual field constitutes a blind spot. Local retinal damage caused by small vascular accidents (retinal stroke) and other localized pathology can produce additional blind spots. As with the normal blind spot, persons are not usually aware of the existence of scotomata in their visual fields unless they encounter problems seeing objects in certain restricted parts of the visual field.

Absences near or in the center of the bilateral visual field can be annoying and even disastrous. Although the hole is not recognized as such, the person finds that a part of a printed page appears or disappears depending on where the fixation point is held. Most persons learn to position their eyes so as to use the remaining central foveal vision for high-acuity tasks. Defects in the peripheral visual field, including the monocular peripheral fields, are less annoying but potentially more dangeous. Often the person is unaware of the defect and, when walking or driving an automobile, does not see cars or bicyclists until their image reaches the functional visual field—sometimes too late to avert an accident. With careful education, an individual can learn to constantly shift the gaze in such a way as to obtain visual coverage of important parts of the visual field. If the damage is at the retinal or optic nerve level, only the monocular field of the damaged eye becomes a problem. A lesion affecting the central foveal vision of one eye can result in complaints of eye strain during reading and other close work, because only one eye is really being used. Localized damage to the optic tracts, LGN, optic radiation, or primary visual cortex will affect corresponding parts of the visual fields of both eyes.

Disorders of the optic pathways. The visual pathway extends from the front to the back of the head. It is much like a telephone line between distant points in that damage at any point along the pathway results in functional defects (Fig. 46-24). Among the disorders that can interrupt the visual pathway are vascular lesions, trauma, and tumors. For example, normal visual system function depends on vascular adequacy in the ophthalmic artery and its branches; the central artery of the retina; the anterior and middle cerebral arteries, which supply the

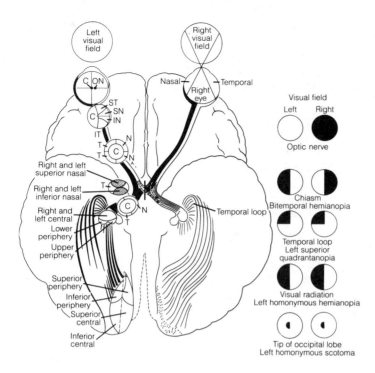

Figure 46-24 *Typical visual field defects that occur with damage to different regions of the optic pathways. Visual fields are diagrammed to reflect the source of the light that stimulates the retina. Light from the temporal side stimulates the nasal portion of the retina, light from above stimulates the lower portion, and so on. Thus, the visual field defect caused by a lesion affecting fibers arising from the nasal half of the retina is diagrammed as a temporal field defect. (From Newell FW: Ophthalmology: Principles and Concepts, 5th ed. St Louis, CV Mosby, 1982)*

intracranial optic nerve, chiasm, and optic tracts; and the posterior cerebral artery, which supplies the lateral geniculate, optic radiation, and visual cortex. In turn, adequacy of the posterior cerebral artery function depends on that of the vertebral and basilar arteries that supply the brain stem. Vascular insufficiency in any one of these arterial systems can seriously affect vision. Examination of the visual system function is of particular diagnostic use because lesions at various points along the pathway have characteristic symptoms that assist in the localization of pathology.

Visual field defects of each eye and of the two eyes together are useful in localizing lesions affecting the system. Blindness in one eye is termed *anopia*. If half of the visual field for one eye is lost, the defect is termed *hemianopia;* loss of a quarter field is called *quadrantanopia*. Enlarging pituitary tumors can produce longitudinal damage through the optic chiasm with loss of retinal ganglion cell axons from the retinas of both eyes. As a result, the lateral half-field of each eye is lost, and a very narrow binocular visual field results, commonly called *tunnel vision*. The loss of different half-fields, in the two eyes is called a *heteronymous* loss, and the abnormality is called *bitemporal heteronymous hemianopia*. Destruction of one or both lateral halves of the chiasm is not uncommon with multiple aneurysms of the circle of Willis. Here the function of the left or both temporal retinas occurs, and the nasal fields of the left or of both eyes are lost. The loss of the nasal fields of both eyes is called *bitemporal heteronymous anopia*. With both eyes open, the person with bilateral defects still has the full binocular visual field.

Loss of the optic tract, lateral geniculate, full optic radiation, or complete visual cortex on one side results in loss of the corresponding visual half-fields in each eye. In left-sides lesions, the right visual field is lost for each eye and is called *complete right homonymous hemianopia. Homonymous* means the same for both eyes. Partial injury to the left optic tract, LGN, or optic radiation can result in the loss of a quarter of the visual field, again the same for both eyes. This is called *homonymous quadrantanopia* and, depending on the lesion, it can involve the upper (superior) or lower (inferior) fields.

Disorders of the visual cortex.   Discrete damage in the binocular portion of the primary visual cortex can also result in scotomas in the corresponding visual fields. If the visual loss is in the central high-acuity part of the field, severe loss of visual acuity and pattern discrimination occur. Such damage is permanent and cannot be corrected with lenses.

The bilateral loss of the entire primary visual cortex, called *cortical blindness,* eliminates all visual experience. Some suggestion remains that crude analysis of visual stimulation exists on reflex levels. Eye-orienting and head-orienting responses to bright moving lights, pupillary reflexes, and blinking at sudden bright light are retained even though vision has been lost.

Testing of visual fields.   Crude testing of the binocular visual field and the visual field of each individual eye (monocular vision) can be accomplished without specialized equipment. In the confrontation method, the examiner stands or sits 2 feet to 3 feet in front of the person to be tested and instructs the person to focus on an object such as a penlight with one eye closed. The object is moved from the center toward the periphery of the person's visual field and from the periphery toward the center, and the person is instructed to report the presence or absence of the object. By moving the object through the vertical, horizontal, and oblique aspects of the visual field, a crude estimate can be made of the visual field. If the test object is kept midway between the examiner and the person being tested, the examiner can close the corresponding eye and compare the person's monocular vision with his or her own. Large field defects can be estimated by the confrontation method, and it may be the only way for testing young children and uncooperative adults.

Accurate determination of the presence, size, and shape of smaller holes, or scotomata, in the visual field of a particular eye can be demonstrated by the ophthalmologist only through the use of a method known as *perimetry*. This is done by having the person look with one eye toward a central spot directly in front of the eye while the head is stabilized by a chin rest or bite board. A small dot of light or a colored object is moved back and forth in all areas of the visual field. The person reports whether or not the stimulus is visible and, if a colored stimulus is used, what the perceived color is. A hemispherical support is used to control and standarize the movement of the test object, and a plot of radial coordinates of the visual field is made (see Fig. 46-9). Perimetry provides a means of determining alterations from normal and, with repeated testing, a way of following the progress of the disease or treatment.

In summary, visual information is carried to the brain by axons of the retinal ganglion cells forming the optic nerve. The two optic nerves meet and fuse in the optic chiasm. The axons of each nasal retina cross in the chiasm and join the uncrossed fibers of the temporal retina of the opposite eye in the optic tract. From the optic chiasm, the crossed fibers of the nasal retina of one eye and the uncrossed temporal fibers of the other eye pass to the LGN and then to the primary visual cortex, which is located in the calcarine fissure of the occipital lobe. Damage to the visual pathways or visual cortex leads to visual field defects that can be identified through visual field testing or perimetry and used to determine the lesion's location.

Eye Movements

Normal vision is dependent on the coordinated action of the entire visual system involving the neural and muscular pathways of the brain. It is through these mechanisms that an object is simultaneously imaged on the fovea of both eyes and perceived as a single image. Strabismus and amblyopia are two disorders that affect this highly integrated system.

Extrinsic eye muscles

Each eyeball can rotate around its vertical axis (lateral or medial rotation in which the pupil moves away from or toward the nose), its horizontal left–right axis (vertical elevation or depression in which the pupil moves up or down), and its longitudinal horizontal axis (intorsion or extorsion in which the top of the pupil moves toward or away from the nose).

Six extrinsic muscles (four rectus and two oblique) control the movement of each eye (Fig. 46-25). The four rectus muscles are named according to where they insert into the sclera on the medial, lateral, inferior, and superior surfaces of the eye. The two oblique muscles insert on the lateral posterior quadrant of the eyeball: the superior oblique on the upper surface and the inferior oblique on the lower. Each of the three sets of muscles in each eye is reciprocally innervated so that one muscle relaxes when the other contracts. The middle and lateral recti contract reciprocally to move the eye from side to side; the superior and inferior recti contract to move the eye up and down. The oblique muscles rotate the eye around its optic axis. Although the origins and insertions of the extrinsic eye muscles would seem to make their role in eye movement predictable, their function is somewhat complex. This is because the muscles insert into a rotatable eyeball.

Inserting approximately on the horizontal plane, the antagonistic medial and lateral recti rotate the eye medially (adduction) or laterally (abduction). When the optical axes of the two eyes are parallel, these muscles provide horizontal conjugate (paired) gaze. Convergence (moving toward a common point) and divergence (moving away from a common point) of the optical axes of the eyes result from the differential contraction of the recti muscles accompanied by coordinated inhibition of the antagonistic muscles. The phrase *being yoked together* is often used to describe such direct antagonism between eye muscles.

The actions of the superior and inferior recti are more complex. Their predominant action is the elevation and depression of the eyeball, usually a conjugate movement. Because of their medial orbit origin, both muscles contribute to medial rotation. In addition, each contributes to some extent to intorsion (superior rectus) and extorsion (inferior rectus). A major function of the oblique muscles is the extorsion (the inferior oblique pulls the inferior surface of the eyeball medially) and the intorsion (the superior oblique pulls the superior surface of the eyeball medially) of the optic globe. These muscles function as antagonists for rotation around the longitudinal axis of the eye. Because of the insertion position

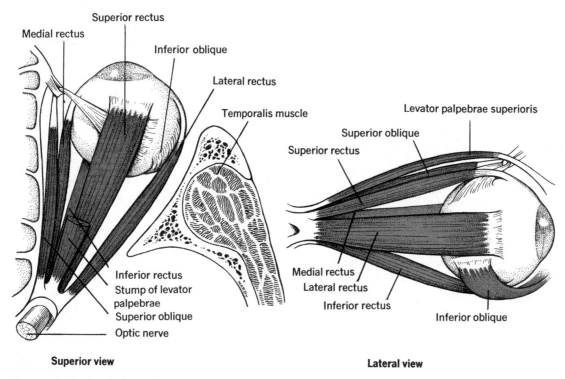

Figure 46-25   *Extrinsic muscles of the right eye:* (left) *viewed from above within the orbital cavity;* (right) *lateral view. (From Chaffee EE, Lytle IM: Basic Anatomy and Physiology, 4th ed. Philadelphia, JB Lippincott, 1980)*

posterior to the equator of the eyeball, the superior oblique pulls the upward-pointed eye downward, assisting the function of the inferior rectus. The inferior oblique, similarly, pulls upward a downward-pointed eye, assisting the superior rectus. When the eye is strongly medially deviated, the oblique muscles function almost entirely as elevator and depressor muscles.

The extraocular muscles are innervated by three cranial nerves: the trochlear (IV) innervates the superior oblique, the abducens (VI) innervates the lateral rectus, and the oculomotor (III) innervates the remaining four muscles. The medial longitudinal fasciculus (MLF) connects the nuclei of these cranial nerves. This important tract system transmits impulses that coordinate conjugate movements of the eye. Eye movements are further influenced by input from control centers in the frontal cortex (frontal premotor area), the visual association area, and the superior colliculus, a midbrain optic reflex center that is concerned with eye movements. Strong signals are also transmitted into the oculomotor system from the vestibular nuclei by way of the MLF (to be discussed later).

Eye movements and gaze

Conjugate movements are those in which the optical axes of the two eyes are kept parallel, sharing the same visual field. *Gaze* refers to the act of looking steadily in one direction. Eye movements can be categorized into fives classes of movement: smooth pursuit, saccadic, vestibular, vergence, and tremor. Smooth pursuit (object following), saccadic (position correcting), and vestibular (nystagmus) movements involve conjugate coordination. *Vergence* (divergence and convergence) movements involve coordinated movements of the eyes in opposite directions. A *tremor* refers to involuntary rhythmic oscillatory (quivering) movements. Small-range optical tremor is a normal and useful independent function of each eye. Eye movements are important motor capabilities that are integrated into vestibular, auditory, and visual reflex and learned functions.

Smooth pursuit movements.   Smooth pursuit movements are tracking movements that serve to maintain an object at a fixed point in the center of the visual fields of both eyes. The object may be moving and the eyes following it, or the object may be stationary and the head of the observer moving. Voluntary pursuit movements are tested by asking the person to follow a finger or another object as it is moved smoothly through the visual field. Successful conjugate following requires a functional optic system communicating to the superior colliculus and to the primary visual cortex. The communication from the primary visual cortex to the superior colliculus must also be functional.

Normal eye posture is a conjugate gaze directed straight forward with the head held in a forward-looking posture. Smooth pursuit movements normally begin from this position. In fact, holding a strongly deviated gaze becomes tiring within about 30 seconds, and most people will make head and body rotation adjustments to bring the eyes to a central position within that time period.

Saccadic movements. Saccadic eye movements are sudden, jerky conjugate movements that quickly change the fixation point. During reading, the fixation pattern involves a focus on a word or short series of words and then a sudden jump of the eyes to a new fixation point on the next word or phrase. These shifts in fixation points are saccadic movements. The neural circuitry that makes coordinated saccadic movements possible remains under study, but certain areas of the midbrain reticular formation are essential for these movements. Saccadic movements are quick readjustments of the binocular fixation point that must occur to accomplish a change in fixation. This readjustment occurs while searching the visual environment. Changes in fixation point must be accomplished quickly in order to provide the individual with a new, stable part of the visual field on which to focus. No sensation of blur is experienced during the period of rapid eye movement, although the mechanism by which the blurred vision is eliminated is not understood.

The visual startle reaction in which the eyes are quickly turned in the direction of a sudden and intense visual stimulus entering the periphery of the visual field, is saccadic movement initiated by the optic system. This reflex occurs in the absence of the cortical portion of the visual system (cortical blindness). The auditory startle reaction (startle reflex) involves rapid saccadic movements in the direction of a sudden auditory stimulus. It is present in the neonate and in persons with impaired cortical auditory apparatus.

The frontal eye fields of the premotor cortex are of critical importance for voluntary saccadic movements such as reading. If this frontal premotor area is not functional, a person can describe objects in the visual field but cannot voluntarily search the visual environment.

Vergence movements. Convergence of the optical axes of the two eyes is an automatic aspect of changing binocular fixation from a distant to a close fixation point. This readjustment of the position of each eye in relation to the other accompanies changes in ciliary muscle activity that affect the lens shape and pupillary dilation that exposes more of the lens refractive surface. All of these adjustments function to permit a closer and sharper binocular retinal image and are included in the function of accommodation. Convergence can occur smoothly as a pursuitlike, continuous adjustment when a moving object approaches the observer. Convergence can also occur as a saccadic movement when fixation is changed from a distant to a near object, or vice versa. Divergence occurs when a fixated object recedes in the visual field. The convergence–divergence aspect of accommodation requires a functional visual cortex and intact projection to the pretectal area and to the parasympathetic efferent neurons of the oculomotor nerve. A region of the midbrain reticular formation near the oculomotor nuclei must also be functional for convergence to occur. Master control is by the depth perception mechanism of the occipital visual association cortex. Voluntary convergence is achieved by altering the fixation point to one close to the eyes, requiring participation of the frontal eye fields.

Optic tremor. Without special equipment, the very fine continuous tremor of each eye is difficult to detect. This tremor is attributed to the inequality in the number of motor units active in opposing extraocular muscles at any moment. Because of the great amplification factor between the minute shifts in eye position relative to the large shifts in a distant fixation point, one might expect eye tremor to be a serious impediment to acuity. Yet, the visual system functions rapidly enough to keep up with these minute shifts in fixation; if the tremor were eliminated, the visual image would quickly fade away through adaptation of the individual cone receptors. The function of the tremor is to keep the retinal image moving over the receptor array so that it is constantly encountering recovered or unadapted receptors.

Horizontal gaze. Lateral conjugate gaze is accomplished through a reflex mechanism involving the medulla, pons, and midbrain, which contain the sixth, fourth, and third cranial nerve nuclei. Lateral rotation of an eye results from the increased activity of the sixth-nerve-innervated lateral rectus muscle accompanied by the corresponding reduced activity of the third-nerve-innervated medial rectus muscle. Synergists of the medial rectus, the third-nerve-innervated superior and inferior recti, also must be inhibited. Communication between the sixth nerve and third nerve nuclei must be rapid and precise. Conjugate (bilateral) side-to-side eye movement involves lateral rotation of one eye and medial rotation of the other. This requires close coordination between the sixth nerve nucleus of one side and the third nerve nucleus of the other. Further, smooth movement in conjugate gaze requires continuous variation in the contractional tone in synergists as well as in opposing eye muscles throughout the full range of dual eye rotation.

Reflex coordination of lateral gaze involves a longitudinal tract system of the brain stem, the medial longitudinal fasciculus (MLF), that interconnects the lower motor neurons of the sixth and third cranial nerves. A region in the reticular formation near the sixth nerve nucleus, called the pontine gaze center, controls this highly coordinated reflex mechanism.

Destruction of the lateral gaze control region on one side results in ipsilateral gaze palsy, that is, there is lateral gaze to the contralateral side but not to the affected side. Interruption of the MLF on one side between the sixth and third nerve nuclei, called internuclear ophthalmoplegia, results in abnormality of the contralateral lateral gaze: the eye on the affected side fails to adduct (cranial nerve III) when the contralateral eye abducts (cranial nerve VI). Bilateral destruction of the MLF results in loss of adduction during lateral gaze to either side. A visual target moving smoothly in the horizontal plane is followed by this conjugate gaze mechanism through the intervention of the superior colliculus, which communicates directly with this gaze center through tectobulbar fibers. Conjugate following of a bright, smoothly moving target occurs automatically, even in the absence of a functional visual cortex. In deep coma, for instance, the presence of visual following indicates that the brain stem, including the midbrain, remains functional. Voluntary control of conjugate following of a horizontally moving object in the visual field requires the function of the primary and associational visual cortices that project axons to the superior colliculus.

When a lateral conjugate following movement exceeds the range of eye rotation, head rotation is often added. The MLF extends down to cervical spinal levels; descending control from the horizontal gaze center by way of this tract is exerted on the spinal accessory and other cervical-level lower motor neurons. By this means the powerful head-turning muscles, the sternocleidomastoid, and other cervical muscles are smoothly brought into play. The major function of the MLF is the coordination circuitry of the lateral gaze mechanism.

Vertical gaze. Vertical gaze, or the upward and downward rotation of an eye, involves four extraocular muscles. The third-nerve-innervated superior rectus and inferior oblique work in concert to rotate the eye upward with coordinated inhibition of the inferior rectus (III) cranial nerve and superior oblique (IV) cranial nerve. Conjugate vertical gaze, upward or downward, with parallel optical axes of the two eyes is coordinated by a vertical gaze center located in the midbrain deep to the rostral end of the MLF. Communication between this center and the innervational nuclei does not use the MLF. Instead, another major longitudinal tract system, the central tegmental fasciculus (CTF), provides longitudinal communication.

Torsional conjugate eye movements. Conjugate twisting, or torsion, of the two eyes occurs when the head is tipped to one side. Exact, appropriate countertorsion of the two eyes serves to preserve a stable visual field in spite of minor head movements. A torsion gaze center, or control region, in the reticular formation of the brain stem has yet to be clearly localized.

Conjugate gaze control is extremely precise, and the central circuits providing this capability are quite complex. The superior colliculus, the midbrain vertical and medullary horizontal gaze centers, and the cerebellum, which add temporal smoothness to these coordinated movements, are all involved.

Disorders of eye movement

Strabismus. Strabismus (heteropsia, or squint) refers to any abnormality of eye coordination that results in loss of binocular eye alignment and focus of a visual image on corresponding points of the two retinas. In standard terminology, the disorders of eye movement are described according to the direction of movement. *Esotropia* refers to medial deviation, *exotropia* to lateral deviation; *hypertropia* to upward deviation, *hypotropia* to downward deviation, and *cyclotropia* to torsional deviation. The term *concomitance* refers to equal deviation in all directions of gaze. A nonconcomitant strabismus is one that varies with the direction of gaze. Strabismus may be divided into (1) paralytic (nonconcomitant) forms, in which there is weakness or paralysis of one or more of the extraocular muscles, or (2) nonparalytic (concomitant), in which there is no primary muscle impairment. Strabismus is termed *intermittent*, or *periodic*, when there are periods in which the eyes are parallel. It is *monocular* when the same eye always deviates and the fellow eye fixates.

Paralytic strabismus. Paralytic strabismus results from paresis (weakness) or plegia (paralysis) of one or more of the extraocular muscles. When the normal eye fixates, the affected eye is in the position of primary deviation. In the case of esotropia, there is weakness of one of the lateral rectus muscles, usually the result of palsy of the abducens (VI) cranial nerve. When the affected eye fixates, the unaffected eye is in a position of secondary deviation. The secondary deviation of the unaffected eye is greater than the primary deviation of the affected eye. This is because the affected eye requires an excess of innervational impulse to maintain fixation; the excess impulses also are distributed to the unaffected eye (Hering's law of equal innervation), causing overaction of its muscles.[3]

Paralytic strabismus is uncommon in children but accounts for nearly all cases of adult strabismus; it can be caused by a number of conditions. Paralytic strabismus is most commonly seen in adults who have had cerebral vascular accidents and may also occur as the first sign of a tumor or inflammatory condition involving the central nervous system. One type of muscular dystrophy exerts its effects on the extraocular muscles. Initially eye movements in all directions are weak, with later progression to bilateral optic immobility. Weakness of eye movement and lid elevation is often the first evidence of myasthenia gravis. The pathway of the oculomotor (III), trochlear (IV), and abducens (VI) cranial nerves through the cavernous sinus and the back of the orbit make them vulnerable to basal skull fracture and tumors of the cavernous sinus (cavernous sinus syndrome) or orbit (orbital syndrome). In infants, paralytic strabismus can be caused by birth injuries affecting either the extraocular muscles or the cranial nerves supplying these muscles. It can also result from congenital anomalies of the muscles. In general, paralytic strabismus in an adult with previously normal binocular vision causes diplopia (double vision). This does not occur in individuals who have never developed binocular vision.

Nonparalytic strabismus. In nonparalytic strabismus there is no extraocular muscle weakness or paralysis, and the angle of deviation is always the same in all fields of gaze. With persistent deviation, secondary abnormalities may develop because of overaction or underaction of the muscles in some fields of gaze. Nonparalytic esotropia is the most common type of strabismus. The disorder may be accommodative, nonaccommodative, or a combination of the two. Accommodative strabismus is caused by disorders such as uncorrected hyperopia, in which the esotropia occurs with accommodation. The onset of this type of esotropia characteristically occurs at between 18 months and 4 years of age (because the accommodation is not well developed until that time). The disorder is most often monocular but may be alternating. About 50% of the cases of esotropia fall into this category. Characteristically the convergent deviation is manifested early in life, usually by the first year and often at birth. The causes of nonaccommodative strabismus are obscure. The disorder may be related to faulty muscle insertion, fascial abnormalities, or faulty innervation. There is evidence that idiopathic strabismus may have a genetic basis; siblings may have similar disorders.

Diagnosis and treatment. Examination by a qualified practitioner is indicated in any infant whose eyes are not aligned at all times during waking hours after 6 months of age.[3] Diagnostic measures emphasize two major areas: (1) ocular deviation and (2) visual acuity. Rapid assessment of extraocular muscle function is accomplished by three methods. First, in a somewhat darkened room and with the child staring straight ahead, a penlight is pointed at the midpoint between the two eyes,

and a bright dot of reflected light can be seen on the cornea of each eye. With normal eye alignment, the reflected light should appear at the same spot on the cornea of each eye. Nonparallelism of the two eyes indicates muscle imbalance because of weakness or paralysis of the deviant eye. With the second method, the person is asked to follow the movement of a small object (a pencil point or lighted penlight) as it is moved through the extremes of what are called the six cardinal positions of gaze. In extreme lateral gaze, normal subjects can show a few quick beats of a jerky or nystagmoid movement (to be discussed). Nystagmoid movement is abnormal if it is prolonged or present in any other eye posture. The third method (called the cover–uncover test) eliminates binocular fusion as a factor in maintaining parallelism between the eyes. The examiner looks at the patient and estimates which eye is used for fixation. The patient's attention is directed toward a fixation object such as a small picture or tongue blade. A light should not be used because it may not stimulate accommodation. If a mild weakness is present, the eye with blocked vision will drift into a resting position, the extent of which depends on the relative strength of the muscles. The eye should snap back when the card is removed. The test is always done for both near and far fixation. Visual acuity is evaluated to obtain a comparison of the two eyes. An illiterate E chart (or similar test chart) can be used for young children.

Treatment of strabismus is directed toward the development of normal visual acuity, the correction of the deviation, and superimposition of the retinal images to provide binocular vision. Both nonsurgical and surgical methods can be used. In children, early treatment is important; the ideal age to begin is 6 months. Nonsurgical treatment includes occlusive patching, pleoptics, and prism glasses. Occlusive patching (alternating between the affected and the unaffected eye) may be used to prevent loss of vision in one eye. Pleoptics is a method used to disrupt eccentric fixation and establish foveal fixation. With one technique, the entire retina around the fovea is stimulated by a ophthalmoscope light source that has a central dark shield to protect the macula from the stimulation. After the light has been removed, the macula stands out as a positive afterimage, followed by a negative afterimage. The patient is taught that the afterimage is in the straight-ahead position, and in this way foveal vision can be gradually restored to the straight-ahead position. Many hours of pleoptic training are required for reorientation of the fovea. Prism glasses compensate for an abnormal alignment of an optic globe. Long-acting miotics in weak strengths (echothiophate iodide solution, Phospholine, or isoflurophate ointment, Floropryl) may be used in treating accommodative esotropia. In young children these drugs can be used instead of glasses. They act by altering the accommodative convergence relationship in a favorable manner so that fusion is maintained despite accommodation. Miosis also allows for clearer vision with less accommodation in both near and far vision. Surgical procedures may be used to strengthen a muscle or weaken a muscle by altering its length or attachment site. Surgery should not be done until maximum visual acuity has been restored by means of patching or pleoptics.

Amblyopia. Amblyopia describes a condition of diminished vision (uncorrectable by lenses) in which no detectable organic lesion of the eye is present. This condition is sometimes referred to as *lazy eye*. It is caused by visual deprivation (conditions such as cataracts) or abnormal binocular interactions (strabismus or anisometropia) during visual immaturity. Normal development of the thalamic and cortical circuitry necessary for binocular visual perception requires simultaneous binocular use of each fovea during a critical period of time early in life (0 to 5 years).[3] In infants with monocular cataracts, this time is before 4 months of age. In conditions causing abnormal binocular interactions, one image is suppressed to provide clearer vision. In esotropia, vision of the deviated eye is suppressed to prevent diplopia. A similar situation exists in anisometropia in which the refractive indexes of the two eyes are different. Even though the eyes are correctly aligned, they are unable to focus together and the image of one eye is suppressed. In experimental animals monocular deprivation results in reduced synaptic density in the LGN and the primary visual cortical areas that process input from the affected eye or eyes.

The reversibility of amblyopia depends on the maturity of the visual system at the time of onset and the duration of the abnormal experience. If esotropia is involved, some individuals will alternate eyes and not experience diplopia. With late-adolescent or adult onset, this habit pattern must be unlearned after correction.

Peripheral vision is less affected than central foveal vision in amblyopia. Suppression becomes more evident with high illumination and high contrast. It is as if the affected eye did not possess central vision and the person learns to fixate with the nonfoveal retina. If bilateral congenital blindness or near blindness (*e.g.,* cataracts) occurs and remains uncorrected during infancy and early childhood, the person will remain without pattern vision and will have only overall field brightness and color discrimination. This is essentially bilateral amblyopia.

Treatment. The treatment of children with the potential for developing amblyopia must be instituted well before the age of 6 to avoid the suppression phenomenon.

Surgery for congenital cataracts and ptosis should be done early. Severe refractive errors should be corrected. In strabismus, alternately blocking vision in one eye and then the other forces the child to use both eyes for form discrimination. The duration of occlusion of vision in the good eye must be short and closely monitored or deprivation amblyopia can develop in the good eye as well. Although amblyopia is not likely to occur after the age of 8 or 9, plasticity in central circuitry is evident even in adulthood. For example, after refractive correction for long-standing astigmatism in adults, visual acuity improves slowly, requiring several months to reach normal levels.

In summary, normal vision depends on coordinated movement of the two eyes. Eye movements depend on the action of six extraocular muscles (four rectus and two oblique) and their cranial (III, IV, and VI) nerve innervation. Conjugate eye movements are those in which the optical axes of the two eyes are kept parallel, sharing the same visual field. There are five types of eye movements: smooth pursuit (tracking movements), saccadic (position correcting), vestibular (nystagmus), vergence (divergence and convergence), and tremor (fine movements). Lateral gaze is used in viewing lateral objects. It involves the coordinated movements of the extraocular muscles and their cranial nerve nuclei, the MLF tract of the brain stem, and the pontine lateral gaze center. Unilateral destruction of the pontine gaze center results in ipsilateral gaze paralysis. Vertical gaze facilitates looking upward and downward. It is controlled by the action of the extraocular mucles and their cranial nerve nuclei, the central tegmental fasciculus pathway, and the midbrain vertical gaze center.

Disorders of eye movements include strabismus (heteropsia, or squint) and amblyopia. Strabismus refers to abnormalities in the coordination of eye movements with loss of binocular eye alignment and focus of a visual image on corresponding parts of the two retinas. Esotropia refers to medial deviation, exotropia to lateral deviation, hypertropia to upward deviation, hypotropia to downward deviation, and cyclotropia to torsional deviation. Paralytic strabismus is caused by weakness or paralysis of the extraocular muscles. Nonparalytic strabismus results from the inappropriate length or insertion of the extraocular muscles or from accommodation disorders. Amblyopia (lazy eye) is a condition of diminished vision that cannot be corrected by lenses and one in which no detectable organic lesion in the eye can be observed. It results from inadequately developed CNS circuitry because of visual deprivation (cataracts) or abnormal binocular interactions (strabismus or anisometropia) during the period of visual immaturity.

■ Hearing

Hearing is a specialized sense whose external stimulus is the vibration of sound waves. The compression waves that produce sound have both frequency and intensity. *Frequency* indicates the rate of change with time (cycles per second [cps] or hertz [Hz]). Most people cannot hear compressional waves that have a frequency higher than 20,000 Hz. Waves of higher frequency are called ultrasonic waves, meaning that they are above the audible range in terms of frequency. In the audible frequency range, the subjective experience correlated with sonic frequency is the pitch of a sound. Waves below 20 Hz to 30 Hz are experienced as a rattle or drum beat rather than a tone. The ear is most sensitive to waves in the frequency range of around 3000 Hz. Wave intensity is represented by either amplitude or units of sound pressure. By convention, the *intensity* (in power units, or ergs per square centimeter) of a sound is expressed as the ratio of intensities between the sound and a reference value. A tenfold increase in pressure is called a *bel,* after Alexander Graham Bell. This representation is often too crude to be of use; the most often used unit is the decibel, or one-tenth of a bel. In the normal sonic environment, approx-imately 1 decibel of increased intensity (loudness) can be detected. The region of intelligible speech sounds falls between 42 decibels and 70 decibels.

Auditory System

The ear receives sound waves, distinguishes their frequency, translates this information into nerve impulses, and transmits them to the central nervous system. The auditory system can be divided into five parts: the external ear, the middle ear, the inner ear, or cochlea, auditory brain stem pathways, and the primary and associational auditory cortex of the brain's temporal lobe.

External ear

The external ear is called the pinna, or auricle. It is supported by elastic cartilage and shaped like a funnel. The funnel shape concentrates high-frequency sound entering from the lateral–forward direction into the external acoustic meatus, or ear canal (Fig. 46-26). The shape also helps prevent front–back confusion of sound sources. The anterior portion of the pinna and external ear canal are innervated by branches of the mandibular division of the trigeminal (V) cranial nerve. The pos-

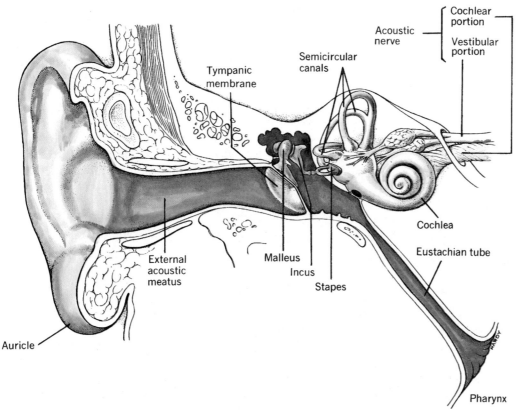

Figure 46-26 *The ear: external, middle, and internal subdivisions. (From Chaffee EE, Lytle IM: Basic Physiology and Anatomy, 4th ed. Philadelphia, JB Lippincott, 1980)*

terior portions, including the back of the external ear as well as the posterior wall of the ear canal, are innervated by auricular branches of the facial (VII), glossopharyngeal (IX), and vagus (X) cranial nerves. Because of the vagal innervation, the insertion of a speculum or an otoscope into the external ear canal can stimulate coughing or vomiting reflexes, particularly in small children.

The external acoustic meatus extends from the auricle to the tympanic membrane, or eardrum. Its outer two-thirds is supported by elastic cartilage, and its inner one-third by the tympanic bone. It is somewhat S-shaped and acts as a resonator, amplifying frequencies around 3500 Hz. It is lined by a thin layer of skin containing fine hairs, sebaceous glands, and ceruminous glands, which secrete protective cerumen or earwax. Earwax has certain antimicrobial properties and is thought to serve a protective function.

Tympanic membrane

The tympanic membrane (or eardrum), which separates the external ear from the middle ear, has three layers: (1) an outer layer of thin skin continuous with the lining of the external acoustic meatus, (2) a middle layer of tough collagenous fibers mixed with fibrocytes and some elastic fibers, and (3) an inner epithelial layer continuous with the lining of the middle ear. It is attached in a manner that allows it to vibrate freely when audible sound waves enter the external auditory canal. When viewed through an otoscope, the tympanic membrane appears as a shallow, almost circular cone pointing inward toward its apex, the umbo (Fig. 46-27). The landmarks include the lightened stripe over the handle of the malleus, the umbo at the end of the handle, the pars tensa, which constitutes most of the drum, and the pars flaccida, the small area above the malleus attachment. Light is usually reflected from the right side of the pars tensa at approximately the 4 o'clock position. Normally, the tympanic membrane is semitransparent, and a small whitish cord, which traverses the middle ear from back to front, can be seen just under its upper edge. This is the corda tympani, a branch of the intermedius component of the facial (VII) cranial nerve.

Middle ear and eustachian tube

The middle ear is a tiny cavity, roughly the shape of a red blood cell set on edge, located in the petrous (stony) temporal bone. Its lateral wall is formed by the tympanic membrane and its medial wall by the bone dividing the middle and inner ear. Two tissue-covered openings in the medial wall, the oval and the round windows, provide for communication between the middle and the inner ear. Posteriorly the middle ear is continuous with small air pockets in the temporal bone called *mastoid air spaces* or *cells* (Fig. 46-28). In early life these air spaces are filled with hematopoietic tissue. Replacement of hematopoietic tissue with air sacs begins during the third year of life and is completed at puberty.

There is a gap in the bone between the anterior and medial walls for a canal, called the *eustachian tube, or auditory canal,* that communicates with the nasopharynx (see Fig. 46-28). The middle ear is filled with the air that reaches it from the nasopharynx by way of the eustachian tube; it is lined with a mucous membrane that is continuous with the pharynx and mastoid air cells. Infections from the nasopharynx can travel from the nasopharynx along the mucous membrane of the auditory tube to the middle ear, causing otitis media. Near the opening of the eustachian tube, the columnar epithelial lining changes to the pseudostratified cilated-columnar surface of the pharynx, which contains occasional mucus-secreting cells. Hypertrophy of the mucus-secreting cells contributes to the mucoid secretions that develop during certain types of otitis media.

The eustachian tube, which connects the middle ear with the nasopharynx, serves three basic functions: (1) ventilation of the middle ear, along with equalization of middle ear and ambient pressures, (2) protection of the middle ear from unwanted nasopharyngeal sound waves and secretions, and (3) drainage of middle ear secretions into the nasopharynx. The entrance to the eustachian tube, which is usually closed, is opened by the action of the tensor veli palatini muscles (Fig. 46-29). Innervation occurs as a part of the swallowing and yawning reflexes

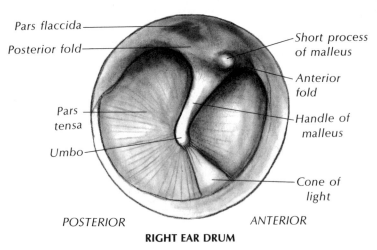

Pars flaccida
Posterior fold
Pars tensa
Umbo
Short process of malleus
Anterior fold
Handle of malleus
Cone of light

POSTERIOR   ANTERIOR

RIGHT EAR DRUM

Figure 46-27 Right eardrum. (From Bates B: A Guide to Physical Examination, 3rd ed. Philadelphia, JB Lippincott, 1983)

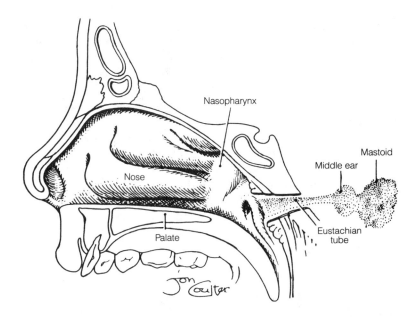

Figure 46-28 *Nasopharynx-eustacian tube-mastoid air cell system. (From Bluestone CD: Recent advances in pathogenesis, diagnosis, and management of otitis media. Pediatr Clin North Am 28, No 4: 36, 1981. Reproduced with permission.)*

and provides the mechanism for equalizing the pressure of the middle ear with that of the atmosphere. This equalization ensures that the pressures on both sides of the tympanic membrane are the same, so that sound transmission is not reduced and rupture does not result from sudden changes in external pressure, such as occurs during plane travel.

Ossicles.   Three tiny bones, the auditory ossicles, are suspended from the roof of the middle ear cavity and connect the tympanic membrane with the oval window. They are connected by synovial joints and are covered with the epithelial lining of the cavity. The malleus (hammer) has its handle firmly fixed to the upper half of the tympanic membrane. The head of the malleus articulates with the incus (anvil) which, in turn, articulates with the stapes (stirrup), which is inserted and sealed into the oval window by an annular ligament. The ossicles are arranged so that their lever movements transmit vibrations from the tympanic membrane to the oval window and from there to the fluid in the inner ear. It is the pistonlike action of the stapes footplate that sets up compression waves in the inner ear fluid. Air and liquid offer different degrees of impedance (resistance) to the transmission of sound waves. Therefore, the bones of the middle ear serve as impedance-matching devices between the low impedance of the air and the high impedance of the cochlear fluid. This matching is accomplished by (1) concentrating the pressure from the large area of the tympanic membrane (43–55 mm²) to the small area of the oval window (about 3 mm²) and (2) amplifying the air-transmitted sound waves into the force required to set up compression waves in the fluid of the inner ear. The latter is accomplished by the ossicular lever system,

which increases the pressures from the tympanic membrane to the oval window.

Two tiny skeletal muscles, the tensor tympani and the stapedius, support the ossicles. The tensor tympani is positioned on the roof of the auditory tube and inserts on the base of the malleus handle. The functional role of this muscle is in dispute. The stapedius muscle alters the movement of the stapes, reducing the displacement of fluid in the inner ear. Reflex contraction of this muscle by

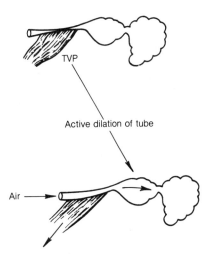

Figure 46-29 *Diagrammatic representation of physiologic pressure regulation of the middle ear by the active opening of the eustachian tube by the tensor veli palatini muscle (TVP). An alternative mechanism is by gradient-activated opening of the eustachian tube. (From Bluestone CD: Recent advances in the pathogenesis, diagnosis, and management of otitis media. Pediatr Clin North Am 28, No 4:727, 1981. Reproduced with permission.)*

means of the facial nerve, the stapedial reflex, provides a protective mechanism for the delicate inner ear structures when high-intensity sound occurs.

Inner ear

The inner ear, or labyrinth, contains the receptors for hearing and position sense. The outer bony wall of the inner ear, the bony labyrinth, encloses a thin-walled, membranous duct system, the membranous labyrinth (Fig. 46-30). Two separate fluids are found in the tiny canals of the inner ear. A fluid called the *perilymph* separates the bony labyrinth from the membranous labyrinth, and one called the *endolymph* fills the membranous labyrinth. The bony labyrinth is divided into three com-

partments: the cochlea, the vestibule, and the semicircular canals. The cochlea, which contains the auditory receptors, is a bony tube shaped like a snail shell that winds around a central bone column called the modiolus. The utricle, saccule, and semicircular canals contain the receptors for position sense and are discussed later in the chapter.

The membranous cochlear duct is a triangular-shaped structure that completely stretches across the cochlear canal, separating it into two parallel tubes, each containing perilymph: the scala vestibuli and the scala tympani (Fig. 46-31). One side of the cochlear duct, the basilar membrane, stretches under tension laterally from the modiolus to an elastic spiral ligament. The second side, the vestibular (Reissner's membrane), is a delicate

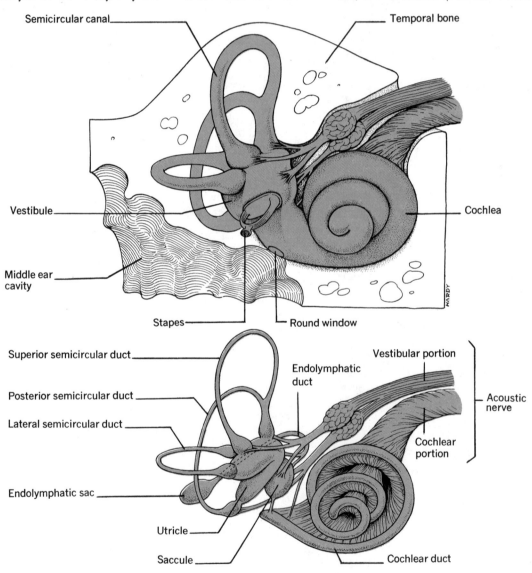

Figure 46-30 (Top) *Diagram of the bony labyrinth;* (bottom) *the membranous labyrinth as seen when removed from the bony labyrinth. (From Chaffee E, Lytle IM: Basic Anatomy and Physiology. Philadelphia, JB Lippincott, 1980)*

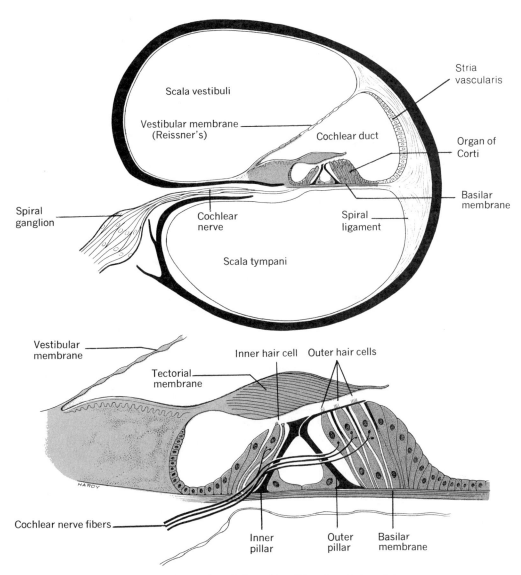

Figure 46-31   (Top) *Drawing of a portion of the cochlea. Note the relation of the cochlear duct to the scala vestibuli and tympani.* (Bottom) *The spiral organ of Corti has been removed from the cochlear duct and greatly enlarged. (From Chaffee EE, Lytle IM: Basic Physiology and Anatomy, 4th ed. Philadelphia, JB Lippincott, 1980)*

layer of squamous epithelial cells. The third side consists of a well-vascularized epithelium, the stria vascularis, that is the source of endolymph. The cochlear duct separates the scala vestibuli and the scali tympani from the base of the cochlear throughout its two and one-half spiral turns to its apex. An opening at the apex, called the helicotrema, permits communication between the two scali. Sound waves delivered by the stapes footplate to the perilymph travel throughout the fluid of the inner ear to the apex of the cochlea.

Perched on the basilar membrane and extending along its entire length is an elaborate arrangement of columnar epithelium called the organ of Corti. Continu-

ous rows of hair cells, separated into inner and outer rows, can be found within the cell arrangement. The cells have hairlike cilia that protrude through openings in an overlying supporting reticular membrane into the endolymph of the cochlear duct. A gelatinous mass, the tectorial membrane, extends from the medial side of the duct to enclose the cilia of the outer hair cells. Vibrations of the organ of Corti cause the hairs to be bent against the fixed tectorial membrane. Each hair cell is supplied by a nerve fiber, some by more than one. It is the bending of the hair fibers that transform (transduce) sound energy, which thus far has been mechanical, into membrane potential changes, transmitter release, and stimulation of nerve endings. It is generally agreed that the inner rows of hair cells, transducing different frequencies, are arranged sequentially with those transducing the higher tones, located on the lower end of the cochlea, and those transducing lower tones, located near its apex. Thus, selective destruction of hair cells in a particular segment of the cochlea can lead to hearing loss of particular tones. The outer rows of hair cells appear to provide the signals upon which the experience of sound loudness is based.

Neural pathways

Afferent fibers from the organ of Corti lead to cell bodies in the spiral ganglion in the central portion of the cochlea. Nerve fibers from the spiral ganglion (acoustic, or vestibulocochlear nerve [VIII]) travel to the cochlear nuclei located in the pons (Fig. 46-32). Many of the secondary nerve fibers from the cochlear nuclei pass to the opposite side of the pons. These secondary fibers may project to cell groups called the trapezoid nuclei, the superior olivary nucleus (or olive), or rostrally toward the inferior colliculus of the midbrain. Ipsilateral projections and interconnections between the nuclei of the two sides occur throughout the central auditory system. Consequently, impulses from either ear are transmitted through the auditory pathways to both sides of the brain stem.

A number of reflexes, initiated by sound stimuli, are integrated in the central auditory pathways. The superior olivary nucleus is involved in basic auditory reflexes, including the stapedial and tensor tympani reflexes. A comparison of impulses from the two sides, which provides the basis for spatial localization of a sound source, occurs at the level of the inferior colliculi. Superior colliculi function is required for auditory startle reflexes, which include rapid saccadic eye movements and turning of the head and body toward the sound source. The superior olivary nuclei, which have extensive connections with the brain stem respiratory and cardiovascular centers, integrate the heart rate, blood pressure, and respiratory changes that occur with the auditory startle reflex.

From the inferior colliculus, the auditory pathway passes to the medial geniculate nucleus of the thalamus, where all the fibers synapse. Considerable evidence supports the capability of this level of organization to provide crude auditory experience, including crude tone and intensity discrimination as well as the directionality of a sound source. From the medial geniculate nucleus, the auditory tract spreads by way of the auditory radiation to the primary auditory cortex (area 41) located mainly in the superior temporal gyrus and insula (see Fig. 46-23). The auditory association cortex (areas 42 and 22) borders the primary cortex on the superior temporal gyrus.

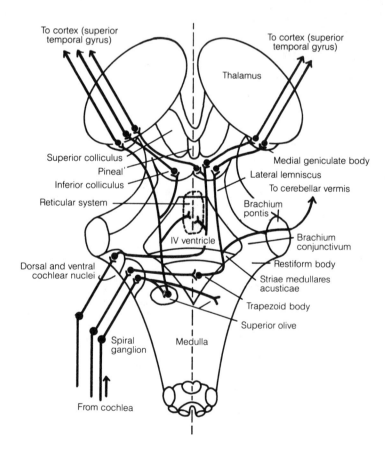

Figure 46-32 Simplified diagram of main auditory pathways superimposed on a dorsal view of the brain stem. Cerebellum and cerebral cortex removed. (Reproduced, with permission, from Ganong W: Review of Medical Physiology, 7th ed. Los Altos, CA, 1975)

This area and its associated high-order thalamic nuclei are necessary for auditory gnosis or the meaningfulness of sound to occur. Past experience, as well as precise analysis of momentary auditory information, is integrated during this process.

Disorders of Auditory Function

Hearing loss may be the most common physical disability suffered by people in the United States. It has been estimated that approximately 8% of the population suffer some hearing handicap, and approximately 3% have a severe handicap.[8]

Alterations in external ear function

The external ear conducts sound waves to the tympanic membrane. The function of the external ear is disturbed when sound transmission is obstructed by excessive amounts of accumulated cerumen or inflammation of the external ear (otitis externa).

Impacted cerumen.   Although the cerumen (earwax) produced by the glands of the ear canal normally dries up and leaves the ear, it can accumulate with excessive dryness, narrowing the canal. Repeated unskilled attempts to remove the wax may pack it more deeply into the ear canal. Usually impacted earwax produces no symptoms until the canal becomes completely occluded, at which point a feeling of fullness, deafness, tinnitus, or coughing because of vagal stimulation develops. On otoscopic examination a mass of yellow, brown, or black wax is visualized.

Removal of earwax can often be accomplished through the otoscope using a dull-ring curet. If this is not possible, the wax may be dislodged using a large syringe or dental irrigating device to produce a water stream. A few drops of baby shampoo, baby oil, or hydrogen peroxide can be instilled into the ear for several days prior to irrigation to soften the wax.

Otitis externa.   Otitis externa may vary in severity from a mild eczematoid dermatitis to severe cellulitis. It can be caused by infectious agents or materials contained in earphones or earrings (contact dermatitis). Infections of the external ear are usually bacterial in origin, with occasional secondary infection by fungi. Predisposing factors include moisture in the ear canal following swimming (swimmer's ear) or bathing, trauma resulting from scratching or attempts to clean the ear, and allergic dermatitis. External otitis is usually accompanied by redness, scaliness, narrowing of the canal because of swelling, itching, and pain. Inflammation of the pinna or canal makes movement of the auricle painful. There may be watery or purulent drainage and intermittent deaf-

ness. Treatment methods include the use of topical antibiotic ointments, eardrops, and topical corticosteroids to reduce inflammation.

Alterations in middle ear function

Otitis media.   Otitis media, or inflammation of the middle ear, is the most common diagnosis made by physicians who care for children. It has been estimated that approximately $2 billion are spent annually on medical and surgical treatment of the disorder.[7] This figure includes the expenses of the estimated 1 million children who receive tympanostomy tubes each year and for the 60,000 children who have tonsillectomies and adenoidectomies annually, many of which are performed to prevent otitis media.

Otitis media can be acute, subacute, or chronic. It may or may not be infectious in origin and may or may not be associated with effusion (fluid collection). Infants and small children are at the highest risk for developing it, the peak prevalence occurring between 6 and 36 months. There are two reasons for the increased risk in infants and small children: (1) the eustachian tube is shorter, more horizontal, and wider in this age group than in older children and adults, and (2) infection can spread more easily through the canal of the infant who spends most of the day lying in bed. Bottle-fed babies have a higher incidence of otitis media than breast-fed babies, probably because bottle-fed babies are held in a more horizontal position during feeding, and swallowing while in the horizontal position facilitates the reflux of milk into the middle ear. Breastfeeding also provides for the transfer of protective maternal antibodies to the infant. The incidence of otitis media is higher among children with craniofacial anomalies (cleft palate and Down's syndrome), Alaskan natives (Eskimos), and American Indians.

Abnormalities of the eustachian tube are important factors in the pathogenesis of middle ear infections. Two major types of eustachian tube dysfunction contribute to otitis media: obstruction and abnormal patency (Fig. 46-33). Obstruction can be either mechanical or functional. Functional obstruction results from the persistent collapse of the eustachian tube because of a lack of tubal stiffness or an abnormal muscular opening mechanism. It is common in infants and small children because the amount and stiffness of the cartilage supporting the eustachian tube is less than in older children and adults. Also, age-related changes in the craniofacial base tends to render the muscle responsible for opening the eustachian tube less efficient in this age group. Mechanical obstruction can be either intrinsic or extrinsic, the most common obstruction being caused by intrinsic swelling resulting from upper respiratory tract infection or allergy. Extrinsic obstruction can result from the enlargement of ade-

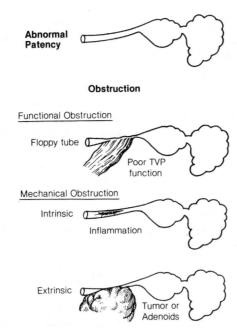

Figure 46-33 *Pathophysiology of the eustachian tube. (From Bluestone CD: Recent advances in pathogenesis, diagnosis, and management of otitis media. Pediatr Clin North Am 28, No 4:737, 1981. Reproduced with permission.)*

noid tissue or a tumor. With obstruction, oxygen in the middle ear is absorbed, causing a negative pressure and the transudation of serous fluid into the middle ear.

The abnormally patent tube either does not close or does not close completely. In children, air and secretions may be pumped into the eustachian tube during nose blowing and crying. Organisms or foreign material from the nasophraynx incite an inflammatory response with exudate, leukocytosis, and hypertrophy of the mucous glands in the eustachian tube and mucous membrane lining the middle ear.

Acute otitis media. Acute otitis is usually suppurative, or purulent, but serous otitis media may also be acute. Most cases of otitis media follow an upper respiratory tract infection that has been present for several days. *Streptococcus pneumoniae* and *Hemophilus influenzae* are the most frequently isolated organisms. Acute suppurative otitis media is characterized by otalgia (earache), fever (up to 104°F), and hearing loss. Occasionally there may be rhinorrhea, vomiting, and diarrhea. Pain usually increases as purulent exudate accumulates behind the tympanic membrane. An infant may cry and rub the infected ear, while an older child will complain of sharp or severe pain in the ear. If the tympanic membrane ruptures because of excessive pressure, the pain will be relieved, and a purulent drainage will be present in the external ear canal.

Acute serous otitis media may also occur following a viral disease, with an allergy, or following sudden changes in atmospheric pressure. If air cannot pass back through the eustachian tube upon descent during an airplane flight, hearing loss and discomfort will develop. This occurs most commonly in those who travel while suffering from an upper respiratory infection. Yawning, swallowing, and chewing gum seem to facilitate the opening of the eustachian tube, which equalizes air in the middle ear. Signs of acute serous otitis media include conductive hearing loss, eardrum retraction, and fluid level or air bubbles visible through the tympanic membrane.

Recurrent otitis media. Recurrent otitis media can occur as an acute episode of otitis media along with almost every respiratory tract infection. Most of these children respond well to treatment and have fewer recurrences with advancing age. However, some children have persistent middle ear effusion with superimposed recurrent episodes of acute otitis media.

Chronic otitis media. Otitis media that persists beyond 3 months is usually considered chronic.[8] Chronic otitis media can occur with or without effusion. Chronic suppurative otitis media is most common in those who have suffered ear problems during early childhood. With the chronic infection permanent perforation of the tympanic membrane often occurs. Ear ossicles may be destroyed, and chronic changes can occur in the mucosa of the ear. The chronic condition is frequently exacerbated by upper respiratory infections.

Diagnosis and treatment. Diagnosis of otitis media is often made by otoscopic examination of the tympanic membrane. A bulging, lusterless eardrum with subsequent obliteration of the bony landmarks and cone of light are observed. Gentle movement of the pinna can help distinguish otitis media from otitis externa. This maneuver does not produce pain in purulent otitis media but causes exquisite discomfort in otitis externa. A culture of middle ear effusion fluid is used for verifying the presence and type of microorganism present. A needle can be inserted through the inferior part of the tympanic membrane to obtain a specimen of effusion fluid, or a culture can be made of the drainage present in the external ear canal when the tympanic membrane has perforated.

Use of the pneumatic otoscope permits the introduction of air into the canal for the purpose of determining tympanic membrane flexibility. The movement of this membrane is decreased in some cases of acute otitis media and absent in chronic middle ear infection. Tympanometry is an important advance in the identification of middle ear disease. A tympanogram is obtained by inserting a small probe into the external auditory canal; a tone of fixed characteristics is then presented through the probe, and the mobility of the tympanic membrane is measured electronically while the external canal pressure is artificially varied.

The treatment of otitis media includes the use of appropriate antibiotic therapy. Oral ampicillin or amoxicillin is commonly prescribed. Additional supportive therapy, including analgesics, antipyretics, and local heat may be indicated. A myringotomy (surgical incision of the tympanic membrane) may be done to relieve pressure on the eardrum, reduce pain and hearing loss, and prevent the ragged opening that can follow spontaneous rupture of the eardrum. The use of antihistamines and decongestants is controversial. They are usually of most benefit to children with serous otitis media of an allergic origin.

Tympanostomy tubes may be used in the treatment of children with recurrent or chronic otitis media. Insertion of the tubes is one of the most commonly performed surgical procedures in the United States; however, the long-term benefits are controversial. Placement of the tubes is usually performed under general anesthesia. The ears of children with the tubes must be kept out of water. Spontaneous extrusion of the tubes usually occurs after 5.5 months to 7 months.[9,10] The side-effects include recurrent otorrhea, persistent perforation, scarring and atrophy of the eardrum, and cholesteatoma.

Complications. Complications of otitis media are not common, but they can follow inadequate treatment. The most common are those associated with the aural cavity and surrounding temporal bone. Intracranial complications are rare but are the most serious complications.

One of the most common complications of otitis media is persistent conductive hearing loss. Fluid may be present in the middle ear for weeks or months after an acute bout of otitis media. This may impair hearing and affect the child's learning of language skills. Fortunately, hearing loss that is associated with fluid retention usually resolves when the effusion clears. Permanent hearing loss may occur as the result of damage to the tympanic membrane or other middle ear structures.

Adhesive otitis media involves an abnormal healing reaction to an inflamed middle ear. It produces irreversible thickening of the mucous membranes and may cause impaired movement of the ossicles and, possibly, conductive hearing loss. Tympanosclerosis involves the formation of whitish plaques and nodular deposits on the submucosal surface of the tympanic membrane with possible adherence of the ossicles and conductive hearing loss. Perforation of the eardrum occurs most often following acute otitis media; although it usually heals spontaneously, tympanoplasty may be necessary.

A cholesteatoma is a saclike mass containing a silvery white debris of keratin, which is shed by the squamous epithelial lining of the eardrum. As the lining of the epithelium sheds and desquamates, the lesion expands and erodes the surrounding tissues. The lesion is insidiously progressive, and erosion may involve the temporal bone, causing intracranial complications. The treatment involves microsurgical techniques to remove the cholesteatoma material.

The mastoid antrum and air cells constitute a portion of the temporal bone and may become inflamed as an extension of an acute or chronic otitis media. Because of the use of antibiotics, acute mastoiditis (a complication of acute otitis media) is unusual. If it does occur, there is necrosis of the mastoid process and destruction of the bony intercellular matrix, which are visible by x-ray examination. Mastoid tenderness and drainage of exudate through a perforated tympanic membrane can occur. Chronic mastoiditis can develop as the result of chronic middle ear infection. The usefulness of antibiotics for this condition is limited. Mastoid or middle ear surgery, along with other medical treatment, may be indicated.

Intracranial complications, though rare, can develop if the infection spreads through vascular channels, by direct extension, or through preformed pathways such as the round window. These complications are seen more often with chronic suppurative otitis media and mastoiditis. They include meningitis, focal encephalitis, brain abscess, lateral sinus thrombophlebitis or thrombosis, labyrinthitis, or facial nerve paralysis. Any child who develops persistent headache, tinnitus (ringing in the ear), stiff neck, or visual or other neurologic symptoms should be investigated for possible intracranial complications.

Otosclerosis. Otosclerosis is a familial, autosomal-dominant disorder that causes conductive deafness, sensorineural hearing loss, and tinnitus. It is a disorder of the otic capsule, which becomes the petrous part of the temporal bone that surrounds the inner ear. Otosclerosis may begin at any time in life but usually does not appear until after puberty, most frequently between the ages of 20 and 30 years. There is an increase in the disease process during pregnancy.

In otosclerosis, the disease process begins with resorption of bone in one or more foci. During active bone resorption, the bone structure appears spongy and softer than normal (osteospongiosis). The resorbed bone is replaced by an overgrowth of new sclerotic bone. The process is slowly progressive, involving more areas of the temporal bone, especially in front of and posterior to the stapes footplate. As it invades the footplate, the pathologic bone increasingly immobilizes the stapes, reducing the transmission of sound. Pressure of otosclerotic bone on inner ear structures or the eighth nerve may contribute to the development of tinnitus, sensorineural hearing loss, and vertigo.

The symptoms of otosclerosis involve an insidious hearing loss. Initially, one is unable to hear a whisper or someone speaking at a distance. In the earliest stages, the bone conduction by which the person's own voice is heard remains relatively unaffected. Therefore, the person's own voice sounds unusually loud and the sound of chewing becomes intensified. Because of bone conduction, these people can usually hear fairly well on the telephone, which provides an amplified signal. Also, they often are able to hear better in a noisy environment (paracusis), probably because the masking effect of background noise causes people to speak louder.

The treatment of otosclerosis can be either medical or surgical. A carefully selected well-fitting hearing aid may allow a person with conductive deafness to lead a normal life. Sodium fluoride has been used in the medical treatment of osteospongiosis. Because much of the conductive hearing loss associated with otosclerosis is due to stapedial fixation, the surgical treatment involves stapedectomy with stapedial reconstruction using either the patient's own stapes or a stapedial prosthesis. The argon lazer beam may be used in the surgical procedure.

Abnormalities of central auditory pathways

The auditory pathways in the brain involve intercommunication between the two sides at many levels. As a result, strokes, tumors, abscesses, and other focal abnormalities rarely produce more than a mild reduction in auditory acuity on the side opposite the lesion. However, when it comes to the intelligibility of auditory language (phagia), lateral dominance becomes very important. On the dominant side, usually the left side, the more medial and dorsal portion of associational auditory cortex is of crucial importance. This area is called *Wernicke's area,* and damage here is associated with auditory receptive aphasia (an agnosia of speech). Persons with damage to this area of the brain can speak intelligibly and can read normally but are unable to understand the meaning of major aspects of heard speech.

Irritative foci affecting the auditory radiation or the primary auditory cortex can produce roaring or clicking sounds, which appear to come from the auditory environment of the opposite side (auditory hallucinations). Focal seizures originating in or near the auditory cortex are often immediately preceded by the perception of ringing or other sounds. Damage to the auditory association cortex, especially if bilateral, results in deficiencies of sound recognition and memory (auditory agnosia). If the damage is in the dominant hemisphere, speech recognition can be affected (sensory aphasia).

Disorders of internal ear function and deafness

More than 13 million people in the United States have some hearing impairment. Of these persons, 6 million are seriously handicapped, and more than 1.7 million are totally deaf.[11] There are many causes of hearing loss or deafness. Most fit into the categories of conductive, sensorineural (perceptive), or mixed deficiencies involving a combination of conductive and sensorineural function deficiencies of the same ear.

Conductive hearing loss. Conductive hearing deficit occurs with external ear or middle ear disorders such as impacted cerumen, perforation of the tympanic membrane, fluid or pus in the middle ear, or ossicle fusion. A partial hearing loss can occur if sonic stimuli are not adequately transmitted to the inner ear through the external acoustic meatus (auditory canal), the tympanic membrane (eardrum), the middle ear, and the chain of ossicles. Otosclerosis is a common familial form of conductive hearing loss.

Sensorineural hearing loss. Sensorineural, or perceptive, hearing loss can occur when disorders affect the inner ear, the acoustic nerve, or the auditory pathways of the brain. With this type of deafness, sound waves are conducted to the inner ear, but abnormalities of the cochlear apparatus or auditory nerve decrease or distort the transfer of information to the brain. Spontaneous ringing of the ears (tinnitus) accompanies cochlear nerve irritation. Abnormal function resulting from damage or malformation of the central auditory pathways and circuitry is included in this category. Sensorineural hearing loss may be congenital as a result of birth trauma, maternal rubella, or malformations of the inner ear. Trauma to the inner ear, vascular disorders with hemorrhage or thrombosis of vessels that supply the middle ear, can also cause sensorineural deafness. Other causes of sensorineural deafness are infections and drugs.

Environmentally induced deafness can occur through direct exposure to excessively intense sound, as in the workplace or at a concert. This type of deafness was once called "boilermaker's deafness" because of the intense reverberating sound to which riveters were exposed when putting together boiler tanks. Noise pollution is often characterized by high-intensity sounds of a specific frequency that cause corresponding damage to the organ of Corti.

Deafness or some degree of hearing impairment is the most common serious complication of bacterial meningitis in infants and children. It has been reported that sensorineural deafness complicates bacterial deafness in 10% of cases and is most likely to follow *S. pneumoniae meningitis.*[12]

Drugs that damage inner ear structures are labeled ototoxic. Several classes of drugs have been identified as having ototoxic potentials: aminoglycoside antibiotics and other basic antibiotics with similar ototoxic potential, antimalarial drugs, loop diuretics, and salicylates. In addition to these drug groups, many other drug groups have been implicated in causing ototoxicity. The risk of ototoxicity depends on the total dose of the drug and its concentration in the bloodstream. The risk is increased in persons with impaired renal functioning and in those previously or currently treated with another potentially ototoxic drug. Table 46-2 lists drugs with the potential for producing ototoxicity.

Old age hearing loss.   Hearing loss is a common disability in the elderly. It has been estimated that 30% of people over age 65 and 50% of people over 85 years of age have significant hearing handicaps.[11] Decreased acuity begins in early adulthood and progresses for as long as the individual lives.[13] This contrasts with other sensory losses in the aged that tend to reach a plateau in functional deficit. High-frequency sounds are affected more than low-frequency sounds. Males are affected earlier and experience a greater loss than females. Individuals also experience what is called phonetic regression, or a word-discrimination loss, which interferes with normal communication.

Hearing tests.   To estimate hearing, each ear is tested separately. Specific procedures used to assess hearing depend on the age and developmental level of the infant and young child (details of procedures can be found in texts on physical assessment).

The ability to hear is tested by occluding first one ear and then the other. The examiner stands 1 foot to 2 feet away and whispers numbers in the direction of the unoccluded ear. Care is taken to prevent lipreading. A ticking watch may also be used, but this only tests the higher frequencies.

Audiogram.   The audiogram is an important method of analyzing a person's hearing. It requires highly specialized sound production and control equipment. Pure tones of controlled intensity are delivered, usually to one ear at a time, and the minimum intensity needed for hearing to be experienced is plotted as a function of frequency. The Bekesy method permits the subject to test himself or herself. The equipment generates continuous pure tones that decrease in intensity as long as the subject presses a button. When the subject releases the button, the equipment then increases the intensity till the button is pressed again. The frequency spectrum is tested by continuous advancement.

Table 46-2   Major Ototoxic Drugs in Order of Decreasing Incidence of Toxicity*

Drug	Cochlear Toxicity	Vestibular Toxicity	Permanent Damage
Minocycline	0	+ + + +	Rare
Kanamycin	+ + +	+	Usual
Amakacin	+ + + +	0	Occasional
Neomycin	+ + +	+	Occasional
Streptomycin	+	+ + +	Usual
Viomycin	+ +	+ +	Occasional
Gentamicin	+	+ + +	Occasional
Tobramycin	+	+ + +	Occasional
Ethacrynic acid	+ + +	+	Rare
Furosemide	+ + + +	0	Rare
Vancomycin	+ + + +	0	Occasional
Quinine	+ + + +	0	Rare
Salicylates	+ + + +	0	Rare
Polymyxin B†	0	+ + + +	Usual
Colistin†	0	+ + + +	Usual

*Ototoxicity is indicated on a scale of 0 to + + + +.
†Applied topically, to the middle ear.
(From Chermak G, Jinks M: Hearing impaired elderly, Drug Intell Clin Pharm 15:379, May 1981)

Tests of conduction versus sensorineural deafness.   If a hearing loss is present, conduction deafness must be distinguished from sensorineural deafness. A tuning fork of 1024 Hz is used to test hearing for two reasons: (1) it tests within the range of human speech (400–5000 Hz), and (2) it does not confuse sound with palpable vibration. The tuning fork may be tapped on the handle to set it into light vibration.

Weber test.   The Weber test evaluates bone conduction by the lateralization of sound. The test is performed by placing the base of a lightly vibrating tuning fork on the middle of the forehead or at the vertex of the patient's head. It can also be placed on the upper (maxillary) incisor teeth. The person is then asked to determine whether sound is heard better in one ear than in the other. With conductive deafness, the bone-conducted sound is heard more loudly and clearly on the side with the conduction deficit because the inner ear structures are functional and remain undisturbed by extraneous environmental sounds.

Rinne test.   The Rinne test compares air and bone conduction of sound. The test is done by placing the base of the lightly vibrating tuning fork on the mastoid process until the sound is no longer heard. The vibrating fork is then quickly placed near the external auditory meatus of the ear to be tested. If the sound is louder when the tuning fork is placed in front of the ear, hearing is normal, or there is no sensorineural component. If the sound is louder when the tuning fork is placed over the mastoid process, conduction hearing loss is indicated. If the sound is heard the same in both places, a mixed hearing loss is possible.

Brain stem–evoked responses.   In recent years a noninvasive method has been developed that permits functional evaluation of certain defined parts of the central auditory pathways. Scalp electrodes and high-gain amplifiers are required to produce a record of the electrical wave activity elicited during repeated acoustic stimulations of either or both ears. Certain of the early waves come from discrete portions of the pons and midbrain auditory pathways, and localized damage can to some extent be correlated with specific sensorineural abnormalities. This method is called the brain stem–evoked response (BSER), and it has advanced from the research laboratory to fairly widespread use in the neurologic and EENT clinic.

Treatment of deafness.   Conduction deafness can be corrected through the use of electrical amplification methods (hearing aids). Hearing aids deliver sonic stimuli directly to the skull bones with sufficient added power to, in turn, directly vibrate the inner ear apparatus. This method bypasses the middle ear conduction apparatus. Amplification is of no assistance with sensorineural hearing loss. With sensorineural deficit a hearing aid serves only to increase the intensity of a signal experienced as distorted. In mixed hearing loss, amplification can provide improvement only for the conduction problems that are part of the syndrome. Although most standard tests for auditory acuity use pure tone stimuli, intelligibility of sound stimuli is not necessarily correlated with pure tone loss, and damage to the very important communicative function of heard speech produces a social isolation that is potentially very damaging to an individual's attitude and motivation for repair and rehabilitation.

Recently, surgically implantable cochlear prostheses for the profoundly deaf have been developed. A number of auditory prostheses have been produced that use electrodes implanted outside or within the cochlea or in the modiolus. A cochlear prosthesis, as presently developed, does not provide normal hearing. Rather, it provides perception of background noises. For example, the cochlear prosthesis allows the person to hear footsteps and become aware that someone is speaking, so that lipreading can be used. It also allows for recognition of protective sounds, such as the sound of an automobile approaching, the sound of a fire alarm, and the opening and closing of doors. Improvements have been made that increase the quality of speech recognition. The method has promise except for those few pathologic conditions in which total labyrinthine destruction or total cochlear nerve degeneration has occurred.

In summary, hearing is a specialized sense whose external stimulus is the vibration of sound waves. The ear receives the sound waves, distinguishes their frequencies, translates this information into nerve impulses, and transmits these to the central nervous system. The auditory system consists of the external ear, middle ear, inner ear, auditory pathways, and central auditory cortex. Among the disorders of the auditory system are infections of the external and middle ear, otosclerosis, and conduction and sensorineural deafness. Otitis externa is an inflammatory process of the external ear. The middle ear is a tiny air-filled cavity located in the temporal bone. The eustachian tube connects the middle ear to the nasopharynx and allows for equalization of pressure between the middle ear and the atmosphere. Infections can travel from the nasopharynx to the middle ear along the eustachian tube, causing otitis media, or inflammation of the middle ear. The eustachian tube is shorter and more horizontal in infants and young children, and infections of the middle ear are a common problem in this age group. Otitis media can be acute, subacute, or chronic. The most common form, acute suppurative otitis media, usually follows an upper respiratory tract infection. It is characterized by otalgia, fever, and hearing loss. The effusion that accompanies otitis media can persist for weeks or months, interfering with hearing and impairing speech development. Otosclerosis is a familial disorder of the otic capsule. It causes bone resorption followed by excessive replacement with sclerotic bone. The disorder eventually causes immobilization of the stapes and conduction deafness. Deafness, or hearing loss, can develop as the result of a number of auditory disorders. Deafness can be conductive, sensorineural, or mixed. Conduction deafness occurs when transmission of sound waves from the external to the inner ear is impaired. Sensorineural deafness can involve cochlear structures of the inner ear or the neural pathways that transmit auditory stimuli.

■ Vestibular Function

The vestibular receptive organs, which are located in the inner ear, and their central nervous system connections contribute to the reflex activity necessary for effective posture and movement in a physical world governed by momentum and a gravitational field. Because the vestibular apparatus is part of the inner ear and is thus located in the head, it is head motion and acceleration that are sensed. The vestibular system serves two general and related functions: (1) it maintains body balance in the presence of forces acting on the head through postural reflexes, and (2) it maintains the steady position of visual objects in spite of marked changes in head position through vestibulo-ocular reflexes.

Vestibular System

The peripheral apparatus of the vestibular system lies embedded in the petrous portion of the temporal bone, adjacent to and continuous with the cochlea of the auditory system. All of the vestibular structures are contained in bony canals called the bony labyrinth. A membranous labyrinth that has the same shape as the bony labyrinth is fitted into the bony canals. The area immediately surrounding the membranous labyrinth is filled with perilymph, in which the membranous labyrinth floats. The composition of the perilymph is very similar to that of the cerebral spinal fluid (CSF), and a tubular perilymphatic duct connects the perilymph fluid with the CSF in the subarachnoid space of the posterior fossa. The membranous labyrinth is filled with endolymph. A small-diameter tubular extension, the endolymphatic sac, connects this system with the subdural space near the jugular foramen, providing an exit for the slowly circulating endolymph into the lymphatic system. The endolymph has a high potassium concentration and is similar to intracellular fluid.

The vestibular apparatus is divided into five prominent divisions: three semicircular canals, a utricle, and a saccule (see Fig. 46-30). The receptors of these structures are differentiated into the angular acceleration–deceleration receptors of the semicircular canals and the linear acceleration–deceleration and static gravitational receptors of the utricle and saccule. The utricle and saccule are two widened membranous sacs within the bony vestibule. The utricle connects the ends of each semicircular canal. The saccule communicates with the utricle through a small duct and with the cochlear duct of the auditory apparatus through the ductus reuniens.

There are small patches of tall columnar ciliated epithelial cells in the floor of the utricle (utricular macula), in the side wall of the sacculus (sacculi macula), at the base of each semicircular canal (cristae), and along the floor of the cochlear duct (organ of Corti, see Fig. 46-31). Each hair cell has several microvilli and one true cilium called a kinocilium. Ganglion cells, homologous with dorsal root ganglion cells, form three afferent ganglia: the superior vestibular ganglion, which innervates the hair cells of the utricular macula and the cristae of the superior and horizontal semicircular canals; the inferior vestibular ganglion, which innervates the saccular macula and the cristae of the inferior semicircular canal; and the spiral (or acoustic) ganglion, which innervates the cochlear duct. The central axons of these ganglion cells become the superior and inferior vestibular nerves and the cochlear auditory nerve. They are often collectively called the eighth cranial nerve, and they enter the side of the nearby medullary-pontine junction of the brain stem.

Semicircular canals

The three semicircular canals, each about two-thirds of a circle, are arranged at right angles to each other, with the horizontal duct tilted at approximately 12° above the normal horizontal plane of the head (see Fig. 46-30). The horizontal ducts of the two sides of the head are in the same plane, so that the superior duct of one side is parallel with the inferior duct of the other side. At each duct and the utricle junction, an enlargement of each semicircular duct, called an *ampulla,* contains the hair cell sensory surface raised into a crest, or crista, at right angles to the duct. The stereocilia of each hair cell extends into a flexible gelantinous mass, the cupula, which essentially closes off fluid flow through the semicircular canal. When the head begins to rotate around the axis of a semicircular duct (*i.e.,* undergoes angular acceleration), the momentum of the endolymph causes an increase in pressure to be applied to one side of the cupula. This is similar to the lagging behind of the water in a glass that is suddenly rotated, except that the endolymph cannot flow past the cupula and instead applies a differential pressure to its two sides, bending it and the cilia of the hair cells. This results in a reduced membrane potential across the hair cell plasma membrane when the hair is bent toward the microvilli and an increased membrane potential when the hair cell is bent in the opposite direction. Impulses from the cristae are transmitted by the vestibular part of the vestibulocochlear (VIII) cranial nerve to the vestibular nuclei of the caudal pons.

Maximal stimulation of the afferents of a semicircular canal results when rotation of the head occurs exactly in the plane of the membranous duct. Because of the orientation of the three semicircular canals, angular accelerations of the head will always result in action potentials in at least one and usually more than one of the vestibular nerve branches to the three cristae. If the angular acceleration reduces to a steady angular velocity, friction between the endolymph and the canal wall gradually results in, first, a reduction of pressure and then a loss of differential pressure on the two sides of the cupula—a form of sensory adaptation. Upon the sudden reduction or cessation of head rotation, the momentum of the endolymph will apply pressure on the cupula from the opposite direction. Thus, the semicircular duct system provides a mechanism for signaling to the CNS the direction and rate of accelerations and decelerations in head rotation.

Utricle and saccule

The hair cell surface (macula) of the utricle is oriented approximately in the horizontal plane. The macula of the sacculus is oriented in the vertical plane. In both instances, the stereocilia of the hair cells extend into a gelantinous mass within the endolymph. Myriad microscopic crystals of calcium carbonate and calcium phosphate, called *otoliths,* are embedded in this gelatinous material, adding considerably to its total mass. The gelatinous mass with its otoliths is called the otolithic membrane. When the head is tilted, the gelatinous mass shifts its position because of the pull of the gravitational field bending the stereocilia of the macular hair cells. Although each hair cell becomes hyperpolarized or hypopolarized depending on the direction in which the cilia are bending, the hair cells are oriented in all directions, making these sense organs sensitive to static or changing head position in relation to the gravitational field. The central connections from the maculae provide the mechanism by which head, body, and eye postural adjustments occur in response to tilting the head and by which a stable visual fixation point ("optic grasp" of the visual field), as well as postural support of a stable head position, is maintained. Projections to the forebrain provide the basis for sensations of head tilt away from the horizontal plane.

In addition to this rather static tilt reception function, the utricle and saccule provide the organism with linear acceleration and deceleration reception. When the head is accelerated in linear fashion, such as the initial or terminal phase of an elevator ride or during automobile acceleration or deceleration, differential movement between the head and the otolithic membranes provides the basis for reflex compensatory bracing of neck, trunk, and limbs. They also provide the input data on which the air-righting reflexes are based. A cat dropped from an upside down position lands on its feet and will do so even if blindfolded. Most vestibular reflexes, including air righting, are functional at birth. If a newborn is supported in the prone position, and the support is momentarily (and with great care) removed, the trunk is extended and all four limbs are extended as falling begins. In the supine position, the trunk is flexed and the limbs are flexed as the fall progresses. On the other hand, the head-on-body vestibular reflexes of the infant are not sufficiently operational during the first 6 weeks or so after birth to maintain head posture. This is why the newborn's head must be supported when the newborn is lifted in the supine position to prevent extreme cervical flexure and possible damage to the cervical segmental nerves.

Central nervous system connections

The nerve fibers from the vestibular receptors travel in the vestibular portion of the acoustic (VIII) cranial nerve (see Fig. 46-30) to the superior, medial, lateral, and inferior vestibular nuclei located at the junction of the medulla and pons. In addition, some of the afferent fibers travel to the ipsilateral cerebellar cortex and a deep cerebellar nucleus called the *fastigial nucleus.* The part of the cerebellum receiving vestibular input is called the *archicerebellum,* or the *flocculonodular lobe.* On the output side, cells in the fastigial nucleus receiving afferent terminals and terminals from cortical neurons send their axons back to the vestibular nuclei of the same and opposite sides of the brain stem.

In addition to complex internal circuitry, neurons from the vestibular nuclei project into the nearby reticular formation and provide powerful control on postural reflexes of the eyes, head, body, and limbs. Projections occur to the pons lateral gaze control center, to the vertical and torsional gaze control regions, to the sixth cranial nerve nuclei, to the MLF, to the fourth and third nerve nuclei, and to cervical-level lower motor neurons innervating the sternocleidomastoid and other neck muscles that control head turning and posture. The MLF projections primarily control horizontal or lateral turning and gaze. In addition, extensive projections into and through the reticular formation follow the central tegmental fasciculus (CTF) pathway controlling the vertical and rotatory (torsion) gaze reflexes.

Postural reflexes

A small group of vestibular nuclei neurons send their axons to make efferent synaptic contact either directly on the hair cells or on afferent terminals at the hair cells. These vestibular efferents appear to be excitatory to afferent activity and to perform a modulatory role that is yet to be understood.

The descending portion of the MLF, essentially a medial vestibulospinal tract, continues at least into thoracic cord levels and provides vestibular control of the muscle tone of axial mucles, including the dorsal back muscles. A rapid-conducting lateral vestibulospinal tract descends the spinal cord to provide powerful vestibular control of the lower motor neurons of the upper and lower limbs. As the head begins to tip (*i.e.,* rotate) on the neck or as a part of general body tipping, the vestibular system activates the appropriate extensor muscles of the neck, trunk, and limbs, opposing the direction of the tilt. These powerful reflex adjustments in muscle tone assist in maintaining stable head and, therefore, body postural support during static posture and during passive or active movement.

The cerebellar connections of the vestibular system are necessary for adjustments of temporally smooth, coordinated movements to ongoing head movement, tilt, or angular acceleration. For instance, accurate grasping can occur during a fall, indicating cerebellar adjustments based on vestibular information during the performance of a smooth, accurate movement.

Vestibular reflexes are quite powerful, and considerable learning is required to inhibit or greatly modify them, as is necessary for acrobatic pilots, divers, and gymnasts. Dancers and skaters who engage in rapid spinning movements also learn to use or at least partially inhibit these reflexes.

Eye movement reflexes

Vestibular control of conjugate eye posture can be understood in terms of complex reflex bilateral (conjugate) eye movements that preserve eye fixation on stable objects in the visual field. As one begins to fall, such visual stability is essential to successful recovery attempts. Thus, as the body and head begin rotation, the eyes in conjugate fashion move in exactly the opposite direction, maintaining the previous fixation point. Compensation for the ongoing head movement is precise. This is called the slow phase of nystagmus. In a sense, central nervous system circuitry provides for an accurate optic grasp of the visual environment. If the rotation continues beyond the range of lateral eye movement, a very quick conjugate eye correction (saccadic return) occurs as if to obtain a new stable fixation point, and then the slow phase continues again. This nystagmus pattern continues as long as angular acceleration continues. When a steady rotational velocity is reached, compensatory nystagmus movements gradually wane as the disparity between the movement of endolymph and the semicircular duct wall is lost, as is the differential pressure on the two sides of the cupula.

Clinically, the direction of this nystagmus pattern is named for the fast, or saccadic, phase. The reflex circuitry is in very precise control of motor units in the nuclei innervating the extrinsic muscles of the eye via cranial nerves III, IV, and VI. In fact, the precision of nystagmus movements is as great in persons with eyes closed and in the congenitally blind as it is in normal-sighted persons. If the eyes are not allowed to move, or if stimulation is strong, the head will also move in nystagmoid fashion as a result of vestibular control of the sternocleidomastoid muscles via cranial nerve XI.

Vestibular-driven nystagmus can occur in any plane. Beginning rotation of the head around a transverse axis in head-over-heels fashion is accompanied by compensatory nystagmus, which has its slow, smooth-pursuit phase in the upward direction and its fast phase in the direction of rotation. Starting rotation around the frontal-occipital axis (*i.e.,* head tilting to the side), is accompanied by compensatory slow-phase torsion eye movements, twisting in the direction opposite to the rotation. The saccadic phase will be in the direction of body rotation. In each instance, nystagmus can be understood in terms of repeated attempts to grasp stable fixed visual fields as the head rotates, with a quick correction to a new, stable fixation point.

Nystagmus can be classified in terms of the direction of eye movement: horizontal, vertical, rotatory, or mixed. Nystagmus derived from a sense organ or vestibular nerve is of the slow phase–fast phase or jerky type described previously. Nystagmus resulting from CNS pathology usually has equal rates in each direction, called pendular nystagmus.

If the visual environment is rotated or appears to rotate past an individual with a normally functioning visual system, a fixation point is selected and a smooth pursuit movement will rotate the eyes to the limit of the binocular field. At this point a saccadic correction quickly moves the eye back to a new fixation point, and the pursuit will occur again. This visually induced, or optokinetic, nystagmus and the associated vertigo are experienced when a neighboring vehicle or train moves past the visual field. The phenomenon demonstrates the ability of visual stimuli to overpower the vestibular end organs' signals that the head is indeed stable in relation to gravitational and inertial forces.

Thalamic and cortical projections

Some of the neurons of the vestibular nuclei project their axons rostrally to the ventrolateral nuclei of the thalamus. In addition to the intrathalamic circuitry, thalamic projections go to the temporal cortex near the primary auditory cortex and to the somesthetic area of the parietal cortex. These thalamic and cortical projections provide the basis for the subjective experiences of position in space, of rotation, and of vertigo that accompanies the onset or sudden cessation of head rotation. Vertigo is often experienced as a result of toxic conditions, such as alcohol toxicity, or of infective conditions. During such episodes, nystagmus is observed.

Severe damage to the forebrain or to the brain stem rostral to the pons often results in loss of rostral control of these static vestibular reflexes. If the patient's head is moved from side to side or up and down, the eyes retain a stable fixation point. Thus, the eyes move in conjugate gaze much as those of a doll with counterweighted eyes. This phenomenon, called "doll's eyes," demonstrates the always-present vestibular static reflexes without forebrain interference or suppression. These static vestibular reflexes are to be contrasted with dynamic vestibular reflexes (nystagmus and the linear acceleration and deceleration reflexes).

Abnormalities of Vestibular Function

Disorders of vestibular function are characterized by a condition called vertigo, in which a hallucination of motion occurs; that is, either the person is stationary and the environment is in motion (objective vertigo), or the person is in motion and the environment is stationary (subjective vertigo). Vertigo should be differentiated from dizziness, which is characterized by light-headedness, fainting, and unsteadiness. Abnormal nystagmus, tinnitus, and hearing loss are other common manifestations of vestibular dysfunction, as are autonomic manifestations such as perspiration, nausea, and vomiting. Disorders of vestibular function can be either peripheral (involving the labyrinth) or central (involving the vestibular connections).

Spontaneous nystagmus is always pathologic. It seems to appear more readily and more severely when fatigue is present and, to some extent, can be influenced by psychological factors. Nystagmus derived from the central nervous system, in contrast with peripheral end organ or eighth cranial nerve sources, is rarely accompanied by vertigo, if present, the vertigo is of mild intensity.

Disorders of peripheral vestibular function

Motion sickness. One of the most common alterations of vestibular function is motion sickness. It is caused by repeated rhythmic stimulation of the vestibular system, such as is encountered in car, air, or boat travel. Vertigo, malaise, nausea, and vomiting are the principal symptoms. Autonomic signs, including lowered blood pressure, tachycardia, and excessive sweating, may occur. Antimotion sickness drugs are often used to ameliorate these symptoms. Motion sickness usually decreases in severity with repeated exposure.

Vestibular system injury or irritation. The inner ear is vulnerable to injury caused by fracture of the petrous portion of the temporal bones; infection of nearby structures, including the middle ear and meninges, and bloodborne toxins and infections. Damage to the vestibular system can occur as a side-effect of certain drugs or from allergic reactions to foods. The aminoglycosides (*e.g.,* streptomycin and gentamicin) have a specific toxic affinity for the vestibular portion of the inner ear. Shellfish seem to be the most common food allergen producing vertigo. Alcohol can also cause transient episodes of vertigo.

Severe irritation or damage of the vestibular end organs or nerves resulting in severe balance disorders reflected by instability of posture, dystaxia, and falling accompanied by vertigo. With irritation, falling is away from the affected side, and with destruction it is toward the affected side. Adaptation to asymmetrical stimulation occurs within a few days, after which the signs and symptoms diminish and are eventually lost. Following recovery, there is usually a slightly reduced acuity for tilt, and the person walks with a somewhat broadened base to improve postural stability. The neurologic basis for this adaptation to unilateral loss of vestibular input is not understood. Following adaptation to the loss of vestibular input from one side, the loss of function of the opposite vestibular apparatus produces signs and symptoms identical to those resulting from unilateral rather than bilateral loss. Within weeks, adaptation is again sufficient for locomotion and even for driving a car. Such a person relies very heavily on visual and proprioceptive input and has severe orientational difficulty in the dark, particularly when traversing uneven terrain.

Meniere's syndrome. Meniere's syndrome is a disorder of vestibular function caused by an overaccumulation of endolymph, also called endolymphatic hydrops. It is characterized by fluctuating episodes of tinnitus, feelings of ear fullness, and violent rotary vertigo that often renders the person unable to sit or walk. There is a need to lie quietly with the head fixed in a comfortable position, avoiding all head movements that aggravate the vertigo. Symptoms referable to the autonomic nervous system, including pallor, sweating, nausea, and vomiting, are usually present. The more severe the attack, the more prominent the autonomic manifestations. A fluctuating hearing loss occurs, and initially there is a return to normal after the episode subsides; but as the disease progresses, it becomes more severe and permanent. Meniere's syndrome is usually unilateral, and since the sense of hearing is bilateral, persons with the disorder are often not aware of the full extent of their hearing loss.

A number of conditions such as allergy, adrenal–pituitary insufficiency, trauma, and hypothyroidism can cause Meniere's syndrome. The most common form of the disease is an idiopathic form thought to be caused by a single viral injury to the fluid transport system of the inner ear.

Methods used in the diagnosis of Meniere's syndrome include audiograms, vestibular testing by electronystagmography, and petrous pyramid x-rays. Administration of hyperosmolar substances, such as glycerin and urea, often produces acute temporary hearing improvement in persons with Meniere's syndrome and is sometimes used as a diagnostic measure of endolymphatic hydrops. The diuretic furosemide may also be used for this purpose.

The treatment of Meniere's syndrome can be either medical or surgical. Medical treatment consists primarily of bed rest, sedation, and antiemetic and antimotion-sickness drugs. Use of a low-salt diet and diuretic therapy may be useful in decreasing the frequency of attacks. Surgical treatment is indicated in persons who do not benefit from medical treatment. Surgical methods include an endolymphatic–subarachnoid shunt in which excess endolymph from the inner ear is diverted into the subarachnoid space. Surgical destruction of labyrinth can be used to eliminate vertigo. This procedure is reserved for persons with severe deafness of the involved ear, in which the disease is unilateral and of more than 2 years' duration. An otic–perotic shunt (cochleosacculotomy) can be performed through the external auditory canal and round window. Cryosurgery involves the application of intense cold to the lateral semicircular canal. This procedure either reduces the sensitivity of the vestibular apparatus or creates a fistula in the membranous labyrinth, causing a shunt between the endolymph and the perilymph. Vestibular nerve resection may also be done.

Disorders of central vestibular function

Nystagmus and vertigo can occur as a result of central nervous system pathology. Compression of the vestibular nuclei by cerebellar tumors invading the fourth ventricle results in progressively severe signs and symptoms. In addition to nystagmus and vertigo, vomiting, and broad-base and dystaxic gait become progressively more evident. Centrally derived nystagmus usually has equal excursion in both directions (pendular). Congenital and lifelong nystagmus is not uncommon, often occurring as part of a number of hereditary syndromes. It can also accompany other motor defects in cerebral palsy and degenerative syndromes such as multiple sclerosis. Nystagmus can make reading and other tasks requiring precise eye positional control very difficult. When assessing for minimal nystagmus in possible brain damage, the patient is asked to fixate on the tester's finger; the tester then moves it laterally within the patient's visual field. At the most extreme limit of lateral deviation, ipsilateral nystagmoid eye flutter enduring longer than three beats and nystagmus upon eye deviation in any other plane indicate hyperexcitability of the vestibular reflex systems.

Diagnostic methods

Diagnosis of vestibular disorders is based on a description of the symptoms, a history of trauma or exposure to agents that are destructive to vestibular structures, and physical examination. Tests of eye movements (nystagmus) and muscle control of balance and equilibrium are often used.

Tests of postrotational nystagmus. If the head is suddenly slowed or stopped from a steady angular velocity of rotation, the same sequence of reflex conjugate eye movements occurs, but in the opposite direction. Because it is easier to observe a person's responses following the cessation of rotation than it is for the observer to rotate with the person, the postrotational nystagmus is usually used to study the adequacy of vestibular reflexes. A rotatable chair (Barany chair), much like a barber's chair, is used for this purpose. The person being tested is strapped into the chair with the head positioned so that the plane of one pair of semicircular canals is in the horizontal plane (plane of rotation). The person is then rotated until a steady rate of rotation is achieved. The chair is suddenly stopped, and the ensuing reflex postrotational nystagmus as well as the compensatory movements of the body and limbs are observed. Each of the three primary planes of the canals can be tested in turn, the corresponding semicircular ducts of both sides being tested simultaneously. Unilateral defects are not clearly detected by this method. After the rotation in the Barany chair is stopped, the person being tested is asked to point toward a fixed visual target. The pointing arm will drift past the target; this is called *past-pointing*. Because of the danger of injury associated with the powerful vestibular reflexes of the body and limbs, only trained personnel should perform the Barany chair tests.

Caloric stimulation. A more commonly performed test of vestibular reflexes involves irrigation of the external meatus of one ear with warm (40°C) or cold (25°C) water. The resulting changes in temperature, as conducted through the petrous portion of the temporal bone, set up convection currents in the otic fluid that mimic the effects of angular acceleration. Maximal stimulation occurs in the semicircular duct that is vertical during irrigation, and the corresponding nystagmoid eye movements can be assessed. An advantage of the caloric stimulation method is the ability to test the vestibular apparatus on one side at a time.

Electronystagmography. The caloric test for evaluating nystagmoid eye movements is based on subjective observation and is therefore subject to error. A more precise and objective diagnostic method of evaluating nystagmus is through the use of electronystagmography (ENG). With this method, the standard caloric stimulus is delivered to the ear canal, and the duration and velocity of eye movements are recorded using electrodes in a manner similar to electrocardiography. Electrodes are placed lateral to the outer canthus of each eye and above and below each eye. A ground electrode is placed on the forehead.

Romberg test. The Romberg test is used to demonstrate disorders of static vestibular function. The person being tested is requested to stand with feet together and arms extended forward so that the degree of sway and arm stability can be noted. The person is then asked to close his or her eyes. When visual clues are removed, postural stability is based on proprioceptive sensation from the joints, muscles, and tendons and from static vestibular reception. Deficiency in vestibular static input will be indicated by greatly increased sway and a tendency for the arms to drift toward the side of deficiency.

If vestibular input is severely deficient, the subject will fall toward the deficient side. Care must be taken, because defects of proprioceptive projection to the forebrain will also result in some arm drift and postural instability toward the deficient side. Only if two-point discrimination and vibratory sensation from the lower and upper limbs are bilaterally normal can the deficiency be attributed to the vestibular system.

Antivertigo drugs

Among the methods used to treat vertigo are the antivertigo or antimotion-sickness drugs. Drugs used in the treatment of vertigo include anticholinergic drugs (scopolamine, atropine), monoaminergic drugs (amphetamine, ephedrine), and antihistamines (meclizine [Antivert]), cyclizine [Marezine], dimenhydrinate [Dramamine], promethazine [Phenergan]. Animal studies have documented that drugs with anticholinergic or monoaminergic activity diminish the excitability of neurons in the vestibular nucleus.[14] Although the antihistamines have long been used in treating vertigo, little is known about their mechanism of action. However, most of these drugs have some anticholinergic activity, and some also enhance sympathetic activity by blocking the reuptake of monoamines at the synaptic nerve terminals.[14] A transdermal scopolamine preparation (Transderm-V) has recently become available for use in treating motion sickness. The medication is prepared on slow-release microporous polypropylene membrane contained in a patch that can be placed behind the ear. A small dose of the drug is released slowly and absorbed over a 3-day period. This method of drug delivery has proven effective in preventing motion sickness with minimal side-effects. To be effective, however, the patch must be in place for several hours before exposure to motion.

In summary, the vestibular system plays an essential role in the equilibrium sense, which is closely integrated with visual and proprioceptive (position) senses. The receptors for the vestibular system, which are located in the semicircular canals of the inner ear, respond to changes in linear and angular acceleration of the head. The vestibular nerve fibers travel in the vestibulocochlear (VIII) cranial nerve to the vestibular nuclei located at the junction of the medulla and pons. Some of the fibers pass through the nuclei to the cerebellum. The cerebellar connections are necessary for temporally smooth, coordinated movements during ongoing head movements, tilt, and angular acceleration. The vestibular nuclei also connect with the nuclei of oculomotor (III), trochlear (IV), and abducens (VI) cranial nerves. Vestibular control of conjugate eye movements serves to preserve eye fixation on stable objects in the visual field during head movement. The term nystagmus is used to describe vestibular-controlled eye movements that occur in response to angular and rotational movements of the head. Neurons of the vestibular nuclei also project to the thalamus, to the temporal cortex, and to the somesthetic area of the parietal cortex. The thalamic and cortical projections provide the basis for the subjective experiences of position in space and of rotation and vertigo. Disorders of the vestibular system include motion sickness and Meniere's syndrome. Meniere's syndrome, which is caused by an overaccumulation of endolymph, is characterized by severe disabling episodes of tinnitus, feelings of ear fullness, and violent rotary vertigo. The diagnosis of vestibular disorders is based on a description of the symptoms, a history of trauma or exposure to agents destructive to vestibular structures, and tests of eye movements (nystagmus) and muscle control of balance and equilibrium. Among the methods used in the treatment of vertigo that accompanies vestibular disorders are the antivertigo, or antimotion-sickness drugs. These drugs act by diminishing the excitability of neurons in the vestibular nucleus.

■ Study Guide

After you have studied this chapter, you should be able to meet the following objectives:

☐ List the three layers of the eyeball.

☐ Differentiate between exophthalmos and proptosis.

☐ Describe the normal characteristics of the lateral and medial canthi.

☐ Cite the difference between marginal blepharitis, a hordeolum, and a chalazion.

☐ Describe eyelid changes that occur with entropion and ectropion.

☐ Explain how the strength of the orbicularis oculi can be tested.

☐ Describe the neural mechanisms associated with Horner's syndrome.

☐ Compare symptoms associated with the redeye caused by conjunctivitis, corneal irritation, acute glaucoma, subconjunctival hemorrhage, and blepharitis.

☐ List at least four causes of dry eye.

☐ Describe the appearance of corneal edema.

☐ List the symptoms of keratitis.

☐ Explain the mechanism of pupillary constriction and dilatation.

☐ Compare closed-angle and open-angle glaucoma.

☐ Define refraction and accommodation.

☐ Describe the visual changes that occur with cataract.

☐ Describe the function of the retina and its photoreceptors.

☐ Differentiate between retinal structures supplied by the choroid capillaries and those supplied by the retinal arteries.

☐ State the value of the fundoscopic examination of the eye using the ophthalmoscope.

☐ State the cause of color blindness.

☐ Relate the phagocytic function of the retinal pigment epithelium to the development of retinitis pigmentosa.

☐ Describe the pathogenesis of background and proliferative diabetic retinopathy and their mechanisms of visual impairment.

☐ Explain the pathology and visual changes associated with macular degeneration.

☐ Discuss the cause of retinal detachment.

☐ Trace the pathways of the nasal and temporal retina from the optic nerve to the primary visual cortex.

☐ Define the term scotoma and discuss its significance.

☐ Describe a method for testing the visual field.

☐ Name the six extraocular muscles and their cranial nerves.

☐ Define smooth pursuit, saccadic, vestibular, vergence, and tremor eye movements.

☐ Describe two causes of strabismus.

☐ Explain the difference between paralytic and non-paralytic strabismus.

☐ Explain the need for early diagnosis and treatment of strabismus in infants and small children.

☐ Define amblyopia and explain its pathogenesis.

☐ List the structures of the external, middle, and inner ear and cite their function.

☐ Cite the impact of damage to Wernicke's area in the brain.

☐ Describe the symptoms of impacted cerumen.

☐ Relate the functions of the eustachian tube to the development of otitis media.

☐ Explain why infants and small children are more prone to develop otitis media.

☐ List three common symptoms of otitis media.

☐ Describe the disease process that occurs with otosclerosis, and relate this to the hearing loss that occurs.

☐ Differentiate between conductive and sensorineural hearing loss.

☐ List at least three drug groups that have potential ototoxicity.

☐ Explain the function of the vestibular system.

☐ Describe normal nystamus eye movements.

☐ List the symptoms of motion sickness.

☐ Describe the pathology associated with Meniere's syndrome.

■ References

1. National Society to Prevent Blindness: Vision Problems in the U.S. New York, 1980
2. Newell FW: Ophthalmology, 5th ed, pp 250, 341. St Louis, CV Mosby, 1982
3. Vaughan D, Asbury T: General Ophthalmology, 10th ed, pp 52, 139. Los Altos, CA, Lange Medical Publications, 1982
4. Wise JB: Long-term control of adult open angle glaucoma by argon laser treatment. Ophthalmology 88:197, 1981
5. Bresler MJ, Hoffman RS: Prevention of iatrogenic acute narrow-angle glaucoma. Ann Emerg Med 10:535, 1981
6. Jaffee NS: The current status of cataract and intraocular lens implant surgery. M Sinai J Med 48:539, 1981
7. Bluestone CD: Otitis media in children: To treat or not to treat. N Engl J Med 306:1399, 1982
8. Parareela MM (moderator): Report of the Ad Hoc Committee on Definition and Classification of Otitis Media and Otitis Media with Effusion. Ann Otolaryngol 89(Suppl):3, 1980
9. Barfold C, Roborg J: Secretory otitis media: Long-term observations after treatment with grommets. Arch Otolaryngol 106:553, 1980
10. Al-Sheikhle ARJ: Secretory otitis media in children. (A retrospective study of 249) J Laryngol Otol 94:1117, 1980
11. Meyerhoff WL: Diagnosis and Management of Hearing Loss, p 1. Philadelphia, WB Saunders, 1984
12. Dodge PR, Hallowell D, Feigin RD et al: Prospective evaluation of hearing impairment as a sequela of acute bacterial meningitis. N Engl J Med 311:879, 1984
13. Brown RD, Wood CD: Vestibular pharmacology. Trends Pharmacol Sci (Feb):150, 1980
14. Baloh RW: The dizzy patient. Postgrad Med 73:317, 1983

■ Additional References

Hearing

Balkany TJ: An overview of electronic cochlear prosthesis: Clinical and research considerations. Otolaryngol Clin North Am 16, No 1:209, 1983

Bentzen O: Otosclerosis, a universal disease. Adv Oto-Rhin-Laryngol 29:151, 1983

Bluestone CD: Recent advances in the pathogenesis, diagnosis, and management of otitis media. Pediatr Clin North Am 28, No 4:727, 1981

Bluestone CD, Klein JO, Paradise JL et al: Workshop on effects of otitis media in the child. Pediatrics 71:639, 1983

Brondbo K, Hawke M, Abel SM et al: The natural history of otosclerosis. J Otolaryngol 13:164, 1983

Cantekin E, Phillips DC, Doyle WJ et al: Gas absorption in the middle ear. Ann Otolaryngol 89 (Suppl):71, 1980

Causse JB, Causse JR: Minimizing cochlear loss during and after stapedectomy. Otolaryngol Clin North Am 15, No 4:813, 1982

Crawford LV, Goode RL, Grundfast KM et al: Otitis media: Selecting the therapy. Patient Care (Sept):108, 1983

D'Alonzo BJ, Cantor AB: Ototoxicity: Etiology and issues. J Fam Pract 16:489, 1983

DiChara E: A sound method for testing children's hearing. Am J Nurs 84:1104, 1984

Dodge PR, Davis H, Feigin RD et al: Prospective evaluation of hearing impairment as a sequela of acute bacterial meningitis. N Engl J Med 311:869, 1984

Ecliachar I, Joachims HZ, Goldsher M et al: Assessment of long-term middle ear ventilation. Acta Otolaryngol 96:105, 1983

Farmer HS: A guide to treatment of external otitis. Am Fam Pract 21:96, 1980

Feigin RD: Otitis media: Closing the information gap. N Engl J Med 306:1417, 1982

Fourcin A, Douek E, Moore B et al: Speech pattern element stimulation in electrical hearing. Arch Otolaryngol 110:145, 1984

From J: Otitis media (clinical review). J Fam Pract 15:743, 1982

Glover G: Management of otosclerotic deafness. Ear Nose Throat J 60:571, 1981

Herzon FS: Tympanostomy tubes. Arch Otolaryngol 106:645, 1980

Hinojosa R, Lindsay JR: Profound deafness. J Otolaryngol 106:193, 1980

Human Communication and Its Disorder. NINDS Monograph No 10. DHEW Publication No (NIH) 76-1090, 1970

Magnuson B, Falk B: Eustachian tube malfunction and middle ear disease in new perspective. J Otolaryngol 12:187, 1983

Paparella MM, Goycoolea MV, Meyerhoff WL: Inner ear pathology and otitis media—A Review. Ann Otolaryngol 89 (Suppl):249, 1980

Paradise JL: Otitis media during early life: How hazardous to development? A critical review of the evidence. Pediatrics 68:869, 1981

Rubin W: Diagnosis: Noise and hearing loss. Hosp Med 19, No 5:77, 1983

Senturia BH, Bluestone CD, Klein JO et al: Report of the Ad Hoc Committee on Definitions and Classification of Otitis Media and Otitis Media with Effusion. Ann Otolaryngol 89 (Suppl):3, 1980

Shea JJ: Otosclerosis and tinnitus. J Laryngol Otol (Suppl) 4:149, 1981

Singh RP: Anatomy of Hearing and Speech. New York, Oxford University Press, 1980

Spellman FA: The cochlear prosthesis: A review of the design and evaluation of electrode implants for the profoundly deaf. CRC Crit Rev Biomed Eng 8, No 5:223, 1982

Square R, Cooper JC, Hearne EM et al: Eustachian tube function. Arch Otolaryngol 108:567, 1982

Sutton D: Cochlear pathology: Hazards of long-term implants. Arch Otolaryngol 110:164, 1984

Teele DW, Klein JO, Rosner BA: Epidemiology of otitis media in children. Ann Otolaryngol 89 (Suppl):5, 1980

Vestibular function

Baldwin RL: The dizzy patient. Hosp Pract 19, No 10:151, 1984

Brooks GB: Meniere's disease: A practical approach. Drugs 25:77, 1983

Condi JK: Types and causes of nystagmus in the neurosurgical patient. J Neurosurg Nurs 15, No 2:56, 1983

Dix MR: Positional nystagmus of the central type and its neural mechanisms. Acta Otolaryngol 95:585, 1983

Gussen R: Vascular mechanisms in Meniere's disease. Arch Otolaryngol 108:544, 1982

Pulec JL: Meniere's syndrome. Hosp Med 19, No 6:81, 1981

Schmidt PH: Pathophysiology of Meniere attack: Facts and theories. Acta Otolaryngol 95:417, 1983

Shea JJ: Intracochlear shunt. Otolaryngol Clin North Am 16, No 1:293, 1983

Tonndorf J: Vestibular signs and symptoms in Meniere's disorder: Mechanical consideration. Acta Otolaryngol 95:431, 1983

Wall CW III, Black FO: Postural stability and rotational tests: Their effectiveness for screening dizzy patients. Acta Otolaryngol 95:235, 1983

Wolfson RJ, Silverstein H, Marlowe FI et al: Vertigo. Clin Symposia 33, No 6, 1981

Vision

Abrahamson IA: Cataract update. Am Fam Pract 24:112, 1981

Beller R, Hoyt CS, Marg E et al: Good visual function after neonatal surgery for congenital monocular cataracts. Am J Ophthalmol 91:559, 1981

Birnbaum MH: Clinical management of myopia. Am J Optom Physiol Opt 58:554, 1981

Calhoun JH: Cataracts in children. Pediatr Clin North Am 30, No 6:1061, 1983

Check WE: New findings in diabetic retinopathy. JAMA 246:2792, 1981

Chew E, Morin JD: Glaucoma in children. Pediatr Clin North Am 30, No 6:1043, 1983

Cotlier E: Senile cataracts: Evidence of acceleration by diabetes and deceleration by salicylate. Can J Ophthalmol 16:113, 1981

Gitschlag G, Scott WE: Strabismus, amblyopia, and dyslexia. Primary Care 9:661, 1982

Grant WM, Burke JF: Why do some people go blind with glaucoma? Am Acad Ophthalmol 89:991, 1982

Greenwald MJ: Visual development in infancy and childhood. Pediatr Clin North Am 30, No 6:977, 1983

Jaffe NS: The current status of cataract and intraocular lens implant surgery. M Sinai J Med 48:539, 1981

Katz IM, Soll DB: Beta blockers and glaucoma. Am Fam Pract 21:150, 1980

Kerns RL: Contact lens control of myopia. Am J Optom Physiol Op 58:541, 1981

Liesegang TJ: Cataracts and cataract operations (subject review). Part 1 and Part 2. Mayo Clin Proc 59:556, 622, 1984

Marcus DF, Bovino JA: Retinal detachment. JAMA 247:873, 1982

Meltzer MA: Diagnosis of eyelid and periorbital abnormalities. Hosp Pract 20, No 9:67, 1984

Michels RG: What role vitrectomy in managing diabetic retinopathy. Hosp Pract 15, No 9:73, 1977

Nelson LB: Diagnosis and management of strabismus and amblyopia. Pediatr Clin North Am 30, No 6:1003, 1983

Nirankari VS, Katzen LE, Richards RD et al: Prospective clinical study of radial keratotomy. Am Acad Ophthalmol 89:677, 1982

Perrin ED: Laser therapy for diabetic retinopathy. Am J Nurs 80:664, 1980

Quinn GE, Schaffer DB, Johnson L: A revised classification of retinopathy of prematurity. Am J Ophthalmol 94:744, 1982

Rand LI: Recent advances in diabetic retinopathy. Am J Med 70:595, 1981

Resler MM, Tumulty G: Glaucoma update. Am J Nurs 83:752, 1983

Rice TA, Michels, Rice EF: Vitrectomy for diabetic rhegmatogenous retinal detachment. Am J Ophthalmol 95:34, 1983

Rice TA, Michels RG, Rice E: Vitrectomy for diabetic traction retinal detachment involving the macula. Am J Ophthalmol 95:22, 1983

Riordan P, Pascoe PT, Vaughan DG: Refractive change in hyperglycemia: hyperopia, not myopia. Br J Opthalmol 66:500, 1982

Shields MB: Combined cataract extraction and glaucoma surgery. Acad Ophthalmol 89:231, 1982

Shin DH: Surgical management of cataract and glaucoma. Ann Ophthamol (Sept):1015, 1981

Sussman EJ, Tsiaras WG, Soper KA: Diagnosis of diabetic eye disease. JAMA 247:3231, 1982

Teisch SA: Retinal manifestations of vascular diseases. Hosp Pract 20, No 8:69, 1984

Wald G: The receptors of human color vision. Science 145:1007, 1964

Wets B, Milot JA, Polomeno RC et al: Cataracts and ketotic hypoglycemia. Am Acad Ophthalmol 89:999, 1982

Wise JB: Long-term control of adult open angle glaucoma by argon laser treatment. Am Acad Ophthalmol 88:197, 1981

Chapter 47

Disorders of Cerebral Function

Mary Wierenga

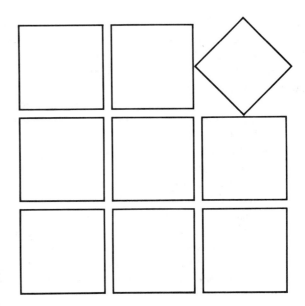

Normally, neurons respond appropriately to changes in stimuli from the internal and external environments. Periods of wakefulness and sleep are regulated by need, and even during sleep, a person can be aroused with relative ease. The threshold of excitation of neurons is such that responses can be controlled. The extremes of normal responses are coma or unconsciousness, which can be considered inappropriate extensions of sleep; confusion, a disturbance in alertness; and seizures and epilepsy, in which neurons become paroxysmally hyperexcitable. Among the causes of the extreme responses are injuries and infections of the nervous system. Increased intracranial pressure (ICP), or intracranial hypertension, which can be caused by injuries or infections, can precipitate coma, confusion, and seizures. This chapter, therefore, contains a discussion of increased intracranial pressure, hydrocephalus, head injury, brain infections, seizures, coma, and organic brain syndrome.

Increased Intracranial Pressure (ICP)

The cranial cavity contains blood, brain tissue, and cerebrospinal fluid (CSF) within a rigid, nonexpandable skull. Each of these substances contributes to the normal intracranial pressure of 50 mm to 300 mm H_2O or 4 mm to 15 mm Hg. Normally, each of these substances may vary slightly in volume, but the intracranial pressure remains relatively constant. Small increases in the volume of one substance can be compensated by a decrease in the volume of the other two. Small increases caused by daily activities, such as straining or coughing, occur frequently and cause little problem unless they are sustained.

Abnormal variation in intracranial volume can be caused by several factors. An increase in tissue volume occurs with a brain tumor, an increase in extracellular fluid develops when edema or bleeding is present, and an increase in blood volume occurs as a result of vasodilatation of cerebral vessels or the obstruction of venous outflow. Cerebral blood flow is greatly affected by the arterial carbon dioxide concentration and, to a lesser degree, by the arterial oxygen concentration. Hypothermia and defective cerebral autoregulation also affect cerebral blood flow. The CSF increases when excess production, decreased reabsorption, or obstructed circulation occurs. When the change in volume is due to a brain tumor, it tends to occur slowly and is usually localized to the immediate area, whereas the volume change resulting from head injury usually increases rapidly and is generalized in one hemisphere. Localized edema because of brain tumors often responds to corticosteroids, but these drugs have little effect on generalized edema.

The impact of increases in blood, brain tissue, or CSF on ICP varies among individuals and depends on the amount of increase that occurs, the effectiveness of compensatory mechanisms, and cerebral elastance. The brain is both plastic (or easily deformed) and elastic (or resistant to deformation), plasticity being its more evident characteristic. The blood vessels provide the major elastic component. Compensation involves a shunting of CSF to the spinal subarachnoid space and, secondarily, a reduction of cerebral blood volume. The ICP remains normal as long as the increase in volume does not exceed the CSF or blood volume that was displaced. The compensation of the brain tissue is determined by the cerebral elastance or its reciprocal compliance. The relationship between volume and pressure is elastance. When elastance is high, even small increases in volume increase the ICP to dangerous levels.

When the CSF and blood can no longer compensate for the increased volume and the excess space in the cranial cavity is filled, the ICP rises sharply and may result in cerebral hypoxia or brain shift. When the pressure in the cranial cavity approaches or exceeds the mean systemic arterial pressure, tissue perfusion becomes inadequate, cellular hypoxia results, and if it is maintained, neuronal death may occur. The highly specialized cortical cells are the most sensitive to oxygen deficit; therefore, a decrease in the level of consciousness is one of the earliest and most reliable signs of increased intracranial pressure. The increasing cellular hypoxia leads to general neurologic deterioration. The level of consciousness may deteriorate progressively from alertness through confusion, lethary, obtundation, stupor, and coma.

There is growing evidence that the other traditional signs and symptoms of increasing ICP—changes in motor function, pupillary dilation, widening of the pulse pressure, and changes in respiration—are due to shifting and herniation, or downward displacement of brain tissue through the tentorial incisura or notch. The most important pupillary change is unilateral dilatation. The third cranial nerve, the oculomotor, controls pupillary constriction and runs along the tentorial ridge. The downward displacement of the cerebral cortex, which exerts pressure on this nerve, causes unilateral pupil dilatation. This is a primary sign of impending herniation. The motor signs include changes in the strength and coordination of voluntary movements. Respiratory changes may also occur, and body temperature may or may not rise. Herniation also interferes with the function of the reticular activating system (RAS) and the control of vital signs. The blood pressure and heart rate should be monitored frequently when there is a possibility of ICP, because these vital signs reflect the body's attempt to compensate for the increased pressure.

One of the late reflexes seen with marked increases in intracranial pressure is the *CNS ischemic response*, which is triggered by ischemia of the vasomotor center. The neurons in the vasomotor center respond directly to ischemia by producing a marked increase in mean arterial blood pressure, sometimes to levels as high as 270 mm Hg. The Cushing reaction is a type of CNS ischemic response. It results from a severely increased intracranial pressure that compresses the blood flow to the brain. If the increase in blood pressure initiated by the CNS ischemic reflex is greater than the pressure surrounding the compressed vessels, blood flow will be reestablished. The CNS ischemic response is a last ditch effort by the nervous system to maintain cerebral circulation. It is accompanied by a widening of the pulse pressure and a reflex bradycardia. This *widening of the pulse pressure* and the *decrease in heart rate* are important but late indicators of increased intracranial pressure.

Intracranial Pressure Monitoring

Herniation through the tentorial notch is a late complication of increased ICP. Therefore, the signs and symptoms traditionally used to detect rising pressure are unreliable for the early recognition and treatment of increased ICP. The recent introduction of intracranial pressure monitoring along with computerized tomography (CT) has facilitated the prompt diagnosis and appropriate treatment of neurologic trauma. ICP monitoring can provide continuous information about the compensatory mechanisms and other dynamics of intracranial pressure. Volume–pressure relationships, compliance, pulse pressure, pressure waves, and cerebral perfusion pressure may be evaluated with ICP monitoring. There are three types of intracranial pressure waves: A, B, and C waves; B and C waves have little clinical significance. The A waves, now called *plateau* waves, are most important and are only seen in advanced stages of increased ICP. The plateau waves represent repeated increases in ICP.[1]

Monitoring of ICP is accomplished through the use of a measuring device (intraventricular catheter, subarachnoid bolt, or implanted transducer) and a recording device. The measurement device can be inserted directly into the ventricles, subarachnoid space, or epidural space. The measurement of CSF pressure is used to indicate the overall ICP, assuming that all the spaces are open between compartments.

Hydrocephalus

One form of increased volume in the cranial cavity is hydrocephalus, which is defined as an abnormal increase in CSF volume within any part or all of the ventricular system. Hydrocephalus is not a disease but the result of a pathologic process that causes production of CSF at a rate greater than its rate of removal. The two causes of hydrocephalus are overproduction of CSF and obstruc-

tion to its flow through the ventricular system, around the brain in the subarachnoid space, or outflow through the arachnoid villi.

There are two types of hydrocephalus: communicating and noncommunicating. *Noncommunicating hydrocephalus* occurs when flow within the ventricular system is obstructed. The obstruction can be caused by congenital malformation, infection, or tumors encroaching on the ventricular system. *Communicating hydrocephalus* occurs when the CSF is not reabsorbed into the arachnoid villi. This can occur if too few villi are formed, if postinfective (meningitis) scarring occludes them, or if the villi become obstructed by fragments of blood or infectious debris. The signs of ICP elevation depend on the type of hydrocephalus, the age of onset, and the extent of increase in CSF pressure. The usual treatment is a shunting procedure, which provides an alternative route for return of CSF to the circulation.

Head Injury

Head injuries are prime examples of the many neurologic conditions in which increased ICP is a major problem. Cerebral edema caused by the head injury is the primary cause of increased ICP. The more criticial an organ or system is to the body as a whole, the more provisions nature makes to protect its structures. The brain is protected by the skull, meninges, and CSF. When the integrity of this protective system is broken, usually as the result of trauma, brain damage may occur; the ultimate results may range from a minor psychomotor deficit to total dependency.[2] Hemiparesis (weakness of one side of the body), aphasia, hemianopia (blindness or defective vision in half of the visual field), unconsciousness, either immediate or delayed, posttraumatic epilepsy, and postconcussion syndrome are common sequelae of head injury.

Although the skull and the CSF provide protection for the brain, they can also contribute to trauma in some injuries, known as *contrecoup injuries.* In this type of injury the side of the brain opposite the side of the head that was struck is injured. This occurs because the brain floats freely in the CSF, while the brain stem is stable. Thus, the skull, being lighter in mass than the brain, is hit first, causing the brain to be thrown against the opposite side of the skull and then to rebound. As the brain strikes the rough surface of the cranial vault, brain tissue, blood vessels, nerve tracts, and other structures are bruised and torn.

Head injury may be due to either penetration (open head injury) or impact (closed head injury), and each affects the brain, meninges, CSF, and skull in different ways.

For descriptive purposes, head injuries are divided into primary, or *direct,* injuries in which damage is due to impact, and *secondary injuries,* in which damage results from the subsequent brain swelling (cerebral edema), intracranial hematomas (blood clots), infection, cerebral hypoxia, and ischemia.[3] Because secondary injuries follow rapidly, usually within hours of the direct injury, it is often difficult to distinguish the damage done by each. The distinction between direct and secondary injuries is crucial, however, because the main objective of treatment is to prevent or minimize secondary brain injury.

Direct injuries

One of the most serious types of direct injury is skull fracture. In one neurosurgical unit, 80% of fatal injuries were associated with fractures of the skull.[4] Skull fractures can be divided into three groups: simple linear, comminuted, and compound. A *simple linear* skull fracture is a break in the continuity of the bone. Multiple linear fractures, which cause splintering or crushing of bone, are classified as *comminuted fractures.* When bone fragments are depressed into the brain tissue, the fracture is said to be *depressed.* When an opening is present through the skull or mucous membrane of the sinuses, the fracture is termed a *compound fracture.* A compound fracture may be linear or comminuted.

Usually, radiologic examination is needed to confirm the presence and extent of a skull fracture. This is important because of the possible damage to the underlying tissues. A frequent complication of fractures is the leakage of CSF from the nose (rhinorrhea) or ear (otorrhea), with resultant infection. One way to differentiate between CSF and mucus drainage from the nose is to collect a specimen and test it for glucose. Glucose is normally present in the CSF but is absent in mucus. There may be lacerations to vessels in the dura, most often to the middle meninges, with resulting intracranial bleeding. Damage to cranial nerves may also result from skull fractures.

Concussion–contusion.   Even if there is no break in the skull, a blow to the head can cause severe and diffuse brain damage. Such closed injury can be classified as (1) mild, moderate, or severe, or as (2) a concussion or contusion. There is some overlap in these classifications. For example, the terms mild head injury and concussion may be used interchangeably.

In *mild head injury,* there may be momentary loss of consciousness without demonstrable neurologic symptoms or residual damage, except for possible residual amnesia. Microscopic changes can usually be detected in the neurons and glia within hours of injury. Although recovery usually takes place within 24 hours, mild symptoms, such as headache, irritability, and insomnia, may persist for months.

Moderate head injury is characterized by a longer period of unconsciousness and may be associated with

neurologic manifestations, such as hemiplegia. In this type of injury, many small hemorrhages and some swelling of brain tissue (cerebral edema) occur.

In *severe head injury,* there is cerebral contusion (bruising of the brain) and tearing and shearing of brain structures. It is often accompanied by symptoms such as hemiplegia. These injuries frequently occur with other types of trauma—to the extremities, the chest, and the abdomen, for example. Extravasation of blood may occur; if the contusion is severe, the blood may coalesce, as in intracerebral hemorrhage.[4] Similarly, when laceration of the brain directly under the area of injury occurs, especially if the skull is fractured, hemorrhage may be so extensive as to merit the designation of *hematoma.* The contusion is often distributed along the rough, irregular inner surface of the brain, and so is more likely to occur in the occipital area than in the frontal lobes.[4] Contusions are usually multiple and may be bilateral.

Frequently ischemic necrosis occurs in the center of a contused area, with eventual scar tissue formation. These scars are predisposing factors in posttraumatic epilepsy.

Secondary injuries

The significance of contusion depends on the extent of secondary injury caused by edema, hemorrhage, and infection. Cerebral edema secondary to the injury is caused by vasogenic, cytotoxic (metabolic), and ischemic processes. In the vascular system, loss of autoregulatory mechanisms and extracellular edema resulting from alterations in capillary permeability may occur. Metabolic toxins may cause disruption of the sodium pump, resulting in intracellular edema. Ischemia leads to the eventual breakdown of cells, including those of the blood–brain barrier.[5,6] Two types of hematomas may result from hemorrhage—epidural and subdural. Each of these processes results in increased ICP, which may proceed to herniation of cranial contents through the tentorial notch.

Epidural hematoma (extradural hematoma).   Epidural hematomas are usually caused by a severe head injury in which the skull is fractured. An *epidural* (extradural) hematoma is one that develops between the skull and the dura, outside the dura (Fig. 47-1). It is usually due to a tear in the middle meningeal artery, and, because the bleeding is of arterial origin, rapid compression of the brain occurs. Epidural hematomas are more common in young persons because in them the dura is not so firmly attached to the skull surface as it is in older persons; as a consequence, the dura can be easily stripped away from the inner surface of the skull, allowing the hematoma to form.[3]

Typically, a person with an epidural hematoma presents the following picture: a history of head injury, a

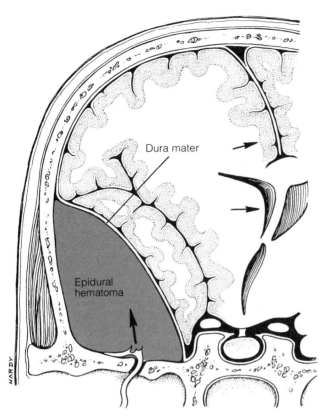

Figure 47-1 *Epidural hematoma. The dark area in the lower left is the hematoma. Note the broken blood vessel and the shift in the midline structures of the brain. (Cosgriff JH, Anderson DL: The Practice of Emergency Nursing. Philadelphia, JB Lippincott, 1975)*

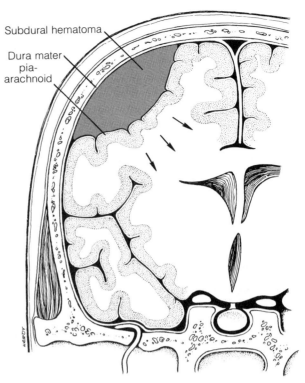

Figure 47-2 *Subdural hematoma. The dark area in the upper left is the hematoma. Note the midline shift of brain structures. (Cosgriff JH, Anderson DL: The Practice of Emergency Nursing. Philadelphia, JB Lippincott, 1975)*

brief period of unconciousness followed by a lucid period in which consciousness is regained, followed by a rapid progression to unconsciousness. The lucid interval is not always present, but when it is, it is of great diagnostic value. With rapidly developing unconsciousness there are focal symptoms related to the area of the brain involved. These symptoms can include ipsilateral (same side) pupil dilatation and contralateral (opposite side) hemiparesis. If the hematoma is not removed, the condition progresses, with increased intracranial pressure, tentorial herniation, and finally death.

Subdural hematoma. The area between the dura and the arachnoid is the subdural space. A subdural hematoma is the result of a tear in the arachnoid that allows blood from the small bridging veins between the dura and the pia mater to collect in the subdural space (Fig. 47-2). It develops more slowly than an epidural hematoma because the tear is in the venous system, whereas epidural hematomas are arterial. Subdural hematomas are classified as acute, subacute, or chronic. Symptoms of acute subdural hematoma are seen within 24 hours of the injury, whereas subacute hematoma does not pro-

duce symptoms until 2 to 10 days following injury. These types of hematoma are frequently discussed together. Symptoms of chronic subdural hematoma may not arise until several weeks after the injury. These classifications are based partially on temporal and partially on pathologic considerations.

Acute subdural hematomas progress rapidly and carry a high mortality because of the severe secondary injuries related to edema and increased intracranial pressure. The high mortality rate has been associated with the uncontrolled intracranial pressure increase, loss of consciousness, decerebrate posturing, and delay in surgical removal of the hematoma.[7] The clinical picture is similar to that of epidural hematoma except that there is usually no lucid interval. In *subacute* hematoma, there may be a period of improvement in the level of consciousness and neurologic symptoms, only to be followed by deterioration if the hematoma is not removed.

Symptoms of *chronic subdural hematoma* develop weeks after a head injury, so much later, in fact, that the person may not remember having had a head injury. This is especially true of older persons with brittle vessels. Seepage of blood into the subdural space occurs very slowly. Because the blood in the subdural space is not absorbed, fibroblastic activity begins and the hematoma becomes encapsulated. Within this encapsulated area, the cells are slowly lysed and a fluid with a high osmotic pressure is formed. This creates an osmotic gradient, with fluid from the surrounding subarachnoid space being pulled into the area; in turn, the mass increases in size, exerting pressure on the cranial contents.

In some instances, the clinical picture is less defined, the most prominent symptom being a decreasing level of consciousness indicated by drowsiness, confusion, and apathy. Headache may also be present.

Postconcussion syndrome

Following a head injury, complaints of headache, dizziness, poor concentration and memory, fatigue, and irritability are usual, although their extent and duration vary considerably. Because these complaints are vague and subjective, they have sometimes been regarded as being of psychological origin. Recent findings, however, support the belief in an organic basis for the postconcussion symptoms.[4] Sequelae that have a definite physical basis include hemiparesis, dysphasia, hemianopia, cranial nerve palsy, and epilepsy.

In summary, the contents of the cranial cavity consist of brain tissue, blood, and CSF. It is the collective volumes of these three intracranial components that determines the ICP. A variation in the volume of any of these three components can cause the ICP to rise, affecting cerebral function. Compensatory mechanisms protect the brain from small variations in the volume of any of these three compartments. Large variations, however, exceed the compensatory mechanisms and may lead to hypoxia, brain herniation, and death. Among the causes of ICP are hydrocephalus and head injuries. Hydrocephalus represents an abnormal increase in CSF volume within a part or all of the ventricular system. It is caused by overproduction of CSF or obstruction to its flow through the ventricular system. Head injuries cause swelling of brain tissue and bleeding into the cranial cavity. They can be classified as direct, resulting from the immediate effects of injury, skull fracture, concussion, or contusion; or as secondary, resulting from edema or hemorrhage and infection. Secondary injury may result from hematoma formation, which if not treated may cause herniation of brain tissue, through the tentorial hiatus, and death.

■ Infections

Infections of the CNS may be classified according to the structure involved: the meninges—meningitis; the brain parenchyma—encephalitis; the spinal cord—myelitis; both brain and spinal cord—encephalomyelitis. They may also be classified by the type of invading organism, whether bacterial, viral, or other. In general, the pathogens enter the CNS through the bloodstream by crossing the blood–brain barrier in a systemic disease or by direct invasion through skull fracture, a bullet hole, or, more rarely, contamination during surgery or lumbar puncture. This section focuses on meningitis and encephalitis.

Meningitis

Meningitis is an infection of the pia mater, the arachnoid, and the subarachnoid space. The annual reported incidence of meningitis in 1978 was 2.9 cases per 100,000 population.[8] Because meningococcal meningitis is the only reportable meningitis, the condition is believed to be underreported by about 30%. The case-fatality rate in the United States for reported cases was 13.6% in 1978. *Hemophilus influenzae* and meningococcal meningitis had significantly lower case fatalities than pneumococcal or neonatal meningitis.[9] Children under 5 years of age account for 70% of all cases of bacterial meningitis.[9] The predominant causes of meningitis in infants under 1 month of age are *Escherichia coli* and group B streptococcus. In infants and children more than 1 month of age, *Hemophilus influenzae* type B, *Neisseria meningitidis* (infectious agent for meningococcal meningitis), and *Streptococcus pneumoniae* account for approximately 90% of cases.

In an adult, the symptoms are those of meningeal irritation: fever, headache, lethargy, stiff neck (nuchal rigidity), and vomiting. The headache is frequently described as "the worst ever." Children may have less specific symptoms, with fever the most common and vomiting the second most frequent. Infants have few specific symptoms. The health professional should consider meningitis whenever these symptoms are present. An analysis of CSF will confirm or rule out meningitis and will identify the organism. Other observations should include (1) the presence of infection, (2) alterations in behavior or level of consciousness, and (3) neurologic symptoms.

As the disease progresses, nausea and vomiting, photophobia, convulsions, petechiae, and arthritis may occur. Kernig's sign and Brudzinski's sign will determine whether or not meningeal irritation is present. *Kernig's sign* is elicited when the leg cannot be extended while the patient is lying with the hip flexed at a right angle. A positive *Brudzinski's sign* is seen when forcible flexion of the neck results in flexion of the hip and knee.

As the pathogens enter the subarachnoid space, they cause inflammation, characterized by a cloudy, purulent exudate. Thrombophlebitis of the bridging veins and dural sinuses may develop, followed by congestion and infarction in the surrounding tissues. Ultimately, the meninges thicken and adhesions form. These adhesions may impinge on the cranial nerves, giving rise to cranial nerve palsies, or may impair the outflow of CSF, giving rise to hydrocephalus.

Encephalitis

Generalized infection of the parenchyma of the brain or spinal cord is almost always caused by a virus. The infection takes one of these forms: (1) inflammation caused by direct invasion, as in encephalitis, (2) a postinfectious noninflammatory process, as in Reye's syndrome, (3) a postinfectious inflammatory process, as in encephalomyelitis, and (4) a slow-growing infection that has a prolonged incubation period and runs a chronic course.[10]

The pathologic picture includes local necrotizing hemorrhage, which ultimately becomes generalized, with prominent edema. There is progressive degeneration of nerve cell bodies. The histologic picture, though rather general, demonstrates some specific characteristics; for example, the poliovirus selectively destroys the cells of the anterior horn of the spinal cord.[11]

Encephalitis, like meningitis, is characterized by fever, headache, and nuchal rigidity. In addition, a wide range of neurologic disturbance is present, such as lethargy, disorientation, seizures, dysphasias, focal paralysis, delirium, and coma. The nervous system is subject to invasion by many viruses, such as arbovirus, poliovirus, and rabies virus. The mode of transmission varies: it may be the bite of a mosquito, tick, or rabid animal; it may be enteral, as in poliomyelitis. A very common cause of encephalitis in the United States is herpes simplex virus.

In summary, infections of the CNS may be classified according to the structures involved (meningitis, encephalitis) or the type of organism causing the infection. The damage caused by infection may predispose to hydrocephalus, seizures, or other neurologic defects.

■ Seizures

A seizure may be defined as a spontaneous, uncontrolled, paroxysmal, transitory discharge from the cortical centers in the brain. This uncontrolled activity causes symptoms based on the location of the involved area—bizarre muscle movements, strange sensations and perception, and loss of consciousness.

A seizure is not a disease but a symptom of an underlying disorder. Seizures can be caused by almost all serious illnesses or injury, including congenital deformities, vascular lesions, head injury, drug or alcohol abuse, infections, and tumors. Although seizures are commonly associated with epilepsy, the two are not necessarily the same. For example, metabolic abnormalities are a major cause of a pathologic condition that gives rise to seizures and that is reversible. Examples include electrolyte imbalance, hypoglycemia, hypoxia, hypocalcemia, and acidosis. Toxemia of pregnancy, water intoxication, uremia, and CNS infections (meningitis, for example) may also precipitate a seizure. The rapid withdrawal of sedative–hypnotic drugs, such as alcohol or barbiturates, is another cause.[12] In children, a high fever (temperature over 104°F) may precipitate a seizure.

Seizure activity may be initiated by abnormal cells within the brain called *epileptogenic foci.* This abnormal activity is believed to be caused by alterations in membrane permeability or in the distribution of ions across the cell membrane.

Epilepsy

Recurrence of seizures without evidence of reversible metabolic activity is called *epilepsy.* These seizures are caused by paroxysmal and transitory disturbance of brain function, caused by the excessive discharge of cerebral neurons, which develops suddenly and disappears spontaneously. Unlike other types of seizure, epilepsy exhibits a definite tendency to recur and is not usually associated with systemic disease. After stroke, epilepsy is the most prevalent neurologic disorder. Two million Americans, or 1 out of every 100 people, have epilepsy.[13] The two chief types of epilepsy are secondary epilepsy, or structurally induced seizure, which has a known cause; and primary epilepsy, also called idiopathic epilepsy, which does not have a known cause.

In secondary epilepsy, seizures result from cerebral scarring due to head injury, cerebral vascular accident, infection, degenerative CNS disease, or recurrent childhood febrile seizures. Head injury is one of the main causes of seizures. Approximately 10% of persons with acute head injury may have seizures, probably because of bleeding, edema, and neuronal death.[6] The incidence of posttraumatic seizures has been reported to be 5% to 50%, depending on the severity of the underlying injury or disease, whether or not unconsciousness was present, and whether or not the dura was penetrated.

The age of onset can be a clue to the type or cause of the seizure. Seizures occurring between birth and 6 months of age are probably due to *congenital defects* or birth injury. Seizures first occurring between the ages of 2 and 18 years with no known cause may be due to the vulnerability of the developing nervous system to seizure activity.[14] Genetic predisposition as a possible cause of idiopathic seizures is currently being investigated. After 20 years of age, seizures are usually due to structural damage or trauma, tumor, or stroke.

Classification

Although a knowledge of the etiology is important, seizure management is usually directed toward seizure activity and its control. In 1969, a classification system was developed by the International League Against Epilepsy that combined clinical and electroencephalographic (EEG) manifestations to describe seizure activity.[15] This classification system was prompted by the need for more accurate diagnosis and quantification of seizure activity for use with new and more specific types of medications. The recent use of videotape to record seizure activity has helped to improve the classification of seizures, and a revised seizure classification system has been proposed by the Commission on Classification and Terminology of the International League Against Epilepsy.[16] The main difference between the 1969 version and the proposed version is the allowance for a description of seizure progression, which would improve descriptive accuracy. Although the revised classification system is not universally accepted, it is used as a basis for discussing seizures in this text. As technology advances and the knowledge of medications and their effects on the various types of seizures increases, the classification system will probably continue to be redefined.

There are two main classifications of seizures, depending on whether one hemisphere (partial) or both hemispheres (generalized) are initially involved. Partial seizures have evidence of a local onset but not a discreet focus, whereas generalized seizures do not exhibit a local onset.

Partial seizures. Partial seizures are classified as simple partial, complex partial, and partial seizures secondarily generalized. Classification depends primarily on whether consciousness, defined as awareness or responsiveness to the environment, is decreased. Seizures are classified as simple partial seizures when consciousness is not impaired. If consciousness is impaired, the seizure is classified as a complex partial seizure. One of the problems with the 1969 classification system was that it failed to account for seizure progression. Simple partial seizures may exist alone or may progress to complex partial seizures or to generalized tonic–clonic seizures. Complex partial seizures may progress to generalized tonic––clonic seizures.

Simple partial seizures usually involve only one hemisphere and are not accompanied by loss of consciousness or responsiveness. These seizures have also been referred to as elementary partial seizures, partial seizures with elementary symptomatology, or focal seizures. The 1981 Commission on Classification and Terminology of the International League Against Epilepsy has classified simple partial seizures according to (1) motor signs, (2)

sensory symptoms, (3) autonomic manifestations, and (4) psychic symptoms. If the motor area of the brain is involved, the earliest symptom is motor movement corresponding to the location of onset on the contralateral side of the body. The motor movement may remain localized or may spread to other cortical areas with sequential involvement of body parts in an epileptic-type "march," known as a Jacksonian seizure. If the sensory portion of the brain is involved, there may be no apparent clinical manifestations. Sensory symptoms correlating with the location on the contralateral side of the brain may be described as numbness, tingling, and crawling sensations or, more commonly, as the sensation of a foul odor or taste in the mouth. When abnormal cortical discharge stimulates the autonomic nervous system, flushing, tachycardia, diaphoresis, hypotension or hypertension, or pupillary changes may be evident. Simple partial seizures with only psychotic symptoms are rare and in the past have been called temporal or psychomotor seizures with consideration of the state of consciousness. The new classification system allows for symptoms such as *déjà vu* (familiarity with seemingly unfamiliar events or environments), *jamais vu* (unfamiliarity with a known environment), and overwhelming fear.

The term *aura* has traditionally meant a warning sign of impending seizure activity or the onset of a seizure that affected persons could describe because they were conscious. It is now thought that the aura itself is the seizure.[14] Because consciousness is maintained and only a small portion of the brain is involved, the aura is a simple partial seizure. Simple partial seizures may progess to complex partial seizures or generalized tonic–clonic seizures that result in unconsciousness. Therefore, the aura, or simple partial seizure, may in fact be a warning sign of impending complex partial seizures.

Complex partial seizures always involve both hemispheres and result in a loss of consciousness. The seizure begins in a localized area but may rapidly progress to both hemispheres. These seizures may also be referred to as temporal lobe seizures or psychomotor seizures. They can give rise to a wide variety of unusual behaviors such as hallucinations, sensations, and automatism. The behavior of a person during complex partial seizures, such as playing with clothing, is not purposeful. A person with complex symptomatology is sometimes misunderstood as requiring hospitalization for a psychiatric disorder.

Generalized seizures. Seizures are classified as primary and generalized when the first EEG and clinical changes indicate involvement of both cerebral hemispheres. The clinical symptoms include unconsciousness and rapidly occurring widespread bilateral symmetrical motor responses without an indication of localization to one hemisphere. These seizures range from minor motor seizures, sometimes called nonconvulsant seizures, such as absence (petit mal) and akinetic seizures, to major motor, or tonic–clonic seizures (grand mal). Almost all primary generalized epilepsies are transmitted genetically; structural lesions are rare.

In a *minor motor* or *nonconvulsive* seizure, abnormal discharge activity occurs throughout the brain, but the manifestations are so subtle that it may pass unnoticed. There is often a brief loss of contact with the environment, but no loss of consciousness. The seizure usually lasts only a few seconds and then the person is able to resume normal activity. Although *absence seizures* have been characterized as a blank stare, motionlessness, and unresponsiveness, motion occurs in about 90% of absence seizures. This motion takes the form of automatisms such as lip smacking, mild clonic motion, usually in the eyelids, increased or decreased postural tone, and autonomic phenomena. The absence seizure typically occurs only in children and either is outgrown or evolves into generalized major motor seizures. In *atonic seizures,* there is a sudden split-second loss of muscle tone leading to slackening of the jaw, dropping of a limb, or falling to the ground. These attacks are also known as drop attacks.

The major motor or convulsive seizures include myoclonic, tonic, clonic, and tonic–clonic seizures. In a myoclonic seizure there is bilateral jerking of muscles, either generalized or confined to the face, trunk, or one or more extremities. Tonic seizures are characterized by a rigid, violent contraction of the muscles fixing the limbs in a strained position. Clonic seizures consist of repeated contractions and relaxations of the muscle-stretch reflex.

The tonic–clonic (grand mal) seizure is the most common major motor seizure. Frequently, the person has a vague warning (probably a simple partial seizure) and then experiences a sharp tonic contraction of the muscles. The person falls to the ground, remains rigid, and may be incontinent. Cyanosis may occur from the tonic contraction of the airway and respiratory muscles. Clonic convulsive movements follow the tonic phase. At the end of the convulsive stage, the person remains unconscious, the muscles relax, and deep respirations occur. The seizure is followed by a deep sleep.

The prevalence of primary tonic–clonic (traditionally called grand mal) seizures has probably been overestimated; most of the tonic–clonic seizures occur as a progression from partial seizures or less dramatic seizures (absence).[14] The tonic–clonic seizure is the only type of seizure activity (primarily from drug or alcohol withdrawal) in fewer than 10% of persons with seizures. In more than half of all forms of epilepsy, tonic–clonic seizures occur secondarily to another form of seizure,

such as a simple partial or complex partial seizure. The classification of epileptic seizures is summarized in Table 47-1.

Diagnosis and Treatment

The diagnosis of epilepsy is based on a thorough history and neurologic examination, including a full description of the seizure. The physical examination helps rule out any metabolic disease that could precipitate seizures. Skull x-ray studies and computerized axial tomograms (CAT scan) help to identify any structural defects. Changes in the brain's electrical activity are recorded on the EEG, and this record is the most useful aid in diagnosis.

The first rule of treatment is to protect the affected person from injury; the next is to treat any underlying disease. Treatment of the underlying disorder may reduce the frequency of seizures. Once the underlying disease is treated, the aim of treatment is to bring the seizures under control with the least possible disruption of the person's life-style and a minimum of side-effects. This is accomplished primarily through anticonvulsant drug therapy. With proper drug management, 60% to 80% of persons with epilepsy can obtain good seizure control.[17] During the last 10 years, the therapy for epilepsy has drastically changed because of the improved classification system, the ability to measure serum anticonvulsant levels, and the availability of potent new anticonvulsant drugs. The principles of anticonvulsant drug therapy are summarized in Table 47-2.

Anticonvulsant medications
The pharmacokinetic parameters of half-life, distribution, and steady state must be understood to provide drug control for epilepsy. Half-life is the period of time

Table 47-1 Classification of Epileptic Seizures

Partial Seizures
  Simple partial seizures
    With motor symptoms
    With sensory symptoms
    With automatic signs
    With psychic symptoms
  Complex partial seizures
    Simple partial onset followed by impaired consciousness
    Impairment of consciousness at onset
Generalized Seizures
  Absence seizures (true petit mal)
  Atonic seizures
  Myoclonic seizures
  Tonic seizures
  Clonic seizures
  Tonic–clonic seizures (grand mal)

Table 47-2   Principles of Anticonvulsant Drug Therapy

General Treatment	1. Treat underlying disease first, if any
	2. Aim is clinical control of seizures with the least curtailment of patient's life and a minimum of side-effects
Pharmacologic Treatment	1. Start with a drug that normally is effective in this kind of seizure; titrate until maximum effect is reached or toxicity occurs; if unable to control with one drug, add another
	2. Use as few drugs as possible; this helps compliance and keeps down unwanted side-effects
Plasma Levels	Plasma levels do NOT indicate whether or not seizure control occurs; they indicate compliance, absorption, and the possibility of drug toxicity

(Courtesy Marilyn Weber, R.N., M.S., Clinical Coordinator Epilepsy Clinic, Mt. Sinai Hospital, Milwaukee, WI)

until the drug concentration falls below the saturation level. Peak time, the amount of time after oral administration at which the peak serum concentration is achieved, is a measure of speed and completeness of absorption and is not affected by half-life. After peak concentrations are reached, serum levels fall rapidly as the drug is distributed to body tissues. Rapidly acting drugs, given in large frequent doses, can cause acute side-effects. With frequent administration, the dose must be decreased. With repeated administration, a balance will eventually develop between absorption and elimination, producing a serum steady-state level. If the interval between doses is longer than the half-life, the drug will not accumulate, and the steady state will not be reached. Several administrations of the drug are required to regain the steady state.[18]

Although some anticonvulsant drugs can be given together, one of the main problems with these drugs is interaction. Whenever possible, a single drug should be used in epilepsy therapy. Adding a second medication raises toxic substrate levels, speeds the metabolism of both drugs through enhanced induction of hepatic enzymes that metabolize the drugs, and increases the possibility of side-effects without either drug reaching sufficient levels to prevent seizures. When more than one drug is required, careful monitoring of plasma levels during induction of therapy is needed to indicate the interactive metabolism and level of each agent.[18] Drugs that produce prominent side-effects (*e.g.*, barbiturates and benzodiazepines) should be avoided when possible. Anticonvulsant medications may also interact with medications given for other medical problems. For example, aspirin impairs the plasma protein binding of phenytoin and increases the unbound (active) levels of the drug and the possibility of side-effects. The discovery of the

powerful new anticonvulsant drug valproic acid, which is structurally related to gamma-aminobutyric acid (GABA), has opened up new research.

Among the drugs used in the treatment of epilepsy are carbamazepine, phenytoin, ethosuximide, and valproate. Carbamazepine and phenytoin, the drugs of choice in partial seizures, are especially effective when used together. They are also used for tonic–clonic seizures secondary to partial seizures. Ethosuximide is the drug of choice for absence seizures but is not effective for tonic–clonic seizures that have progressed from partial seizures. Valproate is helpful for people with many of the minor motor seizures and tonic–clonic seizures. Valproate and ethosuximide can be used together. Atonic seizures are highly resistant to therapy. Table 47-3 describes the drugs that are commonly used in the treatment of seizures, their side-effects, half-life, and distribution speed.

Most anticonvulsant drugs are taken orally, to be absorbed through the intestinal mucosa and metabolized by the liver. Liver damage that is present will affect drug tolerance, as will other factors that alter absorption, distribution, metabolism, and excretion of the drug. Plasma levels are measured to determine absorption, compliance in taking medications, and possibly drug toxicity, but these levels do not indicate whether or not seizures are controlled.

Drug toxicity is manifested in CNS symptoms of diplopia, ataxia, extreme drowsiness, and mental dullness. These symptoms should not be mistaken for the side-effects of drowsiness, rash, and stomach upset often seen during the first days of administration. Drug dosage is generally not reduced unless the side-effects interfere with functional activities. Gingival hyperplasia may occur in children with the continued use of pheny-

Table 47-3   Anticonvulsant Medications

Drug	Types of Seizures	Side-Effects	Half-Life (hours)	Speed of Distribution
Carbamazepine (Tegretol)	Partial, tonic–clonic	Blood dyscrasias, leukopenia, aplastic anemia	12	Medium
Phenytoin (Dilantin)	Partial, tonic–clonic	Hirsutism, gingival hyperplasia, coarsening of features, teratogenic potential	24	Medium
Ethosuximide (Zarontin)	Absence, generalized	Relatively free of side-effects	40	Fast
Valproate (Depakene)	Generalized, absence	Hepatitis, weight gain, hair loss, fine tremor, drug interaction, gastrointestinal irritation	8	Fast

toin (Dilantin). Phenytoin is a suspected teratogenic agent. Nevertheless, it is often necessary to continue the use of the drug during pregnancy to prevent seizures.

Determining the proper dose of the anticonvulsant drug(s) is a long and tedious process, which can become very frustrating to the person with epilepsy. Consistency in taking the medication is essential. Anticonvulsant drugs should never be discontinued rapidly; the dose should be decreased slowly.

Other therapy

Although surgical therapy has limited use in the treatment of seizures, a topectomy—the surgical removal of a single isolated cortical lesion—is helpful if a single lesion can be identified and removed. The most common procedure, the temporal lobectomy, is designated for seizures that originate in the temporal lobe. The use of EEG-operant conditioning methods for biofeedback training to influence the pathophysiologic substrate in motor seizures is being investigated and has potential for future treatment.[18]

Status Epilepticus

Seizure that does not stop spontaneously or in which the person passes from one seizure to another without recovery between attacks is called *status epilepticus*. There are many types of status epilepticus, but when it occurs with major motor seizures such as tonic–clonic, it is a medical emergency and if not promptly treated may lead to respiratory failure and death.

The main causes of status epilepticus are patient failure to take the prescribed dose of medication[19] and severe neurologic or systemic disease in a person with no previous history of epilepsy. If status epilepticus is due to neurologic or systemic disease, the cause needs to be identified and treated immediately, because the seizures probably will not respond until the underlying disturbance is corrected. When status epilepticus is the result of discontinuing medication, the drug regimen should be reinstituted as soon as possible. The prognosis is related to the underlying cause more than to the seizures themselves.

In summary, seizures are caused by spontaneous, uncontrolled, paroxysmal, transitory discharge from the cortical centers in the brain. Seizures may occur as a reversible symptom of another disease condition or as a recurrent condition called epilepsy. Epileptic seizures are classified as partial or generalized seizures. Partial seizures have evidence of local onset, beginning in one hemisphere. They include simple partial seizures, in which consciousness is not lost, and complex partial seizures, which begin in one hemisphere but progress to involve both. Generalized seizures involve both hemispheres and include unconsciousness and rapidly occurring widespread bilateral symmetrical motor responses. They include minor motor seizures such as absence, akinetic seizures, and major motor or grand mal seizures. Control of seizures is the primary goal of treatment and is accomplished with anticonvulsant medications. Anticonvulsant medications interact with each other and need to be monitored closely when more than one drug is used.

■ Consciousness and Unconsciousness

In order to understand alterations in consciousness, the reader must first gain an understanding of the reticular activating system (RAS). The RAS controls overall CNS activity, including sleep and wakefulness. The RAS is not a discrete anatomic structure but a diffuse formation of cells and fibers that extends from the lower brain stem upward through the mesencephalon (midbrain) and thalamus and is projected throughout the cerebral cortex. Axons of the motor and sensory neurons in the RAS bifurcate, with one end extending downward to the spinal cord and one end extending upward to the diencephalon. The RAS is divided into two areas, the bulboreticular facilitatory area and the bulboreticular inhibitory area.

The *bulboreticular facilitatory* area is located in the uppermost and lateral parts of the medulla, and all of the pons, mesencephalon, and diencephalon. The facilitatory area is intrinsically active. If no inhibitory signals are being transmitted from other parts of the body, continuous nerve impulses will be transmitted both downward to the motor areas of the cord and upward toward the brain, producing immediate marked activation of the cerebral cortex. There are two positive feedback loops: (1) to the cerebral cortex and back to the reticular formation and (2) to the peripheral muscles and back to the reticular formation through the spinal cord. Stimulation of the facilitatory area causes an increase in muscle tone in localized areas or throughout the body. Thus, once the RAS becomes activated, the feedback impulses from both the cerebral cortex and the periphery maintain the excitation. After prolonged wakefulness, the neurons in the RAS gradually become fatigued or less excitable. When this happens, neuronal mechanisms give way to lower-level functioning and sleep.

The lower three-fourths of the medulla is known as the *bulboreticular inhibitory* area. Stimulation of this area causes a decrease in muscle tone throughout the body. When both the bulboreticular inhibitory and bulboreticular facilitatory areas are functioning normally, the motor function of the spinal cord is neither excited nor inhibited, and the individual is conscious. Consciousness is a condition in which the individual is fully responsive to stimuli and demonstrates awareness of the environment. The ability to respond to stimuli, arousal, relies on an intact RAS in the brain stem, and the ability to respond to the environment, cognition, relies on an intact cerebral cortex. Therefore, altered forms of consciousness can result from a dysfunction or interruption along the pathway of the reticular formation from the brain stem to the cerebral cortex.

Altered levels of consciousness may be manifested by sleep (the only normal form), confusion, lethargy, obtundation, stupor, and coma. There is little agreement on the definitions of the terms and the less definitive clinical manifestations of the stages of coma. There are, however, some commonly used terms, which are described in Table 47-4. Because there are no accepted definitions of these terms, accurate descriptions of motor responses, pupils, respirations, and vital signs for monitoring patient progress are essential.

Because unconsciousness can be due to many causes, onset, duration, and the extent of damage vary from case to case. Coma may have an extracranial origin involving metabolic toxins or an intracranial origin resulting from structural damage to the brain. In metabolic coma, disruption in the metabolism of the cerebral cortex and brain stem can be caused by the ingestion of exogenous toxins, such as alcohol or drugs, or from diseases such as hepatic and renal failure, which result in production of such endogenous toxins as ammonia and elevated levels of blood urea nitrogen.[6] Interruption of cerebral metabolism may result in the disruption of impulse transmission, nerve injury, and eventually nerve death.

As described in Chapter 45, the tentorium, a tough dural fold, divides the cavity of the skull into the anterior and middle fossae above and the posterior fossa below. There is a large opening, the tentorial hiatus, through which the nerve pathways pass. Structurally, the lesions that cause coma may be divided into two groups: supratentorial lesions, which occur above the tentorium in the cerebral hemispheres, and subtentorial lesions, which occur below the tentorium in the brain stem.

Coma caused by subtentorial lesions, which is rarer than that caused by supratentorial lesions, may result from tumors or hemorrhage involving the cranial nerves, cerebellum, pons, and medulla. Coma occurs if the lesions affect the facilitatory portion of the RAS located

Table 47-4 Terms Used in Description of Unconscious States

Term	Characteristics
Consciousness	Alertness, orientation to person, place, and time; normal speech, voluntary movement; oculomotor activity
Confusion	Alteration in perception of stimuli; disorientation to time, first, and then to place, and eventually to person; shortened attention span
Lethargy	Orientation to person, place, and time; slow vocalization; decreased motor and oculomotor activity
Obtundation	Awakening in response to stimulation; continuous stimulation needed for arousal; eyes usually closed
Stupor	Vocalization only in response to stimuli that cause pain; markedly decreased spontaneous movement; eyes closed
Coma	No vocalization; posturing and respirations dependent on level; no spontaneous eye movement; brain stem reflexes intact

in the central pons and mesencephalon, thereby inhibiting the arousal centers. Subtentorial lesions are usually seen late in the course of a disease and indicate a poor prognosis.

Coma associated with supratentorial lesions may be caused by extensive damage to the cerebral hemispheres even if the brain stem remains intact. The damage may result from tumors, trauma, or hemorrhage in the cerebral cortex that causes direct injury to the areas involved. Supratentorial coma may also be caused by the downward displacement of cerebral tissue into the brain stem. The normal response to injury (edema, vascular dilatation, and invasion of leukocytes) and, in cerebral injuries, proliferation of the glial cells along with expansion of the tumor and blood clot, results in an increased volume within the confined cranial cavity. The rising intracranial pressure created by the increased volume causes displacement of the cerebral tissue toward a less dense area. Above the tentorium, a shift of tissue occurs from one cavity to another and downward through the tentorial incisura; this shift is commonly called herniation. In turn, the herniation may produce compression of adjacent vessels and tissues with resultant edema and ischemia.

If the supratentorial lesion is near the midline, there may be central displacement, which causes expansion and edema of the diencephalon. If the supratentorial mass is lateral, the herniating tissue compresses the third cranial nerve, causing unilateral pupillary dilatation. Arterial occlusion produces ischemia, edema, and infarction. If the cerebrospinal fluid pathway is blocked, and fluid cannot leave the ventricles, the volume will expand, as will the downward displacement through the tentorial notch. The expanding volume will cause all functions at a given level to cease as destruction progresses in a rostral–caudal direction. The result of this displacement is brain stem ischemia and hemorrhage extending from the diencephalon to the pons. If the lesion expands rapidly, displacement and obstruction occur quickly, leading to irreversible infarction and hemorrhage.

Diencephalon

Disruptions affecting the diencephalon, midbrain, pons, and medulla usually cause a predictable pattern of change in the level of consciousness (Table 47-5). The highest level of consciousness is seen in an alert person who is oriented to person, place, and time and is totally aware of the surroundings. The first symptoms of diminution in level of consciousness are decreased concentration, agitation, dullness, and lethargy. With further deterioration, the person may become obtunded and may respond only to vigorous shaking. Early respiratory changes include yawning and sighing with progression to Cheyne–Stokes breathing (Chap. 22). This is indicative of bilateral hemisphere damage with danger of tentorial herniation. Although the pupils may respond briskly to light, the full range of eye movements is seen only when the head is passively rotated from side to side (oculocephalic reflex, or "doll's eyes" maneuver) or when the caloric test (injection of hot or cold water into the ear canal) is done to elicit nystagmus. In the "doll's eyes" test, the eyes move in the direction of rotation rather than rolling in the opposite direction, as occurs normally. There is some combative movement as well as purposeful movement in response to pain. As coma progresses, the bulboreticular facilitatory area becomes more active as fewer inhibitory signals descend from the basal ganglia and cerebral cortex. This results in decorticate posturing with flexion of the upper extremities and adduction and extension of the lower extremities.

Midbrain

With progression continuing in rostral–caudal fashion, the midbrain becomes involved. Cheyne–Stokes respiration changes to neurogenic hyperventilation. Respirations often exceed 40 per minute because of uninhibited stimulation of both the inhibitory and expiratory centers. The pupils are fixed in midposition and no longer respond to stimuli. Muscle excitability increases with

Table 47-5 Rostral–Caudal Progression of Coma

Area Involved	Levels of Consciousness	Pupils	Muscle Tone	Respiration
Diencephalon (thalamus/ hypothalamus)	Decreased concentration, agitation, dullness, lethargy Obtundation	Respond to light briskly Full range of eye movements only on "doll's eyes" or caloric test	Some purposeful movement in response to pain; combative movement Decorticate	Yawning and sighing → Cheyne–Stokes
Midbrain	Stupor → coma	Midposition fixed (MPF)	Decerebrate	Neurogenic hyper-ventilation
Pons	Coma	MPF	Decerebrate	Apneustic
Medulla	Coma	MPF	Flaccid	Atactic

decerebrate posturing, in which the arms are rigid and extended with the palms of the hand turned away from the body.

Pons

As coma advances to involve the pons, the pupils remain in midposition and fixed, and the decerebrate posturing continues. Breathing is apneustic, with sighs evident in midinspiration and with prolonged inspiration and expiration because of excessive stimulation of the respiratory centers.

Medulla

With medullary involvement, the pupils remain fixed in midposition. Respirations are atactic, that is, totally uncoordinated and irregular. Apnea may occur because of the loss of responsiveness to carbon dioxide stimulation. Complete ventilatory assistance should be considered for any person with atactic breathing. Because the medulla has bulboreticular inhibitory neurons but no facilitatory neurons, the hyperexcitability that gave rise to the decorticate and decerebrate posturing disappears, giving way to flaccidity.

In progressive brain deterioration, the patient's neurologic capabilities appear to fall off in stepwise fashion. Similarly, as neurologic function returns, there appears to be stepwise progress to higher levels of consciousness.

Brain Death

As we have learned to maintain circulation of oxygenated blood artificially, the definition of death has had to be reexamined. In 1968, criteria of irreversible coma were published by a Harvard Medical School Ad Hoc Committee.[20] The criteria include the following: (1) unresponsiveness, (2) no spontaneous respirations for a period of 3 minutes without assistance, (3) absence of CNS reflexes and ocular movements and presence of fixed dilated pupils, (4) flat EEG for at least 10 minutes, (5) the same findings during a repeat examination 24 hours later, and (6) no evidence of the use of hypothermia or CNS depressants that may alter these findings.

Since that time, several other criteria have been proposed that modify the Harvard criteria. All have as their fundamental assumption the irreversibility of coma and the absence of responsiveness and respirations. However, some complex movement processes at the spinal level may remain with complete brain destruction. Therefore, all the criteria rely on observation of coma, apnea, cranial nerve reflexes, and the absence of brain stem reflexes. Yet it should not be overlooked that there are legal and moral aspects of brain death, which must be taken into consideration.

In summary, consciousness is a state of mental alertness, orientation, voluntary movement, and oculomotor movement. It exists on a continuum from consciousness and normal sleep to confusion, lethargy, obtundation, stupor, and coma. Consciousness depends on normal function of the facilitatory and inhibitory areas of the RAS. Coma can be metabolic, supratentorial, or tentorial in origin. It usually follows a rostral–caudal progression with characteristic changes in levels of consciousness, pupillary response, muscle tone, and respiratory activity occurring as the diencephalon through the medulla are affected.

■ Organic Brain Syndrome

The term organic brain syndrome refers to deterioration of mental function because of pathologic changes in brain tissue. Any pathologic process that affects the cerebral hemisphere can cause irreversible confusion and impairment of intellect. Several terms are used to describe the confusion and mental deterioration that occurs with organic brain disease, including chronic organic brain syndrome (COBS), dementia, senility, or cerebral atrophy. Based on community surveys, it is estimated that in the United States, 5% of persons above age 65—about 1 million people—have organic brain syndrome. These surveys also indicate that another 2 million persons (10% of that population group) have a mild form of COBS.[21] Just as dementia should not be equated with aging, neither should the changes observed in COBS be considered normal. It is the most common diagnosis among elderly persons in state and county hospitals. COBS is believed to be the cause, whether direct or indirect, of between 90,000 and 97,000 deaths annually.[21] It has been suggested that life expectancy is considerably shortened by the presence of COBS.[22] The most common characteristic of these conditions is cellular atrophy. The diffuse atrophy of the cerebral cortex, especially in the frontal and temporal lobes, is associated with impairment of intellectual functioning. Alzheimer's disease is the most common disorder characterized by cerebral atrophy, but other diseases such as Creutzfeldt–Jakob disease, Pick's disease, Wernicke–Korsakoff's syndrome, Huntington's chorea, and amyotrophic lateral sclerosis (ALS) are also characterized by atrophic changes. Enlargement of the ventricles, senile plaques, and granulovascular degeneration of neurons are usually present with the cerebral atrophy.

The constellation of symptoms associated with COBS is easily remembered by the acronym JAMCO: judgment, affect, memory, confusion, orientation. The syndrome is characterized by impairment of judgment and memory, a flat affect, confusion, and loss of orientation.

The *catastrophic reaction* is a phenomenon commonly seen in COBS. When faced with a task that seems overwhelming, the person may react by withdrawing from the situation or by becoming extremely agitated. The *sundown syndrome* is another behavioral manifestation of COBS, characterized by nocturnal awakening, confusion, agitation, and sometimes psychotic symptoms.[23] Various primitive *reflexes,* such as the sucking and rooting reflexes, may return.[24]

Alzheimer's Disease

Alzheimer's disease has the typical characteristics of COBS—cerebral atrophy, ventricular dilatation, senile plaques, and granulovascular bodies. In addition, neurofibrillary tangles and filaments are wrapped around each other in the neurons of the cerebral cortex. There are apparent reductions in acetylcholinesterase and choline acetyltransferase. The extent of these alterations and their effect on Alzheimer's disease is currently being studied.

At present controversy exists over differentiating between what is sometimes called presenile dementia of Alzheimer's disease and the so-called senile dementia of Alzheimer's type. Most authorities agree that two disorders are probably one and the same disease, comprising 65% of all dementias. The main difference between them is that of age. Alzheimer's disease occurs at an average age of 55, whereas senile dementia occurs at an average age of 75.

The cause of Alzheimer's disease is unknown, and the diagnosis is frequently made by ruling out other possible causes such as drug intoxication, head injury, brain tumor, depression, and nutritional deficiencies. Alzheimer's disease may also be diagnosed on the basis of symptoms. There is usually a progressive loss of intellectual function, from forgetfulness, to confusion, to the senility phase. It affects women more often than men. Its onset is usually characterized by impairment of memory. There is a lack of insight. Usually, cognitive impairment follows within several years, and hyperexcitability, aphasia, apraxia, and agnosia may be associated findings. Gait disorders are prominent. The prognosis is extremely poor; the disease progresses relentlessly for some 5 years to 10 years, ending in death.

Multi-Infarct Dementia

Dementia associated with vascular disease does not result directly from arteriosclerosis, but rather from infarction due to multiple emboli that disseminate throughout the brain[25]—hence the appellation multi-infarct dementia (MID).

It is probable that only some 10% to 20% of all dementias may be caused by MID.[25] The duration of the disease is variable, but within about 4 years most patients die from a cerebral vascular accident or a superimposed infection, such as pneumonia.

Memory impairment is often the first symptom of MID, followed by impairment in judgment. There may be episodes of delirium, possibly accompanied by hallucinations. Catastrophic reaction and nocturnal confusion are also common.

Creutzfeldt–Jakob Disease

Creutzfeldt–Jakob disease is an organic brain disease currently believed to be caused by a transmissible agent, possibly a virus. It is marked by degeneration of the pyramidal and extrapyramidal systems.

Creutzfeldt–Jakob disease is most readily distinguished by its rapid course; the affected persons are usually severely demented within 6 months of onset. The disease is uniformly fatal, with death usually occurring within 7 months.[26] The early symptoms consist of abnormalities in personality and visual/spatial coordination. Extreme dementia and myoclonus follow as the disease advances.

Pick's Disease

Pick's disease is a rare form of COBS. Atrophy of the frontal, temporal, and parietal lobes of the brain occurs. The neurons in the affected areas contain cytoplasmic inclusions called *Pick bodies*.

The average age at onset of Pick's disease is 54 years. It is more common in women than in men. Behavioral manifestations may be noted earlier than memory deficits, taking the form of a striking absence of concern and care, a loss of initiative, echolalia (automatic repetition of anything said to the person), hypotonia, and incontinence.[27] The course of the disease is relentless, with death ensuing within 2 years to 10 years. The immediate cause of death generally is infection.

Normal Pressure Hydrocephalus

Normal pressure hydrocephalus (NPH) is in some cases reversible, or at least treatable. It is due to an obstruction of CSF, with resulting dilatation of the ventricles. It can occur at any age, after head trauma, meningitis, or subarachnoid hemorrhage.

Gait disturbance is the cardinal sign of NPH, followed by incontinence of bowel and bladder. Severe dementia occurs in the late stages. The person has a flat affect and tends to be withdrawn. Treatment of choice is the surgical creation of a shunt that routes the cerebrospinal fluid around the obstructed area and back into the circulation. The improved cerebral blood flow may bring some relief of symptoms.

Table 47-6 Diagnostic Features of Chronic Organic Brain Syndrome

Syndrome	Age at Onset	Mode of Onset	Contributing Factors	Brain Pathology
Alzheimer's disease	Range, 40–60 years; average 55 years	More abrupt than senile dementia	Multiple genetically determined factors	Cortical atrophy and loss of neurons
Senile dementia (of Alzheimer type)	Over 70 years; average, 75 years	Insidious	Same as Alzheimer's disease	Cortical atrophy and loss of neurons
Multi-infarct dementia	Range, 55–70 years; average 65 years	Gradual or acute; insidious with fluctuating states of awareness	Some familial tendency, life-style consistent with atherosclerotic risk factors	Diffuse and/or focal changes due to atherosclerosis; thrombi may be present
Creutzfeldt–Jakob disease	Middle years range, 20–68 years; average, 50 years	Rapid	Thought to be of slow virus etiology; mode of transmission unknown	Presence of status spongiosus (widespread vacuoles) in cerebral cortex and sometimes in basal ganglia
Pick's disease	As early as age 21; range, 40–60 years; average, 54 years	Slow and insidious	Familial incidence; hereditary mode of transmission of dominant type	Cortical atrophy of frontal and temporal lobes; presence of Pick bodies (round cytoplasmic inclusions) in nerve cells of affected brain areas
Normal pressure hydrocephalus	Variable depending on primary etiology	Gradual	Idiopathic, or history of head trauma	Dilated ventricles
Alcoholic encephalopathy, Wernicke's or Korsakoff's syndrome	40–80 years	Gradual	Alcoholic history	*Wernicke's syndrome:* lesions most pronounced in mammillary bodies, consist of small hemorrhages, congestion with brownish gray discoloration; *Korsakoff's syndrome:* involves medial nucleus and sometimes posterior of thalamus

(Courtesy, Janet Krejci)

Characteristics	Course	Prognosis and Outcome
Memory loss Disorientation Agitation Language disturbance Lack of insight Deterioration of social behavior and personal habits	Rapidly progressive	Very poor; death usually due to infection or failure of other body systems
Memory loss Disorientation Agitation Language disturbance Lack of insight Deterioration of social behavior and personal habits	Slow or rapid	Same as Alzheimer's disease
Mental symptoms associated with hemiparesis Pathologic reflexes Pseudobulbar palsy and signs of cerebellar dysfunction	Downward course with intermittent and fluctuating progression of symptoms	Usually poor, but may be variable; death due to cerebral vascular accident, heart disease, or infection such as pneumonia
Cerebellar ataxia Weakness of legs and complaints of neurasthenia and muscle wasting Myoclonic fasciculations Somnolence Abnormalities in visual/spacial coordination	Rapidly progressive; complete dementia in 6 months	Very poor; death due to infection or cardiac or respiratory failure
Speech disturbance, utterance of incomprehensible jargon Lack of anxiety Loss of initiative Flat affect Hypotonia Incontinence	Progressive, more rapid than Alzheimer's disease	Very poor; death usually due to infection or general failure of body systems
Amnesia and confusion Mutism Withdrawal Gait disturbance Urinary incontinence	Progressive	Poor in absence of intervention
Confabulation Loss of memory Paresthesia, ataxia, weakness Deterioration of psychomotor skills	Progressive	Poor unless abstinence from alcohol ingestion; administration of thiamin may arrest symptoms of Wernicke's syndrome

Wernicke–Korsakoff's Syndrome

Wernicke–Korsakoff's syndrome is due to chronic alcoholism. Wernicke's disease is characterized by weakness or paralysis. of the extraocular muscles, nystagmus, ataxia, and confusion. Signs of peripheral neuropathy may be present. The person has an unsteady gait and complains of diplopia. There may be signs attributable to alcohol withdrawal—delirium, confusion, hallucinations, and so on. It is generally agreed that this disorder is caused by a deficiency in thiamin (vitamin B_1), and many of the symptoms are rapidly reversed when nutrition is improved by supplemental thiamin.

The Korsakoff component of the syndrome involves severe impairment of recent memory. There is often difficulty in dealing with abstractions, and the person's capacity to learn is defective. Confabulation is probably the most distinguishing feature of the disease. Polyneuritis is also common. Unlike Wernicke's disease, Korsakoff's psychosis does not improve significantly with thiamin therapy. Features of Wernicke's disease and Korsakoff's syndrome may be found in one person.

In summary, chronic organic brain syndrome is a significant health problem, particularly among the elderly. It is estimated that 80% of elderly persons at first admission to psychiatric units are given a diagnosis of COBS and that it is the most common diagnosis among the elderly in state and county hospitals.

A number of antecedent conditions may give rise to COBS, among which are multi-infarct dementia, Alzheimer's disease, Creutzfeldt–Jakob disease. Pick's disease, and Wernicke–Korsakoff's syndrome (see Table 47-6). A distinction should be made between chronic organic brain syndrome and both acute brain syndrome and functional disorders, of which depression is a representative example.

■ Study Guide

After you have studied this chapter, you should be able to meet the following objectives:

☐ Describe the compensatory mechanisms used to prevent large changes in ICP from occurring when there are changes in brain, blood, or CSF volumes.

☐ Explain the cause of tentorial herniation of the brain and its consequences.

☐ Describe the CNS ischemic response.

☐ Explain the significance of unilateral pupillary dilatation with reference to intracranial pressure.

☐ Describe the importance of measuring vital signs in the assessment of increasing intracranial pressure.

☐ Compare the causes of communicating and noncommunicating hydrocephalus.

☐ Describe the effects of contrecoup injury.

☐ Compare the symptoms of concussion with those of contusion.

☐ Explain why it is important to determine whether or not a head injury has resulted in chronic subdural hematoma.

☐ List the constellation of symptoms involved in the postconcussion syndrome.

☐ Trace the sequence of events that occur in meningitis.

☐ Describe the symptoms that are indicative of encephalitis.

☐ Explain the difference between the terms seizure and epilepsy.

☐ State four or more causes of seizure activity other than epilepsy.

☐ Differentiate between the origin of seizure activity in partial and generalized epilepsy.

☐ Compare the manifestations of simple partial seizures and complex seizures and those of minor motor epilepsy and major motor epilepsy.

☐ Define the terms clonic and tonic as they relate to seizure activity.

☐ Describe the precautions to be followed in prescribing anticonvulsant drugs.

☐ Characterize *status epilepticus*.

☐ Relate the activity of the bulboreticular facilitatory area to level of consciousness.

☐ Define the terms conscious, confusion, lethargy, obtundation, stupor, and coma.

☐ Trace the progression of symptoms from consciousness to unconsciousness.

☐ State the Harvard criteria of irreversible coma.

☐ Define chronic organic brain syndrome.

☐ Cite the origin of the acronym JAMCO.

☐ Describe the manifestations of the catastrophic reaction and the sundown syndrome.

☐ Explain the designation MID for dementia associated with vascular disease.

☐ List the progressive stages in Alzheimer's disease.

☐ Describe the symptoms of the Wernicke–Korsakoff syndrome.

■ References

1. McNamera M, Quinn C: Epidural intracranial pressure monitoring: Theory and clinical application. J Neurosurg Nurs 13, No 5:267, 1981

2. Tindall GT, Fleischer AS: Head injury. Hosp Med 12, No 5:89, 1976

3. Ransoff J, Koslow M: Guide to diagnosis and treatment of cerebral injury. Hosp Med 14, No 5:127, 1978

4. Jeannett B, Teasdale G: Management of Head Injuries. Philadelphia, FA Davis, 1981

5. Grossman RG: Treatment of patients with intracranial hematomas. N Engl J Med 304:1540, 1981

6. Rudy EB: Advanced Neurological and Neurosurgical Nursing. St Louis, CV Mosby, 1984

7. Seelig JM, Becker DP, Miller JD et al: Traumatic acute subdural hematoma: Major mortality reduction in comatose patients treated within four hours. N Engl J Med 304:1511, 1981

8. Center for Disease Control: Bacterial meningitis and meningococcemia: United States—1978. MMWR 28:277, 1979

9. Gold R: Bacterial meningitis—1982. Am J Med 75(1B):98, 1983

10. Murphy FK, Mackowiak R, Luby J: Management of infections affecting the nervous system. In Rosenberg RN (ed): The Treatment of Neurological Diseases. New York, SP Medical & Scientific Books, 1979

11. Robbins SL, Cotran RS, Kumar V: Pathologic Basis of Disease, 2nd ed, p 1385. Philadelphia, WB Saunders, 1984

12. Hawken M: Seizures: Etiology, classification, intervention. J Neurosurg Nurs 11, No 3:166, 1979

13. US Department of Health and Human Services: Epilepsy: Hope through Research. Public Health Services, National Institute of Health, Superintendent of Documents, Washington, DC, US Government Printing Office, NIH Publication No 81-167, 1981

14. Porter RJ: Epilepsy 100 Elementary Principles. Philadelphia, WB Saunders, 1984

15. Gastaut H: Clinical and electroencephalographical classification of epileptic seizures. Epilepsia 11:102, 1970

16. Commission on Classification and Terminology of the International League Against Epilepsy: Proposal for revised clinical and electroencephalographic classification of epileptic seizures. Epilepsia 22:489, 1981

17. Hawken M, Ozuna J: Practical aspects of anticonvulsant therapy. Am J Nurs 79:1062, 1979

18. Engle J Jr, Trouper AS, Crandell PH et al: Recent development of diagnosis and treatment of epilepsy. Ann Intern Med 97:584, 1982

19. Bruya MA, Bolin RH: Epilepsy: A controllable disease. Part 1. Classification and diagnosis of seizures. Am J Nurs 76:388, 1976

20. Black PM: Criteria of brain death. Review and comparison. Postgrad Med 57, No 2:69, 1975

21. Report on the Panel of Inflammatory, Demyelinating and Degenerative Diseases of the National Advisory Neurological and Communicative Disorders and Stroke Council, p 61, US Department of Health, Education, and Welfare, NIH Publication No 79-1916, June 1, 1979

22. Karasu TB, Katzman R: Organic brain syndromes. In Bellak L, Katzman T (eds): Geriatric Psychiatry, p 129, New York, Grune & Stratton, 1976

23. Raskind M: Nocturnal Delirium, pp 4–5. New York, Biomedical Information Corp, 1979

24. Charatan FB: Chronic Brain Syndrome, p 4. New York, Roering, 1979

25. Hachinski V et al: Multi-infarct dementia. Lancet 2:207, 1974

26. Robbins SL, Cotran RS: Pathologic Basis of Disease, p 1549. Philadelphia, WB Saunders, 1979

27. Verwoerdt A: Clinical Geropsychiatry, pp 47–52. Baltimore, Williams & Wilkins, 1976

■ Additional References

Allen N: Prognostic indicators in coma. Heart Lung 8:1075, 1979

Aring CD: Metabolic encephalopathy: Neurologic and psychiatric considerations. Heart Lung 11:516, 1982

Barns EK et al: Guidelines to treatment approaches. Gerontologist 13:513, 1973

Bartol MA: Dialogue with dementia. J Gerontol Nurs 5:21, 1979

Blacker HM: Closed head injury. Primary Care 3:231, 1976

Boss BJ: The dementias. J Neurosurg Nurs 15:87, 1983

Bozian MW, Clark HM: Counteracting sensory changes in aging. Am J Nurs 80:473, 1980

Burnside IM: Alzheimer's disease: An overview. J Gerontol Nurs 5:14, 1979

Caronna JJ: Assessment and management of coma. Consultant 19, No 1:175–184, 1979

Cooper P: Treatment of head injuries. In Rosenberg RN (ed): The Treatment of Neurological Diseases. New York, SP Medical & Scientific Books, 1979

Delgado-Escueta AV et al: The treatable epilepsies. N Engl J Med 308:1508, 1983

Elwes RD, Johnson AL, Shorvon SD et al: The prognosis of seizure control in newly diagnosed epilepsy. N Engl J Med 311:944, 1984

Engel J Jr (moderator): UCLA Conference: Recent developments in the diagnosis and therapy of epilepsy. Ann Intern Med 97:584, 1982

Fischer-Williams M: Partial and generalized seizures associated with cerebral ischemia. In Broughton RJ (ed): Henri Gastaut and the Marseilles School's Contribution to the Neurosciences (EEG Suppl No 35). Amsterdam, Elsevier Biomedical Press, 1982

Gifford RRM, Plant MR: Abnormal respiratory patterns in the comatose patient caused by intracranial dysfunction. J Neurosurg Nurs 7:58, 1975

Hanlon K: Description and uses of intracranial pressure monitoring. Heart Lung 5:277, 1976

Heros RC, Zervas NT: Subarachnoid hemorrhage. Annu Rev Med 34:367, 1983

Leppik IE: Seizures and epilepsy: Understanding the mechanisms, achieving control. Postgrad Med 75:229, 1984

Lipe MP, Mitchell PH: Positioning the patient with intracranial hypertension: How turning and head rotation affect the internal jugular vein. Heart Lung 9:1031, 1980

Lovely MP: Identification and treatment of status epilepticus. J Neurosurg Nurs 12:93, 1980

Norman S: The pupil check. Am J Nurs 82:588, 1982

Norman SE, Browne TR: Seizure disorders. Am J Nurs 81:984, 1981

Paulson GW: Disorders of the central nervous system in the elderly. Med Clin North Am 67, No 2:345, 1983

Schneck MK et al: Overview of current concepts of Alzheimer's disease. Psychiatry 139:165, 1982

Sklar FH: Treatment of increased intracranial pressure. In Rosenberg RN (ed): The Treatment of Neurological Diseases. New York, SP Medical & Scientific Books, 1979

Tucker CA: Complex partial seizures. Am J Nurs 81:996, 1981

Wink DM: Bacterial meningitis in children. Am J Nurs 84:456, 1984

Wright FS: Epilepsy in childhood. Pediatr Clin North Am 31, No 1:177, 1984

Chapter 48

Alterations in Motor Function

Mary Wierenga

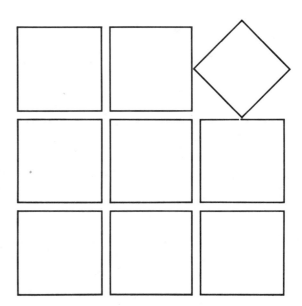

Effective motor function requires not only that muscles move but also that the mechanics of their movement be programmed in a manner that provides for smooth and coordinated movement. In some cases, purposeless and disruptive movements can be almost as disabling as the relative or complete absence of movement. This chapter discusses normal motor activity and its alterations as manifested in stroke, Parkinson's disease, spinal cord injury, multiple sclerosis, and neuromuscular disorders.

▣ Control of Motor Function

Control of motor activity is achieved through the interaction of three systems: the cerebral cortex, the cerebellum, and the basal ganglia. These systems initiate and regulate the two types of motor pathways by which the cerebral cortex exerts influence on the spinal cord and the lower motor neuron pathways. Many fibers from the motor area of the cerebral cortex travel directly to the brain stem or spinal cord. These fibers decussate, or cross over, to the opposite side of the nervous system in the *pyramids* of the medulla. These fibers make up the *pyramidal* system. Other fibers from the cortex project to the *cerebellum* and *basal ganglia* before they descend and innervate the motor neurons. These fibers do not decussate in the pyramids and are considered to be outside (extra) the pyramidal tract, hence the name *extrapyramidal* system. The pyramidal and extrapyramidal tracts have opposing effects on muscle tone. The *pyramidal system* is largely excitatory; it initiates muscle movement. The *extrapyramidal* tract serves to smooth and coordinate muscle movement; it is largely inhibitory. Spinal cord reflex is either facilitated or inhibited by these two levels of control (Table 48-1).

The motor neurons that have their origin in the cortex of the brain and whose fibers remain within the CNS are called upper motor neurons (UMN). The motor neurons that are located in the ventral horns of the cord and that send projections to the motor fibers are called lower motor neurons (LMN). The cranial nerves synapse with UMN in the brain or brain stem and are also LMN (Fig. 48-1).

Table 48-1   Characteristics of Pyramidal and Extrapyramidal Motor Control

Feature	Pyramidal	Extrapyramidal		Peripheral
Nomenclature	(1) Voluntary motor pathway (2) Upper motor neuron (UMN) pathway (3) Corticospinal pathway	(1) Involuntary motor pathway (2) Extracorticospinal		(1) Final common pathway (2) Lower motor neuron (LMN) pathway
Location	From the Betz cells of the frontal lobe motor strip to the anterior horn cell of the spinal cord	Motor cortex with projections into basal ganglia, and communication with the reticular formation	Posterior fossa of cerebellum	From the ventral horn cells of the spinal cord to the neuromuscular junction
Function	Initiates and transmits impulses for smooth voluntary movement to spinal cord	(1) Inhibits muscle tone throughout the body (2) Initiates and regulates gross intentional movements	(1) Coordinate movements by monitoring and making adjustments in motor activity elicited by other parts of the nervous system (2) Dampen muscle movement	Transmits impulses from the spinal cord to the muscles for voluntary movement
Disruption	Hyperactive reflexes and spastic paralysis on the contralateral side—hemiplegia	Muscle rigidity and incoordination Loss of discrete movement Abnormal posture	Incoordination, intention tremors, ataxia, overshooting; inability to progress in orderly sequence from one movement to another	Hypoactive reflexes and paresis or flaccid paralysis, usually monoplegia
Extent of damage	Small amount of damage in important area (*e.g.,* internal capsule) causes extensive decrease in function	If part of basal ganglia is left intact, gross postural and "fixed" movements can still be performed; widespread damage leads to muscle rigidity throughout the body	Depends on the extent of damage to the cerebellum	Extensive damage (several levels) before function is significantly decreased

Pyramidal Tract

The neuronal bodies for the pyramidal, or corticospinal, tract are found in the large pyramidal (Betz) cells of the motor cortex, which is located in the posterior portion of the frontal lobe in the precentral gyrus. Specific areas in this part of the brain are assigned to certain muscle groups on the *opposite* side of the body. The pattern for this motor activity is often depicted in the shape of a *homunculus*, as described in Chapter 45 (see Fig. 45-18). The distortion in shape has a purpose—it represents, by the size of its various segments, body areas according to their motor function. Those that have minimal motor function (*e.g.*, the trunk) have minimal representation; those that have maximal motor function (*e.g.*, the hands) have maximal representation.

The voluntary motor tracts travel downward through the internal capsule (see Chapter 45, Fig. 45-17) where they are pulled closer together (retaining the shape of the homunculus) in preparation for the descent into the brain stem and spinal cord. The majority of nerve pathways decussate in the medulla, moving to the opposite side of the cord to innervate the opposite side of the body. The Betz cells on the right side of the motor cortex control hand movement on the left side of the body. As the pathway descends from the motor area, it sends collaterals to the other parts of the central nervous system, basal ganglia, cerebral cortex, cerebellum, and spinal cord, which help to maintain smooth, voluntary movement.

Disruption of pyramidal tract function

The motor cortex, the pyramidal tract, or both are common sites of damage, especially by stroke (discussed later in this chapter). With damage to the pyramidal tract voluntary motor movement is disrupted, although the LMN pathway is not directly affected. The reflex arc of the spinal cord remains intact but it is not controlled by the higher centers. Among the manifestations of pyramidal tract damage are increased deep tendon reflexes, hypertonia (spasticity) paresis, and Babinski's sign.

Damage to the pyramidal tract can occur in two common sites: the motor cortex and the internal capsule as it courses through the brain toward the spinal cord. For example, damage to a small area of the motor cortex causes a loss of voluntary motor activity in the represented muscles. On the other hand, even minimal damage to an important structure, such as the internal capsule, which carries both sensory and motor fibers, causes extensive dysfunction because all the fibers innervating one side of the body and the basal ganglia are located in this area. If the basal ganglia are not damaged, gross postural and fixed movements will be intact, but discrete function on the opposite side of the body will be

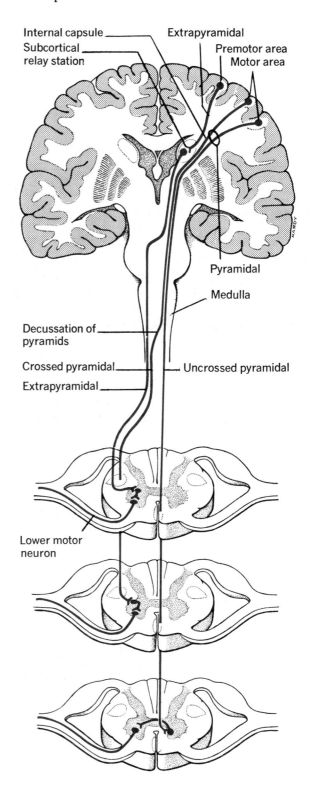

Figure 48-1 *Motor pathways between the cerebral cortex, one of the subcortical relay centers, and lower motor neurons in the spinal cord. Decussation (crossing) of fibers means that each side of the brain controls skeletal muscles on the opposite side of the body. (Chaffee EE, Lytle IM: Basic Physiology and Anatomy, 4th ed, p 244. Philadelphia, JB Lippincott, 1980)*

lost. Thus, even though the damage may seem insignificant in both areas, the resulting dysfunction may be quite different.

Lower motor neurons

The LMN is best understood when compared to the UMN, or voluntary motor, pathway. The LMN begins in the ventral horn cell of the spinal cord and its fibers project to the neuromuscular junction between the large nerve fibers and the muscle fibers. In contrast to UMN injury, which causes hyperreflexia and hypertonicity, injury to the LMN interrupts the reflex, causing hyporeflexia; when damage is extensive, flaccidity results. With LMN dysfunction and flaccid paralysis, muscle atrophy becomes prominent. Because of nerve branching, dysfunction becomes discernible only when several LMN pathways are damaged. Monoparesis (weakness of one extremity) and monoplegia (paralysis of one extremity) are the most common dysfunctions arising from LMN damage.

Extrapyramidal Tract

The extrapyramidal tract arises from the motor cortex and is indirectly routed through the brain with projections into the *basal ganglia* and the *cerebellum*. From the basal ganglia and the cerebellum, the fibers communicate with the next level of control, the reticular formation of the brain stem. The extrapyramidal system is usually considered a functional rather than an anatomic unit because of its many projections. In contrast with the more direct route of the pyramidal tract, the extrapyramidal tract reaches the spinal cord only after many detours and indirect routing. The final pathway is primarily the reticulospinal tract.

Basal ganglia

The basal ganglia are the several large masses that lie caudal to the thalamus and project around the internal capsule. The term corpus striatum (striped body) is sometimes used interchangeably with basal ganglia. The major components of the basal ganglia are the caudate (tailed) nucleus, the putamen, and the globus pallidus (pale body). The globus pallidus and the putamen make up the lenticular nucleus. Although not specifically a part of the basal ganglia, the subthalamic nucleus and substantia nigra are closely related on the basis of function. Neurons arising in the substantia nigra transmit dopamine, an inhibitory neuromediator, to the striatum.

The extrapyramidal tract fibers from the basal ganglia inhibit muscle tone throughout the body by transmitting inhibiting signals. These fibers, which regulate gross postural mechanisms and intentional movements of the body that are normally performed subconsciously, provide the muscle tone needed for movement.

Cerebellar pathway

The cerebellum has both voluntary and involuntary components. It does not initiate activity, but it is responsible for muscle synergy (correlated action) throughout the body. The cerebellum monitors and makes corrective adjustments in the motor activity elicited by other parts of the brain. It receives information continuously from the periphery of the body to assess the status of each body part—position, rate of movement, forces acting on it, and so on. The cerebellum compares what is actually happening with what is intended to happen and transmits appropriate corrective signals back to the motor system, instructing it to increase or decrease the activity of various muscles. In this way, the cerebellum coordinates the action of muscle groups and regulates their contractions so that smooth and accurate movements are performed. Voluntary movements can be performed without cerebellar intervention but the movements will be clumsy and uncoordinated. An extensive feedback system (both input and output) allows the cerebellum to make corrections rapidly while the motor movement is taking place.

A second function of the cerebellum is to dampen muscle movement. All body movements are basically pendular (like a pendulum). As movement begins, momentum develops and must be overcome before movement can be stopped. Because of momentum, all movements have a tendency to overshoot if they are not dampened. In the intact cerebellum, subconscious signals stop movement precisely at the intended point. In providing for this type of control, the cerebellum predicts the future position of moving parts of the body; the rapidity with which the limb is moving is detected from incoming proprioceptive signals as well as the projected time for the course of movement. This allows the cerebellum to inhibit agonist muscles and excite antagonist muscles when movement approaches the point of intention.

The cerebellum functions much the same way in involuntary, postural, and subconscious movements as it does in voluntary movement but through different pathways. Extrapyramidal fibers, which originate in the cerebral cortex, send collaterals to the cerebellum. As the muscle movement occurs, messages from the muscles, joints, and periphery are sent back to the cerebellum, which provides the same "error" control for involuntary movement as it does for voluntary movement.

Disruption of basal ganglia function

Damage to the basal ganglial component of the extrapyramidal tract does not cause paralysis, as does damage to the pyramidal and lower motor neuron tracts. Disruption of these extrapyramidal fibers results instead, in muscle rigidity and incoordination. Remembering that the pyramidal and extrapyramidal tracts have opposing effects on muscle tone, one can understand that damage to either tract may disrupt the delicate balance that ensures smooth muscle movement. If the damage is in the primary motor cortex, there may be no change in muscle tone because the pyramidal and extrapyramidal systems are affected equally. Usually, however, the lesion is large and involves extensive motor areas as well as the basal ganglia, which normally transmit inhibitory signals through the extrapyramidal system. In this case, loss of extrapyramidal inhibition leads to overactivity of the facilitory area with resultant increase in muscle tone.

Several forms of disrupted motor activity occur in impairment of the basal ganglial portion of the extrapyramidal tract. *Chorea* is characterized by quick, jerky, and purposeless movements and is usually associated with damage to the basal ganglia. These random, uncontrolled contractions of different muscle groups interrupt normal progression of movement. *Athetosis* involves continuous slow, writhing, wormlike movements, which exhibit a high degree of spasticity and which make normal voluntary movement difficult to perform. *Hemiballismus* consists of continued wild, violent movements of large body parts.

Disruptions of cerebellar function

Several types of disruption of motor activity occur in impairment of the cerebellar portion of the extrapyramidal tract. The most common dysfunction is an uncoordinated movement of muscles, called *ataxia*. The loss of equilibrium is due to a lack of muscle posture manifested in a staggering, unsteady gait. If there is a lesion in one of the cerebellar hemispheres, the person will fall toward the side on which the lesion is situated. *Dysmetria* is characterized by an inability to predict and measure the endpoint of a movement, resulting in movement past the point of intention, called past-pointing, or overshooting. In this situation, the movement begins too early or too late, disrupting the normal orderly progression of movement; the condition is called *dysdiadochokinesia*. Similarly, a failure in progression of word formation resulting in explosive, slurred, almost unintelligible speech is called *dysarthria*. Failure of the cerebellum to dampen motor movement may give rise to *tremors*, in contrast to *resting* tremors seen in dysfunction of the basal ganglia portion of the extrapyramidal tract. When the cerebellum cannot dampen motor activity appropriately, overshooting occurs. Eventually, consciousness centers of the cerebrum recognize the overshooting and initiate movement in the opposite direction to bring the part into the intended position. But because of momentum, overshooting and correction occur again. The part may oscillate several times, causing intention tremors, before correction is made.

Nystagmus is the rapid, involuntary, horizontal, vertical, or rotatory movement of the eyeball. This cerebellar nystagmus is probably also a result of failure to dampen movements. The tremor is evident when the person attempts to look at a fixed point, especially on the side on which the disturbance is located.

In summary, movement is controlled by three interrelated motor systems: (1) the cerebral cortex, which is responsible for initiating voluntary motor activity, (2) the basal ganglia, which are responsible for maintaining posture, and (3) the cerebellum, which is responsible for coordinating movement. These three systems make up the pyramidal and extrapyramidal tracts, which affect motor movement through the spinal cord and the lower motor neuron (LMN) pathway to the neuromuscular junction.

Injuries or lesions to these areas tend to produce the following neurologic deficits: (1) injury to the pyramidal tract results in paralysis of voluntary motor movement; (2) injury to the basal ganglia of the extrapyramidal tract results in increased muscle tone, postural deficits, and abnormal body positions; and (3) injury to the cerebellum of the extrapyramidal tract results in incoordination. Damage to the LMN results in monoparesis or flaccid monoplegia. Table 48-1 summarizes the characteristics of the three motor systems.

■ Alterations in Cerebral Circulation

Cerebral Circulation

Knowledge of normal cerebral circulation is essential to an understanding of vascular disorders. Blood transports oxygen, nutrients, and metabolic substances to the brain and removes waste products from the brain; thus, it is critical that blood supply to the brain be maintained. Arterial blood flow is supplied to the brain by the two internal carotid arteries (anteriorly) and the two vertebral arteries (posteriorly), which originate in the arch of the aorta (Fig. 48-2). The internal carotid artery branches into several arteries: the ophthalmic, posterior communicating, the anterior communicating, the anterior cerebral, and the middle cerebral arteries (Fig. 48-3). The two vertebral arteries arise from the subclavian artery, ascend into the cranium through the foramen magnum, and join to form the large basilar artery. The basilar artery divides to form the posterior cerebral arteries. Branches of the basilar and vertebral arteries supply the medulla, pons, cerebellum, midbrain, and part of the diencephalon. The posterior cerebral arteries supply the temporal and occipital lobes.

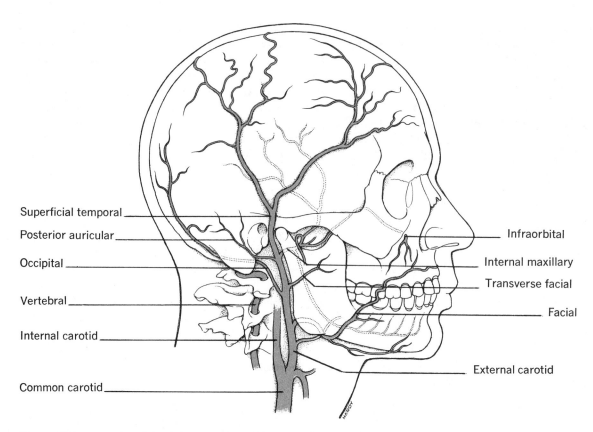

Figure 48-2 *Branches of the right external carotid artery. The internal carotid artery ascends to the base of the brain. The right vertebral artery is also shown as it ascends through the transverse foramina of the cervical vertebrae. (Chaffee EE, Lytle IM: Basic Physiology and Anatomy, 4th ed, p 338. Philadelphia, JB Lippincott, 1980)*

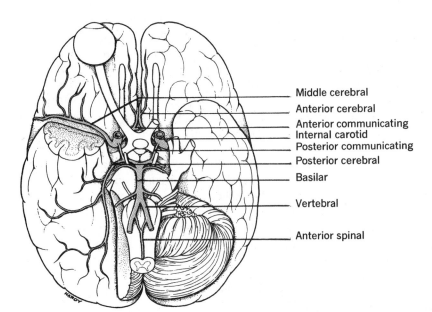

Figure 48-3 *The circle of Willis as seen at the base of a brain removed from the skull. (Chaffee EE, Lytle IM: Basic Physiology and Anatomy, 4th ed. Philadelphia, JB Lippincott, 1980)*

Anastomotic Connections and Collateral Circulation

There are two defense mechanisms that help protect the brain against ischemia: the collateral circulation and autoregulation of blood flow. The internal carotid arteries and the vertebral arteries communicate at the base of the brain through the *circle of Willis*, ensuring continued circulation should blood flow through one of the main vessels be disrupted. There are extensive anastomotic channels in the brain. Under normal circumstances, the anastomotic channels in the circle of Willis are not patent. If blood flow is occluded, however, these connections become patent and can maintain blood supply to the affected area. There are no significant anastomotic connections other than in these large cerebral vessels and the small capillary vessels. Occlusions of adjacent or terminal arteries from the large cerebral vessels may result in neural damage because the anastomotic connections may not be adequate to allow blood to reach the ischemic area in sufficient quantity and with sufficient rapidity to meet the high metabolic needs of the occluded area.

The brain is amazingly able to regulate its own blood supply. Cerebral blood flow is constant within a mean blood pressure range of 60 mm Hg to 140 mm Hg. In persons with hypertension the pressure may be as high as 180 mm Hg to 200 mm Hg, but the cerebral blood flow remains constant.

The remarkable vasodilation mechanism of the brain operates when a high carbon dioxide concentration, a high hydrogen ion concentration, or a low oxygen tension is present in the blood. High concentrations of hydrogen ion or carbon dioxide depress neural activity, and through vasodilation these substances are quickly removed. The brain utilizes oxygen at the rate of 3.5 ml of oxygen per 100 gm of brain tissue per minute.[1] If its blood flow should become insufficient, the vasodilation mechanism will immediately respond bringing blood flow and oxygenation back to near normal.

Stroke

A cerebral vascular accident (CVA) is a sudden, severe episode of neurologic symptoms caused by a deficit in blood supply to areas of the brain. It is manifested in any combination of the following symptoms: hemiplegia (paralysis of one side of the body), hemiparesis (weakness of muscle groups of one side of the body), aphasia (lack of sensory input), incontinence, perceptual deficits, and behavioral aberrations.

Stroke is one of the most common disorders of the cardiovascular system, ranking second only to heart attack. It is the third leading cause of death and the major cause of long-term disability. It was estimated that, in 1978, 172,500 Americans died of stroke and another 750,000 persons experienced a CVA.[2] The incidence of first stroke increases with age from 0.25 per 1000 in the 35-to-44-year-old age group to 20 per 1000 in the 75-to-84-year old age group and 40 per 1000 in those 85 years of age or older.[3] Stroke is more common in men than in women and more common in black than in white persons. The total cost in the United States from direct medical expenses, lost income, and productivity is estimated at $14 billion a year.[4]

As indicated above, stroke is more likely with advancing age. However, the exceptions to this generalization are embolic stroke and some types of hemorrhagic stroke, which are more common in younger persons. Stroke is also linked with atherosclerosis, obesity, cigarette smoking, physical inactivity, positive family history, elevated serum glucose, elevated serum lipids, increased blood volume or viscosity, anemia, and use of oral contraceptives.[3]

The neurologic manifestations of stroke are associated with the deficit in cerebral blood flow. If there is generalized anoxia throughout the brain, symptoms of diffuse cerebral damage will be seen: drowsiness, disorientation, confusion, stupor, and finally loss of consciousness. In most cases the anoxia is localized, and specific neurologic deficits related to the involved area of the brain are noted.

Regardless of the cause, strokes disrupt both the flow of oxygen, nutrients, and metabolic substances to the brain and the removal of waste products from the brain. With deficient cerebral blood flow there is not only cerebral anoxia but also edema and congestion in the surrounding area, which compress the tissue and further impair function. The brain is extremely sensitive to ischemia, and neurologic deficits can be seen when the blood supply is reduced even in small areas. The two mechanisms used to attempt to maintain homeostasis of blood supply—autoregulation of blood flow and collateral circulation—are determined by whether the ischemia occurs rapidly or slowly and by the presence or absence of previous vascular problems. If tissue perfusion is resumed adequately, the cells may survive. As the blood supply to the area is improved and the edema subsides, some functional improvement may be seen. It is possible that the dysfunction may have been due to the edema and not to neuronal damage from the stroke. The necrotic tissue is generally removed by macrophage activity and replaced by glia and vascular scar.

Predisposing factors

Efforts to prevent stroke should be directed toward identifying and treating persons who have hypertension, transient ischemic attacks (TIAs), atherosclerosis, and cardiac disorders, all of which may contribute to stroke.

Hypertension. Hypertension, a major cause of hypertensive and other nonembolic forms of stroke, is a significant but treatable risk factor. Indeed, the declining incidence and mortality of stroke has been attributed to improved control of hypertension. In extreme hypertension, there may be hemorrhage into the meninges or into the subdural, extradural, and subarachnoid spaces. In the present discussion, the term hemorrhage refers to intracerebral or intracranial bleeding into the brain substance, while the phrase primary cerebral hemorrhage excludes causes of hemorrhage other than hypertension (arteriovenous malformation, trauma, hemorrhagic tendency, tumor). The incidence of primary cerebral hemorrhage is as high as 25 per 100,000 of the population.[3]

Transient ischemic attacks. Transient ischemic attacks are characteristic of atherosclerosis of cerebral vessels with thrombosis. Atherosclerotic plaque involves the intima of medium-sized vessels. Gradually the lumen is filled with the sclerotic material. The plaques usually occur where arteries branch or become tortuous. The roughened edges of the plaques cause the platelets to adhere to the plaque. The clumped platelets may break off as an embolism or gradually occlude the artery.

Many TIAs take the form of transient focal neurologic deficits of vascular origin. Focal deficits are symptoms suggestive of the locus of the attack. Episodes of TIA may last for as little as a few minutes to as long as a day and leave no residual damage. They are frequently called "angina of the brain." If the same set of symptoms occurs with each episode of TIA, the pathologic process probably involves one vessel. If the symptoms are variable, different vessels may be involved. Early diagnosis may permit surgical or medical intervention and thus prevent extensive damage.

In contrast to a transient ischemic attack, a neurologic deficit that continues to progress or worsen over a period of 1 or 2 days is called a *stroke-in-evolution*. It is a gradually evolving stroke occurring in a person with a history of TIAs and is most likely due to thrombosis. A *completed stroke* may be described as follows: there has been maximum neurologic deficit due to thrombosis, to embolism, or (rarely) to hemorrhage; the patient's condition has stabilized or is improving; and there is residual neurologic damage. Recovery may take place over days, weeks, or months, and may be only partial.

Cardiac disorders. Various cardiac conditions predispose to formation of emboli. An embolus is a clot or other plug in a blood vessel. Most cerebral emboli have their origin in a thrombus in the left heart, from which they have broken away and been transported by the circulatory system to the cerebrum.

Stroke is associated with myocardial infarction, heart failure, and cardiac arrhythmias, all of which contribute to decreased cardiac output, in turn leading to cerebral ischemia and embolism. Recent advances in the diagnosis and treatment of heart disease can be expected to favorably alter the incidence of embolic stroke.

Subclavian steal syndrome. Although relatively rare, accounting for only 4% of all cerebrovascular diseases and 17% of extracranial carotid disorders, subclavian steal should be considered when there is a complaint of dizziness and lightheadedness,[5] because, with the vascular surgery that is now available to redirect the blood flow, the prognosis for recovery is excellent.

When the subclavian artery is occluded near its origin, the blood flows from the vertebral artery (reverse or retrograde flow), draining from the basilar artery and the circle of Willis, into the arm.[6] (The blood is "stolen" from the subclavian artery.) This subclavian steal syndrome is another cause of cerebral ischemia. Its symptoms include dizziness, lightheadedness, and syncope; the radial pulse is absent or diminished; and there is usually a difference of 20 mm Hg or more in blood pressure between the affected and the unaffected arms.

Types of strokes

Three main processes that affect the cerebral vessels may eventually lead to stroke: hemorrhage, embolism, and thrombosis. They vary in their rapidity of onset and prognosis (Table 48-2). The presence of a concomitant disease will also affect the outcome of stroke.

The most frequently fatal stroke is rupture of the vessel wall—intracerebral *hemorrhage*. With rupture of a blood vessel, hemorrhage into the brain substance or subarachnoid space occurs, resulting in edema, compression of the brain contents, or spasms of the adjacent vessels. The most common predisposing factor is hypertension. Other causes of hemorrhage are aneurysm, trauma, erosion of vessels by tumors, vascular malformations, and blood dyscrasias. A cerebral hemorrhage occurs suddenly, usually when the person is active. The person may complain of a severe headache and stiff neck (nuchal rigidity) because blood has entered the cerebrospinal fluid (CSF). Focal symptoms depend on which vessel is involved. There is usually contralateral hemiplegia, with initial flaccidity progressing to spasticity. The hemorrhage and resultant edema exert great pressure on the brain substance, and the clinical course progresses rapidly to coma and frequently to death.

An embolic stroke is caused by a moving blood clot. Although most cerebral emboli originate in a thrombus in the left heart, they may also originate in an atherosclerotic plaque in the carotid arteries. The embolus travels quickly to the brain and becomes lodged in a small artery through which it cannot pass. Therefore, this

Table 48-2   Causes of Stroke

Cause	Onset	Symptoms	Predisposing Factors	Prognosis
Hemorrhage	Sudden, usually during activity	Rapid hemiplegia and loss of consciousness, severe headache and stiff neck	Hypertension; less often: aneurysm, trauma, erosion of vessels, arteriovenous malformations, blood dyscrasias	Poor
Embolus	Sudden, not related to activity	Immediate maximum deficit, consciousness preserved	Thrombus left heart or atherosclerotic plaque	Fair to good
Thrombus	Gradual, evolving over minutes or days	Slow decrease in function	Atherosclerosis	May see rapid improvement

embolic stroke also has a sudden onset with immediate maximum deficit. The middle cerebral artery is the most common site of embolus formation. Cardiac arrhythmias are frequently noted and serve as a source of emboli. If there is a history of formation of numerous small emboli, the pattern of symptoms will vary depending on which vessels are involved. There may be more extensive tissue death due to emboli than occurs in the more slowly progressing thrombosis, because in the former there is no opportunity for collateral circulation to develop. Nevertheless, the damage is less than occurs in cerebral hemorrhage. If coma ensues, it will not be as deep as hemorrhagic coma, and recovery is more likely.

A *thrombotic* stroke is caused by a thrombus, or blood clot, that forms in a cerebral vessel; it has a much slower onset than embolic stroke, evolving over minutes or hours. The arterial lumen gradually becomes occluded due to atherosclerosis. Usually, thrombosis is seen in older people, and evidence of arteriosclerotic heart disease is frequently present, as is diabetes mellitus. The thrombotic stroke is not associated with activity and may occur in a person at rest. Consciousness may or may not be lost, and improvement may be rapid.

Localized effects by blood vessels

Arterial blood flow to the brain is supplied from the aortic arch by the two internal carotid arteries (anteriorly) and the two vertebral arteries (posteriorly). The carotid arteries are subject to development of atherosclerotic plaques at their site of origin from the aortic arch and at the bifurcations of the common carotid arteries and the proximal portions of the internal carotid arteries. The symptoms of stroke from this cause vary depending on the extent of collateral circulation that is present.

Anterior cerebral artery.   The internal carotid divides into branches, of which the two largest are the anterior

and middle cerebral arteries. The *anterior cerebral artery* supplies the medial portions of the frontal and parietal lobes and the corpus callosum. Since the prefrontal area anterior to the motor strip in the frontal lobe is responsible for many thought processes, the characteristic signs of damage to this area are distractability and inability to plan in an orderly fashion. Confusion is the primary symptom when the frontal lobe is affected, as are other mental changes frequently classified as typical of dementia. The frontal lobe also contains the motor cortex neurons that are concerned with motor function; therefore, contralateral paresis or paralysis, especially of the leg, may be seen. There also may be some sensory deficit because of parietal lobe involvement. Urinary incontinence often occurs.

Middle cerebral artery.   The *middle cerebral artery* supplies most of the lateral surface of the cerebrum and the deeper structures of the frontal, parietal, and temporal lobes, including the internal capsule and basal ganglia. Many major strokes involve the middle cerebral artery, so that a stroke originating at this site is likely to cause extensive damage because the fibers in the motor strip are brought together in the internal capsule. Among the symptoms that stem from middle cerebral artery stroke are (1) contralateral (motor and sensory loss) paralysis, especially of the arm (the leg area is supplied by the anterior cerebral artery); (2) homonymous hemianopia (contralateral blindness), if the stroke involves the optic nerve; (3) aphasia, if the stroke involves the dominant hemisphere where the speech centers are located; (4) agnosia (inability to recognize sensory stimuli), if the stroke involves the sensory cortex, or (5) perceptual deficits, if the stroke involves the nondominant hemispheres.

Posterior cerebral artery.   The *posterior cerebral artery* supplies the occipital lobe and the anterior and medial portions of the temporal lobe. Although the occipital lobe is primarily for vision, the temporal lobe, specifically the angular gyrus, is responsible for memory and some associative function. If occlusion interrupts the blood supply to deeper structures, there may be mild contralateral hemiparesis (weakness on one side of the body), cerebellar ataxia (incoordination), and third nerve palsy. Visual disturbances of hemianopia, visual aphasia, or alexia (word blindness—an inability to recognize words as symbols of ideas) may occur. If both occipital lobes are involved, there may be cortical blindness (the cortical visual center cannot function).

The cerebellum and brain are supplied by branches of the basilar and vertebral arteries. The vertebral arteries may develop plaques at the sites of origin from the subclavian arteries and the first portion of the arteries before they enter the vertebral foramina. Ischemia resulting from disruption of the *vertebral-basilar circulation* may produce a variety of symptoms. These include visual disturbances, such as diplopia due to involvement of the oculomotor, trochlear, and abducens nerves, ataxia due to cerebellar involvement, vertigo due to involvement of the vestibular nuclei, and dysphagia and dysphonia due to involvement of the glossopharyngeal and vagus nerves.

Acute and chronic manifestations

When the patient regains consciousness (if consciousness was lost), characteristically there will be contralateral hemiplegia, with either a speech disturbance or a spatial-perceptual deficit depending on which side of the brain was affected, and possibly incontinence. The specific focal deficits depend on which vessel is involved.

Motor recovery. Initially following a stroke, there is total *flaccidity*, characterized by a decrease in or absence of normal muscle tone. There is a tendency toward foot drop, outward rotation of the leg, and dependent edema in the affected extremities. Putting the extremities through passive range of motion helps to maintain the joint function and to prevent edema, shoulder subluxation (incomplete dislocation), and muscle atrophy. The smooth, sequential movement of the exercises may help to reestablish motor patterns.

Early motor recovery is seen with the beginning of *spasticity*—the resistance of muscle groups to passive stretch, with an increase of muscle tone throughout the body. Spasticity follows the decline in cerebral edema and the initial flaccidity, because inhibition of muscle tone from the basal ganglia is now reduced. With spasticity, the flexor muscles are usually stronger in the upper extremities; the extensor muscles are stronger in the lower extremities.[7] Involuntary muscle contractions are manifested in shoulder adduction, forearm pronation, finger flexion, and knee and hip extension. If spasticity has not begun within 6 weeks (certainly within 3 months), function will probably not return to that extremity. Passive range of motion should be continued and positioning should be directed toward keeping all joints in functional position.

Aphasia. The most common cause of aphasia is vascular disease of the middle cerebral artery of the dominant cerebral hemisphere. In close to 90% of the population, the left hemisphere is dominant. Aphasia, a defect or loss of the power of expression by writing, speech, or signs, is estimated to be present in 40% of cases of stroke.[8] Confusion, anxiety, or memory loss may be present and, if not detected and treated, will seriously hinder rehabilitation.

Aphasia is a general term that encompasses varying degrees of inability to comprehend, integrate, and express speech. This generalization may lead to misinterpretation. Aphasia may be more accurately described as an acquired neurologic disorder of *language* abilities caused by damage in the CNS.[8] The term "language" implies a higher integrative function of perception, integration, and formulation of verbal stimuli; a speech disorder is essentially a neuromuscular problem. For example, a person with dysarthria—an imperfect articulation of speech—still retains some language ability. Two categories are usually used when describing aphasia; expressive and nonexpressive. *Motor,* or *expressive,* aphasia is the loss of the ability to express thoughts and ideas in speech or writing. The person with expressive aphasia may be able, with difficulty, to utter two or three words, usually words having an emotional overlay. Automatic speech and social phrases are usually easier to articulate. Although comprehension is usually intact, in speech some words may be omitted or inappropriate words may be used. *Jargon* aphasia is the utterance of nonexistent words, which the person is unable to recognize as such and believes to be correct and appropriate.

Sensory, or *receptive,* aphasia is the inability to comprehend written or spoken words. Receptive aphasia is also called Wernicke's aphasia or auditory aphasia. Some persons manifest elements of both receptive and expressive aphasia, called *mixed* aphasia. When all language ability is lost—both receptive and expressive—the aphasia is said to be *global* or *total*. Most aphasias are partial, however, and a thorough speech evaluation is essential to determining the type and extent of aphasia and the therapy needed.

One of the most common characteristics of aphasia is distorted spontaneous or conversational speech, which is usually classified as fluent (many) or nonfluent (few) words. Although the terms fluent and nonfluent have been in use for years, they have recently been reemphasized. *Fluency* refers to the characteristics of speech and not to content or ability to comprehend. Fluent output requires little or no effort, is articulate, and is of increased quantity. It is rambling, wordy, yet meaningless—what is sometimes called empty speech. There are three categories of fluent aphasia: Wernicke's, anomic, and conduction aphasia.[8] *Wernicke's* aphasia is characterized by an inability to comprehend the speech, reading, and writing not only of other persons but also of oneself. *Anomic* aphasia is speech that is nearly normal, but in which the person has difficulty selecting appropriate words. Inappropriate word use in the presence of good comprehension is called *conduction* aphasia.

Nonfluent aphasia presents opposite problems: poor articulation, poor modulation, dysarthria, and sparse output of words with considerable effort and limited to short phrases or single words. The words are substantive and have considerable meaning. Nonfluent aphasia may also be called *Broca's* aphasia. If the aphasia-producing lesion affects the anterior and posterior speech areas, a mixed or global aphasia may result, with problems of nonfluent aphasia and the comprehension difficulties of Wernicke's aphasia.

There is a correlation between the anatomic location of cerebral damage and the aphasia syndrome, which was recognized by Broca and Wernicke more than a century ago. Although exceptions exist, most persons with nonfluent aphasia have lesions anterior to the Rolandic fissure, known as anterior Broca's aphasia; people with fluent aphasia have a lesion posterior to the fissure, known as posterior Wernicke's aphasia.[9]

Diagnosis and treatment

Accurate diagnosis is based on a complete history and a thorough physical and neurologic examination. A careful history, including TIAs, their rapidity of onset and focal symptoms, as well as those of any other diseases that may be present, will help to determine the type of stroke that is involved. Several test procedures are essential to diagnosis: arteriography will demonstrate the site of the deficit and afford visualization of most intracranial vascular areas. The brain scan and the electroencephalogram (EEG) also aid in localizing the area. And computerized axial tomography (CAT or CT scan) has become an important tool in diagnosing stroke and in differentiating cerebral hemorrhage and intracranial lesions that may mimic stroke.[10] Positron emission tomography (PET) makes it possible to define the location and size of strokes by providing data on cerebral blood flow and volume and brain cell metabolism.

The treatment of stroke is largely symptomatic. The main goals are to prevent complications and treat any underlying disease. There is some controversy over whether or not effort should be made to lower the blood pressure after a stroke. A chief consideration is to maintain oxygenation of brain tissue, and the possibility exists that a rapid fall in blood pressure could compromise blood flow and oxygenation. There is also controversy over the use of anticoagulants as a means of preventing further occlusion. Anticoagulants represent a double-edged sword because they can precipitate hemorrhage. Although further study is indicated, a significant decrease in recurrent stroke and myocardial infarction has been demonstrated in persons who have been treated with small daily doses of aspirin.[11,12] Surgical attempts at restoring blood supply to the brain focus on removing any clots from the carotid or vertebral arteries or bypassing occluded vessels.

Symptomatic treatment is aimed at preventing complications and promoting the fullest possible recovery of function. During the acute phase, proper positioning and range of motion exercising are essential. Early rehabilitation efforts need to include not only the physician and nurse but other members of the rehabilitation team, such as the speech therapist and occupational therapist, and the family.

In summary, a stroke or cerebral vascular accident is a sudden severe deficit in neurologic function caused by a deficit in the blood supply to areas of the brain. It is the third leading cause of death in the United States and a major cause of disability. Uncontrolled hypertension is a significant risk factor for the development of stroke. Stroke can result from hemorrhage, embolus, or thrombus. The effects of stroke depend on the location of the blood vessel involved and include motor, sensory, and speech manifestations. The treatment is primarily symptomatic, involving the combined efforts of the health care professionals in the rehabilitation team, the patient, and the family.

■ Parkinson's Disease

Parkinson's disease usually begins after age 50 and increases markedly with age, the majority of cases being diagnosed in the sixth and seventh decades of life. Estimates of the incidence of Parkinson's disease in the United States vary from 500,000 to 1,000,000 cases. Men and women appear to be equally affected; a higher prevalence is noted in the white race than in the black race. Although some scientists suggest that there is a genetic susceptibility to the disease, other research findings suggest that heredity is not important.

As was stated earlier, the motor system is composed of two antagonistic components, the excitatory pyramidal system and the inhibitory extrapyramidal system. These components form a single complex system, which is under cortical control but is modulated by the basal ganglia and cerebellum. The extrapyramidal system modifies voluntary movement by adjusting the degree of muscle contraction to make the movement smooth and fluid. In addition, the basal ganglia along with the cerebellum are believed to control certain acquired motor skills usually performed with conscious awareness once they have been learned.

Neurons from the nigrostriatal tract, which originates in the substantia nigra part of the basal ganglia of the extrapyramidal motor system and terminates in the corpus striatum, release the neurotransmitter dopamine. Although the primary etiology of Parkinson's disease is not known, it is known that the nigrostriatal tract is most consistently and severely affected. The reduction in dopamine, an inhibitory neurotransmitter, results in a neurochemical imbalance in which the nerve cells that release acetylcholine, an excitatory neurotransmitter, become predominant.

Parkinsonism may present as a pure syndrome affecting only the extrapyramidal tract or as a more generalized disease. The former is referred to as idiopathic Parkinson's disease and is the most commonly occurring type. Further research is needed on the more generalized form of the disease, which may be related to progressive cerebral atrophy, biochemical changes in the brain, or the normal aging process. It is useful to differentiate between persons whose symptoms are primarily tremor rigidity and akinesias and those with symptoms of more diffuse damage.[13]

Although the majority of cases of Parkinson's disease are idiopathic, the disease appears to be related to (1) encephalitis (postencephalitic parkinsonism, (2) side-effects of medications such as reserpine and the phenothiazines (drug-induced or iatrogenic parkinsonism),[14] (3) other diseases, such as degenerative diseases (parkinsonism-plus) or precursors to other diseases (juvenile parkinsonism), and (4) trauma, hemorrhage, or tumor (secondary parkinsonism or traumatic parkinsonism). Parkinsonlike symptoms are also seen with small strokes known as lacunar infarcts; magnesium, carbon monoxide, or mercury toxicity; and hyperthyroidism or hypothyroidism (pseudoparkinsonism).

Disruption of the extrapyramidal system causes problems associated with inhibition of impulses, gross intentional movements, and body posture. In Parkinson's disease, the chief symptoms are characteristic of damage to the extrapyramidal tract: (1) increase in muscle tone and rigidity, (2) tremor, usually at rest, (3) akinesia (absence of spontaneous movement), and (4) postural difficulties resulting from an uncontrollable gait. The symptoms are progressive.

Clinical Manifestations

The classic picture of a person with an advanced case of Parkinson's disease demonstrates the extrapyramidal nature of the symptoms. Tremor, rigidity, and akinesia are the three cardinal symptoms. Tremor is an early symptom and usually occurs at rest (resting tremor). The rhythmic alternating flexion and contraction of the muscles resembles pill rolling; in fact, it is often referred to as a pill-rolling tremor. The rigidity, a generalized hypertonicity of muscle, results in jerky, cogwheel motions in which considerable energy is needed to move muscle groups. Flexion contractions may result. In addition, spontaneous movement (bradykinesia, slowed voluntary movement) is reduced and unconscious associative movements are lost. People with Parkinson's disease have difficulty initiating walking. When they walk, they take small, shuffling steps, lean forward, head bent, without swinging their arms, and stop only with difficulty as they move faster and faster (propulsion).

The characteristic facial appearance is stiff and masklike. The mouth may be open, with saliva drooling from the corners because the person cannot move the saliva to the back of the mouth and swallow it. The speech is slow, monotonous, without modulation, and poorly articulated. Autonomic symptoms of constipation, urinary incontinence, and lacrimation may be present. Although the person with Parkinson's disease may appear to be affected intellectually, it is not known whether persons with idiopathic Parkinson's disease are more prone to dementia than other persons of the same age. Occasional depression, however, may occur. There are several stages in the progression of Parkinson's disease. The symptoms usually are noted first on one side of the body and progress to bilateral involvement, with early postural changes in 1 to 2 years following onset. Postural changes and gait disturbances continue to become more pronounced until the person has significant disability and requires constant care.

Treatment

Antiparkinsonian drugs act in one of two ways: (1) to increase the functional ability of the underactive dopaminergic system or (2) to reduce the excessive influence of excitatory cholinergic neurons on the extrapyramidal tract. The first group include levodopa (L-dopa, Dopar, Larodopa), amantadine (Symmetrel), and bromocriptine (Parlodel). The second group of drugs are anticholinergic drugs. Administration of L-dopa, a precursor of dopamine which, unlike dopamine, crosses the blood-brain barrier, has demonstrated significant improvement in clinical symptoms.

Prior to the discovery of L-dopa, anticholinergics were the mainstay of treatment. Today, anticholinergics are used primarily in mild cases or when L-dopa is not tolerated. Although the exact mechanism is not known, research indicates that striated structures receive antagonistic cholinergic and dopamine inputs; and the balance between these two inputs determines motor control of the striatum.[15]

Because dopamine transmission is disrupted, it appears that there is a cholinergic preponderance, which is decreased with anticholinergic drugs; this brings about improvement of the symptoms. The dopamine postsynaptic receptors are located on cholinergic cells.[16] They can inhibit the uptake and storage of dopamine, thus potentiating the postsynaptic efficacy of the neurotransmitter. This information also explains why cholinergics tend to exaggerate Parkinson's symptoms.

Trihexyphenidyl hydrochloride (Artane) is an anticholinergic widely used in Parkinson's disease. Other anticholinergics are procyclidine (Kemadrin) and benztropine mesylate (Cogentin). The anticholinergics lessen the tremors and rigidity and afford some functional improvement. Their potency seems to decrease over time, however; increasing the dosage merely increases the side-effects such as blurred vision, dry mouth, bowel and bladder problems, and some mental changes.

L-dopa

The evidence of decreased dopamine in the striatum in Parkinson's disease led to the administration of large doses of L-dopa (L-dihydroxyphenylalanine), which is absorbed from the intestinal tract, crosses the blood-brain barrier, and is converted to dopamine by centrally acting dopa decarboxylase. The main problem with L-dopa, or the synthetic compound levodopa, is that the large dose that is needed to relieve symptoms has many side-effects. Patients are started on very small doses of L-dopa, and the dose is gradually increased until therapeutic levels are reached. Nevertheless, side-effects are seen in almost all of these patients. These may be relatively mild, such as nausea and vomiting, or much more severe, ending in cardiac arrhythmia and death. Other adverse effects of L-dopa include depression, orthostatic hypotension, and involuntary movements of the tongue and lips. Most will disappear with reduction of the dose.

The large L-dopa dose is necessary because most of L-dopa is converted to dopamine (which does not cross the blood-brain barrier) by *peripheral* decarboxylase before it can cross the blood-brain barrier.[17] *Carbidopa*, a dopa-decarboxylase inhibitor, can be given to increase the amount of L-dopa entering the brain and thus reduce the dose of L-dopa. With carbidopa, the patient does not have to eliminate vitamin B_6 from the diet. Vitamin B_6, a cofactor of dopa decarboxylase, has an adverse effect on L-dopa but not when administered with carbidopa. Sinemet is a preparation containing carbidopa and L-dopa.

In summary, Parkinson's disease is a disorder of the basal ganglia of the extrapyramidal system, which modifies the voluntary control of motor function. The disease is characterized by a decrease in dopamine, an inhibitory neurotransmitter, in the dopaminergic neurons of the basal ganglia and substantia nigra. This results in a neurochemical imbalance in which the nerve cells that release acetylcholine, an excitatory neurotransmitter, become dominant. The clinical manifestations of the disease, especially tremor, rigidity, and akinesia, reflect impairment of the modulating effects that the extrapyramidal system exerts on motor function. The treatment consists of medications to replace dopamine with L-dopa or to reduce acetylcholine with anticholinergic agents.

■ Disorders of the Myelin

The myelin sheath is produced by one of the glias, oligodendroglia, in the central nervous system and by the Schwann cells of the peripheral nervous system. All myelin is composed of fat and lipids, but the CNS myelin has lipid solubility because of its major protein, proteolipid.[18] The composition of myelin forms an insulation that allows neural discharge to occur only at the internode, thus speeding the conduction of impulses and reducing the metabolic work required to maintain the necessary ionic gradients for neural conduction. The myelination process starts *in utero* and is not completed until the second year of life. Myelination begins at the cell body and proceeds distally, forming a seam on the back side of the neuron, which may be the first area to break down in demyelinating disease.

Multiple Sclerosis

A large number of neurologic disorders are called demyelinating diseases, because the primary pathology is destruction of the myelin sheath. Multiple sclerosis (MS) is the most common demyelinating disease. Because of the difficulty in diagnosis, an accurate incidence is hard to determine, but estimates of the total number of cases in the United States range from 123,000 to 250,000. Multiple sclerosis is usually diagnosed between the ages of 20 and 40 years, and it affects women twice as often as it does men.

The cause of multiple sclerosis remains unknown. The geographic distribution and migration studies suggest an environmental influence. The prevalence is higher in northern Europe, the northern United States, southern Australia, and New Zealand. There is also a family tendency to multiple sclerosis that may be due to hereditary factors. The most frequently suggested causes of the disease are a slow-growing dormant or long-incubation-period virus or a deficiency of the immune system.

The presence of demyelinated glial patches called plaques, ranging from 1 mm to 4 cm, is macroscopically visible throughout the white matter of the central nervous system.[19] These lesions are usually symmetrical and seem to have a predilection for certain areas, such as the periventricular area. The color of the plaques depends on the age of the lesion: newer plaques are pink; older lesions gray. These plaques represent the end result of acute myelin breakdown.

The characteristic feature of multiple sclerosis, seen microscopically, is the breakdown of myelin sheath with relative sparing of the axons. Oligodendroglia are reduced in number and may be absent, especially in older lesions. The sequence of myelin breakdown is not well understood, although it is known that the lesions contain small amounts of myelin, basic proteins, increased amounts of proteolytic enzymes, macrophages, lymphocytes, and plasma cells. A wallerian degeneration (degeneration of the nerve portion on the side closest to the CNS, with an intact nerve portion on the peripheral side of the lesion) may be present in advanced stages or in severe lesions in the acute stage. Acute, subacute, and chronic sclerotic lesions are scattered throughout the central nervous system.

Histologic evidence supports the clinical picture of remission and exacerbations. There is evidence of remyelination, which supports the thesis that clinical deterioration is followed by periods of apparent tissue healing and remission of symptoms. The healing is rarely able to provide a return to normal function, as is evidenced by misshapen nodes of Ranvier.

The demyelinating fibers have a variety of conduction abnormalities, ranging from decreased conduction velocity to conduction blocks. In the demyelinated fiber, conduction velocity is decreased, so that the threshold is reached very slowly or not at all.[20]

Manifestations and clinical course

The interruption of neural conduction is manifested by a variety of symptoms, depending on the location and duration of the lesion. Areas commonly affected by multiple sclerosis are the optic chiasm, optic nerves, brain stem, cerebellum, corticospinal tracts, and posterior columns of the spinal cord. The most common symptoms are paresthesias, optic neuritis, and motor weakness. Other symptoms frequently seen are abnormal gait, bladder dysfunction, vertigo, and diplopia.

Multiple sclerosis is characterized by slowly progressive weakness starting in the lower extremities. Other pyramidal tract symptoms include spasticity, hyperreflexia, and bilateral Babinski signs. Involvement of the cerebellar and the corticospinal tracts is manifested by cerebellar ataxia, nystagmus, intention tremor, balance disturbance, and dysarthria. Corticospinal tract involvement is responsible for signs of urinary tract dysfunction such as incontinence, urgency, hesitancy, frequency, and retention.

Psychological manifestations, such as mood swings, may represent a psychological reaction to the nature of the disease or, more likely, involvement of the white matter of the cerebral cortex. Depression, euphoria, inattentivenes, apathy, forgetfulness, and loss of memory may occur.

In the majority of multiple sclerosis cases, the disease presents with exacerbations and remissions. Initially, there is normal or near-normal neurologic function between exacerbations. As the disease progresses, there is less improvement between exacerbations and increasing neurologic dysfunction.

A small percentage of people develop an acute form of multiple sclerosis that progresses rapidly with incomplete remissions of short duration. This form of multiple sclerosis can be fatal within a few months or years. There is also a benign form of the disease that has a few mild exacerbations followed by complete recovery. In the benign form, a person remains relatively asymptomatic without neurologic dysfunction for many years. There may also be a subclinical form of the disease, since demyelination has been observed in asymptomatic persons on autopsy.[19] Because of the varied clinical courses of multiple sclerosis, there is justified optimism for recently diagnosed persons.

Diagnosis and treatment

Diagnosis of multiple sclerosis is difficult because there is no specific laboratory test for the disease, manifestations are variable, and there may be long intervals between the first appearance of symptoms and recurrence. The conditions necessary for the diagnosis of multiple sclerosis are lesions that have occurred on more than one occasion and at more than one site and are not explained by other mechanisms. Clinical findings have traditionally been used for documentation. Recently, however, electrophysiologic evaluations and computerized tomography have aided the identification and documentation of lesions; but they still do not provide information about the cause of the lesions. Nuclear magnetic resonance (NMR) imaging has also been used recently to evaluate multiple sclerosis.

Although no laboratory test can be used to diagnose multiple sclerosis, examination of the CSF is helpful. A large percentage of patients with multiple sclerosis have elevated IgG levels and some have oligoclonal patterns (discrete electrophoretic bands) even with normal IgG levels. There may also be a mild increase in total protein or lymphocytes in the CSF.

The variety of symptoms, course of the disease, and lack of specific diagnostic methods have made the evaluation and treatment of multiple sclerosis difficult. Corticotropin (ACTH) and corticosteroids can shorten the duration of an acute attack. The long-term administration of the drug does not, however, appear to alter the course of the disease and may be harmful because of its many side-effects. Other treatments that are currently being studied include use of the transfer factor and interferon (Chap. 9).

The primary treatment of multiple sclerosis is symptomatic. Pharmacologic treatment may include (1) dantrolene (Dantrium), baclofen (Lioresal), or diazepam (Valium) for spasticity, (2) cholinergic drugs for bladder problems, (3) antidepressant drugs for depression, and (4) carbamazepine for paroxysmal attacks. The person should be encouraged to maintain as healthy a life-style as possible, including good nutrition and adequate rest and relaxation. Physical therapy may be helpful for maintaining muscle tone. Every effort should be made to avoid excessive fatigue, physical deterioration, emotional stress, and extremes of environmental temperature, which may precipitate exacerbation of the disease.

In summary, multiple sclerosis is an example of a demylinating disease involving a slowly progressive breakdown of myelin and the formation of plaques, but sparing the axis cylinder of the neuron. The cause of multiple sclerosis remains unknown. The geographic distribution and migration studies suggest an environmental influence. The interruption of neural conduction in multiple sclerosis is manifested by a variety of disabling signs and symptoms depending on the neurons that are affected. The most common symptoms are paresthesias, optic neuritis, and motor weakness. The disease is usually characterized by exacerbations and remissions. Initially, near normal function returns between exacerbations. The variety of symptoms, course of the disease, and lack of specific diagnostic tests make diagnosis and treatment of the disease difficult. At present treatment is largely symptomatic.

■ Spinal Cord Injury (SCI)

A review of the spinal cord demonstrates that the spinal cord, like the brain, has extensive protective mechanisms—the bony protection of the vertebral column, the meninges, and the CSF. These mechanisms protect the structures responsible for innervation of the body, exclusive of the head. In addition to initiating the spinal reflex response, sensory endings relay data originating in the endings to the brain stem and cerebellum, where they are utilized in various circuits, including those that influence motor performance. Sensory information is also relayed to the thalamus and cerebral cortex, where it becomes part of the conscious experience, with the possibility of immediate or delayed behavioral response. Motor neurons in the spinal cord are excited or inhibited by impulses originating at various levels of the brain from the medulla to the cerebral cortex. Vascular supply of the spinal cord comes mainly from the vertebral arteries. The anterior spinal artery from the vertebral arteries supplies the ventral and lateral portion of the spinal cord, including the anterior horns, lateral spinothalamic tracts, and pyramidal tracts. The posterior spinal artery supplies the posterior horns.

In SCI, there is no sensory or motor function below the spinal cord level of the lesion, although there may be reflex activity. A *quadriplegic* has suffered an injury to the cervical (or upper thoracic) area of the spinal cord that involves all four extremities. There may be some function in the upper extremities, depending on the level of the lesion and the area innervated by that spinal cord level. The innervation can be determined by dermatome testing. Below the level of the lesion, there is no sensory input for heat, cold, or pain to warn of impending danger, nor is there any voluntary motor movement. There may be an increase in muscle tone in extensor spasms and hyperactive deep tendon reflexes. High lesions in the cervical or upper thoracic spinal cord usually cause some difficulty with sitting balance and respiratory function. Reflex emptying of bowel and bladder may be established. People who are *paraplegic* have sustained an injury to the lower thoracic, lumbar, or sacral portion of the spinal cord. The paralysis is in the lower extremities, usually involving the bowel and bladder but sparing respiratory function.

Trauma to the spinal cord may result from external or internal stressors. An external stressor is a knife, a bullet, or any other instrument that affords direct entry into the spinal cord from the outside. Internal stressors, which are more common, consist of damage to the vertebral column in which no entry into the spinal canal has occurred, such as fracture, dislocation of the vertebral column, or such violent agitation that the cord suffers injury. Severe flexion-extension, such as is caused by whiplash or a blow to the head, causes squeezing or shearing of the cord.

There are 10,000 new spinal cord injuries each year, most of which are caused by automobile accidents; falls and sports injuries are the second most common cause. Spinal cord injury is more common in males (82%) than in females (18%).[21] Because 80% of injuries occur before 40 years of age, and 50% occur between the ages of 15 and 25 years, the annual cost of caring for someone with SCI may be more than $250,000. In the United States, approximately 200,000 people who have sustained SCI use wheelchairs for mobility, at a cost to the nation of $2 billion per year.[22] The financial cost, however, is minor compared with the social, psychological, and physical cost to the individual and family.

Damage to the spinal cord is frequently due to a sudden narrowing of the spinal canal, in which the cord is caught between the lamina of a lower vertebra and the body of a higher one. Squeezing or shearing of the spinal cord causes destruction of gray matter, which has the highest blood flow, and hemorrhage of varying degree. The anterior spinal artery and vertebral artery hemorrhage, causing ischemic necrosis, edema, hematoma formation, and death of the nerve cells. The maximum effect is at the level of injury and one to two segments above and below the lesion.

Within minutes of the SCI, hypoxia of the gray matter stimulates the release of catecholamines in large quantities. The mechanism of SCI is not well understood but is probably due to either direct vascular injury or norepinephrine-induced vasoconstriction. In severe SCI, the blood flow to the region may cease for long intervals. Researchers have used norepinephrine-blocking agents such as reserpine, cooling, endorphin blockers, and steroids as measures to prevent additional ischemic damage, with varying degrees of success. The duration of compression because of hematoma formation is extremely important in predicting the potential for improvement. Continuous compression causes the death of nerve cells, which leads to gaps in the cord, with the development of scar tissue. Communication between the spinal cord and the brain is destroyed.

Although various terms are used to describe SCI, such as concussion, contusion, and compression, it is more useful to describe the effect of SCI. Injury to the spinal cord may result in complete, partial, or no permanent damage. The terms *severed* and *transected* spinal cord are often used, but rarely is the cord completely severed or transected. More appropriate terms are *complete* SCI, that is, loss of all motor and sensory function below the level of the lesion, and partial or *incomplete* SCI, in which some degree of motor and sensory function is retained. Complete SCI is discussed below.

Hematoma formation causes spinal shock, which lasts from 2 to 6 weeks, until the hematoma has dissolved. In spinal shock, there is a temporary decrease in neuronal excitability. Apparently, the motor neuron pools are dependent on excitation, usually supplied by the internuncial system; when this is no longer present, the motor neurons are depressed.[23] This causes an acute disruption of the corticospinal pathway, with paralysis of voluntary movement, and also temporarily abolishes spinal reflexes. This temporary loss of spinal reflexes is known as *spinal shock*. The resulting muscular flaccidity involves the loss of all motor, sensory, and reflex activity below the level of the lesion. Until spinal shock is resolved, the extent of damage cannot be totally determined. Several autonomic functions are also disrupted in spinal shock, resulting in retention of urine and feces, loss of vasomotor tone, and loss of thermoregulatory sweating below the level of the lesion.

After a few weeks, flaccidity disappears and slowly gives rise to reflex activity initiated with a positive Babinski reflex. The reflex recovery follows a pattern: (1) return of the Babinski reflex (2) minimal reflex activity, (3) flexor spasms, (4) alternate flexor-extensor spasms, and (5) after 6 months, dominant extensor spasms. The reflex spasms are due to the heightened sensitivity of the isolated segment of the cord, which has been released from the control of the higher centers. These flexor and extensor spasms may be evoked by a variety of stimuli in the anesthetic area, occasionally even being stimulated by bedclothes or a draft of air. At the same time, bowel and bladder function improves and, in most lesions except those in the sacral area, automatic control of these functions can be developed.

After 1 year, the clinical picture of spinal cord injury demonstrates complete paralysis below the level of the lesion and loss of motor and sensory function. In addition, the deep tendon reflexes are hyperactive, and bilateral positive Babinski reflexes are present. Reflex sweating occurs below the level of the lesion, but this sweating is not under thermoregulatory control. In higher spinal cord injuries, there is bowel and bladder reflex emptying. With lower lesions, especially those affecting the sacral area, there may be no reflex bowel or bladder emptying.

Alterations in Function

Cervical injury

In the past, a person who experienced a high cervical lesion (C 1,2,3) did not survive the initial injury; with the emergency transportation and treatment now available, however, this is no longer always the case. The main difficulty related to cervical lesions is that there is complete respiratory paralysis, and respiratory assistance is required. In lesions of C_3 to C_5, the phrenic nerve innervating the diaphragm is involved. Lesions between C_4 and T_{12} (thoracic) give rise to respiratory problems due to paralysis of the intercostal muscles, but respirations can be maintained without assistance. Colds and upper respiratory infections need to be vigorously avoided.

A lesion of C_4 results in a lack of voluntary movement in the trunk and the upper and lower extremities. But if C_4 is spared, the deltoids and the biceps are functional. A lesion at C_6 leaves the radial wrist extensors intact, and some flexion movements remain because of gravity. Triceps, finger flexors, and extensors are intact if the damage is at C_7. How much function will remain can be determined by assessing the area innervated by the spinal segment (dermatome).

Thoracic-lumbar injury

Full innervation of upper extremity muscles and varying degrees of innervation of back, abdominal, and intercostal muscles are present with lesions at the thoracic level. In lower thoracic and upper lumbar lesions, full abdominal and upper back control is achieved. In lower lumbar lesions, hip flexors and quadriceps muscles are innervated.

Autonomic nervous system responses

Spinal cord injury interrupts autonomic nervous system function. Problems are particularly severe in quadriplegics because the preganglionic neurons of the sympathetic nervous system are located in the thoracic and lumbar areas of the spinal cord, and the communication between higher centers and these neurons is interrupted in high SCI. This leads to problems with temperature regulation, cardiovascular difficulties, bowel and bladder incontinence, and disturbances in sexual functioning. On the other hand, the preganglionic neurons of the parasympathetic nervous system are located either in the cranial nerves or in the sacral segment of the cord. In any SCI, the cranial portion of the parasympathetic nervous system remains under the control of higher centers.

Thermoregulation. Sweating below the level of the lesion is a cord reflex and does not contribute to thermoregulation. In high lesions, there is very little area for thermoregulation to take place, and excessive sweating is seen on the head and the neck. Excess body heat cannot be released effectively in hot weather, and a controlled environment is important to the patient's well-being.

Cardiovascular response. In intact persons, customary changes in the internal environment do not cause changes in the blood pressure—it remains normal because of baroreceptor-mediated control by the autonomic nervous system. These mechanisms regulate heart rate, cardiac output, and adjustment of blood flow through peripheral and visceral vascular beds. In SCI, the baroreceptors become separated from the neural effector mechanism, so that blood pressure regulation and regional circulation become abnormal. For example, if a person with SCI is positioned so that the head is higher than the body, *postural hypotension* will result. Compensatory mechanisms fail and effective vasoconstriction does not occur; peripheral pooling of blood, decreased venous return, and a lower cardiac output occur.

If lightheadedness or dizziness occurs, the person should be placed in a horizontal position. Ultimately, adaptation takes place and postural hypotension becomes less of a problem. A tilt table and support stockings can help prevent postural hypotension until adaptation is complete.

The adaptation mechanism is not fully understood. However, improvement in adaptation is thought to be related to (1) the development of reflexes arising in the isolated spinal cord, (2) increased levels of urinary excretion of norepinephrine, (3) increased sensitivity of vascular beds to circulatory catecholamines, (4) increased blood volume, and (5) changes in baroreceptors and arterial PO_2 and PCO_2, which may stimulate reflex vasomotor constriction at the cord level.

Normally, cardioacceleration is a result of both a reduction in vagal tone and an activation of sympathetic cardioacceleration stimulation. In the absence of sympathetic stimulation, the heart rate responds only to vagal reduction. Vasoconstrictor tone is also inadequate and cardiac output falls because of inadequate venous return.

Autonomic dysreflexia (hyperreflexia). The parasympathetic section of the autonomic nervous system arises from the craniosacral area of the spinal cord, while the sympathetic nervous system arises from the thoracolumbar region. Autonomic dysreflexia is a disorder of autonomic homeostasis. In a spinal cord lesion above the level of sympathetic outflow—thoracic 6—stimulation of sensory receptors from a distended bladder or bowel sends impulses to the lower spinal cord. These impulses ascend the cord to the level of the lesion, where they are blocked. Because the autonomic reflexes are intact and not inhibited by impulses from higher centers, a reflex arteriolar spasm takes place in the skin and viscera.

The increased sympathetic response causes the blood pressure to rise, and profuse sweating occurs above the level of the lesion. The hypertension is recognized by the baroreceptors in the carotid sinus, aortic arch, and cerebral vessels. These receptors stimulate cranial nerve IX, the glossopharyngeal nerve, and cranial nerve X, the vagus nerve, to transmit afferent impulses to the vasomotor center of the medulla.[24] Normally, efferent impulses from the vagus would be relayed to the sinoatrial node of the heart in order to slow the cardiac rate, and other fibers would stimulate the splanchnic nerves to dilate the peripheral and visceral vasculature and thus lower the blood pressure. In the person with a spinal cord lesion, impulses along the tenth cranial nerve cause bradycardia, but impulses to the sympathetic motor preganglionic neurons in the thoracic and lumbar segments cannot go beyond the SCI. Therefore, compensatory vasodilation cannot occur below the level of the lesion, and severe hypertension persists even though vasodilation occurs above the level of the lesion. Vasodilation above the level of the lesion causes the skin of the neck and face to be hot and reddened, while it is pallid at the level of the lesion.

Sexuality. The desire for sexual activity remains unchanged, although initially the hormonal level may be altered somewhat. Women may not menstruate for up to 7 months following injury; they will then revert to their normal pattern. Pregnant women with high lesions (quadriplegia) may not be aware that they are ready to deliver, and the pregnancy may stimulate an automatic reaction of dysreflexia. In the man, sexual function depends somewhat on the level of the lesion. A person with a high lesion will probably have reflexogenic erections. In lower lesions, especially those of sacral segments 2 through 4, reflex activity is absent. When reflex activity and erection are present, coordination between erection and ejaculation is lost, and semen may be forced back into the bladder retrogradely. Many men with SCI are sterile because of the lower temperature in the testicles.

Bowel and bladder function. Renal disease is an important cause of death in SCI, and care must be taken to prevent infections in these patients. As with general muscle tone, the muscles of the bladder are flaccid immediately following the SCI. Overdistention of the bladder with resulting infection is a too-common problem. Following recovery from spinal shock, reflex bladder emptying may occur if the injury is not in sacral segments 2 to 4 (see Chap 31). Reflex bladder emptying is an automatic spinal cord reflex triggered by stimulation of the lower abdomen, the inner aspects of the thighs, or the genitalia.

Bowel function responds much the same way as bladder function with initial flaccidity and sometimes reflex emptying after recovery from spinal shock. Extensive bowel-training programs promote utilization of reflex activity for bowel evacuation.

Treatment

The treatment includes primary prevention through education about the causes of SCI. With persons who have SCI, the goals are to maintain independence and prevent complications. Electronic aids that allow SCI victims to regulate vital organs when nerve supply has been impaired are helping to increase independence.

Although nerve fiber regeneration that will cross the gap in the spinal cord is not in the immediate future, research is being conducted.

In summary, SCI is a disabling neurologic condition most commonly caused by automobile accidents, falls, and sports injuries. It occurs most frequently in males, and 80% of cases occur in people under 40 years of age. Initially hematoma formation and spinal shock occur, lasting for 2 to 6 weeks. Later manifestations reflect the level of injury and the completeness of the transection. In most cases, communication between the brain and the spinal cord is lost and complete paralysis is present below the level of injury. As recovery occurs, spinal cord reflex activity emerges, uninhibited by higher centers, to take over the control of muscle tone and autonomic reflexes. Reflex muscle spasms may be evoked by a variety of stimuli. Reflex control of bowel and bladder emptying develops and can be used as a means of controlling these functions. Hypersensitivity of sympathetic neurons below the level of injury can produce the life-threatening situation called autonomic hyperreflexia. It is usually triggered by afferent impulses from the bowel or bladder and produces extreme hypertension, bradycardia, and other signs of excessive sympathetic stimulation. Treatment of SCI is symptomatic and is directed toward rehabilitation and prevention of complications.

■ Alterations in Neuromuscular Function

Myasthenia Gravis

Myasthenia gravis is a disorder of the neuromuscular junction that affects the communication between the axonal terminal and the innervated muscle cell. Acetylcholine (ACh) functions as the neuromediator, the mode of communication, at the myoneural junction. In the normal person, each neuromuscular junction contains about 38 million ACh receptor sites. Myasthenia gravis is thought to be due to a deficiency in ACh receptor sites on the muscle side of the neuromuscular junction. In the person with myasthenia gravis the number of receptors may be reduced to levels as low as 20% of normal.[25] This reduction in receptor sites is believed to be caused by an autoimmune response. This immune response has two effects: it blocks the receptor site and causes receptor destruction.

The incidence of myasthenia gravis is about 1 in 10,000 to 1 in 25,000 persons in the United States. The disease is at least twice as common in women as in men, especially during young adulthood. The primary clinical manifestation of myasthenia gravis is weakness of the striated muscles, with specific variations in the degree of weakness and the muscles involved. Because the disease affects the myoneural junction, there are no sensory changes or hyperactive reflexes. The most common manifestations are weakness of the eye muscles, with ptosis (drooping of the eyelids) and diplopia caused by weakness of the extraocular muscles. The clinical course varies. Ocular weakness may progress to generalized weakness, including respiratory muscle weakness. Chewing and swallowing may be difficult. Weakness in limb movement is usually more pronounced in proximal than in distal parts of the extremity, so that climbing stairs and lifting objects are difficult. As the disease progresses, the muscles of the lower face may be affected, causing speech impairment. When this happens, the person often supports the chin with one hand to assist in speaking.

Persons with myasthenia gravis may develop sudden respiratory difficulty, called myasthenia crisis, which is severe enough to require mechanical ventilation. This usually occurs during a period of stress, such as infection or following surgery. The crisis is usually transient and subsides if adequate ventilatory support can be maintained.

Diagnosis and treatment

Muscular weakness without sensory symptoms, changes of consciousness, or autonomic dysfunction are early signs of myasthenia gravis. Because the disease is uncommon, it is frequently not diagnosed until generalized weakness occurs. The diagnosis is based on the Tensilon (edrophonium chloride) test, which is a pharmacologic challenge with edrophonium, a short-acting form of the drug used to treat myasthenia gravis. When weakness is due to myasthenia gravis, a dramatic transitory improvement in muscle function occurs when edrophonium is administered.

There are two treatment methods for myasthenia gravis. One involves the administration of drugs, such as neostigmine and pyridostigmine, that prevent the normally rapid breakdown of ACh. The other form of treatment is designed to halt the immune response and induce a remission in the disease; adrenocorticosteroid and immunosuppressive drugs are included as part of this treatment regimen. Surgical removal of the thymus gland also may be done. Significant improvement has been noted in two-thirds of the myasthenic persons who were so treated.[26]

Muscular Dystrophy

Muscular dystrophy (MD) is a term applied to a number of disorders that produce progressive deterioration of voluntary muscles because of muscle necrosis. As the muscles undergo necrosis, fat and connective tissue replace muscle fibers, which increases the weakness. The increase in muscle size resulting from tissue infiltration is called hypertrophy or pseudohypertrophy. The muscular weakness is insidious in onset but continuously progressive, varying with the type of disorder. Skeletal muscles, especially the postural muscles of the hip and shoulder, are affected first. The nervous system is not involved in the disease.

The most common form of the disease is Duchenne's dystrophy, which has an incidence of 3 per 100,000; the other forms are much rarer. Duchenne's muscular dystrophy is inherited as a recessive sex-linked trait and is transmitted by the mother to her male offspring. A spontaneous form may occur in females. With Duchenne's muscular dystrophy, the child usually grows normally until around 3 years of age, when frequent falling begins. Wheelchairs are usually needed by the preteen years, and death frequently occurs in young adulthood because of respiratory and cardiac muscle involvement.

Diagnosis and treatment

Observation of the child's voluntary movement and a complete family history provide important diagnostic data for the disease. Muscle biopsy, which shows fat in the tissues, electromyograms, and serum levels of the enzyme creatine phosphokinase (CPK), which leaks out of damaged muscle, can be used to confirm the diagnosis.

There is no cure for muscular dystrophy. Management of the disease is directed toward maintaining ambulation and preventing deformities. Deformities are common because of habitual postures, which lead to the development of contractures in some muscles, and because of imbalances between agonist and antagonist muscles. Passive stretching, correct or counter posturing, and splints help to prevent deformities. All precautions should be taken to avoid respiratory infections.

In summary, myasthenia gravis is a disorder of the myoneural junction, most likely resulting from a deficiency of acetylcholine, that causes weakness of the striated muscles. Because the disease affects the myoneural junction, there is no loss of sensory function. The most common manifestations are weakness of the eye muscles, with ptosis and diplopia. The muscles of the jaw may be affected, making chewing and swallowing difficult. Usually the proximal muscles of the extremities are involved, making it difficult to climb stairs and lift objects. Myasthenia crisis, in which there is sudden and transient weakness of the respiratory muscles, may also occur and may necessitate temporary mechanical ventilatory assistance. The treatment is directed toward preventing the rapid breakdown of acetylcholine or halting the immune response that is thought to contribute to the disorder.

Muscular dystrophy is a term used to describe a number of disorders that produce progressive deterioration of skeletal muscle. Muscle necrosis with fat and connective tissue replacement is seen. The disease usually strikes children. One form, Duchenne's muscular dystrophy, is inherited as a recessive sex-linked trait and is transmitted by the mother to her male offspring. At present there is no cure for the disease, which follows a progressive course. Management is directed toward maintaining ambulation and preventing deformities.

■ Study Guide

After you have studied this chapter, you should be able to meet the following objectives:

☐ Describe the function of the pyramidal tract versus the extrapyramidal tract.

☐ Describe the effects of lower motor neuron injury.

☐ Describe cerebellar control of motor activity and muscle movement.

☐ Describe the effects of damage to the basal ganglial portion of the extrapyramidal tract.

☐ Describe the disruptions that occur when the cerebellar portion of the extrapyramidal tract is injured.

☐ Define the terms chorea, athetosis, hemiballismus, dysdiadochokinesia, tremor, and nystagmus.

☐ Describe the collateral circulation to the brain.

☐ List the clinical manifestations of a CVA.

☐ Characterize TIAs.

☐ Describe the subclavian steal syndrome.

☐ Compare stroke due to hemorrhage, embolus, and thrombosis.

☐ Describe the effects of a stroke involving the anterior, middle, and posterior cerebral arteries, respectively.

☐ Compare the manifestations of motor aphasia with those of sensory aphasia.

☐ Explain the symptoms of Parkinson's disease with reference to the extrapyramidal system.

☐ Explain the rationale underlying the use of anticholinergics and dopamine in Parkinson's disease.

☐ Explain the significance of demyelination and plaque formation in multiple sclerosis.

☐ Describe the rationale for the clinical picture of multiple sclerosis.

☐ Relate the function of higher neural centers to muscle spasms that occur following recovery from acute SCI.

☐ Describe the events that culminate in spinal shock.

☐ Describe the effects of SCI on the cardiovascular system.

☐ Explain the occurrence of hypertension following SCI.

☐ Explain the probable cause of myasthenia gravis.

☐ Describe the clinical picture of myasthenia gravis.

☐ Describe what happens to the muscles in muscular dystrophy.

☐ State the primary goals of muscular dystrophy management.

■ References

1. Guyton AC: Textbook of Medical Physiology, 6th ed, p 347. Philadelphia, WB Saunders, 1981
2. Heart Facts. American Heart Association, Dallas, 1981
3. Sahs AL, Hartman EC, Aronson SM: Cause, Prevention, Treatment and Rehabilitation. London, Castle House Publications Ltd, 1980
4. Stroke hope through research. National Institute of Health, National Institute of Communicative Disorders and Stroke, US Department of Health and Human Services, NIH Publication No 83-2222, 1983
5. DeLaria GA, Javid H: Evaluating subclavian steal syndrome. Consultant 20, No 2:88-98, 1980
6. Burch GE, DePasquale NP: Axioms on cerebrovascular disease. Hosp Med 11, No 6:8-22, 1975
7. Bobath B: Adult Hemiplegia: Evaluation and Treatment, 2nd ed, London, William Heinemann Medical Books, 1978
8. Palmer EP: Language dysfunction in cerebrovascular disease. Primary Care 6, No 4:827-842, 1979
9. Holland AL: Treatment for aphasia following stroke. Current concepts of cerebrovascular disease. Stroke 14, No 2:5-8, 1979
10. Campbell JK: Use of computerized tomography and radionuclide scan in stroke. Current concepts of cerebrovascular disease. Stroke 12, No 3:11-16, 1977
11. Canadian Cooperative Study Group: Randomized trial of aspirin and sulfinpyrazone in threatened stroke. N Engl J Med, 299:53-59, 1978
12. Fields WS, Lemark NA, Frankowski RF, Hardy RJ: Controlled trial of aspirins on cerebral ischemia. Stroke, 8:301-316, 1977
13. Morris JGL: The management of Parkinson's disease. Aust NZ J Med, 12:195-205, 1982
14. Rodman MJ, Smith OW: Clinical Pharmacology in Nursing, pp 117-187. Philadelphia, JB Lippincott, 1984
15. Cotzias GG, Papavasilious PS, Genos SZ, Tolosa ES: Treatment of Parkinson's disease and allied conditions. In

Tower DB (ed): The Nervous System. Volume 2. The Clinical Neurosciences. New York, Raven Press, 1975

16. Crawford I: Neurotransmitters: Relevance to neurologic disease and therapy. In Rosenberg RN (ed): The Treatment of Neurological Diseases. New York, S P Medical & Scientific Books, 1979

17. Stewart RM: Treatment of movement disorders. In Rosenberg RN (ed): The Treatment of Neurological Diseases. New York, S P Medical & Scientific Books, 1979

18. Pollard T: Neuroglia: The forgotten cells of neurology. J Neurosurg Nurs 12, No 3:114-120, 1980

19. McFarlin DE, McFarland HF: Multiple sclerosis. N Engl J Med, 307, No 19:1183-1187, 1983

20. Waxman SG: Membranes, myelin and the pathophysiology of multiple sclerosis. N Engl J Med, 306, No 25:1529-1533, 1982

21. Zejdlek CM: Management of Spinal Cord Injury. Monterey, CA, Wadsworth, 1983

22. Spinal Cord Injury Hope through Research. National Institute of Health, National Institute of Neurological and Communicative Disorders and Stroke, US Department of Health and Human Services, NIH Publication No 81-160, 1981

23. Newman PP: Neurophysiology. New York, SP Medical & Scientific Books, 1979

24. Feustel D: Autonomic hyperreflexia. Am J Nurs 76, No 2:228-239, 1976

25. Report of the Panel on Convulsive and Neuromuscular Disorders to the National Advisory Neurological and Communicative Disorders and Stroke Council, p 53. US Department of Health, Education, and Welfare, PHS, NIH Publication No 79-1913, 1979

26. Rowland LP: Diseases of the muscle and neuromuscular junction. In Beeson PB, McDermott W, Wyngaarden JB (eds): Cecil Textbook of Medicine, p 928. Philadelhia, WB Saunders, 1979

■ Additional References

Adelstein W, Watson P: Cervical spine injuries. J Neurosurg Nurs 15:65, 1983

Anand R: Cellular membranes in Duchenne muscular dystrophy. Int J Biochem 15:1211, 1983

Berkmayer W, Riederer P: Parkinson's Disease: Biochemistry, Clinical Pathology, and Treatment. New York, Springer-Verlag, 1983

Booth K: Subclavian steal syndrome: Treatment with proximal vertebral to common carotid artery transposition. J Neurosurg Nurs 12:28, 1980

Boshes B: Sinemet and the treatment of Parkinsonism. Ann Intern Med 94, No 3:364-370, 1981

Calne DB: Current views on Parkinson's disease. Can J Neurol Sci 10, No 1:11, 1983

Cormarr AE: Sex among patients with spinal cord and/or cauda equina injuries. Med Aspects Human Sexuality 7:222, 1973

Cormarr AE, Gunderson BB: Sexual function in traumatic paraplegia and quadriplegia. Am J Nurs 75:250, 1975

Doolittle N: Arteriovenous malformations: The physiology, symptomatology, and nursing care. J Neurosurg Nurs 11:221, 1979

Drachman DB: The biology of myasthenia gravis. Annu Rev Neurosci 4:195, 1981

Dubowitz V, Heckmatt J: Management of muscular dystrophy. Br Med J 36, No 2:139, 1980

Fishbach FT: Easing adjustment to Parkinson's disease. Am J Nurs 78:66, 1978

Hirsch LF: Modern treatment of intracranial aneurysms. Postgrad Med 67, No 3:153, 1980

Kess R: Suddenly in crisis—Unpredictable myasthenia. Am J Nurs 84:994, 1984

Johnson M, Quinn J: The subarachnoid screw. Am J Nurs 77:448, 1977

Jones HR: Disease of the vertebral system. Primary Care 6:733, 1979

Kestler JP: Cardiac embolic cerebrovascular disease. Primary Care 6:745, 1979

Larrabee JH: Physical care during early recovery. Am J Nurs 7:1320, 1977

Lisak RP: Myasthenia gravis: Mechanisms and management. Hosp Pract 18, No 3:101, 1983

Medwin DG: Clinical features and classification of the muscular dystrophies. Br Med Bull 36, No 2:109, 1980

Mesulam MM: Acute behavioral derangements without hemiplegia in cerebrovascular disease. Primary Care 6:813, 1979

Norman S: Diagnostic categories for the patient with a right hemisphere lesion. Am J Nurs 79:2126, 1979

Norman S, Baratz R: Understanding aphasia. Am J Nurs 79:2135, 1979

Pacheco PM: Cerebral artery vasospasm and current trends of treatment. J Neurosurg Nurs 11:171, 1979

Polhopek M: Stroke: An update on vascular disease. J Neurosurg Nurs 12:81, 1980

Renne UK: Parkinson's disease as a model for changes in dopamine receptor dynamics in aging. Gerontology 28 (Suppl 1): 35, 1982

Scadding GK, Havard CW: Pathogenesis and treatment of myasthenia gravis. Br Med J 283:1008, 1981

Seybold ME: Myasthenia gravis: A clinical and basic science review. JAMA 250:2516, 1983

Stanley M: Cerebral vasospasm: Pathophysiology and nursing care. Crit Care Nurs 4, No 6:39, 1984

Webb PH: Neurological deficit after carotid endarterectomy. Am J Nurs 79:654, 1979

Weiner M: Update on antiparkinsonian agents. Geriatrics 37, No 9:81, 1982

Chapter 49

Pain

Sheila M. Curtis

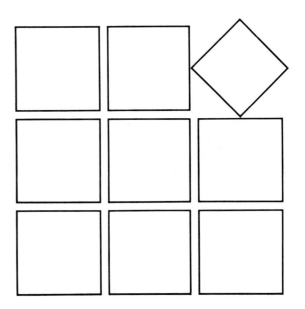

Pain is a complex and personal phenomenon. It involves not only anatomic structures and physiologic behaviors but psychological, social, cultural, and cognitive factors as well. It has been demonstrated repeatedly that learning is an important factor in a person's response to painful stimuli. Pain can be a prepotent or overwhelming experience, often disruptive to customary behavior. When severe, pain demands and directs all of one's attention to it. Because pain is common to so many diseases, a full chapter is devoted to it in this text, centering on its mechanisms, theories, manifestations, disorders, and treatment.

Pain Mechanisms and Responses

In spite of its unpleasantness, pain can serve a useful purpose, for it warns of impending tissue injury and causes the individual to seek relief. An inflamed appendix, for example, would progress in severity, could rupture, and eventually might cause death were it not for the warning afforded by the pain. Pain is probably the most common symptom that motivates an individual to seek professional help; its location, radiation, duration, and severity give important clues about its etiology. Indeed, it probably sends sufferers to the physician's office more often and with greater speed than any other symptom. Pain may be an indication of depression or dependency. It may also be used for secondary gain, whether consciously or unconsciously.

Definitions and Theories

Historically, pain has often been looked on as a punishment or a means of atonement. The term itself—Greek, *poinē;* Latin, *poena;* French, *peine*—means punishment. Some Western cultures have viewed pain as something to be avoided at all costs. Aristotle regarded pain as the antithesis of pleasure, whereas Freud discussed the pleasure principle in relation to the avoidance of pain. It is impossible to really separate the pain sensation from emotion, because the sensation itself is only a part, and perhaps not even the main part, of the total pain experience. Responses to pain are patterned according to the norms of the person's cultural group. Zborowski, in his studies of Italian and Jewish women, found that both groups had low levels of pain tolerance and complained loudly when in pain. Interestingly, this behavior occurred for different reasons. The Italian women were relatively satisfied once their pain was relieved, whereas the Jewish women pursued the matter further, demanding to know its meaning.[1]

But what is pain? What is its purpose? Is it of any use? Does it help or harm? Scientific disciplines have attempted to answer these and other questions about pain. The many definitions of pain flowing from these efforts serve to highlight its complex nature. Yet, in the face of intense interest in and research on pain, we still have much to learn about this very human, very common experience. The puzzle of pain persists.

Sternbach describes pain as "an abstract concept which refers to (1) a personal, private sensation of hurt; (2) a harmful stimulus which signals current and impending tissue damage; (3) a pattern of responses which operate to protect the organism from harm."[2] Useful as this definition is, it fails to describe all facets of the experience called pain.

Margo McCaffery, a nurse in private practice with more than 20 years of experience in the management of pain, has provided one of the most clinically useful definitions to date. She states, "Pain is whatever the experiencing person says it is, existing whenever he says it does."[3] Clinically, there are advantages to this definition. It is broad enough to cover the client's expression of pain, verbal or nonverbal; but perhaps more important, it indicates that the client is believed, which is critical to developing the trust relationship so important in managing pain. Merskey[4] believes that if pain is accepted as a psychological phenomenon with physiologic correlates, rather than vice versa, some clinical problems can be prevented (*i.e.,* the patient will not be considered a malingerer or a liar if no objective cause for the pain can be found).

One of the difficulties in arriving at a workable definition of pain is the lack of research findings that adequately support clinical observations. Traditionally, there have been two opposing theories of pain: specificity and pattern theories. Those who proposed the specificity theory regarded pain as a separate sensory modality evoked by the activity of specific receptors that transmit information to pain centers in the brain. Pattern theorists propose that pain receptors share endings or pathways with other sensory modalities, but the different pattern of activity (spatial or temporal) in the same neuron can be used to signal painful and nonpainful stimuli. Both theories focus on the neurophysiologic basis of pain but fail to consider the motivational–cognitive, cultural, and affective components of pain.

The gate control theory, which was originally proposed by Melzak and Wall in 1965, is a modification of the specificity theory. They postulated the presence of neural-gating mechanisms at the segmental spinal level to account for interactions between pain and other sensory modalities.[5] The gate control theory proposes a network of transmitting (t) cells and internuncial neurons that can inhibit the t cells to form a gate at the segmental level of the spinal cord. The internuncial fibers are activated by the large-diameter, faster-propagating fibers that carry touch information. Thus, the simultaneous firing of large-diameter fibers that transmit tactile information and small-diameter myelinated and unmyelinated fibers that transmit pain information can block the transmission of pain impulses by creating an inhibitory gating circuit. Pain therapists have long known that pain intensity can be temporarily reduced during active tactile stimulation.

Pain modulation is now known to be a much more complex phenomenon than that proposed by the original gate control theory. Tactile information is transmitted by small- as well as large-diameter fibers. Also, major interactions between sensory modalities occur at levels other than the input segment. Other extremely important factors are endogenous opioids and their receptors, descending feedback modulation, altered sensitivity, and learning culture. In spite of this, the Melzak and Wall theory has served a useful purpose. It excited interest in pain and stimulated research and clinical activity related to the pain-modulating systems. For example, gate control theory has been cited as an explanation for such pain control techniques as transcutaneous electrical nerve stimulation (TENS), which activates tactile receptors.

Pain Receptors

The mechanisms of pain are many and complex. There are receptors that monitor the stimuli for pain, the pathways that project pain information, the integration and modulation of the pain information in the thalamus and cortex, and finally the subjective reaction to pain.

The receptors for pain are termed *nociceptive* receptors, which means that they are capable of responding to stimuli that cause tissue damage. These receptors are widely distributed to the skin, dental pulp, some internal organs, periosteum, and meninges. Structurally, pain receptors are free nerve endings that are part of small afferent myelinated A-delta fibers and unmyelinated C fibers. Receptors that have pain as their lowest intensity threshold stimulus are known as pain receptors. Considerable controversy remains regarding the recruitment of pain by the overstimulation of other receptors, such as those of temperature and pressure. The available evidence seems to support the idea that noxious stimuli lead to the release of pain-producing substances, such as plasmakinins and bradykinin. Plasmakinins have been shown to cause edema by increasing capillary permeability during inflammation. Bradykinin is one of the most potent examples; it causes pain when extremely low doses are injected intra-arterially or intraperitoneally. It is broken down relatively rapidly and therefore may be involved primarily in acute pain. Other pain-producing substances that have been implicated are substance P, acetylcholine, 5-hydroxytryptamine, and histamine. Prostaglandins may increase the sensitivity of pain receptors by enhancing bradykinin's pain-provoking effect.[6]

Pain Pathways

The A-delta and C fibers enter the spinal cord in the lateral division of each dorsal (and ventral) root. They ascend and descend one or two segments and project collaterals into the dorsal horn of these segments.

Activated circuits function in several ways; they project pain information to the forebrain and trigger the flexor withdrawal and other reflexes. The withdrawal reflex is designed to remove endangered tissue from a damaging stimulus.

Fast and slow pain components

Both fast and slow components of the pain response have been identified. When, for example, one's finger gets caught in a car door, the first component of the pain experience is a sharp, bright, and localized unpleasant sensation known as first, or fast, pain. This is followed by a dull, aching, diffuse, and extremely unpleasant sensation known as second, or dull, pain. The presence of two fiber groups seems to explain the two components of pain. The farther the stimulus from the brain, the more time separates the fast and slow components. It is generally accepted that first, or fast, pain is primarily carried by the A-delta pain fibers, which are $2\mu m$ to $5\mu m$ in diameter and which transmit at a rate of 12 m to 30 m per second. Second, or slow, pain is thought to be primarily transmitted by the small C fibers, which are $0.4\mu m$ to $1.2\mu m$ in diameter and which transmit at a rate of 0.5 m to 2 m per second.

Although pain pathways to the brain are diffuse, the main pathways are the neospinothalamic, the paleospinothalamic, and the spinoreticular systems (Fig. 49-1). The A-delta fibers of the neospinothalamic tract are mainly associated with the spatial and temporal aspects of sharp, bright, or fast pain. Small unmyelinated C fibers of the slow-conducting paleospinothalamic tract are associated with diffuse dull, aching, and extremely unpleasant pain. The spinoreticular system in conjunction with the collaterals of the paleospinothalamic system facilitates avoidance reflexes at all levels. All three systems facilitate the functioning of the ascending reticular activating system in electroencephalogram (EEG) activation, wakefulness, and selective attention.

Pain perception

The basic sensation of hurtfulness, or pain, occurs at the level of the thalamus. In the neospinothalamic system, interconnections between the lateral thalamus and the

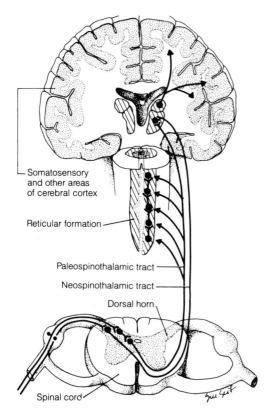

Figure 49-1 *The spinothalamic system, one of the several ascending systems that carry pain impulses. One spinothalamic tract runs to the thalamic nuclei and has fibers that project to the somatosensory cortex. Another tract sends collateral fibers to the reticular formation and other structures, from which further fibers project to the thalamus. These fibers finally influence the hypothalamus and limbic system, as well as the cerebral cortex. (Rodman MJ, Smith DW: Pharmacology and Drug Therapy in Nursing, 2nd ed, p 263. Philadelphia, JB Lippincott, 1979)*

somatosensory cortex are necessary to add precision and discrimination to the pain sensation. Association areas of the parietal cortex are essential to the perception, or learned meaningfulness, of the pain experience. For example, if a mosquito bites a person's index finger on the left hand and only the thalamus is functional, the person will complain of pain somewhere on the hand. With the primary sensory cortex functional, the person can localize the pain to the precise area on the index finger. The association cortex, on the other hand, is necessary in order to interpret the buzzing and the sensation that preceded the pain as being related to the mosquito bite.

The paleospinothalamic system projects diffusely from the intralaminar nuclei of the thalamus to large areas of the cortex and is associated with wakefulness and attention. This may explain the tremendous arousal effects of certain pain stimuli.

The area in the medial thalamus (nucleus submedius), along with its projections into the limbic system, is also thought to be a possible pain center. It appears to be involved in the affective, arousal, or motivational aspects of pain.

The reticulospinal system projects bilaterally to the reticular formation of the brain stem. This system, in conjunction with the collaterals of the paleospinothalamic system, facilitates avoidance reflexes at all levels. It also contributes to an increase in the EEG activity associated with alertness and indirectly influences hypothalamic functions.

Endogenous Analgesic Mechanisms

Focal stimulation of the midbrain central gray region was reported by Reynolds 4 years after the introduction of gate control theory. The analgesic level was sufficient to permit abdominal surgery, although levels of consciousness and reactions to auditory and visual stimuli remained unaffected. A few years later opiate receptors were found to be highly concentrated in regions of the CNS where electrical stimulation produced analgesia. This led to a search for natural body substances capable of interacting with these receptors. The natural ligands, or binding molecules, for these opiate receptors are the endogenous opioid peptides (the endorphins and enkephalins), which were discovered in 1975. New therapeutic approaches to the treatment of pain were envisioned when (1) it was discovered that these peptides exert inhibitory modulation of pain transmission and (2) the release of endogenous opioids following CNS stimulation was correlated with patient reports of pain relief.

Endorphins (morphinelike substances) are found primarily in the amygdala, limbic system, hypothalamic–pituitary axis, and other brain stem structures. They have increased resistance to enzymatic degradation, compared with the enkephalins, and function like neurohormones. The enkephalins (in the head) are found primarily in short interneurons of the periaqueductal gray (PAG) of the midbrain, limbic system, basal ganglia, hypothalamus, and spinal cord, where they undergo rapid enzymatic degradation and may function in a manner similar to neurotransmitters.

The presence of these morphinelike substances tends to mimic the peripheral and central effects of morphine and other opiate drugs. Opiate receptors have been identified in nervous tissue of various parts of the CNS and in the plexuses of the gastrointestinal tract. The amygdala has the greatest density of opiate receptors, followed, in decreasing order, by the hypothalamus, thalamus, and PAG of the midbrain and diencephalon.[7,8]

Classification

Types of pain can be classified according to their source, duration, objective signs, and referral.

Source

The sources of pain are commonly divided into three general categories: cutaneous, deep somatic, and visceral. Cutaneous pain arises from superficial structures, such as the skin and subcutaneous tissues. A paper cut on the finger is an example of easily localized superficial, or cutaneous, pain. It tends to be a sharp, bright pain with a burning quality and may be either abrupt or slow in onset. It can be accurately localized and may be distributed along the dermatomes. Because there is an overlap of nerve fiber distribution between the dermatomes, the boundaries of pain frequently are not as clear-cut as the dermatomal diagrams indicate.

A second type of pain is related to the deep somatic structures, such as the periosteum, muscles, tendons, joints, and blood vessels. Deep somatic pain tends to be more diffuse than cutaneous pain. Various stimuli, such as strong pressure exerted on bone, ischemia to a muscle, or tissue damage, can produce deep somatic pain. This is the type of pain one experiences from a sprained ankle. The pain can radiate from the original site of injury. For example, damage to a nerve root can cause the person to experience pain radiating along its fiber distribution.

A third type of pain, called *visceral,* or *splanchnic,* pain, originates in the viscera. Common examples of visceral pain are renal colic, pain resulting from cholecystitis, pain associated with acute appendicitis, and ulcer pain. Although the viscera are diffusely and richly innervated, cutting or burning of the viscera, in contrast with similar noxious stimuli applied to cutaneous or superficial structures, is unlikely to cause pain. Instead, strong abnormal contractions of the gastrointestinal sys-tem, distention, or ischemia affecting the walls of the viscera can induce severe pain. Anyone who has suffered from either severe gastrointestinal distress or ureteral colic can readily attest to the misery involved. We are most accustomed to thinking of visceral pain as emanating from the abdominal cavity. However, visceral pain tends to be diffuse, especially in its early stages.

Visceral pain is transmitted by small unmyelinated pain fibers that travel with the nerves of the autonomic system; consequently, visceral pain is often accompanied by autonomic responses such as nausea, vomiting, sweating, pallor, and possibly shock. Pain from the lower end of the esophagus and pain below the midtransverse colon tends to travel the course of cranial nerves IX and X and the parasympathetic nerves entering the sacral region of the spinal cord. Pain fibers entering the thoracolumbar region of the spinal cord travel the course of the sympathetic nerves.

Duration

Pain can also be classified as acute or chronic pain depending on its duration. The pain research of the past 25 years has emphasized the importance of differentiating acute pain from chronic pain and dealing with them separately. This is because these types of pain differ in etiology, mechanisms, pathophysiology, and function and because the diagnosis of and therapy for each is distinctive (Table 49-1).

Acute pain is usually defined as pain of less than 6 months' duration. It consists of unpleasant sensory, perceptual, and emotional components with associated somatic, autonomic, psychological, and behavioral

Table 49-1 Characteristics of Acute and Chronic Pain

Characteristic	Acute Pain	Chronic Pain
Onset	Recent	Continuous or intermittent
Duration	Short duration	6 months or more
Autonomic responses	Consistent with sympathetic fight or flight response* Increased heart rate Increased stroke volume Increased blood pressure Increased pupillary dilation Increased muscle tension Decreased gut motility Decreased salivary flow (dry mouth)	Absence of autonomic responses
Psychological component	Associated anxiety	Increased irritability Associated depression Somatic preoccupation Withdrawal from outside interests Decreased strength of relationships
Other types of response		Decreased sleep Decreased libido Appetite changes

*Responses are approximately proportional to intensity of the stimulus.

responses. Acute pain is caused by noxious, or tissue-damaging stimuli; its purpose is to serve as a protective, or warning, system. It alerts the individual to the existence of actual or impending tissue damage and prompts the person to seek professional help. The pain's location, intensity, duration, and radiation, as well as those factors that aggravate or relieve it, are essential diagnostic clues. Unlike chronic pain, acute pain is very rarely due to psychological factors alone. Acute pain is often accompanied by anxiety and autonomic responses, which usually disappears when the pain is relieved.

Chronic pain is defined as pain of 6 months' duration or longer. The pain may be continuous (*e.g.,* arthritis) or intermittent (*e.g.,* angina or intermittent claudication). Unlike acute pain, persistent pain usually serves no useful function. To the contrary, it imposes severe physiologic, psychological, familial, and economic stresses and may exhaust the resources of the person. In contrast with the case of acute pain, with chronic pain and the development of behaviors associated with it, psychological and environmental influences often play a significant role. Chronic pain is often associated with depression and despair rather than anxiety. Amazingly, this depression is often relieved spontaneously when the pain is removed.

It is extremely important to appreciate that persons suffering chronic pain may not exhibit the somatic, autonomic, or affective behaviors associated with acute pain. One reason for this is that the stress response cannot be maintained for long periods of time. As was described earlier, either parasympathetic rebound or adaptation occurs. Then, too, certain behaviors viewed as acceptable in patients with severe but short-lived pain would not be expected or considered appropriate in the chronic situation. With chronic pain, it is important to heed the person's own description of the pain because the expected psychophysiologic responses may or may not be present.

One proposed classification of chronic pain divides the affected persons into two broad groups according to life expectancy (brief versus normal). This classification assumes importance primarily if a decision must be reached concerning long-term use of narcotics for pain relief.

Behaviors

Organic or *somatogenic* pain is that which originates in the body, or the soma. *Functional* or *psychogenic* pain is that which is attributed to the psyche or emotions. In both situations, the physical sensation of pain is the same. The individual may be unaware that the origin of the pain is emotional and may experience it as if the pain were truly originating from an organic disorder. Many persons who suffer from pain of psychogenic origin have had developmental difficulties during adolescence. It is important to

note that persons in pain usually experience both its physical and its emotional aspects. It is difficult to conceive of pain as being either purely organic or purely functional. McCaffery's statement that "pain is whatever the experiencing person says it is and exists whenever he says it does" is particularly applicable here.[3]

Positive placebo reactors (those who experience pain relief from such measures as pills containing inert or ineffective substances) may be found among those suffering from either organic or functional pain. Research has demonstrated the importance of higher central nervous system control over sensory input. Whereas in the past there was no adequate explanation for the behavior of positive placebo reactors, and in fact such persons sometimes were regarded as malingerers, the discovery of endogenous modulators of pain, such as endorphins and enkephalins, suggests that placebos may trigger the release of pain-modulating substances, which cause the pain to diminish. (See "Placebo Response" later in this chapter.)

Referral

Referred pain is that pain perceived at a site on the skin surface distant from its point of origin but innervated by the same spinal segment. Pain originating in the abdominal or thoracic viscera tends to be diffuse and poorly localized and is often perceived at a site far removed from the affected area. For example, the pain associated with myocardial infarction is often referred to the left arm and neck.

Referred pain may arise alone or concurrently with pain located at the origin of the noxious stimulus. Although the term *referred* is usually applied to pain originating in the viscera and experienced as if originating from the body wall, it may also be applied to pain arising from somatic structures. An example would be pain for which the stimulus arises in the peripheral diaphragm but which is referred to the chest wall.

An understanding of pain reference is of great value in diagnosing illness because afferent neurons from visceral or deep somatic tissue enter the spinal cord at the same level as those from the cutaneous areas to which the pain is referred.

This relationship can be demonstrated by tracing the development of organ systems in the embryo (Fig. 49-2). Let us say that the client has peritonitis but complains of pain in the shoulder. Internally, there is irritation or inflammation of the central diaphragm. In the embryo, the diaphragm originates in the neck, and its central portion is innervated by the phrenic nerve, which enters the cord at the level of the fifth to seventh cervical segment (C5–7). As the fetus develops, the diaphragm descends to its adult position between the thoracic and abdominal cavities, innervated by the phrenic nerve. Therefore, fibers entering the spinal cord at the C5–7 level carry information from the neck area, as well as from the diaphragm. Although *visceral* pleura, pericardium, and peritoneum are said to be relatively free of pain fibers, *parietal* pleura, pericardium, and peritoneum *do react* to nociceptive stimuli. Visceral inflammation can involve parietal or somatic structures, and this in turn may give rise to diffuse local or referred pain. For example, irritation of the parietal peritoneum resulting from appendicitis often gives rise to pain directly over the inflamed area in the right lower quadrant. Also, such stimuli can evoke pain *referred* to the umbilical area.

Another type of pain is *muscular spasm*, or guarding, when somatic structures are involved. *Guarding* is a protective-reflex rigidity and its purpose is to protect the affected body parts (*e.g.,* an abscessed appendix or a sprained muscle). This protective guarding may give rise to the pain of muscle *ischemia* causing both local and referred pain.

Pain from the viscera may be localized only with difficulty. There are several explanations for this. First, innervation of visceral organs is very poorly represented at forebrain (sensation) levels. A second explanation, held by some researchers, is that the brain does not easily learn to precisely localize sensations originating from organs that at best are only imprecisely visualized. For example, a cut on the third finger of the right hand can be readily seen, identified, and localized, whereas an inflamed internal organ can be localized only vaguely. A third explanation is that sensory information from thoracic and abdominal viscera can travel by two pathways to the central nervous system. The first route is called the *visceral,* or *true visceral, pathway.* According to this hypothesis, the pain information travels with the fibers of the autonomic nervous system; and the pain is felt at a site on the surface of the body distant to the pain locus. Pain felt along the inner left arm following a myocardial infarction is an example.

The second route, the parietal pathway, which is somatic, is not usually considered to be a pathway for visceral pain, but may be the pain route in inflammation of *parietal* pleura, pericardium, or peritoneum. Sensations traveling along this pathway can be localized directly over the affected part, a common example being pain in the right lower quadrant or in the umbilical area associated with an inflamed appendix.

It is always possible that referred pain can be one of the consequences of an anatomic anomaly; therefore, the reader should guard against jumping to conclusions. Needless to say, although pain may be the stimulus that prompts the person to seek professional help, a careful history and examination are needed to correctly assess the problem.

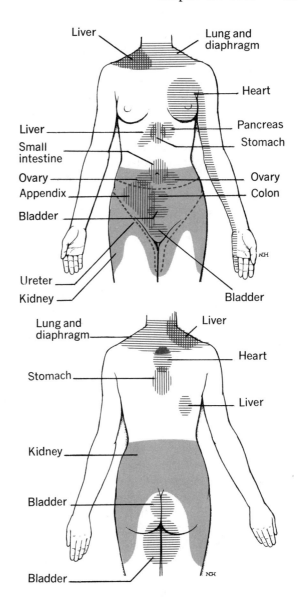

Figure 49-2 *Areas of referred pain:* (Top), *anterior view;* (bottom) *posterior view. (Chaffee EE, Lytle IM: Basic Anatomy and Physiology, 4th ed, p 266. Philadelphia, JB Lippincott, 1980)*

Reactions to Pain

Reactions to pain are affected by pain threshold and tolerance. Although the terms are often used interchangeably, pain threshold and pain tolerance are not the same. The former is more closely associated with nociceptive (*i.e.,* tissue damaging) stimuli, whereas the latter relates more to the total pain experience. Separation and identification of the role of each of these concepts continues to pose fundamental problems for the pain management team as well as pain researchers.

Pain threshold.   Pain threshold is usually defined as the least intense stimulus that will cause pain. Although pain threshold is still controversial, it is generally accepted that the threshold is similar in most normal persons, particularly under controlled experimental situations. For example, upon exposure to heat of increasing intensity, most people state that the sensation of heat converts to a sensation of pain at approximately 45°C.

Pain tolerance. Pain tolerance is usually defined as the maximum intensity or duration of pain that the subject is willing to endure—the point beyond which the person wants something done about the pain. Tolerance is not necessarily indicative of the severity of the pain. Psychological, familial, cultural, and environmental factors significantly influence the intensity of pain an individual is willing to tolerate.

Physical reactions. Physical reactions to pain may be manifested in biting of lips, clenching of teeth, and facial expressions, such as frowning or wrinkling the brows. Protective body movements can be both involuntary and voluntary. The flexor withdrawal reaction, as discussed in Chapter 44, moves the part away from the pain source; it is involuntary. Voluntary movements are those such as changes in posture and relaxation exercises, which often relieve discomfort.

Physiologic responses. Physiologic responses to pain involve activation of the *sympathetic* nervous system, which evokes the "fight or flight" response, with catecholamine release from the adrenal medulla. What happens is this: as blood is shifted from nonvital or vital parts of the body, the vessels of the skin and the abdominal viscera (spleen, kidney, intestine) constrict, while those of the heart, skeletal muscles, lungs, and brain dilate. The face is pallid, the pupils dilated. Respiration, heart rate, and strength of contraction increase. Muscle tension rises, and energy stores are mobilized to supply blood glucose. A relative decline in parasympathetic activity may result in a loss of appetite, nausea, and vomiting. Gastrointestinal motility and digestive gland secretion also diminish. After a period of time, there occurs a *parasympathetic,* or rebound, response in which respiration, pulse rate, and blood pressure may fall below the prepain level. This is likely when pain is intense but of short duration.

Pain that persists or is repetitive calls up *adaptation of response,* with observable reductions in sympathetic signs and symptoms. Pain receptors show little if any adaptation; on the contrary, reactions to long-term pain tend to be centrally mediated. With time, physiologic and psychological coping mechanisms evolve, but these behavioral responses do not necessarily indicate pain relief. The person may merely be too fatigued to respond.

Occasionally, pain is associated with *neurogenic shock* (Chap. 21) resulting from inhibition of the medullary vasomotor center with decreased vasomotor tone. This mechanism is not well understood; it is believed that it might cause circulatory collapse, despite the presence of sympathetic activity.

During rapid eye movement (REM) or dream sleep, the EEG records very great brain activity. Certain disorders in which pain predominates—such as angina and ulcer—appear to be exacerbated during this stage of sleep.

Psychosocial reactions. *Psychosocial reactions* to pain are deeply influenced by the same factors that affect pain tolerance, including past experiences with pain. A verbally competent person may be able to accurately describe the location, duration, and intensity of the pain, as well as the ability or willingness to tolerate it. A change in the tone of voice may be as revealing as the words spoken. Previous personal and family experiences with certain diseases, such as cancer, can significantly affect the degree of fear, anxiety, and depression associated with pain and, consequently, the individual's reaction to it.

Pain that necessitates absence from work will probably be of greater importance to one who is paid an hourly wage than to one who has ample health insurance and sick time available.

Vocalizations include a group of responses such as crying, groaning, grunting, and gasping. Their frequency, loudness, and duration can assume greater significance in situations in which the person is either young or too confused to be verbally competent. These manifestations are particularly important in young children and the elderly.

Age factors. Pain is multidimensional, and each individual is affected differently. When the problems of pain are addressed, the elderly and children may require special attention in certain areas, compared with young or middle-aged adults.

The literature regarding pain in the elderly is sparse, and more studies are needed. Several aspects require particular attention.[9] The elderly may receive inappropriate dosages of medications because of tissue changes resulting from the normal aging process. Abrupt hospitalization may result in disorientation, decreased exercise, loss of control over one's life, inability to express pain, and regression. Depression and fear of death may also cause special problems. These problems must be considered when dealing with pain in the elderly.

The literature on the pain experience in children is also meager. More systematic research in this area is needed. The special problems of children in pain may often be found in references related to specific health problems, such as under headaches. Several investigators have reported that, contrary to a widely held belief, children can and often do suffer considerable pain. In addition, they do have a remarkable ability to report their pain accurately. A combination of pain measurement techniques is helpful. The use of a painometer, a diagram of a thermometerlike device with ten gradations and five verbal descriptions from no pain to intense pain, has been quite successful.

One startling finding has been that children, unlike adults, are often permitted to suffer intense postoperative pain even when pain medication has been ordered and is available. The factors resulting in this behavior on the part of caregivers need to be investigated and addressed. Some of these factors include inappropriate beliefs that (1) children suffer less intense pain than adults because of their immature nervous systems, (2) children recover quickly, (3) children should not have narcotics because they may become addicted, (4) respiratory depression is a particular threat, (5) children are unable to identify where they hurt, and (6) the nurse who uses the needle will get negative feedback.[10] In children, complex relationships may occur between previous threats or experiences with pain and their current response. The developmental level of the child, his or her position in the family, and his or her understanding of what happened or is happening, and why, are only a few of the variables that need study.

Like adults, children appear to be better able to cope with pain when they are informed about what is happening to them and helped to develop appropriate coping strategies. Doll play, a variety of sensory inputs, films, and videotapes may help them cope. Distraction, hypnosis, relaxation-guided imagery, and various other techniques can be used effectively depending on the child's age.

Children who have an inaccurate understanding of what is happening may develop fantasies of mutilation, become extremely anxious, and doubt their ability to cope. Realistic reassurance measures that promote their sense of control and coping abilities are recommended.[3,10–12]

In summary, pain is an elusive and complex phenomenon; it is a symptom common to many illnesses. Pain is a highly individualized experience that is shaped by a person's culture and previous life experiences and, thus, is very difficult to measure. Traditionally there have been two opposing theories of pain: specificity and pattern theories. However, neither theory accounts for the motivational–cognitive, cultural, and affective components of pain. Pain can be classified according to source, duration, objective signs, and reference. Reactions to pain, which are affected by pain threshold, pain tolerance, and age factors, are manifested through physical, physiologic, and psychosocial responses.

■ Pain Disorders

Alterations in Pain Sensitivity and Perception

Sensitivity to pain varies among people, as well as in the same person, under different circumstances and in different parts of the body. *Analgesia* is a lack of pain without loss of consciousness. *Hyperalgesia* is an increased sensitivity to pain, which may be one of two types, primary or secondary. Tenderness in an area of infection and inflammation is an example of primary hyperalgesia; an abnormality of the central nervous system is an example of secondary hyperalgesia. *Hypoalgesia* is a decreased sensitivity to pain. *Hyperpathia* is a situation in which the pain threshold is normal but the subjective response is not; pain is more unpleasant or prolonged when it does occur.

Inherited insensitivity to pain may take the form of congenital indifference or congenital insensitivity to pain. In the former, transmission of nerve impulses appears normal but appreciation of painful stimuli at higher levels appears to be absent. In the latter, a peripheral nerve defect apparently exists such that transmission of painful nerve impulses does not result in perception of pain. Whatever the cause, in either case there may be severe and extensive tissue damage without the person's being aware of it. Obviously, pain is not serving its protective function in these circumstances.

Pain may occur with or without an apparently *adequate stimulus;* on the other hand, even in the presence of an *adequate* noxious stimulus, pain may be absent. Most familiar to us is pain following adequate noxious stimulation. For example, a hand touched by a flame will be quickly withdrawn. The interesting feature of this reaction, known as local sign, is that the hand is moved away from the painful stimulus in whichever direction is appropriate—up, down, or to either side, as demanded by the situation. In each such situation, the response serves to remove the limb or other body part from the noxious stimulus. Local sign and a response long outlasting the stimulus are characteristics of polysynaptic, multisegmental spinal reflexes.

Pain without an apparently adequate stimulus is puzzling. It may be that an area is hypersensitive because of inflammation or another cause, and a normally subthreshold stimulus is sufficient to trigger the sensation of pain. This response is thought to be chemically mediated, possibly the result of tissue damage in the surrounding area.

As stated earlier, persons who lack the ability to perceive pain are at constant risk. Trauma, infection, even loss of a body part or parts may be the eventual outcome of this lack.

Persons with diabetes mellitus may develop neurologic deficits, most commonly in the nerves that supply the feet. As a consequence, the diabetic may have no sensation in the feet—which explains why diabetics are constantly cautioned about the necessity of meticulous foot care to prevent trauma. In other disease processes, pain pathways may be accidentally or deliberately destroyed to prevent noxious stimuli from relaying messages to the forebrain.

Cultural and environmental factors may play a role in pain perception, too. For example, a Native American who values stoicism is unlikely to cry out in public when subjected to a painful stimulus, whereas this may be an acceptable response in an Italian–American.

Pain can provide reassurance. In one study, the members of a group of men, matched as to injuries, gave very different responses depending on the circumstances of their wounding.[13] Trauma inflicted on the battlefield evoked denial of pain and refusal of medications; the same types of injuries inflicted in civilians evoked complaints of pain and requests for pain relief. These striking differences have been attributed to the high emotional state at the time of injury as well as to the significance each person attached to the injuries. For the soldier, being wounded afforded a face-saving escape from unpleasant, life-threatening situations. It meant being transported to a relatively safe environment, perhaps even home. But a civilian with the same type of injury felt that life-style as well as income were threatened.

Head Pain

Headache

Headache is discussed here because it is a type of pain that is recognized almost universally. Although headache is extremely common, its cause is frequently not known. There are many types of headache, of which the most common appear to be muscle contraction, or tension, headache and migraine headache. Hypertension, as well as traction on intracranial pain-sensitive structures by tumors, subdural hemorrhages, or the weight of the brain after CSF removal, can also induce headaches. Depression can result in headache and is a serious and frequently overlooked cause in children. Nonmigrainous vascular headaches include those related to systemic infections with fever, convulsive states, and hypoxic conditions such as cyanotic heart disease and severe asthma.

It is estimated that 50% to 90% of adult Americans experience headache at some time, at a cost of millions of workdays lost and billions of dollars spent on headache relief.[14] Physicians estimate that at least 20% of the complaints they receive are related to headache.[15] Bille's study revealed that 40% of children have experienced headache by the age of 7, and 75% by the age of 15.[11,12]

Tension headache. The most common form of headache in adults and adolescents is the tension headache resulting from sustained contraction of the muscles of the neck and scalp.[11,16] Contraction of these muscles causes pressure on the nerves in the area, and it can also constrict blood vessels at the base of the neck. When these mechanisms increase pressure, waste products (*e.g.*, lactic acid) also accumulate, causing more pain. The usual source of this tensing of muscles is an unconscious reaction to stress. However, any activity that requires the head to be held in one position, such as typing, repairing jewelry, or using a microscope, can cause muscle contraction headache. Even sleeping in a cold room or with the neck in an inappropriate or strained position can cause a tension headache.

Prevention and treatment are best approached by identifying and removing precipitating factors. This can include such measures as sleeping in a warm room, wearing a scarf to avoid muscle spasms when exposed to the cold, and using a small pillow under the neck for sleeping. Proper eye care, light, and posture during reading, as well as exercising the neck and shoulders frequently, should lower the incidence of muscle spasms. Sleep, deep relaxation exercises, and massage of sore or tense muscles can help to reduce or eliminate painful headaches.

Biofeedback, which provides information about the current status of certain bodily functions, can be used to relax the neck, as well as other muscles of the body. In addition to monitoring the degree of muscle contraction, biofeedback can provide signals related to hand temperature and sweat responses, which are indicators of stress or tension.

Use of medication can often be reduced or eliminated by successfully employing one or more of the above alternative approaches to pain relief.

Migraine headache. Migraine headache is a vascular disorder characterized by paroxysmal attacks of vasoconstriction, usually followed by vasodilatation. This type of headache affects between 12 million and 16 million Americans. It occurs in all age groups, even young infants. Sex incidence is equal in young children, but in adolescents and adults, three to ten times more females are affected. In 70% to 80% of cases there is a positive family history.[11] Although there are several types of migraines, for the purposes of this text they are discussed in general.

Throbbing unilateral pain, photophobia, anorexia, pallor, and nausea and vomiting frequently accompany these headaches. Such neurologic deficits as hemiparesis and hemisensory defects may sometimes be noted. In children, migraines may be associated with other periodic disorders such as cyclic vomiting and benign paroxysmal vertigo.

Most such headaches are thought to be due to change in blood flow and, therefore, changes in oxygen availability. The pain receptors are sensitive to this diminution of oxygen. There may be two phases to the migraine experience. During the prodromal stage, vascular spasm, decreased cerebral blood flow, and sensory or motor alterations can occur. An aura, typically visual and consisting of flashing lights, blind spots, double vision, or hallucinations, can occur 10 minutes to 20 minutes before the onset of headache. During the headache phase, there is vasodilatation and increased cerebral blood flow. Certain vasoactive substances such as serotonin, catecholamines, peptide kinins, and prostaglandins are released. The result is inflammation around the blood vessels. This, combined with the vasodilatation, causes throbbing head pain. Blocking serotonin has been shown to prevent headache. An antagonist to prostaglandin E (a potent vasodilator) also reduces the intensity and duration of attacks.

Migraine headache sufferers are advised to moderate caffeine intake and to avoid large fluctuations in estrogen levels by eliminating oral contraceptives and postmenopausal hormones. Reducing psychological and environmental stresses can also decrease the precipitation of attacks. Dietary changes include avoiding tyramine-containing foods, cured meats, and monosodium glutamate (see Chart 49-1). Smoke-filled rooms and hypoglycemia, whether early morning or fast-induced, can increase migraine attacks.

When dietary and life-style changes and nonpharmacologic approaches, such as biofeedback and relaxation techniques, fail to achieve relief, medications may be necessary. The goal is prevention, because it is much more effective than treatment. Administration of ergotamine tartrate at the onset of symptoms is effective in the majority of cases including adults, adolescents, and children more than 10 years of age. This drug should not be used in pregnancy because of its oxytocic effect. Tolfenamic acid, a prostaglandin E antagonist, is a new and effective medication and may result in fewer side-effects than ergotamine. This drug is still being investigated and is not advised for children. Other drugs used for preventive therapy are propranolol (a beta-adrenergic blocker), anticonvulsants, and amitriptyline. The latter is frequently used for treating childhood depression that

---

Chart 49-1   *Foods That Cause Migraine Headache*

Tyramine-containing
  Red wine
  Strong or aged cheese
  Smoked herring
  Chicken livers
  Canned figs
  Broad bean pods
Sodium nitrate-containing cured meats
  Bacon
  Hot dogs
  Salami
Monosodium glutamate
Chocolate
Nuts, peanut butter
Fruits
  Avocados
  Bananas
  Citrus fruits
Fermented, pickled, and marinated foods
Onions
Dairy products
  Yogurt
  Sour cream
Bakery
  Fresh bread
  Coffee cake
  Doughnuts

---

presents as headache. Clonidine, cyproheptadine, and methysergide are also used, although methysergide is not recommended for children. Midrin is a good substitute for ergotamine; it contains a mild vasoconstrictor, sedative, and acetaminophen. Other drugs used are monoamine oxidase (MAO) inhibitors, platelet antagonists, and steroidal and nonsteroidal anti-inflammatory drugs.

Temporomandibular joint pain

Temporomandibular joint (TMJ) syndrome is now known to be one of the major causes of headache. It is usually caused by an imbalance in the joint movement because of poor bite, bruxism (teeth grinding), or joint problems such as inflammation, trauma, or degenerative changes. The pain is almost always referred. Headache associated with this syndrome is common in both adults and children and can cause chronic pain problems. The treatment of TMJ pain is aimed at correcting the problem, and in some cases this may be difficult.

Dysautonomia
Causalgia

Causalgia is an extremely painful condition that follows sudden and violent deformation of peripheral nerves.

This problem is often initiated in combat by nerve damage caused by high-velocity missiles (*e.g.,* bullets or metal fragments). The nerve is typically damaged but not severed. The classic syndrome was described by Mitchell in 1864 for men sustaining gunshot wounds in the extremities. The median and sciatic nerves are most commonly affected. The pain is characteristically burning and can be elicited with the slightest movement or touch to the affected area. It is excruciating, and even clothing or puffs of air are sufficient to set it off in severe cases. It can be exacerbated by emotional upsets or any increased peripheral sympathetic nerve stimulation. Sympathetic components are part of all variations of causalgia. These are characterized by vascular and tropic (nutritive) changes in the skin, soft tissue, and bone. Reflex sympathetic dystrophy (RSD) is a disorder of the sympathetic nervous system characterized by rubor or pallor, sweating or dryness, edema, pain, or skin atrophy.

Treatment by sympathetic block is usually successful, which may be why this condition is considered a dysautonomia (*i.e.,* a dysfunction of the autonomic nervous system). In some cases, electrical stimulation of the large myelinated fibers innervating the area from which the pain arises is effective. Controversy remains regarding the mechanisms involved in these pain relief measures. The long-term use of narcotics is discouraged because of the danger of addiction. Effective treatment is imperative to prevent invalidism and, in severe cases, suicide.

Neuralgia

Neuralgia is characterized by severe, brief, often constantly recurring attacks of lightninglike or throbbing pain. It occurs along the distribution of a spinal or cranial nerve and is usually precipitated by stimulation of the cutaneous region supplied by that nerve.

Trigeminal neuralgia

Trigeminal neuralgia, or tic douloureux, is one of the most common and severe neuralgias. It is manifested by facial tics or grimaces. It is characterized by stabbing, paroxysmal attacks of pain usually limited to the unilateral sensory distribution of one or more branches of the trigeminal nerve, most often the maxillary division. Victims describe the pain as excruciating. It may be triggered by light touch, eating, swallowing, shaving, talking, chewing gum, washing the face, or sneezing or have no apparent cause. Stimulation of small-diameter afferent fibers is more effective in provoking attacks than are cold, warm, or noxious stimuli. Abnormalities of facial sensation are not likely between attacks. Neurologic deficits are rare, as are neuralgias of cranial nerves VII, IX, and X. Surgical release of vessels, dural struc-

tures, or scar tissue surrounding the semilunar ganglion or root in the middle cranial fossa often eliminates the symptoms. If not, transection or blocking peripheral branches of cranial nerve V produces loss of all sensation, including pain. A more satisfactory treatment is sectioning the descending spinal tract of nerve V in the brain stem. This may be effective because it removes background inflow of impulses on which spontaneous attacks depend. Dissociation of facial sensation occurs, in that pain and temperature disappear, but only a slight decrease in tactile activity occurs. This neurosurgical procedure provided evidence that the nucleus caudalis of the trigeminal complex is necessary for the transmission of facial pain. Considerable controversy remains regarding the pathophysiology of trigeminal neuralgia. The drug carbamazepine (Tegretol), originally developed as an anticonvulsant, may control the pain of trigeminal neuralgia and may delay or eliminate the need for surgery.

Postherpetic neuralgia

The pain associated with postherpetic neuralgia (herpes zoster, or shingles) characteristically follows infection of a dorsal root ganglion and spinal nerves of corresponding ganglia of cranial nerves by herpes zoster virus. It most often affects thoracic spinal nerves. The ophthalmic division of the trigeminal nerve, which innervates the upper face and eye, is the cranial nerve most often affected. The DNA-type virus appears in chickenpox (varicella) and may remain dormant for many years. When immunity falls, the virus can replicate again, causing reddened skin with vesicles and hyperpathia (abnormally exaggerated subjective response to pain). Local or segmental distribution is characteristic and is believed to be due to a rapid rise in immunity. In the acute infection, proportionately more of the large nerve fibers tend to be destroyed. Regenerated fibers appear to have smaller diameters. Older patients tend to have pain, dysesthesia, and hyperesthesia after the acute phase; these are increased by minor stimuli. Because there is a relative loss of large fibers with age, the elderly tend to be particularly prone to suffering because of the shift in the proportion of large- to small-diameter nerve fibers.

Postherpetic neuralgia is extremely distressing and is most efficaciously treated early (*i.e.,* in the first 3 months) before the condition becomes established. Idoxuridine (Herpid), which inhibits a portion of cases with DNA virus infections, is painted on as soon as the rash appears. Steroids have been used, but widespread dissemination can occur, so they are not favored. Pain and vesiculation have been reduced by sympathetic block. Idoxuridine appears to be the best treatment, because vesicles heal and pain is reduced in about 75% of patients receiving it.[17]

Phantom Limb Pain

This type of neurologic pain follows amputation of a limb or part of a limb. At first it is characterized by sensations of tingling, heat and cold, or heaviness. The pain that follows is burning, shooting, or crushing. It may disappear spontaneously or persist for many years. The basic mechanisms involved remain controversial. Terminal neuromas can form, and their fine nerve endings are exquisitely sensitive to pressure or vibration. There is evidence that multiple areas, both peripheral and central, are involved in generating phantom limb pain. One theory is that abnormal sensory input secondary to limb amputation or trauma alters the pattern of information processing in the central nervous system. A closed self-exciting neuronal loop in the posterior horn of the spinal cord is postulated to send impulses to the brain, resulting in pain. Even the slightest irritation of the amputated limb area can initiate this cycle. Treatment has been accomplished by the use of sympathetic blocks, TENS, and relaxation training of the large myelinated afferents innervating the area.[18] Controversy continues as to the precise mechanisms responsible for the usefulness of these methods. Many of the complications following limb amputation can be alleviated by the immediate fitting of a prosthesis and conscientious nursing care of the stump.

In summary, pain, as well as pain disorders, is a universal experience; headache is so common that it is experienced by 75% of the population by the age of 15. Pain may occur with or without an adequate stimulus, or it may be absent in the presence of an adequate stimulus—either of which describes a pain disorder. There may be analgesia (lack of pain without loss of consciousness), hyperalgesia (increased sensitivity to pain), hypoalgesia (decreased sensitivity to pain), or hyperpathia (an unpleasant and prolonged response to pain).

■ Treatment of Pain

It is often not possible to eliminate the cause of pain, and efforts to relieve it may take any of several forms—physical, psychological, pharmacologic, surgical, stimulation-induced analgesia, or a multidisciplinary approach. The decision about which approach should be tried is based on the duration, characteristics, cause, and mechanisms of the pain, if known; the age and social responsibilities of the individual; the prognosis; any previous therapy; and psychological considerations.

Ideally, removal of the sources of noxious stimuli, including anything that causes exacerbation, would be effective. When this is not possible, attempts are made to moderate the reaction to pain. Distraction, imagery, relaxation therapy, hypnosis, biofeedback, and counterirritation methods have all been found useful in some cases. Focal electrical stimulation of PAG has also been shown to decrease pain in the specific body area represented. Drug therapy can include pharmacologic agonists or antagonists working at opioidergic or serotoninergic synapses. Anti-inflammatory and vasoconstrictive agents, antidepressants, antianxiety drugs, and sometimes even anticonvulsant drugs have been used successfully. If none of these approaches is effective, then it may be necessary to interrupt pain pathways by such methods as spinal blocks, use of local anesthetics, surgical interruption of pain fiber tracts, or removal of the pituitary. The latter has been remarkably effective, but the reason for this is unknown at present.

Stimulation-Induced Analgesia

Chapman has called the early 1970s the "stimulation-induced analgesia (SIA) period of investigation."[19] Electrical acupuncture and transcutaneous electrical nerve stimulation are included under this term.

Acupuncture

Electrical stimulation may gradually increase the pain threshold to almost double.[19] This stimulation-induced analgesia is one of the oldest known pain relief methods. It consists of brief, intense stimulation of trigger points by the injection of normal saline, dry needling, or intense cold, which in many cases brings prolonged relief. The Chinese have practiced acupuncture—insertion of needles into certain body areas followed by manual manipulation—for centuries. In the mid-1970s, interest in this modality peaked as a result of reports of complete surgical analgesia by use of acupuncture alone. However, later findings indicate that complete analgesia is unlikely. The Chinese are now practicing electroacupuncture, in which electrical impulses are passed through the needles. Acupressure over the same sites has also been done. Analgesic effects are reported to be greater over specifically designated sites. Pain relief from acupuncture and electroacupuncture has been shown to be reversible by the morphine antagonist naloxone.[20,21] Inconsistencies in some experimental results indicate that further experimental work is needed.[22,23]

Transcutaneous electrical nerve stimulation

Transcutaneous electrical nerve stimulation (TENS) units have been developed that are convenient and relatively economical to use. These units, the size of a small transistor radio or a cigarette package, deliver a measurable amount of current to a target and can be transported and operated easily.

The system usually consists of three parts, *electrodes* connected by *lead wires* to a *stimulator*. The electric current delivered by the generator can be varied in *frequency* and *intensity*. It increases the activity in the large-diameter afferent fibers, which have a lower stimulation threshold and hence relay information more quickly than the small-diameter nociceptive afferent fibers.

As discussed earlier, pain information is transmitted by small-diameter A-delta and C fibers. Large-diameter afferent A fibers as well as small-diameter fibers carry tactile information mediating touch, pressure, and kinesthesis. Transcutaneous electrical nerve stimulators function on the basis of preferentially firing off impulses in the large fibers that carry nonpainful information. According to the gate control theory, increased activity in these large fibers closes the gate—to block or modulate transmission of painful information to the forebrain. Although this theory is in disfavor now because of new evidence that provides alternative explanations, it unfortunately continues to be used as the primary explanation for this phenomenon. The idea of counterirritation has not been put to rest, however, because clinically it works for some patients.

It is known that TENS can activate opioid- and nonopioid-mediated analgesic systems.[24-26] In addition, an opioid-mediated spinal circuit has been implicated. Naloxone does not antagonize pain suppression produced by low-frequency, high-intensity stimulation.[24,25] This may mean that a nonopioid-mediated system is in operation or that an alternative set of receptors is involved.[27]

TENS has the advantages that it is noninvasive, is easily regulated by the individual or health professional, and is quite effective in some forms of acute and chronic pain. Its use can be taught preoperatively, affording a reduction in both hospital days and postoperative analgesic medication. Mannheimer and Lampe provide a good discussion of the scientific data related to this modality, as well as its uses and limitations.[18] Some investigators have reported poor results using TENS with narcotic addicts, indicating the possibility of cross-tolerance (reduced susceptibility because of acquired tolerance for one or more narcotics).

Psychological Techniques

Distraction and imagery

Distraction, that is, focusing one's attention on stimuli other than painful stimuli, is often helpful. It could be considered a type of sensory shielding whereby attention to pain is sacrificed for attention to objective or physical stimuli that are already present or easily obtained. Examples are counting, repeating phrases or poems, engaging in activities that require concentration such as projects, activities at work, conversation, describing slides, and rhythmic breathing. Television, adventure movies, music, and humor can also provide diversion. It is often a mistake to assume that an individual who appears to be able to cope with pain by the use of distraction does not have pain. This individual should not be punished for his or her efforts by the withholding of appropriate medication.[3]

Imagery consists of using one's imagination to develop a mental picture—a visual image. In pain management, therapeutic guided imagery (goal-directed imaging) is used. It can be employed in conjunction with relaxation techniques, biofeedback, and other management methods to develop sensory images that can decrease the perceived intensity of pain. It can also be used to lessen anxiety and reduce muscle tension. Further descriptions of distraction, imagery, and relaxation techniques can be found elsewhere.[3]

Biofeedback

Biofeedback basically involves providing feedback to an individual concerning the current status of some body function (*e.g.,* finger temperature, temporal artery pulsation, blood pressure, muscle tension). It is a process of learning designed to make the individual aware of certain of his or her own body functions for the purpose of modifying these functions at a conscious level (Chap. 6). Interest in this modality rose with the possibility that biofeedback could be used in the management of migraine and tension headache. At this point, there is conflicting evidence on the usefulness of this method in treating migraine headaches. The results are better for electromyographic (EMG) biofeedback training for treating muscle tension, or contraction, headaches.

Pharmacologic Treatment

The use of drugs to control pain is only one aspect of the overall program for pain relief. These agents have been used for many years to relieve pain of short duration, enabling the person to achieve mobility, for example, after surgery, when exercises such as coughing and deep breathing may be required.

An analgesic is defined as a drug that acts on the nervous system to decrease or eliminate pain without inducing loss of consciousness. In general, analgesics have no powerful curative effects.

Analgesics are categorized as narcotic or nonnarcotic, addictive or nonaddictive, prescription or over-the-counter, strong or weak, and peripherally or contrally acting.

The ideal analgesic would be potent yet nonaddicting and would have few side-effects. It would be effective yet would not alter the state of awareness. Tolerance would not occur. Finally, it would not be expensive.

Nonnarcotic oral analgesics

Aspirin, or acetylsalicylic acid (ASA), is an example of a nonnarcotic, nonaddictive, over-the-counter medication that is effective both peripherally and centrally. ASA also has antipyretic and anti-inflammatory properties and, like steroids, is known to inhibit prostaglandins, which make the nerve endings more sensitive to chemicals such as bradykinin. It does have the well-known side-effect of producing bleeding as a result of local and systemic effects. Locally it causes irritation of the gastrointestinal tract; systemically it causes prolonged bleeding time by inhibiting platelet aggregation. Because the latter effect may last for several days, regular daily doses should be avoided at least 1 week prior to surgery. Severe liver disease, vitamin K deficiency, hypoprothrombinemia, or any type of bleeding disorder, such as hemophilia, can be a contraindication to the use of aspirin in some individuals. McCaffery suggests several ways to give aspirin that will minimize its side-effects.[3]

Acetaminophen (Tylenol, Datril, Tempra) may be an effective alternative to aspirin in some individuals. It does not have the side-effects of aspirin, but it can cause liver damage. Children under 5 years of age appear to be less susceptible to this hepatotoxicity. Because there is controversy regarding prolonged use or large doses, it should be used with caution.

Another group of drugs with aspirinlike properties are the nonsteroidal anti-inflammatory drugs (NSIADs). The NSIADs include ibuprofen (Motrin, Rufen), naproxen (Anaprox, Naprosyn), fenoprofen (Nalfon), and indomethacin (Indocin). These drugs act mainly through the inhibition of prostaglandin biosynthesis. They decrease the sensitivity of blood vessels to bradykinin and histamine, affect lymphokine production from T lymphocytes, reverse vasodilation, and decrease the release of inflammatory mediators from granulocytes, mast cells, and basophils. To varying degrees all of the NSIADs are inhibitors of prothrombin synthesis, and all are analgesic, anti-inflammatory, and antipyretic. They are all gastric irritants, but to a lesser extent than aspirin. Nephrotoxicity has also been observed. In addition to their use in rheumatoid and osteoarthritis, the NSIADs (ibuprofen and naproxen) have proved useful in treatment of primary dysmenorrhea.

The relative analgesic potencies of these and other medications can be found in several publications.[3] Combinations of nonnarcotic and narcotic medications to increase effectiveness at lower dosages are also addressed.

Narcotic analgesics

The group of drugs known as narcotics, or opiates, is composed of various naturally occurring alkaloids of the opium poppy. Morphine is the most familiar example. Some synthetic drugs with similar actions include heroin, levorphanol, meperidine, and pentazocine. The pain-relieving (analgesic) and psychopharmacologic properties of morphine have been known for centuries. However, the discovery that the brain contains its own (endogenous) analgesic, morphinelike chemicals that include a group of peptides known as endorphins, is very recent. The principal endogenous opioids found in the brain, spinal fluid, and pituitary gland are the two small peptides called *leu-enkephalin and met-enkephalin.* A larger molecule called *beta endorphin,* which is found in large amounts in the pituitary gland, incorporates the structure of met-enkephalin in its peptide structure.

Opiates and endorphins act on opiate receptors on the surface of certain CNS neurons. These receptors are particularly concentrated in areas of the brain where the enkephalins have also been found to be localized. Research has indicated that there are at least two and possibly more types of opiate receptors in the CNS. One type, called *mu-receptor,* preferentially binds opiates (morphinelike drugs). Another type, called *delta-receptors,* preferentially binds enkephalin. It is generally agreed that the analgesia of the opioids is mediated by mu-receptors. Another recently discovered morphinelike substance, dynorphin, has been found to be several hundred times more potent than enkephalin. It may be the true endogenous opioid for the mu-receptor, because in low concentrations, morphine and the enkephalins bind only to their own receptors.

Pain reactions reflect complex cognitive and emotional responses elicited by noxious stimuli. Beecher distinguished pain sensations from a variety of pain reactions and influenced concepts of the past 20 years regarding the actions of narcotics, or opiates, in the relief of pain.[10] Until this time, clinical analgesia produced by opiates was presumed to result primarily from a decrease in the unpleasantness of the pain reactions rather than in the intensity of the pain sensation. Recent reports seriously question this as the principal action of opiates. Morphine and heroin have mood-changing properties, but these form only part of the complex psychological and physiologic effects that these drugs can induce.

Addiction and overdose.   Morphine and other narcotics are addictive. When used for temporary relief of severe pain, such as that occurring postoperatively, there is strong evidence that narcotics are far more effective when given routinely before the pain becomes extreme than when given sporadically; patients seem to require fewer doses and are better able to resume regular activities earlier. Spinal injection of drugs has been attempted to provide regional specificity of analgesic action in certain types of cancer. Those of high-lipid solubility are rapidly absorbed and produce systemically active concentrations. Morphine is highly hydrophilic, and profound, sustained analgesia can be produced by maintaining high CSF levels over a reasonable time period. One problem is that rostral flow of CSF may produce serious central depression.

In the clinical setting, excessive fear of opiate dependency has been demonstrated repeatedly to result in undertreatment rather than overtreatment of pain, especially of acute pain. This appears to be because of inadequate knowledge of pain relief measures and of the appropriate use of medications, especially narcotics.

Life expectancy may be an important factor in the use of narcotic analgesics for pain control. Because there is undue concern about the possibility of addiction, many chronic pain sufferers with a short life expectancy receive inadequate pain relief. Though social factors rather than medical treatment are the primary cause of drug addiction, many patients do not get enough medication of the proper strength to meet their needs. Many pain experts agree that it is quite appropriate to provide as much narcotic as is necessary to patients with severe, intractable pain whose life expectancy is very limited.

Ambulatory infusion pumps have been used for continuous administration of morphine.[28] These pumps allow advanced cancer patients some control over their own pain within their own homes and without excessive sedation. Subcutaneous infusion, intermittent intrathecal (into the subarachnoid space of the spinal cord) injections, and intravenous infusion of morphine sulfate have all been shown to assist the patient in preserving his or her physical and emotional resources. The result is that the patient is better able to cope with the remainder of life, as well as impending death.

One views the chronic pain sufferer with a normal life expectancy somewhat differently. For example, if a person suffers from low back pain, sciatica, or some other condition that is not life-threatening, it would not ordinarily be appropriate to prescribe narcotics. Such a person is more likely to feel a need to gradually increase the amount and frequency of medication; hence the possibility of addiction exists.

Naloxone, an opiate antagonist, is frequently used in the treatment of narcotic overdose. It competes for opiate receptor binding sites. Administration of this drug can reverse the effects of morphine immediately.

Placebo response

An interesting phenomenon that deserves comment is the placebo response (*placebo,* "I will please"). A placebo is an inert substance. At one time "placebo reactors" were thought to be malingerers or to have psychogenic or functional pain that was more imaginary than real. Newer research indicates that most individuals are, to a greater or lesser degree, placebo reactors.

The analgesic effect of the placebo was postulated to be mediated by the release of endogenous opioids when it was discovered that naloxone reversed its effects in patients with postoperative dental pain.[29] Response to the placebo, like that to opiates, appears to be more effective for moderate or severe pain. There is some evidence to suggest that a certain pain intensity must be reached before the endogenous opioid-mediated analgesic system can be activated.[30] Naloxone has been found to enhance the effect of placebos in some instances. Some postulate that two separate mechanisms may be responsible for the observation of positive and negative placebo reactions.[31] Further research regarding the properties of the endogenous analgesic system is needed to clarify these observations.

Placebos are not recommended as a test to determine whether pain is imaginary or real, mild or severe; nor are they recommended as a means of assessing other physiologic or psychological reactions, such as changes in blood pressure, respiration, heart rate, gastrointestinal activity, or temperature.

Surgical Intervention

Surgery for severe, intractable pain of either peripheral or central origin has met with some success. It can be used to remove the cause or block the transmission of pain. Persons with phantom limb pain, severe neuralgia, inoperable cancer of certain types, or causalgia sometimes suffer so intensely that they consider suicide as their only means of escape. In these extreme cases, surgery may be the only remaining treatment that seems to offer relief from the agony. Nevertheless, surgical methods to relieve pain are usually considered a last resort because damage to nerve cell bodies is irreversible. In addition, a penalty is paid because of damage to other systems, predisposing the patient to other problems. Although severed axons may regenerate, full recovery is highly unlikely. After a few weeks or months the pain often returns and may be more disturbing than before the surgery was done. Regenerating nerve fibers may give rise to dysesthesias (extremely uncomfortable sensations); but if survival time is short, surgery may be warranted. However, in some cases, such as removal of a tumor pressing on nerve fibers or removal of an inflamed appendix, pain is completely relieved.

Surgery to block the transmission of pain signals along peripheral or central pathways may be successful. Peripherally, nerve section (*neurotomy*) or section of a dorsal root ganglion (*rhizotomy*) is not uncommon; some success has been reported for this type of surgery, particularly in tic douloureux.

At the spinal cord level, *cordotomy* and *tractotomy* may require very deep incisions into the cord to give adequate relief. With such deep surgery, bladder function may be affected. The success of these types of surgery depends on the source of the pain and the cord level involved. Electrical stimulation or pharmacologic agents, or both, are often used either to determine the appropriate surgical site or to eliminate the need for surgery.

Hypophysectomy, the removal of the pituitary, has an interesting history. It was done originally in efforts to prevent metastasis in certain hormone-dependent malignancies, including some breast cancers. It was found, rather unexpectedly, that the pain was often immediately and totally relieved. Hypophysectomy, now employed to relieve intractable pain from other sources, has been particularly helpful for severe bone pain. The mechanism of pain relief is not yet understood. It is particularly mysterious because the pituitary is a rich source of endogenous opioids.

Multidisciplinary Approach

More than 30 years ago, the notion of a *multidisciplinary approach* to complex chronic pain problems was first put into practice. It has been found to be particularly effective. Today, a number of pain clinics have been established. This team approach utilizes the knowledge and expertise of many health professionals to diagnose and manage complex types of pain. Besides being useful clinically, the team approach is effective both in teaching and in collaborative research. The acute pain model assumes an objective cause that can be treated and diminished or eliminated within a short time, but, unfortunately, the most perplexing difficulties are those related to chronic pain. This approach has demonstrated its value in addressing many of the chronic pain problems simultaneously from the physical, physiologic, and psychosocial aspects.

In summary, pain can be either acute or chronic, and the latter is particularly difficult to manage. Controversy continues about whether chronic pain should be viewed as a physiologic phenomenon with psychological correlates or as a psychological phenomenon with physiologic correlates. A growing body of data suggests that the latter definition may eliminate many of the chronic pain management problems.

Current treatment modalities include physical, psychological, pharmacologic, neurosurgical, and stimulation-induced analgesic methods, singly or in combination. The last 4 to 5 years have seen a tremendous increase in the available information related to the endogenous opioid analgesic systems. This information has answered some previous questions and raised many more that need to be explored.

It is becoming apparent, however, that even with chronic pain, the most effective approach is early treatment or even prevention. Once pain is present, the greatest success in the management of related problems is achieved with the use of multidisciplinary teams.

■ Study Guide

After you have studied this chapter, you should be able to meet the following objectives:

☐ Differentiate between specificity and pattern theories of pain.

☐ Explain gate control theory.

☐ Describe the action of nociceptors in response to pain information.

☐ Trace the transmission of pain signals with reference to the neospinothalamic, paleospinothalamic, and reticulospinal pathways.

☐ Differentiate *chronic* pain from *acute* pain.

☐ Give examples of visceral, cutaneous, and somatic pain.

☐ Describe the mechanism of referred pain and list the common sites of referral for cardiac and other types of visceral pain.

☐ Compare pain threshold and pain tolerance.

☐ Explain the cultural factors that may influence a person's response to pain.

☐ State how the pain response may differ in children and the elderly.

☐ Define the terms analgesia, hyperalgesia, hypoalgesia, and causalgia.

☐ Give examples of alterations in sensitivity to pain or its perception that may place the affected person at risk.

☐ Describe the reaction of the sympathetic nervous system to a painful stimulus.

☐ Differentiate between causes of tension headache and migraine headaches and their treatment.

☐ State possible causes of migraine headache.

☐ List at least five foods commonly associated with the occurrence of migraine headaches.

☐ Cite the most common cause of TMJ pain.

☐ Describe the cause and characteristics of pain associated with tic douloureaux.

☐ Explain the cause of postherpetic neuralgia and its relationship to pain location.

☐ Cite a possible mechanism of phantom limb pain.

☐ Relate the concept of imagery to pain relief.

☐ Describe the phenomenon called stimulation-induced analgesia.

☐ Explain the rationale underlying the use of TENS.

☐ Cite the actions of nonnarcotic analgesic agents in terms of pain relief.

☐ Define the terms narcotic, exogenous opioid peptide, and opiate.

☐ Discuss factors that are considered when prescribing and administering pain medications for persons with short-term acute pain, long-term chronic pain, and those with prolonged pain due to a terminal illness.

☐ Name the drug used to treat narcotic overdose and explain its mechanism of action.

☐ Cite an explanation for pain relief resulting from the administration of a placebo.

☐ Describe three surgical interventions that can be used for pain control.

☐ Describe the advantages of a multidisciplinary approach to the treatment of pain disorders.

■ References

1. Zborowski M: Cultural components in response to pain. J Soc Issues 8:16, 1952
2. Sternbach R (ed): The Psychology of Pain. New York, Raven Press, 1978
3. McCaffery M: Nursing Management of the Patient with Pain, 2nd ed. Philadelphia, JB Lippincott, 1979
4. Mersky H: Pain and personality. In Sternbach RA: The Psychology of Pain, pp 123–124. New York, Raven Press, 1978
5. Melzak R, Wall PD: Pain mechanisms: A new theory. Science 150:971, 1965
6. Ottoson D: Physiology of the Nervous System, pp 462–463. New York, Oxford University Press, 1983
7. Kuhar M, Pert C, Snyder S: Regional distribution of opiate receptor binding in monkey and human brain. Nature 245:447, 1973
8. Pert A, Yaksh T: Sites of morphine induced analgesia in the primate brain: Relation to pain pathways. Brain Res 80:135–140, 1974
9. Wachter-Shikora NL: The elderly patient in pain and the acute care setting. Nurs Clin North Am 18, No 2 (June):395–401, 1983
10. Beecher HK: Measurement of Subjective Responses. New York, Oxford University Press, 1959
11. Shinnar S, D'Souza BJ: The diagnosis and management of headaches in children. Pediatr Clin North Am 29, No 1 (Feb):79–103, 1982
12. Billie B: Migraine in school children. Acta Paediatr Scand 51 (Suppl 136):1–15, 1962
13. Beecher HK: Relationship of significance of wound to pain experienced. JAMA 161:1609–1613, 1956
14. The interagency Committee on New Therapies for Pain and Discomfort: Report of the White House, IV-38. National Institute of Health, Public Health Service, US Department of Health, Education, and Welfare, May 1979
15. Diamond S: In Kahn AP: Headaches, p 4. Chicago, Contemporary Books, 1983
16. Diamond S, Delessio DJ: The Practicing Physician's Approach to Headache, 2nd ed, p 1. Baltimore, Williams & Wilkins, 1978
17. Lipton S: The Control of Chronic Pain, p 83. Chicago, Year Book Medical Publishers, 1979
18. Mannheimer JS, Lampe GN: Clinical Transcutaneous Electrical Nerve Stimulation. Philadelphia, FA Davis Company, 1984
19. Chapman CR: Contribution of research on acupuncture and transcutaneous electrical stimulation to the understanding of pain mechanisms and pain relief. In Roland F, Beers J, Bassett EG: Mechanisms of Pain and Analgesic Compounds, pp 7–183. New York, Raven Press, 1979
20. Sjolund BH, Terenius L, Erickson MBE: Increased cerebrospinal fluid levels of endorphin after electroacupuncture. Acta Physiol Scand 100:382, 1977
21. Sjolund BH, Erickson MBE: Stimulation techniques in the management of pain. In Kosterlitz HW, Terenius LY (eds): Pain and Society. Life Sciences Report No 17. Deerfield Beach, FL, Weinheim, 1980
22. Sherman JE, Liebeskind JC: An endorphinergic centrifugal substrate of pain modulation: Recent findings, current concepts and complexities. In Banica JJ (ed): Pain. New York, Raven Press, 1980
23. Buchsbaum MS, Davis GC, Bunney WE Jr: Naloxone alters pain perception and somatosensory evoked potentials in normal subjects. Nature 270:620, 1977
24. Chapman CR, Benedetti C: Analgesia following transcutaneous electrical stimulation and its partial reversal by a narcotic antagonist. Life Sci 21:740–741, 1977
25. Pertovaara A, Kemppainen P: The influence of naloxone on dental pain. Threshold elevation produced by peripheral conditioning stimulation at high frequency. Brain Res 215:426–429, 1981
26. Woolf CJ, Barrett GD, Mitchell D, Myers RA: Naloxone-reversible peripheral electroanalgesia in intact and spinal rats. Eur J Pharmacol 45:311–314, 1977
27. Terenius L: Families of opioid peptides and classes of opioid receptors. Plenary Session (527). Annual Meeting of the International Pain Society, Seattle, WA, 1984
28. Dennis EMP: An ambulatory infusion pump for pain control: A nursing approach to home care. Cancer Nurs 7 (Aug):309–313, 1984
29. Levine JD, Gordon NC, Fields HL: The mechanism of placebo analgesia. Lancet 2:654–657, 1978

30. Levine JD, Gordon NC, Fields HL: Naloxone dose dependently produces analgesia and hyperalgesia in postoperative pain. Nature 278:740–741, 1979
31. Levine J: Pain and analgesia: The outlook for more rational treatment. Ann Intern Med 100, No 2 (Feb):269–276, 1984

▌ Additional References

Abu-Saad H: Assessing children's responses to pain. Pain 19:163–171, 1984

Barber J, Adrian C (eds): Psychological Approaches to the Management of Pain. New York, Brunner/Mazel, 1982

Bogin M: The Path to Pain Control. Boston, Houghton Mifflin, 1982

Bonica JJ: Current status of pain therapy. In The Interagency Committee on New Therapies for Pain and Discomfort. Report to the White House, May 1979

Bonica JJ: Important clinical aspects of acute and chronic pain. In Beers RF, Bassett EG (eds): Mechanisms of Pain and Analgesic Compounds. New York, Raven Press, 1979

Boyd DB, Merskey H, Nielsen JS: The pain clinic: An approach to the problem of chronic pain. In Smith WL, Merskey H, Gross SC (eds): Pain: Meaning and Management. New York, SP Medical & Scientific Books, 1980

Brenner JI, Berman MA: Chest pain in childhood and adolescence. J Adolesc Health Care (Review) 3, No 4 (Jan):271–276, 1983

Brown JK: Migraine and migraine equivalents in children. Med Child Neurol 19:683–692, 1977

Cohen FL: Postsurgical pain relief: Patients' status and nurses' medication choices. Pain 9, No 2:265–274, 1980

Davis GC: Endorphins and pain (Review). Psychiatr Clin North Am 6, No 3(Sept):473–487, 1983

Diamond S: Headaches: common but not ordinary. Part 1. Migraine. Emerg Med 16 (July 15):32–42, July 15, 1984

Donovan M: Cancer pain . . . you can help! Nurs Clin North Am 17, No 4 (Dec):713–728, 1982

Emmers R: Pain: A Spike-Interval Coded Message in the Brain. New York, Raven Press, 1981

Ferreira SH: Site of analgesic action of aspirin-like drugs and opioids. In Beers RF, Bassett EG (eds): Mechanisms of Pain and Analgesic Compounds. New York, Raven Press, 1979

Fitz RD: Therapeutic traction: A review of neurologial principles and physical applications. J Manipulative Physiol Ther 7, No 1 (March):39–49, 1984

Graves DA, Foster TS, Batenhorst RL, Bennett RL, Baumann TJ: Patient-controlled analgesia. Am Ann Intern Med 99, No 3 (Sept):360–366, 1983

Hawley DD: Postoperative pain in children: Misconceptions, descriptions, and interventions. Pediatr Nurs 16, No 1(Feb):10–14, 1984

Hendler NH, Long DM, Wise TN (eds): Diagnosis and Treatment of Chronic Pain. Bristol, England, John Wright and Sons Ltd, 1982

Herz A, Sculz R, Blasig J: Changes in neuronal sensitivity in opiate tolerance dependence. In Beers RF, Bassett EG (eds): Mechanisms of Pain and Analgesic Compounds. New York, Raven Press, 1979

Ignelzi RJ, Atkinson JH: Pain and its modulation. Part 1. Afferent mechanisms. Neurosurgery 6, No 5:577–583, 1980

Jacox AK: The assessment of pain. In Smith WL, Merskey H, Gross SC (eds): Pain: Meaning and Management. New York, SP Medical & Scientific Books, 1980

Janko M, Trontelj JV: Transcutaneous electrical nerve stimulation: A microneurographic and perceptual study. Pain 9, No 2:219–230, 1980

Jasinski DR: Morphine and nonaddicting analgesics: A current prospective. In Beers RF, Bassett EG (eds): Mechanisms of Pain and Analgesic Compounds. New York, Raven Press, 1979

Kahn A: Headaches. Chicago, Contemporary Books, 1983

Kim S: Pain: Theory, research and nursing practice. Adv Nurs Sci 2, No 2:43–59, 1980

Knox VJ, Handfield-Jones CE, Shum K: Subject expectancy and the reduction of cold pressor pain with acupuncture and placebo acupuncture. Psychosom Med 41 (Oct):477–485, 1979

Kotarba JA: Chronic Pain. Beverly Hills, Sage Publications, 1983

Levine JD, Gordon NC: Pain in prelingual children and its evaluation by pain-induced vocalizations. Pain 14, No 2 (Oct):85–93, 1982

Mannheimer JS, Lampe GN: Clinical Transcutaneous Electrical Nerve Stimulation. Philadelphia, FA Davis, 1984

Meinhart NT, McCaffery M: Pain, A Nursing Approach to Assessment and Analgesia. East Norwalk, CT, Appleton-Century-Crofts, 1983

Melzack R: The Puzzle of Pain. New York, Basic Books, 1973

Melzack R, Dennis SG: Neurophysiological foundations of pain. In Merskey H, Gross SC (eds): Pain: Meaning and Management. New York, SP Medical & Scientific Books, 1980

Neri M, Agazzani E: Aging and right-left asymmetry in experimental pain measurement. Pain 19:43–48, 1984

Pearce S: A review of cognitive-behavioral methods for the treatment of chronic pain. J Psychosom Res 27, No 5:431–440, 1983

Porges P: Local anesthetics in the treatment of cancer pain (Review). Recent Results Cancer Res 89:127–136, 1984

Rogers AG: Nursing education in the management of pain. No 437. Workshop, World Congress on Pain of the International Association for the Study of Pain. Seattle, WA, August 31–September 5, 1984

Ross DM, Ross SA: The importance of type of question, psychological climate and subjective set in interviewing children about pain. Pain 19:71–79, 1984

Roy R, Tunks E: Chronic Pain. Baltimore, Williams & Wilkins, 1982

Smith WL, Merskey H, Gross SC (eds): Pain: Meaning and Management. New York, SP Medical & Scientific Books, 1980

Unit VIII

Alterations in Skeletal Support and Movement

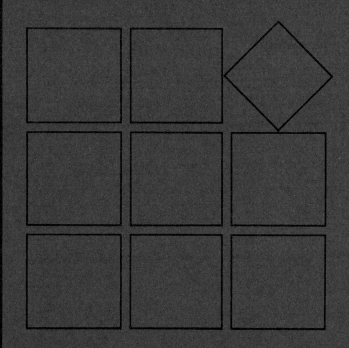

Chapter 50

Structure and Function of the Skeletal System

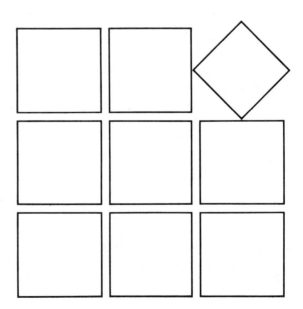

Without the skeletal system, movement in the external environment would not be possible. Bones of the skeletal system serve as a framework for the attachment of muscles, tendons, and ligaments. The skeletal system protects and maintains soft tissues in their proper position, provides stability for the body, and maintains the body's shape. The bones act as a storage reservoir for calcium, and the central cavity of some bones contains the hematopoietic connective tissue in which blood cells are formed.

The skeletal system consists of the axial and appendicular skeleton (Fig. 50-1). The axial skeleton, which is composed of the bones of the skull, thorax, and vertebral column, forms the axis of the body. The appendicular skeleton consists of the bones of the upper and lower extremities, including the shoulder and hip. For our purposes, the skeletal system is considered to include the bones and cartilage of the axial and appendicular skeleton as well as the connective tissue structures (ligaments and tendons) that connect the bones and join muscles to bone.

■ Characteristics of Skeletal Tissue

The tissues found in bones, cartilage, tendons, and ligaments have many things in common. Each of these connective tissue types consists of living cells, nonliving intercellular protein fibers, and an amorphous, or shapeless, ground substance. The tissue cells are responsible for secreting and maintaining the intercellular substances in which they are housed. These substances provide the structural characteristics of the tissue. For example, the intercellular matrix of bone is impregnated with calcium salts, providing the hardness that is characteristic of this tissue.

Two main types of intercellular fibers are found in skeletal tissue: collagenous and elastic. Collagen is an inelastic and insoluble fibrous protein. Because of its molecular configuration, collagen has great tensile strength; the breaking point of human collagenous fibers found in tendons is reached with a force of several hundred kilograms per square centimeter.[1] Fresh collagen is colorless, and tissues that contain large numbers of collagenous fibers generally appear white. It is the collagen fibers in tendons and ligaments that give these structures their white color. Elastin is the major component of elastic fibers that allows them to stretch several times their length and rapidly return to their original shape when the tension is released. Ligaments and structures that must undergo repeated stretching contain a large amount of elastic fibers.

Bone

Bone is connective tissue in which the intercellular matrix has been impregnated with inorganic calcium salts so that it has great tensile and compressible strength but is light enough to be moved by coordinated muscle movements. The intercellular matrix is composed of two types of substances—organic matter and inorganic salts. The organic matter, including bone cells, blood vessels, and nerves, constitutes about one-third of the dry weight of bone; the inorganic salts make up the other two-thirds.

The organic matter consists primarily of collagen fibers embedded in an amorphous ground substance. The inorganic matter consists of hydroxyapatite, an insoluble macrocrystalline structure of calcium phosphate salts, and small amounts of calcium carbonate and calcium fluoride. Bone may also take up lead and other heavy metals, thereby removing these toxic substances from the circulation. This can be viewed as a protective mechanism. The antibiotic tetracycline drugs are readily bound to calcium deposited in newly formed bones and teeth. When tetracycline is given during pregnancy, it can be deposited in the teeth of the fetus, causing discoloration and deformity. Similar changes can occur if the drug is given for long periods to children under 6 years of age.

Types of bone

There are two types of mature bones, cancellous and compact bone (Fig. 50-2). Both types are formed in layers and are therefore called lamellar bone. Cancellous, or spongy, bone is found in the interior of bones and is composed of trabeculae, or spicules, of bone, which form a latticelike pattern. These latticelike structures are lined with osteogenic cells and filled with either red or yellow bone marrow. Cancellous bone is relatively lightweight, yet its structure is such that it has considerable tensile strength and weight-bearing properties. Compact (cortical) bone has a densely packed calcified intercellular matrix that makes it more rigid than cancellous bone. The relative quantity of compact and cancellous bone varies in different types of bones throughout the body and in different parts of the same bone, depending on the need for strength and lightness. Compact bone is the major component of tubular bones. It is also found along the lines of stress on long bones and forms an outer protective shell on others.

Bone cells

Four types of bone cells participate in the formation and maintenance of bone tissue: (1) osteogenic cells, (2) osteoblasts, (3) osteocytes, and (4) osteoclasts (see Table 50-1).

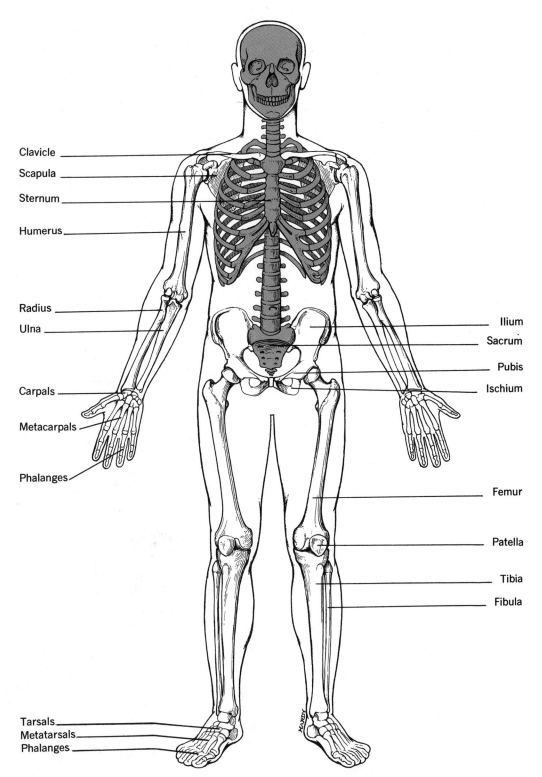

Figure 50-1 *The skeleton. The bones of the head and the trunk that form the axial skeleton are shown in color, and those of the extremities forming the appendicular skeleton are uncolored. (From Chaffee EE, Lytle IM: Basic Physiology and Anatomy, 4th ed. Philadelphia, JB Lippincott, 1980)*

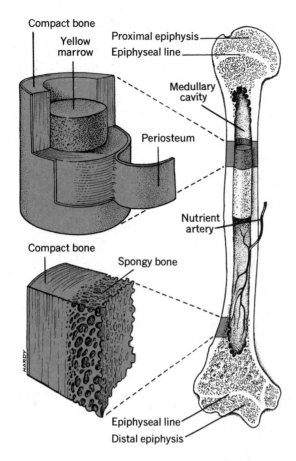

Figure 50-2   *A long bone shown in longitudinal section. (From Chaffee EE, Lytle IM: Basic Physiology and Anatomy, 4th ed. Philadelphia, JB Lippincott, 1980)*

Osteogenic cells.   The undifferentiated osteogenic cells are found in the periosteum, endosteum, and epiphyseal plate of growing bone. These cells differentiate into osteoblasts and are active during normal growth; they may also be activated in adult life during healing of fractures and other injuries. Osteogenic cells also participate in the continual replacement of worn-out bone tissue.

Osteoblasts.   The osteoblasts, or bone-building cells, are responsible for the formation of the bone matrix. Bone formation occurs in two stages: ossification and calcification. Ossification involves the formation of osteoid, or prebone. Calcification of bone involves the deposition of calcium salts in the osteoid tissue. The osteoblasts synthesize collagen and other proteins that make up osteoid tissue. They also participate in the calcification process of the osteoid tissue, probably by

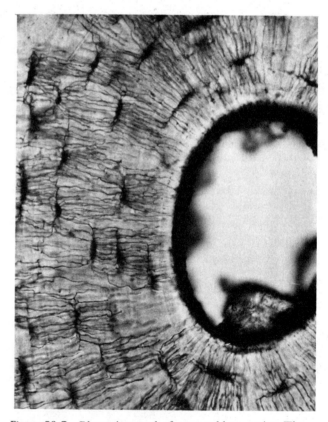

Figure 50-3   *Photomicrograph of a ground bone section. The lacunae in which osteocytes reside appear as dark flattened ovals. The fine lines (canaliculi) connect the lacunae to each other and to the canal on the right. In life, this canal contained blood vessels that supplied interstitial fluid to the canaliculi. (Reprinted from Ham A, Cormack DH: Histology, 8th ed. Philadelphia, JB Lippincott, 1979)*

Table 50-1   Function of Bone Cells

Type of Bone Cell	Function
Osteogenic cells	Undifferentiated cells that differentiate into osteoblasts. They are found in the periosteum, endosteum, and epiphyseal growth plate of growing bones.
Osteoblasts	Bone-building cells that synthesize and secrete the organic matrix of bone. Osteoblasts also participate in the calcification of the organic matrix.
Osteocytes	Mature bone cells that function in the maintenance of bone matrix. Osteocytes also play an active role in releasing calcium into the blood.
Osteoclasts	Bone cells responsible for the resorption of bone matrix and the release of calcium and phosphate from bone.

controlling the availability of calcium and phosphate. Osteoblasts secrete the enzyme alkaline phosphatase, which is thought to act locally in bone tissue to raise calcium and phosphate levels to a point at which precipitation occurs. The activity of the osteoblasts undoubtedly contributes to the rise in serum levels of alkaline phosphatase that occurs following bone injury and fractures.

Osteocytes.   The osteocytes are mature bone cells that are actively involved in the maintenance of the bony matrix. Death of the osteocytes results in the resorption of this matrix. The osteocytes lie in a small lake filled with extracellular fluid, called a lacuna, and are surrounded by a calcified intercellular matrix (Fig. 50-3). Extracellular fluid-filled passageways permeate the calcified matrix and connect with the lacunae of adjacent osteocytes. These passageways are called canaliculi. Because diffusion does not occur through the calcified matrix of bone, the canaliculi serve as communicating channels for the exchange of nutrients and metabolites between the osteocytes and the blood vessels on the surface of the bone layer.

The osteocytes, together with their intercellular matrix, are arranged in layers, or lamellae. In compact bone, 4 to 20 lamellae are arranged concentrically around a central haversian canal, which runs essentially parallel to the long axis of the bone. Each of these units is called a haversian system, or osteon. The haversian canals contain blood vessels that carry nutrients and wastes to and from the canaliculi (Fig. 50-4). The blood vessels from the periosteum enter the bone through tiny open-

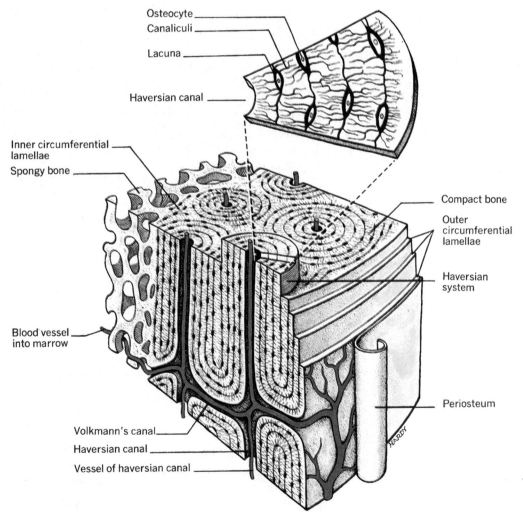

Figure 50-4   *Haversian systems as seen in a wedge of compact bone tissue. The periosteum has been peeled back to show a blood vessel entering one of Volkmann's canals. (Upper right) Osteocytes lying within lacunae; canaliculi permit interstitial fluid to reach each lacuna. (From Chaffee EE, Lytle IM: Basic Physiology and Anatomy, 4th ed. Philadelphia, JB Lippincott, 1980)*

ings called Volkmann's canals and then connect with the haversian systems. Cancellous bone is also composed of lamellae, but its trabeculae are usually not penetrated by blood vessels. Instead, the bone cells of cancellous bone are nourished by diffusion from the endosteal surface through canaliculi, which interconnect their lacunae and extend to the bone surface.

Osteoclasts.   Osteoclasts are bone cells that function in the resorption of bone, removing both the mineral content and the organic matrix. Unlike the osteoblasts, which originate in osteogenic cells, the osteoclasts are formed by the fusion of blood-derived monocytes. Although the mechanism of osteoclast formation and activation remains elusive, it is known that parathyroid hormone increases the number and resorptive function of the osteoclasts. Calcitonin, on the other hand, is thought to reduce the number and resorptive function of the osteoclasts. The mechanism whereby osteoclasts exert their resorptive effect on bone is also unclear. These cells may secrete an acid that removes calcium from the bone matrix, thus releasing the collagenic fibers for digestion by either osteoclasts or mononuclear cells.

Classification of bones
Bones are classified, on the basis of their shape, as (1) long bones, (2) short bones, (3) flat bones, and (4) irregular bones. Long bones are found in the upper and lower extremities. Short bones are irregularly shaped bones located in the ankle and the wrist. Except for their surface, which is compact bone, these bones are spongy throughout. Flat bones are composed of a layer of spongy bone between two layers of compact bone. They are found in areas such as the skull and rib cage, where extensive protection of underlying structures is needed or, as in the scapula, where a broad surface for muscle attachment must be provided. Irregular bones, because of their shapes, cannot be classified in any of the previous groups. This group includes such bones as the vertebrae and the bones of the jaw.

A typical long bone has a shaft, or diaphysis, and two ends, called epiphyses. Long bones are usually narrow in the midportion and broad at the ends so that the weight they bear can be distributed over a wider surface. The shaft of a long bone is formed mainly of compact bone roughly hollowed out to form a marrow-filled medullary canal. The ends of long bones are covered with articular cartilage that rests on a bony plate, the subchondral bone.

In growing bones the part of the bone shaft that funnels out as it approaches the epiphysis is called the metaphysis (Fig. 50-5). It is composed of bony trabeculae that have cores of cartilage. In the child, the epiphysis is separated from the metaphysis by the cartilaginous growth plate. After puberty, the metaphysis and epiphysis merge, and the growth plate is obliterated.

Bone marrow
Bone marrow occupies the medullary cavities of the long bones throughout the skeleton and the cavities of cancellous bone in the vertebrae, ribs, sternum, and flat bones of the pelvis. The cellular composition of the bone marrow varies with both age and skeletal location. Red bone marrow contains developing red blood cells and is the site of blood cell formation. Yellow bone marrow is composed largely of adipose cells. At birth, nearly all of the marrow is red and hematopoietically active. As the need for red blood cell production decreases during postnatal growth red marrow is gradually replaced with yellow bone marrow in most of the bones. In the adult, red marrow persists in the vertebrae, ribs, sternum, and ilia.

Periosteum and endosteum
Bones are covered, except at their articular ends, by a membrane called the periosteum (see Fig. 50-2). The periosteum has an outer fibrous layer and an inner layer that contains the osteogenic cells needed for bone growth and development. The periosteum contains blood vessels and acts as an anchorage point for vessels as they enter and leave the bone. The endosteum is the membrane that lines the spaces of spongy bone, the

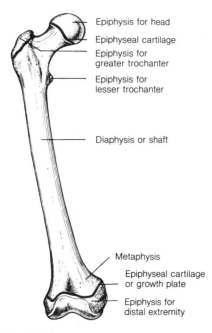

Epiphysis for head
Epiphyseal cartilage
Epiphysis for greater trochanter
Epiphysis for lesser trochanter

Diaphysis or shaft

Metaphysis
Epiphyseal cartilage or growth plate
Epiphysis for distal extremity

Figure 50-5 *A femur, showing epiphyseal cartilages for the head, metaphysis, trochanters, and distal end of the bone. (Adapted from Chaffee EE, Lytle IM: Basic Physiology and Anatomy, 4th ed. Philadelphia, JB Lippincott, 1980)*

marrow cavities, and the haversian canals of compact bone. It is composed mainly of osteogenic cells. These osteogenic cells contribute to the growth and remodeling of bone and are necessary for bone repair.

Cartilage

Cartilage is a firm but flexible type of connective tissue consisting of cells and intercellular fibers embedded in an amorphous gel-like material. It has a smooth and resilient surface and a weight-bearing capacity exceeded only by that of bone.

Cartilage is essential for growth both before and after birth. It is able to undergo rapid growth while maintaining a considerable degree of stiffness. In the embryo, most of the axial and appendicular skeleton is formed first as a cartilage model and is then replaced by bone. In postnatal life, cartilage continues to play an essential role in the growth of long bones and persists as articular cartilage in the adult.

There are three types of cartilage: elastic cartilage, hyaline cartilage, and fibrocartilage. *Elastic cartilage* contains some elastin in its intercellular substance. It is found in areas, such as the ear, where some flexibility is important. Pure cartilage is called *hyaline cartilage* (from the Greek meaning glass) and is pearly white. It is the type of cartilage seen on the articulating ends of fresh soup bones found in the supermarket. *Fibrocartilage* has characteristics that are intermediate between dense connective tissue and hyaline cartilage. It is found in the intervertebral disks, in areas where tendons are conected to bone, and in the symphysis pubis.

Hyaline cartilage is the most abundant type of cartilage. It forms much of the cartilage of the fetal skeleton. In the adult, hyaline cartilage forms the costal cartilages, which join the ribs to the sternum and vertebrae, many of the cartilages of the respiratory tract, the articular cartilages, and the epiphyseal plates.

Cartilage cells, which are called *chondrocytes,* are located in small spaces called *lacunae.* These lacunae are surrounded by an uncalcified gellike intercellular matrix of collagen fibers and ground substance. Cartilage is devoid of blood vessels and nerves. The free surfaces of most hyaline cartilage, with the exception of articular cartilage, is covered by a layer of fibrous connective tissue called the *perichondrium.*

It has been estimated that about 75% of the wet weight of cartilage is water held in its gel structure.[2] Because cartilage has no blood vessels, this tissue fluid allows for the diffusion of gases, nutrients, and wastes between the chondrocytes and blood vessels outside the cartilage. Diffusion cannot take place if the cartilage matrix becomes impregnated with calcium salts. Therefore, cartilage dies if it becomes calcified.

Tendons and Ligaments

In the skeletal system, tendons and ligaments are dense connective tissue structures that connect muscles and bones. Tendons connect muscles to bone, and ligaments connect the movable bones of joints. Tendons can appear as cordlike structures or flattened sheets, called aponeuroses, such as in the abdominal muscles.

The dense connective tissue found in tendons and ligaments has a limited blood supply and is composed largely of intercellular bundles of collagen fibers arranged in the same direction and plane. This type of connective tissue provides great tensile strength and can withstand tremendous pulls in the direction of fiber alignment. At the sites where tendons or ligaments are inserted into cartilage or bone, a gradual transition from pure dense connective tissue to either bone or cartilage occurs. In cartilage this transitional tissue is called fibrocartilage.

Tendons that might rub against bone or other friction-generating surfaces are enclosed in double-layered sheaths. An outer connective tissue tube is attached to the structures surrounding the tendon, and an inner sheath encloses the tendon and is attached to it. The space between the inner and outer sheath is filled with a fluid similar to synovial fluid.

In summary, skeletal tissue includes bone, cartilage, ligaments, and tendons. These skeletal structures are composed of similar tissue types; each has living cells and nonliving intercellular fibers and ground substance that is secreted by the cells. The characteristics of the various skeletal tissue types are determined by the intercellular matrix. In bone, this matrix is impregnated with calcium salts to provide hardness and strength. There are four types of bone cells: osteocytes, or mature bone cells; osteoblasts, or bone-building cells; osteoclasts, which function in bone resorption; and osteogenic cells, which differentiate into osteoblasts. A typical long bone has a shaft, or diaphysis, and two ends called epiphyses. Densely packed compact bone forms the outer shell of a bone, and latticelike cancellous bone forms the interior. Cartilage is a firm, flexible type of skeletal tissue that is essential for growth both before and after birth. There are three types of cartilage: elastic, hyaline, and fibrocartilage. Hyaline cartilage, which is the most abundant type, forms the costal cartilages that join the ribs to the sternum and vertebrae, many of the cartilages of the respiratory tract, and the articular cartilages. Tendons and ligaments are dense connective skeletal tissue that connect muscles and bones. Tendons connect muscles to bones and ligaments connect the movable bones of joints.

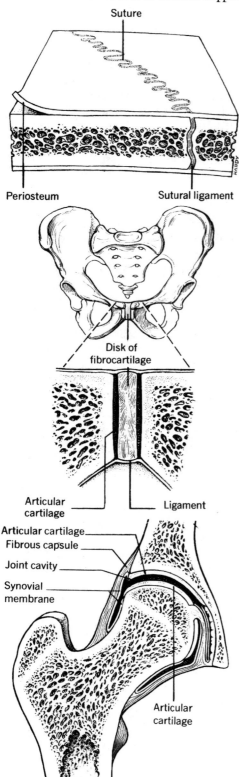

Figure 50-6 *Three types of joints. (Top) Synarthrosis, which is joined by a fibrous suture ligament; (center) amphiarthrosis, symphysis type, which is joined by a disk of fibrocartilage; (bottom) diarthrosis, or synovial joint, in which bones are joined by ligaments and a fibrous joint capsule. (From Chaffee EE, Lytle IM: Basic Physiology and Anatomy, 4th ed. Philadelphia, JB Lippincott, 1980)*

■ Joints and Articulations

Articulations, or joints, are areas where two or more bones meet. The term *arthro* is the affix used to designate a joint. For example, *arthrology* is the study of joints and *arthroplasty* is the repair of a joint. There are three classes of joints based on movement and the type of tissue present in the joint: synarthroses, amphiarthroses, and diarthroses (Fig. 50-6).

Synarthroses

Synarthroses are immovable joints in which the surfaces of the bones come in direct contact with each other and are fastened together by fibrous tissue, cartilage, or bone. The bones of the skull are joined by synarthroses.

Amphiarthroses

Amphiarthroses are slightly movable joints connected by cartilage. There are two types of amphiarthrotic joints: symphyses, which are connected by fibrocartilage disks, and synchrondroses, which have cartilages that are temporarily replaced by bone. The symphysis pubis of the pelvis and the bodies of the vertebrae that are joined by intervertebral disks are examples of symphysis articulations. The normal process of bone elongation in bones with epiphyses involves synchrondrosis between the end and the shaft of the bone. After growth is completed, the synarthroses become ossified.

Diarthroses

Diarthrodial joints (synovial joints) are freely movable joints. Most joints in the body are of this type. Although they are classified as freely movable, their movement actually ranges from almost none (sacroiliac joint) to simple hinge movement (interphalangeal joint), to movement in many planes (shoulder or hip joint). The bony surfaces of these joints are covered with thin layers of articular cartilage, and the cartilaginous surfaces of these joints slide past each other during movement. As will be discussed in Chapter 53, diarthrodial joints are the joints most frequently affected by rheumatic disorders.

In a diarthrodial joint the articulating ends of the bones are not connected directly but are indirectly linked by a strong fibrous capsule (joint capsule) that surrounds the joint and is continuous with the periosteum. This capsule supports the joint and helps to hold the bones in place. Additional support may be provided by ligaments that extend between the bones of the joint. The joint capsule consists of two layers: an outer fibrous layer and an inner membrane, the synovium. The synovium surrounds the tendons that pass through the joints as well as the free margins of other intra-articular structures such as ligaments and menisci. The synovium forms folds that surround the margins of articulations but do not cover the weight-bearing articular cartilage. These folds permit stretching of the synovium so that movement can occur without tissue damage.

Synovium and synovial fluid

The synovium secretes a slippery synovial fluid with the consistency of egg white. This fluid acts as a lubricant and facilitates the movement of the articulating surfaces of the joint. Normal synovial fluid is clear, is colorless or pale yellow, does not clot, and contains fewer than 200 cells/mm.[3] The cells are predominantly mononuclear cells derived from the synovium. The composition of the synovial fluid is altered in many inflammatory and pathologic joint disorders. Aspiration and examination of the synovial fluid plays an important role in the diagnosis of joint diseases.

Articular cartilage

The articular cartilage is an example of hyaline cartilage and is unique in that its free surface is not covered with perichondrium. It has only a peripheral rim of perichondrium, and calcification of the portion of cartilage abutting the bone may limit or preclude diffusion from blood vessels supplying the subchondral bone. Articular cartilage is apparently nourished by the diffusion of substances contained in the synovial fluid bathing the cartilage. Regeneration of most cartilage is slow; it is accomplished primarily by growth that requires the activity of perichondrium cells. In articular cartilage, which has no perichondrium, superficial injuries heal very slowly.[3]

Blood supply

The blood supply to a joint arises from blood vessels that enter the subchondral bone at or near the attachment of the joint capsule and form an arterial circle around the joint. The synovial membrane has a rich blood supply, and constituents of plasma diffuse rapidly between these vessels and the joint cavity. Because many of the capillaries are near the surface of the synovium, blood may escape into the synovial fluid following relatively minor injuries.[2] Healing and repair of the synovial membrane is usually rapid and complete. This is important because synovial tissue is injured in many surgical procedures that involve the joint.

Innervation

The nerve supply to joints is provided by the same nerve trunks that supply the muscles that move the joints. These nerve trunks also supply the skin over the joints. As a rule, each joint of an extremity is innervated by all the peripheral nerves that cross the articulation; this accounts for the referral of pain from one joint to another.[4] For example, hip pain may be perceived as pain in the knee.

The tendons and ligaments of the joint capsule are sensitive to position and movement, particularly stretching and twisting. These sructures are supplied by the large sensory fibers that form proprioceptor endings (Chap. 45). The proprioceptors function reflexly to adjust the tension of the muscles that support the joint and are particularly important in maintaining muscular support for the joint. For example, when a weight is lifted, there is a proprioceptor-mediated reflex contraction and relaxation of appropriate muscle groups to support the joint and protect the joint capsule and other joint structures. Loss of proprioception and reflex control of muscular support leads to destructive changes in the joint.

The synovial membrane is innervated only by autonomic fibers that control blood flow. It is relatively free of pain fibers, as is evidenced by the fact that surgical procedures on the joint are often done under local anesthesia. The joint capsule and the ligaments of joints have pain receptors; these receptors are more easily stimulated by stretching and twisting than the other joint structures. Pain arising from the capsule tends to be diffuse and poorly localized.

Bursae

In some diarthrotic joints, the synovial membrane forms closed sacs that are not part of the joint. These sacs, called *bursae,* contain synovial fluid. Their purpose is to prevent friction on a tendon. Bursae occur in areas where pressure is exerted because of close approximation of joint structures (Fig. 50-7). Such situations occur when tendons are deflected over bone or where skin must move freely over bony tissue. Bursae may become injured or inflamed, causing discomfort, swelling, and limitation in movement of the involved area. A bunion is an inflamed bursa of the metatarsophalangeal joint of the great toe.

Intra-articular menisci

Intra-articular menisci are fibrocartilage structures that develop from portions of the articular disk that occupied the space between the articular cartilage during fetal development. Menisci may have a free inner border (as at the lateral and medial articular surfaces of the knee), or they may extend through the joint, separating it into two separate cavities (as in the sternoclavicular joint). The menisci of the knee joint may be torn as the result of an injury. The detached portion may interfere with joint motion and cause recurring pain and locking or giving way of the joint. When this happens, the injured structure is often removed surgically. Following removal, a new structure sometimes grows in from the fibrous capsule of the joint. The new meniscus is almost a complete duplicate of the old except that it is made up of dense

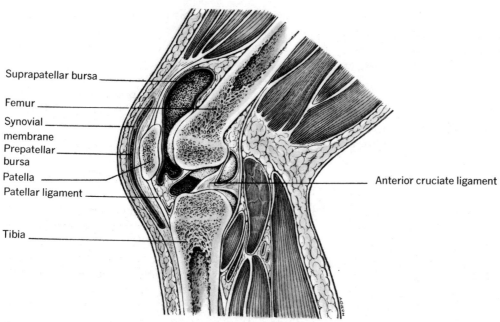

Suprapatellar bursa

Femur

Synovial
membrane

Prepatellar
bursa

Patella

Patellar ligament

Tibia

Anterior cruciate ligament

Figure 50-7 *Sagittal section of knee joint, showing prepatellar and suprapatellar bursae. (From Chaffee EE, Lytle IM: Basic Physiology and Anatomy, 4th ed. Philadelphia, JB Lippincott, 1980)*

connective tissue rather than the fibrocartilage of the original structure.

In summary, articulations, or joints, are areas where two or more bones meet. Synarthroses are immovable joints in which bones are joined together by fibrous tissue, cartilage, or bone. Amphiarthroses are slightly movable joints connected by cartilage. Most joints in the body are diarthrodial, or synovial, joints, which are freely movable joints. The surfaces of these joints are covered with a thin layer of articular cartilage. The articulating ends of bones in a diarthrodial joint are linked by the fibrous joint capsule. The joint capsule consists of two layers: an outer fibrous layer and an inner membrane, the synovium. A slippery fluid called the synovial fluid, which is secreted by the synovium and is present in the joint capsule, acts as a lubricant and facilitates movement of the joint's articulating surfaces. Bursae, which are closed sacs containing synovial fluid, prevent friction in areas where tendons are deflected over bone or where skin must move freely over bony tissue. Menisci are fibrocartilaginous structures that develop from portions of the articular disk that occupied the space between the articular cartilage during fetal development. The menisci may have a free inner border, or they may extend through the joint separating it into two cavities. The menisci in the knee joint may be torn as a result of injury.

■ Study Guide

After you have studied this chapter, you should be able to meet the following objectives:

☐ List the common components of bone, cartilage, and the dense connective tissue of ligaments and tendons.

☐ Compare the properties of the intercellular collagen and elastic fibers of skeletal tissue.

☐ Name and state the function of the four types of bone cells.

☐ Draw a long bone, and label the diaphysis, epiphysis, and metaphysis.

☐ State the location and function of the periosteum and the endosteum.

☐ Compare bone and cartilage in terms of their structure and function.

☐ Cite the characteristics and name at least one location of elastic cartilage, hyaline cartilage, and fibrocartilage.

☐ Define a tendon and a ligament.

☐ Name the three kinds of joints, and give one example of each type.

☐ Describe the source of blood supply to a diarthroidal joint.

☐ Explain why the pain experience is often reflected in all joints of an extremity when only a single joint is affected by a disease process.

☐ Describe the structure and function of a bursa.

☐ Explain the pathology associated with a torn miniscus of the knee.

◼ References

1. Bloom W, Faucett DW: A Textbook of Histology, p 160. Philadelphia, WB Saunders, 1975
2. Ham AW, Cormack DH: Histology, 8th ed, pp 373, 441, 476. Philadelphia, JB Lippincott, 1979
3. Hooker H: Histology of cartilage and synovium. In Wilson FC (ed): The Musculoskeletal System: Basic Processes and Disorders, 2nd ed, p 213. Philadelphia, JB Lippincott, 1980
4. Rodman GP, Schumacker HR (eds): Primer on Rheumatic Diseases, 8th ed, p 15. Atlanta GA, Arthritis Foundation, 1983

Chapter 51

Alterations in Skeletal Function: Trauma and Infection

Kathleen E. Gunta

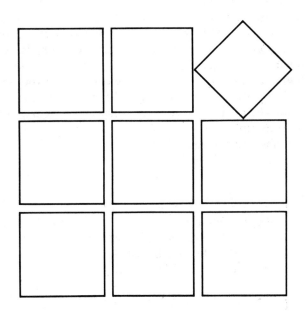

The musculoskeletal system includes the bones, joints, and muscles of the body together with associated structures such as ligaments and tendons. This system, which constitutes more than 70% of the body, is subject to a large number of disorders. These disorders affect people in all age groups and walks of life, causing pain, disability, and deformity. The discussion in this chapter focuses on trauma and infections of skeletal structures.

■ Injury and Trauma of Musculoskeletal Structures

Trauma, which commonly includes injury to musculoskeletal structures, is the third leading cause of death in the United States. A broad spectrum of injuries result from numerous physical forces. Injuries to the musculoskeletal system include blunt tissue trauma, disruption of tendons and ligaments, and fractures of bony structures.

Many of the external physical agents that cause injury to the musculoskeletal system are typical of a particular environmental setting, activity, or age group. In the home, common accidents include tripping over cords or falling on wet floors. In sports injuries, an athlete's conditioning, protection, and movement often determine the outcome of trauma-producing events. Specific injuries are associated with each type of sport, such as tennis elbow, jogger's heel, and injuries to tendons, cartilage, and ligaments seen in contact sports. Trauma resulting from high-velocity motor accidents is now ranked as the number one killer of adults under the age of 35. Motorcycle accidents are especially common in young men, with fractures of the distal tibia, midshaft femur, and radius occurring most often.

The elderly are at particular risk for injuries caused by falls. Visual difficulties, impaired hearing, dizziness, and unsteadiness of gait contribute to falls in the older person. Falls in the elderly are often compounded by osteoporosis, or bone atrophy, which makes it easier for fractures to occur. Fractures of the vertebrae, proximal humerus, and hip are particularly common in this age group. Adrenocorticosteroid medications used for the treatment of diseases such as asthma and rheumatoid arthritis can lead to decreased bone density. Fractures of the ribs and vertebrae are common types of fractures associated with bone loss in these persons.

Soft Tissue Injury

Most skeletal injuries are accompanied by soft tissue injuries. These injuries include contusions, hematomas, and lacerations. They are discussed here because of their association with skeletal injuries.

A *contusion* is an injury to soft tissue that results from direct trauma and is usually caused by striking a body part against a hard object. With a contusion, the skin overlying the injury remains intact. Initially the area becomes ecchymotic (black and blue) because of local hemorrhage; later the discoloration gradually changes to brown and then to yellow as the blood is reabsorbed.

A large area of local hemorrhage is called a *hematoma* (blood tumor). With a hematoma, pain occurs as blood accumulates and causes pressure on nerve endings. The pain increases with movement or when pressure is applied to the area. The pain and swelling of a hematoma takes longer to subside than that accompanying a contusion. A hematoma may become infected because of bacterial growth. Unlike a contusion, which does not drain, a hematoma may eventually split the skin because of increased pressures and subsequently produce drainage.

The treatment for both a contusion and a hematoma consists of elevating the affected part and applying cold for the first 24 hours to reduce the bleeding into the area. A hematoma may need to be aspirated. After the first 24 hours, heat or cold should be applied intermittently for periods of 20 minutes at a time.

A *laceration* is an injury in which the skin is torn or its continuity disrupted. The seriousness of a laceration depends on the size and depth of the wound and on contamination of the object causing the injury. Puncture wounds from nails or rusted material may cause growth of very toxic bacteria, resulting in gas gangrene or tetanus.

Lacerations are usually treated by wound closure, which is done once the area is sufficiently cleansed; the closed wound is then covered with a sterile dressing. It is important to minimize contamination of the wound and control bleeding. Contaminated wounds and open fractures are copiously irrigated and debrided, and the skin is usually left open to heal in order to prevent the development of an anaerobic infection or a sinus tract.

Strains and sprains

Tendons and ligaments, which connect bones and muscles, can be severed by cutting injuries or damaged by forcible twisting or stretching. A *strain* is a stretching injury to a muscle or a musculotendinous unit caused by mechanical overloading. This type of injury may result from either an unusual muscle contraction or an excessive forcible stretch. Although there is usually no external evidence of a specific injury, pain, stiffness, and swelling are present. The most common sites for muscle strain are the lower back and the cervical region of the spine. The elbow and the shoulder are also supported by musculotendinous units that are subject to strains. Foot strain is associated with the weight-bearing stresses of the feet; it may be caused by inadequate muscular and ligamentous support, overweight, or excessive exercise such as standing, walking, or running.

A *sprain,* which involves the ligamentous structures surrounding the joint, resembles a strain, but the pain and swelling subside more slowly (Fig. 51-1). It is usually caused by abnormal or excessive movement of the joint. With a sprain the ligaments may be incompletely torn or, as in a severe sprain, completely torn or ruptured. The signs of sprain are pain, rapid swelling, heat, disability, discoloration, and limitation of function. Any joint may be sprained, but the ankle joint is most commonly involved. Other common sites of sprain are the knee and elbow (on the ulnar side). As with a strain, the soft tissue injury that occurs with a sprain is not evident on x-ray. Occasionally, however, a chip of bone is evident when the entire ligament, including part of its bony attachment, has been ruptured or torn from the bone.

Healing of the dense connective tissues in tendons and ligaments is similar to that of other soft tissues. Following injury, they usually heal with the restoration of their original tensile strength if treated properly. Repair is accomplished by fibroblasts from the inner tendon sheath or, if the tendon has no sheath, from the loose connective tissue that surrounds the tendon. Capillary infiltration occurs in the injured area during the initial healing process and supplies the fibroblasts with the materials needed for the production of large amounts of collagen. Formation of the long collagen bundles begins within 4 to 5 days, and although tensile strength increases steadily thereafter, it is not sufficient to permit strong tendon pulls for 4 to 5 weeks.[1] During the first 3 weeks, there is danger that muscle contraction will pull the injured ends apart; should this occur, the tendon will heal in the lengthened position. There is also danger that adhesions will develop in areas where tendons pass through fibrous channels, such as those that appear in the distal palm of the hands, rendering the tendon useless.

The treatment of muscle strains and ligamentous sprains is similar in several ways. For an injured extremity, elevation of the part followed by local application of cold may be sufficient. Compression, accomplished through the use of adhesive wraps or a removable splint, helps reduce swelling and provides support. A cast is applied for severe sprains, especially those severe enough to warrant surgical repair. Immobilization for a muscle strain is continued until the pain and swelling have subsided. In a sprain, the affected joint is immobilized for several weeks. Immobilization may be followed by graded active exercises. In the lumbar and cervical spine regions, muscle strains are more common than sprains. For these strains, treatment usually consists of bed rest, traction, application of heat, and massage. Occasionally cold may be substituted during the first 24

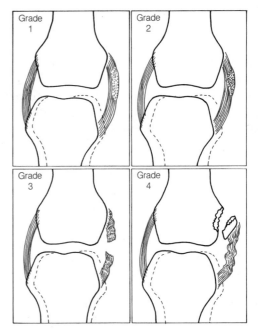

Figure 51-1 *Degrees of sprain on the medial side of the right knee: grade 1, mild sprain of the medial collateral ligament; grade 2, moderate sprain with hematoma formation; grade 3, severe sprain with total disruption of the ligament; and grade 4, severe sprain with avulsion of the medial femoral condyle at the insertion of the medial collateral ligament. (Adapted from Spickler LL: Knee injuries of the athlete. Orthop Nurs 2, No 5:12–13, 1983)*

hours to reduce pain and swelling of the affected area. Exercises, correct posture, and good body mechanics help to reduce the potential for reinjury.

Dislocations

Dislocation of a joint is the loss of articulation of the bone ends within the joint capsule caused by displacement or separation of the bone end from its position in the joint. It usually occurs after a very severe trauma that disrupts the holding ligaments. Dislocations are seen in the shoulder and acromioclavicular joints, occasionally in the hip, and rarely in the knee. A *subluxation* is a partial dislocation in which the bone ends within the joint are still in partial contact with each other.

Dislocations can be congenital, traumatic, or pathologic. Congenital dislocations occur in the hip and knee. Traumatic dislocations occur after falls, blows, or rotational injuries. In the shoulder and patella, dislocations may become recurrent, especially in athletes. They recur with the same motion but require less and less force each time. Pathologic dislocation in the hip is a late complication of infection, rheumatoid arthritis, paralysis, and neuromuscular diseases. Dislocations of the phalangeal joints are not serious and are usually reduced by manipulation. Less common sites of dislocation, seen mainly in young adults, are the wrist and midtarsal region. They are usually the result of violent force.

Diagnosis of a dislocation is made by physical examination and confirmed by x-ray. The symptoms are pain, deformity, and limited movement. With recurrent dislocations, the person often senses the impending dislocation and may have a look of apprehension when range of joint motion is tested.

The treatment depends on the site, mechanism of injury, and associated injuries such as fractures. Dislocations that do not reduce spontaneously usually require manipulation or surgical repair. Various surgical procedures can also be used to prevent redislocation of the patella, shoulder, or acromioclavicular joints. Immobilization is necessary for several weeks following reduction of a dislocation; this allows for healing of the joint structures. In dislocations affecting the knee, isometric quadriceps-strengthening exercises may be used alone or with a temporary brace instead of surgery. Surgical procedures, such as joint replacement, may be necessary in certain pathologic dislocations.

Recurrent subluxation and dislocation of the patella are common injuries in young adults. They account for about 10% of all athletic injuries and are more common in females. Sports such as skiing or tennis may cause stress on the patella. These sports involve external rotation of the foot and lower leg with knee flexion, a position that exerts rotational stresses on the knee. There is often a sensation of the patella "popping out" when the dislocation occurs. Other complaints include the knee giving out, swelling, crepitus, stiffness, and loss of range of motion. Congenital knee variations are predisposing factors. Treatment can be difficult, but nonsurgical methods are used first. They include immobilization with the knee extended, bracing, salicylates, and isometric quadriceps-strengthening exercises. Surgical intervention may be necessary in many cases.

Chondromalacia

Chondromalacia, or softening of the articular cartilage, is seen most commonly on the undersurface of the patella and occurs most frequently in young adults. It can be the result of recurrent subluxation of the patella or overuse in strenuous athletic activities. Patients with this disorder typically complain of pain, particularly when climbing stairs or sitting with the knees bent. Occasionally there is weakness of the knee. The treatment consists of rest, isometric exercises, and application of ice after exercise. Part of the patella may be surgically removed in severe cases. In less severe cases, shaving of the soft portion is accomplished using a saw through the arthroscope.

Loose Bodies

Loose bodies are small pieces of bone or cartilage inside the joint. These can be the result of trauma to the joint or may occur when cartilage has worn away from the articular surface, causing a part of the surface bone to die. When this happens, a piece of bone separates and becomes free floating. The symptoms are painful catching and locking of the joint. Loose bodies are commonly seen in the knee, elbow, hip, and ankle. The treatment consists of surgical removal. The loose body repeatedly gets caught in the crevice of a joint, pinching the underlying healthy cartilage; unless the loose body is removed, it may cause osteoarthritis and restricted movement.

Fractures

Normal bone can withstand considerable compression and shearing forces and, to a lesser extent, tension forces. A fracture is any break in the continuity of bone that occurs when more stress is placed on the bone than it is able to absorb. Grouped according to their etiology, fractures can be divided into three major categories: (1) fractures caused by sudden injury, (2) fatigue or stress fractures, and (3) pathologic fractures. The most frequently occurring fractures are those resulting from sudden injury. The mechanism of force causing the fracture may be direct, from a fall or blow, or indirect, resulting from a massive muscle contraction or from trauma transmitted along the bone. For example, the head of the radius or clavicle can be fractured from the indirect forces that result from falling on an outstretched hand. A fatigue, or stress, fracture results from repeated wear on a bone. This type of fracture commonly occurs in the metatarsal bones as a result of marching or running. A pathologic fracture occurs in bones that are already weakened by disease or tumors. Fractures of this type may occur spontaneously with little or no stress. The underlying disease state can be local, as with infections, cysts, or tumors, or it can be generalized, as in osteoporosis, Paget's disease, or disseminated tumors.

Classification

Fractures are usually classified according to (1) type, (2) location, and (3) direction of the fracture line (Fig. 51-2).

Types. The type of fracture is determined by its communication with the external environment, the degree of break in continuity of the bone, and the character of the fracture pieces. A fracture can be classified as either open or closed. When the bone fragments have broken through the skin, the fracture is called an *open or compound fracture*. Open fractures are often complicated by infection, osteomyelitis, delayed union, or nonunion. In a *closed fracture* there is no communication with the outside skin.

The degree of a fracture is described in terms of a partial or complete break in the continuity of bone. A *greenstick fracture,* which is seen in children, is an example of a partial break in bone continuity and resembles that of a freshly cut sapling. This occurs because children's bones, especially until about age 10, are more resilient than the bones of adults.

A fracture is also described by the character of the fracture pieces. A *comminuted fracture* has more than two pieces. A *compression fracture,* such as occurs in the vertebral body, involves two bones that are crushed or squeezed together. A fracture is called *impacted* when the fracture fragments are wedged together. This type usually occurs in the humerus and is often less serious and generally treated without surgery.

Pattern. The direction of the trauma or mechanism of injury produces a certain configuration or pattern of fracture. Reduction is the restoration of a fractured bone to its normal anatomic position. The pattern of a fracture indicates the nature of the trauma and provides information regarding the easiest method for reduction. Transverse fractures are caused by simple angulatory forces. A spiral fracture results from a twisting motion, or torque. A transverse fracture is not likely to become displaced or lose its position after it is reduced. On the other hand, spiral, oblique, and comminuted fractures are often unstable or may change position following reduction.

Location. A long bone is divided into three parts: proximal, midshaft, and distal (see Fig. 51-2). A fracture of the long bone is described in relation to its position in the bone. Other descriptions are used when the fracture affects the head or neck of a bone, involves a joint, or is near a prominence such as a condyle or malleolus.

Signs and symptoms. The signs and symptoms of a fracture include pain, tenderness at the site of bone disruption, swelling, loss of function, deformity of the affected part, and abnormal mobility. The deformity varies according to the type of force applied, the area of the bone involved, the type of fracture produced, and the strength and balance of the surrounding muscles. In long bones, three types of deformities—angulation, shortening, and rotation—are seen. Severely angulated fracture fragments may be felt at the fracture site and often push up against the soft tissue to cause a tenting effect on the skin. Bending forces and unequal muscle pulls cause angulation. Shortening of the extremity occurs as the bone fragments slide and override each other because of the pull of the muscles on the long axis of the extremity

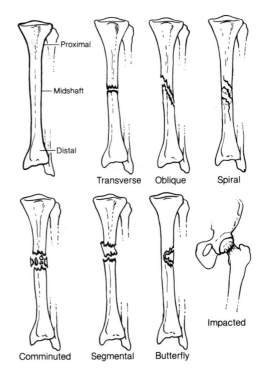

Figure 51-2 *Classification of fractures. Fractures are classified according to location (proximal, midshaft, or distal), the direction of fracture line (transverse, oblique, spiral), and type (comminuted, segmental, butterfly, or impacted).*

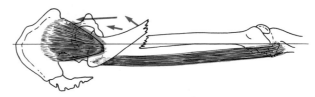

Figure 51-3 *Displacement and overriding of fracture fragments of a long bone (femur) caused by severe muscle spasm.*

(Fig. 51-3). Rotational deformity occurs when the fracture fragments rotate out of their normal longitudinal axis; this can result from rotational strain produced by the fracture or unequal pull by the muscles that are attached to the fracture fragments. A crepitus or grating sound may be heard as the bone fragments rub against each other. In the case of an open fracture, there is bleeding from the wound where the bone protrudes.

Shortly after the fracture has occurred, nerve function at the fracture site may be temporarily lost. The area may become numb and the surrounding muscles flaccid. This condition has been termed *local shock*. During this period, which may last for a few minutes to half an hour, fractured bones may be reduced with little or no pain. Following this brief period, pain sensation returns, and with it muscle spasms and contractions of the surrounding muscles.

Healing

Bone healing occurs in a manner similar to soft tissue healing. It is, however, a more complex process and takes longer. Although the exact mechanisms of bone healing are open to controversy, five stages of the healing process have been identified: (1) hematoma formation, (2) cellular proliferation, (3) callus formation, (4) ossification, and (5) consolidation and remodeling (Fig. 51-4). The degree of response during each of these stages is in direct proportion to the extent of trauma.

Hematoma formation. Hematoma formation occurs during the first 48 hours to 72 hours following fracture. It develops as blood from torn vessels in the bone fragments and surrounding soft tissue leaks between and around the fragments of the fractured bone. As a result of hematoma formation, clotting factors remain in the injured area to initiate the formation of a fibrin meshwork, which serves as a framework for the ingrowth of fibroblasts and new capillary buds. Granulation tissue, the result of fibroblasts and new capillaries, gradually invades and replaces the clot. When a large hematoma develops, healing is delayed because macrophages, platelets, oxygen, and nutrients for callus formation are prevented from entering the area.

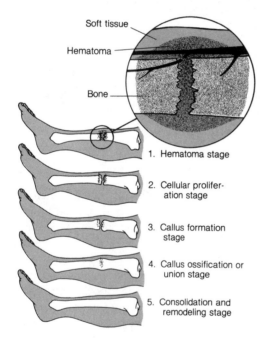

Figure 51-4 Healing of a fracture. During hematoma formation (1) a locally formed clot serves as a fibrin network for subsequent cellular invasion. Cellular proliferation (2) involves the invasion of the hematoma area by fibroblastic and endothelial cells. During callus formation (3), osteoblasts enter the area and produce the osteoid matrix. Callus formation is followed by union (4). The remodeling of the healed fracture is the last stage of the healing process (5).

Cellular proliferation. Three layers of bone structure are involved in the cellular proliferation that occurs during bone healing following a fracture: the periosteum or outer covering of the bone, the endosteum or inner covering, and the medullary canal, which contains the bone marrow. During this process the osteoblasts, or bone-forming cells, multiply and differentiate into a fibrocartilaginous callus. The fibrocartilaginous callus is softer and more flexible than callus. Cellular proliferation begins distal to the fracture, where there is a greater supply of blood. After a few days, a fibrocartilage "collar" becomes evident around the fracture site. The collar edges on either side of the fracture eventually unite to form a bridge, which connects the bone fragments.

Callus formation. During the early stage of callus formation the fracture becomes "sticky" as osteoblasts continue to move in and through the fibrin bridge to help keep it firm. Cartilage forms at the level of the fracture where circulation is less. In areas of the bone with muscle insertion, periosteal circulation is better, bringing in the nutrients necessary to bridge the callus. The bone calcifies as mineral salts are deposited. This stage occurs in 3 to 4 weeks.

Ossification. Ossification involves the final laying down of bone. This is the stage at which the fracture has been bridged and the fracture fragments are firmly united. Mature bone replaces the callus, and the excess callus is gradually reabsorbed by the osteoclasts, or cells that reabsorb bone. The fracture site now feels firm and nonmovable and appears united on x-ray. At this point, it is safe to remove the cast.

Remodeling. Structural remodeling occurs only in children and is the stage during which the bone resumes its near-normal appearance; it may go on for years. It continues according to Wolff's law of stress—bone responds to stress by becoming thicker and stronger and formed in relation to its function.

Healing time. Healing time depends on the site of the fracture, the condition of the fracture fragments, hematoma formation, and other local and host factors. In general, fractures of long bones, displaced fractures, and fractures with less surface area heal slower. Function usually returns within 6 months after union is complete. However, return to complete function may take longer.

Factors affecting healing. The factors that influence bone healing are local factors and those specific to the patient. Local factors include (1) the nature of the injury or the severity of the trauma, including fracture displacement and edema; (2) the degree of bridge formation that develops during bone healing; (3) the amount of bone loss (*e.g.*, it may be too great for the healing to bridge the gap); (4) the type of bone that is injured (*e.g.*, cancellous bone heals faster than cortical bone); (5) the degree of immobilization that is achieved (movement disrupts the fibrin bridge and cartilage forms instead of bone); (6) local infection, which retards or prevents healing; (7) local malignancy, which must be treated before healing can proceed; (8) bone necrosis, which prevents blood flow into the fracture site; and (9) intra-articular fractures (those through a joint), which may heal slower and eventually produce arthritis. Individual factors that may delay bone healing are the patient's age, current medications, debilitating diseases, such as diabetes and rheumatoid arthritis, local stress around the fracture site, circulatory problems, coagulation disorders, and poor nutrition.

Diagnosis and treatment

A *splint* is a device for immobilizing the movable fragments of a fracture. When a fracture is suspected, the injured part should always be splinted before it is moved. This is essential for preventing further injury.

Diagnosis is the first step in the care of fractures and is based on history and physical manifestations. X-ray examination is used to confirm the diagnosis and direct the treatment. The ease of diagnosis varies with the location and severity of the fracture. In the trauma patient, the presence of other more serious injuries may make diagnosis more difficult. A thorough history includes the mechanism, time, and place of the injury, first recognition of symptoms, and any treatment initiated. A complete history is important because a delay in seeking treatment or weight bearing on a fracture may have caused further injury or displacement of the fracture.

Treatment of fractures depends on the general condition of the patient, the presence of associated injuries, the location of the fracture, its displacement, and whether the fracture is open or closed. There are three objectives for treatment of fractures: (1) reduction of the fracture, (2) immobilization, and (3) preservation and restoration of the function of the injured part.

Reduction. Reduction of a fracture is directed toward replacing the bone fragments to as near a normal anatomic position as possible. This can be accomplished by closed manipulation or surgical (open) reduction. Closed manipulation uses methods such as manual pressure and traction. Fractures are held in reduction by external or internal fixation devices. Surgical reduction involves the use of various types of hardware to accomplish internal fixation of the fracture fragments (Fig. 51-5).

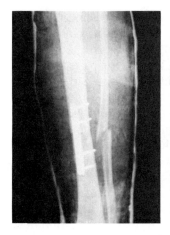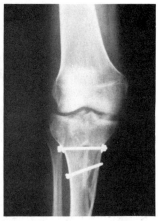

Figure 51-5 (Left) *Internal fixation of the tibia with compression plate.* (Right) *Internal fixation of an intra-articular fracture of the upper tibia with a screw and bolt.* (From Farrell J: *Illustrated Guide to Orthopedic Nursing*, 2nd ed. Philadelphia, JB Lippincott, 1982)

Immobilization. Immobilization prevents movement of the injured parts and is the single most important element in obtaining union of the fracture fragments. Immobilization can be accomplished through the use of external devices, such as splints, casts, external fixation devices, or traction, or by means of internal fixation devices inserted during surgical reduction of the fracture.

Splints. Spints are made from many different materials. Metal splints or air splints may be used during transport to a health care facility as a temporary measure until the fracture has been reduced and another form of immobilization instituted. Plaster of paris splints, which are molded to fit the extremity, work well. Splinting should be done if there is any suspicion of a fracture because motion of the fracture site can cause pain, bleeding, more soft tissue damage, and nerve or blood vessel compression. If the fracture has sharp fragments, movement can cause perforation of the skin and conversion of a closed fracture into an open one. When a splint is applied to an extremity, it should extend from the joint above the fracture site to the joint below it.

Casts. Casts (plaster or synthetic material) are commonly used to immobilize fractures of the extremities. They are often applied with a joint in partial flexion to prevent rotation of the fracture fragments. Without this flexion, the extremity, which is essentially a cylinder, tends to rotate within the cylindrical structure of the cast.

The application of a cast brings the risk of impaired circulation to the extremity because of blood vessel compression. A cast applied shortly after a fracture may not be large enough to accommodate the swelling that inevitably occurs in the hours that follow. Therefore, after a cast is applied, the peripheral circulation must be observed carefully until this danger has passed. Should the circulation become inadequate, the parts that are exposed at the distal end of the cast (*e.g.,* the toes with a leg cast and the fingers with an arm cast) may become cold and cyanotic or pale. An increase in pain may occur initially, followed by paresthesia (tingling or abnormal sensation) or anesthesia as the sensory neurons that supply the area are affected. There will be a decrease in the amplitude or absence of the pulse in areas where the arteries can be palpated. Capillary refill time, which is assessed by applying pressure to the fingernail and then observing the rate of blood return, is prolonged to greater than 3 seconds. This condition demands immediate measures, such as splitting the cast, to restore the circulation and prevent permanent damage to the extremity.

External fixation devices.   With external fixation devices, pins or screws are inserted directly into the bone above and below the fracture site. They are then secured to a metal frame and adjusted to align the fracture. The Hoffman device (Fig. 51-6) is often used for this purpose. Meticulous care is needed at the pin sites to prevent infection. This method of treatment is primarily used for open fractures of the tibia. It is also used in the treatment of other open fractures, infections such as osteomyelitis and septic joints, and unstable closed fractures and for limb lengthening.

Traction.   Another method for achieving immobility and maintaining reduction is *traction.* Traction is a pulling force applied to an extremity or part of the body

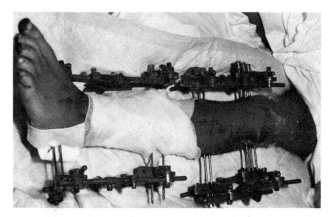

Figure 51-6 *Hoffman device (a form of external fixation) applied to a 19-year-old male with compound comminuted fractures of the tibia and fibula. Note the demarcation of the toes due to vascular insufficiency.*

while a counterforce, or countertraction, pulls in the opposite direction. Countertraction is usually exerted by the body's weight on the bed. Traction is used to maintain alignment of the fracture fragments and reduce muscle spasm.

Effective traction prevents movement of the fracture site. When fractures occur from trauma, there is associated muscle spasm to soft tissue. The muscle contractions cause overriding and displacement of the bone fragments, particularly when fractures affect long bones. The five goals of traction therapy are to (1) correct and maintain the skeletal alignment of either entire bones or joints, (2) reduce pressure on a joint surface, (3) correct, lessen, or prevent deformities such as contractures and dislocations, (4) decrease muscle spasm, and (5) immobilize a part in order to promote healing. Traction may be used as a temporary measure prior to surgery or as a primary treatment method.

There are three types of traction: manual traction, skin traction, and skeletal traction (Fig. 51-7). *Manual traction* consists of a steady, firm pull that is exerted by the hands. It is a temporary measure used to manipulate a fracture during closed reduction, for support of a neck injury during transport when cervical-spine fracture is suspected, or for reduction of a dislocated joint.

Skin traction is a pulling force applied to the skin and soft tissue. It is accomplished by strips of adhesive, flannel, or foam secured to the injured part. Skin traction is used to treat strains (cervical and pelvic traction), hip dislocation (Bryant's or Buck's extension traction), and femoral fractures in children (Russell's traction) and as a temporary or primary treatment for hip fractures (Buck's extension traction).

Skeletal traction is a pulling force applied directly to the bone. Pins, wires, or tongs are inserted through the skin and subcutaneous tissue into the bone distal to the fracture site. Muscles, tendons, arteries, and nerves are identified during the insertion process so that they are not penetrated. Pins are not inserted into joints or open areas. Skeletal traction provides an excellent pull. It can be used for long periods of time and with large amounts of weight. It is commonly used for fractures of the femur, of the humerus, and the cervical spine (Crutchfield tongs). Skeletal traction is also used in maintaining alignment of fractures that are casted and in certain types of reconstructive foot surgery.

Pin tract infection is a complication of skeletal traction. Pin insertion sites should be inspected daily for redness, drainage, and shifting of the traction device. Larger pins need to be cleansed daily with hydrogen peroxide or an antibiotic solution.

Three forces always operate with traction: (1) the pull of the traction itself, (2) countertraction, and (3) friction. Because these are vector forces, they have magnitude and direction. The forces are calculated by using weights to create a pull on different lengths of *rope* between *pulleys* of different *angles*. The number of pulleys used in the traction set-up affects the total pulling force, for example, two pulleys in the line of pull double the pulling force of the weight. Ropes are secured to the traction device and weight hanger. The ropes should be free of friction and hang unimpeded in the pulley grooves, while the weights attached to the pulling ropes should hang freely and not be removed unless traction is intermittent. Weights are prescribed according to the site of the fracture, the strength of the muscle mass, and the age and weight of the patient. Ten or fewer pounds are used with skin traction. Skeletal traction may require more weight.

The angles of traction are determined by the placement of bars on the bedframe holding the pulleys and the position of the affected body part. The resultant line of pull should be along the axis of the bone.

Preservation and restoration of function. During the period of immobilization required for fracture healing, the *preservation and restoration* of function of muscles and joints is an ongoing process in the unaffected as well as affected extremities. Exercises designed to preserve function, maintain muscle strength, and reduce joint stiffness should be started early. Active range of motion, in which the individual moves the extremity, is done on unaffected extremities; and isometric, or muscle tensing, exercises are done on the affected extremities. After the fracture has healed, a program of physical therapy may be necessary. However, the most important factor in restoring function is the person's own active exercises.

Lack of use during immobilization tends to result in muscle atrophy. Joints stiffen as muscles and tendons contract and shorten. The degree of muscle atrophy and joint stiffness depends on several factors. In adults, the degree of atrophy and muscle stiffness are directly related to the length of immobilization, with longer periods of immobility resulting in greater stiffness. Children have a natural tendency to move on their own, and this movement maintains muscle and joint function. Therefore, they usually have less atrophy and recover sooner once the source of immobilization has been removed. Associated soft tissue injury, infection, and preexisting joint disease increase the risk of stiffness. Even though limbs are immobilized in a functional position, casts are removed as soon as fracture healing has taken place.

Complications of fractures

The complications of fractures can be divided into two groups: (1) early complications associated with loss of skeletal continuity, injury from bone fragments, pressure due to swelling and hemorrhage, or development of fat

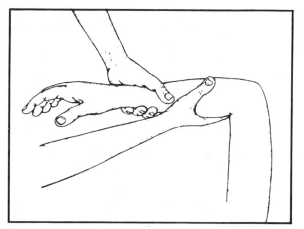

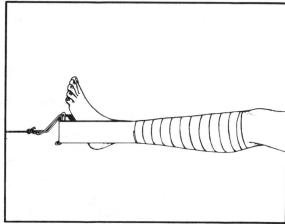

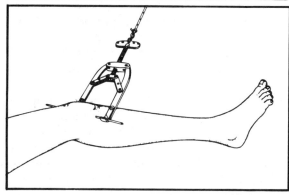

Figure 51-7 *Three types of traction. (Top) Manual traction, in which the hands are used to exert a pulling force on the bone to be realigned; (middle) skin traction, in which strips of tape or some type of commercial skin traction strips are applied directly to the skin; (bottom) skeletal traction, in which the traction force is applied directly to the bone using pins, wires, or screws. (Courtesy of Zimmer, Inc., Warsaw, Indiana)*

emboli, and (2) complications that are associated with fracture healing. The early complications of fractures depend on the severity of the fracture and the area of the body that is involved. For example, bone fragments from a skull fracture may cause injury to brain tissue or multiple rib fractures may lead to a flail chest and respiratory insufficiency. With flail chest, the chest wall on the fractured side becomes so unstable that it may move in the opposite direction of the chest wall when the patient breathes.

Compartment syndrome. Compartment syndrome is the compression of nerves and blood vessels that can occur after a fracture. It is caused by excessive swelling around the fracture site resulting in increased pressure (30 mm Hg or more) within a closed compartment. This occurs because fascia, which covers and separates muscles, is inelastic and unable to compensate for the extreme swelling. It causes severe pain because of passive stretching of soft tissue and skin. There may be a change in sensation, paresthesia such as burning or tingling, diminished reflexes, and eventually loss of motor function resulting from nerve compression. Compression of blood vessels may cause muscle ischemia and loss of function. Permanent muscle and nerve damage may occur if the pressure is not relieved. In contrast with ischemia caused by a tight bandage or cast, in the compartment syndrome the peripheral pulses are normal. The compartment syndrome is more common with crushing type injuries, in closed fractures, and when external compression of a limb produces a tourniquet effect. Treatment is directed at reducing the compression of blood vessels and nerves. Constrictive dressings and casts are loosened, and the involved area is elevated. A fasciotomy, or transection of the fascia that is restricting the muscle compartment, may be required when the pressure in the area rises above 30 mm Hg, which is about equal to the perfusion pressure in the capillary beds. Peripheral nerve damage may also result from injury or entrapment of nerve fibers by bone fragments, stretching of tissues and nerves, or the external compression of compression dressings or casts.

Fat emboli. Fat emboli result from the introduction of intracellular fat globules into the pulmonary and systemic circulation. There are two theories regarding the origin of fat emboli. One theory is that fat globules are released from the bone marrow or subcutaneous tissue at the fracture site into the venous system through torn veins.[2] The second theory postulates that the fat emboli develop intravascularly secondary to an alteration in lipid stability caused by increased tissue lipases, catecholamines, glucagon, or other steroid hormones that are released in response to the stress of injury.[3]

Fat emboli travel throughout the circulation, but their presence in the lung presents the greatest danger to the person's life. The emboli may also pass through the lung and enter the cerebral circulation. Emboli in the cerebral circulation combined with respiratory depression accounts for the mental confusion often seen in patients with the disorder. There are three possible outcomes when fat emboli enter the pulmonary circulation: (1) small emboli may mold to vessel caliber, pass through the lung, and then enter the systemic circulation where they are either trapped in the tissues or eliminated through the kidney, (2) the fat particles may be broken down by alveolar cells and eliminated through sputum, and (3) local lipolysis may occur with release of free fatty acid.[4] Free fatty acids cause direct injury to the alveolar capillary membrane, which leads to hemorrhagic interstitial pneumonitis with disruption of surfactant production and development of the adult respiratory distress syndrome. In addition, the fat globules become coated with platelets, causing a thrombocytopenia. Sequestered platelets release serotonin, resulting in bronchospasm and vasodilatation.

Clinically, the incidence of fat embolization is related to fractures of bones containing the most marrow, for example, long bones and bones of the pelvis. Initial symptoms begin to develop from within a few hours to 3 to 4 days following injury and do not appear beyond 1 week following the injury. The first symptoms include a subtle change in behavior and signs of disorientation. There may be complaints of substernal chest pain and dyspnea accompanied by tachycardia and a low-grade fever. Diaphoresis, pallor, and cyanosis become evident as respiratory function deteriorates. A petechial rash that does not blanch with pressure often occurs 2 to 3 days following the injury. This rash is usually found on the anterior chest, axillae, neck, and shoulders. It may also appear on the soft palate and conjunctiva. The rash is thought to be related to embolization of the skin capillaries or thrombocytopenia.

An important part of the treatment of fat emboli is detecting them. The treatment is directed toward correcting hypoxemia and maintaining adequate fluid balance. Mechanical ventilation may be required. Administration of corticosteroid drugs is used to reduce the inflammatory response of lung tissues, decrease the edema, stabilize the lipid membranes to reduce lypolysis, and combat the bronchospasm.

Impaired healing. *Union* of a fracture has occurred when the fracture is solid enough to withstand normal stresses and it is clinically and radiologically safe to remove the external fixation. In children, fractures generally heal within 4 to 6 weeks; in adolescents, they heal within 6 to 8 weeks; and in adults, they heal within 10 to 18 weeks.

Delayed union is the failure of a fracture to unite within the normal time period (*e.g.,* 20 weeks for a fracture of the tibia or femur in an adult). The treatment for delayed union is determining and correcting the cause of the delay. *Malunion* is healing with deformity, angulation, or rotation that is visible on x-ray. It is usually treated by surgery.

Nonunion is failure to produce union and cessation of the processes of bone repair. It is characterized by mobility of the fracture site and pain on weight bearing. Muscle atrophy and loss of range of motion may also be present. Nonunion is usually established 6 to 12 months after the time of the fracture. The complications of fracture healing are summarized in Table 51-1. Treatment methods for impaired bone healing include surgical interventions, bracing, or electrical stimulation of the bone ends. Electrical stimulation is thought to stimulate the osteoblasts to lay down a network of bone. Three types of commercial bone growth stimulators are available: a noninvasive model, which is placed outside the cast; a seminoninvasive model, in which pins are inserted around the fracture site; and a totally implantable type, in which a cathode coil is wound around the bone at the fracture site and is operated by a battery pack implanted under the skin. Figure 51-8 depicts a noninvasive type of electrical stimulator.

In summary, trauma to the musculoskeletal system results from a number of external physical agents. Factors within the individual can place him or her at greater risk for injury. Some soft tissue injuries such as contusions, hematomas, and lacerations are relatively minor and easily treated. Muscle strains and ligamentous sprains are caused by mechanical overload on the connective tissue. They heal slower than the minor soft tissue injuries and

require some degree of immobilization. Healing of soft tissue begins within 4 to 5 days of the injury and is primarily the function of fibroblasts, which produce collagen. Joint dislocation occurs because of trauma to the supporting structures. Repeated trauma to the joint can cause articular softening (chondromalacia) or the separation of small pieces of bone or cartilage, called loose bodies, within the joint.

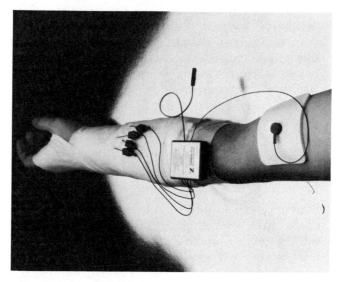

Figure 51-8 *One type of electrical stimulator used in the treatment of nonunion (Zimmer, Inc., Warsaw, Indiana. From Farrell J: Illustrated Guide to Orthopedic Nursing, 2nd ed. Philadelphia, JB Lippincott, 1982)*

Table 51-1 Complications of Fracture Healing

Complication	Manifestations	Contributing Factors
Delayed union	Failure of fracture to heal within predicted time as determined by x-ray	Large displaced fracture Inadequate immobilization Large hematoma Infection at fracture site Excessive loss of bone Inadequate circulation
Malunion	Deformity at fracture site Deformity or angulation on x-ray	Inadequate reduction Malalignment of fracture at time of immobilization
Nonunion	Failure of bone to heal before the process of bone repair stops Evidence on x-ray Motion at fracture site Pain on weight bearing	Inadequate reduction Mobility at fracture site Severe trauma Bone fragment separation Soft tissue between bone fragments Infection Extensive loss of bone Inadequate circulation Malignancy Bone necrosis Noncompliance with restrictions

Fractures occur when the stress placed on a bone is greater than what the bone can absorb. The nature of the stress determines the type of fracture and the character of the bone fragments. Healing of fractures is a complex process that takes place in five stages: hematoma formation, cellular proliferation, callus formation, ossification, and consolidation and remodeling. For satisfactory healing to take place, the affected bone has to be reduced and immobilized. This is accomplished by either surgically implanted internal fixation devices or external fixation devices such as splints, casts, or traction. The complications associated with fractures can occur early when damage to soft tissue, blood vessels, and nerves is present or later when the healing process is interrupted. Local factors related to the healing environment and the individual's general physical condition affect the healing process.

Bone Infections

Bone infections are difficult to treat and eradicate. Their effects can be devastating; they can cause pain, disability, and deformity. Chronic bone infections may drain for years because of a sinus tract. This occurs when a passageway develops from an abscess or cavity within the bone to an opening through the skin.

Iatrogenic Bone Infections

Iatrogenic bone infections are those inadvertently brought about by surgery or other treatment. These infections include complications such as pin tract infections in skeletal traction, septic (infected) joints in joint replacement surgery, and wound infection following any surgery. Preparation of the skin to reduce bacterial growth prior to surgery or insertion of traction devices or wires, strict operating room protocols, prophylactic use of antibiotics, and maintenance of sterile technique when working with drainage tubes and dressing changes are measures used to prevent these infections. Because of the danger of infection, orthopedic wounds are kept covered with a sterile dressing until they are closed.

Osteomyelitis

Osteomyelitis represents an acute or chronic pyogenic infection of the bone. The term *osteo* refers to bone and *myelo* to the marrow cavity, both of which are involved in this disease. It can be caused by hematogenous seeding, direct extension, or direct contamination of an open fracture or wound. In 60% to 70% of the cases, *Staphylococcus aureus* is the infecting organism.[5]

The most common cause of osteomyelitis is the direct contamination of bone from an open wound. It may be the result of an open fracture, a gunshot wound, or a puncture wound. The introduction of foreign material into the wound plus extensive tissue injury are factors that make the bone susceptible to infection. If the infection is not adequately treated, the acute infection may become chronic.

Acute hematogenous osteomyelitis

Acute hematogenous osteomyelitis is almost always limited to those under age 21. It affects, in order of frequency, the femur, tibia, humerus, and radius.[5] The condition usually manifests itself as an acute febrile systemic illness accompanied by the signs of the local bone lesion. The infection generally begins in the metaphysis of the bone where the nutrient artery channels terminate and the blood flow is sluggish. Because of the bone's rigid structure, there is little room for swelling; the pus that forms finds its way to the surface of the bone to form a subperiosteal abscess. The blood supply to the bone may become obstructed by septic thrombi, in which case the ischemic bone becomes necrotic. It then separates from the viable surrounding bone to form a fragment of bone known as a sequestrum (Fig. 51-9).

In children, acute hematogenous osteomyelitis is usually preceded by staphylococcal or streptococcal infections of the skin, sinuses, teeth, or middle ear. There is a history of trauma in one-third of the cases; the trauma apparently reduces the bone's ability to respond to infection.

The signs and symptoms of acute hematogenous osteomyelitis are those of bacteremia accompanied by symptoms referable to the site of the bone lesion. There is often pain on movement of the affected extremity, loss of movement, and local tenderness followed by heat and swelling. X-rays may be normal initially, but they will show evidence of periosteal elevation and increased osteoclastic activity once an abscess has formed. Changes will be evident on a bone scan 10 to 14 days before any radiographic changes are seen.

In the adult, hematogenous osteomyelitis usually affects the axial skeleton and the irregular-shaped bones in the wrist and ankle. It is most common in debilitated patients and in those with a history of chronic skin infections, chronic urinary tract infections, and intravenous drug use.

The treatment of acute osteomyelitis begins with identification of the causative organism through blood cultures, aspiration cultures, and Gram stains. Antibiotics are given for several weeks, usually intravenously. Local rest of the affected limb and pain relief are based on symptomatology. Debridement and surgical drainage may also be necessary.

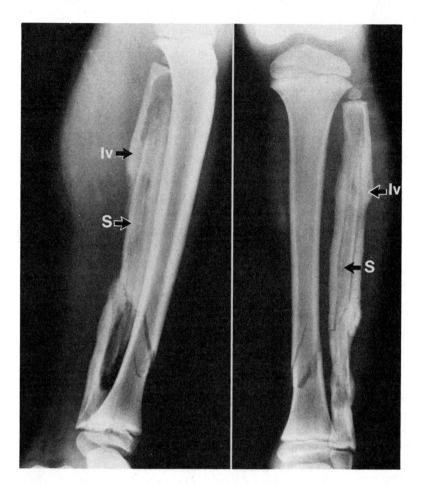

Figure 51-9 Hematomogenous osteomyelitis of the fibula of 3 months' duration. The entire shaft has been deprived of its blood supply and has become a sequestrum (S) surrounded by new immature bone, involucrum (Iv). Pathologic fractures are present in the lower tibia and fibula. (From Wilson FC: The Musculoskeletal System: Basic Processes and Disorders, 2nd ed, p 150. Philadelphia, JB Lippincott, 1980)

Chronic osteomyelitis

Chronic osteomyelitis has long been recognized as a disease. The incidence, however, has decreased in the last century because of improved surgical techniques and antibiotic therapy. Chronic osteomyelitis includes all inflammatory processes in the bone, excluding those in rheumatic diseases, that are caused by microorganisms. It may be the result of delayed or inadequate treatment of acute hematogenous osteomyelitis or osteomyelitis caused by direct contamination of bone. Acute osteomyelitis is considered chronic when the infection persists either beyond 6 to 8 weeks or when the acute process has been adequately treated and expected to resolve. Chronic osteomyelitis can persist for years; it may appear spontaneously, after a minor trauma, or when resistance is lowered. The hallmark feature of chronic osteomyelitis is the presence of infected dead bone, a sequestrum, that has separated from the living bone. A sheath of new bone called the involucrum, forms around the dead bone. Radiologic techniques such as x-rays, bone scans, and sinograms are used to identify the infected site.

Treatment

The treatment of bone infections begins with wound cultures to identify the microorganism and its sensitivity to antibiotic therapy. This is followed by surgery to remove foreign bodies (*e.g.*, metal plates or screws) or sequestrum and long-term antibiotic therapy. Wounds may be left open and packed or closed with a continuous wound-irrigation system in place for several days to several weeks postoperatively. The irrigation system consists of an antibiotic or sodium chloride solution that is flushed directly into the site of the infection and suctioned out by means of a closed drainage system. Immobilization of the affected part is usually necessary, with restriction of weight bearing on a lower extremity.

Hyperbaric oxygenation. Chronic refractory osteomyelitis that has been resistant to other forms of treatment may be treated with hyperbaric oxygenation. Hyperbaric oxygenation, which is the intermittent, short-term administration of 100% oxygen at a greater than normal atmospheric pressure, increases tissue oxygenation and vascularity and reduces edema by releasing pressure on the capillary bed. The improvement of local vascularity enhances bone and soft tissue healing and produces a bacteriocidal effect by facilitating the host's leukocyte defense response function. The increased oxygen also creates a favorable environment for the removal of bony debris and the remnants of the infectious process by osteoclasts. Hyperbaric oxygenation is known to increase the rate of granulation tissue but has not been proven effective in all forms of osteomyelitis. It is thought to be best utilized for anaerobic infections. Not all hospitals and medical centers have facilities for hyperbaric oxygenation treatment.

Tuberculosis

Tuberculosis can spread from one part of the body, such as the lungs or occasionally the lymph nodes, to the bones and joints. It is caused by *Mycobacterium tuberculosis*. The disease is localized and progressively destructive. It affects the vertebrae in about half of the cases, but it is also frequently seen in the hip and knee. The disease is characterized by bone destruction and abscess formation. Local symptoms include pain, immobility, and muscle atrophy; joint swelling, mild fever, and leukocytosis may also be present. Diagnosis is confirmed by a positive culture. The most important part of the treatment is antituberculosis drug therapy. Because of improved methods to prevent and treat tuberculosis, its incidence has diminished in recent decades. Unfortunately, however, the diagnosis of tuberculosis in the bones and joints may be missed because it is not often seen in clinical practice.

In summary, bone infections occur because of either the direct or the indirect invasion of the skeletal circulation by microorganisms, most commonly the bacterium *Staphylococcus aureus*. Osteomyelitis, or infection of the bone and marrow, can be an acute or chronic disease. Acute osteomyelitis is seen most often as a result of the direct contamination of bone by a foreign object. Chronic osteomyelitis is a long-term process that can recur spontaneously at any time throughout a person's life. The incidence of all types of bone infection has been dramatically reduced since the advent of antibiotic therapy.

■ Study Guide

After you have studied this chapter, you should be able to meet the following objectives:

☐ Describe the physical agents responsible for soft tissue trauma.

☐ Name the three types of soft tissue injuries.

☐ Compare muscle strains and ligamentous sprains.

☐ Describe the healing process of soft tissue injuries.

☐ State three causes of joint dislocation.

☐ Name three causes of fractures.

☐ Differentiate between open and closed fractures.

☐ List the signs and symptoms of a fracture.

☐ Describe the fracture healing process.

☐ Relate individual and local factors to the healing process in bone.

☐ Differentiate between internal and external fixation methods used in the treatment of fractures.

☐ Explain the importance of immobilization for fracture healing.

☐ Define traction.

☐ Cite the five goals of traction.

☐ Name the three types of traction.

☐ Explain how traction provides a pulling force.

☐ Describe the rationale for maintenance of muscle and joint function during fracture healing.

☐ Describe the pathogenesis of the compartment syndrome.

☐ Explain the origin and development of fat embolization.

☐ Differentiate between the early complications of fractures and later complications of fracture healing.

☐ Explain the implications of bone infection.

☐ Describe how an acute form of osteomyelitis becomes chronic.

■ References

1. Wright PH, Brashear HR: The local response to trauma. In Wilson FC (ed): The Musculoskeletal System: Basic Processes and Disorders, 2nd ed, p 264. Philadelphia, JB Lippincott, 1980
2. Oh WH, Mital MA: Fat embolism: Current concepts of pathogenesis, diagnosis, and treatment. Orthop Clin North Am 9:767, 1976
3. Maylan JA, Evenson MA: Diagnosis and treatment of fat embolism. Annu Rev Med 28:885, 1979
4. Oldman GL, Weise W: Fat embolism. Ariz Med 36, No 12:885, 1979
5. Robins SL, Cotran RS: Pathologic Basis of Disease, p 1484. Philadelphia, WB Saunders, 1979

■ Additional References

Adinhoff AD, Hollister JR: Steroid induced fractures and bone loss in patients with asthma. N Engl J Med 309:265, 1983

Blockey NJ: Chronic osteomyelitis an unusual variant. J Bone Joint Surg 65-B, No 2:120, 1983

Bolton ME: Hyperbaric oxygen therapy. Am J Nurs 81:1199, 1981

Christianson F: Closed wound irrigation in orthopedics. ONA J 6:359, 1979

Cole WG, Dalziel RE, Leitl J: Treatment of acute osteomyelitis in childhood. J Bone Joint Surg 64-H, No 2:218, 1982

Farrell J: Orthopedic pain: What does it mean. Am J Nurs 84:466, 1984

Gill KP et al: External fixation: The erector sets of orthopedic nursing. Can Nurs 80:29, 1984

Kilcoyne RF et al: Acute osteomyelitis of the lower extremity. Nurs Mirror 155:7, 1982

Kuska BM: Acute onset compartment syndrome. J Emerg Nurs 8:75, 1982

Lupien AE: Head off compartment syndrome before its too late. RN:39, 1980

Miller MC: Nursing care of the patient with external fixation therapy. Orthop Nurs 2:11, 1980

Morrey BF et al: Hyperbaric oxygen and chronic osteomyelitis. Clin Ortho 144:121, 1979

Nade S: Acute hematogenous osteomyelitis in infancy and childhood. J Bone Joint Surg 65-B, No 2:109, 1983

Patterson DC, Lewis GN, Cass CA: Treatment of delayed union and nonunion with implanted direct current stimulator. Clin Orthop 140:117, 1980

Searls K et al: External fixation: General principles of patient care. CCQ 6:45, 1983

Septimus EJ, Musher DM: Osteomyelitis: Recent clinical and laboratory aspects. Orthop Clin North Am 10, No 2:347, 1979

Sisk TD: General principles and techniques of external skeletal fixation. Clin Orthop 180:96, 1983

Special supplement on traction. Amer J Nurs 79:1771, 1979

Taylor JF: Osteomyelitis the acute form. Nurs Times 72:486, 1976

Taylor JF: Osteomyelitis the chronic form. Nurs Times 72:535, 1976

Valerz JM: Surgical implants: Orthopedic devices. AORN J 37:1341, 1983

Yasuda I: Fundamental aspects of fracture treatment. Clin Orthop 124:5, 1977

Chapter 52

Alterations in Skeletal Function: Congenital Disorders, Metabolic Bone Disease, and Neoplasms

Kathleen E. Gunta

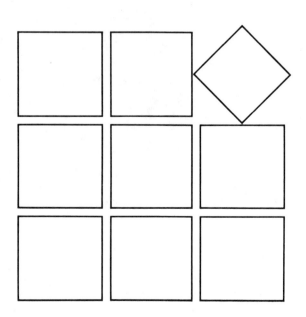

During childhood skeletal structures grow in both length and diameter with a large increase in bone mass. The term modeling refers to the formation of the macroscopic skeleton, which ceases at maturity (age 18 to 20 years). Bone remodeling functions to replace existing bone and occurs in both children and adults. It involves both resorption and formation of bone. With aging, bone resorption and formation are no longer perfectly coupled, and there is loss of bone. Alterations in musculoskeletal structure and function may develop as a result of normal growth and developmental processes or impairment of skeletal development as a result of hereditary or congenital influences. Other skeletal disorders can occur later in life as a result of metabolic disorders or neoplastic growth.

■ Alterations in Skeletal Growth and Development

Bone Growth and Remodeling

Embryonic development
The skeletal system develops from the mesoderm, the thin middle layer of embryonic tissue, by two different ossification processes: endochondral or intramembranous. Endochondral ossification involves ossification of a cartilaginous bone model. Intramembranous ossification occurs where there is no preexisting cartilage model. In the skull, it involves ossification of the loose layer of mesenchymal tissue that fills the space between the brain and the skin.

Development of the vertebrae of the axial skeleton begins at about the fourth week in the embryo; during the ninth week, ossification begins with the appearance of ossification centers in the lower thoracic and upper lumbar vertebrae. The limb buds of the appendicular skeleton make their appearance late in the fourth week. The hand pads are present on day 33, and the finger rays are evident on day 41 of embryonic development.[1]

Bone growth in childhood
During the first two decades of life general overall growth of the skeleton occurs. The long bones of the skeleton, which grow at a relatively rapid rate, are provided with a specialized structure called the epiphyseal growth plate. As long bones grow in length, the deeper layers of cartilage cells in the growth plate multiple and

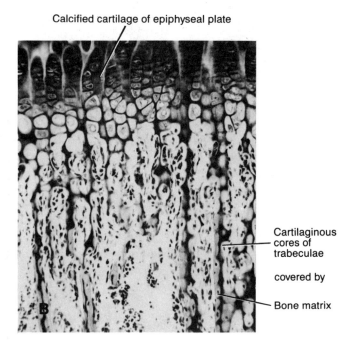

Figure 52-1   (A) *Low-power photomicrograph of one end of a growing long bone (rat). Osteogenesis has now spread from the epiphyseal center of ossification so that only the articular cartilage above and the epiphyseal disk below remain cartilaginous. On the diaphyseal side of the epiphyseal plate (disk), metaphyseal trabeculae extend down into the diaphysis.* (B) *Medium-power photomicrograph of the area indicated in A, showing trabeculae on the diaphyseal side of the epiphyseal plate (disk). These have cores of calcified cartilage on which bone has been deposited. The cartilaginous cores of the trabeculae were formerly partitions between columns of chondrocytes in the epiphyseal plate (disk).* (From Ham AW, Cormack DH: *Histology,* 8th ed, p 429. Philadelphia, JB Lippincott, 1979)

enlarge, pushing the articular cartilage further away from the metaphysis and diaphysis of the bone. As this happens, the mature and enlarged cartilage cells at the metaphyseal end of the plate become metabolically inactive and are replaced by bone cells (Fig. 52-1). This process allows bone growth to proceed without changing the shape of the bone or causing disruption of the articular cartilage. The cells in the growth plate stop dividing at puberty, at which time the epiphysis and metaphysis fuse.

A number of factors can influence the growth of cells in the epiphyseal growth plate. Epiphyseal separation can occur in children as the result of accidents. The separation usually occurs in the zone of the mature enlarged cartilage cells, which is the weakest part of the growth plate. The blood vessels that nourish the epiphysis, which pass through the growth plate, are ruptured with the separation of the growth plate. This can cause cessation of growth and a shortened extremity.

The growth plate is also sensitive to nutritional and metabolic changes. Scurvy (vitamin C deficiency) impairs the formation of the organic matrix of bone with slowing of growth at the epiphyseal plate and cessation of diaphyseal growth. In rickets (vitamin D deficiency) calcification of the newly developed bone on the metaphyseal side of the growth plate is impaired. Thyroid and growth hormones are both required for normal growth. Alterations in these and other hormones can affect growth (see Chap. 38).

Growth in the diameter of bones occurs by oppositional growth of new bone on the surface of existing bone with an accompanying resorption of bone on the endosteal surface; in this manner the shape of the bone is maintained. Figure 52-2 illustrates how bone is deposited and resorbed during structural remodeling at the ends of growing long bones. As a bone grows in diameter, concentric rings are added to the bone surface, much like the rings of a tree trunk. Osteocytes, which develop from osteoblasts, become buried in these rings forming the lamellar structure of mature bone. Haversian channels form as periosteal vessels running along the long axis become surrounded by bone.

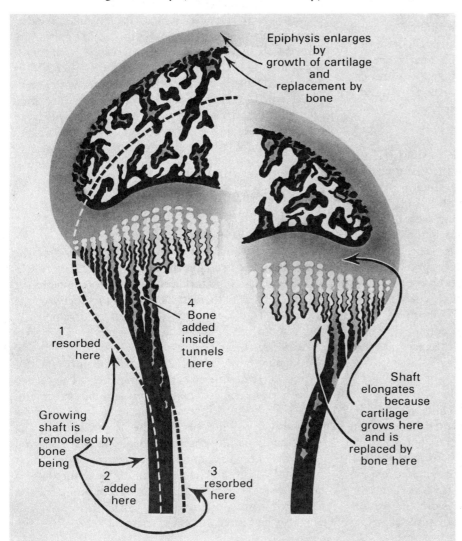

Figure 52-2 *Diagram illustrating the surfaces where bone is deposited or resorbed during remodeling at the ends of growing long bones with flared extremities. (From Ham AW, Cormack DH: Histology, 8th ed, p 436. Philadelphia, JB Lippincott, 1979)*

Alterations Occurring During Normal Growth Periods

Infants and children undergo changes in muscle tone and joint motion during growth and development. These changes usually cause few problems and are corrected during normal growth processes. The normal folded position of the fetus *in utero* causes physiologic flexion contractures of the hips and a froglike appearance of the lower extremities. The hips are externally rotated and the patellae point outward, while the feet appear to point forward because of the internal pulling force of the tibiae. During the first year of life the lower extremities begin to straighten out in preparation for walking. Internal and external rotation become equal, and the hips extend. Flexion contractures of the shoulders, elbows, and knees are also commonly seen in newborns, but they should disappear by 3 months of age.[2]

All infants and toddlers have lax ligaments that become tighter with age and assumption of the weight-bearing posture. The hypermobility that accompanies joint laxity along with torsional, or twisting, forces exerted on the limbs during growth are often responsible for a number of variants seen in young children. Torsional forces caused by intrauterine positions or sleeping and sitting patterns twist the growing bones and can produce the deformities seen with growth and development.

Femoral anteversion

Femoral anteversion (internal femoral torsion) is a normal variance commonly seen during the first 6 years of life, especially in 3- and 4-year-old girls. Internal rotation of the hips exceeds external rotation by 30 degrees or more. It is related to children sleeping with their toes pointing toward each other and sitting in the "M" position, with the hips between the heels. When the child stands, the knees turn in while the feet appear to point straight ahead; when the child walks, both knees and toes point in. Children with this problem are encouraged to sit in the so-called Indian chief, or "W," position. If left untreated, the tibiae compensate by becoming externally rotated so that by 8 to 12 years of age the knees may turn in but the feet no longer do.

Toeing-out

Toeing-out is a common problem in children caused by external femoral torsion. This occurs when the femur can be rotated externally to about 90 degress but internally only to a neutral position or slightly beyond. When a child habitually sleeps in the prone position, the femoral torsion will persist, and an external tibial torsion may also develop. If external tibial torsion is present, the feet point lateral to the midline of the medial plane. External tibial torsion rarely causes toeing-out; it only intensifies the condition. Toeing-out usually corrects itself as the child becomes proficient in walking. Occasionally a night splint is used.

Toeing-in

Toeing-in (pigeon toe) may be caused by torsion in the feet, lower legs, or entire leg. Toeing-in because of adduction of the forefoot is usually due to the fetal position maintained *in utero*. A supple deformity can be passively manipulated into a straight position and requires no treatment. On the other hand, treatment consisting of serial casting, followed by special outflare shoes (or wearing shoes on the opposite feet), is usually required in a fixed deformity, that is, one in which the forefoot cannot be passively manipulated into a straight position.

Internal tibial torsion

Internal tibial torsion (bowing of the tibia) is a rotation of the tibia that makes the feet appear to turn inward. It is present at birth and fails to correct itself if children either sleep on their knees with the feet turned in or sit on in-turned feet. In 80% of cases, it will resolve itself by the time the child is 18 months of age.[3] In the other 20% of cases, the Denis Browne splint (a bar onto which shoes are attached) may be used to put the feet into mild external rotation while the child is sleeping. This treatment stimulates the proximal growth plate of the tibia to grow in a spiral fashion and correct the defect. Surgery may be necessary if tibial torsion persists beyond age 3, but only if the condition is severe and significantly interferes with walking and running.

Genu varum and genu valgum

Genu varum (bowlegs) is an outward bowing of the knees when the medial malleoli of the ankles are touching. Most infants and toddlers have some bowing of their legs up to age 2. If there is a large separation between the knees after age 2, the child may require bracing. The child should also be evaluated for diseases such as rickets or tibia vara (Blount's disease).

Genu valgum (knock-knees) is a deformity in which there is decreased space between the knees. The medial malleoli in the ankles cannot be brought in contact with each other when the knees are touching. It is seen most frequently in children between the ages of 2 and 6. The condition is usually the result of lax medial collateral ligaments of the knee and may be exacerbated by sitting in the "M" position. Genu valgum can be ignored up to age 7, unless it is more than 15 degrees, unilateral, or associated with short stature. It usually resolves spontaneously and rarely requires treatment.

Flatfoot

Flatfoot is a deformity characterized by the absence of the longitudinal arch of the foot. Infants normally have a wider and fatter foot than adults. The fat pads that are normally accentuated by pliable muscles create an illusion of fullness often mistaken for flatfeet. Until the longitudinal arch develops at age 2 to 3 years, all children have flatfeet. The true criteria for flatfoot (pes planus) is that the head of the talus points medially and downward, so that the heel is everted and the forefoot must be inverted (toed in) in order for the metatarsal heads to be planted equally on the ground. With weight bearing, pain may occur in the longitudinal arch and extend up the leg.

There are two types of flatfeet—supple and rigid. Supple flatfeet are always bilateral, occur more often in black people, and tend to be familial.[3] In supple flatfeet, the arch disappears only with weight bearing. The rigid flatfoot is fixed with no apparent arch in any position.

The treatment of flatfeet is conservative and aimed at relieving fatigue, pain, and tenderness. Supportive, well-fitting shoes may be all that is needed to relieve the symptoms. Women may complain of pain in the forefoot when wearing poorly fitting high heels. Surgery may be done in cases of severe and persistent symptoms.

Juvenile Osteochondroses

The term juvenile osteochondroses is used to describe a group of children's diseases that have similar radiologic characteristics. This group of conditions was first differentiated from the septic necrosis caused by tuberculosis of the bone and referred to as aseptic necrosis. The osteochondroses are now separated into two groups according to their etiologies. The first group is called true osteonecrotic osteochondroses because the diseases are caused by localized osteonecrosis of an apophyseal or epiphyseal center (Legg–Calvé–Perthes disease, Freiberg's bone infarction or necrosis, Panner's disease, and Kienbock's disease). The diseases of the second group of juvenile osteochondroses occur because of abnormalities of endochondral ossification, caused either by a genetically determined normal variation or trauma (Osgood–Schlatter disease, Blount's disease, Sever's disease, and Scheuermann's disease). The discussion in this section focuses on Legg–Calvé–Perthes disease from the first group and Osgood–Schlatter disease from the second group.

Legg–Calvé–Perthes

Legg–Calvé–Perthes disease is an osteonecrotic disease of the proximal femoral (capital) epiphysis, which is the growth center for the head of the femur. It affects children between 3 and 12 years of age with an incidence of 1 in 1200 of the general population.[4] It occurs primarily in boys and is much more common in whites than in blacks. Although no definite genetic pattern has been established, it occasionally affects more than one family member.

The cause of Legg–Calvé–Perthes disease is unknown. The disorder is usually insidious in onset and occurs in otherwise healthy children. It may, however, be associated with acute trauma. The children usually affected have a shorter stature and 80% are boys. When girls are affected, they usually have a poorer prognosis than boys because they are skeletally more mature. This means that they would have a shorter period for growth and remodeling than boys of the same age.[5] Although both legs can be affected, in 85% of the cases only one leg is involved.

The primary pathologic feature of Legg–Calvé–Perthes disease is an avascular necrosis of the bone and marrow involving the epiphyseal growth center in the femoral head. The disorder may be confined to part of the epiphysis, or it may involve the entire epiphysis. In severe cases, there is a disturbance in the growth pattern that leads to a broad, short femoral neck. The necrosis is followed by a slow absorption of the dead bone that occurs over a 2- to 3-year period of time. Although the necrotic trabeculae are eventually replaced by healthy new bone, the epiphysis rarely regains its normal shape. The process occurs in four predictable stages, each with its distinctive radiologic characteristics:

1. The incipient or synovitis stage, which is characterized by synovial inflammation and increased joint fluid. This stage usually lasts from 1 to 3 weeks.
2. The aseptic or avascular stage, during which the ossification center becomes necrotic. This stage may last from several months to a year. Damage to the femoral head is determined by the degree of necrosis that occurs during this stage.
3. The regenerative or fragmentation stage, which involves the resorption of the necrotic bone. This stage lasts for 1 to 3 years during which time the necrotic bone is gradually replaced by new immature bone cells and the contour of the bone develops.
4. The healed or residual stage, characterized by the formation and replacement of immature bone cells by normal bone cells. Remodeling of the femoral head continues throughout the growing years but is ultimately determined by the amount of collapse that has occurred during the avascular stage.

Legg–Calvé–Perthes disease has an insidious onset with a prolonged course. The main symptoms are pain in the groin, thigh, or knee and difficulty walking. During the synovitis stage, hip motion may be limited and a hip contracture may occur. The age of onset is important because young children have a greater potential for remodeling, and thus less flattening of the femoral head will occur. Early diagnosis is important and is based on the correlation of physical symptoms and x-ray findings related to the stage of the disease.

The goal of treatment is to reduce deformity and preserve the integrity of the femoral head. Both conservative and surgical interventions are used in the treatment of Legg–Calvé–Perthes disease. Children under 4 years of age with little or no involvement of the femoral head may require only periodic observation. In all other children, some intervention is needed to relieve the force of weight bearing, the muscular tension, and subluxation of the femoral head. It is important to maintain the femur in a well-seated position in the concave acetabulum in order to prevent deformity. This is done by keeping the hip in abduction and mild internal rotation.

The initial treatment usually involves bed rest with traction or with a device to keep the legs separated in abduction with mild internal rotation (*e.g.*, hip spica cast or abduction brace). Once the inflammatory stage has subsided (usually several weeks), the child is allowed up but is not permitted to bear weight on the femoral head. The child walks with crutches and may be required to wear a brace, splint, or walking cast.

Surgery may be done to contain the femoral head within the acetabulum. This treatment is usually reserved for children older than 6 years who at the time of diagnosis have more serious involvement of the femoral head. Several sources indicate that the best surgical results are obtained when surgery is done early, before the epiphysis becomes necrotic.[6,7]

Osgood–Schlatter disease

Osgood–Schlatter disease is a partial separation of the tibial tuberosity caused by sudden or continued strain on the patellar tendon during growth. It occurs most frequently in boys between the ages of 10 and 16 years. The disorder is characterized by pain in the front of the knee associated with inflammation and thickening of the patellar tendon. Both knees are involved in about half of the cases.[8] It is unclear whether or not this disease is truly an osteochondrosis, because the disturbance in circulation and the subsequent necrosis of the tibial tubercle may simply be the result of extraordinary stress placed on the knee during a critical growth period. Follow-up studies have indicated that the disorder may really be a mechanical tendonitis with partial avulsion of the tibial tubercle.[8]

With Osgood–Schlatter disease, pain is usually associated with specific activities such as kneeling, running, bicycle riding, or stair climbing. The symptoms are self-limiting and usually disappear within 1 to 2 years or

at about age 18.[4,8] In some cases limited activity, braces, and even a plaster cast to immobilize the knee may be necessary to relieve the pain. Occasionally minor symptoms or an increased prominence of the tibial tubercle may continue into adulthood.

Slipped Capital Femoral Epiphysis

Normally, the proximal femoral epiphysis unites with the neck of the femur between ages 16 and 19 years. Before this (10 to 17 years in girls and 13 to 16 years in boys), the femoral head may slip from its normal position directly at the head of the femur, becoming displaced medially and posteriorly.[8] This produces an adduction, lateral rotation, and extension deformity.

The etiology of slipped capital femoral epiphysis is obscure, but it may be related to the child's susceptibility to stress on the femoral neck as a result of genetics or abnormal structure. Boys are affected twice as often as girls, and in 30% to 70% of cases the condition is bilateral.[8] Affected children are often overweight with poorly developed secondary sex characteristics or, in some instances, are extremely tall and thin. In many cases there is a history of rapid skeletal growth preceding displacement of the epiphysis.

There are often complaints of referred knee pain in children with the condition, accompanied by reports of difficulty walking, fatigue, and stiffness. X-rays are normal. The diagnosis is confirmed with x-ray when the degree of slipping can be determined on a lateral view. Early treatment is imperative to prevent lifelong crippling. Nonweight bearing on the femur and bed rest are essential parts of the treatment. Traction or gentle manipulation under anesthesia are used to reduce the slip. Surgical insertion of pins to keep the femoral neck and head of the femur aligned is a common method of treatment for children with moderate or severe slips. Crutches are used for several months following surgical correction to prevent full weight bearing until the growth plate is sealed by the bony union.

Scoliosis

Scoliosis is a lateral deviation of the spinal column that may or may not include rotation or deformity of the vertebrae. It has been estimated that more than 1 million Americans have a significant degree of scoliosis.[9] It is most commonly seen during adolescence and is eight-times more common in girls than in boys.

Scoliosis can develop as the result of another disease condition or without known cause. Idiopathic scoliosis, or scoliosis of unknown cause, accounts for 75% to 80% of the total cases of the disorder and affects between 2% and 8% of the total population in the United States.[10]

The other 20% to 25% of cases are caused by more than 50 different etiologies including poliomyelitis, congenital hemivertebrae, neurofibromatosis, and cerebral palsy.

Scoliosis is classified as either postural or structural. With postural scoliosis there is a small curve that corrects with bending. It can be corrected with passive and active exercises. Structural scoliosis does not correct with bending. It is a fixed deformity classified within three categories based on etiology: idiopathic scoliosis, congenital scoliosis, and neuromuscular scoliosis.

Idiopathic scoliosis is a structural spinal curvature for which no etiology has been established. It occurs primarily in male infants of the United Kingdom and Europe during the first 3 years of life. Its usual effect is a curve in the thoracic area that is convex and to the left. Juvenile idiopathic scoliosis occurs between 5 and 6 years of age and is quite rare. Adolescent idiopathic scoliosis is the most common type of scoliosis and usually appears in girls beginning at about age 10.[11]

Congenital scoliosis is caused by disturbances in vertebral development during the third to fifth week of embryologic development.[12] The child may have other anomalies and neurologic complications if the spine is involved.

Neuromuscular scoliosis develops from neuropathic or myopathic diseases. Neuropathic scoliosis is seen with cerebral palsy and poliomyelitis. A long, C-shaped curve from the cervical to the sacral region is often present. In cerebral palsy severe deformity may make treatment and management quite difficult. Myopathic neuromuscular scoliosis develops with muscular dystrophy and is usually not severe.

Scoliosis is usually first noted because of the deformity it causes. A high shoulder, prominent hip, or projecting scapula may be noticed by a parent or in a school screening program. In girls, difficulty in hemming or fitting a dress may call attention to the deformity. Pain is present in severe cases, usually in the lumbar region, which may be caused by pressure on the ribs or the crest of the ilium. There may be shortness of breath caused by diminished chest expansion and gastrointestinal disturbances from crowding of the abdominal organs. A mild backache may occur in adults with less severe deformity. If scoliosis is left untreated, the curve may progress to the point that cardiopulmonary function is compromised and risk of neurologic complications occurs.

Early diagnosis of scoliosis is important in the prevention of severe spinal deformity. School screening programs are an excellent means of early detection of scoliosis in adolescents. Screening should be done yearly in the fifth through tenth grades. School nurses and physical education teachers can be specially trained to carry out the examination, which takes about 30 seconds to complete. Students are examined from the front, back, and sides while standing and bending with arms both at their sides and out in front with palms touching. The cardinal signs of scoliosis are (1) asymmetry of the shoulders and hips with children in a standing position and (2) rib and lumbar humps with children in the forward bending position (Fig. 52-3).

Diagnosis is made by physical examination and confirmed by x-ray. The curve is measured by determining the amount of lateral deviation present on x-ray and is labeled right or left for the convex portion of the curve. Several different methods are used.

The treatment of scoliosis depends on the severity of the deformity (Table 52-1). A conservative approach includes periodic assessment and either an exercise program or some form of external bracing. An exercise program is designed to promote the maximum degree of correction possible based on the degree of flexibility present at the time of diagnosis. The pelvic tilt exercise is an example of an exercise done both with and without a brace.

A brace is used to control the progression of the curvature during growth and also provides some correction. The most commonly used brace is the Milwaukee brace, which was developed by Doctors Blount and Schmitt in 1946 (Fig. 52-4). This was the first brace to

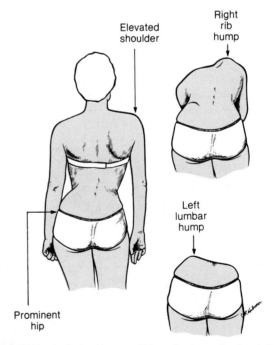

Figure 52-3 *Scoliosis. Abnormalities to be determined at initial screening examination. (From Gore DR, Passehl R, Sepic S, Dalton A: Scoliosis screening: Results of a community project. Pediatrics 67, No 2 (Feb.) 1981. Copyright © 1981 by the American Academy of Pediatrics.)*

provide some degree of active correction. Its use is the treatment of choice for curvatures of 40 degrees or less in adolescents with idiopathic scoliosis. The brace is worn for 23 hours a day, with removal permitted only for personal hygiene purposes. Lateral pads apply pressure to the apex of the curve (*i.e.,* the point most deviated from the vertical axis) on the convex side.

Exercises are done both when the brace is off and when it is on. Good skin care is essential to prevent breakdown under the brace. It is important for health care professionals to work with the adolescent to ensure their compliance with the treatment program. This is particularly important because the brace may present an additional stress to an already threatened body image. Adolescents at greatest risk for noncompliance with treatment regimens are those with (1) lower intelligence and academic skills, (2) a need for acting out their frus-

trations, (3) lowered feelings of personal power or potency, (4) less tension in the presence of physicians, (5) very active personal and family life-styles.[13]

Surgical intervention with instrumentation and spinal fusion is done in severe cases, when the curvature has progressed to 40 degrees or beyond at the time of diagnosis or when curves of a lesser degree are compounded with imbalance or rotation of the vertebrae. Three methods of instrumentation are used (1) Harrington rod and posterior spinal fusion, (2) Dwyer instrumentation and anterior spinal fusion, or (3) segmental (Luque) spinal instrumentation and posterior spinal fusion. With the Harrington rod instrumentation and posterior spinal fusion, a distraction rod is attached to the posterior aspect of the spinal column on the concave side of the curvature. A second, more flexible rod may be used to compress the convex side. With the Dwyer instrumentation method, a wire cable is threaded through screw and staple units inserted directly into the vertebral body as a means of exerting tension on the convex side of the curve. The spine is then fused anteriorly. This is usually followed with a posterior fusion, which is done several weeks later for added correction and stability. A Dwyer instrumentation procedure is difficult because the anterior fusion requires a transthoracic and retroperitoneal approach (through the rib cage and pulmonary cavity). With the segmental instrumentation method, a posterior fusion is used along with the Luque instrumentation. Wire loops are attached to the lamina as a means of securing rods to both sides of the spine. This provides a rigid internal fixation at the level of each vertebrae.

Postoperatively, patients who have had a Harrington rod inserted or a Dwyer procedure performed are immobilized in a body cast or Milwaukee brace.

Table 52-1   Treatment Parameters for Scoliosis

Treatment	Indicators
I. Periodic assessment and exercise	Curvature of less than 20 degrees; resolving infantile curve; mild curve in adults
II. External bracing: Milwaukee brace Orthoplast jacket Body cast	Curvature of 15 degrees to 25 degrees; skeletally immature curvature of 20 degrees to 40 degrees
III. Surgery: Harrington rod instrumentation Dwyer cable instrumentation Segmental (Luque) spinal instrumentation	Some curvatures of 20 degrees to 40 degrees; most curvatures of greater than 40 degrees

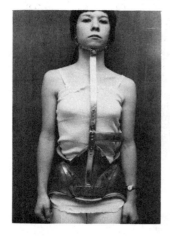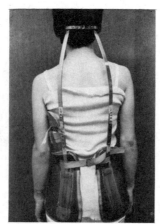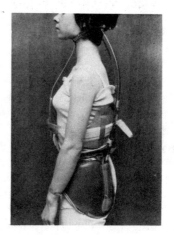

Figure 52-4 *The Milwaukee brace as seen from front, back, and side. (From Farrell J: Illustrated Guide to Orthopedic Nursing, 2nd ed, p 172. Philadelphia, JB Lippincott, 1982)*

Traction may be used initially, applied directly to the Milwaukee brace. A circoelectric bed, Stryker frame, or Foster frame may be used to assist with turning. Patients with a Harrington rod or Dwyer instrumentation require a longer period of postoperative bed rest than those that have the segmental (Luque) spinal instrumentation procedure.

Hereditary and Congenital Deformities

Congenital deformities are abnormalities that are present at birth. They can be caused by hereditary influences or disturbances in embryonic development. They range in severity from mild limb deformities, which are relatively common, to major limb malformations, which are relatively rare. There may be a simple webbing of the fingers or toes (syndactyly) or the presence of an extra digit (polydactyly). Joint contractures and dislocations produce more severe deformity as does the absence of entire bones, joints, or limbs. An epidemic of limb deformities occurred from 1957 to 1962 as a result of the maternal ingestion of thalidomide. This drug was withdrawn from the market in 1961.

Congenital deformities are caused by many factors, some as yet unknown. These factors include genetic influences, external agents that injure the fetus (*e.g.,* radiation, alcohol, medications, and viruses), and *in utero* environmental factors. As discussed in Chapter 4, the fourth to the seventh week of gestation is the most vulnerable period for development of limb deformities.

Congenital dislocation of the hip

Congenital dislocation of the hip is seen in 1.6 out of every 1000 live births. It occurs most frequently in first-born children and is six times more common in female than in male infants.[14] It is thought that the instability of the hip is a consequence of laxity of the ligaments, which is genetically determined, and displacement is the result of environmental factors such as fetal position or breech delivery.[14]

In a child with congenital dislocation of the hip, the head of the femur is located superior to the acetabulum. In less-severe cases, the hip joint may be either unstable or subluxed, so that there are separation of the joint surfaces and a partial dislocation. Hip dislocation may be associated with ligamentous laxity and environmental influences such as intrauterine positioning or breech presentation during delivery.

Normal development of the hip requires that a normal positional relationship exists between the femoral head and the acetabulum. If this relationship is not maintained, there may be a delay in the maturity, size, and development of both the femoral head and the acetabulum. Early diagnosis of congenital hip dislocation is important because treatment is easiest and most effective if begun during the first 6 months of life. Clinical examinations to detect dislocation of the hip should be done at birth and every several months during the first year of life.

Several examination techniques are used to screen for congenital hip dislocation. In infants, signs of dislocation include asymmetry of the hip or gluteal folds, shortening of the thigh so that one knee (on the affected side) is higher than the other, and limited abduction of the affected hip (Fig. 52-5). The asymmetry of gluteal folds is not definitive but indicates the need for further evaluation. A specific examination involves an attempt to manually dislocate and then reduce the abnormal hip while the infant is in the supine position with both knees flexed. With gentle downward pressure being applied to the knees, the knee and thigh is manually abducted as an

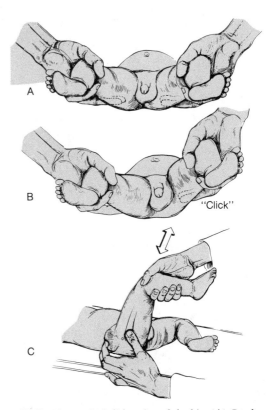

Figure 52-5 *Congenital dislocation of the hip. (A) In the newborn, both hips can be equally flexed, abducted, and externally rotated without producing a "click." (B) A diagnosis of a congenital dislocation of the hip may be confirmed by the Ortolani "click" test. The involved hip cannot be abducted as far as the opposite one, and there is a "click" as the hip reduces. (C) Telescoping of the femur to aid in the diagnosis of a congenitally dislocated hip. (From Hoppenfeld's Physical Examination of the Spine and Extremities. New York, Appleton-Century-Croft, 1976)*

upward and medial pressure is applied to the proximal thigh. In infants with the disorder, the initial downward pressure on the knee produces a dislocation of the hip, which is followed by a palpable or audible click (Ortolani's sign) as the hip is reduced and moves back into the acetabulum. In an older child, instability of the hip may produce a delay in standing or walking and eventually a characteristic waddling gait. With the thumbs over the anterior iliac crest and hands over the lateral pelvis in examination, the levels of the thumbs are not even; the child is also not able to elevate the opposite side of the pelvis (positive Trendelenburg's test). Diagnosis is confirmed with x-ray.

The treatment of congenital hip dislocation is begun as soon as the diagnosis has been made. The best results are obtained if the treatment is begun before there is weight bearing on the hip and the hip is reduced by 1 year of age. Treatment at any age includes reduction of the dislocation and immobilization of the legs in an abducted position. With children under age 3, gentle traction is the primary course of treatment, followed by several months of immobilization in a hip spica cast or on an abduction splint such as a Frejk pillow or Pavlik harness.

Congenital clubfoot

Congenital clubfoot can affect one or both feet. Like congenital dislocation of hip, its occurrence follows a multifactorial inheritance pattern. The condition has an incidence of 1 in every 1000 live births, and it occurs twice as often in males as in females.[14] There is an 8% chance that a sibling will have the defect and an 8% to 11% chance that the offspring of an affected person will have the disorder.[14]

In the most common form of clubfoot (95% of cases), the foot is plantar flexed and inverted.[14] This is the so-called *equinovarus* type, in which the foot resembles a horse's hoof (Fig. 52-6). The other 5% of cases are of the

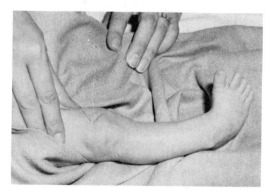

Figure 52-6 *Talipes equinovarus deformity. Note the internal tibial torsion. (From Turek SL: Orthopaedics: Principles and Their Application, 4th ed. Philadelphia, JB Lippincott, 1984)*

calcaneovalgus type, in which the foot is dorsiflexed and everted.

At birth, the feet of many infants assume one of these two positions, but they can be passively overcorrected or brought back into the opposite position. If the foot cannot be overcorrected, some type of correction may be necessary. Although the cause of clubfoot is unknown, three theories are generally accepted: (1) an anomalous development occurs during the first trimester of pregnancy; (2) the leg fails to rotate inward and move from the equinovarus position at about the third month; and (3) the soft tissues in the foot do not mature and lengthen.

Clubfoot varies in severity from a mild deformity to one in which the foot is completely inverted. The treatment is begun as soon as the diagnosis is made. When treatment is initiated during the first few weeks of life, a nonoperative procedure is effective within a short period of time. The foot is either taped and manipulated or put in a cast with frequent cast changes. The treatment is continued until the foot is in a normal position with full correction evident clinically and on x-ray. Surgery may be required for severe deformities or when nonoperative treatment methods are unsuccessful.

Osteogenesis imperfecta

Osteogenesis imperfecta is a rare hereditary disease characterized by defective synthesis of connective tissue, including bone matrix. It is perhaps the most common hereditary bone disease, occurring in approximately 1 in 40,000 births.[15] Although it is usually transmitted as an autosomal dominant trait, a distinct form of the disorder with multiple lethal defects is thought to be inherited as an autosomal recessive trait. In the latter case, as many as 25% of the offspring may be affected while the parents are normal.[16]

The disorder is characterized by thin and poorly developed bones, leading to multiple fractures. Other problems associated with defective connective tissue synthesis include short stature, thin skin, blue sclera, loose jointedness, scoliosis, and a tendency for hernia formation. There may also be deafness because of otosclerosis of the middle and inner ear.

The most serious defects occur when the disorder is inherited as a recessive trait. Severely affected fetuses may die at birth or shortly after. Less severe affliction occurs when the disorder is inherited as a dominant trait. The skeletal system is not so weakened and fractures often do not appear until the child becomes active and starts to walk. These fractures heal rapidly, but with a poor-quality callus. In some cases, parents may be suspected of child abuse when the child is admitted to the health care facility with mutiple fractures.

At present there is no known medical treatment for

correction of the defective collagen synthesis that is characteristic of osteogenesis imperfecta. Instead, current treatment modalities focus on the prevention and treatment of fractures. Surgical intervention is often needed to correct deformities.

In summary, skeletal disorders can occur as the result of congenital or hereditary influences or of factors that occur during normal periods of skeletal growth and development. Newborn infants undergo normal changes in muscle tone and joint motion, causing conditions such as femoral anteversion and toeing-in. Many of these conditions are corrected as skeletal growth and development take place. Other childhood skeletal disorders such as the osteochondroses, slipped capital femoral epiphysis, and scoliosis are not corrected by the growth process. These disorders are progressive, can cause permanent disability, and require treatment. Disorders such as congenital dislocation of the hip and congenital clubfoot are present at birth. Both of these disorders are best treated during infancy. Regular examinations during the first year of life are recommended as a means of achieving early diagnosis of such disorders. Osteogenesis imperfecta is a rare autosomal hereditary disorder that is characterized by defective synthesis of connective tissue including bone matrix. It results in poorly developed bones that fracture easily.

■ Metabolic Bone Disease

The process of bone resorption and formation is continuous throughout life. This process is called *bone remodeling*. There are two types of bone remodeling: structural and internal remodeling.[17] Structural remodeling involves deposition of new bone on the outer aspect of the shaft at the same time that bone is resorbed from the inner aspect of the shaft. It occurs during growth and results in a bone having adult form and shape. Internal remodeling involves the replacement of bone. In the adult skeleton, remodeling involves formation of new packets of bone on trabecular surfaces and is important in replacing existing bone. Internal remodeling involves a coupled sequence of bone cell activity (Fig. 52-7). The sequence is activated by one of many stimuli, including the actions of parathyroid hormone. It begins with relocation of osteoclastic resorption of existing bone, during which both the organic and inorganic components are removed. The sequence then proceeds to the formation of new bone by osteoblasts. In the adult, the length of one sequence (bone resorption and formation) takes about 4 months.[17] Ideally, the replaced bone should equal the absorbed bone. If this does not occur, there is a net loss of bone. In the elderly,

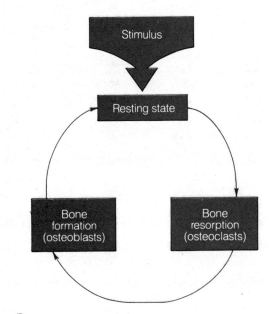

Figure 52-7 *Coupled sequence of bone resorption and formation.*

for example, bone resorption and formation are no longer perfectly coupled, and there is a loss of bone mass.

Three major factors are responsible for maintaining the equilibrium of bone tissue: (1) mechanical stress, which helps stimulate osteoblastic activity and formation of the organic matrix, (2) the level of calcium and phosphate ions in the extracellular fluid, and (3) the effect of hormones and local factors on bone resorption and formation. Mechanical stress stimulates osteoblastic activity and formation of organic matrix. It is important in preventing bone atrophy and in healing fractures. Bone serves as a storage site for extracellular calcium and phosphate ions. Consequently, alterations in the extracellular levels of these ions affect their deposition in bone (Chap. 25).

Hormonal Control of Bone Formation and Metabolism

The process of bone formation and mineral metabolism is complex. It involves the interplay between the action of parathyroid hormone, calcitonin, and vitamin D. Other hormones such as cortisol, growth hormone, thyroid hormone, and the sex hormones influence bone formation either directly or indirectly. The actions of parathyroid hormone, calcitonin, and vitamin D are summarized in Table 52-2.

Parathyroid hormone

Parathyroid hormone (PTH) is one of the important regulators of blood calcium and phosphate levels. The hormone is secreted by the parathyroid glands, which are located on the posterior outer surface of the thyroid gland.

Table 52-2 Actions of Parathyroid Hormone, Calcitonin, and Vitamin D

Actions	Parathyroid Hormone	Calcitonin	Vitamin D
Intestinal absorption of calcium	Increases indirectly through increased activation of vitamin D	Probably not affected	Increases
Intestinal absorption of phosphate	Increases	Probably not affected	Increases
Renal excretion of calcium	Decreases	Increases	Probably increases but less effect than PTH
Renal excretion of phosphate	Increases	Increases	Increases
Bone resorption	Increases	Decreases	$1,25(OH)_2D_3$ increases
Bone formation	Decreases	Uncertain	$24,25(OH)_2D_3$ increases
Serum calcium levels	Produces a prompt increase	Decreases with pharmacologic doses	No effect
Serum phosphate levels	Prevents an increase	Decreases with pharmacologic doses	No effect

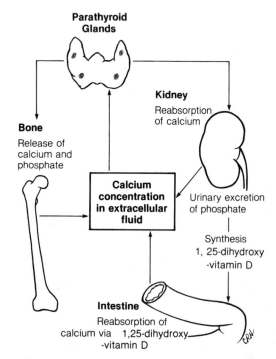

Figure 52-8 Regulation and actions of parathyroid hormone.

Parathyroid hormone acts to prevent serum calcium levels from falling below and serum phosphate levels from rising above normal physiologic concentrations. The secretion of PTH is regulated by negative feedback according to serum calcium levels. PTH, which is released from the parathyroid gland in response to a decrease in plasma calcium, acts to restore the concentration of the calcium ion to just above the normal set point. This, in turn, inhibits further secretion of the hormone. Other factors such as serum phosphate and arterial blood *p*H indirectly influence parathyroid secretion by altering the amount of calcium that is complexed to phosphate or bound to albumin.

PTH functions to maintain serum calcium levels by initiating the (1) release of calcium from bone, (2) conservation of calcium by the kidney, (3) enhanced intestinal absorption of calcium through activation of vitamin D, and (4) reduction of serum phosphate levels (Fig. 52-8). PTH also increases the movement of calcium and phosphate from bone into the extracellular fluid. Calcium is immediately released from the canaliculi and bone cells; a more prolonged release of calcium and phosphate is mediated by increased osteoclast activity. In the kidney, PTH stimulates tubular reabsorption of calcium while reducing the reabsorption of phosphate. The latter effect ensures that increased release of phosphate from bone during mobilization of calcium does not produce an elevation in serum phosphate levels. PTH increases intestinal absorption of calcium because of its ability to stimulate production of 1,25-dihydroxyvitamin D_3 by the kidney.

Calcitonin

Whereas PTH acts to increase blood calcium levels, the hormone calcitonin acts to lower blood calcium levels. Calcitonin (sometimes called thyrocalcitonin) is secreted by the parafollicular, or C, cells of the thyroid gland.

Calcitonin inhibits the release of calcium from bone into the extracellular fluid. It is thought to act by causing calcium to become sequestered in bone cells and by inhibiting osteoclast activity. Calcitonin also reduces the renal tubular reabsorption of calcium and phosphate; the decrease in serum calcium that is observed following administration of pharmacologic doses of calcitonin may be related to this action.[18]

The major stimulus for calcitonin synthesis and release is a rise in serum calcium. The actual role of calcitonin in the overall mineral homeostasis is unclear. There are no clearly definable syndromes of calcitonin deficiency or excess, which suggests that calcitonin does not directly alter calcium metabolism. It has been suggested that the physiologic actions of calcitonin are related to the postprandial handling and processing of dietary calcium.[18] This theory proposes that calcitonin's postprandial presence maintains parathyroid secretion at a time when it normally would be reduced by calcium entering the blood from the digestive tract. Although excess or deficiency states associated with alterations in physiologic levels of calcitonin have not been observed, it has been shown that pharmacologic doses of the hormone reduce osteoclastic activity. Because of this action, calcitonin has proven effective in the treatment of Paget's disease. The hormone is also used to reduce serum calcium levels during hypercalcemic crises.

Vitamin D

It is now recognized that vitamin D and its metabolites are not vitamins but steroid hormones. There are two forms of vitamin D: vitamin D_2 (ergocalciferol) and vitamin D_3 (cholecalciferol). The two forms differ by the presence of a double bond, yet have identical biological activity. The term vitamin D is used to indicate both forms.

Vitamin D has little or no activity until it has been metabolized to compounds that mediate its activity. Figure 52-9 depicts sources of vitamin D and pathways for activation. The first step of the activation process occurs in the liver where vitamin D is hydroxylated to form the metabolite 25-hydroxyvitamin D_3 (25-OH D_3). From the liver, 25-OH D_3 is transported to the kidneys were it undergoes conversion to either 1,25-dihydroxyvitamin D_3 [1,25-$(OH)_2D_3$] or 24,25-dihydroxyvitamin D_3 [24,25-$(OH)_2D_3$]. Other metabolites of vitamin D have been and are still being discovered.

There are two sources of vitamin D: intestinal absorption and skin production. Intestinal absorption occurs mainly in the jejunum and includes both vitamin D_2 and vitamin D_3. The most important dietary sources of vitamin D are fish, liver, and irradiated milk. Because vitamin D is fat soluble, its absorption is mediated by bile salts and occurs by means of the lymphatic vessels. In the skin, ultraviolet radiation from sunlight spontaneously converts 7-dehydrocholesterol previtamin D_3 to vitamin D_3. A circulating vitamin D–binding protein provides a mechanism to remove vitamin D from the skin and make it available to the rest of the body. With adequate exposure to sunlight, the amount of vitamin D that can be produced by the skin is usually sufficient to meet physiologic requirements. The importance of sunlight exposure is evidenced by population studies that report lower vitamin D levels in countries such as England, which has less sunlight than the United States.[19] Sea-

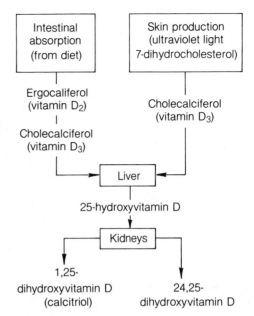

Figure 52-9   *Sources and pathway for activation of vitamin D.*

sonal variations in vitamin D levels probably reflect changes in sunlight exposure.

The most potent of the vitamin D metabolites is 1,25-$(OH)_2$ D_3. This metabolite increases intestinal absorption of calcium and resorption of calcium and phosphate from bone. Bone resorption by the osteoclasts is increased and bone formation by the osteoblasts is decreased; there is also an increase in acid phosphatase and a decrease in alkaline phosphatase. Both intestinal absorption and bone resorption increase the availability of calcium and phosphorus to the bone mineralizing surface. The role of 24,25-$(OH)_2D_3$ is less clear. There is increasing evidence that 24,25-$(OH)_2D_3$, in conjunction with 1,25-$(OH)_2D_3$, may be involved in normal bone mineralization.[20]

The regulation of vitamin D activity is influenced by several hormones. Parathyroid hormone and prolactin stimulate 1,25-$(OH)_2D_3$ production by the kidney. States of hyperparathyroidism are associated with increased levels of 1,25-$(OH)_2D_3$, whereas hypoparathyroidism leads to lowered levels of the metabolite. Prolactin may have an ancillary role in regulating vitamin D metabolism during pregnancy and lactation. Calcitonin inhibits 1,25-$(OH)_2D_3$ production by the kidney. In addition to hormonal influences, changes in the concentration of ions such as calcium, phosphate, hydrogen, and potassium exert an effect on both 1,25-$(OH)_2D_3$ and 24,25-$(OH)_2D_3$ production. Under conditions of deprivation of phosphate and calcium, 1,25-$(OH)_2D_3$ is increased, whereas hyperphosphatemia and hypercalcemia decrease the metabolite.

Disorders of Bone Metabolism

Osteopenia

Osteopenia is a condition that is common to all metabolic bone diseases. It is characterized by a reduction in bone mass greater than expected for age, race, or sex, and it occurs because of a decrease in bone formation, inadequate bone mineralization, or excessive bone deossification. Osteopenia is not a diagnosis but a term used to describe an apparent lack of bone on x-ray. The major causes of osteopenia are osteoporosis, osteomalacia, malignancies such as multiple myeloma, and endocrine disorders such as hyperparathyroidism and hyperthyroidism.

Osteoporosis

Osteoporosis is a disorder in which the rate of bone resorption is greater than the rate of bone formation. There are parallel losses of both the organic matrix and mineral content of the bone. The total composition of bone remains the same; there is just too little of it. Osteoporotic bone is brittle, fragile, and fractures easily. Osteoporosis can occur as the result of an endocrine disorder or malignancy but is most often associated with the aging process. Loss of bone mass begins at about age 25. After age 40, the rate of bone loss is approximately 0.5% per year and increases to about 1% per year or more in menopausal women.[21] It has been estimated that osteoporosis currently affects about 14 million women in the United States. Age-related bone losses in men are seen 15 to 20 years after that in women and occur at a slower rate.[22] It has also been shown that bone mass positively correlates with the amount of skin pigmentation; whites have the least amount of bone mass and blacks have the most.[22] Although osteoporosis is uncommon among black women, many cases are seen among postmenopausal women with brown and yellow skin. One of the reasons for the increased risk in postmenopausal women of white or Asian descent may be that their original bone mass is less and therefore the losses associated with aging affect them sooner.

With osteoporosis, changes occur in both the diaphysis and the metaphysis. The diameter of the bone enlarges with age, causing the outer supporting cortex to become thinner. In severe osteoporosis, the vertebrae and hip bones begin to resemble the fragile structure of a fine china vase. There is loss of trabeculae from cancellous bone and thinning of the cortex to such an extent that fractures can occur with minimal stress.

The development of osteoporosis involves many factors. It is related to hormone levels, physical fitness, and general nutrition. It is thought that an indirect action of estrogen is the suppression of bone resorption. This action is reduced after menopause. Exercise helps to prevent involutional bone loss and may serve to prevent or delay the progression of osteoporosis.[23] Poor nutrition or an age-related decrease in intestinal absorption of calcium because of deficient activation of vitamin D may contribute to osteoporosis, particularly in the elderly. Other factors found to be associated with osteoporosis are a diet high in protein, cigarette smoking, alcohol ingestion, and a family history of osteoporosis.[24]

Osteoporosis in children is rare. When it does occur, it is related to causes such as the excess corticosteroid levels associated with Cushing's syndrome, colon disease, prolonged immobility, or osteogenesis imperfecta. The cardinal features occur at the onset or just before puberty and may include pain in the back and extremities and multiple fractures. There is evidence on x-ray of new bone that is osteoporotic. Idiopathic juvenile osteoporosis, which is more common in children, resembles rickets.

Little is known about the true etiology of osteoporosis, but most data suggest that the primary problem is an acceleration of bone resorption. The serum alkaline phosphatase, a measure of osteoblastic activity, is increased slightly.[22] There may also be a lower level of calcitonin and a decreased response to a calcium stimulus.[21] Decreases in sex hormone levels, which seem to act as an intermediate to prevent bone loss, in both men and women are somehow important in the pathogenesis of osteoporosis. In postmenopausal women, these changes can be reversed by estrogen therapy.

The clinical manifestations of osteoporosis are skeletal fractures, primarily of the hip and vertebrae, deformity, and pain. One out of every five women who reach the age of 90 has had a fractured hip.[22] There are loss of height in the vertebral body and increased kyphosis in the dorsal spine. Usually, no generalized bone tenderness is present. When pain occurs, it is related to fractures.

The initial diagnosis of osteoporosis is usually made on x-ray. However, radiologic evidence of decreased bone density is nonspecific. Unfortunately, the only true measure of bone density and calcium level is through bone biopsy, which is not practical as a routine diagnostic measure. A bone density study may be helpful, but at present, there is no way to assess the rate of bone breakdown, bone repair, or skeletal strength. Even a bone scan, which measures osteoblastic activity and blood pooling, cannot diagnose osteoporosis.

In all cases of osteoporosis, clinical examination and x-ray findings must be compared, along with various blood chemistry levels. Blood chemistry levels of calcium, phosphorus, and alkaline phosphatase and protein electrophoresis should be done before treatment is started. These levels may all be within normal range in postmenopausal osteoporosis, with only a slight rise in serum calcium and phosphate reflecting the increased bone destruction.

Prevention and early detection of osteoporosis are essential to the prevention of deformities and fractures associated with its presence. It is important to identify persons in high-risk groups as a means of beginning treatment early. Postmenopausal women, women of small stature or lean body mass, and those with sedentary life-style, poor calcium intake, and diseases that demineralize bone are at greatest risk. Regular exercise and adequate calcium intake are important factors in preventing osteoporosis. The average daily requirement for calcium is approximately 800 mg in adults. Women need more than 1 gm of calcium daily.[8] This means that adults should drink three to four glasses of milk daily or substitute other foods that are high in calcium. Unfortunately, dietary calcium levels of the general population are estimated to be between 600 mg and 800 mg, and only 10% of this calcium is absorbed from the intestine.

At present, the efficacy of treatment methods for osteoporosis is questionable. A combination of fluoride, calcium, and vitamin D is most often used. Administration of fluoride leads to widespread formation of new bone. Because the new bone is laid down on existing bone, the treatment must be started while there is still adequate bone onto which the fluoride bone can be built. There is evidence that deficient activation of vitamin D may be an important factor in the impaired intestinal absorption of calcium in the elderly. Based on this evidence, calcitriol (1,25-dihydroxyvitamin D_3) is being studied as a treatment for osteoporosis.[25]

The use of estrogen therapy in postmenopausal women in the United States, although relatively common, is still controversial. Several studies have shown a reduction in postmenopausal bone loss in women using estrogen therapy, particularly those treated within the first 3 years of menopause.[23] However, there is strong evidence that women who have not undergone a hysterectomy are at increased risk for developing endometrial cancer when taking estrogens.[23] This risk appears to be related to the length of treatment, dose, and concomitant use of progestins.

Persons with osteoporosis have many special needs. In treating fractures, it is important to minimize immobility. Bed rest is imposed only after recent fractures. The use of leg braces is avoided. Walking and swimming are encouraged. Unsafe conditions that predispose individuals to falls and fractures should be corrected or avoided.

Osteomalacia and rickets

In contrast with osteoporosis, which causes a loss of total bone mass and results in brittle bones, osteomalacia and rickets produce a softening of the bones and do not involve the loss of bone matrix. About 60% of bone is mineral content, about 30% is organic matrix, and the rest is living bone cells. Both the organic matrix and the inorganic mineral salts are needed for normal bone consistency. As an example, placement of a fresh bone in dilute nitric acid will remove the inorganic mineral salts. The organic matrix that remains will still resemble a bone, but it will be so flexible that it can be tied in a knot. On the other hand, when a bone is placed over a hot flame, the organic material is destroyed and the bone becomes very brittle.

Osteomalacia. Osteomalacia is a generalized bone condition in which inadequate mineralization of bone matrix results from a calcium or phosphate deficiency (or both). It is sometimes referred to as the adult form of rickets.

There are two main causes of osteomalacia: (1) insufficient calcium absorption from the intestine because of either a lack of calcium or resistance to the action of vitamin D and (2) increased renal phosphorus losses. As discussed previously, vitamin D is a fat-soluble vitamin that is either derived from the intestinal absorption of the intact vitamin or produced in the skin as a result of ultraviolet irradiation of 7-dehydrocholesterol. Vitamin D that is absorbed from the intestine or synthesized in the skin is inactive. Vitamin D is activated in a two-step process that begins in the liver and is completed in the kidney. The most common cause of vitamin D deficiency are due to reduced vitamin D absorption resulting from biliary tract or intestinal diseases that impair fat and fat-soluble vitamin absorption. Lack of vitamin D in the diet is rare in the United States because many foods are fortified with the vitamin. Anticonvulsant medications, such as phenobarbital and phenytoin, induce hepatic hydroxylases that accelerate breakdown of the active forms of vitamin D. The long-term use of antacids, such as aluminum hydroxide, which bind dietary forms of phosphate and prevent their absorption, is another cause of phosphate deficiency. A form of osteomalacia, called renal rickets, occurs with chronic renal failure. It is caused by the inability of the kidney to activate vitamin D and excrete phosphate and is accompanied by hyperparathyroidism, increased bone turnover, and increased bone resorption. Another form of osteomalacia is due to renal tubular defects that cause excessive phosphorus loses. This form of osteomalacia is commonly referred to as vitamin D–resistant rickets and is often a familial disorder. It is inherited as an x-linked dominant gene, being passed by mothers to half of all their children and by fathers to their daughters only. This form of osteomalacia affects boys more severely than girls.

The incidence of osteomalacia is high among the elderly because of diets deficient in both calcium and vitamin D and is often compounded by intestinal malabsorption problems that occur with aging. Osteomalacia is often seen in cultures in which the diet is deficient in vitamin D, such as in northern China, Japan, and northern India. Women in these areas have a higher incidence of the disorder than men because of the combined effects of pregnancy, lactation, and more indoor confinement. There is also a greater incidence of osteomalacia in colder regions of the world, particularly during the winter months, probably because of lessened exposure to sunlight.

The clinical manifestations of osteomalacia are bone pain, tenderness, and fractures as the disease progresses. In severe cases, muscle weakness is often an early sign. The cause of muscle weakness is unclear, although experimental evidence suggests that vitamin D deficiency affects muscle metabolism.[16] The combined effects of gravity, muscle weakness, and bone softening contribute to the development of deformities. There may be a dorsal kyphosis in the spine, rib deformities, a heart-shaped pelvis, and marked bowing of the tibiae and femurs. Osteomalacia predisposes an individual to pathologic fractures in the weakened areas, especially in the distal radius and proximal femur. There may be delayed healing and poor retention of internal fixation devices.

Osteomalacia is usually accompanied by a compensatory hyperparathyroidism stimulated by low serum calcium levels. Parathyroid hormone reduces renal absorption of phosphate and removes calcium from the bone. Thus, calcium levels are only slightly reduced in osteomalacia.

Diagnostic measures are directed toward identifying osteomalacia and establishing its cause. Diagnostic methods include x-ray, laboratory workup, bone scan, and bone biopsy. X-ray findings typical of osteomalacia are the development of transverse lines or pseudofractures called Looser's zones. These are apparently caused by pulsations of the major arteries where they cross the bone.[16]

The treatment of osteomalacia is directed at the underlying cause. If the problem is nutritional, restoring adequate amounts of calcium and vitamin D to the diet may be sufficient. The elderly with intestinal malabsorption may also benefit from vitamin D. The least expensive and most effective long-term treatment is a diet rich in vitamin D (fish, dairy products, and margarine) along with careful exposure to the midday sun. Vitamin D is specific for adult osteomalacia and vitamin D–resistant rickets, but large doses are usually needed to overcome the resistance to its calcium absorption action and to prevent renal loss of phosphate. The biologically active form of vitamin D, calcitriol, is available for use in the treatment of osteomalacia resistant to vitamin D (*e.g.,* osteomalacia resulting from chronic liver disease and kidney failure). If osteomalacia is due to malabsorption, the treatment is directed toward correcting the primary disease condition. For example, adequate replacement of pancreatic enzymes is of paramount importance in pancreatic insufficiency. In renal tubular disorders, the treatment is directed at the altered renal physiology.

Rickets.   Vitamin D deficiency rickets, seen in children, is called infantile or nutritional rickets. It is a skeletal disease evidenced by osteomalacia and varying and widespread bony deformities. Rickets occurs primarily in underdeveloped areas of the world and in urban areas where pigmented ethnic groups have migrated from sunny to cloudy climates. It is seen most often in infants from 6 to 24 months of age.

Nutritional rickets is caused by either a lack of vitamin D in the diet or malabsorption diseases. Inadequate amounts of calcium and phosphorus in the diet also play a part in the development of rickets. The bony changes are a result of inadequate absorption of calcium.

The pathology of rickets is the same as that of osteomalacia seen in adults. Because rickets affects children during periods of active growth, some different structural changes are seen in the bone. Bones become deformed; ossification at epiphyseal plates is delayed and disordered. This results in widening of the epiphyseal cartilage plate. Any new bone growth that does occur is unmineralized bone.

The symptoms of rickets are usually seen near the end of the child's first year. Early symptoms are lethargy and muscle weakness, which may be accompanied by convulsions or tetany related to hypocalcemia. Irritability is common. In severe cases, children lose their skin pigment, develop flabby subcutaneous tissue, and have poorly developed musculature. The ends of long bones and ribs are enlarged. The thorax may be abnormally shaped with prominent rib cartilage (rachitic rosary). Either bowlegged (varus) or knock-kneed (valgus) deformities of the legs occur. The skull is enlarged and soft with a delay in closure of the fontanels. The child is slow to develop teeth and may have difficulty standing.

Rickets is treated with a balanced diet sufficient in calcium, phosphorus, and vitamin D. Exposure to sunshine is also important. Supplemental vitamin D in excess of normal requirements is given for several months. Maintaining good posture, positioning, and bracing in older children are used to prevent deformities. Once the disease is controlled, deformities may have to be surgically corrected as the child grows.

Paget's disease (osteitis deformans)

Paget's disease is discussed separately because it is not a true metabolic disease. It is a progressive skeletal disorder that involves excessive bone destruction and repair and is characterized by increasing structural changes of the long bones, spine, pelvis, and cranium. The disease affects about 3% of the population over age 40 and 10%

of those over age 70.[26] It is rarely diagnosed before age 40. In children, a rare inherited disorder, hyperostosis corticalis deformans juvenilis, hyperphosphatemia, and diseases that cause diaphyseal stenosis may mimic Paget's disease and are sometimes referred to as juvenile Paget's disease. The etiology of Paget's disease is unknown. Recent studies propose that it may be caused by a virus with osteoclastic capability.[27]

The disease usually begins insidiously and progresses slowly over many years. An initial osteolytic phase is followed by an osteoblastic sclerotic phase. During the initial osteolytic phase, abnormal osteoclasts proliferate. Bone resorption occurs so rapidly that new bone formation cannot keep up, and the bone is replaced by fibrous tissue. The bones actually increase in size and thickness because of accelerated bone resorption followed by abnormal regeneration. Irregular bone formation results in sclerotic and osteoblastic lesions. The result is a thick layer of coarse bone with a rough and pitted outer surface that has the appearance of pumice. Histologically, the Paget's lesions show increased vascularity and bone marrow fibrosis with intense cellular activity. The bone has a somewhat mosaic pattern caused by areas of density outlined by heavy blue lines, called cement lines.

The disease varies in its severity and may be present long before it is clinically detected. The clinical manifestations of Paget's disease depend on the specific area involved. About 20% of those persons with the disorder are totally asymptomatic, and the disease is discovered accidentally.[27] Involvement of the skull causes headaches, intermittent tinitus, vertigo, and eventual hearing loss. In the spine, collapse of the anterior vertebrae causes kyphosis of the thoracic spine. The femur and tibia become bowed. Softening of the femoral neck can cause coxa vara (reduced angle of the femoral neck). Coxa vara, in combination with softening of the sacral and iliac bones, causes a waddling gait. When the lesion affects only one bone, it may cause only mild pain and stiffness. Because of progressive deossification, the normal bone structure is weakened. The deossification process begins along the inner cortical surfaces and continues until the substance of the bone disappears. The bone becomes weak and distorted. Pathologic fractures may occur, especially in the bones subjected to the greatest stress (*e.g.*, the upper femur, lower spine, and pelvic bones). These fractures often heal poorly, with excessive and poorly distributed callus.

Other manifestations of Paget's disease include nerve palsy syndromes from lesions in the upper extremities, mental deterioration, and cardiovascular disease. Cardiovascular disease is the most serious complication and is listed as the most common cause of death in advanced generalized Paget's disease. It is caused by vasodilation of the vessels in the skin and subcutaneous tissues overlying the affected bones. When one-third to one-half of the skeleton is affected, the increased blood flow may lead to high-output cardiac failure.[27] Ventilatory capacity may be limited by rib and spine involvement.

Sarcoma occurs in about 7% of persons with Paget's disease, with a slight predominence in men. The bones most often affected, in order of frequency, are the femur, humerus, pelvis, and tibia. The fact that the cellular activity seen in sarcoma (*e.g.*, these tumors have a large number of osteoclasts and atypical osteoblasts) seems to be an exaggeration of the remodeling process of Paget's disease gives credence to the theory that both diseases have a viral origin.[28]

Diagnosis and treatment. Diagnosis of Paget's disease is based on characteristic bone deformities and x-ray changes. Elevated levels of serum alkaline phosphatase and urinary hydroxyproline support the diagnosis and may be used to monitor the effectiveness of treatment. Bone biopsy may be done to differentiate the lesion from osteomyelitis or a primary or metastatic bone tumor.

The treatment of Paget's disease is based on the degree of pain and the extent of the disease. Pain can be reduced with either nonsteroidal or other anti-inflammatory agents. Suppressive agents such as calcitonin, mithramycin, and diphosphate compounds are used to prevent further spread of the disease and neurologic defects. Calcitonin and etidronate disodium (a phosphate compound) decrease bone resorption. Mithramycin is a cytotoxic agent that causes osteoclasts to reduce their resorption of bone. Because this drug is very toxic, it is reserved for resistant cases. Decreases in serum alkaline phosphatase and urinary hydroxyproline along with radiologic improvement indicate the effectiveness of the treatment. However, symptomatic improvement is usually considered the best measure of success.

In summary, metabolic bone diseases such as osteoporosis, osteomalacia, rickets, and Paget's disease are the result of a disruption in the equilibrium of bone formation and resorption. Osteoporosis, which is the most common of the metabolic bone diseases, occurs when the rate of resorption is greater than that of bone formation. It is seen frequently in postmenopausal women and is the major cause of fractures in people over 45 years of age. Osteomalacia and rickets are caused by inadequate mineralization of bone matrix, primarily because of a deficiency of vitamin D. Paget's disease results from excessive osteoclastic activity and is characterized by the formation of a poor quality of bone. The success rate of the various drugs and hormones that are used to treat metabolic bone diseases varies. Further research is needed to clarify the etiology, pathology, and treatment of these diseases.

■ Neoplasms

Neoplasms in the skeletal system are usually referred to as bone tumors. Primary malignant tumors of the bone are uncommon, constituting about 1% of all cancers.[29] Metastatic disease of the bone, however, is relatively common. Primary bone tumors may arise from any of the skeletal components, including osseous bone tissue, cartilage, and bone marrow. The discussion in this section focuses on primary benign and malignant bone tumors of osseous or cartilaginous origin and metastatic bone disease. Tumors of bone marrow origin (leukemia and multiple myeloma) are discussed in Chapter 10.

As with other types of neoplasms, bone tumors may be either benign or malignant. The benign types, such as osteochondromas and giant cell tumors, tend to grow rather slowly and usually do not destroy the supporting or surrounding tissue or spread to other parts of the body. Malignant tumors, such as osteosarcoma and Ewing's sarcoma, grow rapidly and can spread to other parts of the body through the bloodstream or lymphatics.

Specific types of bone tumors affect different age groups. Adolescents have the highest incidence, with a rate of 3 cases per 100,000. In children less than 15 years of age, only 3.2% of all malignancies are primary bone tumors.[29] The two major forms of bone cancer in children and young adults is osteogenic sarcoma and Ewing's sarcoma. It is unusual for either condition to be seen after age 25. The incidence of bone tumors declines in young adults to a rate of 0.3 per 100,000 between the ages of 30 and 35 years and then slowly begins to rise until the incidence at age 60 equals that of adolescence.[29] The classification of benign and malignant bone tumors is described in Table 52-3.

Characteristics of Bone Tumors

There are three major symptoms of bone tumors: *pain, presence of a mass,* and *impairment of function* (Chart 52-1).[30] Pain is a feature common to almost all malignant tumors but may or may not be present in benign tumors. For example, a benign bone cyst is usually asymptomatic until a fracture occurs. Pain that persists at night and is not relieved by rest is suggestive of malignancy. A mass or hard lump may be the first sign of a bone tumor. A malignant tumor is suspected when a painful mass exists that is enlarging or eroding the cortex of the bone. The discovery of a mass is often dictated by the location of the tumor. A small lump arising on the surface of the tibia is easy to detect, whereas a tumor that is deep in the medial portion of the thigh may grow to considerable size before it is noticed. Both benign and malignant tumors may cause erosion of the bone, so that it cannot with-

---

Chart 52-1 *Symptoms of Bone Cancer*

Bone pain in an adult or child that lasts for as long as a week, is constant or intermittent, and is usually worse at night

Unexplained swelling over the knee, thigh, or other bone

Skin over the bone that feels considerably warmer than the rest of the body, or veins that are noticeably prominent

(Adapted from Facts on Bone Cancer. American Cancer Society, 1978. The American Cancer Society suggests that persons with these symptoms see their physician.)

Table 52-3   Classification of Primary Bone Neoplasms

Tissue Type	Benign Neoplasm	Malignant Neoplasm
Bone	Osteoid osteoma	Osteosarcoma
	Benign osteoblastoma	Parosteal osteogenic sarcoma
	Osteoma	
Cartilage	Osteochondroma	Chondrosarcoma
	Chondroma	
	Chondroblastoma	
	Chondromyxoid fibroma	
Bone marrow		Multiple myeloma
		Reticulum cell sarcoma
Unknown	Giant cell tumor	Ewing's sarcoma
	Fibrous histiocytoma	Malignant giant cell tumor
		Malignant fibrous histiocytoma
		Adamantinoma

stand the strain of ordinary use. In such situations, even a small amount of bone stress or trauma precipitates a pathologic fracture. A tumor may produce pressure on a peripheral nerve causing decreased sensation, numbness, a limp, or limitation of movement.

Benign Neoplasms

Benign bone tumors usually are found to be limited to the confines of the bone, have well-demarcated edges, and are surrounded by a thin rim of sclerotic bone. The four most common types of benign bone tumors are (1) osteoma, (2) chondroma, (3) osteochondroma, and (4) giant cell tumor.

An *osteoma* is a bony tumor found on the surface of a long bone, flat bone, or the skull. It is usually composed of hard, compact (ivory osteoma), or spongy (cancellous) bone. It may be either excised or left alone.

A *chondroma* is a tumor composed of cartilage. It either grows outward from the bone (ecchondroma) or within the bone (enchondroma). These tumors may become large and are especially common in the hands and feet. At times a chondroma may persist for many years and then take on the attributes of a malignant chondrosarcoma. A chondroma is usually not treated unless it becomes unsightly or uncomfortable.

An *osteochondroma* is the most common form of benign tumor in the skeletal system. It grows only during periods of skeletal growth, originating in the epiphyseal cartilage plate and growing out of the bone like a mushroom. An osteochondroma is composed of both cartilage and bone and usually occurs singly but may affect several bones in a condition called multiple exostoses. Malignant changes are rare, and excision of the tumor is done only when necessary.

A *giant cell tumor*, or osteoclastoma, is a benign tumor of multinucleated cells that often behaves like a malignant tumor, metastasizing through the bloodstream and recurring locally following excision. It occurs most often in young adults, and is most commonly found in the knee, wrist, or shoulder. The tumor begins in the metaphyseal region, grows into the epiphysis, and may extend into the joint surface itself. Pathologic fractures are common because the tumor destroys the bone substance. Clinically pain may occur at the tumor site, with gradually increasing swelling. X-rays show destruction of the bone with expansion of the cortex.

The treatment of giant cell tumors depends on the tumors' site. If the affected bone can be eliminated without loss of function, such as the clavicle or fibula, the entire bone or part of it may be removed. When the tumor is near a major joint, such as the knee or shoulder, a local excision is done. Irradiation may be used in an attempt to prevent recurrence of the tumor.

Malignant Bone Tumors

In contrast with benign tumors, malignant tumors tend to be ill defined, lack sharp borders, and extend beyond the confines of the bone, showing that it has destroyed the cortex. Although malignant bone tumors are rare, they have a high mortality rate. In addition, there is much morbidity and trauma from the often mutilating surgical excision. Surgery often leads to amputation or removal of a large part of the bone, which causes disability.

Methods used in the diagnosis of bone tumors include roentgenography (x-ray), computed tomography, bone scanning, and biopsy of the tumor. Biopsy can be performed by means of a large needle or open surgical methods.

The treatment of malignant bone tumors primarily involves surgical removal of the tumor with amputation of the affected limb. Radiation therapy is used as a definitive and adjuvant treatment to slow the progression of the cancer, prevent pathologic fractures, and reduce bone pain. Because high-grade bone and soft tissue sarcomas produce clinically nondetectable metastases called micrometastases, immunotherapy, irradiation, and chemotherapy are often used in combination as adjuvant therapy. Chemotherapy is the most effective modality for controlling metastases. Extremely aggressive drug combinations have been developed, particularly in the pediatric and young adult age groups. Many conservative limb salvage surgical procedures are now being used as an alternative to limb amputation. They are most often used in younger individuals in an attempt to increase their function and mobility.

Osteogenic sarcoma

An osteogenic tumor is one arising from or having genesis within bone tissue. Osteogenic sarcoma involves proliferation of osteoid or immature bone.

Osteogenic sarcoma is the most common and most fatal primary malignant bone tumor, with the exception of multiple myeloma. It is a disease primarily of children and young adults between the ages of 10 and 20 years, with males being affected slightly more often than females. The tumor occurs most frequently during periods of peak skeletal growth, with the growth potential of each long bone determining the frequency of tumor occurrence. The most common sites of occurrence are the distal femur (41.5%), proximal tibia (16%), and proximal humerus (15%).[31] Occasionally, malignancies arise from the middle portion of the long bones. Persons affected with osteogenic sarcoma are usually tall and are found to have a high plasma level of somatomedin. Osteogenic sarcoma is an aggressive tumor that grows rapidly. It moves from the metaphysis of the bone out to the periosteum much like the process of acute hematogenous osteomyelitis. The causes of osteogenic carcinoma are unknown. It has been shown that viruses can induce sarcomas in laboratory animals. In addition, radiation from either an internal source, such as the radioactive pharmaceutical technetium used in bone scans, or an external source, such as x-rays, may also be a causative factor.

The primary clinical feature of osteosarcoma is severe pain in the affected bone, usually of sudden onset. There is a wide variation in the hardness of osteogenic tumors. Osteosarcoma usually begins as a firm white or reddish mass and later becomes softer with a viscous interior. Swelling is often present over the area. The skin overlying the tumor may be very shiny and stretched, with prominent superficial veins. There may be restricted range of motion of the adjacent joint.

Sarcomas infrequently metastasize to the lymph nodes because the cells are unable to grow within the node. Most often the tumor cells exit the primary tumor through the venous end of the capillary and early metastasis to the lung occurs. In osteosarcoma, the cause of death in 60% to 80% of cases is metastasis to the lungs.[29] Lung metastases, even if massive, are usually relatively asymptomatic. The prognosis depends on the aggressiveness of the malignancy, radiologic features, presence or absence of pathologic fracture, size of the tumor, rapidity of growth, and sex of the individual. There is some suggestion that females have a better survival rate than males.[30]

Chemotherapy, using various drug combinations, is the most effective treatment for metastatic osteosarcoma. The tumor is almost always resected by means of a high amputation of the affected limb. Even though this type of tumor extends through the medullary cavity, there is no evidence on x-ray. Microscopic examination has shown that the extension may be 1 in. to 3 in. or more beyond the cortical bone.[32] Because of this, the level of amputation is "as much as necessary, but as little as possible."[31] Surgical treatment alone for localized primary osteogenic sarcoma yields a poor prognosis, with a 3-year survival rate of about 20% to 30%. In the case of an inoperable tumor or widespread metastasis, chemotherapy with or without irradiation may be used. Pulmonary irradiation is being utilized with increasing success to reduce pulmonary metastasis in children under age 12. The use of immunotherapy, including interferon, is still in the experimental stages, as it is with other types of cancers.

Chondrosarcoma

Chondrosarcoma, a malignant tumor of cartilage, is the second most common form of malignant bone tumor. It is about half as common as osteosarcoma. It accounts for about 13% of bone tumors,[29] and affects males slightly more often than females. It is found in an older age group than osteogenic sarcoma, with the peak incidence occurring around 45 years of age.[29] It arises from points of muscle attachment to bone, particularly the knee, shoulder, hip, and pelvis. Cartilaginous tumors that are nearer to the trunk are apt to be malignant.

Chondrosarcomas, are slow growing, metastasize late, and are often painless. They can remain hidden in an area like the pelvis for a long time. This type of tumor, like many primary malignancies, tends to destroy bone and extend into the soft tissues beyond the confines of the bone of origin. Often, irregular flecks and streaks of calcification are a prominent radiographic finding.

Early diagnosis is important because chondrosarcoma responds well to early radical surgical excision. It is generally resistant to radiation therapy and current available chemotherapeutic agents.

Ewing's sarcoma

Ewing's sarcoma is the third most common type of primary bone tumor and is highly malignant, often with only a 3- to 5-year survival rate.[29] It is seen in people under age 30 with the highest incidence in the second decade of life. Ewing's tumor arises from cells in the bone marrow and causes bone destruction from within. It can occur in any bone.

Manifestations of Ewing's tumor include pain, tenderness, fever, and leukocytosis. Pathologic fractures are common because of bone destruction. The current treatment of Ewing's sarcoma is radiation along with combination chemotherapy. Ewing's sarcoma is more radiosensitive than other primary bone tumors. The use of central nervous system radiation is being investigated. Radical amputation is often necessary, especially because of the aggressiveness of the tumor.

Metastatic Bone Disease

Metastatic tumors are the most common malignancy of osseous tissue, accounting for 60% to 65% of all skeletal tumors.[33] Metastatic lesions are seen most frequently in the spine and pelvis and are less common in anatomic sites that are further removed from the trunk of the body. Tumors that frequently spread to the skeletal system are those of the breast, lung, kidney, thyroid, and prostate, although any cancer can ultimately involve the skeleton. It has been reported that 80% of bone metastases come from the breast, lung, and kidney.[33] The peak incidence of metastatic bone disease occurs in persons over age 40. In 90% of cases, bony metastases are multiple, with or without metastatic spread to other organs. Because of the effectiveness of current cancer treatment modalities, cancer patients are living longer, so that the incidence of clinically apparent skeletal involvement appears to be increasing in the long run. These skeletal metastases are sources of great pain; they increase the risk of fractures and the disability of the cancer patient. Therefore, orthopedic surgeons have become more aggressive in treatment of the pathologic condition.

Metastasis to the bone frequently occurs without involving other organs. This is because the blood flow to the veins of the skeletal system is sluggish. There are thin-walled veins without valves with many storage sites along the way. If metastasis is limited to the skeletal system, without other major organ involvement, a person can live for many years. The control of metastasis, along with treatment of the primary tumor, is essential because death is usually a consequence of metastasis to vital organs rather than of the primary tumor itself.

The major symptom of bone metastasis is pain with evidence of an impending pathologic fracture. X-ray examinations are used along with computerized tomography or bone scans to detect, diagnose, and localize metastatic bone lesions. About one-third of persons with skeletal metatases have positive bone scans without radiologic findings, and about 28% have metastatic lesions on x-ray with a negative bone scan.[34] Arteriography, using a radiopaque contrast medium, may be helpful in outlining the tumor margins. Serum levels of alkaline phosphatase and calcium are often elevated in persons with metastatic bone disease. A bone biopsy is usually done when there is a question regarding the diagnosis or treatment.

The primary goals in treatment of metastatic bone disease are to prevent pathologic fractures and promote maximum functioning along with survival in order to help maintain the quality of life, with as much mobility and pain control as possible. The treatment methods include surgery, chemotherapy, and irradiation. The discovery of new and more effective drugs along with the use of combination protocols have increased the effectiveness of chemotherapy in the treatment of metastatic bone disease secondary to tumors of the breast, prostate, and lung.[35] Surgery is used to prevent or treat pathologic fractures. Radiation therapy is primarily used as a palliative treatment to alleviate pain and prevent pathologic fractures.

Pathologic fractures occur in about 10% to 15% of persons with metastatic bone disease. The affected bone appears on x-ray to be eaten away and, in severe cases, crumbles on impact, much like dried toast. Many pathologic fractures occur in the femur, humerus, and vertebrae. In the femur, fractures occur because the proximal aspect of the bone is under great mechanical stress. Surgery or radiation therapy may be done prophylactically when a lesion is detected to prevent pathologic fractures from occurring. When a pathologic fracture has occurred, traction, intramedullary nailing, casting, or bracing is used. Because adequate fixation is often difficult with diseased bone, bone cement (methyl methacrylate) is often used with internal fixation devices to stabilize the bone. The selection of a treatment modality to either prevent or treat pathologic fractures depends on the severity of the lesion, the degree of pain, and the life expectancy of the patient. The goal is to give people flexibility, mobility, and pain relief. A certain degree of aggressiveness is used by surgeons in treating metastatic lesions so that patients can function as normally as possible.

In summary, bone tumors, as any other type of neoplasms, may be either benign or malignant. Benign bone tumors grow slowly and usually do not destroy the surrounding tissues. Malignant tumors can be either primary or metastatic. Primary bone tumors are relatively rare, grow rapidly, metastasize to the lungs and other parts of the body through the bloodstream, and have a high mortality rate. Metastatic bone tumors are usually multiple, originating primarily from cancers of the breast, lung, and kidney. The incidence of metastatic bone disease is probably increasing because the improved treatment methods enable people with cancer to live longer. Recent advances in chemotherapy, radiation therapy, and surgical procedures have substantially increased the survival and cure rates for many types of bone cancers. A primary goal in metastatic bone disease is the prevention of pathologic fractures.

■ Study Guide

After you have studied this chapter you should be able to meet the following objectives:

☐ Differentiate between the processes of endochondral and intramembranous ossification that occur during embryonic development.

☐ Describe the function of the epiphysis in terms of skeletal growth.

☐ Cite at least three factors that can affect epiphyseal growth.

☐ Explain how an infant's limbs differ from those of an adult.

☐ Define femoral anteversion.

☐ Differentiate between toeing-in and internal tibial torsion.

☐ Define genu varum and genu valgum.

☐ Name one treatment for flatfeet.

☐ Identify two childhood diseases that are classified as osteochondroses.

☐ Describe the pathology of Legg–Calvé–Perthes disease.

☐ List the symptoms of Osgood–Schlatter disease.

☐ Explain why it is important to treat a slipped capital femoral epiphyseal as soon as it is diagnosed.

☐ Cite the incidence of scoliosis.

☐ List the cardinal signs of scoliosis that serve as a basis for school screening programs.

☐ Contrast the conservative and surgical treatments of scoliosis.

☐ Describe the physical appearance of an infant with congenital dislocation of the hip.

☐ Cite the recommended schedule for clinical examination to detect congenital hip dislocation.

☐ Explain the treatment for a newborn with clubfoot.

☐ List the problems that occur because of defective tissue synthesis in osteogenesis imperfecta.

☐ Name the three factors that are responsible for maintaining the equilibrium of bone tissue.

☐ Compare structure remodeling of bone with internal remodeling.

☐ Cite the functions of parathyroid hormone, vitamin D, and calcitonin in bone metabolism.

☐ Trace the activation of vitamin D in the body.

☐ Define the term osteopenia.

☐ Describe the primary features of osteoporotic bone.

☐ Cite the sex, race, and age groups of persons most frequently affected by osteoporosis.

☐ List three factors that contribute to the development of osteoporosis.

☐ Cite the action of fluoride in the treatment of osteoporosis.

☐ Contrast osteomalacia, rickets, and osteoporosis.

☐ Relate vitamin D deficiency to the inadequate mineralization of bone that occurs in osteomalacia and rickets.

☐ Describe the appearance of bone affected by Paget's disease (osteitis deformans).

☐ List the clinical manifestations of Paget's disease.

☐ Differentiate between the properties of benign and malignant bone tumors.

☐ Name the three major symptoms of bone cancer.

☐ Describe the population primarily affected by osteogenic sarcoma.

☐ Contrast osteogenic sarcoma and chondrosarcoma.

☐ List the primary sites of tumors that frequently metastasize to the bone.

☐ Explain why metastasis to the bone frequently occurs without involving other organs.

☐ State the three primary goals for treatment of metastatic bone disease.

■ References

1. Moore KL: Before We Are Born, pp 2–3. Philadelphia, WB Saunders, 1983
2. Hopper WC: Genetics in orthopedics. Orthop Nurs 1:38, 1983
3. DeAngles C: Pediatric Primary Care, pp 289, 292. Boston, Little, Brown, 1984
4. Hilt C, Cogburn SB: Manual of Orthopedics, pp 303, 303. St Louis, CV Mosby, 1980
5. Greshuni DH: Preliminary evaluation and prognosis in Legg–Calvé–Perthes disease. Clin Orthop 150, No 4:16, 1980
6. Axer A et al: Indications for femoral osteotomy in Legg–Calvé–Perthes disease. Clin Orthop 150, No 4:78, 1980
7. Jani LFH, Dick W: Results of three different types of therapeutic groups in Perthes disease. Clin Orthop 150, No 4:88, 1980
8. Rodman GP, Shumacker HR (eds): Primer on Rheumatic Disorders, pp 145, 147, 170. Atlanta, Arthritis Foundation, 1983
9. Harrel J, Meehan PL: School screening in spinal deformity. ONAJ 6, No 5:201, 1977
10. Harrington PR: The etiology of idiopathic scoliosis. Clin Orthop 126, No 4:17, 1977
11. Segil C: Current concepts in management of scoliosis. Nurs Clin North Am 11, No 4:692, 1976
12. Holt deToledo C: The patient with scoliosis: The defect, the classification, and detection. Am J Nurs 79, No 9:1588, 1979
13. Wickers FC et al: Psychological factors in failure to wear the Milwaukee brace for treatment of idiopathic scoliosis. Clin Orthop 126, No 4:62, 1977
14. Hooker CW, Greene WB: Congenital malformations. In Wilson FC (ed): The Musculoskeletal System, 2nd ed, p 27. Philadelphia, JB Lippincott, 1983
15. Duncan C: Osteogenesis imperfecta. ONAJ 6, No 5:193, 1979
16. Robbins SL, Cotran RS: Pathologic Basis of Disease, ed. 2, pp 1480, 1491. Philadelphia, WB Saunders, 1979
17. Ham AW, Cormack DH: Histology, 8th ed, p 441. Philadelphia, JB Lippincott, 1979
18. Talmadge RV, Grubb SA, VanderWeil CJ: Physiological processes in bone. In Wilson FC (ed): The Musculoskeletal System, 2nd ed, p 123. Philadelphia, JB Lippincott, 1983
19. Stamp TCB, Round JM: Seasonal changes in human plasma levels of 25-dihydroxyvitamin D. Nature 247:563, 1974
20. Bickle DD: The vitamin D endocrine system. Ann Intern Med 27:45, 1982

21. Raisz LG: Osteoporosis. J Am Geriat Soc 30, No 2:127–138, 1982
22. Gordon GS, Vaughn C: Osteoporosis: Early detection, prevention, and treatment. Consultant 25, No 1:64, 1980
23. Aloia JF: Estrogen and exercise in prevention and treatment of osteoporosis. Geriatrics 37, No 6:81–85, 1982
24. Spencer H: Osteoporosis: Goals of therapy. Hosp Pract 17, No 3:131, 1982
25. Slovik DM, Adams JS, Neer RM et al: Deficient production of 1,25 dihydroxyvitamin D in elderly osteoporotic patients. N Engl J Med 305:372, 1981
26. Aroncheck JM, Haddad JG. Paget's disease. Orthop Clin North Am 14, No 1:3, 1983
27. Wallach S: Treatment of Paget's disease. Adv Intern Med 27:1, 1982
28. Schajowicz F, Arauyo ES, Bernestein M: Sarcoma complicating Paget's disease of bone. J Bone Joint Surg 65-B, No 3:299–307, 1983
29. Rubin R (ed): Clinical Oncology: A Multidisciplinary Approach. New York, American Cancer Society, 1983
30. Facts on Bone Cancer. New York, American Cancer Society, 1978
31. Huvos AG: Bone Tumors: Diagnosis, Treatment and Prognosis. Philadelphia, WB Saunders, 1979
32. Brashear HR: Tumors and tumorlike conditions of bone. In Wilson FC (ed): The Musculoskeletal System, 2nd ed, p 158. Philadelphia, JB Lippincott, 1980
33. Sherry HS, Levy RN, Siffert RS: Metastatic disease of bone in orthopedic surgery. Clin Orthop 169:44, 1982
34. Bhardwaj S, Holland JF: Chemotherapy of metastatic cancer in bone. Clin Orthop 169:28, 1982
35. Schocker JD, Brady LW: Radiation therapy for bone metastasis. Clin Orthop 169:38, 1982

■ Additional References

Albright JA: Management overview of osteogenesis imperfecta. Clin Orthop 159:80, 1981
Aloia JF: Estrogen and exercise in prevention and treatment of osteoporosis. Geriatrics 37, No 6:81, 1982
Alvioli LV: Management of osteomalacia: Hosp Pract 14, No 1:109, 1979
Binder H, Hawks L, Graybill G et al: Osteogenesis imperfecta: Rehabilitation approach with infants and young children. Arch Phys Med Rehabil 65:537, 1984
Bowen JR, Foster BK, Hartzell CR: Legg–Calvé–Perthes disease. Clin Orthop 185:97, 1984
Brewer V, Meyer BM, Keele MS et al: Role of exercise in prevention of involutional bone loss. Med Sci Sports Exerc 15:445, 1983
Dalinka MK, Aronchick JM, Haddad JG: Paget's disease. Orthop Clin North Am 14, No 1:3, 1983
Gordon GS, Vaughn C: Osteoporosis: Early detection, prevention, and treatment. Consultant 20, No 1:64, 1980
Jackson MA et al: Etiology and medical management of acute suppurative joint infections in pediatric patients. J Pediatr Orthop 2, No 3:313, 1982

Kane WJ: Early detection of scoliosis. Orthop Dig (May):13, 1977
Kaplan FS: Osteoporosis. Clin Symp 35, No 5, 1983
Lahde RE: Luque rod instrumentation. AORN J 38:35, 1983
Lukert B: Osteoporosis—A review and update. Arch Phys Med Rehabil 63:480, 1982
Madigan RR, Wallace SL: What's new in scoliosis. J Tenn Med Assoc 76:292, 1983
Mann RA: Acquired flat foot in adults. Clin Orthop 181:46, 1983
Marcus R: The relationship of dietary calcium to maintenance of skeletal integrity in man—An interface of endocrinology and nutrition. Metabolism 31:93, 1982
Marx JL: Osteoporosis: New help for thinning bones. Science 207:628, 1980
Nasca RJ: Newer concepts in diagnosis and treatment of scoliosis. Ala J Med Sci 19:284, 1982
Pitt M: Osteopenic bone disease. Orthop Clin North Am 14, No 1:65, 1983
Raisz LG: Osteoporosis. J Am Geriatr Soc 30:127, 1982
Schock CC: Progress in treatment of adolescent idiopathic scoliosis. J Arkansas Med Soc 79:319, 1983
Siris ES, Jacobs TP, Canfield RE: Paget's disease of bone. Bull NY Acad Med 56:285, 1980
Slovik DM, Adams JS, Neer RM et al: Deficient production of 1,25-dihydroxyvitamin D in elderly osteoporotic patients. N Engl J Med 305:372, 1981
Spencer H: Osteoporosis: Goals of therapy. Hosp Pract 17, No 3:131, 1982
Victoria-Diaz A, Victoria-Diaz V: Pathogenesis of idiopathic club foot. Clin Orthop 185:14, 1984
Wallack S: Treatment of Paget's disease. Adv Intern Med 27:1, 1982
Werner P, Metz L, Dubowski F: Nursing care of an osteogenesis imperfecta infant and child. Clin Orthop 159:108, 1981
Whedon GD: Osteoporosis. N Engl J Med 305:397, 1981
Wynne-Davies R, Gormley J: Clinical and genetic patterns in osteogenesis imperfecta. Clin Orthop 159:26, 1981

Chapter 53

Alterations in Skeletal Function: Rheumatic Disorders

Pamela M. Schroeder

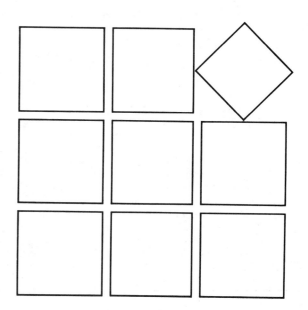

Arthritis, or inflammation of the joint, is a rheumatic disorder characterized by inflammatory and degenerative joint changes. More than 100 different types of arthritis affect one in every seven individuals.[1] The disease affects individuals of all age groups and is the second leading cause of disability in the United States.[2] The disabling effects may be manifested in an individual's personal, professional, and social activities.

There is a wide spectrum of perceptions about arthritis. Some individuals perceive arthritis as a minor ache or pain; others envision being in a wheelchair within a matter of months. Because arthritis is not often perceived as life threatening, frequently treatment is not sought until the disorder has made a significant impact on a person's life.

Some forms of arthritis may develop as a primary joint disorder, while other forms may occur as a secondary disorder resulting from another disease condition. Table 53-1 provides a classification of rheumatic diseases. The discussion in this chapter is limited to rheumatoid arthritis, osteoarthritis, spondyloarthropathies, and crystal-induced arthropathies.

Table 53-1 Classification of the Rheumatic Diseases

I. Diffuse connective tissue diseases
    A. Rheumatoid arthritis
    B. Juvenile arthritis
       1. Systemic onset
       2. Polyarticular onset
       3. Oligarticular onset
    C. Systemic lupus erythematosus
    D. Progressive systemic sclerosis
    E. Polymyositis/dermatomyositis
    F. Necrotizing vasculitis and other vasculopathies
       1. Polyarteritis nodosa group (includes hepatitis B associated arteritis and Churg–Strauss allergic granulomatosis)
       2. Hypersensitivity vasculitis (includes Schönlein-Henoch purpura)
       3. Wegener's granulomatosis
       4. Giant cell arteritis (temporal arteritis, Takayasu's arteritis)
       5. Mucocutaneous lymph node syndrome (Kawasaki's disease)
       6. Behcet's disease
    G. Sjögren's syndrome
    H. Overlap syndromes (includes mixed connective tissue disease)
    I. Others (includes polymyalgia rheumatica, panniculitis (Weber–Christian disease), erythema nodosum, relapsing polychondritis, and others)
II. Arthritis associated with spondylitis
    A. Ankylosing spondylitis
    B. Reiter's syndrome
    C. Psoriatic arthritis
    D. Arthritis associated with chronic inflammatory bowel disease

III. Degenerative joint disease (osteoarthritis, osteoarthrosis)
    A. Primary (includes erosive osteoarthritis)
    B. Secondary
IV. Arthritis, tenosynovitis, and bursitis associated with infectious agents
    A. Direct
       1. Bacterial (staphylococcus, gonococcus, mycobacteria, treponemes, and others)
       2. Viral
       3. Fungal
       4. Parasitic
       5. Unknown, suspected (Whipple's disease)
    B. Indirect (reactive)
       1. Bacterial (includes acute rheumatic fever, intestinal bypass, postdysenteric—shigella, yersinia)
       2. Viral (hepatitis B)
V. Metabolic and endocrine diseases associated with rheumatic states
    A. Crystal-induced conditions
       1. Monosodium urate (gout)
       2. Calcium pyrophosphate dihydrate (pseudogout, chondrocalcinosis)
       3. Hydroxyapatite
    B. Biochemical abnormalities
       1. Amyloidosis
       2. Vitamin C deficiency (scurvy)
       3. Specific enzyme deficiency states (includes Fabry's, Farber's, alkaptonuria, and Lesch–Nyhan)
       4. Hyperlipidemias (types II, IIa, IV)
       5. Mucopolysaccharides
       6. Hemoglobinopathies (SS disease and others)
       7. True connective tissue disorders (Ehlers–Danlos, Marfan's, and pseudoxanthoma elasticum)
       8. Others
    C. Endocrine diseases
       1. Diabetes mellitus
       2. Acromegaly
       3. Hyperparathyroidism
       4. Thyroid disease (hyperthyroidism, hypothyroidism)
    D. Immunodeficiency diseases
    E. Other hereditary disorders
       1. Arthrogryposis multiplex congenita
       2. Hypermobility syndromes
       3. Myositis ossificans progressiva
VI. Neoplasms
    A. Primary (*e.g.*, synovioma, synoviosarcoma)
    B. Metastatic
VII. Neuropathic disorders
    A. Charcot joints
    B. Compression neuropathies
       1. Peripheral entrapment (carpal tunnel syndrome and others)
       2. Radiculopathy
       3. Spinal stenosis
    C. Reflex sympathetic dystrophy
    D. Others
VIII. Bone and cartilage disorders associated with articular manifestations
    A. Osteoporosis
       1. Generalized
       2. Localized (regional)
    B. Osteomalacia
    C. Hypertrophic osteoarthropathy
    D. Diffuse idiopathic skeletal hyperostosis (includes ankylosing vertebral hyperostosis—Forrestier's disease)

E. Osteitis
1. Generalized (osteitis deformans—Paget's disease of bone)
2. Localized (osteitis condensans ilii; osteitis pubis)
F. Avascular necrosis
G. Osteochondritis (osteochondritis dissecans)
H. Congenital displasia of the hip
I. Slipped capital femoral epiphysis
J. Costochondritis (includes Tietze's syndrome)
K. Osteolysis and chondrolysis
IX. Nonarticular rheumatism
A. Myofascial pain syndromes
1. Generalized (fibrositis, fibromyalgia)
2. Regional
B. Low back pain and intervertebral disk disorders
C. Tendinitis (tenosynovitis) and/or bursitis
1. Subacromial/subdeltoid bursitis
2. Bicipital tendinitis, tenosynovitis
3. Olecranon bursitis
4. Epicondylitis, medial or laterial humeral
5. DeQuervain's tenosynovitis
6. Adhesive capsulitis of the shoulder (frozen shoulder)
7. Trigger finger
D. Ganglion cysts
E. Fascitis
F. Chronic ligament and muscle strain
G. Vasomotor disorders
1. Erythromelalgia
2. Raynaud's disease or phenomenon
H. Miscellaneous pain syndromes (includes weather sensitivity, psychogenic rheumatism)
X. Miscellaneous disorders
A. Disorders frequently associated with arthritis
1. Trauma (the result of direct trauma)
2. Lyme arthritis
3. Pancreatic disease
4. Sarcoidosis
5. Palindromic rheumatism
6. Intermittent hydarthrosis
7. Villonodular synovitis
8. Hemophilia
B. Other conditions
1. Internal derangement of joints (includes chondromalacia patella, loose bodies)
2. Familial Mediterranean fever
3. Eosinophilic fasciitis
4. Chronic active hepatitis
5. Other drug-induced rheumatic syndromes

(From Primer on the Rheumatic Diseases, 8th ed. Atlanta, Arthritis Foundation, 1983)

■ Rheumatoid Arthritis

Rheumatoid arthritis is a systemic inflammatory disease that affects 1% to 2% of the population, women being affected two to three times more frequently than men.[2] Although rheumatoid arthritis occurs in all age groups, its prevalence increases with age. In women the peak incidence is between ages 40 and 60.

Although the cause of rheumatoid arthritis remains somewhat of a mystery, there is evidence that immunologic events may play an important role. About 70% of individuals with the disease have the rheumatoid factor (RF), which is considered to be an antibody to an autologous (self-producing) immunoglobin in their blood.[2]

Why the body would begin to produce antibodies against its own IgG cannot be answered as yet. It is possible that an infectious agent, such as a virus, could alter the immunoglobulin so that it is recognized as foreign. Another possibility is that genetic predisposition plays a role in the development of the response. A large number of persons with rheumatoid arthritis have been found to have the histocompatibility antigen HLA-DR4 (discussed in Chap. 9).[3]

The rheumatoid factor has been found not only in the blood, but also in the synovial fluid and synovial membrane of affected persons. In fact, it has been shown that much of the RF is produced by lymphocytes in the inflammatory infiltrate of the synovial tissue.[2] To partially explain the destructive changes that occur in rheumatoid arthritis, it has been suggested that the RF reacts with IgG or other types of antibodies to form immune complexes. These immune complexes activate the complement system, which, in turn, initiates the inflammatory reaction. Polymorphonuclear leukocytes, monocytes, and lymphocytes are attracted to the area. These cells phagocytize the immune complexes and, in the process, release lysosomal enzymes capable of causing destructive changes in the joint cartilage. The inflammatory response that follows attracts additional lymphocytes and plasma cells, setting into motion a chain of events that perpetuates the condition.

Pathologic Changes

In rheumatoid arthritis the pathologic changes begin with inflammatory changes in the synovial membrane. The synovial cells and the subsynovial tissue undergo a reactive hyperplasia. Vasodilation and increased blood flow cause warmth and redness. Swelling results from the increased capillary permeability that accompanies the inflammatory process.

Characteristic of rheumatoid arthritis is the development of a destructive vascular granulation tissue called *pannus,* which extends from the synovium to involve the articular cartilage (Fig. 53-1). The inflammatory cells found in the pannus have a destructive effect on the adjacent cartilage and bone. Eventually, the pannus develops between the joint margins, leading to reduced joint motion and the possibility of eventual ankylosis. With the progression of the disease, joint inflammation and the resulting structural changes can lead to joint instability, muscle atrophy from disuse, stretching of the ligaments, and involvement of the tendons and muscles. The effect of the pathologic changes in the joint is related to the disease activity, which can change at any time. The destructive changes are irreversible.

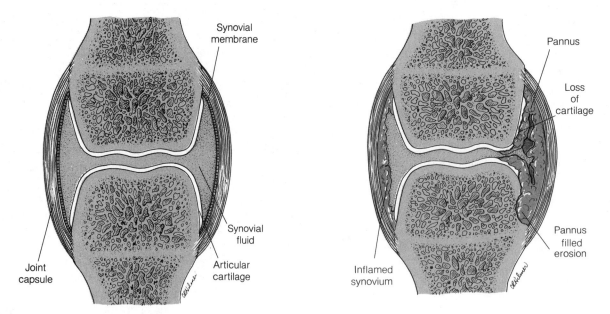

Figure 53-1 (Left) *Normal joint structures;* (right) *joint changes in rheumatoid arthritis. The left side denotes early changes occurring within the synovium, and the right side shows progressive disease that leads to erosion and the formation of pannus.*

Clinical Manifestations

Rheumatoid arthritis is often associated with extra-articular as well as articular manifestations. The disease, which is characterized by exacerbations and remissions, may involve only a few joints for brief durations or it may be relentlessly progressive and debilitating. About 15% of persons with the disease have a progressive, unremitting form of rheumatoid arthritis, which can lead to crippling.[2]

Joint manifestations

Rheumatoid arthritis usually has an insidious onset marked by systemic manifestations such as fatigue, anorexia, weight loss, and generalized aching and stiffness. Joint involvement is usually symmetrical and polyarticular. Any diarthroidal joint can be involved. The individual may complain of joint pain and swelling in addition to stiffness. Morning stiffness usually lasts 30 minutes and frequently for several hours. The limitation of joint motion that occurs early in the disease is usually

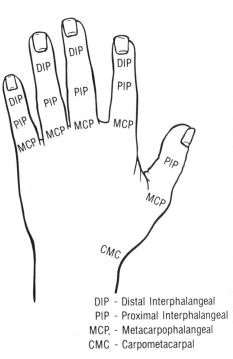

DIP - Distal Interphalangeal
PIP - Proximal Interphalangeal
MCP - Metacarpophalangeal
CMC - Carpometacarpal

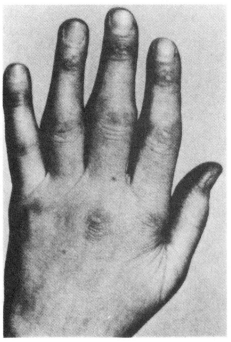

Figure 53-2 (Left) *Diagram of the joints of the hand;* (right) *early rheumatoid arthritis—spindling of the fingers. (Photograph reprinted from the Revised Clinical Slide Collection on the Rheumatic Diseases, © 1972. Used by permission of the Arthritis Foundation.)*

due to pain; later it is due to fibrosis. The most frequently affected joints initially are the fingers, hands, wrists, knees, and feet. Later, other diarthroidal joints may become involved. Spinal involvement is usually limited to the cervical region.

In the *hands* there is usually symmetrical involvement of the proximal interphalangeal (PIP) and metacarpophalangeal (MCP) joints in the early stages of rheumatoid arthritis; the distal interphalangeal (DIP) joints are rarely affected. The fingers often take on a spindle-shaped appearance because of inflammation of the proximal interphalangeal joints (Fig. 53-2).

Progressive joint destruction may lead to subluxation and instability as well as limitation in movement. Swelling and thickening of the synovium can result in stretching of the joint capsule and ligaments. When this occurs, muscle and tendon imbalance develop, and mechanical forces applied to the joints through daily activities produce joint deformities. In the metacarpophalangeal joints, the extensor tendons can slip to the ulnar side of the metacarpal head, causing ulnar deviation of the fingers. Subluxation of the metacarpophalangeal joints may develop when this deformity is present (Fig. 53-3). Hyperextension of the proximal interphalangeal joint and partial flexion of the distal interphalangeal joint is called a *swan neck deformity* (Fig. 53-4). Once this condition becomes fixed, severe loss of function occurs, because the person can no longer make a fist. When flexion of the proximal interphalangeal joint with hyperextension of the distal interphalangeal joint occurs it is called a *boutonnière deformity* (Fig. 53-5).

In rheumatoid arthritis a condition called *carpal tunnel syndrome* can occur when the median nerve is compressed as a result of synovial hypertrophy and tenosynovitis on the volar aspect of the wrist. Carpal tunnel syndrome is an entrapment neuropathy and is a common cause of paresthesias of the hand in rheumatoid arthritis as well as other conditions. Burning pain and tingling of the hands occurs, often at night. Numbness of the middle or three radial fingers is common. Occasionally the pain spreads above the wrist into the arm. As the condition progresses, muscle weakness may develop and there may be difficulty in abducting the thumb or opposing the thumb to the index finger.

The knee is one of the most commonly affected joints and is responsible for much of the disability associated with the disease.[2] Active synovitis may be apparent as visible swelling that obliterates the normal contour over the medial and lateral aspects of the patella. The bulge sign, which involves milking fluid from the lateral to the medial side of the patella, may be used to determine the presence of excess fluid when it is not visible. Joint contractures, instability, and valgus deformity are further manifestations that can occur (Fig. 53-6). There is often severe quadriceps atrophy, which contributes to

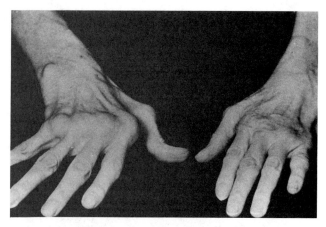

Figure 53-3 *Swelling and atrophy of the metacarpophalangeal joints in both hands. Ulnar deviation and subluxation of the metacarpophalangeal joints in the right hand occur. (Reprinted from the Arthritis Teaching Slide Collection, © 1980. Used by permission of the Arthritis Foundation).*

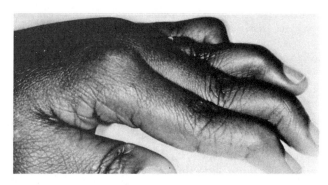

Figure 53-4 *Swan neck deformity, in which the proximal interphalangeal* (middle) *joint is hyperextended and the distal interphalangeal joint is in flexion. (Reprinted from the Arthritis Teaching Slide Collection, © 1980. Used by permission of the Arthritis Foundation.)*

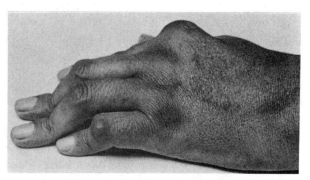

Figure 53-5 *Boutonnière deformity, which is characterized by flexion of the proximal interphalangeal joint, hyperextension of the distal interphalangeal joint, and inability to straighten the joint. (Reprinted from the Arthritis Teaching Slide Collection, © 1980. Used by permission of the Arthritis Foundation).*

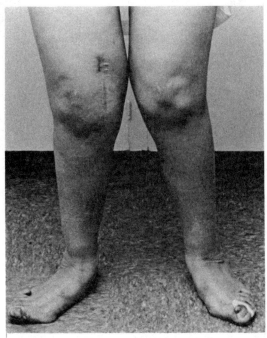

Figure 53-6   *Genu valgum (knock knees). This abnormal position is the result of a gradual wearing of cartilage and weakened ligaments in the knee joint. (Reprinted from the Arthritis Teaching Slide Collection, © 1980. Used by permission of the Arthritis Foundation.*

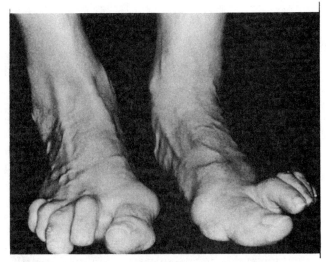

Figure 53-7   *Hallus valgus and hammer toes. The "cock-up" toe deformities are associated with subluxation at the metatarsophalangeal joints. Painful corns and bunions are made worse by irritation caused by faulty shoes. (Reprinted from the Arthritis Teaching Slide Collection, © 1980. Used by permission of the Arthritis Foundation.)*

disability. A Baker's cyst may occur behind the knee. This is caused by bursa enlargement and usually does not cause symptoms unless the cyst ruptures, in which case symptoms mimicking thrombophlebitis occur.

Disease activity can limit flexion and extension of the ankle, which can create difficulty in walking. Involvement of the metatarsophalangeal joints can cause subluxation, hallux valgus, and cock-up toe deformities (Fig. 53-7).

Neck discomfort is common. In rare cases, long-standing disease can lead to neurologic complications. Dislocation of the first cervical vertebra or subluxation of the odontoid process of the second vertebra into the foramen magnum are uncommon but potentially fatal complications.

Extra-articular manifestations

Although characteristically a joint disease, rheumatoid arthritis can affect a number of other tissues. The extra-articular manifestations probably occur with a fair degree of frequency but are usually mild enough that they cause few problems. They are most likely to be present in persons with a positive RF.

Because rheumatoid arthritis is a systemic disease, it may be accompanied by the previously mentioned complaints of fatigue, weakness, anorexia, weight loss, and low-grade fever during periods when the disease is active. The erythrocyte sedimentation rate (ESR), which is commonly elevated during inflammatory processes, has been found to correlate with the amount of disease activity.[2] Anemia associated with a low serum iron or low iron-binding capacity is common.[2]

Rheumatoid nodules are granulomatous lesions that develop around small blood vessels. The nodules may be tender or nontender, movable or nonmovable. The size is variable. Typically they are found over pressure points such as the extensor surfaces of the ulna (Fig. 53-8). The nodules may remain unless surgically removed, or they may resolve spontaneously.

Vasculitis is an uncommon manifestation of rheumatoid arthritis seen in individuals with a long history of active arthritis and high titers of rheumatoid factor. It is possible that some individuals have vasculitis that remains silent. Vasculitis is caused by the inflammatory process affecting the small and medium-sized arterioles. Manifestations include ischemic areas in the nailfold and digital pulp that appear as brown spots. Ulcerations may occur in the lower extremities, particularly around the malleolar areas. These ulcerations may be difficult to distinguish from other forms of skin ulcerations.[4] In some individuals, neuropathy may be the only symptom of vasculitis. The visceral organs, such as the heart, lungs, and gastrointestinal tract may also be affected.

Sjögren's syndrome is present in about 10% to 15% of individuals with rheumatoid arthritis.[2] It may also be present with other connective tissue diseases or be a disorder without an accompanying disease process. The primary symptoms are reduced lacrimal and salivary gland secretion, frequently referred to as the sicca complex. The eyes may feel sandy or gritty, as if foreign bodies are in them. The mouth feels dry, and the individual usually feels the need for frequent fluid consumption. The individual is more prone than normal to dental caries and halitosis because saliva is not present to reduce these problems. The dryness associated with Sjögren's syndrome can affect any of the mucous membranes. The treatment is generally symptomatic. Artificial tears, or 0.5% methylcellulose eye drops, provide temporary relief of dry eyes. Sugarless hard candy, artificial saliva products, and the use of a home humidifier can help reduce mouth and throat dryness. The use of water-soluble lubricants during sexual activity can be helpful if vaginal dryness is a problem.

Other extra-articular manifestations include eye lesions such as episcleritis and scleritis, hematologic abnormalities, pulmonary disease, cardiac complications, infection, and Felty's syndrome (leukopenia with or without splenomegaly).

Diagnosis and Treatment

The diagnosis of rheumatoid arthritis is based on history, physical examination, and laboratory tests. The diagnostic criteria developed by the American Rheumatism Association are used in establishing the diagnosis (see Table 53-2). At least seven of the criteria must be present to make a definite diagnosis, three for probable rheumatoid arthritis, and two for possible rheumatoid arthritis. Some of the criteria require minimum periods of observation by a physician.

In the early stages, the disease is much more difficult to diagnose. On physical examination the affected joints show signs of inflammation, swelling, tenderness, and possibly warmth and reduced motion. The joints have a soft spongy feeling because of the synovial thickening and inflammation. Body movements may be guarded to prevent pain. Changes in joint structure are usually not visible early in the disease. Information should be elicited regarding the duration of symptoms, systemic manifestations, stiffness, and family history.

The RF may be used as a diagnostic test, but is inconclusive, because 1% to 5% of healthy individuals have rheumatoid factor. The presence of RF seems to be more common with advancing age. It is important to note than an individual can have rheumatoid arthritis without the rheumatoid factor being present. X-ray findings are not diagnostic in rheumatoid arthritis because joint erosions are not often seen on x-ray in the early stages of the disorder.[2]

Synovial fluid analysis can be helpful in the diag-

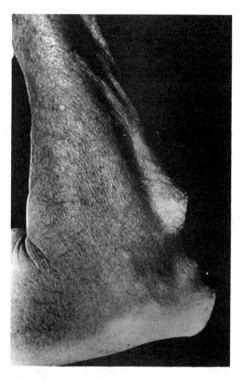

Figure 53-8   *Rheumatoid nodules on the elbow. (Reprinted from the Clinical Slide Collection on the Rheumatic Diseases, © 1972. Used by permission of the Arthritis Foundation.)*

nostic process. The fluid has a cloudy appearance because the white blood cell count is elevated as a result of inflammation, while the complement components of the synovial fluid are depressed.

The treatment goals for a person with rheumatoid arthritis are to reduce pain, minimize stiffness and swelling, maintain mobility, and become an informed health care consumer. The treatment plan includes education about the disease and its treatment, rest, therapeutic exercises, and medications. Because of the chronicity of the disease and the need for continuous long-term adherence to the prescribed treatment modalities, it is important that the treatment be integrated with the individual's life-style.

Basic education is fundamental in removing misconceptions. The knowledge that although arthritis cannot be cured, much can be done to control the disease process is needed by not only the individual with arthritis but also the general population. Fear of crippling is a major concern that should be addressed, so that the disease is perceived within a realistic context. All aspects of the treatment require that the individual with arthritis accept responsibility for the health care program. Family members should be included in education programs; their support in integrating prescribed treatment regimens is very important. Because many unproven reme-

Table 53-2 Criteria for the Classification of Rheumatoid Arthritis

A. Classic rheumatoid arthritis

This diagnosis requires seven of the following criteria. In criteria 1 through 5 the joint signs or symptoms must be continuous for at least six weeks.

1. Morning stiffness.

2. Pain on motion or tenderness in at least one joint (observed by a physician).

3. Swelling (soft tissue thickening or fluid, not bony overgrowth alone) in at least one joint (observed by a physician).

4. Swelling (observed by a physician) of at least one other joint (any interval free of joint symptoms between the two joint involvements may not be more than three months).

5. Symmetric joint swelling (observed by a physician) with simultaneous involvement of the same joint on both sides of the body (bilateral involvement of proximal interphalangeal, metacarpophalangeal, or metatarsophalangeal joints is acceptable without absolute symmetry). Terminal phalangeal joint involvement will not satisfy this criterion.

6. Subcutaneous nodules (observed by a physician) over bony prominences, on extensor surfaces, or in juxta-articular regions.

7. Roentgenographic changes typical of rheumatoid arthritis (which must include at least bony decalcification localized to or most marked adjacent to the involved joints and not just degenerative changes). Degenerative changes do not exclude patients from any group classified as having rheumatoid arthritis.

8. Positive agglutination test—demonstration of the "rheumatoid factor" by any method which, in two laboratories, has been positive in not over 5% of normal controls, or positive streptococcal agglutination test. [The latter is now obsolete.]

9. Poor mucin precipitate from synovial fluid (with shreds and cloudy solution). (An inflammatory synovial effusion with 2000 or more white cells/mm^3, without crystals can be substituted for this criterion.)

10. Characteristic histologic changes in synovium with three or more of the following: marked villous hypertrophy; proliferation of superficial synovial cells often with palisading; marked infiltration of chronic inflammatory cells (lymphocytes or plasma cells predominating) with tendency to form "lymphoid nodules"; deposition of compact fibrin either on surface or interstitially; foci of necrosis.

11. Characteristic histologic changes in nodules showing granulomatous foci with central zones of cell necrosis, surrounded by a palisade of proliferated mononuclear and peripheral fibrosis and chronic inflammatory cell infiltration.

B. Definite rheumatoid arthritis

This diagnosis requires five of the above criteria. In criteria 1 through 5 the joint signs or symptoms must be continuous for at least 6 weeks.

C. Probable rheumatoid arthritis

This diagnosis requires three of the above criteria. In at least one of criteria 1 through 5 the joint signs or symptoms must be continuous for at least 6 weeks.

(From Primer on the Rheumatic Diseases, 8th ed. © 1983. Used by permission of the Arthritis Foundation.)

dies are tried for arthritis, there is a need for information on how to determine the validity of available treatments. The Arthritis Foundation provides information and community services to people with arthritis and their families.

Both physical and emotional rest are important aspects of care. Physical rest reduces joint stress. Rest should include total body rest of 8 hours to 10 hours at night and one to two naps or rest periods during the day. Rest of specific joints is recommended to relieve pain. For example, sitting reduces the weight on an inflamed knee and the use of lightweight splints reduces undue movement of the hand or wrist. Emotional rest is also important. Some individuals find that discomfort increases with emotional stress; with emotional rest, muscles relax and discomfort is reduced.

Although rest is essential, therapeutic exercises are important in maintaining joint motion and muscle strength. Range of motion exercises involve the active and passive movement of joints. Isometric (muscle tensing) exercises may be used to strengthen muscles. These exercises are frequently taught by a physical therapist and then performed on a daily basis at home. There is also a need to emphasize the difference between normal activity and therapeutic exercise.

Instruction in the safe use of heat and cold modalities to relieve discomfort and the use of relaxation techniques are also important. Proper posture, positioning, body mechanics, and the use of supportive shoes can provide further comfort. Information about the principles of joint protection and work simplification is often needed. Assistive devices are necessary for some individuals to reduce pain and improve the ability to perform activities of daily living.

Strategies to aid in symptom control also involve regulating activity by pacing, establishing priorities, and setting realistic goals. Support groups and group education experiences benefit some individuals. The home and work environments should be assessed and interventions incorporated as the situation warrants.

Aspirin remains the medication of choice in the treatment of rheumatoid arthritis. The dose required for treatment is within a range that will reduce inflammation. The analgesic dose of aspirin is often smaller than the dose required to suppress inflammation, and individuals should be instructed that the anti-inflammatory dose needs to be maintained to control symptoms. The exact mechanism of aspirin's action is not completely understood, but it is known to inhibit prostaglandin synthesis. Enteric-coated and buffered forms of aspirin are available and are sometimes better tolerated in persons who are prone to gastrointestinal side-effects. Tinnitus and decreased hearing are common side-effects that resolve when the medication dosage is reduced or discontinued. Sometimes other aspirin preparations are better tolerated, such as magnesium salts, choline conjugates, salicylic acid, and mixtures of these.[3] If the individual cannot tolerate or does not receive benefit from aspirin, other nonsteroidal anti-inflammatory drugs (NSAID) may be tried. These include fenoprofen, ibuprofen, meclofenamate, naproxen, piroxicam, sulindac, indomethacin, phenylbutazone, and tolmetin. These medications have analgesic and anti-inflammatory properties similar to those of aspirin. Individuals with active peptic ulcers or blood coagulation problems should not be given these preparations, because, like aspirin, they have gastrointestinal side-effects.

A slow-acting type of drug may be added to the medication regimen of the disease if it is not sufficiently controlled by aspirin or the nonsteroidal anti-inflammatory drugs. The exact mechanism of action for the slow-acting medications such as gold compounds, hydroxychloroquine, or penicillamine is unknown. Their beneficial effects do not usually become evident until after 2 months of therapy. These drugs and some of their side-effects are summarized in Table 53-3.

Corticosteroid drugs may be used to reduce discomfort, but only in specific situations for short-term therapy at a low dose level to avoid long-term side-effects. They may be used for unremitting disease with extra-articular manifestations. These medications do not modify the disease and thus are unable to prevent joint destruction. Intra-articular corticosteroid injections can provide rapid relief of persistent inflammation in a few joints with a low incidence of systemic side-effects.

Immunosuppressant drugs, such as azathioprine, cyclophosphamide, chlorambucil, and methotrexate, have the potential for modifying the disease process in rheumatoid arthritis. Plasmapheresis, leukopheresis, lymphapheresis, thoracic-duct drainage, and total body irradiation are procedures that are currently considered experimental. Levamisole, a T-lymphocyte stimulator, is an experimental medication. These treatments may hold promise for the future.

Surgery may be indicated as part of the treatment of rheumatoid arthritis. Synovectomy may be indicated to reduce pain and joint damage when synovitis does not respond to medical treatment. The most common soft tissue surgery is tenosynovectomy (repair of damaged tendons) of the hand to release nerve entrapments. Total

Table 53-3 Slow-type Medications Used in the Treatment of Rheumatoid Arthritis

Medication	Side-Effects
Gold Compounds	
Intramuscular	Skin rash, pruritus
Sodium thiomalate (myochrysine)	Stomatitis (may be preceded by metallic taste)
Aurothioglucose (solganal)	Nephrotic syndrome
	Glomerulitis with hematuria
Oral	Albuminuria
Auranofin	Blood dyscrasias
	Granulocytopenia
	Thrombocytopenia
	Hypoplasic and aplastic anemia
	Reduction of hemoglobin
	Leukopenia
	Nitritoid reaction: flushing, dizziness, fainting, sweating
	Nausea, vomiting, diarrhea
	Hair loss
Antimalarial	
Hydroxychloroquine	Retinopathy, corneal changes,
Chloroquine	Visual field defects
	Alopecia
	Skin rashes, pruritus
	Gastrointestinal disturbances
Penicillamine	Dermatitis, pruritus
	Fever, lymphadenopathy
	Gastrointestinal disturbances
	Loss of taste
	Stomatitis
	Bone marrow depression and blood dyscrasias
	Proteinuria and hematuria

joint replacements may be indicated to reduce pain and increase motion.

Although the course of rheumatoid arthritis is unpredictable, the past 20 years have brought more effective treatment for the disease. Individuals are now being diagnosed and treated earlier.

Juvenile Rheumatoid Arthritis

Juvenile rheumatoid arthritis is a chronic disease that affects approximately 60,000 to 200,000 children in the United States.[5] It is characterized by synovitis and can influence epiphyseal growth by stimulating growth of the affected side. Generalized stunted growth may also occur.

Systemic onset (Still's disease) affects about 20% of children with juvenile rheumatoid arthritis.[5] The symptoms include a daily intermittent high fever, which is usually accompanied by a rash, generalized lymphadenopathy, hepatosplenomegaly, leukocytosis, and anemia. Most of these children also have joint involvement. Systemic symptoms usually subside in 6 to 12 months. This form of juvenile rheumatoid arthritis can also make an initial appearance in adulthood. Infections, heart disease, and adrenal insufficiency may cause death.

Pauciarticular juvenile rheumatoid arthritis affects no more than four joints. This subgroup affects 40% of children with juvenile rheumatoid arthritis.[5] The pauciarticular arthritis affects two distinct groups. The first group generally consists of females less than 6 years of age with chronic uveitis. Antinuclear antibody testing in this group is usually positive. The second group have a late onset arthritis seen most commonly in males. The HLA-27 testing is positive in over half of this group. Sacroiliitis is present and the arthritis is usually in the lower extremities.

The third subgroup, which affects about 40% of children with rheumatoid arthritis, is polyarticular onset disease. It affects more than four joints during the first 6 months of the disease. This form of arthritis more closely resembles the adult form of the disease than the other two subgroups. A positive rheumatoid factor is sometimes present and may indicate a more active disease process. Systemic features include a low-grade fever, weight loss, malaise, anemia, stunted growth, slight organomegaly (*e.g.*, hepatosplenomegaly), and adenopathy.[5]

The prognosis for most children with rheumatoid arthritis is good. Aspirin is the main medication used. Although some nonsteroidal anti-inflammatory drugs are available, not all have been approved by the FDA for use in children. Intramuscular gold therapy is often used when aspirin or nonsteroidal anti-inflammatory drugs have proven ineffective. Other aspects for treatment of children with juvenile rheumatoid arthritis are similar to those used for the adult with rheumatoid arthritis. Children are encouraged to lead as normal a life as possible.

In summary, rheumatoid arthritis is a systemic inflammatory disorder that affects 1% to 2% of the population. Women are affected more frequently than men. This form of arthritis, the cause of which is unknown, has a chronic course and is usually characterized by remissions and exacerbations. Joint involvement is symmetrical and begins with inflammatory changes in the synovial membrane. As joint inflammation progresses, structural changes can occur, leading to joint instability. Systemic manifestations include weakness, anorexia, weight loss, and low-grade fever. Some extra-articular features include rheumatoid nodules, vasculitis, and Sjögren's syndrome. The treatment goals include reducing pain, stiffness, and swelling, maintaining mobility, and assisting the individual in becoming an informed health care consumer.

■ Osteoarthritis

Osteoarthritis, also referred to as degenerative joint disease, is the most common form of arthritis. It is a chronic disease of unknown etiology that can lead to loss of mobility and chronic pain. It often causes significant disability, especially when the involved joints are critical to the performance of daily activities. The occurrence of osteoarthritis increases with age and affects most individuals over age 65, with women developing osteoarthritis twice as frequently as men.[6] It is estimated that 50% of the population have x-ray evidence of osteoarthritis.[7]

The joint changes associated with osteoarthritis are progressive and are characterized by the development of joint pain, stiffness, limitation of motion, and possibly joint instability and deformity. The disease is usually not considered to be an inflammatory type of arthritis (*i.e.*, no local redness or heat or systemic manifestation of the inflammatory response is present). Although there may be periods when mild inflammation is present, it is not the severe type seen in the inflammatory forms of rheumatic diseases such as rheumatoid arthritis.

Osteoarthritis may occur as a primary or a secondary disorder. Primary osteoarthritis occurs without an obvious reason and is the most common form. The secondary form of the disease develops for some identifiable reason. For example, osteoarthritis can occur secondary to joint instability caused by injury to a knee ligament or a meniscus cartilage tear. Other joint disorders such as rheumatoid arthritis, damage due to metabolic alterations of the cartilage, congenital abnormalities, childhood changes in joint structure, and crystal deposition may also cause secondary arthritis.

Several additional factors warrant mention. Although aging does not cause osteoarthritis *per se*, it does cause alterations in chondrocyte function, which may contribute to the development of the disease.[6] There may be a genetic predisposition to some forms of osteoarthritis, as in Heberden's nodes, which affect the distal interphalangeal joints of the hand. Because osteoarthritis is more prevalent in women, hormonal factors are another consideration. The relationship of obesity to the development of osteoarthritis is still unknown.

Pathologic Changes

Osteoarthritis affects the articular cartilage and subchondral bone (Fig. 53-9). Normally, cartilage is a translucent, white, smooth material. In osteoarthritis, the cartilage softens and acquires a yellowish appearance early in the disease process; as the disease progresses, the joint becomes rough because of fissuring and pitting and is followed by the development of focal and eventually diffuse ulcerations. Eventually erosion of the cartilage occurs, leading to thinning and destruction of cartilage down to the bone. Although this process is occurring in the cartilage, changes are also taking place in the subchondral bone underlying the cartilage. Sclerosis, or formation of new bone, usually occurs in the juxta-articular bone, that is, the bone near the joint. Cyst formation in juxta-articular bone is common. Formation of new bone occurs at the joint margins and is called osteophyte spur formation.

Mild synovitis may also occur. This is more likely to be seen in advanced disease. In certain cases, the synovitis may be related to the release of calcium pyrophosphate dihydrate from the cartilage or calcium hydroxyapatite crystals from synovial tissues.

It has been suggested that the cellular events responsible for the development of osteoarthritis begin with some type of insult involving the chondrocytes. According to this theory, the affected chondrocytes either die or release destructive enzymes, or they begin to divide, which increases the number of cells and predisposes to the formation of abnormal clones.[6] With an increase in cells, synthesis of an abnormal intercellular matrix occurs, and the production of lysosomal and other enzymes that degrade the intercellular matrix increases. As the disease progresses, the erosive loss of cartilage leads to proliferative changes in subchondral bone marked by thickening, sclerotic changes, osteophyte spur formation, and structural joint changes.

Clinical Manifestations

The manifestations of osteoarthritis may occur suddenly or insidiously. Initially, pain may be described as aching and may be somewhat difficult to localize. Pain usually occurs after the use of the involved joints and is relieved by rest. As the disease advances, pain may occur with minimal activity. Pain usually increases throughout the day, causing most discomfort in the evening; overactivity can also increase pain.

The most frequently affected joints are the hips, knees, lumbar and cervical vertebrae, proximal and distal interphalangeal joints of the hand, and first carpometacarpal joint and the first metatarsophalangeal joints of the feet. Stiffness is localized to the involved joints. It is usually present in the morning, upon awakening, and lasts until the individual can "work it out" by moving about. Usually, morning stiffness is reduced in about 30 minutes. Stiffness also occurs after sitting, so that individuals need to limit the duration of sitting to avoid prolonged stiffness. Pain may occur with passive motion of the involved joint. Crepitus and grinding may also be evident when the joint is moved.

Other clinical features include limitations in joint

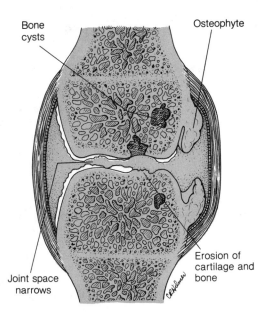

Figure 53-9 *Joint changes in osteoarthritis. The left side denotes early changes, joint space narrowing with cartilage breakdown. The right side shows more severe disease progression with lost cartilage and osteophyte formation.*

motion or joint instability. Joint enlargement is usually due to new bone formation, so that the joint feels hard in contrast with the soft spongy feeling characteristic of rheumatoid arthritis. Sometimes mild synovitis or increased synovial fluid are present, which can also cause joint enlargement.

Diagnosis and Treatment

The diagnosis of osteoarthritis is usually determined by history and physical examination, x-ray, and laboratory findings that exclude other diseases. Table 53-4 identifies the joints that are commonly affected by osteoarthritis and the common clinical features correlated with the disease activity of each particular joint. Although pain and stiffness are common features of the disease, the impact of the disease will vary with each person.

In osteoarthritis, the most beneficial method of diagnosis is radiography. If pathologic changes are mild, the x-rays may be normal. Characteristic x-ray changes include joint space narrowing, osteophyte formation, subchondral bony sclerosis, and cyst formation. Laboratory studies are usually normal because the disorder is not a systemic disease. The sedimentation rate may be slightly elevated in generalized osteoarthritis or erosive inflammatory variations of the disease. If inflammation is present, there may be a slight increase in cell count. The synovial fluid is also usually normal. However, calcium pyrophosphate dihydrate or hydroxyapatite crystals may be seen in the synovial fluid.

Table 53-4 Clinical Features of Osteoarthritis

Joint	Clinical Features
Distal interphalangeal joint (DIP) Heberden's nodes	Occurs more frequently in women; usually involves multiple DIPs, lateral flexor deviation of joint, spur formation at joint margins, pain and discomfort following joint use
Proximal interphalangeal joint (PIP) Bouchard's nodes	Same as for distal interphalangeal joint disease
First carpometacarpal joint (CMC)	Tenderness at base of thumb; squared appearance to joint
First metatarsal phalangeal joint (MTP)	Insidious onset; irregular joint contour; pain and swelling aggrevated by tight shoes
Hip	Most common in older male adults; characterized by insidious onset of pain, localized to groin region or inner aspect of the thigh; may be referred to buttocks, sciatic region, or knee; reduced hip motion; leg may be held in external rotation with hip flexed and adducted; limp or shuffling gait; difficulty getting in and out of chairs
Knee	Localized discomfort with pain on motion; limitation of motion; crepitus; quadricep atrophy due to lack of use; joint instability; genu varus or valgus; joint effusion
Cervical spine	Localized stiffness; radicular or nonradicular pain; posterior osteophyte formation may cause vascular compression*
Lumbar spine	Low back pain and stiffness; muscle spasm; decreased back motion; nerve root compression causing radicular pain*; spinal stenosis*

*Rare complication.

The treatment of osteoarthritis is directed toward the relief of pain and the maintenance of mobility and is individualized to meet the needs of the patient. Education about the disease and type of treatment methods is important. The treatment continuum may range from no treatment to very extensive forms of treatment. Excessive stress on the affected joints should be avoided. Pain and stiffness may be controlled by a balance of activity and rest of the affected joints. A cane or walker may be helpful for weight-bearing joints; weight control also reduces the stress placed on the weight-bearing joints. The work environment should be evaluated to reduce repetitive movements and allow for joint rest when possible. The individual should be instructed in activity pacing, planning, priority setting, and simplification of movement that involves the affected joint. Instruction in proper posture and positioning may also be warranted. Heat treatments and therapeutic exercises are directed toward improving and reducing pain and stiffness. Application of cold, provided it is not contraindicated by other medical conditions, may also be used if the individual finds heat uncomfortable.

Analgesics, such as acetaminophen and propoxyphene derivatives, may be used as needed. Narcotics are rarely used except in instances of severe disease exacerbation. Aspirin may be used as an analgesic or as an anti-inflammatory medication. If the individual cannot tolerate aspirin, a nonsteroidal anti-inflammatory drug may be used. The exact mechanism of these medications on the osteoarthritic process is unknown. Local corticosteroid injections are used during the acute stages of the disease to reduce pain. These injections are used only after considering other conservative measures, as their use may accelerate joint destruction. The destruction occurs because pain is reduced after the injection and then the joint may be overused. Corticosteroid injections are used infrequently, especially in weight-bearing joints. Further studies are needed to determine the effectiveness of transcutaneous electrical stimulation (see Chap. 48) and acupuncture.[7-9]

Surgery is considered when the individual is having severe pain and joint function is severely reduced. For individuals with early osteoarthritis in the hip or knee, an osteotomy may be done to redirect the forces of weight bearing. Total hip replacements have provided effective relief of symptoms for many individuals, as have total knee replacements, although the latter procedure has produced less consistent results.[9] Joint replacement has recently been developed for the first carpometacarpal joint. An arthrodesis is used in advanced disease to reduce pain; however, this results in loss of motion. Specific treatments are determined by the extent of the disease, the joints involved, and the response to previous and current treatment regimens.

In summary, osteoarthritis is the most common form of arthritis; it occurs as either a primary or a secondary disorder. It is a localized condition affecting primarily the weight-bearing joints. The disorder is characterized by degeneration of the articular cartilage and subchondral bone. Joint enlargement is usually due to new bone formation, which causes the joint to feel hard. Pain and stiffness are primary features of the disease. The treatment is directed toward the relief of pain and maintenance of mobility.

■ Spondyloarthropathies

The spondyloarthropathies include ankylosing spondylitis, Reiter's syndrome, and spondylitis associated with psoriatic arthritis or inflammatory bowel disease. These disorders affect the axial skeleton and have many common clinical features. However, the etiology remains unknown. Inflammation in the axial skeleton is more difficult to identify than that in the peripheral joints. The inflammation develops at sites where ligaments insert into bone (entheses). There is a familial tendency toward the development of spondyloarthropathy.

Ankylosing Spondylitis

Ankylosing spondylitis is an inflammatory disease of the axial skeleton, including the sacroiliac joints, intervertebral disk spaces, and the apophyseal and costovertebral articulations. Bilateral sacroiliitis is a primary feature of the disease. Occasionally large synovial joints may be involved, usually the hips, knees, and shoulders. Small peripheral joints are usually not affected. This disorder is more common than was once believed; it probably affects about 1% to 2% of the population, which is comparable to the prevalence of rheumatoid arthritis.[10] At one time this disease was thought to occur four to ten times more frequently in men than in women. It now appears that the prevalence in women is probably the same or only slightly less than in men, but the disease is not usually as severe in women.[11] Although ankylosing spondylitis can occur in individuals of any age, it is usually diagnosed in the second or third decade of life. The disease is seen frequently in North American Native Americans and is rarely seen in blacks and Orientals.[10]

There are primary and secondary forms of ankylosing spondylitis. The individual with primary ankylosing spondylitis does not have signs or symptoms of other rheumatic diseases. In contrast, the secondary form is diagnosed when another spondyloarthropathy is responsible for the sacroiliitis.

The etiology of ankylosing spondylitis is unknown. However, during recent years a strong association has been identified between HLA-B27 antigen and ankylosing spondylitis. The HLA-B27 antigen is found in 90% of white individuals with the disorder but only in 6% to 8% of the general population.[3] This provides some information supporting the familial tendency of the disease, although, in contrast, only 20% of individuals with HLA-B27 are symptomatic.[4] Further genetic and environmental factors are being explored as possible causes of the disease. There has been speculation about the role of infection because some exacerbations of

Reiter's syndrome seem to follow certain infections. Recently there has been speculation that ankylosing spondylitis may be an immunologic disease. Research has cited such immunologic changes as increased levels of complement inactivation products, evidence of antiglobins of the IgG class, elevations of C4 of which complement is an acute phase reactant, elevated levels of IgA, and evidence of immune complex formation. It is unclear whether the disease is caused by the presence of HLA-B27 alone or whether an associated immune response gene needs to be present.

Ankylosing spondylitis may cause the development of fibrosis calcification and ossification of joints with progression to ankylosis. The disease generally brings to mind an image of an individual with a rigid bamboolike spine. Fortunately, however, few individuals develop a progressive disease pattern that leads to this outcome. The disease spectrum ranges from an asymptomatic sacroiliitis to a progressive disease that can affect many body systems. When a progressive disease pattern does develop, it is usually in men.

Clinical manifestations

The individual with ankylosing spondylitis will typically complain of low back pain, which may be persistent or intermittent. The pain may initially be blamed on muscle strain or spasm from physical activity. Lumbosacral pain may also be present with discomfort in the buttocks and hip areas. Sometimes pain can radiate to the thigh in a manner similar to that of sciatic pain. Although the pain is usually in the lower back, some individuals may complain of pain at a higher vertebral level as an initial symptom. In some individuals, other problems such as tendonitis and peripheral joint changes may precede problems of back pain. Prolonged stiffness is present in the morning and after periods of rest. Mild activity helps reduce pain and stiffness. It is understandable that sleep patterns are frequently interrupted because of these manifestations. Walking or exercise may be needed to provide the comfort needed in order to return to sleep. Muscle spasm may also contribute to discomfort.

Loss of motion in the spinal column is characteristic of the disease. The severity and duration of disease activity have an effect on the individual's degree of mobility. Motion can be lost in anterior or lateral flexion, extension, and rotation of the spinal column. Loss of lumbar lordosis occurs as the disease progresses and is followed by kyphosis of the thoracic spine and extension of the neck.

Because ankylosing spondylitis is a disorder that affects the sites of enthesis, or sites of muscular or tendinous attachment to bone, recurrent tendonitis may develop. This usually occurs at the achilles tendon or the areas of intercostal muscle insertion, and as plantar fasciitis. Little residual damage is done in these situations.

Peripheral arthritis occurs in 35% of individuals with ankylosing spondylitis.[11] Women seem to have peripheral joint disease more frequently than men.[12] Involvement is usually asymmetric and affects hip, shoulder, and knee joints. Hip pain can be a major cause of disability. Heel pain is commonly seen as a result of plantar fasciitis.

The disease process varies considerably among individuals. Exacerbations and remissions are common; their unpredictability can create uncertainty in planning daily activities as well as future goals and expectations. Fortunately, most individuals are able to lead productive lives.

Systemic features of weight loss, fever, and fatigue may be apparent. Thoracic involvement including manubriosternal and sternoclavicular inflammation can create symptoms similar to those of other medical conditions such as angina or esophageal dysfunctions. Acute iritis may develop and be recurrent in 25% of individuals.[13] Osteoporosis can occur, especially in the spine, which contributes to the risk of spinal fracture. Fusion of the costovertebral joints can lead to reduced lung volume.

Complications of ankylosing spondylitis, although infrequent, include spinal fracture in ankylosed areas of the spine, atlantoaxial subluxation (the atlas is the first cervical vertebra that articulates above with the occipital bone and below with the axis), spinal cord compression, aortic regurgitation, apical fibroses of the lung, and cauda equina syndrome with bowel and bladder dysfunction. The complications are more likely to occur in long-standing disease.

Diagnosis and treatment

The diagnosis of ankylosing spondylitis is based on history, physical examination, and x-ray examination. Several methods are available to determine mobility and sacroiliitis. Although these measures alone do not provide a diagnosis of ankylosing spondylitis or other spondyloarthropathies, they can provide useful measurements for monitoring the disease status. Sacroiliitis can be detected by having the individual lean forward over a table and pressing firmly on the sacroiliac joints. Pain or tenderness may be elicited and spinal muscle spasm may also be detected.

General fitness and hip mobility can be measured by having the individual flex forward from the waist with the knees straight and extend the arms to touch the floor. The distance from the fingertips to the floor is then measured.

The modified Schober's test is also used to determine lumbar spine involvement. With this test, an imaginary perpendicular line is drawn from a mark placed midpoint between the postiliac spines to 10 cm above this point. The individual is then asked to bend forward; the distance between the two points is noted. The distance increases to 15 cm or more with flexion in normal individuals. To determine lateral flexion, the top point of the midaxillary line serves as one reference point, and a point 20 cm below is a second reference point. An increase in distance between these two points to 25 cm to 30 cm is normal with contralateral flexion.

Chest expansion may be used as an indirect indicator of thoracic involvement, which usually occurs late in the disease. Measurements are taken at the fourth intercostal space. Normally chest expansion increases 4 cm to 5 cm with inspiration. This measurement is more difficult to obtain in women. Measurement may also be taken at the xyphoid process.

The measurement of the occiput to the wall is determined by having the individual stand erect with the back against the wall and measuring the distance from the occiput to the wall. This is most appropriate to provide the parameters for monitoring late disease, to show loss of normal vertebral structure, and to expose hip flexion contractures.

Laboratory findings frequently show elevation in erythrocyte sedimentation rate. A mild normocytic anemia may also be present. Slight and intermittent elevations in serum alkaline phosphatase related to bone reabsorption may occur. HLA typing is not diagnostic of the disease.

Radiologic evaluations will help differentiate sacroiliitis from other diseases. Symmetric sacroiliitis is usually identified when the first x-ray changes are noted; however, in early disease x-rays may be normal. Vertebrae are normally concave on the anterior border. In ankylosing spondylitis the vertebrae take on a squared appearance. This occurs because of erosion of the upper and lower margins of the vertebrae at the site of insertion of the anulus fibrosis. Syndesmophyte formation occurs as a result of the inflammatory process in the outer layers of the anulus fibrosis. Progressive ossification can occur. Spinal changes usually follow a progressive ascending pattern up the spine.

Treatment is directed at controlling pain and maintaining mobility. Patient education is essential, because regimens require that the individual take responsibility for self-care activities. Instruction should address proper posture and positioning. This includes sleeping in a supine position on a firm mattress using one small pillow or no pillow. Sleeping in extension may reduce the possibility of flexion contractures. A bed board may be used to supply additional firmness. Some individuals find the most comfort by sleeping on the floor. Therapeutic exercises are important to assist in maintaining motion in peripheral joints and in the spine. Muscle strengthening exercises for extensor muscle groups are also prescribed.

Heat applications or a shower or bath may be beneficial before exercise to improve ease of movement. These strategies can also be used in the morning or at bedtime to reduce stiffness and pain. Immobilizing joints is not recommended.

Following general health principles such as the maintenance of ideal weight reduces the stress on weight-bearing joints. Smoking should be discouraged because it can exacerbate respiratory problems. Swimming is an excellent general conditioning exercise that avoids joint stress and enhances muscle tone. Occupational counseling or job evaluation may be warranted because of postural abnormalities.

Aspirin or nonsteroidal anti-inflammatory medications are used to reduce inflammation, which in turn helps to control pain and reduce muscle spasm. In cases of severe pain, phenylbutazone or indomethacin may be the medications of first choice.

Most peripheral joint pain and limitations of motion occur in the hip. Total hip replacement surgery has contributed to pain reduction. Anesthesia can be problematic for individuals with cervical rigidity or with reduced chest expansion. These factors need to be weighed before surgery is considered.

Other Types of Spondyloarthropathies

Reiter's syndrome usually occurs as a postvenereal disease or after a bacterial dysentery infection involving enteric pathogens. Urethritis is ordinarily the first feature of the disease; conjunctivitis and arthritis usually follow. Not all individuals exhibit this triad of features; some individuals may only have one or two of them. In addition, other mucocutaneous manifestations may be present, including mouth ulcerations, circinate balanitis, and skin rashes. Back pain may be present. Spinal radiologic changes are similar to those of ankylosing spondylitis but may be more asymptomatic.

Several patterns of psoriatic arthritis are recognized. Both large joints and small peripheral joints can be affected. The metatarsophalangeal joints and the interphalangeal joints are usually affected. The fingers and toes may take on a sausagelike appearance. The display of joint involvement is usually asymmetric and may involve only two or three joints. Spondylitis may also be present, in which case the changes are consistent with those seen in Reiter's syndrome.

Spondyloarthritis is also associated with inflammatory bowel disease such as Crohn's disease and ulcerative colitis. When ankylosing spondylitis is present, it has usually developed before the bowel disease and follows the same disease process as that described for ankylosing spondylitis. The activity of the bowel disease is not related to the activity of the arthritis.

In summary, spondyloarthropathies affect the axial skeleton. Inflammation develops at sites where ligaments insert into bone. Ankylosing spondylitis is considered a prototype of this classification category. Bilateral sacroiliitis is the primary feature of ankylosing spondylitis. The disease spectrum ranges from asymptomatic sacroiliitis to that of a progressive disorder affecting many body systems. The etiology remains unknown; however, a strong association between HLA-B27 antigen and ankylosing spondylitis has been identified. Loss of motion in the spinal column is characteristic of the disease. Peripheral arthritis may occur in some individuals. Other forms of spondyloarthritis include Reiter's syndrome and spondyloarthritis associated with inflammatory bowel disease.

■ Crystal-Induced Arthropathies

Crystal deposition within joints has been shown to produce arthritis. The term gout is derived from a Latin word meaning "a drop." It reflects the ancient belief that the condition was caused by a malevolent humor falling by drops into the joint.[14] In gout, uric acid crystals are found in the joint cavity; in another condition called pseudogout, calcium pyrophosphate dihydrate (CPPD) crystals are found in the joint. In this section the two most common forms of crystal deposition, gout and pseudogout, will be discussed.

Gout

Gout is characterized by acute attacks of arthritis caused by the presence of monosodium urate crystals in the joint. The disorder is accompanied by hyperuricemia, which results from either overproduction of uric acid or the reduced ability of the kidney to rid the body of excess uric acid. Gout tends to affect men seven times as frequently as women and is the most common form of inflammatory joint disease in men over age 40.[14] However, the incidence of gout in women tends to increase after menopause.

Uric acid formation

Uric acid is a metabolite of the purines, adenine and guanine, which serve as the nitrogenous base for the biosynthesis of nucleotides. Nucleotides serve a number of functions in the body. They are precursors of DNA and RNA, ATP, which serves as the energy currency of the cell, and cyclic AMP, another adenine nucleotide that mediates the action of many hormones. Other nucleotides are components of the major coenzymes (NAD, FAD, and CoA) involved in energy metabolism.

The nucleotides of a cell undergo continuous turnover requiring a continuous supply of purine bases for their renewal. Two pathways supply the purine bases needed for synthesis of the nucleotides: one is the salvage pathway in which the purine bases are saved as the nucleotides are broken down, and the second is the new, or *de novo*, pathway in which the purine nucleotides are synthesized from a compound called 5-phosphoribosyl-1-pyrophosphate (PRPP) and the amino acid glutamine. Production of the purines by the *de novo* pathway is regulated through negative feedback by the presence of products from the salvage pathway, for example, when increased purine products are formed by means of the salvage pathway, the activity of the *de novo* pathway is decreased and vice versa (Fig. 53-10).

The purine bases that are not reused by means of the salvage pathway to form nucleotides are broken down to form uric acid (Fig. 53-10). In the degradation process adenine is broken down to hypoxanthine, then xanthine, and finally into uric acid. Xanthine is also an intermediate in the formation of uric acid from the breakdown of the guanine nucleotides. Most of the uric acid production takes place in the liver where the enzyme xanthine oxidase, needed for conversion of xanthine to uric acid, is present in the greatest quantity.

Elimination of uric acid by the kidney

Normally about two-thirds of the uric acid produced each day is excreted through the kidneys; the rest is

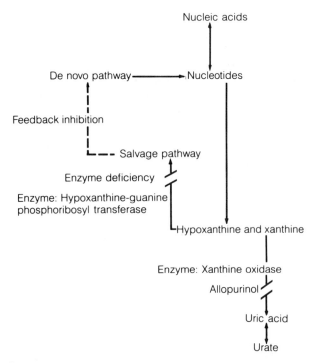

Figure 53-10 *Pathways for the production of uric acid.*

eliminated through the gastrointestinal tract. Normal renal handling of uric acid involves three steps: (1) filtration, (2) reabsorption, and (3) secretion. Uric acid is freely filtered across the glomerulus, is completely reabsorbed in the proximal tubule, and then is secreted back into the tubular fluid by another mechanism for the transport of organic acids in the distal end of the proximal tubule or distal tubule. The tubular secretion and postsecretory reabsorption determine the final concentration of uric acid in the urine. Another anion with a high affinity for the transport carrier may alter the reabsorption or secretion of uric acid. Small doses of uricosuric agents may preferentially reduce secretion and have a uric acid retaining effect, whereas therapeutic doses block reabsorption and increase uric acid elimination. The salicylates reduce secretion and cause net retention of uric acid when given at doses used for pain relief; very large doses are needed to both block reabsorption and secretion. Consequently, aspirin and other salicylates are not recommended for use as analgesics in persons with gout. Some of the diuretics, including the thiazides, which are weak acids, are secreted by the proximal tubular cells and can also interfere with the excretion of uric acid.

Most individuals with gout have a reduced urate clearance. In order to excrete a normal amount of urate, the serum urate level becomes elevated, this achieves urate homeostasis in these individuals. In most individuals with increased production of urate the excretion of uric acid will be increased. However, if kidney damage is present, an increased amount of uric acid will be eliminated by the gastrointestinal tract.

Mechanisms of hyperuricemia

Monosodium urate crystal deposition usually develops when hyperuricemia is present. However, most individuals with hyperuricemia do not develop gout. Attacks of gout seem to be related to sudden increases or decreases in serum uric acid levels. Hyperuricemia may occur because of an overproduction of uric acid, underexcretion of uric acid, or combination of both. Primary and secondary forms of hyperuricemia exist. Primary causes are related to genetic defects in purine metabolism. A deficiency of the enzyme hypoxanthine-guanine phosphoribosyltransferase, which is essential to the salvage pathway for synthesis of the adenine nucleotides, leads to marked acceleration of purine biosynthesis by the *de novo* pathway. Another form of primary hyperuricemia results from increased activity of phosphoribosyl pyrophosphate (PRPP) synthesase. Secondary forms of hyperuricemia are related to certain disease conditions and medications. Table 53-5 lists some common causes of hyperuricemia.

An attack of gout occurs when the monosodium urate crystals precipitate within the joint and initiate an inflammatory response. This may occur after a sudden rise in the serum urate levels. The excess urate is not soluble, so that precipitation occurs. Gout can also occur with a sudden drop in the urate level. In either situation crystals are released into the synovial fluid and an inflammatory response is initiated.

Phagocytosis of urate crystals by the polymorphonuclear leukocytes occurs, which leads to cell death and the release of lysosomal enzymes. As this process continues, the inflammation causes destruction of the cartilage and subchondral bone. Occasionally deposits of monosodium urate crystals (tophi) can occur in the cartilage and bone; this produces further destruction. Crystal deposition usually occurs in peripheral areas of the body such as the great toe and pinnae of the ear. Sodium urate is less soluble at temperatures below 37°C.[15] The peripheral tissues are cooler than other parts of the body, and this may at least partially explain why gout occurs most frequently in peripheral joints.[15]

The typical acute attack of gout is monoarticular and usually affects the first metatarsophalangeal joint. The tarsal joints, ankles, and knees may also be initial sites of involvement.[16] The onset of pain is usually abrupt, with redness and swelling, and frequently occurs at night. It may last for days or weeks. Pain may be severe enough to be aggravated even by the weight of the bedsheet covering the affected area. Attacks of gout may be precipitated by certain medications, foods, or alcohol. After the first attack, it may be months or years before another attack occurs. The attacks usually become more frequent, and as they do, more joints are affected.

In the early stages of gout, after the initial attack has subsided, the individual is asymptomatic, and joint abnormalities are not evident. This is referred to as intercritical gout. As attacks recur with increased frequency, joint changes occur and become permanent. Erosions occur in the cartilage and subchondral bone because of the inflammatory response elicited by the urate crystals.

Tophi are usually large, hard nodules that have an irregular surface and are most commonly found in the synovium, subchondral bone, olecranon bursa, Achilles tendon, and extensor surface of the forearm. Tophi usually do not appear until an average of 10 years or more after the first gout attack. This stage of gout, called chronic tophaceous gout, is characterized by more frequent and prolonged attacks, which are often polyarticular.

Diagnosis and treatment

A definitive diagnosis of gout can be made only when monosodium urate crystals are present in the synovial fluid or in tissue sections of tophaceous deposits. Synovial fluid analysis is useful in ruling out other conditions, such as septic arthritis, pseudogout, and rheumatoid arthritis. The presence of hyperuricemia cannot be equa-

Table 53-5   Some Causes and Mechanisms of Secondary Hyperuricemia

Causes	Mechanisms

Neoplastic disorders
   Lymphoma
   Leukemia
   Myeloproliferative
      disease
	Rapid turnover of purines

Polycythemia vera	Increased bone marrow activity or increased cell (and purine) turnover at other sites
Metabolic acidosis	Competition of lactic acid and ketones with uric acid for secretion
Renal failure	Reduced glomerular filtration of uric acid
Psoriasis	Large turnover of nucleoproteins
Sarcoidosis	Mechanisms unknown
Paget's disease	Mechanism unclear
Parathyroid gland disorders	Mechanism unclear
Drugs Cancer chemotherapy drugs	Excess production of uric acid because of rapid cell turnover
Diuretics	Interference with tubular secretion of urate, dehydration
Aspirin	Inhibition of urate secretion at low doses
Penicillin	Interference with normal uric acid secretion
Prednisone	Possibly because of increased cell breakdown resulting in increased purine metabolism

ted with gout because many individuals with this condition never develop gout. In some situations, individuals with gout are not hyperuricemic because they are taking medications that lower serum urate levels.

Secondary gout is clinically similar to primary gout. Usually the serum urate levels and uric acid excretion are both higher than in primary gout. This form of gout is usually seen in myeloproliferative diseases, such as the leukemias.

Individuals with gout are usually evaluated to determine if the disorder is related to overproduction or underexcretion of uric acid. Blood is drawn to determine the uric acid levels and a 24-hour urine sample is collected. Ideally, the individual should be on a purine-free diet during the time that the urine specimen is being collected, in which case the normal urate values range from 350 to 590 mg/day compared with values below 1000 mg/day when there are no dietary restrictions of purines. Values above these levels indicate an overproduction of uric acid.[3] The normal serum urate concentration is 5.1 ± 1.0 mg/dl in men and 4.0 ± 1.0 mg/dl in women.

The acute disease state management is directed toward the reduction of joint inflammation. Hyperuricemia and the related conditions of tophi, joint destruction, and renal problems are treated after the acute inflammatory process has subsided. Treatment with colchicine is used early in the acute stage. Although the drug is usually given orally, a more rapid response is obtained when cholchicine is given intravenously. The fact that the drug causes nausea and diarrhea when large doses are given orally is often a limiting factor in oral therapy. These side-effects are, however, essentially eliminated when the drug is given intravenously. The acute symptoms of gout usually subside within 48 hours after treatment with oral colchicine has been instituted and 12 hours following intravenous administration of the drug.

Although pain relief may not occur as rapidly, nonsteroidal anti-inflammatory medications are sometimes preferred to colchicine because they have fewer toxic side-effects. Phenylbutazone is usually very effective but is generally only used on a short-term basis because bone marrow suppression can occur with long-term use. Indomethacin is also effective and does not cause bone marrow suppression, although gastrointestinal disturbances and headache can occur. Other nonsteroidal anti-inflammatory drugs are effective during the acute stage when used at their maximal dosage. The actions and side-effects of medications used in the treatment of acute gout are described in Table 53-6.

The corticosteroid drugs are not recommended for the treatment of gout unless all other medications have

Table 53-6 Medication Used in Treatment of Acute Gout

Medication	Action	Side-Effects
Colchicine	Inhibits production and release of chemotactic factors from polymorphonuclear leukocytes	Oral administration Abdominal cramping Nausea, vomiting and diarrhea
	Other actions unknown	Potential of developing leukopenia with intravenous administration
	May be used as an interval therapy to prevent acute attacks of gout	Precaution: should not be given if inflammatory bowel, hepatic, or renal disease is present
Phenylbutazone	Inhibits prostaglandin synthesis	Gastrointestinal complaints
	Inhibits leukocyte migration	Increased fluid retention in individuals with a potential for cardiac decompensation Rare cases of bone marrow suppression
	Inhibits the release and/or activity of lysosomal enzymes	Precaution: should not be given if active ulcer disease is present
Indomethacin	Inhibits prostaglandin synthesis	Gastrointestinal complaints, headache, dizziness, drowsiness, depression, fatigue, tinnitus
	Mode of action unknown	Precautions: should not be given if active ulcer disease is present Should be used with caution in persons with epilepsy and Parkinson's disease
Other nonsteroidal anti-inflammatory drugs	Inhibit prostaglandin synthesis Mode of action unkown	Gastrointestinal complaints Precaution: should not be given if active ulcer disease is present

been proven unsuccessful. Intra-articular injections of corticosteroid agents may be used when only one joint is involved and the individual is unable to take colchicine or nonsteroidal drugs.

After the acute attack has been relieved, the hyperuricemia is treated. One method is to reduce hyperuricemia through the use of a uricosuric agent. These medications prevent the tubular reabsorption of urate. The serum urate concentrations are monitored to determine the efficiency and dosage needed. Uricosuric agents include probenecid and sulfinpyrazone, a phenylbutazone derivative. These drugs are usually started in small doses and gradually increased over 7 to 10 days. Low-dose aspirin should not be used with these medications because it reduces the urinary excretion of uric acid.

Hyperuricemia can also be treated with allopurinol, which inhibits the production of uric acid. Allopurinol inhibits xanthine oxidase, an enzyme needed for the conversion of hypoxanthine to xanthine and xanthine to uric acid. There is a slight possibility that xanthine kidney stones can develop if allopurinol is used for many years. It is usually used for the individual who does not have an adequate response or is unable to tolerate other forms of treatment. The actions and side-effects of drugs used in the treatment of hyperuricemia are described in Table 53-7.

Treatment of hyperuricemia is aimed at maintaining normal uric acid levels and requires life-long treatment. Prophylactic colchicine or nonsteroidal anti-inflammatory drugs may be used between gout attacks. If the uric acid level is normal and the individual has not had recurrent attacks of gout, these medications may be discontinued.

Education about the disease and its management is fundamental to the treatment and management of gout. The individual should be aware that the prognosis is very good and that the disease, although chronic, can be controlled in almost all cases. Some life-style changes may need to be incorporated, such as maintenance of ideal weight and moderation in alcohol consumption. The application of cold to the affected joint, joint rest, and joint protection are used during active disease. The application of cold provides a cooling effect and distracts from the pain but probably has little if any effect on the inflammatory process. Adequate fluid intake of at least 2 liters per day may help to prevent the development of uric acid renal calculi (Chap. 29). Although certain foods cause an elevation in purine levels, the amount is usually too insignificant to require modification. Adherence to the life-long use of medications may be the only major life-style change for many individuals.

Table 53-7   Medications Used in Treatment of Hyperuricemia

Medication	Action	Side-Effects
Allopurinol	Inhibits xanthine oxidase, needed for conversion of hypoxanthine to xanthine and xanthine to uric acid	Gastrointestinal complaints, drug rash, transient leukopenia, and changes in liver function Precautions: should not be given to individuals with liver disease or bone marrow depression. Dose must be adjusted when given with cytotoxic drugs
Probenecid	Inhibits the tubular reabsorption of urate, increases uric acid excretion	Gastrointestinal complaints, headache, fever, drug rash, urinary frequency Precautions: predisposes to kidney stones. Not recommended for persons with blood dyscrasias (may cause aplastic anemia)
Sulfinpyrazone	Inhibits the tubular reabsorption of urate, increases uric acid excretion	Gastrointestinal complaints Precautions: not recommended for persons with peptic ulcer, gastrointestinal inflammation, or blood dyscrasias

Pseudogout

Pseudogout is an acute, inflammatory arthritis caused by the deposition of calcium pyrophosphate dihydrate crystals within the joint. The inflammation can occur in one or several joints and lasts for several days. Joint degeneration may occur simultaneously or be apparent before and after the diagnosis of pseudogout. Because degenerative changes and inflammation are present, the disorder can mimic other forms of arthritis, leading to difficulty in establishing a diagnosis. The knee is the most common joints to be involved. As in gout, the individual with pseudogout may be asymptomatic between attacks.

Pseudogout is more common in men than in women, with a 4:1 ratio. There may be an inherited tendency toward the disorder. It is commonly seen in metabolic disorders such as hyperparathyroidism. The diagnosis is confirmed by x-ray, synovial fluid analysis, or biopsy. Nonsteroidal anti-inflammatory drugs are used to reduce inflammation. The intra-articular injection of corticosteroids is sometimes used to treat affected large joints. To date there are no drugs that can remove the crystals from the joints. The degenerative changes associated with this disorder are treated in a manner similar to the treatment of osteoarthritis.

In summary, crystal-induced arthropathies are characterized by crystal deposition within the joint. Gout is the prototype of this group. Acute attacks of arthritis occur with gout and are characterized by the presence of monosodium urate crystals in the joint. The disorder is accompanied by hyperuricosemia, which results either from overproduction of uric acid or from the reduced ability of the kidney to rid the body of excess uric acid. Acute disease management is directed, first, toward the reduction of joint inflammation, and then the hyperuricemia is treated. Hyperuricemia is treated with uricosuric agents that prevent the tubular reabsorption of urate, or it may be treated with medication that inhibits the production of uric acid. Although gout is chronic, in most cases it can be controlled.

■ Study Guide

After you have studied this chapter, you should be able to meet the following objectives:

☐ Describe the pathologic changes that may be found in the joint of an individual with rheumatoid arthritis.

☐ List the extra-articular manifestations of rheumatoid arthritis.

☐ State the components of a basic treatment program for rheumatoid arthritis.

☐ Compare rheumatoid arthritis and osteoarthritis in terms of joint involvement, level of inflammation, and local and systemic manifestations.

☐ Describe the pathologic joint changes that occur with osteoarthritis.

☐ Cite the primary features of ankylosing spondylitis.

☐ Describe how the site of inflammation differs in spondyloarthropathies from that of rheumatoid arthritis.

☐ Cite the common features in the management of rheumatoid arthritis, osteoarthritis, and ankylosing spondylitis.

☐ Differentiate between the type of crystals found in the joint of an individual with acute gout and in that of an individual with pseudogout.

☐ Trace the pathway for the production of uric acid.

☐ Describe renal mechanisms for the elimination of uric acid.

☐ State four causes of hyperuricemia and the mechanism by which uric acid levels become elevated.

☐ List three drugs that are used in the treatment of gout and describe their mechanisms of action.

■ References

1. Meeman RF, Liang MH, Handler NM, Disability Task Force of the Arthritis Foundation: Social security disability and the arthritis patient. Bull Rheum Dis 33, No 1, 1983
2. Harris ED: Rheumatoid arthritis: The clinical spectrum. In Kelly WN, et al (eds): Textbook of Rheumatology, Vol 1. Philadelphia, WB Saunders, 1981
3. Rodman GP, Schumacher HR (eds): Primer on the rheumatic diseases, 8th ed, pp 38, 85. Atlanta, Arthritis Foundation, 1983.
4. Hunder GG, Beench T: Treatment of rheumatoid arthritis. Bull Rheum Dis 32, No 1, 1982
5. Rodman GP, Schumacher HR (eds): Primer on the Rheumatic Diseases, 8th ed, p 104. Atlanta, Arthritis Foundation, 1983
6. Hoskisson EC: Osteoarthritis: Changing concepts in pathogenesis and treatment. Postgrad Med 65, No 3:97–104, 1979
7. Moskowitz R: Management of osteoarthritis. Hosp Pract 14, No 7:75, 1979
8. Moskowitz R: Management of osteoarthritis. Bull Rheum Dis 31, No 6:31–34, 1981
9. Calin A: Anklylosing spondylitis. In Kelly WN, Harris E, Ruddy S et al (eds): Textbook on Rheumatology, Vol II, pp 1017–1030. Philadelphia, WB Saunders, 1981
10. Felts W: Ankylosing spondylitis: The challenge of early diagnosis. Postgrad Med 72, No 3:184–195, 1982

11. Calin A, Marks S: Management of ankylosing spondylitis. Bull Rheum Dis 31, No 6:35–38, 1981
12. Rodman G, Schumaacher R (eds): Primer on the Rheumatic Diseases, 8th ed, p 85. Atlanta, Arthritis Foundation, 1983
13. Bluestone R: Seronegative spondyloarthropathies. Hosp Pract 14, No 10:87–97, 1979
14. Resnick D, Niwayama G: Diagnosis of Bone and Joint Disorders, Vol 2. Philadelphia, WB Saunders, 1981
15. McCarty D: The management of gout. Hosp Pract 14, No 9:75, 1979
16. Boss DR, Geegmiller JE: Hyperuricemia and gout: Classification, complicatins and management. N Engl J Med 300, No 26: 1459, 1979

■ Additional References

Rheumatoid arthritis

Bardwick PA, Swezey RL: Physical therapies in arthritis. Postgrad Med 72, No 3:223, 1982
Bernstein RM, Hughes GRV: Rheumatoid arthritis: Current concepts. Inter Rehab Med 4, No 3:119, 1983
Britton MC: Rheumatoid arthritis: A two-component disease. Consultant 20, No 10:25, 1980
D'Cunha JV, Kochar AS, Huang T: Felty's syndrome. Clin Rheum Pract 1, No 2:91, 1983
Fink CW: Predicting the outcome of JRA. Consultant 19, No 10:40, 1979
Frank ST: Rheumatoid arthritis: A multi-system disease. Consultant 20, No 12:171, 1980
Garber E, Bluestone R: Rheumatic disease: The most useful tests. Consultant 20, No 9:79, 1980
Hunder GG: Check for its systemic manifestations. Consultant 22, No 5:33, 1982
Hunder GG, Bunch T: Treatment of rheumatoid arthritis. Bull Rheum Dis 32, No 1:1, 1982
Irby WR, Owen DS: Drug therapy in the management of rheumatoid arthritis: A review. Clin Rheum Pract 1, No 1:10, 1983
Miller ML, Glass DN: The major histocompatibility complex antigens in rheumatoid arthritis and juvenile arthritis. Bull Rheum Dis 31, No 6:21, 1981
Mullin GT: Gold for rheumatoid arthritis. Postgrad Med 72, No 3:205, 1982
Navarro AH: Physical therapy in the management of rheumatoid arthritis. Clin Rheum Pract 1, No 3:125, 1983
Scott RD: Arthritic knees: Help can range from pain relief to total knee replacement. Consultant 22, No 3:149, 1982
Smith RD, Polley HF: Rest therapy for rheumatoid arthritis. Mayo Clin Proc 53:141, 1978
Strodthoff C: Pathophysiology of rheumatoid arthritis. Nurs Pract 7:32, 1982
Todd B: For arthritis: Plain aspirin or an aspirin alternative. Geriatr Nurs 3:191, 1982
Waring NP, DeSharp RD: JRA diagnosis: Why it can be confusing even for the experts. Consultant 23, No 5:93, 1981
Williams RC: Rheumatoid arthritis. Hosp Pract 14, No 6:57, 1979, 1983

Juvenile arthritis

Alipa FP: Juvenile rheumatoid arthritis. Ariz Med 38, No 2:115, 1981
Ansell BM: Chronic arthritis in childhood. Ann Rheum Dis 37:107, 1978
Ansell BM: Management of juvenile chronic arthritis. Int Rehabil Med 4, No 3:128, 1983
Baum J: Juvenile arthritis. Am J Dis Child 135:55, 1981
Blau SP: How to spot rheumatoid arthritis in youngsters. Consultant 19, No 7:74, 1979
Fink CW: Clinical, genetic, and therapeutic aspects of juvenile arthritis. Clin Rheum Pract 1, No 3:100, 1983

Spondyloarthropathies

Calin A, Marks S: Management of ankylosing spondylitis. Bull Rheum Dis 31, No 6:35, 1981
Gorman TK, Mayo EM: Arthritis at an early age. Am J Nurs 84:1472, 1984
LeVine HI: The many faces of Reiter's syndrome. Consultant 20, No 8:61, 1979

Osteoarthritis

Bland JH: The reversibility of osteoarthritis. Am J Med 74, No 6-A:16, 1983
Weiss TE, Quinett RJ: Clinical concepts of osteoarthritis: Part 1. Clin Rheum Pract 1, No 6:269, 1983
Weiss TE, Quinett RJ: Clinical concepts of osteoarthritis: Part 2. Clin Rheum Pract 2, No 1:4, 1984

Crystal-induced arthropathies

Agus B: Hyperuricemia: When you should start therapy. Curr Prescribing 12:55, 1979
Agus B: Hyperuricemia: What to do about it. Consultant 19, No 12:19, 1979
Diamond H: The kidney in hyperuricemia. Clin Rheum Pract 1, No 5:205, 1983
Duffy BW, Senwekjian HO, Knight TF, Weinman EJ: Management of asymptomatic hyperuricemia. JAMA 246, No 19:2215, 1981
Fox IH, Kelly WN: Management of gout. JAMA 242, No 4:361, 1979
Gall EP: Hyperuricemia and gout—A modern approach to diagnosis and treatment. Postgrad Med 65, No 4:163, 1979
Holmes EW: A rational approach to gout. Drug Therapy 11, No 2:117, 1981
Rodman GP: Treatment of gout and other forms of crystal-induced arthritis. Bull Rheum Dis 32, No 5:43, 1982
Schmacher RH: Gout and Pseudogout: Discussions in Patient Management. New York, Medical Examination Publishing, 1978
Talbott JH: Fifteen questions physicians most often ask about gout and its treatment. Consultant 20, No 11:41, 1980
Yu T: A rational approach to gouty arthritis. Consultant 20, No 5:150, 1980

Rheumatic disease in the elderly

Davison SD: Rheumatic disease in the elderly. Mt Sinai J Med 47, No 2:175, 1980
Garber E, Bluestone R: Evaluating arthritis in the elderly. Consultant 19, No 7:97, 1980

Unit IX

Alterations in Skin Defenses

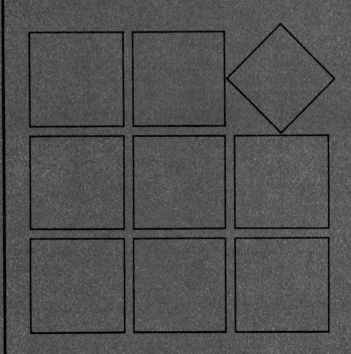

Chapter 54

Alterations in Skin Function and Integrity

Gladys Simandl

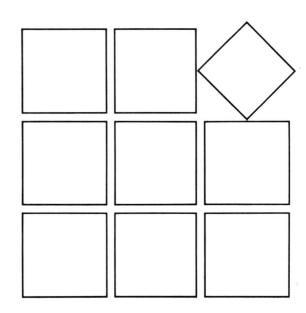

The skin is primarily an organ of protection. It is the largest organ of the body and forms the major barrier between the internal organs and the external environment. The skin of an average-sized adult covers approximately 18 square feet and weighs 6 pounds to 9 pounds.[1,2] As the body's first line of defense, the skin is continuously subjected to potentially harmful environmental agents including solid matter, liquids, gases, sunlight, and microorganisms. Although the skin may become bruised, lacerated, burned, or infected, it has remarkable properties that allow for a continuous cycle of healing, shedding, and cell regeneration.

In addition to protection, the skin serves several other important functions. The skin is richly innervated with pain, temperature, and touch receptors. Skin receptors relay the numerous qualities of touch, such as pressure, sharpness, dullness, pleasure, and fine localization of touch to the central nervous system (CNS) for fine discrimination (Chap. 45). Further, the skin is important in regulating body temperature (Chap. 8). Through CNS control, blood vessels in the skin are dilated or constricted to maintain thermoregulation and the amount of perspiration secreted at any given time. The skin also plays an essential role in vitamin D synthesis and fluid and electrolyte balance. Finally, a less well known property of the skin may be its ability to store glycogen and contribute to glucose metabolism.[3]

■ Structure of the Skin

Because of the great variations in structure in different parts of the body, normal skin is difficult to describe.[4] Corresponding variations are found in the properties of the skin, such as the thickness of skin layers, the distribution of sweat glands, and the number and size of hair follicles. For example, the skin is thicker on the palms and soles of the feet, hair follicles are densely distributed in the scalp, and apocrine sweat glands are confined to the axillae and the anogenital area. Nevertheless, certain structural properties are common to all skin in all areas of the body. The skin is composed of two layers: the epidermis (outer layer) and the dermis (inner layer). A basement membrane zone (BMZ) divides the two layers. The subcutaneous tissue, a layer of loose connective and fatty tissues, binds the dermis to the underlying tissues of the body (Fig. 54-1).

Epidermis

The functions of the skin depend on the properties of its outermost layer, the epidermis. The epidermis not only covers the body, but is also specialized to form the various skin appendages: hair, nails, and glandular structures. Its cells produce a fibrous protein called *keratin*, which is essential to the protective function of skin, and a pigment called melanin, which protects against ultraviolet radiation. The epidermis contains two types of glands: sweat glands, which produce watery secretions, and sebaceous glands, which produce an oily secretion called *sebum*. The epidermis is composed of stratified squamous epithelium, which when viewed under the microscope is seen to consist of five distinct layers, or strata, that represent a progressive differentiation of epidermal cells: stratum germinativum, or basal layer; stratum spinosum; stratum granulosum; stratum lucidum; and stratum corneum (see Fig. 54-1).

The first layer, the stratum corneum, consists of dead, keratinized cells. This layer contains the most cell layers and the largest cells of any zone of the epidermis. It ranges from 15 layers thick in areas such as the face to 25 layers or more on the arm.[5] In specialized areas, such as the palms of the hands or soles of the feet, 100 or more layers are present.[5]

The stratum lucidum, or second layer, is thin and transparent. It consists of transitional cells that retain some of the functions of living skin cells from the layers below and resemble the cells of the stratum corneum. This layer can be seen on the palms of the hands and soles of the feet.

The stratum granulosum, the third layer of the epidermis, consists of granular cells that are the most differentiated cells of the living skin. The cells in this layer are unique in that two polar functions are occurring simultaneously. While some cells are losing cytoplasm and DNA structures, other continue to synthesize keratin.

The fourth layer, the stratum spinosum, is formed as the progeny of the basal cell layer move upward. This layer is two to four layers thick, and its cells become more differentiated as they migrate upward (Fig. 54-2). Keratinocytes, Langerhans' cells, and melanocytes are present in this layer. The cells of this layer are commonly referred to as *prickle cells* because they develop a spiny appearance as their cell borders retract.

The stratum germinativum, or stratum basale, is the deepest layer of the epidermis. It consists of a single layer of basal cells that are attached to the basement membrane. The basal cells produce new skin cells that move upward to replace cells lost during normal skin shedding.

The major cells of the epidermis are the keratinocytes, melanocytes, Langerhans' cells, and Merkel's cells. The five layers of the epidermis arise from these basal-layer cells. These cells do not move upward but remain stationary in the stratum germinativum.

The keratinocyte is the major cell of the epidermis. It is able to synthesize DNA and produce keratin. The keratinocyte changes morphologically as it is pushed toward the outer layer of the epidermis. For example, in

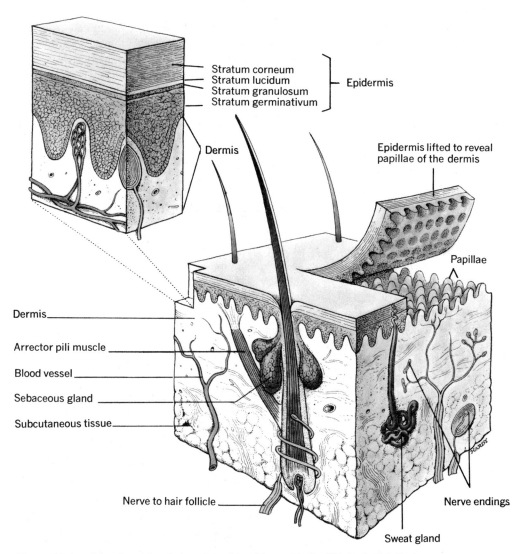

Figure 54-1   *Three-dimensional view of the skin. (From Chaffee EE, Lytle IM: Basic Anatomy and Physiology, 4th ed. Philadelphia, JB Lippincott, 1980)*

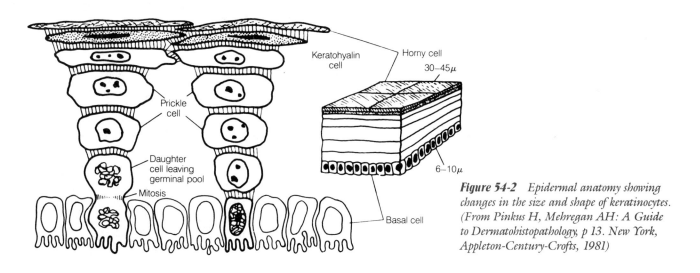

Figure 54-2   *Epidermal anatomy showing changes in the size and shape of keratinocytes. (From Pinkus H, Mehregan AH: A Guide to Dermatohistopathology, p 13. New York, Appleton-Century-Crofts, 1981)*

the basal layer, the keratinocyte is round. As it is pushed into the stratum spinosum, the keratinocyte becomes multisided; it becomes flatter in the granular layer and is flattened and elongated in the stratum corneum (see Fig. 54-2). Keratinocytes also change cytoplasmic structure and composition as they are pushed outward. This transformation from viable cells to the dead cells of the stratum corneum is called keratinization.

Melanocytes are pigment-synthesizing cells. They are almost always located in the basal layer. They function to produce pigment granules called melanosomes, which contain melanin, the brown substance that gives skin its color. Although melanocytes remain in the basal layer, the melanosomes are transferred to the keratinocytes through a dendritic process. During this process, the normally round melanocytes become dendritic in shape. The dendrite tip of the melanocyte is engulfed by a nearby keratinocyte, and the melanosomes are transferred (Fig. 54-3). Each melanocyte is capable of supplying several keratinocytes with melanin. It is the amount of melanin in the keratinocytes that determines a person's skin color. Color protects the skin from the ultraviolet sun rays, and conversely, the ultraviolet rays increase the production of melanin. Black-skinned and white-skinned people have the same amount of melanocytes; however, the number of melanosomes produced differs greatly among individuals.

Langerhans' cells are located in the suprabasal layers of the epidermis and become established among the keratinocytes. They are few in number compared with the keratinocytes. They are derived from precursor cells originating in the bone marrow and continuously repopulate the epidermis.[6] Like melanocytes, they are dendritic in shape and have clear cytoplasms. Microscopically, they resemble a tennis racquet and are there-

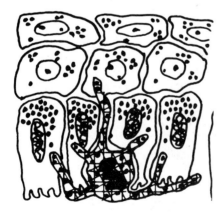

Figure 54-3 *Melanocyte. Note the dendrites passing melanosomes to the nearby keratinocytes. (From Pinkus H, Mehregan AH: A Guide to Dermatohistopathology, p 36. New York, Appleton-Century-Crofts, 1981)*

fore easy to differentiate from other skin cell types. The exact origin of these cells remains unknown, as does their function. Research has indicated that they may play a role in the cutaneous immune response and serve as a possible source of prostaglandins.[7,8]

Merkel's cells consist of free nerve endings attached to modified epidermal cells. Their origin remains unknown, and they are the least densely populated cell of the epidermis. It is generally agreed that Merkel's cells function as mechanoreceptors, or touch receptors.[9]

Basement Membrane Zone

The BMZ is a layer of tissue that connects the epidermis to the dermis, both structures contributing to its formation. Characteristics of the BMZ have become more defined over the past few years. Essentially, the BMZ contains collagen fibers and glycoproteins and consists of four distinct layers, all contributing to the adhesion and elasticity of the skin. The collagen fibers provide the skin with tensile strength, anchorage, and elasticity. The glycoproteins are believed to be associated with cohesion. The function of the BMZ as a barrier remains debatable, as many substances are able to penetrate it. Lymphocytes, neutrophils, and Langerhans' cells easily penetrate the BMZ; however, the BMZ has been found to bar larger molecules.

Dermis

The dermis is the connective tissue layer that separates the epidermis from the subcutaneous fat layer. It supports the epidermis and serves as the primary source of nutrition for the epidermis. The two layers of the dermis, the papillary dermis and the reticular dermis, are composed of cells, fibers, and ground substances as well as nerves and blood vessels. The pilar (hair) structures and glandular structures are embedded in this layer and elaborated upon in the epidermis.

The papillary dermis (pars papillaris) is a thin superficial layer that lies adjacent to the epidermis. It consists of collagen fibers and ground substance. The basal cells of the epidermis project into the papillary dermis, forming dermal papillae (see Fig. 54-1). Dermal papillae contain capillary venules, which serve to nourish the epidermal layers of the skin. This layer of the dermis is well vascularized. Lymph vessels and nerve tissue are also found in this layer.

The reticular dermis (pars reticularis) is the thicker area of the dermis and forms the bulk of the dermis. This is the layer from which tough leather hides are made. The reticular dermis is characterized by a mesh of three-dimensional collagen bundles interconnected with large elastic fibers and ground substance. The collagen fibers are oriented parallel to the body's surface in any given area. These collagen bundles may be organized lengthwise, as on the abdomen, or in round blocks, as in the heel. The direction of surgical incisions is often determined by this organizational pattern. The epidermis extends deep into the reticular dermis and either terminates there or extends into the subcutaneous layer. Blood vessels, lymph vessels, and nerve fibers are found in this area. Extremely small nerve endings extend into the papillary dermis.

Cells found in the dermis include fibroblasts, macrophages, and mast cells. Limited numbers of lymphocytes are found around dermal blood vessels. Fibroblasts synthesize the connective tissue matrix. They also secrete enzymes needed to break down and thereby remodel the matrix. Macrophages are abundant in the dermis and serve to synthesize certain enzymes that enhance or suppress lymphocyte activity, certain prostaglandins, and interferon. Mast cells are also abundant, but their exact function remains unknown.

The microvasculature of the dermal papillae is linked to the larger vessels that exist between the dermal papillae. These vessels transport epidermal nutrients and waste products and also function in thermoregulation. The lymphatic system of the skin, which controls certain infectious skin processes, is also limited to the dermis.

The innervation of the skin is complex. The skin, with its accessory structures, serves as an organ for receiving sensory information from the environment. Accordingly, it is well supplied with sensory nerves. In addition, it contains nerves that supply the blood vessels, sweat glands, and arrector pili muscles. The receptors for touch, pressure, heat, cold, and pain are widely distributed in the skin. Because of the variation in function among the different types of nerve endings, it is generally agreed that sensory modalities are not associated with a particular type of receptor. For example, the sensations of pain, touch, and pressure probably result from multiple stimuli. The final sensation is the result of central summation in the CNS, which mediates patterned responses.

Most of the skin's blood vessels are under sympathetic nervous system control. The sweat glands are innervated by cholinergic fibers but controlled by the sympathetic nervous system. Likewise, the sympathetic nervous system controls the arrector pili (piloerector) muscles that cause hairs on the skin to stand up. Contraction of these muscles tends to cause the skin to dimple, producing "goose pimples."

Subcutaneous Tissue

The subcutaneous tissue layer consists primarily of fat and connective tissues that lend support to the vascular and neural structures supplying the outer layers of the skin. There is controversy about whether or not the subcutaneous tissue should be considered an actual layer of the skin. However, the eccrine glands and deep hair follicles extend to this layer, and several skin diseases involve the subcutaneous tissue.

Skin Appendages

The skin houses a variety of appendages including hair, nails, and sebaceous and sweat glands. The distribution as well as the function of the appendages varies.

Hair

Hair is a structure that originates from hair follicles in the dermis. Most hair follicles are associated with sebaceous glands, and these structures combine to form the pilosebaceous apparatus. The entire hair structure consists of the hair follicle, sebaceous gland, hair muscle (arrector pili), and, in some instances, the apocrine gland (Fig. 54-4). Hair is a keratinized structure that is pushed upward from the hair follicle. Growth of the hair is centered in the bulb (base) of the hair follicle and the hair undergoes changes as it is pushed outward. Hair has been found to go through cyclic phases identified as anagen (the growth phase), catagen (the atrophy phase), and telogen (the resting phase). A vascular network at the site of the follicular bulb nourishes and maintains the hair follicle. Melanocytes are found in the bulb and are responsible for the color of the hair. The arrector pili muscle, located under the sebaceous gland, provides a thermoregulation function by contracting and reducing the skin surface area that is available for the dissipation of body heat.

Sebaceous glands

The sebaceous glands (see Fig. 54-4) secrete a fatty material called *sebum*, which lubricates hair and skin. Sebum prevents undue evaporation of moisture from the stratum corneum during cold weather and helps to conserve body heat. It is also thought to possess some bactericidal and fungicidal properties. It is the sebaceous glands that are most involved in the development of acne (to be discussed).

Sweat glands

There are two types of sweat glands: eccrine and apocrine (see Fig. 54-4). Eccrine sweat glands are simple tubular structures that originate in the dermis and open directly to the skin surface. They vary in density and are located over the entire body surface. Their purpose is to transport sweat to the outer skin surface to regulate body temperature.

Apocrine sweat glands are fewer in number than eccrine sweat glands. They are larger and located deep in

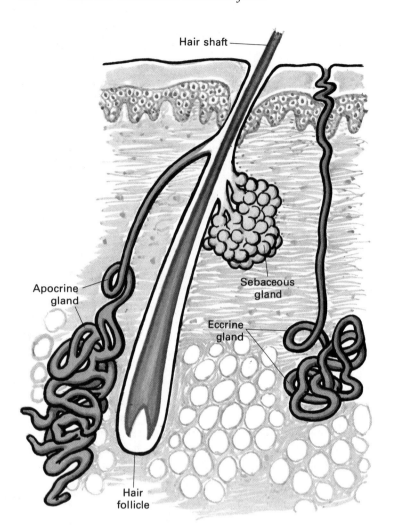

Hair shaft

Apocrine gland

Sebaceous gland

Eccrine gland

Hair follicle

Figure 54-4   *The sweat glands. Note that the apocrine type of gland opens into the hair follicle, whereas the eccrine gland opens directly onto the surface of the skin. (From Chaffee EE, Lytle IM: Basic Anatomy and Physiology, 4th ed. Philadelphia, JB Lippincott, 1980)*

the dermal layer. They open through a hair follicle, even though a hair may not be present, and are found primarily in the axillae and groin. The major difference between these glands and the eccrine glands is that they secrete an oily substance. In animals, apocrine secretions give rise to distinctive odors that enable animals to recognize the presence of others. In humans, apocrine secretions are sterile until mixed with the bacteria on the skin surface and then they produce what is commonly known as body odor.

Nail

The nail is a hardened keratinized plate that protects the fingers and toes and enhances dexterity. The nail is the end product of dead matrix cells that grow from the nail plate. Unlike hair, nails grow continuously unless permanently damaged or diseased.

In summary, the skin is primarily an organ of protection. It is the largest organ of the body and forms the major barrier between the internal organs and the external environment. In addition, the skin is richly innervated with pain, temperature, and touch receptors; it synthesizes vitamin D and plays an essential role in fluid and electrolyte balance. It contributes to glucose metabolism through its glycogen stores. The skin is composed of two layers, the epidermis and the dermis, separated by a basement membrane zone. A layer of subcutaneous tissue binds the dermis to the underlying organs and tissues of the body. The epidermis contains five layers, or strata, and is the outermost layer of the skin. The major cells of the epidermis are the keratinocytes, melanocytes, Langerhans' cells, and Merkel's cells. These cells, which remain in the stratum germinativum (or basal layer) of the epidermis, are the source of the cells in all five layers of the epidermis. The keratinocytes, which are the major cells of the epidermis, are transformed from viable keratinocytes to dead keratin as they move from the innermost layer of the epidermis (stratum germinativum) to the outermost layer (stratum corneum). The melanocytes are pigment-synthesizing cells that give skin its color. The dermis provides the epidermis with support and nutrition and is the source of blood vessels, nerves, and skin appendages (hair follicles and sebaceous glands, nails, and sweat glands).

Manifestations of Skin Disorders

The skin is a unique organ in which numerous signs are immediately observable. These signs contribute to accurate diagnosis and treatment. In many cases, the skin may relay signs of other organic dysfunction. The most common manifestations of skin disorders are rashes, lesions, and pruritus (itching).

Lesions and Rashes

Rashes are temporary eruptions of the skin, such as those associated with childhood diseases, heat rash, diaper rash, or drug-induced eruptions. The term lesion usually refers to a traumatic or pathologic loss of normal tissue continuity, structure, or function. Sometimes the components of a rash are referred to as lesions. The various types of lesions are described in Tables 54-1, 54-2, and 54-3. Rashes and lesions may range in size from a fraction of a millimeter (as in petechiae) to many centimeters (as in a decubitus ulcer, or pressure sore). They may be blanched (white), reddened (erythematous), hemorrhagic or purpuric (containing blood), or pigmented. Skin lesions may be vascular in origin (Table 54-1); they may occur as primary lesions arising in previously normal skin (Table 54-2); or they may develop as secondary lesions resulting from primary lesions (Table 54-3).

Pruritus

Pruritus, or itching, is a symptom common to many skin disorders. Pruritus may be present with dry skin and often accompanies major skin disorders. Itching may also be symptomatic of other organ disorders, such as diabetes or biliary disease, when no skin anomaly exists. Physiologically, two theories exist regarding itch. The first is that an anatomically distinct itch receptor exists, although none has been found to date, perhaps because of their scarcity and small size.[10] The second theory is that itching is the sensation experienced by an individual when multiple nerve fibers in the skin are stimulated. The central nervous system interprets these sensations as itch through central summation. In other words, no single nerve fiber is responsible for a single sensation called itch; the itch sensation is the result of multiple-fiber stimulation.

The well-known response to an itch is scratching; this can cause skin excoriations. Excoriated skin is much more susceptible to infectious processes, and measures to reduce pruritus and prevent scratching should therefore be taken. Because vasodilatation increases itching, a common method of reducing pruritus is the use of cold applications. Application of topical corticosteroids may be helpful in some situations. Administration of systemic antihistamines and corticosteroids may be indicated in severe pruritus. Phototherapy may be used with the chronic forms of itching associated with internal organic disease processes.

In summary, skin lesions, rashes, and pruritus are common manifestations of skin disorders. Rashes are temporary skin eruptions. Lesions result from traumatic or pathologic loss of the normal continuity, structure, or function of the skin. Lesions may be vascular in origin; they may occur as primary lesions in previously normal skin; or they may develop as secondary lesions resulting from primary lesions. Pruritus, or itching, is a symptom common to many skin disorders. Scratching because of pruritus can lead to excoriation, infection, and other complications.

Developmental Skin Problems

Many skin problems occur more commonly in certain age groups. Because of aging changes, common skin problems of the infant, adolescent, and elderly person are different.

Infancy and Childhood

Infancy connotes the image of perfect, blemishless skin. For the most part, this is true; however, several congenital skin lesions, such as mongolian spots, hemangiomas, and nevi are associated with the early neonatal period. Mongolian spots are caused by selective pigmentation. They usually occur on the buttocks or sacral area and are commonly seen in the yellow or black race. Hemangiomas are vascular disorders of the skin. Two types of hemangiomas are commonly seen in infants and small children: bright red raised strawberry hemangiomas and flat reddish-purple, port-wine stain hemangiomas. The strawberry hemangiomas begin as small red lesions that are noted shortly after birth. They may remain as small superficial lesions or extend to involve the subcutaneous tissue. Strawberry hemangiomas usually disappear before 5 to 7 years of age without leaving an appreciable scar. Port-wine stain hemangiomas are rare, usually occur on the face, and are disfiguring. They do not disappear with age, and there is no satisfactory treatment. Usually cover-up cosmetics are used in an attempt to conceal their disfiguring effects. The term nevus, discussed later in this chapter, is used to

Table 54-1   Vascular and Purpuric Lesions of the Skin

	Vascular			Purpuric	
	Cherry Angioma	*Spider Angioma*	*Venous Star*	*Petechia*	*Ecchymosis*
Color	Bright or ruby red; may become brownish with age	Fiery red	Bluish	Deep red or reddish purple	Purple or purplish blue, fading to green, yellow, and brown with time
Size	1–3 mm	Very small up to 2 cm	Variable, from very small to several inches	Usually 1–3 mm	Variable, larger than petechiae
Shape	Round, sometimes raised, may be surrounded by a pale halo	Central body, sometimes raised, surrounded by erythema and radiating legs	Variable, may resemble a spider or be linear, irregular, cascading	Round, flat	Round, oval, or irregular; may have a central subcutaneous flat nodule
Pulsatility	Absent	Often demonstrable in the body of the spider, when pressure with a glass slide is applied	Absent	Absent	Absent
Effect of Pressure	May show partial blanching, especially if pressure is applied with a pinpoint's edge	Pressure over the body causes blanching of the spider	Pressure over center does not cause blanching	None	None
Distribution	Trunk, also extremities	Face, neck, arms, and upper trunk, almost never below the waist	Most often on the legs, near veins; also anterior chest	Variable	Variable
Significance	None; increase in size and numbers with aging	Liver disease, pregnancy, vitamin B deficiency, occurs in some normal people	Often accompanies increased pressure in the superficial veins, as in varicose veins	Blood extravasated outside the vessels; may suggest increased bleeding tendency or emboli to skin	Blood extravasated outside the vessels; often secondary to trauma; also seen in bleeding disorders

(From Bates B: A Guide to Physical Examination, 3rd ed. Philadelphia, JB Lippincott, 1983)

Table 54-2   Primary Lesions (May Arise from Previously Normal Skin)

Circumscribed, Flat, Nonpalpable Changes in Skin Color	Palpable Elevated Solid Masses	Circumscribed Superficial Elevations of the Skin Formed by Free Fluid in a Cavity within the Skin Layers
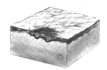	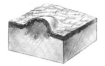	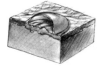
Macule—small, up to 1 cm.* Example: freckle, petechia	*Papule*—up to 0.5 cm. Example: an elevated nevus	*Vesicle*—up to 0.5 cm; filled with serous fluid. Example: herpes simplex
Patch—larger than 1 cm. Example: vitiligo	*Plaque*—a flat, elevated surface larger than 0.5 cm, often formed by the coalescence of papules	*Bulla*—Greater than 0.5 cm; filled with serous fluid. Example: 2nd degree burn
	Nodule—0.5 cm to 1–2 cm; often deeper and firmer than a papule	*Pustule*—filled with pus. Examples: acne, impetigo
	Tumor—larger than 1–2 cm	
	Wheal—a slightly irregular, relatively transient, superficial area of localized skin edema. Example: mosquito bite, hive	

(From Bates B: A Guide to Physical Examination, 3rd ed. Philadelphia, JB Lippincott, 1983)
*Authorities vary somewhat in their definitions of skin lesions by size. The dimensions given in this table should be considered approximate, not rigid.

---

denote any congenital colored lesion.[11] Nevi may vary in shape or size and they may be present at birth or develop later in life.

Because of its newness, infant skin is also subject to irritation, injury, and extremes of temperature. Prolonged exposure to a warm humid environment can lead to prickly heat, and too frequent bathing can cause dryness and lead to skin problems. The contents of soiled diapers, if not changed frequently, can lead to contact dermatitis and bacterial infections. Cradle cap is usually attributed to infrequent and inadequate washing of the scalp. Table 54-4 summarizes common skin problems of the infant and small child.

The primary factor in preventing infant skin disorders is careful attention to the skin. Baby lotions are helpful in maintaining skin moisture, while baby powder acts as a drying agent. Both are useful aids when used selectively and according to the nature of the skin problem (excessive moisture or dryness). Baby powders containing talc can cause serious respiratory problems if inhaled; therefore, containers should be kept out of the reach of small children. Cornstarch works well for this purpose, and baby powders containing cornstarch are now available on the market. Unnecessary bathing should be avoided, and clothing appropriate to the environment should be worn.

Table 54-3 Secondary Lesions (Result from Changes in Primary Lesions)*

Loss of Skin Surface

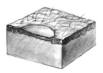

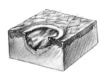

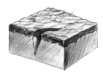

Erosion—loss of the superficial epidermis; surface is moist but does not bleed. Example: moist area after the rupture of a vesicle, as in chickenpox

Ulcer—a deeper loss of skin surface; may bleed and scar.
Examples: stasis ulcer of venous insufficiency, syphilitic chancre

Fissure—a linear crack in the skin.
Example: athlete's foot

Material on the Skin Surface

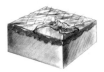

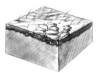

Crust—the dried residue of serum, pus, or blood. Example: impetigo

Scale—a thin flake of exfoliated epidermis. Examples: dandruff, dry skin, psoriasis

Miscellaneous

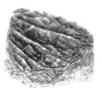

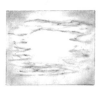

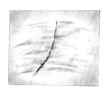

Lichenification—thickening and roughening of the skin and increased visibility of the normal skin furrows. Example: atopic dermatitis

Atrophy—thinning of the skin with loss of the normal skin furrows; the skin looks shinier and more translucent than normal.
Example: arterial insufficiency

Excoriation—a scratch mark

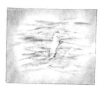

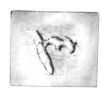

Scar—replacement of destroyed tissue by fibrous tissue

Keloid—a hypertrophied scar

(From Bates B: A Guide to Physical Examination, 3rd ed. Philadelphia, JB Lippincott, 1983)
*Authorities vary somewhat in their definitions of skin lesions by size. The dimensions given in this table should be considered approximate, not rigid.

Table 54-4 Common Skin Lesions of Infants and Small Children

Lesion	Appearance
Congenital Dermatoses	
Hemangiomas	
Strawberry	Bright red raised and rounded lesions; may enlarge with growth of infant and then regress; usually disappear by 5 to 7 years of age
Port-wine stain	Flat reddish purple disfiguring lesion; usually found on the face; does not disappear with age
Mongolian spot	Light blue, gray-green to slate gray macule; commonly located in the lumbosacral area; usually disappears with age
Nevi (moles)	Vary in size, shape, and location; usually brown-black, flat or raised macules or papules; borders are usually well defined and rounded
Irritative and Inflammatory Dermatoses	
Cradle cap	Yellowish, greasy, and crusted collection of vernix and shedding skin on scalp
Prickly heat	Tiny vesicles usually located on the neck, back, chest, trunk, abdomen, and folds of skin; pruritus is common
Diaper rash	Erythematous macular rash; blister formation, excoriation, and infection may develop

Diaper rash results from a combination of ammonia and alkaline media (breakdown products of urine). The treatment includes frequent change of diapers with careful cleansing of the irritated area to remove the ammonia. This is important particularly in hot weather. Exposing the irritated area to air is helpful. Use of plastic pants should be discouraged. Disposable diapers or diapers washed in gentle detergent and thoroughly rinsed to remove all traces of ammonia and alkali help to reduce the risk of diaper rash.

Prickly heat results from constant maceration of the skin because of prolonged exposure to a warm and humid environment; this leads to midepidermal obstruction and rupture of the sweat glands. The treatment includes the removal of excessive clothing, cooling the skin with warm water baths, drying the skin with powders, and avoiding hot humid environments.

Cradle cap is usually treated by mild shampooing and gentle combing to remove the scales. Application of oil is no longer recommended, as this can compound the problem.

As children become mobile and interact with the environment, they become susceptible to the myriad of skin disorders affecting people of all age groups. Children, because of their physiologic development, are also more prone to accidents that may result in major skin trauma, such as lacerations and burns. Careful activity supervision consistent with the developmental needs of children is the prime factor in the prevention of these traumas. Besides interacting with the environment, children are frequently in close contact with other children. As a result, diseases such as head lice, tinea capitis, and impetigo are more frequently seen in chidren. Epidemiologically, the incidence of roseola, rubeola, rubella, and chickenpox is also highest in this age group; hence, these diseases have become known as the childhood diseases.

Rashes associated with childhood diseases

Roseola infantum.   Roseola infantum is a contagious viral disease that generally affects children under 4 and usually children about 1 year of age. It produces a characteristic maculopapular rash covering the trunk and spreading to the appendages. A rapid rise in temperature to 105°F and coldlike symptoms accompany the disease. Unlike in rubella, no cervical or postauricular lymph node adenopathy occurs. The symptoms usually subside within 3 days to 5 days. Roseola infantum is frequently mistaken for rubella. Rubella can usually be ruled out by the age of the child as well as the absence of lymph node adenopathy. Generally, children under 6 months to 9 months do not develop rubella because of maternal antibodies. Blood antibody titers may be taken to determine the actual diagnosis. In most cases, there are no long-term effects from this disease.

Treatment for roseola infantum is palliative; there is no vaccine for prevention. Antipyretic drugs such as acetaminophen (Datril or Tylenol) and cooling baths are used to reduce the fever. Rest and fluid are recommended for recuperation and body rehydration. Pruritus may accompany the other symptoms, but this is rare. If severe, pruritus can be treated with topical lotions such as Caladryl.

Rubeola.   Rubeola (hard measles, 7-day measles) is a communicable viral disease caused by morbillivirus. The characteristic rash is macular and blotchy; sometimes the macules become confluent. The rubeola rash usually begins on the face and spreads to the appendages. There are several accompanying symptoms: a fever of 100°F or greater, Koplik's spots (small irregular red spots with a bluish white speck in the center) on the buccal mucosa, and mild to severe photosensitivity. Coldlike symptoms and general malaise and myalgia are often present. In severe cases, the macule may hemorrhage into the skin tissue or to the other body surface. This is called hemorrhagic measles. Measles is more severe in malnourished children. Complications include otitis media, pneumonia, and encephalitis.

Rubeola is a disease preventable by vaccine, and immunization is required by law in most states. Immunization is accomplished by injection of a live-virus vaccine. Two doses during infancy, followed by booster doses a year later and before school are sufficient to produce immunity. For a positive diagnosis of rubeola, most states require antibody titers. Blood titers are usually drawn during the disease process and 6 weeks after the symptoms have resided.

The treatment for rubeola is symptomatic. Children are kept in darkened rooms; antipyretic medications are given to reduce the fever; and rest and fluids are encouraged. If marked dehydration exists or the symptoms are severe, the physician should be consulted.

Rubella.   Rubella (3-day measles, German measles) is a childhood disease caused by the rubella virus. It is characterized by a diffuse, punctate, macular rash that begins on the trunk and spreads to the arms and legs. Mild febrile states occur; generally the fever is less than 100°F. Postauricular, suboccipital, and cervical lymph node adenopathy are common. Coldlike symptoms usually accompany the disease in the form of cough, congestion, and coryza.

Rubella generally has no long-lasting sequelae; however, the transmission of the disease to pregnant women early in the gestation period may result in severe teratogenic effects in the unborn fetus. Among the teratogenic effects are cataracts, microcephaly, mental retardation, deafness, patent ductus arteriosus, glaucoma, purpura, and bone defects. Most states require immunization by law to prevent the transmission of rubella to pregnant women. Immunization is accompanied by live-virus injection. Two injections during infancy followed by two booster doses, one a year later and one before the child begins school, are considered adequate in the prevention of rubella. Cases of rubella in unimmunized children are rare. As with rubeola, the treatment is symptomatic.

Chickenpox.   Chickenpox is a common communicable childhood disease. It is caused by the herpes zoster virus, which is also the agent in shingles. The characteristic skin lesion occurs in three stages: macule, vesicle, and granular scab. The macular stage is characterized by rapid development (within hours) of macules over the trunk of the body, spreading to the limbs, buccal mucosa, scalp, axillae, upper respiratory tract, and conjunctiva. During the second stage, the macules vesiculate (become filled with water, or blister) and may become depressed or umbilicated (raised blisters with depressed centers). The vesicles break open, and a scab forms during the third stage. Crops of lesions occur successively, so that all three forms of the lesion are usually visible by the third day of the illness. Mild to extreme pruritus accompanies these lesions and can be a complicating factor by leading to scratching and subsequent development of secondary bacterial infections. Other symptoms that accompany chickenpox are coldlike symptoms including cough, coryza, and sometimes photosensitivity. Mild febrile states usually occur. Side-effects, such as pneumonia, septic complications, and encephalitis are rare.

The treatment, as in most of the other childhood diseases, is palliative. To date, no vaccine is available to prevent chickenpox. Antipyretic drugs such as acetaminophen are given for fever reduction; they may also relieve local discomfort. Pruritus is relieved with lukewarm baths and applications of topical antipruritics such as Caladryl lotion. Home remedies, such as baking soda baths, also relieve itching. The physician should be notified in cases of severe pruritus. Oral administration of diphenhydramine (Benadryl) or other antihistamines may be prescribed. Rest and fluids are important in recuperation and rehydration.

Scarlet fever.   Scarlet fever is a systemic reaction to the toxins produced by the group A beta-hemolytic streptococci. It occurs when the person is sensitized to the toxin-producing variation of streptococci. It frequently occurs in association with streptococcal sore throat (strep throat); but it may also be associated with a wound, skin infection, or puerperal infection. Scarlet fever is characterized by a pink punctate skin rash on the neck, chest, axillae, groin, and thighs. When palpated, the rash feels like fine sandpaper. There is flushing of the face with circumoral pallor. Other symptoms include high fever, nausea and vomiting, strawberry tongue, raspberry tongue, and skin desquamation. Complications of scarlet fever inlude otitis media, peritonsillar abscess, rheumatic fever, acute glomerulonephritis, and cholera. Penicillin is the drug of choice for treatment.

Adolescence and Young Adulthood

The most common disorder of adolescence and young adulthood is acne vulgaris (to be discussed). The increased production of sex hormones and oils contribute to this problem. The problems associated with childhood diseases are less common in this age group;

however, diseases such as pityriasis rosea are more commonly seen. Also, chronic skin diseases may exacerbate or change with the aging process.

Old Age

The elderly person may experience a variety of skin disorders as well as exacerbation of earlier skin problems because of the aging process. Physiologically, in the skin of the elderly person the dermal-epidermal junction is flattened; dermal and subcutaneous mass is lost; the capillary loops are shortened; and the number of melanocytes, Langerhans' cells, and Merkel's cells is reduced. This results in less padding, thinning of the skin, and color and elasticity changes. The skin is much less resilient to environmental and mechanical trauma, and tissue repair takes longer. Similarly, there is less hair and nail growth, and the hair loses pigment.

Dry skin and pruritus associated with dry skin are common in the elderly. Reduced activity of the sebaceous glands and sweat glands contributes to this problem. For some elderly persons, these changes may be a great help in clearing a lifelong struggle with acne.

Common skin problems*

The most common skin problems in the elderly are skin tags, keratoses, lentigines, and vascular lesions (Table 54-5). Many of these problems reflect continued exposure to sun and weather over the years.

Skin tags. Skin tags are soft, pedunculated, brown or flesh-colored papules appearing on the front or side of the neck or in the axilla. Ranging in size from a pinhead to the size of a pea, the tags have the normal color and texture of the skin.

Keratoses. A keratosis is a horny growth or a condition characterized by an abnormal growth of the keratinizing cells of the epidermis. *Seborrheic keratoses* are sharply circumscribed, wartlike lesions that seem to rest on top of the skin. They usually begin as yellow to brown flat lesions of less than 1 cm and may become larger, dark brown to coal black lesions with a greasy appearance.

Keratoses are usually found on the face or trunk, sometimes in the form of a solitary lesion or in other cases as literally hundreds of lesions. Although seborrheic keratoses are benign, they must be differentiated from nevi, or moles, which are formed from clusters of melanocytes, because a change in the color, texture, or size of a nevus may indicate malignant transformation to a melanoma.

*This section is reprinted from Porth C, Kapke K: Aging and the skin. Geriatric Nursing 3:160-161, 1983. Copyright American Journal of Nursing Company. Reprinted by permission.

Table 54-5 Skin Lesions Common Among Elders

Lesion	Appearance
Skin tags	Small protrusions (pinhead to size of pea), color and texture of normal skin
Seborrheic keratoses	Raised, sharply circumscribed, wartlike growths, yellow-brown to brown-black color, often multiple, usually on face or trunk
Actinic keratoses	Premalignant, slightly raised, light-to-dark-brown, scaly lesions on "weathered" areas, scale is adherent and returns each time it is removed
Senile lentigines	Flat, tan-to-brown macules, usually on face or hands, often called liver spots
Malignant lentigines	Premalignant lesions; slow growing, flat, light-to-dark-brown mottled "freckles"; usually larger than senile lentigines
Senile angiomas	Small ruby red or purplish vascular tumors; usually on the trunk
Telangiectases	Dilatations of capillaries or terminal arteries; located on the skin surface, often on face, particularly around the nose
Venous lakes	Flat, small, bluish blood vessels, frequently seen on the back of hands, ears, and lips

(From Porth C, Kapke K: Aging and the skin. Geriatr Nurs (May/June) 3:161, 1983. Copyright American Journal of Nursing Company. Reprinted by permission.)

Actinic (solar) keratoses are premalignant skin lesions that develop on sun-exposed areas. The lesions, ranging in size from 0.1 to 1 cm or larger, usually appear as dry, brown, and scaly areas, although some may have a shiny surface. A slight erythematous area often encircles the lesion.

Actinic lesions are often multiple and more easily felt than seen. When scale is present, it is extremely adherent, and efforts at removal often cause capillary bleeding. The scale tends to recur when it is removed. Characteristics of actinic keratoses is the "weathered" appearance of the surrounding skin. Enlargement, induration, or ulceration of the lesions suggests malignant transformation.

Lentigines. Senile lentigines are the brown, so-called liver spots often seen on sun-exposed areas. Over-the-counter (OTC) creams and lotions containing hydroquinone (Eldoquin, Solaquin, others) may be used to temporarily bleach these spots. This agent interferes with the synthesis of new pigment but does not destroy existing pigment.

In the concentration approved for OTC preparations, however, hydroquinone has limited usefulness. In the higher concentrations available in prescription preparations, hydroquinone may cause inflammation with burning, tingling, and stinging. Despite the limited usefulness of OTC preparations, their effects may make some people feel less self-conscious about skin discoloration. The success of treatment depends on avoiding sunlight completely or consistently applying a high-potency sunscreen.

Malignant lentigines, sometimes referred to as Hutchinson's melanotic freckles, begin as premalignant lesions arising from the melanocytes and are usually larger than the senile lentigenes. They start as a small, light to dark brown mottled area that is flat with the surface of the skin and grows laterally. Growth may continue at a variable rate over many years. As malignant changes occur, the area grows vertically and becomes elevated.

Vascular lesions.   Vascular lesions consist of vascular tumors and chronically dilated blood vessels. *Senile angiomas* are small, ruby red or purplish vascular tumors, usually compressible and found mainly on the trunk. *Senile ectasia* refers to a slightly raised erythematous papule that is composed of dilated capillaries. They are usually 2 mm to 5 mm in diameter and located on the trunk. *Telangiectases* are single dilated blood vessels (capillaries or terminal arteries) that appear most frequently on the cheeks and the nose—areas long exposed to excessive sunlight and harsh weather.

Venous lakes are usually seen on the exposed body parts, particularly the backs of the hands, ears, and lips. They consist of small, flat, bluish blood vessels that have a lakelike appearance. The color of the lesion can usually be blanched when sustained pressure is applied to one side. Senile angiomas and venous lakes can be removed by fulguration if a person desires.

In summary, many skin problems occur in specific age groups. Common to infants are diaper rash, prickly heat, and cradle cap. Rashes associated with childhood diseases such as roseola, rubeola, rubella, and chickenpox are common in young children. Acne vulgaris is a common disorder of adolescence and young adulthood. Skin changes that occur as a part of the aging process predispose the elderly to dry skin, keratosis, lentigines, and vascular skin lesions.

■ Primary Disorders of the Skin

Primary skin disorders are those originating in the skin. They include infectious processes, inflammatory conditions, allergic reactions, parasitic infestations, overexposure or hypersensitivity to sunlight, and neoplasms. Although most of these disorders are not life threatening, they can affect the quality of life.

Infectious Processes

The skin is subject to attack by a number of microorganisms. Normally the skin flora, sebum, immune responses, and other protective mechanisms guard the skin against infection. Depending on the virulence of the infecting agent and the competence of the host's resistance, infections may result.

Fungal infections

Fungal infections of the skin are classified as superficial and deep types. The superficial infections are called dermatophytoses; they are commonly known as *tinea*, or *ringworm*. Different forms of tinea affect different body areas. Tinea can affect the body (tinea corporis), scalp (tinea capitis), beard (tinea barbae), hands (tinea manus), feet (tinea pedis),nails (onychomycosis), or groin and upper aspects of the thigh (tinea cruris; see jock itch, Chap. 33). Deep fungal infections involve the epidermis, dermis, and subcutis. Infections that are typically superficial may exhibit deep involvement in immunosuppressed individuals.

A fungus is a parasitic plant composed of chlorophyll-lacking cells (Chap. 7). Certain strains of fungi are considered normal flora. Fungi causing superficial skin infections live on the dead, keratinized cells of the epidermis. They emit an enzyme that enables them to digest keratin, which results in superficial skin scaling, nail disintegration, and hair structure breakage. An exception to this is the invading fungus of tinea versicolor, which does not produce a keratolytic enzyme. Individual species of three genera have been identified as the invading fungi in most forms of tinea: *Microsporum, Epidermophyton,* and *Trichophyton.*

Diagnosis of fungal infections is primarily done by microscopic examination of skin scrapings. Hyphae are threadlike filaments that grow from spores and are visible microscopically. Mycelia refers to the macroscopic aggregation of hyphae. The fungal spores, the reproducing bodies of fungi, are rarely seen on skin scrapings. Potassium hydroxide (KOH) preparations are used to prepare slides of skin scrapings. The KOH disintegrates human tissue and leaves behind the hyphae for examination. With another method of diagnosis a Wood's light (ultraviolet light) is directed onto the affected area; under the light, many fungi will fluoresce a green to yellow-green color.

Tinea corporis.   Tinea corporis (ringworm of the body) can be caused by any of the fungal agents. Usually, it is caused by *Microsporum canis* or *M. audouini*; less frequently it is caused by *Trichophyton rubrum* or *T. mentagrophytes*. The lesions are round, oval, or circular scaly patches (Fig. 54-5). There is central clearing of the patches with raised red borders consisting of vesicles, papules, or pustules. The lesion begins as a red papule and enlarges with central healing. The borders are sharply defined; lesions may coalesce. Pruritus, a mild burning sensation, and erythema frequently accompany the skin lesion.

Tinea corporis affects all ages; however, children seem most prone to infection. Transmission is most commonly from kittens, puppies, and other children who have infections. Less common forms are from foot and groin infections.

Treatment of mild cases is generally with over-the-counter antifungal preparations containing tolnaftate or undecylenic acid. Tinactin contains a 1% tolnaftate base, whereas Desenex and other name brands contain undecylenic acid. Both of these topical agents are effective if used correctly. Griseofulvin, a pharmaceutically controlled oral antifungal agent, is warranted in severe cases.

Tinea capitis.   Tinea capitis (ringworm of the scalp) is separated into two types: primary (noninflammatory) and secondary (inflammatory). Primary lesions characteristically present as grayish round hairless patches, or balding spots, on the head. The lesion varies in size and is most commonly seen on the back of the head (Fig. 54-6). Mild erythema, crust, or scale may be present. The child is usually symptomless, although occasionally pruritus may exist. The primary form of tinea capitis is caused by *M. audouini* and *M. canis* transferred from kittens, puppies, and other humans. Epidemics have occurred from

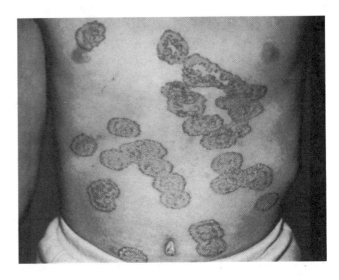

Figure 54-5   *Tinea corporis. (From Sauer GC: Manual of Skin Diseases, 4th ed. Philadelphia, JB Lippincott, 1980)*

Trichophyton tonsurans and *M. audouini* and represent human-to-human transmission.

Children aged 3 to 8 are primarily affected. Tinea capitis seldom occurs in an adult; this has been partially attributed to the higher content of fatty acids in the sebum after puberty, a finding that has generated the development of several antifungal agents with fatty acid bases. These antifungal agents revolutionized the old remedies in which children were often subjected to head shavings and harsh shampoos and salves.

The inflammatory type of tinea capitis is caused by a virulent strain of *Trichophyton mentagrophytes, T. verrucosum,* and *Microsporum gypseum*. The onset is acute, and lesions are usually localized to one area. The initial lesion consists of a pustular scaly round patch with bro-

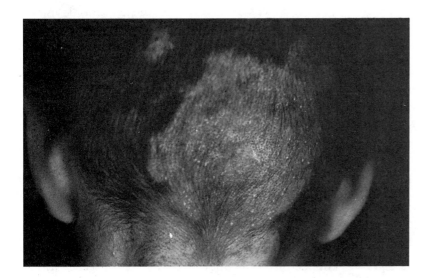

Figure 54-6   *Tinea capitis. (From Sauer GC: Manual of Skin Diseases, 4th ed. Philadelphia, JB Lippincott, 1980)*

ken hairs. A secondary bacterial infection is common and may lead to a painful circumscribed, boggy, and indurated lesion called a *kerion*. The highest incidence is in children and farmers who are around infected animals.

The treatment for both forms of tinea capitis is primarily griseofulvin, an oral antifungal agent. Topical ointments, in addition to oral therapy, are sometimes indicated. Wetpacks and medicated shampoos along with antibiotics may be prescribed for the secondary types of infection.

Tinea pedis. Tinea pedis (athlete's foot, ringworm of the feet) is a common skin disorder primarily affecting the spaces between the toes, the soles of the feet, or the sides of the feet. It is caused by *T. mentagrophytes* and *T. rubrum*. The lesions vary from a mild scaling lesion to a painful exudative, erosive inflamed lesion with fissuring. Lesions are often accompanied by pruritus and foul odor.

Evidence suggests that athlete's foot occurs in two forms, simple and complex. Simple forms of tinea pedis have high fungal populations and low bacterial growths. They are characterized by mild to moderate skin peeling and are largely asymptomatic. Complex tinea pedis has a higher bacterial count (*Proteus* and *Pseudomonas*) with a receding fungal count. Complex forms involve maceration of tissue, inflammation, and fissuring. Pruritus and pain are often present.[12]

Some people are prone to chronic conditions of athlete's foot. Mild forms are more common during dry environmental conditions. Exacerbations in the mild form occur as a result of hot weather, sweating, and exercise, or when the feet are exposed to more moisture. Tinea pedis may occur alone or in combination with other infections such as tinea corporis or tinea cruris. Patches on the hands may occur; this is known as the intradermal, or dermatophytid, reaction.

Simple forms of tinea pedis are treated with topical application of antifungals such as tolnaftate. In the past, complex forms have been treated with oral griseofulvin and topical antifungal agents. Based on their study, Klingman and Leyden[12] now suggest the combination of antibiotics (neomycin sulfate) and tolnaftate in the treatment of complex forms. Other treatment and preventive modalities include scrupulous cleansing and drying of affected areas, clean dry socks, and changing of socks daily. When bathed, the feet should be dried after other parts of the body to prevent spread of the disease.

Onychomycosis. Onychomycosis (tinea unguium, ringworm of the nails) is a chronic fungal infection of the nails of the hands or feet. Tinea of the toenails is common; tinea of the fingernails is less common. Toenail infection is common in people prone to chronic infec-

tions of tinea pedis. Often, the infection in the toenails becomes a ready resource for future infections of the foot. It may begin from a crushing injury to a toenail or from the spread of tinea pedis. Usually onychomycosis is caused by *T. rubrum* or *T. mentagrophytes*. The infection usually begins at the tip of the nail where the fungus digests the keratin of the nail. Initially, the nail appears opaque, white, or silvery. The nail then turns yellow or brown. This condition remains unchanged for years and may involve only one or two nails. Generally, there is no discomfort. Gradually, the nail thickens and becomes frail as the infection spreads to the entire nail and nail plate. The nail cracks and thickens, and the nail plate separates from the nail bed as the nail becomes permanently discolored and distorted. Spreading to other nails may occur.

The prognosis for fungal infections of the toenail is poor. The treatment usually involves oral griseofulvin for up to 1 year. It rarely produces a cure, and some authorities recommend not using griseofulvin or only using the drug with removal of the infected toenails. Even with this therapy, recurrence is frequent. Fingernail infections are more easily treated. Oral griseofulvin therapy for 6 months to 1 year has been successful but is dependent on the persistence of both the therapist and the patient.

Tinea manus. Tinea manus (ringworm of the hands) is rarely the primary site of infection. More frequently it occurs with tinea pedis. A diagnostic differentiation among hand diseases is that tinea manus usually occurs only on one hand, whereas other infectious processes, such as contact dermatitis and psoriasis, affect both hands.

The same fungal agents responsible for tinea pedis are found active in tinea manus, *T. rubrum* and *T. mentagrophytes*. The characteristic lesion is a blister on the palm or finger surrounded by erythema. Chronic lesions are scaly and dry. Cracking and fissuring may occur. The lesions may spread to the plantar surfaces of the hand; if chronic, tinea manus may lead to tinea of the fingernails. The treatment of choice is oral griseofulvin therapy for approximately 3 months.

Tinea barbae. Tinea barbae (ringworm of the beard) is rare. It occurs primarily in farmers, who contract it from infected cattle. It is usually caused by *T. verrucosum*, found in cattle, or *T. mentagrophytes*, found in dogs and horses.

The milder form of tinea barbae involves lesions similar to those found in tinea corporis or tinea capitis. A macule spreads into a patch with raised borders and central clearing. Vesicles and papules may be found. Alopecia accompanies involved areas. Severe forms include pustule formation with bacterial infection. The beard hairs break off close to the skin surface and are easily pulled out.

The usual mode of treatment is oral griseofulvin therapy with or without topical antifungal applications. Boric acid wet packs are sometimes indicated. The benefits of antibiotic therapy are limited to secondary bacterial infections.

Tinea versicolor.   Tinea versicolor is a fungal infection involving the upper chest, back, and sometimes arms. The causative agent is *Malassezia furfur*. The infection occurs primarily in young adults in tropic and temperate regions; however, cases have been reported in the northern states.

The characteristic lesion is a yellow, pink, or brown sheet of scaling skin. The name versicolor is derived from the multicolored variations of the lesion that exist. The patches are depigmented and do not tan when exposed to ultraviolet light, and the skin has an overall appearance of being "dirty." This cosmetic defect often brings the patient to the physician in the summer months. The theory is that the fungus filters the ultraviolet light, thus preventing tanning. In darker-skinned persons, the depigmented areas are more apparent.

Although there is no specific drug that will prevent the recurrence of tinea versicolor, selenium sulfide, found in several shampoo preparations, has been a most effective treatment measure. Boiling or steam-pressing clothes may prevent recurrence.

Dermatophytid reaction.   A secondary skin eruption may occur in persons allergic to one of the dermatophytes and is called a dermatophytid, or intradermal (ID), reaction. It may occur during an acute episode of a fungal infection. The most common reaction occurs on the hands, in response to tinea pedis. The lesions are vesicles with erythema extending over the palms and fingers of the hand; extension to other areas may occur. Less commonly, a more generalized reaction involving papule or vesicle eruption on the trunk or extremities occurs. These eruptions may resemble tinea corporis and may become excoriated and infected with bacteria. Treatment revolves around treating the primary site of infection. The ID reaction will resolve in most cases without intervention if the primary site is cleared.

Candidal (monilial) infections.   Candidiasis (moniliasis)is a fungal infection caused by *Candida albicans*. This yeastlike fungus is a normal inhabitant of the gastrointestinal tract, mouth, and vagina (see genital *C. albicans*, Chap. 36). The skin problems that result are due to the release of toxins on the skin surface that irritate the skin. Some conditions predispose a person to can-

didal infections, such as diabetes mellitus, antibiotic therapy, pregnancy, use of birth control pills, poor nutrition, and immunosuppressed diseases.

C. albicans thrives in warm, moist intertriginous areas of the body. The rash is red with well-defined borders. Patches erode the epidermis, and there is scaling (Fig. 54-7). Severe forms of infection may involve pustules or vesiculopustules. A differential diagnostic feature of candidal in comparison with tinea infection is the presence of satellite lesions. These satellite lesions are maculopapular and are found outside the clearly demarcated borders of the candidal infection. The appearance of candidal infections varies according to the site; Table 54-6 summarizes site characteristics.

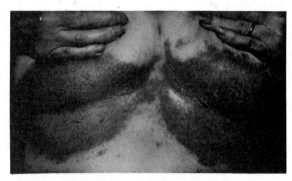

Figure 54-7 *Submammary candidiasis. Note the satellite lesions beyond the border of the eruption. (From Demis DJ (ed): Clinical Dermatology. Philadelphia, Harper & Row, 1985)*

Table 54-6   Candidal Infections: Location and Appearance of Lesions

Location	Appearance
Breasts, groin, axillae, anus, umbilicus, toe or fingerwebs	Red lesions with well-defined borders and presence of satellite lesions; lesions may be dry or moist
Vagina	Red, oozing lesions with sharply defined borders and inflamed vagina; cervix may be covered with moist, white plaque; cheesy, foul-smelling discharge; presence of pruritus and burning
Glans penis (balanitis)	Red lesions with sharply defined borders; penis may be covered with white plaque; presence of pruritus and burning
Mouth (thrush)	Creamy white flakes on a red, inflamed mucous membrane; papillae on tongue may be enlarged
Nails	Red, painful swelling around nail bed; common in people who often have their hands in water

Treatment measures vary according to the location. Prevention measures, such as wearing rubber gloves, are encouraged for people with infections of the hands. Intertriginous areas are often separated with clean cotton cloth. Nystatin (Mycostatin), an antibiotic available in tablets, powder, or vaginal suppositories, is effective in control of infection.

Bacterial infections

Bacteria are considered normal flora of the skin. Most bacteria are not pathogenic; however, when pathogenic bacteria invade the skin, superficial or systemic infections may develop. Bacterial infections are classified as primary, or superficial, and secondary, or deep. Impetigo is an example of a primary bacterial infection and infected ulcers of a secondary bacterial infection.

Bacterial infections are usually cultured for diagnosis. In addition to antibiotic therapy, the treatment of bacterial infections often includes hygiene education, general isolation procedures, and diet control.

Impetigo. Impetigo is a common superficial bacterial infection caused by staphylococci or beta-hemolytic streptococci. It is most common among young infants and children, although older children and adults occasionally contract the disease. It is highly communicable in the younger population.

Initially, impetigo appears as a small vesicle or pustule, or a large bulla. The primary lesion ruptures, leaving a denuded area that discharges a honey-colored serous liquid; the liquid hardens on the skin surface and deposits a honey-colored crust with a stuck-on

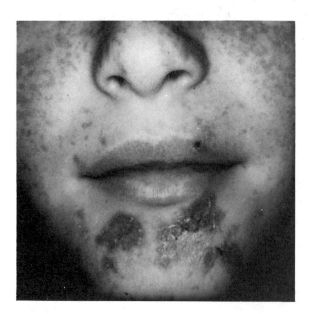

Figure 54-8 *The crusted lesions of impetigo. (From Demis DJ (ed): Clinical Dermatology. Philadelphia, Harper & Row, 1985)*

appearance (Fig. 54-8). New vesicles erupt within hours. Pruritus often accompanies the disease, and the skin excoriations that result from scratching multiply the infection sites. Lesions are most often found on the face, but they can occur anywhere on the body. Untreated, impetigo can last for weeks and may continue to spread and become a deeper bacterial infection requiring emergency medical attention. A complicaton of unreated impetigo is chronic glomerulonephritis.

Treatment measures vary among physicians. Some physicians treat the lesions locally: crusts are removed with soaks, infected areas are washed with bacteriostatic soaps, and topical antibiotics are applied. Other physicians believe that impetigo should be treated systemically with antibiotics to prevent glomerulonephritis.

Ecthyma. Ecthyma is an ulcerative form of impetigo, usually secondary to minor trauma. It frequently occurs on the buttocks and thighs of children. The lesions are similar to those of impetigo. A vesicle or pustule ruptures, leaving a skin erosion or ulcer that weeps and dries to a crusted patch, often resulting in scar formation. With extensive ecthyma, there is a low-grade fever and extension of the infection to other organs. The treatment is the same as for impetigo. When other organs are involved, oral or intramuscular penicillin is indicated.

Viral infections

Viruses resemble live cells in that they contain RNA and DNA and have cell walls. Viruses, however, rely completely on live cells for reproduction. DNA-containing viruses are more frequently seen in skin lesion disorders. Viruses invade the keratinocyte, begin to reproduce, and cause cellular proliferation or cellular death. The rapid increase in viral skin diseases has been attributed to the use of birth control medication and corticosteroid drugs, which have immunosuppressive qualities, and the use of antibiotics, which alter the bacterial flora of the skin.[13] As the number of bacterial infections has decreased, there has been a proportional rise in viral skin diseases.

Verrucae. Verrucae, or warts, are common benign papillomas caused by DNA-containing papovaviruses. Although warts vary in appearance depending on their location, the histology of all lesions is similar (Table 54-7). The wart is not a mass of uniform tumor cells but is similar to other skin diseases in that it is an exaggeration of the normal skin composition. There is an irregular thickening of the stratum spinosum and greatly increased thickening of the stratum corneum. The human papilloma viruses (HPVs), the subgroup of the papovaviruses that cause human warts, are not found in animals and invade only the skin and mucous membrane of humans.

Table 54-7   Types and Characteristics of Verrucae (Warts)

Type	Location	Appearance
Verruca vulgaris (common warts)	Anywhere on the skin, usually on the hands	Ragged dome-shape with above-the-skin-surface growth
Verruca filiformis	Eyelids, face, neck	Long fingerlike projections
Verruca plana (flat wart)	Forehead, dorsum of hand	Small flat tumors, may be barely visible
Verruca plantaris (plantar wart)	Sole of foot	Flat to slightly raised growth extending deep into skin; painful; bleeding occurs with superficial trimming; coalesced plantar warts are referred to as mosaic warts
Condyloma acuminata	Mucous membrane of the penis, female genitalia, perianal areas, and rectum	Large moist projections with rough surfaces; usually pink or purple in color

Warts resolve spontaneously when immunity to the virus develops. The immune response may be delayed for years; after 5 years, 95% of warts left untreated will have disappeared. In earlier years, treatment measures were directed at eradicating all wart tissue, primarily by excision. Since this frequently left scars, current treatment is directed at irritation of the wart with liquid nitrogen or acid chemicals. Cryotherapy and salicylic acid paint or plasters have also been effective.

Herpes simplex (cold sore, fever blister).   Herpes simplex virus (HSV) infections of the skin and mucous membrane are common (Fig. 54-9). Two types of herpesvirus infect humans, type I and type II. Most of the HSV I infections occur above the waist. HSV I may result when external infection is spread to other parts of the body through the occupational hazards that exist in professions such as dentistry and medicine, and some athletics. Type II is responsible for most infections in the genital region (Chap. 36).

Herpesvirus lesions usually begin with a burning or tingling sensation. Vesicles and erythema follow and progress to pustules, ulcers, and crusts before healing. The lesion is most common on the lips, face, and mouth. Pain is common, and healing takes place within 10 to 14 days. Following an initial infection, the herpesvirus persists in the trigeminal and other ganglia in the latent state. Recurrent lesions are common in a small percentage of people; precipitating factors may be stress, sunlight exposure, menses, or injury.

There is no cure for herpes simplex; most treatment measures are palliative. Lidocaine (Xylocaine) or diphenhydramine (Benadryl) application and aspirin help relieve pain. Cold compresses help in the acute stages. Severe forms have been treated with idoxuridine (IDI, Stoxil), which prevents certain aspects of DNA synthesis and thereby inhibits viral reproduction without causing cell injury.

Herpes zoster.   Herpes zoster (shingles) is an acute localized inflammatory disease of a dermatomal segment of the skin. It is caused by the same herpesvirus that causes chickenpox, varicella-zoster. It is believed to be the

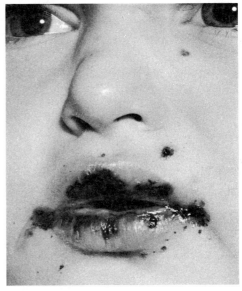

Figure 54-9 *Primary herpes simplex in a two-year-old child. (From Sauer GC: Manual of Skin Diseases, 4th ed. Philadelphia, JB Lippincott, 1980)*

result of reactivation of a latent varicella-zoster virus that has been present in the sensory dorsal ganglia since childhood infection. During an attack of shingles, the reactivated virus travels from the ganglia to the skin of the corresponding dermatome.

The clinical picture of herpes zoster is the eruption of vesicles with erythematous bases that are restricted to skin areas supplied by sensory neurons of a single or associated group of dorsal root ganglia. Eruptions are generally unilateral in the thoracic region, trunk, and face. In immunosuppressed persons, the lesions may extend beyond the dermatome. New crops of vesicles erupt for 3 to 5 days along the nerve pathway. The lesions are deeper and more confluent that those of chickenpox. The vesicles dry, form crusts, and eventually fall off. The lesions usually clear in 2 to 3 weeks. Severe pain and paresthesia are common. In the elderly, herpes zoster is a particularly serious condition that may be long-lasting and eventually lead to death. Pain reports from elderly individuals indicate an increased severity and lengthy episodes of up to 1 year. Postherpetic neuralgia is the most important complication occurring in people over the age of 50. Eye involvement can result in permanent blindness and occurs in 50% of the cases involving the ophthalmic division of the trigeminal nerve (Fig. 54-10).

Treatment is primarily palliative except when complications occur. Topical agents used are Burow's compresses or aqueous alcohol shake lotions. Pain medication is indicated in severe cases. Systemic corticosteroids

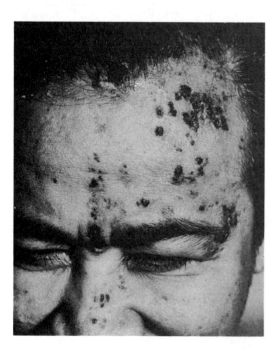

Figure 54-10 *Herpes zoster involving the ophthalmic branch of the trigeminal nerve. (From Sauer GC: Manual of Skin Disease, 5th ed. Philadelphia, JB Lippincott, 1985)*

have been effective in healthy patients over 50 years old with severe pain. High doses of interferon, an antiviral glycoprotein, have been effective in people with cancer when the lesions are limited to the dermatome.

Inflammatory Skin Diseases

The inflammatory skin diseases listed here are generally of unknown cause or etiology. They are usually localized to the skin and are rarely associated with a specific internal disease. They produce marked variations in normal skin, usually papulosquamous in nature. Inflammation and erythema are common. These disorders, which include acne, lichen planus, psoriasis, and pityriasis rosea, are among the most common skin disorders.

Acne

There are several forms of acne: acne vulgaris, acne conglobata, and acne rosacea. Acne vulgaris is the most common form among adolescents and young adults; acne conglobata develops later in life, and acne rosacea occurs in older adults.

Acne vulgaris. Acne vulgaris develops in about 80% to 90% of all people in adolescence and young adulthood and accounts for 25% of all dermatologic visits. In women, acne may persist up to 30 years of age; however, it is more common in men. The cause of acne vulgaris is still unknown, but it is probably multifactorial. Several contributing factors have been determined: (1) the sebaceous follicles, which are influenced by androgens, open onto the skin surface in a widened pore; (2) there is a greater production of keratinized cells in the follicular canal; (3) there is greater production of sebum in relation to the severity of the disease; (4) there may be a decreased amount of linoleic acid; and (5) the primary follicular canal organism is *Propionbacterium acnes*. The *P. acnes* organism seems to be involved in the inflammatory process and lipolysis, and it does not respond well to antibiotic therapy.[14]

Acne lesions form primarily on the face and neck and, to a lesser extent, on the back, chest, and shoulders (Fig. 54-11). Under normal conditions, sebaceous glands do not excrete onto the skin surface, and acne lesions are the result of pilosebaceous gland plugging. Acne lesions consist of comedones (whiteheads and blackheads), papules, pustules, and in severe cases, cysts. Noninflammatory acne consists primarily of comedones, whereas inflammatory acne consists of erythematous-based pustules and cysts. Blackheads are plugs of material that accumulate in sebaceous glands that open to the skin surface. The color in blackheads results from melanin that has moved into the sebaceous glands from adjoining epidermal cells. Whiteheads are pale, slightly elevated papules with no visible orifice. The inflammatory lesions are believed to develop from the escape of sebum into the dermis. Sebum is made up of fatty acids; these fatty acids may also play a role in skin irritation.

Preventive measures as a child nears puberty cannot be overstated. These include frequent washing of the involved areas, avoiding touching the face with the hands, shampooing hair and scalp regularly, keeping hair away from the face, avoiding the use of creams and moisturizers, and using water-based, rather than oil-based, makeup. Exposure to sunlight is helpful. Squeezing, rubbing, or picking of comedones should be avoided. A balanced diet is recommended, and stressful or fatigue-producing activities should be minimized.

Preventive measures are also those used in the treatment of acne. Mild forms of acne respond well to stringent hygiene measures in addition to the topical applications of acne creams, ointments, or lotions. Numerous commercial products are available that contain peeling, drying, or antibiotic agents. Products with resorcinol, salicylic acid, or sulfur bases are helpful in drying and peeling the skin. Oil-based preparations should be avoided, because they contribute to the problem.

Treatment of severe acne is based on four objectives supported by current knowledge of the disease. The first treatment objective is to correct the defect in keratinization. Many acne creams and lotions contain keratolytic agents such as sulfur, salicylic acid, and resorcinol that act as chemically abrasive agents to loosen comedones and exert a peeling effect on the skin. Tretinoin (Retin-A), an acid derivative of vitamin A, is a stronger keratolytic agent, but it is irritating. Because tretinoin is applied topically, it remains chiefly on the epidermis with minimal absorption into the circulation. Surgical aspiration of comedone contents removes bacteria as well as excess keratinized material. The second objective is to lessen sebaceous gland activity. Oral estrogens (oral contraceptives) help some women with acne. Isotretinoin (Accutane), an orally administered synthetic retinoid or acid form of vitamin A, reduces sebum secretion and has proven useful in the treatment of cystic acne. Although acne remissions are extended with this drug, the drug has many side-effects and must be used with extreme caution. The third objective is to reduce the *P. acnes* population. Benzoyl peroxide, a topical antimicrobial agent, has been used successfully. Oral tetracycline has also been effective but requires a sufficient treatment period to establish effective blood levels. The fourth objective is to produce the anti-inflammatory effect. Intralesion injection of adrenocorticosteroids has proved effective in nodulocystic acne.

Acne conglobata. Acne conglobata occurs later in life and is a chronic form of acne. Comedones, papules,

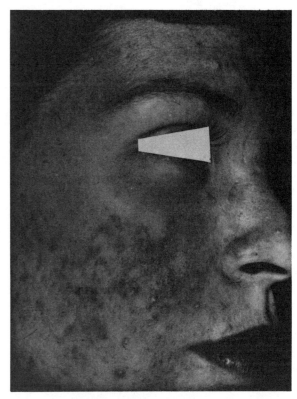

Figure 54-11 *Acne vulgaris. (From Demis DJ (ed): Clinical Dermatology. Philadelphia, Harper & Row, 1985)*

pustules, nodules, abscesses, cysts, and scars occur on the back, buttocks, and chest, and to a lesser extent on the abdomen, shoulders, neck, face, upper arms, and thighs. The comedones have multiple openings and their discharge is odoriferous, serous, and purulent or mucoid. Healing leaves deep keloidal lesions. Afflicted persons have anemia and increased white blood cell counts, sedimentation rates, and neutrophil counts. The treatment is difficult and stringent. It often includes debridement, systemic corticosteroid therapy, oral retinoids, and systemic antibiotics.

Acne rosacea. Acne rosacea is a chronic acne that occurs in middle-aged and older adults. The characteristic lesion is an erythema or telangiectasia with or without acneiform components (comedones, pustules, nodules). The cause is unknown, and the onset is insidious. It begins with redness over the nose and cheeks and may extend to the chin and forehead. After years of affliction, acne rosacea may develop into an irregular, bullous hyperplasia (thickening) of the nose, known as *rhinophyma*. The sebaceous follicles and openings enlarge, while the skin color changes to a purple-red. Treatment measures are similar to those for acne vulgaris; there is no specific treatment. Patients are told to avoid vascular-stimulating agents such as heat, cold, sunlight, hot liquids, highly seasoned foods, and alcohol. Rhinophyma can be treated surgically.

Lichen planus

Lichen planus is a relatively common, chronic, pruritic disease involving inflammation and papular eruption of the skin and mucous membranes. Idiopathic lichen planus is of unknown etiology; but, like other diseases, it can be stimulated by a variety of drugs and chemicals in susceptible persons. The characteristic lesion is a shiny white-topped purple polygonal papule. Lesions appear on the wrist, ankles, and trunk (Fig. 54-12). Mucous membrane lesions are white and lacy and may become bullous. Pruritus is severe, and new lesions develop as a result of scratching. The nails are affected in approximately 10% of the people with lichen planus.

In the majority of people, lichen planus is a self-limiting disease. Treatment measures include discontinuing all medications followed by treatment with topical corticosteroids and occlusive dressings. Systemic corticosteroids may be indicated in severe cases. Antipruritic agents are helpful in reducing itch.

Psoriasis

Psoriasis is a common, chronic papulosquamous disease characterized by various-sized white scaling patches. Lesions occur most frequently on the elbows, knees, and scalp (Fig. 54-13). The primary lesions are papules that vary in shape. The papules form into plaques with thick and silvery scales. Plaques bleed from minute points when removed. Secondary lesions are uncommon, but there can be excoriation, thickening, or oozing. In the black person, plaques may appear purple.

The etiology of psoriasis is unknown. His-tiologically, the migration time of the keratinocyte from the basal cell layer to the stratum corneum decreases from the normal 14 days to approximately 4 to 7 days. This process is called hyperkeratosis. Thinning of the suprapapillary plate and clubbing of the dermal papillae occurs. Capillary beds show permanent damage even when the disease is in remission or has resolved.

The disease is classified as a chronic ailment, yet cases have been known to clear and not recur. There is often a background of psoriasis in a family, indicating a hereditary factor. There also seems to be some association between psoriasis and arthritis, as 5% of persons with arthritis have psoriasis and 5% of psoriasis victims have arthritis. The exact nature of the relationship is unknown. The fingers of persons with psoriasis demonstrate an erosive, destructive process. The nails are often involved.

Topical, systemic, and intralesionally applied corticosteroids are used in the treatment of psoriasis. Topical corticosteroids are most effective if they are potent and used under occlusive dressings. Severe cases or acute exacerbations of the disease may warrant the use of systemic corticosteroid therapy. Intralesional injections of the corticosteroid drug triamcinolone are effective in resistant lesions. Coal tar preparations have been used for years and are highly effective. The Goeckerman regimen consists of combining the therapeutic effects of coal tar and ultraviolet light.

Other treatment modalities include the use of the drug methotrexate and photochemotherapy using a psoralen drug plus ultraviolet-A (UVA) rays in the 320-nm to 400-nm wavelength range (PUVA). Methotrexate is a antimetabolite that inhibits DNA synthesis and thus prevents cells from being biochemically able to undergo cell mitosis. Cell reproduction of the psoriasis lesion is slowed, giving the skin a more normal appearance. This is a remission state and not a cure. Methotrexate has been effective in many cases, but the drug has many side-effects including nausea, malaise, leukopenia, thrombocytopenia, and liver function abnormalities. Psoralens are drugs that must be photoactivated by long-length UVA rays to exert their action. Methoxsalen (8-MOP), the psoralen used in the treatment of psoriasis, is given orally prior to UVA exposure. Activated by UVA, methoxsalen inhibits DNA synthesis and cell mitosis, thereby decreasing the hyperkeratosis that occurs with psoriasis. Even though there has been a high success rate with PUVA treatment, it must be used cautiously, as accelerated aging of exposed skin, skin cancer, development of cataracts, and alterations in immune function may occur. In addition, the skin remains sensitive to sunlight until the methoxsalen is excreted, so that persons receiving PUVA treatment must be cautioned to avoid sun exposure for 8 hours following treatment.

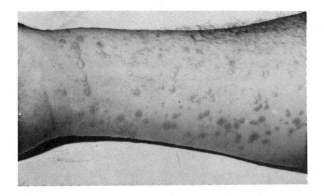

Figure 54-12 *Lichen planus. Note the discrete papules on the forearm. On the wrist, the papules have a linear configuration. (From Demis DJ (ed): Clinical Dermatology. Philadelphia, Harper & Row, 1985)*

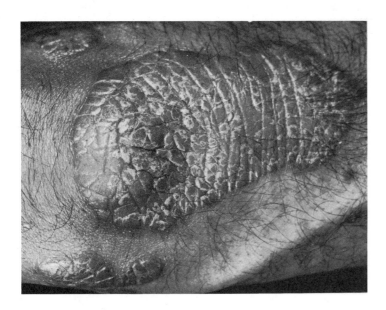

Figure 54-13 *Psoriasis on the elbow. (From Sauer GC: Manual of Skin Diseases, 5th ed. Philadelphia, JB Lippincott, 1985)*

Pityriasis rosea

Pityriasis rosea is a skin rash of unknown origin that primarily affects young adults. The incidence is highest in spring and fall. The belief is that it could be viral, but to date no virus has been isolated. The characteristic lesions is a macule or papule with surrounding erythema. The lesion spreads with central clearing much like tinea corporis. This initial lesion is a solitary lesion called the herald patch and is usually on the trunk or neck. As the lesion enlarges and begins to fade away (2–10 days), successive crops of lesions appear on the trunk and neck. The extremities, face, and scalp may be involved, and mild to severe pruritus may occur. The disease is self-limiting and usually disappears within 6 weeks to 8 weeks. Treatment measures are palliative and include topical steroids, antihistamines, and colloid baths. Systemic corticosteroids may be indicated in severe cases.

Allergic Skin Responses

Allergic skin responses involve the body's immune system and are caused by hypersensitivity reactions (Chap. 9 and 10). They include contact dermatitis, atopic and nummular eczema, and drug reactions.

Contact dermatitis

Contact dermatitis is a common inflammation of the skin. There are two types of contact dermatitis—irritant and allergic. Irritant contact dermatitis occurs in people who are in contact with a sufficient amount of the irritant to cause a reaction (Fig. 54-14). It can occur from mechanical means such as rubbing (wool, fiberglass), chemical irritants (those found in common household cleaning products), or environmental irritants (plants, urine). Allergic contact dermatitis is the cell-mediated allergy response brought about by sensitization of an allergen. It is a type IV sensitivity (Chap. 10). This type is dependent on hapten migration into the skin to produce an immune reaction. Many contact allergens are capable of producing the inflammatory skin response (Table 54-8). The crude forms of many naturally occurring substances are rarely allergenic; additives, builders, dyes, and perfumes account for the major sources of known allergens. Additional examples are poison ivy, chemicals, and metal sources such as jewelry.

The initial contact dermatitis lesion ranges from a mild erythema with edema to vesicles or large bullae. Secondary lesions from bacterial infection may occur. Lesions can occur almost anywhere on the body. The

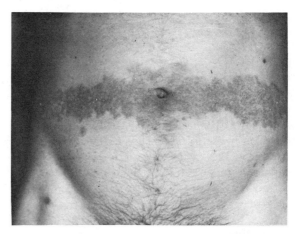

Figure 54-14 *Contact dermatitis resulting from a component of rubber. (From Demis DJ (ed): Clinical Dermatology. Philadelphia, Harper & Row, 1985)*

Table 54-8 Sources of Contact Dermatitis Allergens

Sources	Possible Allergens
Clothing	Raw material such as wool, polyester, cotton; dyes and sizers in new fabrics and clothing; detergents used to wash clothing
Cosmetics	Dyes, perfumes, oils (e.g., lanolin, coconut oil, olive oil, palm oil)
Cleaning products (soaps, detergents)	Fats, alkali, perfumes, dyes, formaldehyde, hydrochloric acid, sodium carbonate, ammonium hydroxide, and germicidal agents
Occupational exposure	Metals, metal salts, and alloys (nickel); resin, natural and synthetic; tung oil, linseed oil, turpentine; usually the allergens are from the processing of rubber rather than crude rubber (acids, alkalies, solvents, soaps, dust, heat) and are more common from rubber products (gloves, footwear, condoms)
Plants and woods	Ragweed; lichens; poison ivy, oak, and sumac; pine (more from resin and turpentine); caterpillars; and growth on trees and plants
Soap ingredients	
Fats	Coconut oil, olive oil, palm oil, rosin, and fish or whale oil
Alkali	Sodium hydroxide, potassium hydroxide, sodium carbonate, trisodium phosphate, sodium tripolyphosphate, pyrophosphate, sodium silicate
Perfumes	Seed oil, oil of bergamot, bitter almond oil, eucalyptus oil, geranium oil, lavender oil, peppermint oil, rosemary oil, musk
Coloring agents	D&C yellow No. 11, esosin, rhodamine, fuchsin, ultramarine green

typical poison ivy lesion consists of vesicles or bullae in a linear pattern. The vesicles and bullae break and weep, leaving an excoriated area.

Treatment measures are aimed at removing the source of the irritant. In some cases, this may mean that the person needs to modify his or her behavior in the home or workplace to avoid the irritant. The actual treatment regimen differs according to the type of irritant and the severity of the reaction. Minor cases are treated by washing the affected areas to remove further sources of irritation; antipruritic creams and lotions are applied, and exposed areas are bandaged. More extreme cases are treated with wet dressings, systemic corticosteroids, and oral antihistamines.

Eczema

There are two forms of eczema, atopic and nummular. Atopic eczema (also called atopic dermatitis) is a common skin disorder that occurs in two clinical forms, infantile and adult. It is associated with a type I hypersensitivity reaction (Chap. 10). There is usually a family history of asthma, hay fever, or atopic dermatitis. The infantile form is characterized by vesicle formation, oozing, and crusting with excoriations. It usually begins in the cheeks and may progress to involve the scalp, arms, trunk, and legs (Fig. 54-15). The infantile form usually becomes milder and often disappears after the age of 3 or 4 years. Adolescents and adults generally have dry, leathery, and hyperpigmented or hypopigmented lesions located in the antecubital and popliteal areas that may spread to the neck, hands, feet, or eyelids, and behind the ears. Itching may be severe with both forms, and secondary infections are common.

The treatment measures are designed around the chronic nature of the disease. Exposure to environmental irritants and foods that cause exacerbation of the symptoms is avoided. Wool and lanolin (wool fat) often aggravate the condition. Dryness of the skin often causes the condition to become worse. For this reason, bathing and the use of soap and water should be reduced. Avoidance of temperature changes and stress helps to minimize abnormal and cutaneous vascular and sweat responses.

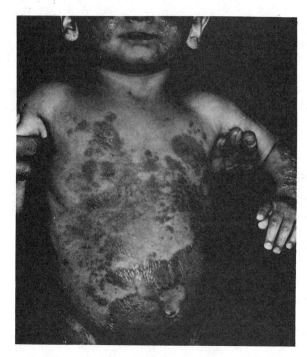

Figure 54-15 *Severe infantile atopic dermatitis. (From Demis DJ (ed): Clinical Dermatology. Philadelphia, Harper & Row, 1985)*

Acute weeping lesions are treated with soothing lotions, soaps, baths, or wet dressings. Subacute or subsiding lesions may be treated with lotions containing mild antipruritic agents. Chronic dry lesions are treated with ointments and creams containing lubricating, keratolytic, and antipruritic agents as indicated. Topical or systemic corticosteroid therapy may be indicated for severe cases.

The exact etiology of nummular eczema is unknown. There is usually a history of asthma, hay fever, or atopic dermatitis. Lesions consist of coin-shaped (nummular) papulovesicular patches mainly involving the arms and legs. The disease is chronic and most often occurs in elderly men. Lichenification and secondary bacterial infections are common. Ingestion of iodides and bromides usually aggravates the condition. The treatment is pallative. Frequent bathing and foods rich in iodides and bromides should be avoided. Topical corticosteroids and antibiotics are prescribed as necessary.

Drug-induced skin eruptions

Without exception, any drug can cause a localized or generalized skin eruption. Generally, topical drugs are responsible for a localized contact dermatitis type of rash, whereas systemic drugs cause generalized skin lesions. Table 54-9 describes the characteristics of selected drug-induced skin eruptions.

The diagnosis of a drug sensitivity depends almost entirely on accurate reporting from the patient because the lesions from drug sensitization differ greatly. Drug reactions mimic almost all other skin lesions described in this chapter. The treatment is aimed at eliminating the offending drug. Mild skin eruptions are treated symptomatically, whereas severe systemic drug eruptions often require systemic corticosteroid therapy and antihistamines.

Insect Bites, Vectors, Ticks, and Parasites

The skin is susceptible to a variety of disorders as a result of an invasion or infestation by bugs, ticks, or parasites. The rash, or sometimes singular lesion, differs depending on the causative agent.

Scabies

Scabies is caused by a mite (*Sarcoptes scabiei*) that burrows into the epidermis. After a female mite is impregnated, she burrows into the skin and lays two to three eggs each day for 4 or 5 weeks. Three to 5 days later, the eggs hatch and the larvae migrate to the skin surface. At this point, they burrow into the skin only for food or for protection. The larvae molt and become nymphs;

they molt once more to become adults. Once they are impregnated, the cycle is repeated.

The characteristic lesion is a small burrow, approximately 2mm long, that may be red to red-brown in color. Small vesicles may cover the burrows. The most common areas affected are the interdigital webs of the fingers; the flexor surface of the wrist; the inner surface of the elbows, axillae, female nipples, penis, belt line, and gluteal creases (Fig. 54-16). Pruritus is common and may

Table 54-9 Types of Rashes Associated with Drug-Induced Skin Eruptions

Drugs	Type of Rash
Barbiturates, arsenic, sulfonamides, quinine	Resembles measles
Barbiturates, arsenic, codeine, morphine	Resembles scarlet fever
Bismuth, gold, barbiturates	Resembles pityriasis rosea
Quinine, procaine, antihistamines	Eczematous
Isoniazid, para-aminosalicylic acid combinations	Resembles nummular eczema
Penicillin, salicylates, opium	Urticaria
Bromides, iodides, testosterone, ACTH	Pustular (acne)
Sulfonamides, penicillin, phenylbutazone	Vesicular, bullous
Quinacrine, arsenic, gold	Lichen planus
Contraceptive drugs, quinacrine	Pigment changes
Arsenic, mercury	Keratosis and epitheliomas

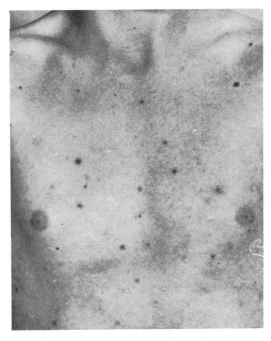

Figure 54-16 *Scabies on the chest (K.C.G.H.). (From Sauer GC: Manual of Skin Diseases, 5th ed. Philadelphia, JB Lippincott, 1985)*

be the result of the burrows, the fecal material of the mite, or both. Excoriations may develop from scratching, and secondary bacterial infections and severe skin lesions may occur if the condition is untreated.

Scabies affects all people in all socioeconomic classes. Usually more prevalent in times of war and famine, it reached pandemic proportions in the 1970s, perhaps as a result of poverty, sexual promiscuity, and worldwide travel.

Diagnosis is done by skin scrapings. Mineral oil is applied to the skin and a scraping is obtained. A positive diagnosis relies on the presence of the mite or its feces. The treatment is simple and curative. Lindane lotion or cream (Kwell) is applied over the entire skin surface for 12 hours. Repeat applications may be recommended in certain cases, but one treatment is usually sufficient. Controversy exists over bathing before the treatment. Some physicians no longer recommend bathing before the treatment, perhaps to enhance full drug effectiveness.[15] Clothes and towels are disinfected with hot water and detergent. Treatment of outer clothing and furniture is unnecessary because the mite cannot live away from the body for more than a few hours. If symptoms persist following treatment, the patient should be advised not to retreat without the physician's consultation. A red-brown nodule, thought to be an allergic response from the mite parts left on the skin, may form after treatment.

Pediculosis

Pediculosis is the term for infestation with lice (genus *Pediculus*). Lice are gray, gray-brown, or red-brown oval and wingless insects that live off the blood supply of humans and animals. Lice are host specific; lice that live on animals do not transfer to humans, and vice versa. Lice are also host dependent; they cannot live apart from the host beyond a few hours. Similar to that of scabies, the incidence of pediculosis increased in the 1970s to pandemic levels and was probably due to poverty, sexual promiscuity, and worldwide travel.

Three types of lice affect humans: *Pediculus humanis corporis* (body lice), *Pediculus pubis* (pubic lice), and *Pediculus humanis capitis* (head lice). Although these three types differ biologically, they have similar life cycles. The life cycle of a louse consists of an unhatched egg or "nit," three molt stages, adult reproductive stage, and death. Before adulthood, lice live off the host and are incapable of reproduction. After fertilization, the egg is laid by the female louse along a hair shaft. These nits appear pearl gray to brown. Depending on the site, a female louse can lay anywhere between 150 and 300 nits in her life. The life span of a feeding louse is 30 to 50 days. Lice are equipped with stylets that pierce the skin. Their saliva contains an anticoagulant that prevents host blood from clotting while the louse is feeding. A louse takes up to 1 mg of blood during a feeding.

Pediculosis corporis.   Pediculosis corporis is infestation with *Pediculus humanis corporis*, or body lice, which are chiefly transferred through contact with infested clothing and bedding. The lice live in the clothes fibers, coming out only to feed. Unlike the pubic louse and the head louse, the body louse can survive 10 days to 14 days without the host. The typical lesion is a macule at the site of the bite. Papules and wheals may develop. The infestation is pruritic and evokes scratching that brings about a characteristic linear excoriation. Eczematous patches are frequently found. Secondary lesions may become scaly and hyperpigmented and leave scars. Areas typically affected are the shoulders, trunk, and buttocks. The presence of nits in the seams of clothes confirms a diagnosis of body lice. Treatment measures consist of eradicating the louse and nits both on the body and clothing. Washing clothes in hot water and steam pressing or dry cleaning them is recommended. Special attention is given to the seams. Merely storing clothing in plastic bags for 2 weeks will rid clothes of lice. Many physicians prefer not to treat the body unless nits are in evidence on hair shafts. If treatment is indicated, lindane shampoo or topical preparations containing gamma benzene hexachloride, pyrethrym, or malathion are recommended.

Pediculosis pubis.   Pediculosis pubis (the infestation known as crabs, or pubic lice) is a nuisance disease that is uncomfortable and embarrassing. The disease is spread by intimate contact with someone harboring *Phithirus pubis*. Lice and nits are located in the pubic area of males and females. Occasionally they may be found in secondary sex sites such as the beard in males or the axilla in males and females. Symptoms include intense itching and irritation of the skin. Diagnosis is made on the basis of symptoms and microscopic examination. The treatment is the same as that used for head lice.

Pediculosis capitis.   Pediculosis capitis, or infestation with head lice, primarily affects white-skinned people; it is relatively unknown in darker-skinned persons. In addition, the incidence is higher in female children, although hair length has not been indicated as a contributing factor. Infestations of head lice are usually confined to the nape of the neck and behind the ears. Less frequently, head lice are found on the beard, pubic areas, eyebrows, and body hairs.

Head lice are primarily transmitted by human-to-human contact. A positive diagnosis depends on the presence of firmly attached nits on hair shafts. Crawling adults are rarely seen. Pruritus and scratching of the head are the primary indicators that head lice may be present. The scalp may appear red and excoriated from scratching. In severe cases, the hair becomes matted together in a crusty foul-smelling "cap." An occasional morbilliform rash, which may be misdiagnosed as rubella, may occur with lymphadenopathy.

Head lice is treated with gamma benzene hexachloride preparations (Kwell). The medicated shampoo is applied to dry hair in a sufficient quantity to wet the hair and skin. After the hair and head are massaged, small amounts of water are added to produce a lather. The head is scrubbed for 4 minutes, rinsed, and dried. The treatment may be repeated after 1 week to eliminate the hatching nits. Dead nits may be removed with a fine-toothed comb.

Bedbugs

The common bedbug, *Cimex lectularius*, is a reddish brown insect, 3 mm to 6 mm long, that turns purple after feeding. Like lice, bedbugs feed on human blood. Unlike lice, bedbugs can alternate hosts from human to animal, and they live up to and sometimes beyond 1 year. When not feeding, bedbugs stay hidden in the cracks and crevices of furniture, mattresses, wallpaper, picture frames, baseboards, flooring, door locks, or any darkened area. They are nocturnal feeders, and when squashed, they emit a foul odor.

The *Cimex* bite is painless. The characteristic lesion is a pruritic oval or oblong wheal with a small hemorrhagic punctum at the center. Bullous lesions are not uncommon. Usually, lesions are multiple and arranged in rows or clusters on the face, neck, hands, and arms. No area is exempt. The wheal is probably a type I sensitivity reaction to the anticoagulant saliva of the bedbug. Secondary excoriation and bacterial infections may occur.

Diagnosis is dependent on the time of the day when the lesions appear. Because of the painless bite, it is not uncommon for the victim to awake to one or several pruritic papules. Topical antipruritics are used in the treatment. The source of the bedbug must be eliminated or recurrence is inevitable. Professional extermination is advised because of the many hiding places of *Cimex*. Bedbugs have been known to feed from animal populatons when forced from their living quarters. Upon rehabilitation in the same quarters, the bedbug will once again find the unsuspecting human host.

Ticks

Ticks are insects that live in woods and underbrush. They attach themselves to human and animal hosts and burrow into the epidermis where they feed on blood. The tick bite itself is not problematic; it is the infectious bacteria or viruses that they carry to human hosts. There are many tick-borne illnesses including Central European encephalitis, Q fever, babesiasis, and relapsing fever. The disease most common to the United States is Rocky Mountain spotted fever (RMSF), which is caused by a tick that carries *Rickettsia rickettsii*. RMSF used to be localized to the Rocky Mountain area, but by 1982 most states had reported a case of RMSF.

The initial tick bite appears as a papule or macule with or without a central punctate. The tick burrows in and enlarges as it feeds. The tick must be attached to the human host for 4 hours to 6 hours before the rickettsiae are activated by the blood. Rickettsiae are found in the tick feces and body parts. The rickettsiae then enter the bloodstream and multiply in the body tissues. Within 4 days to 8 days the patient experiences fever, headache, muscle aches, nausea, and vomiting. A rash that starts on the wrist or ankle follows. The characteristic rash is a macular or maculopapular rash that spreads to the rest of the body. Other symptoms include generalized edema, conjunctivitis, petechial lesions, photophobia, lethargy, confusion, and cranial nerve deficits.

The treatment for RMSF requires hospitalizaton and antibiotic therapy. The most important measure is to prevent tick bites by using insect repellents while engaged in activities in the woods. Once a tick has attached itself, it is important to remove all the body parts to limit the possibility of infection. Ticks may be removed by slowly pulling them, dousing them with mineral oil or alcohol before removing them with a tweezers, or applying a hot match to the end of the tick. The latter method is not the most effective, as the tick may regurgitate into the open wound.

Mosquitoes

Most people are aware of the bite of the mosquito. The typical lesion is a raised wheal on an erythematous base accompanied by pruritus that occurs within 45 minutes of the bite. A second type of reaction is the delayed response. Eight to 12 hours after the bite, the lesion becomes raised, erythematous, and indurated with extensive pruritus or pain. This reaction peaks 24 hours to 72 hours after the bite. The saliva of the mosquito is believed to be the source of the skin reaction. Although severe skin reactions are possible, they are rare. Insect repellents are encouraged for prevention; local antipruritics are used for treatment.

Chiggers

Chiggers are common in the southern United States but can be found as far north as Canada. The chigger resides in grasses and bushes. The mite attaches to legs and thighs and punctures the skin to obtain food. Chigger bites are pruritic papules seen wherever the chigger encounters resistance, such as the top of socks, at the beltline, or around the neckband area. Secondary lesions are excoriations from scratching that have become infected by bacteria. The treatment is palliative, and insect repellent is encouraged for prevention.

Fleas

The source for human fleas is usually dogs and cats. Geographically, specific fleas have been identified that seem to pester newcomers rather than natives of an area. The characteristic lesion is a highly pruritic papule with a central punctum and is generally seen on covered parts of the body. The treatment measures are symptomatic; insect repellents are advised.

Photosensitivity and Sunburn

Physical and mechanical stimuli such as fire, electromagnetic radiation, and ionizing radiation can cause skin burns (Chap. 2). Many of these burns occur accidentally in the home or workplace. Ultraviolet light, or sunlight, also causes skin changes. The obvious and desired skin change is tanning; yet most forms of skin cancer are directly related to sun exposure. Besides cancerous lesions, several skin alterations such as senile lentigines have been linked to sun exposure. Exposure to the sun, as well as harsh weather, has also been linked to early wrinkling and aging of the skin. Some drugs are classified as photosensitive drugs because they produce an exaggerated response to ultraviolet light when the drug is taken in combination with sun exposure (Chart 54-1).

The skin, as an organ, is the protective shield against harmful ultraviolet sun rays. Living epidermal cells are damaged when 280-nm to 310-nm wavelengths penetrate the skin. The cells release vasoactive and injurious chemicals, resulting in vasodilation and sunburn. The melanin content of the stratum corneum protects the skin by absorbing the ultraviolet rays and the skin responds to sunlight exposure by increasing its melanin content as a means of preventing destruction of the lower skin layers.

Sunburn ranges from mild to severe. A mild sunburn consists of varying degrees of redness 2 hours to 12

Chart 54-1 Drugs That Induce Photosensitivity

Sulfonamides
Thiazide diuretics
Furosemide
Sulfonylurea hypoglycemia agents
Tetracycline (particularly demeclocycline)
Phenothiazine, antipsychotic drugs
Nalidixic acid

---

hours after exposure to the sun. Varying degrees of inflammation, vesicle eruption, weakness, chills, fever, malaise, and pain accompany more severe forms of sunburn. Scaling and peeling follow any sunlight overexposure. Black skin also burns, but the occurrence is much less frequent. Sunburned black skin may appear grayish or gray-black.

If the desired outcome of sun exposure is a good suntan, prevention is the best policy for tanning. Early morning and late afternoon sun exposure are less harmful because the ultraviolet rays are longer. Although long rays are less apt to cause severe sunburn, they, too, have been implicated in the development of skin cancers. The FDA now requires a rating on all commercial suntan preparations based on the ability to occlude the ultraviolet light. Para-aminobenzoic acid (PABA) is the most effective blocking ingredient in many of these suntan creams. Suntan creams should be used diligently and according to the individual's tendency to burn rather than tan.

Severe sunburns are treated with boric acid soaks and topical creams to limit pain and maintain skin moisture. Extensive second- and third-degree burns require hospitalization and specialized burn care techniques.

Neoplasms

A number of premalignant and malignant skin lesions can occur. Most of these are found on the skin surfaces exposed to sun and harsh weather. Nevi are common benign tumors of the skin. Cancer of the skin is the most common of all cancers. With the exception of malignant melanoma, the overall cure rate for skin cancer is higher than 90%.[16]

Nevi

Nevi, or moles, are common congenital or acquired tumors of the skin. Almost all adults have nevi, some in greater numbers than others. Nevi can be pigmented or nonpigmented, flat or elevated, and hairy or nonhairy. Pigmented nevi are derived from neural crest-derived cells (nevocellular nevi) that include modified melanocytes of various shapes. Histologically, most nevi begin as aggregates of well-defined cells located within the lower epidermal layer that lies adjacent to the dermis. These nevi are called *junctional nevi*. Eventually, nevus cells begin to grow into the dermis. *Compound nevi* contain both epidermal and dermal components. *Dermal nevi* are located within the dermis.

Generally, nevocellular nevi are tan-to-deep brown, uniformly pigmented, small papules with well-defined and rounded borders. Blue nevi have a blue-black color.

Moles are important because of their capacity for transformation to malignant melanomas. The relationship between preexisting benign nevi and malignant melanoma is unclear. Although the average person has about 20 moles, only 4 people out of 100,000 develop a malignant melanoma.[16] It is known that two types of pigmented nevus are associated with malignant transformation; these are the congenital melanocytic nevi and the large atypical or dysplastic nevi (to be discussed). Because of the possibility of malignant transformation, any mole that undergoes a change in size, thickness, or color, causes itching, or bleeds warrants immediate medical attention.

Basal cell carcinoma

Basal cell carcinoma is the most common form of skin cancer (Fig 54-17). Light-skinned people are more susceptible; blacks and Orientals are rarely affected. It is a nonmetastasizing tumor that will extend wide and deep if left untreated. These tumors are most frequently seen on the head and neck and, less commonly, on the skin surfaces unexposed to the sun.

The most common type of basal cell carcinoma is the noduloulcerative basal cell epithelioma. It begins as a small, smooth, shiny nodule that enlarges over time. Telangiectatic vessels are frequently seen beneath the surface. Over the years, a central depression forms that progresses to an ulcer surrounded by the original shiny, waxy border.

The second most frequently occurring basal cell carcinoma is the superficial form that is more commonly seen on the chest or back. It begins as a flat, nonpalpable erythematous plaque. The red scaly areas slowly enlarge with nodular borders and telangiectatic bases. This type is difficult to diagnose because it mimics other dermatologic problems.

In both cases, tumors are biopsied for diagnosis. The treatment depends on the site and extent of the lesion. Curettage with electrodesiccation, surgical excision, irradiation, and chemosurgery are effective in removing all cancerous cells. Patients should be checked at regular intervals for recurrence.

Squamous cell carcinoma

Squamous cell carcinomas are malignant tumors of the outer epidermis. The lesion begins as a rapidly growing nodule. The center of the nodule ulcerates accompanied by a raised border that is erythematous. These lesions occur on sun-exposed areas of the skin, particularly the nose, forehead, helixes of the ears, lower lip, and back of the hands (Fig. 54-18). The lesions rarely metastasize except in immunosuppressed persons or when the lesion forms on the mucous membranes.

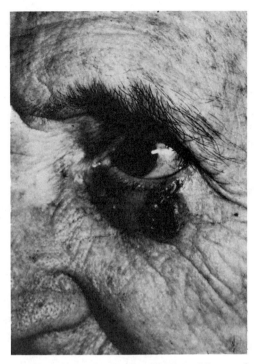

Figure 54-17 *Nodular basal cell carcinoma with central ulceration. (From Demis DJ (ed): Clinical Dermatology. Philadelphia, Harper & Row, 1985)*

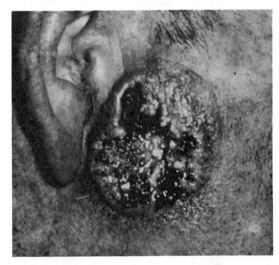

Figure 54-18 *Squamous cell carcinoma. (From Demis DJ (ed): Clinical Dermatology. Philadelphia, Harper & Row, 1985)*

Malignant melanoma

Malignant melanoma is a malignant neoplasm of the melanocytes. It is a rapidly progressing, metastatic form of cancer that accounts for 1% to 3% of all cancers.[11] Early diagnosis and knowledge of precursor lesions has led to earlier intervention and increased survival rates in people who have malignant melanoma.

Malignant melanomas differ in size and shape (Fig. 54-19). The vast majority seem to arise from preexisting benign nevi or as new molelike growths.[17] Usually they are slightly raised and black or brown. Borders are irregular and surfaces are uneven. Periodically, melanomas ulcerate and bleed; there may be surrounding erythema, inflammation, and tenderness. Dark melanomas are often mottled with red, blue, and white shades. These three colors represent three concurrent processes: melanoma growth (blue), inflammation and the body's attempt to localize and destroy the tumor (red), and scar tissue formation (white). Malignant melanomas can appear anywhere on the body; they are most frequently found on sun-exposed areas. In men, they are frequently found on the trunk, head, neck, and arms; in women, they are found on the leg, arm, trunk, head, and neck.

Three precursor lesions have been identified in the development of melanoma: lentigo maligna, congenital melanocytic nevi, and dysplastic nevi. Recognition of these precursors is important to the early diagnosis and treatment of melanoma. Lentigo maligna is a flat lesion that looks like an irregular freckle. The lesion is tan-brown to black with irregular pigmentation and borders; it spreads and may look like a stain. Lentigo malignas frequently occur in elderly patients on sun-exposed areas. Congenital melanocytic nevi are large, brown to black hyperpigmented nevi that are present at birth. Generally, they are found on the hands, shoulders, buttocks, entire arm, or trunk of the body. Some involve large areas of the body in garmentlike fashion. These nevi darken with age, and hairs that are present in the lesion become coarser. Malignant changes often occur at an early age (generally by age 10[11]). Dysplastic nevi are flat to slightly raised lesions consisting of neural crest-derived cells (nevocellular nevi) and often have a diameter greater than 1 cm. A person may have hundreds of these lesions; typically, they are in sun-exposed as well as non-sun-exposed areas of the body. They vary in shades from brown and red to flesh tones with irregular borders. There is some familial tendency to develop dysplastic nevi.

The prognosis of malignant melanoma depends on the depth of the lesion and the extent of the disease process. Stage I patients have no evidence of tumor growth in regional lymph nodes, and the disease process is limited to the localized lesion area. Survival rates for these people with surgical intervention is uncertain but is longer than either of the other two stages. Stage II melanomas have metastasized to the regional lymph nodes. Five-year to 10-year survival rates have been reported. Stage III malignant melanoma involves metastasis to distant organs in the body. The prognosis has been poor, with survival rates of up to 16 months.[18]

The best treatment is early detection. Patients should be taught to watch for changes in existing nevi or the development of new nevi. Color changes, irregular borders, bleeding, and growth of nevi should be brought to the attention of a dermatologist. Treatment measures vary depending on the severity. Deep and wide excisions with skin grafts are used. Systemic immunotherapy, chemotherapy, and radiation therapy are indicated when the disease becomes systemic.

In summary, primary disorders of the skin include infectious processes, inflammatory conditions, allergic reactions, parasitic infestations, skin reactions to sunlight, and neoplasms. Superficial fungal infections are called dermatophytoses and are commonly known as tinea, or ringworm; they include tinea corporis, tinea capitis, tinea barbae, tinea manus, tinea pedis, onychomycosis, and tinea versicolor. Impetigo, which is caused by staphylococci or beta-hemolytic streptococci, is the most common superficial bacterial infection. Viruses are responsible for verrucae (warts), herpes simplex I lesions (cold sores or fever blisters), and herpes zoster (shingles). Noninfectious inflammatory skin conditions such as acne, lichen planus, psoriasis, and pityriasis rosea are generally of unknown etiology. They are usually localized to the skin and are rarely associated with specific internal disease. Allergic skin responses involve the body's immune system and are caused by hypersensitivity reactions to allergens, environmental agents, drugs, and other substances. The skin is sensitive to a number of disorders resulting from invasion or infestation by bugs, ticks, or parasites. The rash or bite from such invasion is

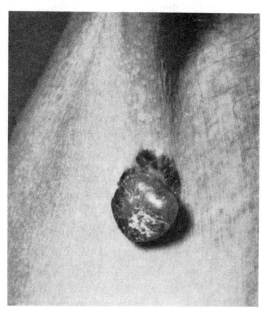

Figure 54-19 *Malignant melanoma. On posterior axillary fold* (K.C.G.H.). *(From Sauer GC: Manual of Skin Diseases, 4th ed. Philadelphia, JB Lippincott, 1980)*

usually singular and varies with the agent. Neoplasms of the skin include basal cell carcinoma, squamous cell carcinoma, and melanoma, with basal cell carcinoma being the most common form. Repeated exposure to the ultraviolet rays of the sun is the principal cause of skin cancer.

■ Black Skin

There are several skin disorders common to blacks that are not commonly found in whites. Similarly, many skin disorders that affect white-skinned peoples do not affect darker-skinned persons, such as skin cancers. Literature related specifically to black skin disorders is rare; frequently, common occurrences in black skin are mistaken for anomalies.

The number of melanosomes produced and transferred to the keratinocyte is responsible for the darker pigmentation in blacks. In other words, blacks do not have more melanocytes, but the production of pigment is increased. Skin pallor, cyanosis, and erythema are more difficult to see in black people. Also, normal variations in skin structure and skin tones make evaluation of black skin difficult (Table 54-10). Often, verbal histories must be relied on to indicate skin changes. Hypopigmentation refers to a loss of pigmentation, and hyperpigmentation refers to excessive melanin production. Often these signs accompany black skin disorders and are important to accurate diagnosis. The appearances of skin disorders

listed in Table 54-11 are common to the American black who represents a blend of African Negro, European Caucasian, and Native American.

Table 54-10 Common Normal Variations in Black Skin

Variation	Appearance
Futcher's (Voigt's) Line	Demarcation between darkly pigmented and lightly pigmented skin in upper arm; follows spinal nerve distribution; common in black and Japanese populations
Midline hypopigmentation	Line or band of hypopigmentation over the sternum, dark or faint, lessens with age; common in Latin American and black populations
Nail pigmentation	Linear dark bands down nails or diffuse nail pigmentation, brown, blue, or blue-black
Oral pigmentation	Blue to blue-gray pigmentation of oral mucosa; gingivae also affected
Palmar changes	Hyperpigmented creases, small hyperkeratotic papules and tiny pits in creases
Plantar changes	Hyperpigmented macules, can be multiple with patchy distribution, irregular borders, and variance in color

(Developed from information in: Rosen T, Martin S: Atlas of Black Dermatology. Boston, Little, Brown, 1981)

Table 54-11 Appearance of Common Disorders of Black Skin

Disorder	Appearance
Hot-comb alopecia	Well-defined patches of scalp alopecia on crown; extends down; decreased number of follicular orifices; hair loss irreversible; due to use of hot comb with petroleum, more common with Afro hairstyles
Infantile acropustulosis	Crops of vesicopustules for 7 to 10 days, followed by a 2 to 3 week remission before recurrence; pruritus; affects palms and soles of feet in children 2 to 10 months of age; resolves by 3 years of age
Keloids	Firm, smooth, shiny hairless elevated scars, sometimes hyperpigmented; often with symptomatic pruritus, tenderness, or pain; extremely common even with simple wounds on ears, neck, jaw, cheeks, upper chest, shoulders, and back
Mongolian spot	Very common; ill-defined light blue to slate gray macule in lumbosacral area; usually disappears, but may persist through adulthood
Atopic dermatitis	Follicular lesion development that progresses to a lichenification stage; hyperpigmented lichenifications are interspersed with excoriated pink patches; common in blacks
Pityriasis rosea	Lesions are salmon pink, dull, red, or dark brown; profuse fine scales, not commonly seen in white skin; postinflammatory pigmentary changes are more common in blacks
Psoriasis	Does not commonly occur in blacks; distribution is similar, but the plaques are bright red, violet, or blue-black; pigment changes may persist after treatment
Tinea versicolor	Common in blacks, increased incidence in tropical climates; hypopigmented or extremely hyperpigmented patches, gray to dark brown; occurs more often on the face in blacks than in whites
Lichen planus	Papules are deep purple from pigmentary leakage; oral lesions are uncommon; hypertrophic lesions are more common in blacks than in whites

(Developed from information in: Rosen T, Martin S: Atlas of Black Dermatology. Boston, Little, Brown, 1981)

Vitiligo

Vitiligo is a pigmentary problem of concern to darkly pigmented people of all races. It also affects whites, but not as often. The lesion is a macular depigmentaiton with definite borders on the face, axillae, neck, or extremities. The borders are smooth. The patches vary in size from small to large macules involving great skin surfaces. The large macular type is much more common. Depigmented areas, which burn in sunlight, appear white or flesh colored or sometimes grayish blue. Vitiligo appears at any age, in men and women alike, and usually occurs before the age of 21 years. It has been on the rise in India, Pakistan, and Far Eastern countries. Although the cause is unknown, inheritance and autoimmune factors have been implicated. Vitiligo also seems to be implicated as a cutaneous expression of a systemic disorder, especially thyroid disease.[19] The areas affected spread over time.

Treatment regimens for vitiligo remain experimental, Psoralen administration in conjunction with ulraviolet radiation (PUVA) has been successful in patients who have involvement of 40% or more of the skin surface. Cosmetics and sunscreens are used for camouflage.

In summary, black skin has an increased number of melanosomes. Thus, skin pallor, cyanosis, and erythema are more difficult to evaluate. Some skin disorders that are common to blacks are not common in whites, and vice versa. The manifestations of common skin disorders are also different. Vitiligo, a condition of depigmentation, is a problem of concern to darkly pigmented people of all races.

■ Study Guide

After you have studied this chapter, you should be able to meet the following objectives:

☐ List five functions of the skin.

☐ Explain the development of the keratin layer of the epidermis.

☐ Describe the function of the melanocytes.

☐ List the structures of the dermis.

☐ State the function of the dermis.

☐ Describe the innervation of the sweat glands and the arrector pili (piloerector) muscles.

☐ Compare the distribution and secretory activity of the eccrine and apocrine sweat glands.

☐ State the location and function of the sebaceous glands.

☐ Describe the following skin rashes and lesions: macule, patch, papule, plaque, nodule, tumor, wheal, vesicle, bulla, pustule, erosion, crust, ulcer, scale, fissure, lichenification, petechiae, ecchymosis.

☐ Cite two theories used to explain the physiology of pruritus.

☐ Differentiate between a strawberry hemangioma and a port-wine stain hemangioma in terms of appearance and outcome.

☐ Describe the distinguishing features of rashes associated with roseola infantum, rubeola, rubella, chickenpox, and scarlet fever.

☐ Define the term keratosis and compare the seborrheic and actinic keratoses.

☐ Relate the behavior of fungi to the production of superficial skin lesions associated with tinea or ringworm.

☐ Explain the dermatomal distribution of herpes zoster lesions.

☐ Compare acne vulgaris, acne conglobata, and acne rosacea in terms of appearance and location of lesions.

☐ State three contributing factors in acne vulgaris.

☐ Cite three goals of acne treatment and one example of a treatment method for each goal.

☐ Describe the appearance of psoriasis lesions.

☐ Explain the action of the drug methoxsalen that is used in the PUVA treatment for psoriasis.

☐ Differentiate between lesions seen in infantile and adult forms of eczema.

☐ Relate the life cycle of the *Sarcoptes scabiei* to the skin lesions seen in scabies.

☐ Utilize knowledge of the life cycles of *Pediculus humanis corporis* and *P. humanis capitis* to explain the lesions associated with body and head lice.

☐ Explain methods used in treating pediculosis and eradicating lice and their nits from bedding and clothing.

☐ Compare the life cycles of bedbugs and ticks.

☐ List three drugs that produce photosensitivity.

☐ State the relationship between sun exposure and skin cancer.

☐ Compare the appearance of basal cell carcinoma, squamous cell carcinoma, and malignant melanoma.

☐ Cite changes in a mole that are suggestive of cancerous transformation.

☐ Provide a physiologic explanation for the red, white, and blue mottled appearance of malignant melanoma.

☐ Compare the appearance of atopic dermatitis, pityriasis rosea, psoriasis, tinea versicolor, and lichen planus in white and black skin.

■ References

1. Arey LB: Human Histology, p 186. Philadelphia, WB Saunders, 1974
2. Jacob SW, Fracone CA, Lossow WJ: Structure and Function in Man, 4th ed, p 75. Philadelphia, WB Saunders, 1978
3. Arndt KA, Jick H: Rates of cutaneous reactions to drugs. JAMA 235:918, 1976
4. Pinkus H, Mehregan AH: A Guide to Dermatohistopathology, 3rd ed, p 5. New York, Appleton-Century-Crofts, 1981
5. Holbrook KA, Odland GF: Regional differences in the thickness (cell layers) of the human stratum corneum: An ultrastructural analysis. J Invest Dermatol 62:415, 1974
6. Katz SI, Tamaki K, Sachs DH: Epidermal Langerhans cells are derived from cells originating in the bone marrow. Nature 282:324, 1979
7. Silberberg-Sinakin I, Baer RL, Thorbekke GJ: Langerhans cells: A review of their nature with emphasis on their immunologic functions. Prog Allergy 24:268, 1978
8. Tamaki K, Stingl G, Katz SJ: The origin of Langerhans cells. J Invest Dermatol 74:309, 1980
9. Hartschuh W, Grube D: The Merkel cell—A member of the APUD cell system: Fluorescence and electron microscopic contribution to the neurotransmitter function of the Merkel cell granules. Arch Dermatol Res 265:115, 1979
10. Herndon JH: Pruritus. In Moschella SL (ed): Dermatology Update, pp 185-196. New York, Elsevier Biomedical, 1982
11. Robbins SL, Cotran RS, Kumar V: Pathologic Basis of Disease, 3rd ed, pp 1275, 1279, 1298. Philadelphia, WB Saunders, 1984
12. Klingman AM, Leyden J: The interaction of fungi and bacteria in the pathogenesis of athlete's foot. In Maibach HI, Aly R (eds): Skin Microbiology: Relevance to Clinical Infection, pp 203-219. New York, Springer-Verlag, 1981
13. Nasemann T: Viral diseases of the skin, mucous membrane and genitalia. Philadelphia, WB Saunders, 1977
14. Strauss JS: Biology of the sebaceous gland and the pathophysiology of acne vulgaris. In Soter NA, Baden HP (eds): Pathophysiology of Dermatologic Disases, pp 159-173, 1984
15. Parish LC, Witkowski JA, Cohen HB: Clinical picture of scabies. In Parish LC, Nutting WB, Schwartzman RM (eds): Cutaneous Infestations of Man and Animal, pp 70-78. New York, Praeger, 1983
16. Facts on Skin Cancer. New York, American Cancer Society, 1978
17. Sherman CD, McCune CS, Rubin P: Malignant melanoma. In Rubin P (ed): Clinical Oncology, 6th ed, p 190. New York, American Cancer Society, 1983
18. Sober AJ, Rhodes AR, Day CL, Fitzpatrick TB, Mihm MC: Primary melanoma of the skin: Recognition of precursor lesions and estimation of prognosis in Stage I. In Fitzpatrick TB, Eisen AZ, Wolff K, Freedburg IM, Austen KF (eds): Update: Dermatology in General Medicine. New York, McGraw-Hill, 1983
19. Mosher DB, Pathak MA, Fitzpatrick TB: Vitiligo: Etiology, pathogenesis, diagnosis, and treatment. In Fitzpatrick TB, Eisen AZ, Wolff K, Freedburg IM, Austen KF (eds): Update: Dermatology in General Medicine. New York, McGraw-Hill, 1983

■ Additional References

Abel E: Psoriasis: Problems with PUVA therapy. Cutis 33:255, 1984

Adams RM: Occupational Skin Disease. New York, Grune & Stratton, 1983

Benenson AS (ed): Control of Communicable Diseases in Man. Washington, DC, American Public Health Association, 1981

Bruno NP, Beacham BE, Burnett, JW: Adverse effects of isotretinoin therapy. Cutis 33:484, 1984

Cohen S: Skin rashes in infants and children. Am J Nurs 78:1, 1978

Connolly SM: Allergic contact dermatitis: When to suspect it and what to do. Postgrad Med 74:227, 1983

Dilaimy MS, Owen WR, Sima B: Keratosis punctata of the palmar creases. Cutis 33:394, 1984

DiLorenzo PA: The clinical approach to pruritus. Cutis 3:1087, 1967

Domonkos AN, Arnold HL, Odom RB: Andrew's Diseases of the Skin: Clinical Dermatology, 7th ed. Philadelphia, WB Saunders, 1982

Epstein E, Epstein E (eds): Skin Surgery, 5th ed. Springfield, IL, Charles C Thomas, 1982

Farber EM, Cox AJ (eds): Psoriasis: Proceedings of the Third International Symposium. New York, Grune & Stratton, 1981

Fitzpatrick TB, Eisen AZ, Wolff K, Freedberg IM, Austen KF (eds): Update: Dermatology in Medicine. New York, McGraw-Hill, 1983

Fraser MC, McGuire DB: Skin cancer's early warning system. Am J Nurs 84:1232, 1984

Gunnoe RE: Diseases of the nails: How to recognize and treat them. Postgrad Med 74:357, 1983

Halder RM: Hair and scalp disorders in blacks. Cutis 32:378, 1983

Halder RM, Grimes PE, McLaurin CI, Kress MA, Kenny JA: Incidence of common dermatoses in a predominantly black dermatologic practice. Cutis 32:388, 1983

Hanifin JM: Atopic dermatitis. Postgrad Med 74:188, 1983

Henderson AL: Skin variations in blacks. Cutis 32:376, 1983

Kaplan AP: Chronic urticaria. Postgrad Med 74:209, 1983

Knopf AW, Bart RS, Rodriguez-Sains RS, Ackerman AB: Malignant Melanoma. New York, Masson Publishing, 1979

Lynch PJ: Sunlight and aging of the skin. Cutis 18:451, 1976

McLaurin CI: Unusual patterns of common dermatoses in blacks. Cutis 32:352, 1983

Miller LH: Herpes zoster in the elderly. Cutis 18:427, 1976

Orkin M, Maibach HI: Current views of scabies and pediculosis pubis. Cutis 33:85, 1984

Orkin M, Maibach HI: Scabies, a current pandemic. Postgrad Med 66:53, 1979

Ragozzino MW, Melton LJ, Kurland LT, Chu CP, Perry HO: Population-based study of herpes zoster and its sequelae. Med 61:310, 1982

Rosen T, Martin S: Atlas of Black Dermatology. Boston, Little, Brown, 1981

Waisman M: A clinical look at the aging skin. Postgrad Med 66:87, 1979

Weller TH: Varicella and herpes zoster: Changing concepts of the natural history, control, and importance of a not-so-benign virus. N Engl J Med 309:1362, 1983

Wilson BL: Skin problems common to blacks: A nursing perspective. In Gorline LL, Stegbauer CC (eds): Common Problems in Primary Care. St Louis, CV Mosby, 1982

Zugerman C: Dermatology in the workplace. Am Fam Pract 26:103, 1982

INDEX

Page numbers followed by f indicate illustration; t following a page number indicates tabular material.

ISBN 0-397-54481-2

90000